CLINICAL
NEUROLOGY

CLINICAL NEUROLOGY

Edited by

John W. Scadding MD FRCP
National Hospital for Neurology and Neurosurgery, London

Nicholas A. Losseff MD FRCP
National Hospital for Neurology and Neurosurgery, London

FOURTH EDITION

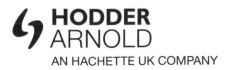
HODDER
ARNOLD
AN HACHETTE UK COMPANY

First published in Great Britain in 1989
Second edition 1998
Third edition 2003

This fourth edition published in 2012 by
Hodder Arnold, an imprint of Hodder Education, Hodder and Stoughton Ltd,
a division of Hachette UK

338 Euston Road, London NW1 3BH

http://www.hodderarnold.com

Hachette UK's policy is to use papers that are natural, renewable and recyclable products and
made from wood grown in sustainable forests. The logging and manufacturing processes are
expected to conform to the environmental regulations of the country of origin.

Whilst the advice and information in this book are believed to be true and accurate at the date
of going to press, neither the author[s] nor the publisher can accept any legal responsibility
or liability for any errors or omissions that may be made. In particular (but without limiting the
generality of the preceding disclaimer) every effort has been made to check drug dosages;
however it is still possible that errors have been missed. Furthermore, dosage schedules are
constantly being revised and new side-effects recognized. For these reasons the reader is
strongly urged to consult the drug companies' printed instructions before administering any of
the drugs recommended in this book.

British Library Cataloguing in Publication Data
A catalogue record for this book is available from the British Library

Library of Congress Cataloging-in-Publication Data
A catalog record for this book is available from the Library of Congress

ISBN-13   978-0-340-99070-4

1 2 3 4 5 6 7 8 9 10

Commissioning Editor:	Caroline Makepeace
Project Editor:	Jenny Wright
Production Controller:	Francesca Wardell
Cover Design:	Julie Joubinaux
Index:	Mary Collier

Cover image © MEDICAL BODY SCANS/SCIENCE PHOTO LIBRARY

Typeset in 9.5 on 12pt Rotis Serif by Phoenix Photosetting, Chatham, Kent
Printed and bound in Great Britain by MPG Books, Bodmin, Cornwall

What do you think about this book? Or any other Hodder Arnold title?
Please visit our website: www.hodderarnold.com

CONTENTS

CONTRIBUTORS

James Allibone BSC FRCS (SN)
Consultant Spinal Neurosurgeon, National Hospital for Neurology and Neurosurgery, London

Roshni Beeharry MA MRCP
Consultant in Rehabilitation Medicine, National Hospital for Neurology and Neurosurgery, London

Martin Brown MA MD FRCP
Professor of Stroke Medicine, Institute of Neurology, UCL, London

Helen Cross PhD FRCP FRCPH
Reader in Paediatric Neurology, Institute of Child Health, UCL, London

Nicholas Davies PhD MRCP
Consultant Neurologist, Chelsea & Westminster Hospital, London

Vivian Elwell MA MBBS MRCS
Specialist Registrar in Neurosurgery, National Hospital for Neurology and Neurosurgery, London

Naomi Fersht PhD MRCP FRCR
Consultant Clinical Oncologist, University College London Hospital, London

Simon Fleminger PhD FRCP FRCPsych
Consultant Neuropsychiatrist, Blackheath Brain Injury Rehabilitation Centre, Kings College, London

Nicholas Fletcher MD FRCP
Consultant Neurologist, Walton Centre NHS Foundation Trust, Liverpool

Timothy Fowler DM FRCP
Formerly Consultant Neurologist, Maidstone and Tunbridge Wells NHS Trust and Kings College Hospital, London

Carolyn Gabriel MD FRCP
Consultant Neurologist, St Mary's Hospital, London

Sonia Gandhi PhD MRCP
NIHR Lecturer in Neurology, University of California, San Francisco

Peter Goadsby MD PhD DSc FRACP FRCP
Professor of Neurology, University of California, San Francisco

Nicholas Hirsch MBBS FRCA
Consultant Anaesthetist, National Hospital for Neurology and Neurosurgery, London

Robin Howard PhD FRCP
Consultant Neurologist, National Hospital for Neurology and Neurosurgery, London

Elaine Hughes FRCP FRCPCH
Consultant Paediatric Neurologist, Kings College Hospital and Evelina Children's Hospital, London

Raju Kapoor DM FRCP
Consultant Neurologist, National Hospital for Neurology and Neurosurgery, London

Gareth Llewelyn MD FRCP
Consultant Neurologist, Royal Gwent Hospital, Swansea

Nick Losseff MD FRCP
Consultant Neurologist, National Hospital for Neurology and Neurosurgery, London

Andrew McEvoy MD FRCS (SN)
Consultant Neurosurgeon, National Hospital for Neurology and Neurosurgery, London

Catherine Mummery PhD FRCP
Consultant Neurologist, National Hospital for Neurology and Neurosurgery, London

Robert Powell PhD MRCP
Consultant Neurologist, Morriston Hospital, Swansea

Niall Quinn MA MD FRCP FAAN
Emeritus Professor of Clinical Neurology, Institute of Neurology, UCL, London

Jeremy Rees MD FRCP
Reader in Neurology, Institute of Neurology, UCL, London

Philip Rich BSc FRCS FRCR
Consultant Neuroradiologist, St George's Hospital,
London

Ley Sander MD PhD FRCP
Professor of Neurology, Institute of Neurology,
UCL, London

John Scadding MD FRCP
Honorary Consultant Neurologist, National
Hospital for Neurology and Neurosurgery, London

Anthony Schapira MD DSc FRCP FMedSci
Professor of Clinical Neurology, Royal Free and
University College Medical School, UCL, London

Katherine Sidle PhD MRCP
Consultant Neurologist, National Hospital for
Neurology and Neurosurgery, London

Sarah Tabrizi PhD FRCP
Professor of Clinical Neurology, Institute of
Neurology, UCL, London

Veronica Tan MD FRCP
Consultant Clinical Neurophysiologist, St Thomas'
Hospital, London

Christopher Turner PhD MRCP
Consultant Neurologist, National Hospital for
Neurology and Neurosurgery, London

Matthew Walker PhD FRCP
Professor of Neurology, Institute of Neurology,
UCL, London

Laurence Watkins MA FRCS (SN)
Senior Lecturer in Neurosurgery, Institute of
Neurology, UCL, London

David Werring MD FRCP
Senior Lecturer in Neurology, Institute of
Neurology, UCL, London

Nicholas Wood PhD FRCP FMedSci
Galton Professor of Genetics, Institute of
Neurology, UCL, London

PREFACE

The clinical neurosciences continue to move forward at a great pace, with impact in numerous areas of clinical practice. In the last few years there have been advances in both basic neuroscience and the understanding of disease, and their translation into clinical practice. We hope that the fourth edition of *Clinical Neurology* reflects these and provides an up-to-date account of the specialty.

However, we have not lost sight of the fact that the essential clinical skills needed to practise competently and safely remain as important as ever. This cannot be over-emphasised and the early chapters again provide detailed descriptions of the assessment of neurological symptoms and the conduct of the neurological examination.

One of the two founder editors of *Clinical Neurology*, Tim Fowler, has decided to stand down as editor. While we are saddened by his departure in this role, we are delighted that he has contributed to the fourth edition as an author. Indeed, his influence continues to be strongly felt in this edition. The establishment of *Clinical Neurology* as a successful and widely read text owes a great deal to his vision, expertise and wide clinical experience.

We welcome many new authors for existing chapters, and in addition to the disease and topic based chapters in the third edition, we have introduced a new stand-alone chapter on Clinical Neurophysiology, and new chapters on Craniofacial Pain and Neuro oncology.

Neurology has become a vast and rich specialty within internal medicine. The aim of this book remains to provide a succint but comprehensive and readable neurology text, which we hope will appeal as a primary source for neurologists, clinical neurophysiologists, general physicians, trainees in these disciplines, for GPs with a special interest in neurology, and indeed as an approachable introduction to the breadth and complexity of clinical neurology for medical students wishing to explore the specialty. We hope that it will continue to be of help in those preparing for examinations, both at the stage of entry to higher medical training, and for more senior examinations including the recently introduced Specialty Certificate Examination in neurology.

We wish to express our indebtedness to our patients, from whom we learn constantly and who provide the stimulus and challenge to improve the understanding and treatment of their neurological disorders.

John Scadding and Nick Losseff
London, 2011

ACKNOWLEDGEMENTS

We wish to thank all the authors of the chapters in this book, both those who have contributed to previous editions and those who have contributed for the first time. They bring a very wide range of clinical and research experience to the disease and system based chapters that make up the greater part of this book. They have given generously and enthusiastically of their time.

We again thank those individuals and publishers who have allowed us to reproduce figures and tables previously published elsewhere. They are acknowledged in the appropriate places in the text.

We repeat the debt we owe to our patients, and wish to thank also our many colleagues and students.

At Hodder, Sarah Penny, Jenny Wright and Caroline Makepeace have provided patient encouragement, expertise and great help at every stage of bringing this edition to publication. We are most grateful to them.

INTRODUCTION

John Scadding and Nick Losseff

Clinical neurology is often considered to be difficult. It is true that the structure of the nervous system is complex, but the knowledge and skills needed to localize most lesions and to perform a reliable examination are relatively easily acquired. The applied anatomy and physiology needed for the competent practice of clinical neurology is relatively straightforward, the essential requirement being a logical and consistent approach to history taking and examination. For the student of neurology, there is no substitute for taking histories and examining patients as frequently as possible; familiarization with the sequence will eventually bring fluency, accuracy and consistency.

The first chapters of this book place great emphasis on neurological clinical skills. While taking the history and during the examination, the clinician needs to have two questions in mind. First, **'where is the lesion?'** (anatomy). The distribution of the symptoms will indicate the anatomical site of the patient's problem in the great majority of cases. And second, **'what is the lesion?'** (causative pathology). The timing of the onset and the evolution of symptoms will provide important clues as to the nature of the underlying pathology. The importance of accurate assessment of the patient's symptoms is such that it is no exaggeration to say that if, by the time the history has been taken, the clinician has no idea either where the problem lies, or what type of pathological process might be responsible, then the physical examination is unlikely to be very rewarding.

The clinician needs to follow the trail of clues presented by the patient. History taking needs to be focused and logical, and not simply take the form of a rigid and mechanical comprehensive enquiry of a catalogue of symptoms. First, the presenting complaints need to be pursued, with supplementary questions about important related symptoms that the patient, devoid of neurological knowledge, may not have connected with the presenting symptoms. However, while advocating a directed approach to neurological diagnosis, it is essential to undertake a screening enquiry about a range of symptoms and perform an examination that systematically and efficiently covers the nervous system, in a systematized order, or there is a danger that important signs and diagnoses will be missed.

It is important to recognize also that many patients, particularly those seen in outpatient clinics, have no abnormal signs on examination. This is true of the majority of patients presenting with headache, dizziness and episodes of loss of consciousness, and in patients with a variety of other complaints, for example facial pain. In such patients, the diagnosis rests entirely on the clinician's ability to take a detailed and accurate history. Of course, an examination must be performed in all patients.

Chapters 2 and 3 are devoted to neurological symptoms and examination. It is worth making the point that despite the enormous advances in diagnostic technology in recent years, clinical skills remain the starting point and cornerstone of all neurological diagnosis. Chapters 4 and 5 outline the principles of neurological imaging and clinical neurophysiology. These core investigative arms of neurology are followed by consideration of neurogenetics, which has an increasingly wide relevance to the understanding and management of neurological disease. The remaining chapters of the book are devoted mainly to a systematic description of the many neurological disorders. Although this textbook deals principally with the clinical neurology of adults, there is a chapter on some of the neurological disorders of childhood. The later chapters in the book cover the generic topics of neurorehabilitation, respiratory problems seen in neurological disease, and the special characteristics and management of pain seen in many neurological conditions. An understanding of neuropsychiatry is essential to the competent practice of clinical neurology, and the psychiatric syndromes commonly seen in patients with neurological symptoms are succinctly but comprehensively described in the final chapter.

Major advances have been made in the assessment and treatment of numerous neurological conditions and these are described throughout the book. The previous frequent criticism of neurologists, that while they were good at making diagnoses, they could not offer treatment for their patients, is no longer justified. On the contrary, a great deal can now be done for very many patients. It is of course unfortunately true that neurological disease can lead to disability that is sometimes severe and may be irreversible. A sensitive, caring and compassionate approach in helping patients come to terms with the effects of their neurological illnesses, and offering means of amelioration of symptoms, together with support, sometimes over many years, are also essential qualities and responsibilities of the clinical neurologist.

EPIDEMIOLOGY

The epidemiological study determines how often a disease occurs in the population, why it occurs and why different populations may show variable patterns. An understanding of the frequency with which different neurological disorders present both to general practitioners and to hospital clinics is a great help to the doctor concerned. Furthermore, some 20 per cent of acute medical admissions to a general district hospital arise as a result of neurological disorders. Table 1.1 gives an indication of the prevalence of some common neurological disorders and Table 1.2 an approximate annual incidence of some neurological conditions in England and Wales.

A number of surveys have provided figures for the 'top 20' and percentage of new patient consultations with neurologists in outpatient clinics in the UK (Table 1.3). It can be seen that headaches (including migraine and tension-type) and blackouts (including epilepsy) top the presenting symptom list, while at the head of the diagnostic categories are cerebrovascular disease, peripheral nerve disorders, multiple sclerosis, spine and disc problems and Parkinson's disease. Psychological diagnoses are common and may overlap with many neurological disorders.

Advances in our understanding of genetics have led to better recognition of some inherited diseases. A list of more common single-gene neurological disorders is given in Table 1.4. Selected inherited disorders can now be diagnosed by laboratory testing (Box 1.1): furthermore the detection of carriers

Table 1.1 Prevalence of some neurological disorders in the UK (adapted from Warlow C (1991) *Handbook of Neurology*. Oxford: Blackwell Scientific Publications, with the permission of the author and publishers)

Disorder	Cases per 100 000	Cases per GP
Migraine	2000	40
Stroke	800	16
Epilepsy	500	10
Parkinson's disease	150[a]	3
Multiple sclerosis	100	2
Trigeminal neuralgia	100–150[a]	2
Primary tumour	46	1
Subarachnoid haemorrhage	50	1
Schizophrenia	10–50	1
Cerebral metastases	10	<1
Motor neurone disease	6	<1
Myasthenia gravis	5	<1
Polymyositis	5	<1
Friedreich's ataxia	2	<1
[a]Increases with age.		
GP, general practitioner.		

Table 1.2 Approximate annual incidence of some common neurological disorders in the UK (adapted from Warlow C (1991) *Handbook of Neurology*. Oxford: Blackwell Scientific Publications, with the permission of the author and publishers)

Condition	Cases per 100 000
Dementia (<age 70 years)[a]	1000
Head injuries requiring hospitalization	200–300
Migraine	150–300
Stroke	200
Major depressive illness	80–200
Acute lumbar disc prolapse	150
Carpal tunnel syndrome	100
Epileptic seizures	50
TIAs	35
Bell's palsy	25
Essential tremor	25
Parkinson's disease	20
Cerebral metastases	15
Subarachnoid haemorrhage	15
Bipolar depression	10–15
Primary cerebral tumours	15
Bacterial meningitis	5
Trigeminal neuralgia	5
Multiple sclerosis	5
Motor neurone disease	2–3
Guillain–Barré syndrome	2
Meningioma	1.0–2.5
Polymyositis	1

[a]>age 70 years the incidence rises to c. 50%.
TIA, transient ischaemic attack.

Table 1.3 Top 20 diagnoses in a sample of 6940 patients. Reproduced with permission from Perkin GD (1989) with permission from BMJ Publishing Group Ltd.

Diagnosis	Proportion of sample (%)
No diagnosis	26.5
Blackouts	12.5
Epilepsy	10.4
Vasovagal attacks	2.1
Headache	12.5
Tension headache	7.5
Migraine	5.0
Cerebrovascular disease	7.4
Entrapment neuropathy	4.4
Conversion hysteria	3.8
Anatomical	3.7
Multiple sclerosis	3.5
Hyperventilation	2.0
Parkinson's disease	1.9
Post-traumatic syndrome	1.8
Dementia	1.5
Peripheral neuropathy	1.4
Depression	1.4
Non-neurological	1.3
Cervical radiculopathy/myelopathy	1.2
Lumbar spondylosis	1.0
Essential tremor	0.9

Table 1.4 Prevalence of single-gene neurological disorders in South East Wales (Reproduced from JC Macmillan, PS Harper. Clinical genetics in neurological disease. 1994, 57: 7–15, with permission from BMJ Publishing Group Ltd.)

Disorder	Prevalence per 100 000
Neurofibromatosis I	13.3
Hereditary motor and sensory neuropathy I, II, III and V	12.9
Duchenne dystrophy[a]	9.6
Huntington's disease	8.4
Myotonic dystrophy	7.1
Becker dystrophy[a]	5.0
Hereditary spastic paraplegia	3.4
Facioscapulohumeral dystrophy	2.9
Tuberous sclerosis	1.6

[a]Males.

and the presymptomatic diagnosis of some conditions may occasionally prove possible; for example, the dominant inherited disorder Huntington's disease can be shown by detection of an expansion in the trinucleotide repeat sequences in the DNA of the affected gene (chromosome 4). The disease can now be confirmed by blood tests and those who will develop the disease can be diagnosed before they show clinical signs. The rapidly expanding field of neurogenetics has led to an increasing need for adequate provision of counselling services for individuals and their families.

Box 1.1 Some inherited neurological conditions that can now be identified using laboratory tests

Duchenne/Becker muscular dystrophy
Myotonic dystrophy
Huntington's disease
Dentatorubropallidoluysian atrophy
X-linked spinobulbar muscular atrophy (Kennedy's disease)
Spinal muscular atrophy (autosomal recessive, proximal)
Hereditary motor and sensory neuropathy or Charcot-Marie-Tooth disease (aided by conduction velocity values)
Hereditary neuropathy with liability to pressure palsy
Fragile X syndrome
DYT1 dystonia
Mitochondrial encephalomyopathies
Facioscapulohumeral dystrophy
Familial motor neurone disease
Friedreich's ataxia
Spinocerebellar ataxia

ANATOMICAL DIAGNOSIS

Anatomical diagnosis
The details of the patient's complaints as the history unfolds will direct attention to the part or parts of the nervous system involved. A few very simple rules will help to focus attention on the likely site of trouble.

Seizures

Seizures (fits), disturbances of intellect and memory, and certain disorders of speech all point to disease of the cerebral cortex.

Seizures are the result of spontaneous discharges in cerebral cortical neurones, and do not occur with diseases of deep cerebral structures, the brainstem or cerebellum, unless the cerebral cortex is also involved. Intellect, reasoning and memory all depend upon the normal function of the cerebral cortex, and any decline in these faculties points to damage in this part of the brain.

Disturbances of speech fall into three categories:
1 **Dysphasia**, in which the content of speech is impaired, although articulation and phonation are intact;
2 **Dysarthria**, in which articulation of speech is abnormal as a result of damage to the neuromuscular mechanisms controlling the muscles concerned with speech production;
3 **Dysphonia**, in which the function of the larynx is impaired.

Dysphasia points to a disorder of the cerebral cortex, particularly that of the dominant hemisphere (see Figure 3.7).

Disturbances of vision are common neurological problems. Loss of visual acuity points to damage to the eye itself, or to the optic nerve. Lesions behind the optic chiasm produce loss of vision in the opposite half of the visual field (hemianopia), but leave intact at least the ipsilateral half of central macular vision, and this is sufficient to provide a normal visual acuity (Figure 1.1). Patients with hemianopias complain of difficulty reading, or of bumping into objects in the blind half-field. Double vision (diplopia) occurs when the axes of the two eyes are out of alignment. This happens when one eyeball is displaced by some mass in the orbit, or if the ocular muscles are weak because of either primary muscle disease or damage to external ocular nerves (Figure 1.2).

Vertigo (a true sense of imbalance) is an illusion of movement and occurs with damage to the peripheral vestibular system, the vestibular nerve,

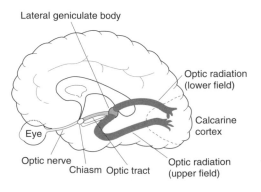

Figure 1.1 Medial sagittal view of the brain to show visual pathways; these traverse the brain from front to back.

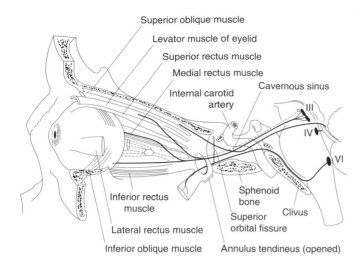

Superior oblique muscle
Levator muscle of eyelid
Superior rectus muscle
Medial rectus muscle
Cavernous sinus
Internal carotid artery
III
IV
VI
Inferior rectus muscle
Sphenoid bone
Clivus
Superior orbital fissure
Lateral rectus muscle
Inferior oblique muscle
Annulus tendineus (opened)

Figure 1.2 Course of the ocular motor nerves from the brainstem to the orbit (reproduced with permission from P Duus *Topical Diagnosis in Neurology*, Stuttgart: Georg Thieme Verlag).

or its brainstem connections. A combination of vertigo and diplopia suggests a lesion in the posterior fossa or brainstem, particularly when associated with bilateral motor or sensory disturbances.

Dysphagia and dysarthria are usually caused by either primary muscle disease, defects at the neuromuscular junction, or bilateral involvement of the neural mechanisms controlling the muscles of mastication and speech.

> Weakness may result from primary muscle disease or defective neuromuscular transmission, damage to the peripheral motor nerves or anterior horn cells in the spinal cord (lower motor neurone lesion), or from damage to the corticomotorneurone pathways (Figure 1.3) responsible for the cerebral control of movement (upper motor neurone lesion).

Such weakness may affect all four limbs (quadriplegia), the arm and leg on one side (hemiplegia), or both legs sparing the arms (paraplegia). A quadriplegia in an alert patient who can talk is usually a result of either primary muscle disease, a generalized peripheral neuropathy, or a high cervical cord lesion. Hemiplegia suggests damage to the opposite cerebral hemisphere, particularly if the face is involved. Paraplegia is most often the result of spinal cord damage, particularly when there is also disturbance of sphincter control. Isolated weakness of one limb (monoplegia) is frequently caused by damage to its motor nerves, although sometimes a monoplegia may arise from lesions in the cerebral cortex.

The pattern of **sensory symptoms** usually follows that of motor disturbance. Thus, a distal sensory loss in all four limbs suggests peripheral nerve disease. Sensory disturbance in a hemiplegic distribution suggests damage to the opposite cerebral hemisphere, particularly of the capsular sensory pathways, in which case the face is often involved. Hemiplegic sensory disturbance on one side of the body with involvement of the face on the opposite side suggests damage in the brainstem (Figures 1.4, 1.5 and 1.6). If the cranial nerves are not involved, sensory disturbances on one side of the body, with motor disturbances on the opposite side of the body, suggest damage to the spinal cord (Figures 1.3 and 1.5). Sensory disturbance in both legs extending onto the trunk also points to a lesion of the spinal cord. Sensory loss affecting parts of one limb only is most often caused by a local peripheral nerve or root lesion.

> These simple rules for interpretation of symptoms usually give the first clue to the likely anatomical site of damage responsible for the patient's complaints. Of course they are not infallible and many exceptions to such generalizations will be encountered in practice. However, they provide the easiest means of the first steps in analysis of the anatomical site of the patient's lesion. The next stage is the physical examination.

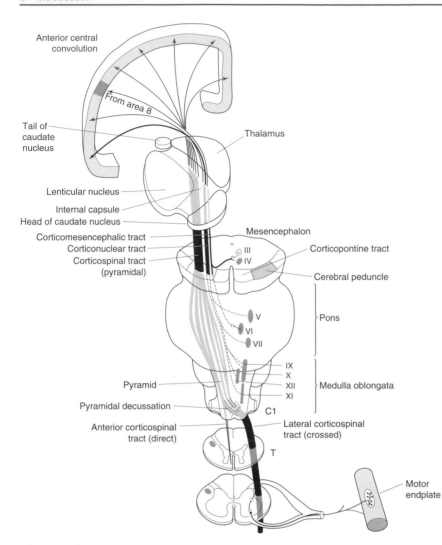

Anterior central convolution

From area 8

Tail of caudate nucleus

Thalamus

Lenticular nucleus

Internal capsule

Head of caudate nucleus

Corticomesencephalic tract

Corticonuclear tract

Corticospinal tract (pyramidal)

Mesencephalon

III
IV

Corticopontine tract

Cerebral peduncle

V

VI

VII

Pons

IX
X
XII
XI

Medulla oblongata

Pyramid

Pyramidal decussation

C1

Anterior corticospinal tract (direct)

Lateral corticospinal tract (crossed)

T

Motor endplate

Figure 1.3 Course of corticospinal, pyramidal tract (reproduced with permission from P Duus *Topical Diagnosis in Neurology*, Stuttgart: Georg Thieme Verlag).

Neurological examination is described in depth in Chapter 3, but some simple principles will be stated here.

When students approach a neurological patient for the first time, a comprehensive examination is a lengthy business, tiring for both examiner and patient. By contrast, an experienced neurologist will complete the task in 10 minutes or less. The secret of the art is to know what one is looking for.

In fact, neurologists divide the clinical examination conceptually into two halves. The first is a detailed evaluation of those parts of the nervous system to which attention has been drawn in the course of taking the patient's history. The second is a general screen of other sections of the nervous system which, from the history, do not seem likely to be involved, but which have to be examined in every patient to ensure that nothing is missed.

To facilitate this method, neurological trainees perfect a routine of clinical examination sufficient to act as a simple screen of the nervous system, onto which they graft the extra detailed investigation of those sections to which their attention has been drawn by the history. The routine screening examination, which can be undertaken very briefly in a matter of minutes, is learnt by repetition of the same sequence over and over again until it becomes second nature. For convenience, most start with a brief assessment of the mental faculties of the patient in the course of the interview, then move to the cranial nerves starting at the top and work-

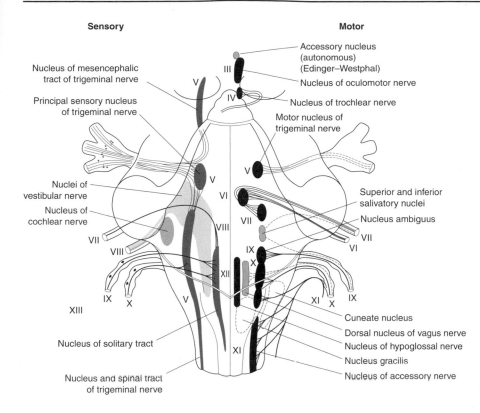

Sensory

Nucleus of mesencephalic
tract of trigeminal nerve

Principal sensory nucleus
of trigeminal nerve

Nuclei of
vestibular nerve

Nucleus of
cochlear nerve

Nucleus of solitary tract

Nucleus and spinal tract
of trigeminal nerve

Motor

Accessory nucleus
(autonomous)
(Edinger–Westphal)

Nucleus of oculomotor nerve

Nucleus of trochlear nerve

Motor nucleus of
trigeminal nerve

Superior and inferior
salivatory nuclei

Nucleus ambiguus

Cuneate nucleus

Dorsal nucleus of vagus nerve

Nucleus of hypoglossal nerve

Nucleus gracilis

Nucleus of accessory nerve

Figure 1.4 Cranial nerve nuclei viewed from behind. Sensory nuclei are on the left and motor nuclei are on the right (reproduced with permission from P Duus *Topical Diagnosis in Neurology*, Stuttgart: Georg Thieme Verlag).

ing downwards. They then assess motor function of the limbs, including stance and gait. Finally, the sensory system is examined.

One of the first problems that neurological beginners encounter is the ease with which apparent abnormalities are detected on careful examination. Frequently it is difficult to decide on the significance of minor degrees of apparent weakness, fleeting and inconsistent sensory signs, slight asymmetry of the tendon reflexes, slightly less facility of repetitive movements of the left hand in a right-handed patient, or a few jerks of the eyes on extreme lateral gaze. To build a neurological diagnosis on minor deficits such as these is courting disaster.

It is a useful exercise to classify each abnormality discovered as a 'hard' or 'soft' sign. 'Hard' signs are unequivocally abnormal – an absent ankle jerk even on reinforcement, a clear-cut extensor plantar response, definite wasting of the small muscles of the hand, or absent vibration sense. Any final anatomical diagnosis must provide an explanation of such 'hard' signs. 'Soft' signs, on the other hand, such as those described above, are unreliable and best ignored when initially formulating a diagnosis. Base your conclusions on the 'hard' signs, and

then see if any of the 'soft' signs that you have discovered may put the diagnosis into doubt. If so, go back and repeat that section of the examination and make up your mind again whether or not the 'soft' sign is real. Students will find that neurology becomes increasingly easy the more confident they become in discarding unwanted 'soft' signs, as they become more experienced in determining the range of normal. They will only achieve this by constant repeated routine examination of the normal human nervous system.

As already mentioned, the interpretation of physical signs found on examination depends heavily upon a practical knowledge of neuroanatomy. It is worth emphasizing which parts of neuroanatomy are of greatest value to the clinical neurologist.

The visual system spans the whole of the head from the front to back and so is commonly involved by intracranial lesions (Figure 1.1). The mechanisms controlling eye movements range from the cortex through the brainstem and external ocular nerves to the eye muscles themselves. Consequently, ocu-

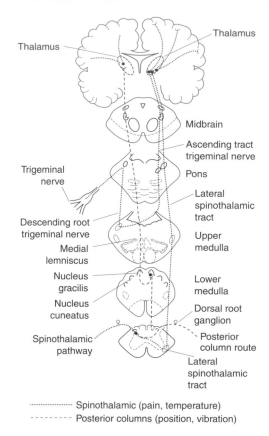

Thalamus

Thalamus

Midbrain

Ascending tract trigeminal nerve

Trigeminal nerve

Pons

Lateral spinothalamic tract

Descending root trigeminal nerve

Upper medulla

Medial lemniscus

Nucleus gracilis

Lower medulla

Nucleus cuneatus

Dorsal root ganglion

Spinothalamic pathway

Posterior column route

Lateral spinothalamic tract

············· Spinothalamic (pain, temperature)
– – – – – Posterior columns (position, vibration)

Figure 1.5 Ascending sensory pathways.

lar motor function is frequently damaged by intracranial lesions. A detailed anatomical knowledge of the visual and ocular motor pathways is essential. So, too, is an understanding of the individual cranial nerves in the brainstem, their course through the basal cisterns and exits through the foramina in the skull (Figure 1.6), and their course and distribution to their extracranial target organs.

In as far as the motor system is concerned, it is essential to be able to distinguish between the characteristics of primary muscle disease, a lower motor neurone lesion and an upper motor neurone lesion. Likewise, it is important to be able to detect the characteristic pattern of weakness in a patient with a hemiplegia, and to be able to distinguish this from the pattern of weakness that occurs with lesions affecting individual nerve roots or peripheral nerves. In the case of sensory findings, it is crucial to be able to recognize the pattern of sensory loss associated with damage to the spinal cord, or to individual nerve roots and peripheral nerves.

Clinicians should be thoroughly familiar with a cross-section of the spinal cord (Figure 1.7) in order to be able to interpret the motor and sensory consequences of spinal cord damage. Likewise, they should know the segmental distribution of motor and sensory roots, and the characteristic motor and sensory consequences of damage to individual large peripheral nerves (see Figure 3.19).

These are the minimum fundamentals of neuroanatomy required for neurological practice. Without them, clinicians will be lost trying to interpret the results of their examinations. A short period spent refreshing the memory on these basic items prior to neurological training will be time well spent. It will allow the student to enjoy that period of neurological apprenticeship in learning about neurological disease, rather than being held back through ignorance of the essential first steps that must be mastered before any sensible discussion about neurological illness can be entered into.

From this brief introduction, it will be seen that the first stage of neurological diagnosis, the anatomical site of the lesion, is deduced initially from the history, which points towards the likely parts of the nervous system to examine in detail, and from the neurological examination itself, which confirms and elaborates, or refutes, the initial impression gained after hearing the patient's symptoms.

> At the end of history taking and clinical examination, neurologists should, with confidence, be able to state what part or parts of the nervous system are affected. They can then pass to the second stage of defining the likely pathological cause.

PATHOLOGICAL DIAGNOSIS

The site of damage to the nervous system will usually give some clue as to the possible pathological cause.

An example of pathological diagnosis is evidence of a lesion affecting the optic chiasm, indicated by the presence of a bitemporal hemianopia, which suggests the possibility of a pituitary tumour.

However, the time-course of the illness gives the greatest clue to the likely pathology responsible.

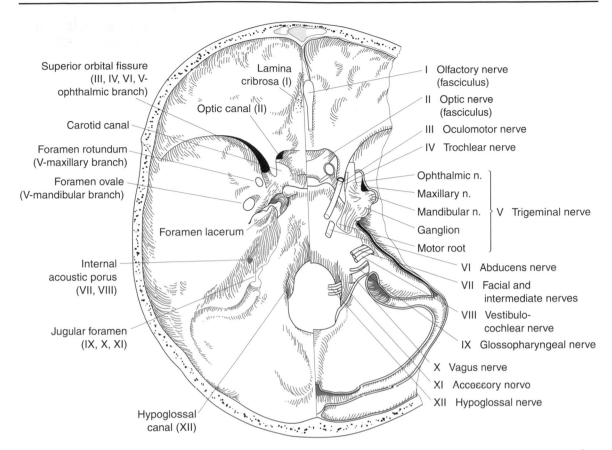

Figure 1.6 View of the skull base. On the left side are shown the exit and entry foramina and on the right side the stumps of the cranial nerves (n.) (reproduced with permission from P Duus *Topical Diagnosis in Neurology*, Stuttgart: Georg Thieme Verlag).

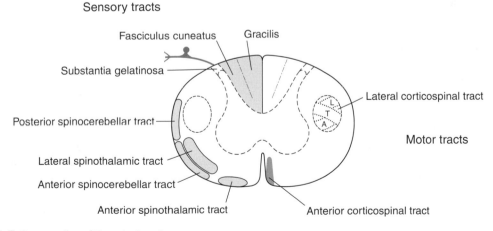

Figure 1.7 Cross-section of the spinal cord.

Neurologists take great care to establish during history taking whether the onset of symptoms was sudden or gradual, and whether the subsequent course has been one of recovery, persistence with stable deficit, or progression of disability. Attention to these simple points provides the best guide to the likely pathology.

History

- An illness of sudden, abrupt onset followed by subsequent gradual recovery is likely to be a result of vascular disease.
- An illness of gradual onset but relentless progression is likely to be caused by a tumour or degenerative condition.
- An illness characterized by episodes of neurological deficit lasting days or weeks, followed by subsequent partial or complete recovery, is suggestive of multiple sclerosis.
- An illness consisting of brief episodes of neurological disability lasting minutes or hours is typical of transient ischaemic attacks, migraine, or epilepsy.

Other factors that will help to define the likely pathological cause of a neurological illness are the age and sex of the patient. Thus, the sudden onset of a focal cerebral deficit lasting half an hour or less in an otherwise healthy 20-year-old woman taking the oral contraceptive pill is almost certainly migraine. A similar cerebral deficit of acute onset lasting an hour or so in a 65-year-old man with diabetes who is a heavy smoker, suggests that cerebrovascular disease is the cause.

In general, attention to these three main categories of information, the site of the lesion, its mode of onset and subsequent course, and the age and sex of the patient, will point to the likely cause of the illness.

An important rule of thumb that is worth emphasizing at this point is that any neurological illness that is progressive must be considered to be the result of a tumour until proven otherwise. One major task of neurology is to detect those benign tumours that can compress the brain, cranial nerves, or spinal cord to cause progressive neurological deficit, which can be halted or reversed by appropriate neurosurgical treatment. Thus progressive blindness not caused by local eye disease, progressive unilateral deafness, a progressive hemiparesis, or a progressive spastic paraparesis all warrant full investigation to exclude a treatable tumour or other compressive lesion as the cause.

NEUROLOGICAL INVESTIGATIONS

From the information obtained from the patient's history and examination, the neurologist will formulate a provisional anatomical and pathological diagnosis. With common neurological diseases, no further investigation is required; for example, migraine is diagnosed solely on the basis of the history and the absence of any abnormal neurological signs on examination. Other patients, however, require investigation to confirm, refute or refine the provisional clinical diagnosis. Major advances have been made in recent years in both neuroimaging and clinical electrophysiology and these are described in Chapters 4 and 5, respectively. However, it has to be recognized that the results obtained from either imaging or electrophysiology must be interpreted in the individual clinical context. These investigations do not in any way remove the need for accurate clinical assessment. Imaging the wrong part of the nervous system, or failure to present correct clinical information in a request for electromyography and nerve conduction studies is likely to yield information that will simply mislead the clinician and lead to diagnostic delay or worse, erroneous diagnosis. Advances in investigative technology have not obviated the need for competent clinical diagnosis, based on the history and examination, which are discussed in detail in the next two chapters.

In many branches of medicine, histological investigation of affected tissues and organs is relatively straightforward, through examination of biopsy specimens. In contrast, access to nervous tissue is very limited and biopsy of the central nervous system is rarely performed, for obvious reasons. Biopsy of peripheral sensory nerves is carried out only in highly selected patients (see Chapter 16), while muscle biopsy is a more routine investigation (see Chapter 18). These techniques are outlined below.

CEREBROSPINAL FLUID

There are many indications for examination of cerebrospinal fluid (CSF), and it is important that this is done competently, by lumbar puncture. The technique requires some practice, but once mastered is simple and usually painless.

However, when there is an intracranial or intraspinal mass lesion, lumbar puncture carries a serious risk of causing rapid deterioration in function as a result of shifts of intracranial or intraspinal contents. Because of the risks involved, lumbar puncture must not be performed in any patient in whom there is clinical suspicion of an intracranial or spinal mass lesion, In such patients, the diagnosis will often be obtained without the need for CSF examination, and lumbar puncture in the presence of an intracranial mass lesion may prove fatal.

Indications for brain imaging prior to lumbar puncture

- Signs or symptoms of raised intracranial pressure
- Focal neurological deficit
- A fixed dilated or poorly reactive pupil
- Coma or a rapidly deteriorating consciousness level
- Signs of posterior fossa lesion (e.g. dysarthria, ataxia).

Lumbar puncture is also contraindicated in the presence of local skin sepsis in the lumbar region. Lumbar puncture is essential to the diagnosis of meningitis, in some patients with subarachnoid haemorrhage, and is a valuable adjunct to the diagnosis of a number of inflammatory conditions such as multiple sclerosis (MS) or encephalitis.

For **lumbar puncture** the patient is best positioned lying on the side, flexed and with the spine horizontal (Figure 1.8). The needle is usually introduced at the L3/4 interspace, which is indicated by a line drawn joining the tips of the iliac crests (Figure 1.8a). It is worth recalling in adults that the spinal cord usually ends at the lower border of L1 so a needle inserted into the subarachnoid space below this level will enter the sac containing the cauda equina floating in CSF. Local anaesthetic is used for the skin and immediate tissues. After allowing time for this to be effective, a sharp, disposable fine lumbar puncture needle (22 gauge) with stilette in position is introduced through the skin and advanced through the space between the two spinous processes. The needle point usually

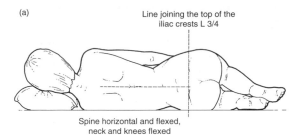

(a) Line joining the top of the iliac crests L 3/4

Spine horizontal and flexed, neck and knees flexed

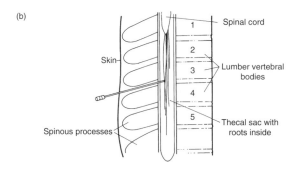

(b) Spinal cord — 1

Skin — 2

3 — Lumber vertebral bodies

4

5 — Thecal sac with roots inside

Spinous processes

Figure 1.8 (a) Position of patient for lumbar puncture. (b) Diagram to show correctly positioned needle within the subarachnoid space.

needs to be directed slightly forwards (anteriorly). At a depth of about 4–7 cm, firmer resistance may be encountered as the ligamentum flavum is reached. Beyond this, there is a slight 'give' as the needle punctures the dura. The stilette is then removed and clear CSF will drip out of the needle if this has been correctly positioned. If no fluid appears or bone is encountered, it is probable that the needle is not in the correct place. The stilette should be reinserted, the needle partially withdrawn and then advanced at a slightly different angle. The most common causes of failure are that the needle is not in the midline, or is at too great an angle with the skin (Figure 1.8b).

Complications of lumbar puncture

- Low pressure headache – postural, worse erect occurs in approximately 20 per cent
- Backache
- Introduced infection
- Precipitation of pressure cone with a cranial or spinal mass lesion
- Subarachnoid or epidural haemorrhage (anticoagulants, bleeding disorder)
- Cranial nerve palsies – diplopia from CN VI
- Dermoid formation

The CSF findings characteristic of specific conditions will be discussed later in this book, but a few general principles will be mentioned now. It is always crucial to obtain the maximum information from examination of the CSF.

Normal cerebrospinal fluid (CSF) values

Clear colourless fluid

Pressure	40–180 mm
Cells	0–5 lymphocytes/mm^3
Sugar	2.5–4.4 mmol/L
	(>60% of blood glucose)
Lactate	<2.8 mmol/L
Protein	0.2–0.5 g/L
IgG	<14% of total protein
	(70% of serum globulin)
Volume (adult)	150 mL

If the presence of blood is suspected, three sequential tubes of CSF should be collected to establish whether the fluid is uniformly and consistently bloodstained, or whether the initial bloody CSF gradually clears, as occurs as a result of a traumatic tap. Likewise, when haemorrhage is suspected, the sample should be centrifuged and the supernatant examined for the presence of xanthochromia, which indicates pathological bleeding rather than the consequences of trauma at the time of lumbar puncture. If infection is suspected, the CSF sugar may be an invaluable guide to the presence of bacterial or fungal inflammation. However, the CSF glucose can only be interpreted in the light of the blood level obtained at the same time. Thus, bacterial or fungal meningitis is suggested if the CSF contains an excess of cells in the presence of a glucose concentration of 2 mmol/L or less than 40 per cent of the blood glucose concentration (Table 1.5). If there are red cells in significant numbers resulting from a traumatic tap, a rough guide suggests that about ten white cells may be allowed for every 7000 red cells.

Specific abnormalities of CSF protein content may be invaluable in diagnosis, particularly the excess gammaglobulin found in many patients with MS, who also commonly exhibit the presence of oligoclonal bands of gammaglobulin on electrophoresis. Nowadays, these are most reliably demonstrated by isoelectric focusing. The synthesis of immune globulins in the central nervous system is not pathognomonic of MS and may occur in a

Table 1.5 Abnormal cerebrospinal fluid findings

Finding	Interpretation
Elevated polymorph count low glucose	meningitis: bacterial TB early fungal viral (uncommon) parameningeal infection
Elevated lymphocyte count low glucose	meningitis: partially treated bacterial TB listeriosis fungal viral carcinomatous meningitis sarcoidosis
Elevated lymphocyte count normal or low glucose	meningitis: partially treated bacterial TB listeriosis spirochaetal – syphilis, *Borrelia burgdorferi* *Mycoplasma pneumoniae* viral – mumps, enterovirus, HIV, HSV fungal – cryptococcus
Atypical aseptic meningitis	sarcoidosis SLE vasculitis drug-induced – NSAIs (ibuprofen, naproxen, sulindac) post-traumatic lumbar puncture post serial major epileptic seizures

HIV, human immunodeficiency virus; HSV, herpes simplex virus; NSAIDs, non-steroidal anti-inflammatory drugs; TB, tuberculosis.

number of inflammatory/infective disorders, for example sarcoidosis, syphilis, Behçet's disease. The CSF immunoglobulin G (IgG) index is a means of evaluating the rate of IgG synthesis in the CSF. The CSF IgG index = (IgG CSF × albumin serum)/(albumin CSF × IgG serum). Normally the value ranges from 0 to 0.77. Higher values suggest increased IgG synthesis, as in MS.

The CSF may also give useful information in a

number of disorders: for example the CSF angiotensin-converting enzyme levels may be raised in neurosarcoidosis or the measurement of 14-3-3 protein in patients suspected of having Creutzfeldt–Jakob disease. In patients with pineal region germ cell tumours, markers may be found in the CSF, such as alpha-fetoprotein in yolk sac tumours, beta-human chorionic gonadotropin in choriocarcinoma and human placental alkaline phosphatase in germ cell tumours.

Examination of CSF for specific bacteria or fungi, such as the tubercle bacilli or cryptococcus, or for malignant cells requires considerable care and experience. The immunodetection of specific bacterial antigens and antibodies has also aided diagnosis of infections, particularly in some patients who have already been started on an antibiotic prior to examination of their CSF. Latex agglutination tests for bacterial antigens may detect *Haemophilus influenzae* B, *Streptococcus pneumoniae* and *Neisseria meningitidis* in over two-thirds of patients. Polymerase chain reactions to detect bacterial DNA may also be useful, for example in tuberculous meningitis or neurological Lyme disease.

It will be apparent that thought must be given before lumbar puncture to what information is to be sought from the material obtained, and care must be exercised in ensuring that the samples are delivered to the appropriate laboratories and individuals. Finally, lumbar puncture provides an opportunity to record CSF pressure using simple manometry, which should be undertaken routinely.

Muscle and nerve biopsy

Muscle biopsy is undertaken routinely in most patients suspected of primary muscle disease, the sample being removed from a weak muscle that has not previously been subjected to electromyographic needling. Routine histology is supplemented by histochemistry, to type muscle fibre populations, and by biochemical investigation of muscle energy metabolism. Electron microscopy may also be necessary. Special staining with immunolabelling may also add information: for example, the use of dystrophin in Duchenne muscular dystrophy. Muscle biopsy also affords the opportunity to examine small blood vessels in patients suspected of inflammatory diseases, such as polyarteritis nodosa.

Nerve biopsy is used less frequently, but it is simple and safe to biopsy the sural nerve at the ankle, which leaves no motor deficit and only a small patch of sensory loss. In a few patients there may be complaints of pain from the biopsy site. Examination of nerve biopsies in patients with peripheral nerve disease will confirm the presence of axonal damage, demyelination, or a combination of these, though nerve biopsy is usually only performed when there is clinical suspicion of arteritis, or of infiltration by substances such as amyloid or lymphoma (see Chapter 16). Quantitative studies can be undertaken, which look at the size and type of the nerve fibres involved in the disease process, and teased fibre preparations may show the presence of segmental or generalized demyelination. Special staining techniques may be useful in evaluating certain patterns of neuropathy in association with dysproteinaemias or immune-mediated diseases.

Other investigations

Many other investigations are employed in individual patients with neurological disease; for instance, skin, liver, rectal, or marrow biopsy may be required for the diagnosis of a number of storage diseases that cause progressive encephalopathy in childhood. Biopsy of lymph glands may be useful in the diagnosis of a number of disorders, particularly in lymphomas, in carcinomatosis and in sarcoidosis. Occasionally, biopsy of the brain itself or the meninges is required to establish the diagnosis in progressive obscure cerebral disorders. Image-linked stereotactic brain biopsies now allow very precise sampling of areas of abnormal signal within the brain substance.

Many metabolic and hormonal diseases may affect the nervous system, so that a wide range of biochemical tests, such as examination of serum electrolytes, liver, renal and bone function, may be required, as will tests of thyroid, parathyroid, pancreas, adrenal and pituitary function. Neurosyphilis, Lyme disease and now AIDS are the great mimics of neurological disorders so that serological tests such as a *Treponema pallidum* haemagglutination test, tests for IgG antibodies for *Borrelia* and human immunodeficiency virus titres are essential to exclude these disorders. A wide range of immunological tests may also be used to assess a variety of connective tissue disorders and an increasing number of neurological conditions where antibodies may be detected to aid diagnosis; for example, anti-acetylcholine receptor antibodies are found in most patients with generalized myasthenia gravis (seropositive) and muscle specific kinase antibodies may be found in many seronegative myasthenic patients. IgG antibodies to P- or Q-type voltage-gated calcium channels may be found in patients with the Lambert–Eaton syndrome.

REFERENCES AND FURTHER READING

Duus P (1998) *Topical Diagnosis in Neurology*, 3rd revised edn. Stuttgart: Georg Thieme.

Fishman GA, Birch DG, Holder GE, Brigell MG (2001) *Electrophysiologic Testing in Disorders of the Retina, Optic Nerve, and Visual Pathway*, 2nd edn. Ophthalmology Monograph 2. San Francisco: The Foundation of the American Academy of Ophthalmology.

Greenstein B, Greenstein A (2000) *Color Atlas of Neuroscience – Neuroanatomy and Neurophysiology*. Stuttgart: Georg Thieme.

Mills KR (1999) *Magnetic Stimulation of the Human Nervous System*. Oxford: Oxford University Press.

Perkin GD (1989) An analysis of 7835 successive new out-patient referrals. *Journal of Neurology, Neurosurgery and Psychiatry*, 52:447–448.

Wood NW (ed.) (2011) *Neurogenetics for Clinicians*. Cambridge: Cambridge University Press.

CHAPTER 2

SYMPTOMS OF NEUROLOGICAL DISEASE

Tim Fowler, Nick Losseff and John Scadding

INTRODUCTION

The symptoms that patients describe are largely responsible for the direction of the clinical examination and it is the tempo of the onset and progression of these symptoms that points to the type of pathology causing them. The combination of symptoms and signs leads to the anatomical diagnosis. Indeed '*where is the problem?*' is the first and independent question a neurologist must ask, the second distinct question being '*what is the problem?*'.

The most common symptoms in neurological practice are shown in Box 2.1. This is by no means exhaustive, but it does account for the majority of complaints encountered.

In addition to the patient's presenting complaint and further details about this, it is worth obtaining answers to a series of routine direct questions (Table 2.1). If answers to these are positive then further exploration will be necessary.

It is not our purpose here to describe in detail the individual diseases causing the various symptoms discussed. We shall concentrate on the approach to the differential diagnosis of selected important symptoms, and the practical management of such patients. Further detailed description of the various disorders discussed is found in the subsequent chapters of this book.

HEADACHE

Headache is one of the most common symptoms encountered in primary care, and certainly is the most common complaint of patients attending the neurologist. It is estimated that one in five of the general population may suffer from headache of sufficient severity to consult a doctor at some time. The majority of these patients will have no abnormal physical signs on examination, and diagnosis depends entirely on the history. One of the most important distinctions is for how long the patient has suffered headache.

Box 2.1 Common symptoms in neurological disorders

Pain
    Headache
    Facial pain
    Spinal pain – cervical, lumbar
    Limb pain – often accompanied by weakness and
        tingling
Loss of consciousness
    Epileptic seizures
    Syncope
    Impaired cerebral perfusion – cardiac causes
    Non-epileptic seizures
Disturbances of the senses
    Visual upsets – impaired acuity, blurred, double
        vision
    Deafness
    Dizziness
    Impaired smell, taste
Motor
    Weakness
        Limbs – often with pain and tingling
        Bulbar muscles – swallowing, speech
        Respiratory muscles – breathless
    Stiffness – spasticity and rigidity
    Clumsiness – incoordination and ataxia
    Imbalance and walking problems
    Tremor
    Involuntary movements
Sensory
    Loss of feeling – numbness
    Distorted – tingling, paraesthesiae, bizarre
        sensations, hyperaesthesiae
    Loss of position sense – sensory ataxia
Autonomic
    Disturbances of bowel, bladder, sexual function
    Faintness – postural hypotension
Disturbances of higher functions
    Memory impairment – dementia
    Confusion
    Changes in mood, behaviour
    Changes in speech – aphasia
    Visuo-spatial disturbance
    Disordered thinking – psychiatric

Table 2.1 Symptoms to aid neurological diagnosis.

A suitable range of ten routine neurological questions is:	
1	Have you noticed any change in your mood, memory or powers of concentration?
2	Have you ever lost consciousness or had a fit or seizure?
3	Do you suffer unduly from headaches?
4	Have you noticed any change in your senses: (i) smell; (ii) taste; (iii) sight; (iv) hearing?
5	Do you have any difficulty in talking, chewing or swallowing?
6	Have you ever experienced any numbness, tightness, pins and needles, tingling or burning sensation in the face, limbs or trunk?
7	Have you noticed any weakness, stiffness, heaviness or dragging of arms or legs?
8	Do you have any difficulty in using your hands for skilled tasks, such as writing, typing or dressing?
9	Do you have any unsteadiness or difficulty in walking?
10	Do you ever have any difficulty controlling your bladder or bowels?

The diagnosis and management of someone with an acute onset of their first severe headache, 'first and worst', is entirely different from that of someone who has suffered from chronic daily headache for a matter of years, though patients often interpret this differently saying that because it has been going on a long time 'it must be due to something bad'.

Acute sudden headache

The sudden onset of severe headache over a matter of minutes or hours often poses a medical emergency, as this may be the presenting symptom of intracranial haemorrhage or infection (Box 2.2a) Most patients with subarachnoid haemorrhage (SAH) from an aneurysm or vascular malformation present with a sudden dramatic and explosive onset of devastating headache which rapidly becomes generalized and is accompanied by neck stiffness; 'It was as if I had been hit on the head with a hammer'.

Some patients with SAH lose consciousness and some may develop focal neurological signs. Patients with primary intracerebral haemorrhage often complain of headache and vomiting and then

Box 2.2 Causes of acute headache

(a) 'First and worst'
Subarachnoid haemorrhage
Intracerebral haemorrhage
Migraine – particularly first episode
Infections – meningitis
    Encephalitis
    Secondary to systemic infections, e.g. 'flu,
      psittacosis
Sudden rise in intracranial pressure – mass lesions –
    obstructive hydrocephalus
Hypertensive crises (accelerated hypertension),
    pheochromocytoma, reversible posterior
    leukoencephalopathy syndrome
Exertional headache, coitus
Cerebral venous thrombosis
Pituitary apoplexy
Drugs, alcohol – vasodilators, cocaine, 'hangover'
Toxic – carbon monoxide poisoning

(b) Causes of headache (based on ICHD)
Primary headaches
    Migraine
    Tension-type headache
    Cluster headache and other trigeminal autonomic
      cephalgias
Secondary headaches
    Following head trauma
    Linked to cranial or cervical vascular disorder
      Ischaemic stroke, AVM, aneurysms, angiitis,
        GCA, arterial dissection, reversible
        angiopathy, pituitary apoplexy
    Associated with raised intracranial pressure
      Tumours and other mass lesions, obstructive
        hydrocephalus
      Idiopathic intracranial hypertension
    Associated with low intracranial pressure
      Following lumbar puncture, trauma,
        spontaneous
    Associated with infections
      Meningitis, encephalitis, abscess, empyema
      Systemic infections
    Associated with toxic and metabolic upsets
      Hypoxia, hypercapnia, sleep apnoea, CO
        poisoning
      Hypoglycaemia, myxoedema; alcohol, cocaine
        use
    Associated with facial pains, eye upsets, sinus
      infections, dental and temporo-mandibular
      upsets

    Cervicogenic disturbances
      Cervical spine degenerative disease, discs,
        occipital neuralgia
    Associated with psychiatric upsets
    Cranial neuralgias and central causes of facial
      pain
      Trigeminal and glossopharyngeal neuralgia,
        atypical facial pain

AVM, arteriovenous malformation; CO, carbon monoxide; GCA, giant cell arteritis; ICHD, International Classification of Headache Disorders.

may rapidly lose consciousness. Commonly they are hypertensive. They may also show a dense neurological deficit due to brain destruction, and often do not have a stiff neck.

If SAH is suspected, immediate CT brain scan should be undertaken (Figure 2.1) and this will detect blood in the vast majority of patients scanned within the first 48 hours. The sensitivity is closely related to the skill of the radiologist. If the scan is normal, then the cerebrospinal fluid (CSF) should be examined to confirm the diagnosis in the small number of patients (approximately 5 per

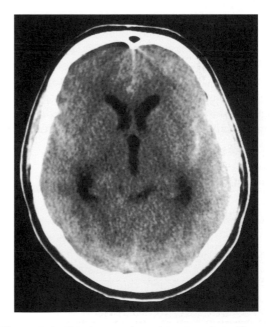

Figure 2.1 CT brain scan of a patient presenting with an acute severe headache following a subarachnoid haemorrhage. There is blood in the sylvian fissure and slight enlargement of the ventricles.

cent) where blood has not been shown on the scan. Xanthochromia of the spun supernatant of the CSF is present for about ten days after a bleed but takes 12 hours to form. Patients who have bled from an intracranial aneurysm, which is the most common cause of SAH, are at serious risk of a second bleed in the ensuing 2 weeks, which may be fatal. Early surgical clipping or endovascular occlusion of the aneurysm can prevent rebleeding.

Those in whom SAH is confirmed by CT scanning or lumbar puncture should be referred urgently to a local neurosurgical centre for further treatment. CT angiography will now detect some 96 per cent of aneurysms >3 mm in diameter.

The most common condition which may be confused with SAH is the acute onset of migraine (Box 2.2a). Migraine usually builds up over minutes or hours, but on occasion may start suddenly, so-called 'benign thunderclap' headache. Some patients may have photophobia and even some neck stiffness as part of a severe migraine, but examination of the CSF and a CT brain scan will reveal no blood or other abnormality.

The headache of meningitis and encephalitis does not start with such a dramatic onset, but builds up over a matter of hours. Such patients also are likely to have fever, confusion and, in the case of meningitis, severe neck stiffness.

In some elderly patients, the very young or the very sick, meningitis may be present without neck stiffness. In the case of encephalitis, neck stiffness is less conspicuous, but confusion, early coma and seizures are characteristic. Any patient suspected of meningitis or encephalitis requires lumbar puncture if not contraindicated to establish the diagnosis and the cause. Systemic infections may cause acute headache, e.g. 'flu, psittacosis, mumps.

Subacute headache

Headache that has been present for a few weeks or months in an individual not previously a headache sufferer must always be taken seriously, though such headaches usually turn out to be the onset of more chronic problem such as tension-type headache or migraine.

In the elderly patient, or in anyone aged over 50 years, **cranial or giant cell arteritis (GCA)** must always be considered.

Such patients are usually systemically unwell with symptoms of malaise, depression, weight loss and generalized aches and pains. Their main symptom, however, is persistent headache, often throbbing or burning, often with tenderness of the scalp, as when brushing the hair. The cranial arteries, particularly the superficial temporal arteries, may be visibly enlarged, tortuous and tender to touch. There may be reddening of the overlying skin. Patients with GCA are at risk of losing vision due to serial ischaemic damage to the optic nerves. Suspicion of the diagnosis should lead to an urgent erythrocyte sedimentation rate (ESR) or C-reactive protein (CRP). These will be raised, the ESR usually above 40 mm/hour, and a biopsy of a temporal artery should follow. Patients thought clinically to have GCA should be urgently started on steroids prior to biopsy.

The headache of raised intracranial pressure (ICP) of whatever cause, be it tumour, subdural haematoma or obstructive hydrocephalus, characteristically has been present for a matter of some weeks or months. Frequently it may awaken the patient from sleep and is often intermittent. It is made worse by coughing, bending or straining at stool, all of which increase ICP, although it is noteworthy that patients with migraine and sometimes other types of headache also report mild exacerbation with these factors. It may be accompanied by vomiting. There may be papilloedema and focal neurological signs on examination but these may also be absent. Occasionally, patients with an intermittent obstructive hydrocephalus may have episodes of acute crescendo headache (Figure 2.2).

The vast majority of patients with isolated cough headache, or isolated headache at orgasm (sex or orgasmic headache) do not have brain tumours.

Persistent headache after minor concussive head injuries (post-traumatic headache) is a very common complaint and is often accompanied by other symptoms such as postural dizziness, impaired memory and concentration, fatigue and depression. These common post-traumatic symptoms are well recognized in the law courts as one of the common sources of claims for compensation for injury. However, similar symptoms frequently develop in stable individuals after a head injury where there is no compensation claim. It has now been shown that minor head injuries may be followed by impairment of some cognitive functions and vestibular disturbances. However, very pro-

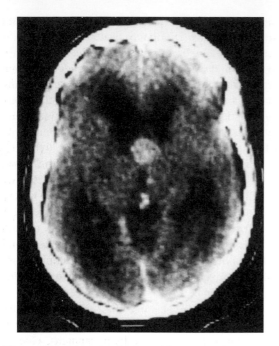

Figure 2.2 This patient had a sudden crescendo headache. This was the result of the colloid cyst shown in the third ventricle causing an intermittent obstructive hydrocephalus, as shown on this CT scan.

longed symptoms may be linked with psychological processes, as the poor prognostic factors for recovery appear independent of the injury severity and relate more to psychosocial factors.

Chronic headache

The most common causes of chronic headache are migraine and tension-type headache (Chapter 10). A headache that occurs on 15 or more days a month is described as a chronic daily headache (CDH). In population-based studies, some 4–5 per cent have primary CDH.

Migraine is very common; approximately 20 per cent of the population are likely to suffer one or more migrainous episodes in their life. It is a periodic disorder with episodes of headache separated by periods in which the subject is entirely well. Migraine with aura (classical migraine) is easily recognized by the characteristic warning symptoms in the half hour or so prior to the onset of the headache. The most common are visual, in the form of flashing lights or zig-zags due to a spreading depression in the occipital cortex. Other warning symptoms are hemisensory disturbances, alarming dysphasia and diplopia with dysarthria and

ataxia. These warning symptoms can occur without a subsequent headache. The headache is usually severe, throbbing and may be hemicranial or more generalized. During the headache, the patient feels ill, nauseated and anorexic, photophobic and drowsy. Frequently they vomit; following which the headache may subside and the patient sleeps. Such headaches usually last several hours (4–72). Once the headache disappears the patient soon returns to normal. The frequency of migraine attacks is variable (from <1 to >5/month).

Although migraine is commonly intermittent, patients may develop chronic symptoms which merge into the persistent, continuous so-called **tension-type headache**. These patients complain of a constant aching or pressure sensation, often like a band around the head, and varying in severity. Some patients claim they are never free from pain and that it interferes with sleep and their daily activities, although in others it is episodic. The pain may worsen with anxiety, noise and when tired. It may spread into the back of the head and down into the neck. There is undoubtedly an overlap between migraine (transformed migraine) and tension-type headaches but as these are clinical diagnoses, one neurologist's transformed migraine may be another's 'tension headache'. Both may be aggravated by medication overuse. There is a link with anxiety and depression: about one-third of depressed patients complain of headache so it is important to be aware of a primary depressive illness.

A group of patients describe the sudden onset of headache on a specific day which then persists: this may be 'new daily persistent headache'. Some of these are secondary to a defined cause, e.g. head trauma, raised intracranial pressure, meningitis. The headache of spontaneous low intracranial pressure may also have a specific onset time.

Uncommon causes of headache

Headache may arise in patients with accelerated hypertension, and with rises in blood pressure linked to a phaeochromocytoma. Acute sinusitis may cause facial and head pain and this may be increased lying flat, bending, coughing or sneezing. Eye disease, such as glaucoma or iritis, causes intense local pain often with tenderness in the eye and some headache. These symptoms are usually accompanied by a change in visual acuity and often reddening of the eye itself. Double vision, eye pain and headache may arise from an oculomotor palsy, a cavernous sinus lesion or pituitary disturbances.

PAIN IN THE FACE

As with headache, patients complaining of pain in the face frequently show no neurological signs so the history is all important (Chapter 11). With a complaint of pain in the face it is worth recalling the local structures that may be involved: eyes, sinuses, teeth, jaw and referred pain from involvement of the trigeminal nerve. In the latter, there may be signs of altered sensation in the trigeminal territory.

Other disorders with minimal or no abnormal physical signs or minimal signs include trigeminal and glossopharyngeal neuralgia, cluster headache (migrainous neuralgia) and other trigeminal autonomic cephalgias, and atypical facial pain. Facial pain (a post-herpetic neuralgia) following a herpes zoster infection in the fifth nerve territory is self-evident from the skin eruption preceding it.

Trigeminal neuralgia (tic douloureux) is a common cause of intermittent severe pain in the face, usually in older patients. The pain is unilateral and usually arises in the second and third divisions of the fifth nerve. It has two absolute characteristics: the individual spasms of pain are extremely brief, like a knife jabbing into the cheek or jaw; and these spasms are triggered. The triggers include touch, eating, washing the face, cleaning the teeth, talking, shaving, a cold wind. The paroxysms of intense pain last a few seconds to minutes and often shoot from a site of onset in the cheek, side of the nose or gums to another part of the face. The illness is intermittent with bouts lasting days or weeks followed by long periods of freedom. These may tend to shorten.

Glossopharyngeal neuralgia is analogous to trigeminal neuralgia but in the territory of the ninth nerve. The severe paroxysms of pain are felt at the back of the throat and tongue, or deep in the ear and are triggered by swallowing.

In some patients orbital pain and headache may be associated with obvious vasomotor/**autonomic symptoms**. These include tearing, eye redness, nasal stuffiness or rhinorrhoea, eyelid swelling, ptosis, miosis and excess sweating.

Cluster headache (migrainous neuralgia) describes a unilateral headache with intense stab-

bing or boring eye pain most often in the orbit and temple most commonly lasting 45–90 minutes (15–180). These bouts of intense pain recur both in sleep and in the day over days or weeks. There are accompanying autonomic symptoms. The bouts may be triggered by alcohol and exercise. The condition is more common in men and is characterized by restlessness and pacing as opposed to migraine where the sufferer lies still with sensory dislike.

Paroxysmal hemicrania has some resemblance to migrainous neuralgia with repeated short-lived (10–20 minutes) attacks of knife-like pain in one side of the face occurring from one to 30 times a day. It responds specifically to indometacin.

Short-lasting unilateral neuralgiform headache attacks with conjunctival injection and tearing (SUNCT) are a further rare form of trigeminal autonomic neuralgia. Here, intense stabbing pain in and around one eye lasting 5–250 seconds (usually about 1 minute) is described. The pains may be triggered by touch and vary in frequency. If you are not sure whether it is cluster headache or trigeminal neuralgia you are dealing with, it may be SUNCT.

There is also a group of patients who complain of a constant pain in the face who show no abnormal physical signs. The description of the pain does not fit into any well recognized category and often is said to be a deep aching involving the eye, nose, cheek, temple or jaw. It is usually unilateral but is sometimes bilateral, often widespread and at times may be described as being much more severe – tearing, ripping, pulling. This may be **atypical facial pain**.

BLACKOUTS, FITS AND FAINTS

Patients commonly use the term 'blackout' to describe loss of consciousness, when it really means loss of vision, so it is always important to establish carefully the nature of this reported symptom. The common causes of blackouts are faints, fits and psychogenic attacks (Chapter 13).

In a faint (neurogenic/vasovagal syncope), there is a sudden drop in blood pressure leading to a drop in cerebral perfusion. The patient may fall to the ground from a loss of muscle tone. With the altered perfusion, the vision goes black before consciousness is lost.

The doctor rarely has the opportunity to witness the episode of loss of consciousness (LOC) so the diagnosis rests on the history. If the patient has LOC without warning, they will have no memory of the episode.

Thus a **description** of events from an independent **witness** is absolutely essential in coming to the correct conclusion about the cause of many such episodes.

The circumstances in which the attack occurred, details of what happened during the attack and afterwards, must be obtained. Eye witnesses often describe what they think they saw, e.g. by concluding that the patient had a fit, but are not trained to distinguish between epilepsy, syncope and non-epileptic psychogenic attacks. Precipitants are also important, e.g. prolonged standing, flickering lights or during an injection.

Epilepsy

Many patients presenting with sudden, unexplained episodes of LOC will turn out to have epilepsy, but many other causes can provoke such events.

Epilepsy itself takes many forms, some of which do not cause LOC.

Major epileptic seizures

A major seizure consists of a period of tonic muscle contraction during which the subject becomes anoxic, followed by repetitive generalized whole body jerking in the clonic phase. The whole event lasts less than 5 minutes, when the subject stops fitting and either drifts into sleep or recovers.

Focal or simple partial epileptic seizures arising in one temporal lobe or in some other cortical area, may not cause LOC. More extensive focal discharges may cause loss of awareness, as in complex partial seizures, which may then propagate to involve both hemispheres to become generalized (secondary generalization). The patient will then go into a typical tonic-clonic or grand mal seizure.

If such grand mal fits are due to secondary generalization from some primary focal cortical source, then they may be preceded by an aura that the patient remembers.

The aura is appropriate to the focal source of the seizure, e.g. a discharge arising in the sensorimotor cortex will provoke contralateral motor and sensory phenomena for a short period prior to the LOC and the commencement of the generalized fit. Details of the characteristics of focal seizures arising from different cortical areas are discussed later.

However, many patients with epilepsy develop major grand mal seizures without any focal onset or aura. They are said to have primary generalized epilepsy of grand mal type.

Another form of epilepsy causing temporary LOC, occurring in children, is also a form of primary generalized seizure discharge causing a brief **absence attack**, called **petit mal**. For a few seconds or so, the child ceases to speak or move, appearing stunned with open flickering eyes, and then rapidly recovers back to normal.

Brief loss of awareness, often accompanied by purposeless movements, chewing, lip smacking or fumbling with clothing may also occur in complex focal seizures arising from the temporal lobe. Sometimes these attacks may be accompanied by psychic symptoms, e.g. memory disturbances, affective symptoms, dreamy states, illusions and even hallucinations.

The old term temporal lobe seizure has largely been replaced by complex partial seizure as a significant number of such attacks arise in other areas of the brain, e.g. the frontal lobes. However, some 60 per cent of symptomatic focal seizures arise from the temporal lobe.

In **complex partial seizures, the term complex refers to** impairment of awareness during attacks. By contrast, in **simple partial seizures**, a focal discharge may occur without loss of awareness so that in a simple partial motor seizure there may be contralateral jerking of the thumb spreading into the arm and perhaps the corner of the mouth on the same side, without disturbance of consciousness. After such a focal motor attack, there may be a temporary weakness in the affected limb – a **Todd's paresis**.

Sometimes, following generalized tonic-clonic seizures, particularly spreading from temporal lobe foci, or after complex partial seizures, the patient may enter into a period of **automatic behaviour** for about 1 hour, but usually much shorter (minutes).

During this phase of **post–epileptic automatism**, the patient may undertake relatively coordinated action for which they subsequently have no memory, amnesia. In such a state, epileptic patients may travel some distance and arrive at their destination with no idea as to how they got there.

Diagnosis of epilepsy

The criteria that contribute to a confident diagnosis of epilepsy are:

1 The sudden, unexpected onset in an otherwise apparently healthy individual of a brief period of LOC not exceeding 5 minutes.
2 The episode of LOC may be prefaced by a characteristic aura in which the same events occur in every attack.
3 If the seizure is of generalized tonic-clonic type, witnesses will say the patient fell, went stiff and blue, and shook. The patients may find afterwards that they have injured themselves, bitten their tongue or been incontinent.
4 If it was an absence seizure or a complex partial seizure, witnesses will remark that the patient suddenly lost contact with the world and was inaccessible for a short period, during which they may have undertaken some crude motor automatisms.
5 The attacks are always brief (unless the patient goes into repeated attacks as in status epilepticus), and the patient returns to normal between the episodes.

Finally, it should be noted that many patients complaining of 'blackouts' may be suspected of suffering from epilepsy, but the evidence initially is insufficient to be certain of that diagnosis. As has already been stated, the EEG cannot be used to establish a certain diagnosis of epilepsy. In this situation, it is usually best to avoid a firm diagnosis and to await events. To mislabel someone as epileptic on insufficient evidence may be catastrophic for the patient's livelihood and there is little risk in seeing what happens.

If the patient's attack of LOC is confidently diagnosed as due to epilepsy, the next stage is to determine the cause (Box 2.3).

Box 2.3 Causes of epilepsy

Focal (partial) seizures – often **symptomatic** of an underlying brain lesion
  Tumour – benign, malignant; metastatic
  Infections – meningo-encephalitis, abscess, subdural empyema, parasitosis, tuberculoma
  Trauma – particularly severe or penetrating
  Vascular – thromboembolic infarct, haemorrhage, cortical venous thrombosis; angioma, cavernoma, hypertensive encephalopathy
  Degenerative – Alzheimer's disease (c. 15% of patients late in the disease)
  Developmental abnormalities – focal cortical dysplasia, malformations
  Hippocampal sclerosis
Systemic disorders
  Hypoxia – adult and pre- and perinatal
  Metabolic – uraemic, hepatic failure, hypoglycaemia
  Drugs – amphetamines, cocaine, baclofen, isoniazid, high-dose penicillin (intrathecal)
  Alcohol – include withdrawal
Generalized seizures – often idiopathic
  Include major tonic-clonic, absence (petit mal), myoclonic, atonic

Some focal seizures spread to become generalized.

The cause of epilepsy changes with age

A simple but important principle is that the aetiology of epilepsy changes with age. Epilepsy in the infant indicates some serious metabolic, structural or infective cause. Epilepsy in the child usually is of unknown cause (idiopathic) or due to some static cerebral pathology, such as that produced by a birth injury or head trauma. Epilepsy beginning in the younger adult often is the first sign of a cerebral tumour (Figure 2.3). Epilepsy commencing for the first time in the elderly frequently is due to vascular or other degenerative disease.

Focal (partial) epilepsy usually has a structural cause

A second useful simple principle is that focal (partial) epilepsy commonly is due to some identifiable structural lesion (Figure 2.4) while primary generalized grand mal or petit mal frequently appears idiopathic in origin.

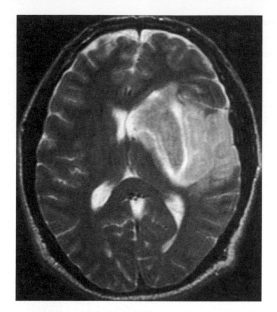

Figure 2.3 T2-weighted axial view MRI scan showing a left frontal tumour. This patient presented with complex partial seizures with secondary generalization.

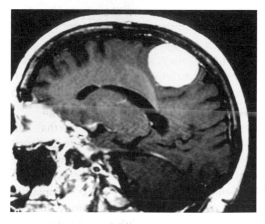

Figure 2.4 Sagittal view MRI scan showing a large convexity meningioma. This was causing simple partial seizures with a focal onset in the face and arm on the opposite side.

These principles guide the subsequent management of the patient whose episodes of LOC are diagnosed as being due to epilepsy.

Epilepsy must be distinguished from other causes of LOC, in particular from fainting (syncope), sleep attacks of narcolepsy, hypoglycaemia, cerebrovascular disease and psychogenic illness.

Syncope

Syncope is defined as a transient loss of consciousness caused by an acute drop in cerebral blood flow (Box 2.4). It is accompanied by a loss of postural tone. In neurogenic/vasovagal syncope (fainting), there is usually a profound drop in systemic systolic blood pressure, below about 60 mmHg from a combination of sudden bradycardia and peripheral vasodilatation in skeletal muscle and internal organs.

Box 2.4 Causes of syncope

Vasovagal
   Simple faint
   Cough, micturition – variants with specific triggers
Orthostatic, postural hypotension
   Autonomic neuropathy, dysautonomia, spinal cord lesions
   Drugs
      Hypotensive, e.g. beta blockers, ACE inhibitors, vasodilators; antipsychotics, antidepressants
   Endocrine
      Hypopituitarism
      Addisonian
Cardiac
   Arrhythmias – too fast, too slow
   Prolonged QT interval, heart block
   Outflow obstruction; aortic stenosis, obstructive cardiomyopathy, left atrial mobile mass
   Cardiomyopathy
Hypovolaemic
   Blood loss, dehydration
Vascular
   Carotid sinus sensitivity; vertebrobasilar TIAs; anaemia
Metabolic
   Hypoglycaemia; hypocalcaemia; hyperventilation
Psychogenic
   Anxiety, panic attacks
   Non-epileptic attack disorder

ACE, angiotensin converting enzyme; TIAs, transient ischaemic attacks.

There are often familiar precipitants, e.g. prolonged standing, the sight of blood, needles, intense pain or emotion. The term vasovagal indicates the two components – vagal slowing of heart rate and peripheral vasodilatation. Such patients 'come over queer', feel dizzy and swimmy, their eyesight dims and hearing recedes, their face goes pale, and they slump forward or fall to the ground. Provided they are laid flat, consciousness soon returns, usually within 15–45 seconds, although patients may feel sick and break out in a heavy sweat.

Somewhat similar symptoms can be triggered in men getting up in the night to empty their bladders (**micturition syncope**), or by pressure over the carotid bifurcation in older patients with excess sensitivity of the carotid sinus (**carotid sinus syndrome**): the last may be the mechanism for syncope in some 15 per cent of elderly patients. Repeated coughing in those with chronic lung disease also can provoke fainting by obstructing the venous return and perhaps by baroceptor stimulation (**cough syncope**). A similar mechanism is probably responsible for the syncope seen in trumpet playing and weight-lifting.

Another cause of fainting is damage to peripheral or central autonomic pathways (**areflexic, orthostatic or paralytic syncope**). In this situation, patients faint when they stand upright, because they are unable to adjust heart rate and the resistance of peripheral blood vessels to cope with the rapid shift of blood to the legs and viscera that occurs with the sudden change in position. A fall of systolic blood pressure of more than 20 mmHg supports the diagnosis. Such postural syncope occurs in any type of peripheral neuropathy affecting the autonomic nervous system, but particularly in diabetics. In addition, many drugs such as hypotensive agents, alcohol, barbiturates, dopamine agonists and phenothiazines may all interfere with the operation of normal baroceptor reflexes to cause postural faintness. Age in itself leads to some loss of efficiency of baroceptor reflexes and many elderly patients experience transient dizziness on rising quickly from a bed or chair. Such patients are particularly sensitive to relatively small doses of hypotensive agents.

Cardiogenic syncope is also relatively common in the elderly and may account for some 25 per cent of patients presenting as an emergency. Cardiac syncope can occur in any position. Symptoms typical of a faint may occur in those with cardiac dysrhythmias (conduction defects – prolonged QT interval and brady- and tachy-arrhythmias), aortic stenosis or congenital heart disease. However, many patients with heart block lose consciousness abruptly (Stokes–Adams attack) probably as a result of cardiac arrest. Cardiac causes of syncope carry a worse prognosis, particularly in the elderly.

In general, a careful history will distinguish syncope from epilepsy, but a complication arises if a failure of cerebral perfusion during a syncopal attack persists for longer than a minute, for in these circumstances the patient who faints may go on to have a fit. The situation may occur if someone faints in a position where they are unable to lie with their head lower than their heart, as may happen on the stairs, in the lavatory or if the patient is supported upright by well-wishers. If unconsciousness lasts longer than 20 seconds, convulsive features may occur (convulsive syncope). Asynchronous myoclonic jerks are common during neurogenic syncope and may be interpreted as a 'fit' by an independent witness. In addition, if the bladder is full during a faint, incontinence may occur.

Other causes of episodic loss of consciousness

Spontaneous **hypoglycaemia** can lead to LOC and many patients may not recall the premonitory symptoms of anxiety, palpitations and sweating. It may also cause bizarre behaviour. The diagnosis can be confirmed by a blood glucose estimation during an attack: a value of <2 mmol/L is diagnostic. Any patient found unconscious for no apparent reason must have blood withdrawn immediately for estimation of glucose and insulin levels, and 50 g of glucose should be given intravenously: it can do no harm and may save a life. Spontaneous hypoglycaemia is very rare (usually due to an islet cell pancreatic tumour) but hypoglycaemia in insulin-treated diabetics is relatively common.

Cerebrovascular disease very rarely causes episodic LOC without other obvious neurological symptoms, particularly when transient ischaemia occurs in the territory of the vertebrobasilar arterial system. However, such patients virtually always suffer other symptoms such as diplopia, dysarthria and ataxia, indicating brainstem ischaemia. Some patients with diffuse cerebrovascular disease affecting the medial portions of the cerebral hemispheres may experience prolonged periods of loss of awareness. Such **transient global amnesia** may last minutes to hours and is very similar to the benign transient global amnesia provoked by immersion in cold water/straining/emotion, etc. During such an episode, the patients are disorientated, unable to recall what they are doing, where they are, or when it is, but can undertake simple automatic tasks, such as washing, dressing or cooking. Subsequently they have no memory for the event, i.e. they are amnesic. Likewise, patients with **migraine** in the vertebrobasilar territory may occasionally describe episodes of loss of awareness for up to 30 minutes although they too often describe other symptoms of brainstem ischaemia and severe occipital headache. Rarely, transient global amnesia may arise in the context of a form of complex partial seizure.

Patients with intense vertigo may also complain of LOC, although they usually have recall of the acute distressing symptom prior to the episode and the LOC is in fact a drop attack with preserved consciousness. Some patients with epilepsy may have a vertiginous aura prior to the onset of their seizure. The sleep attacks characteristic of **narcolepsy** should not be confused with epilepsy or syncope. Sufferers describe an irresistible desire to lapse into otherwise typical sleep, from which they can be awoken, at inappropriate moments.

Prolonged overbreathing, **hyperventilation**, may produce respiratory alkalosis with symptoms of paroxysmal tingling in the extremities and around the mouth (circumoral). These are usually accompanied by giddiness, and rarely by LOC. If the attack persists, carpopedal spasm and muscular twitching may appear. A proportion of these patients complain of headache and visual upset. Many are young women and a trial of overbreathing may provoke similar symptoms.

Finally, it will rapidly become apparent to any student attending neurological outpatients that some patients complaining of blackouts cannot easily be allocated to one of the diagnostic categories. Often this is because there is insufficient information on the circumstances of the attack, or a witness is not available. However, many of these patients describe attacks of altered awareness occurring in relation to emotional provocation. As usual, marital discord, family tensions, job dissatisfaction and other such stresses may provoke acute episodes of phobic anxiety in which the subject is distraught, breathless and incoherent, a state of affairs for which they claim subsequent amnesia. Often it is obvious that such patients have an underlying anxiety state, and careful and gentle enquiry will unearth the usual precipitating circumstances.

In other patients, non-epileptic seizures (non-epileptic attacks, also called pseudo-seizures) occur as a physical manifestation of underlying psychological distress. Frequently these are adolescent females and they may exhibit other conversion symptoms. Careful enquiry into the circumstances and character of their attack may indicate a psychogenic origin. For example, sexual abuse may sometimes be the provocation. Unfortunately, some people (10–15 per cent) who also suffer from epilepsy may be prone to non-epileptic attacks as well. In some circumstances, these non-epileptic attacks are attention-seeking in nature. In some individuals, it may take prolonged observation and careful searching through every facet of the history to establish the true situation. As a general principle, it is best not to commit oneself to a certain diagnosis in those with attacks of uncertain origin. Non-epileptic attack disorder (NEAD) or dissociative seizures are the terms used to describe some of these episodes of uncertain origin. If the episodes are frequent (several weekly) then video-telemetry with EEG recording may establish a clear diagnosis.

LOSS OF VISION

The patient complaining of disturbance of vision either may have disease of the eye, or may have damage to the optic nerve or posterior parts of the visual pathways.

Local eye disease is common, and it is necessary to exclude refractive errors, corneal damage, cataract, glaucoma and obvious retinal lesions by appropriate ophthalmological investigation. These will not be considered in detail here, but most refractive errors are due to short-sightedness (myopia), which can be corrected with a pin-hole. This simple test should be employed in all complaining of visual loss, before considering other causes. A neurological cause of visual failure can only be assumed if vision cannot be improved to normal by correction of refractive error, the ocular media are clear and there is no gross retinal abnormality.

Visual sensitivity or acuity depends upon intact central or macular vision.

Lesions of the optic nerve cause loss of central macular vision (scotoma) and reduced visual acuity. Most show a relative afferent pupillary defect.

However, lesions placed further back in the visual pathways, in the optic chiasm, or radiations, or in the occipital cortex, only produce loss of vision in one half of the visual field (hemianopia) (see later). Visual acuity is normal in patients with such posteriorly placed lesions because, although they have lost vision in the opposite half field, the remaining intact half of central macular vision is sufficient to preserve normal acuity. Patients with visual failure due to anteriorly placed lesions of the optic nerve complain of loss of visual perception for detail of distant objects or reading print, and can be demonstrated to have reduced visual acuity which cannot be improved by correcting refractive error. In contrast, patients with posteriorly placed visual pathway damage complain of difficulty in perceiving objects in the affected opposite field of vision, but retain sensitivity in the remaining intact visual field so that they can make out detail and read print, and show a normal visual acuity on formal testing. Patients with posteriorly placed lesion do complain of difficulties reading, but they are of different character. Those with loss of the right half field of vision have difficulty seeing the next word in a sentence, while those with loss of the left half field have difficulty in moving from one line to the next. The significance of such hemianopic field defects will be discussed later. Here, the problem of visual failure due to a reduced visual acuity that cannot be attributed to local eye disease is considered.

> The most valuable aid in distinguishing different causes of neurological visual failure is the tempo of the illness (Box 2.5).

Visual deficit may be present from early life and static (amblyopia); sudden and transient; sudden but persistent; or progressive. Usually it is possible to distinguish between these patterns of visual loss, but one problem is that of the patient who discovers visual impairment in one eye accidentally when rubbing the other, whereupon the onset is thought acute. In fact, many patients with progressive unilateral visual failure are unaware of their problem until, for some reason or another, they occlude the vision of the opposite intact eye.

Box 2.5 Causes of persistent visual loss

> Acute
>   Ophthalmic
>   Retinal artery occlusion
>   Retinal vein occlusion
>   Retinal detachment
>   Angle closure glaucoma
>   Vitreous haemorrhage
>   Maculopathy – central serous retinopathy
>   Inflammatory – uveitis
>   Neurological
>   Optic neuritis
>   Ischaemic optic neuropathy (include giant cell arteritis)
>   Optic nerve compression
>   Pituitary apoplexy
>   Bilateral occipital lobe infarction
> Subacute/progressive
>   Ophthalmic
>   Cataracts
>   Cone dystrophies
>   Glaucoma
>   Macular degeneration
>   Paraneoplastic retinopathy
>   Retinitis pigmentosa
>   Neurological
>   Leber's optic neuropathy
>   Optic nerve compression – pituitary tumours, gliomas, meningiomas, aneurysms, orbital masses
>   Metabolic – diabetic neuropathy, raised intracranial pressure (late)
>   Toxic – tobacco-alcohol
>   Drugs – chloramphenicol, chloroquine, ethambutol, vigabatrin
>   Vitamin A, vitamin B_{12} deficiency

Amblyopia

Ocular defects in early life, particularly muscle imbalance, cause suppression of visual acuity in one eye to prevent continuing double vision. Such visual suppression is known as amblyopia, which is not progressive after about 6–8 years of age, and which does not affect perception of colour or pupillary responses. Amblyopia as a cause of reduced visual acuity is suggested by visual loss since early childhood, evidence of a squint or severe refractive error.

Sudden transient visual loss

Sudden, but temporary loss of vision occurs in a number of circumstances. **Obscurations of vision**, due to raised ICP, consist of episodic visual loss affecting one or both eyes and lasting for a few seconds to one-quarter of a minute. Obscurations may be provoked by any manoeuvre that increases ICP, such as straining, coughing, sneezing or bending. Examination will reveal swollen optic discs and further investigation and treatment are a matter of urgency, for obscurations may herald impending permanent visual loss.

Amaurosis fugax refers to episodic unilateral visual loss due to vascular disturbance in ophthalmic artery territory. The patient commonly describes a curtain ascending or descending to occlude the lower or upper half of vision due to involvement of the superior or inferior branches of the ophthalmic artery. These field defects respect the vertical meridian. Such episodes may last minutes to hours, but are followed by recovery of vision. Amaurosis fugax is a transient ischaemic attack (TIA) in ophthalmic artery distribution, and in the middle-aged or elderly subject is likely to indicate the existence of cerebrovascular disease.

Uhtoff's phenomenon describes dimness or loss of vision provoked by a rise in body temperature, such as occurs when taking a hot bath, or on vigorous exercise, and is a feature of optic nerve demyelination produced by MS.

Sudden persistent visual loss

Sudden persistent visual loss is nearly always the result of either acute optic neuritis (most commonly due to MS) in the younger subject, or a vascular cause (ischaemic optic neuropathy) in the middle-aged or elderly.

Occasionally, a tumour or cyst compressing the optic nerve expands suddenly to cause abrupt visual failure.

Progressive visual loss
In the absence of ocular pathology, a history of progressive visual loss in one or both eyes must be taken to suggest compression of the anterior visual pathways until proven otherwise by appropriate investigations.

Many such progressive lesions turn out to be benign tumours, such as pituitary adenomas or suprasellar meningiomas, which can be surgically removed with restoration of sight. Toxic damage to the optic nerve by drugs and alcohol/tobacco, and hereditary optic neuropathies, are less common than compressive lesions, which must always be excluded in a patient with progressive visual failure.

In practice, patients complaining of visual loss must be assessed by an ophthalmologist and, if the eyes are found to be normal, by a neurologist. Acute loss of vision must be treated as an emergency, and progressive loss of vision must always be investigated fully to establish the cause.

DIZZINESS

Patients use the words 'giddiness, dizziness, light-headedness and unsteadiness' to describe a variety of sensations due to many causes. Patients with postural syncope will describe giddiness on standing up, while patients with cerebellar ataxia of gait may say they are dizzy and unsteady.

Vertigo refers to a sensation of unsteadiness or disequilibrium that is felt in the head. It is an illusion of movement.

Patients with a cerebellar ataxia know that they are unsteady when trying to walk, but the sensation of disequilibrium is not felt in the head so it is not vertigo.

The sensation of vertigo is one of disequilibrium whatever its nature: it may be a sensation of rotation, of falling, as if on a pitching boat moving up and down, or of swaying. All are sensations of disequilibrium which, if felt in the head, may be described as vertiginous. Thus vertigo is an illusory movement of oneself or one's surroundings. It implies a defect of function in the vestibular system, either of the labyrinthine end-organ or of its central connections, particularly those in the brainstem. Lesions of the cerebral hemispheres rarely cause vertigo, although it may form an uncommon symptom in occasional patients with temporal lobe epilepsy.

The first step in the diagnosis of a patient with vertigo is to decide whether the cause lies peripherally in the labyrinth, or centrally in the brainstem (Box 2.6).

Box 2.6 Causes of dizziness

Peripheral
    Acute labyrinthine failure
        Vestibular neuronitis, vascular
    Benign paroxysmal positional vertigo
    Ménière's disease
    Perilymph fistula
    Post-traumatic vertigo
    Local infection
        Bacterial, viral; mastoiditis
Central
    Brainstem
        Ischaemia, infarction, haemorrhage
        Demyelination (MS)
        Migraine (peripheral – channelopathy)
        Tumours – primary, secondary
        Cerebellopontine angle tumours
        Seizures (rare)
Systemic
    Drugs
        Vestibulotoxic – aminoglycosides, gentamicin;
        Hypotensives, hypnotics, alcohol, tranquillizers,
            analgesics, anticonvulsants
Hypotension
    Orthostatic
    Cardiac arrhythmias
    Endocrine – myxoedema, diabetes mellitus
    Vascular – PRV, anaemia, vertebro-basilar TIAs,
        vasculitis, SLE, giant cell arteritis
    Infective systemic infection, syphilis
    Sarcoidosis
    Psychogenic
        Agoraphobia, acrophobia
        Anxiety states, panic attacks, hyperventilation
        Phobic postural vertigo
        Post-traumatic dizziness - often linked with
            benign positional vertigo

MS, multiple sclerosis; PRV, polycythaemia rubra vera; SLE, systemic lupus erythematosus; TIA, transient ischaemic attack.

Acute peripheral lesions causing vertigo also commonly cause intense nausea, vomiting, sweating and prostration. Because of the proximity of auditory to vestibular fibres in the eighth cranial nerve, deafness sometimes accompanies the vertigo. Conductive deafness due to middle ear disease suggests a peripheral lesion, but perceptive deafness due to damage to the cochlear end-organ or vestibular nerve may be due to peripheral or central lesions. If peripheral, perceptive deafness is often less severe with loud sounds (loudness recruitment), and also causes severe speech distortion. Central lesions of the eighth nerve rarely show loudness recruitment, but exhibit auditory fatigue in that the intensity of sound has to be increased progressively to maintain a constant noise level. Vertigo due to vestibular damage is also often accompanied by nystagmus, a to-and-fro movement of the eyes due to interrupted visual fixation. Different patterns of nystagmus will be described later.

Suffice to say here that peripheral vestibular lesions causing vertigo are usually accompanied by horizontal jerk nystagmus in one direction that gets worse with loss of fixation (as in the dark), while central lesions produce nystagmus that changes direction depending upon the patient's gaze, and which is often rotatory and vertical as well as horizontal.

Differential diagnosis of vertigo
The differential diagnosis of causes of vertigo is aided by considering the time course of the symptoms. The duration of the actual sensation of spinning is important. Benign paroxysmal positional vertigo lasts seconds, that of vertebrobasilar ischaemia or migraine minutes, that of Ménière's disease hours, and that of acute vestibular failure, days. Some diseases produce a single episode of vertigo, others produce recurrent attacks (and of course, any single episode may be the first of such attacks), while others produce persistent vertigo.

Acute single attack of vertigo

An acute episode of vertigo may be provoked by the sudden loss of unilateral labyrinthine function, or by sudden brainstem damage.

Either may cause the sudden onset of severe vertigo, nausea, vomiting and great distress because the patient is unable to move without provoking further severe vertigo. The patient will usually lie with the affected ear uppermost. The episode commonly lasts days, sometimes as long as 2–3 weeks, and then gradually eases because central adaptation to vestibular failure occurs. During the recovery phase, which may last 3–4 weeks, any sudden head movement may cause brief vertigo and unsteadiness. Acute vestibular failure due to sudden unilateral labyrinthine damage may develop in the course of middle ear disease when infection gains access to the labyrinth. Such a course of events is an emergency. If the middle ear is normal, acute peripheral vestibular failure may be attributed to a viral infection (vestibular neuronitis) or to ischaemia in the territory of the internal auditory arteries. However, in many such cases the cause remains uncertain. Acute brainstem lesions that may provoke an attack of vertigo include a plaque of demyelination (from MS), or a vascular lesion, such as an infarct or haemorrhage in the brainstem or part of the cerebellum. Such lesions will usually also produce definite brainstem symptoms and signs including diplopia, dysarthria, weakness, ataxia and sensory disturbances.

Recurrent attacks of vertigo

If the patient describes repeated attacks of vertigo with recovery between episodes, they may be suffering from peripheral vestibular disease such as Ménière's syndrome, from migrainous vertigo or from repeated brainstem ischaemia.

Migrainous vertigo may arise from basilar artery migraine in the younger subject (sometimes in rather poorly defined episodes), or as vertebrobasilar transient ischaemic attacks in the middle-aged and elderly. Very rarely, such recurrent episodes of vertigo may indicate epilepsy. There is a general association between migraine without aura and vestibular failure, indeed many adult migraine sufferers were travel sick as children. Vague disequilibrium is commonly reported in patients who also have a history of migraine and remote for the attacks of migrainous headache.

More commonly, patients may describe recurrent fleeting episodes of vertigo provoked by a sudden change of position. This is usually most striking when lying down at night, or when moving the head suddenly. Such benign paroxysmal positional vertigo may be due to damage arising from otoconia being displaced from the utricle and ending in the posterior semicircular canal. Positional testing will establish the diagnosis. Positional vertigo may follow trauma to the head or infections but often is of undetermined origin. It may also arise from central causes as a brainstem disturbance.

Persistent vertigo

Chronic persistent vertigo is uncommon, due to the rapid compensation that occurs with vestibular deficits. Those patients complaining of persistent dizziness usually are not really describing vertigo proper, but are drawing attention to minor degrees of true instability or a sense of insecurity. However, drug damage to the vestibular nerves (streptomycin, gentamicin), brainstem demyelination or infarction, and occasionally posterior fossa tumours, all may cause persistent vertigo, although this often proves to be ataxia. Many of those with complaints of persistent vertigo may have a phobic anxiety state, with fear of falling. This can be triggered by an episode of true vertigo, by insecurity due to ataxia, or even by a fall or trip. Such patients may become housebound (agoraphobic) or unable to leave the security of walls or furniture (space phobia). In addition, once the vestibular system is damaged, symptoms may re-emerge in the absence of new 'damage' but secondary to the phenomena of breakdown in central compensation. This usually occurs in the setting of unrelated intercurrent illness or stress.

PAIN IN THE ARM

The painful, tingling or weak arm

Acute pain in the arm is most often caused by trauma or local disease of muscle, joint or bone. Only after these are excluded should neurological causes be considered (Box 2.7). Damage to the peripheral nerves, brachial plexus or cervical roots causes sensory disturbance and muscle wasting with weakness in a characteristic distribution, which must be learnt (see later) in order to diagnose the site of damage to these structures. Pain due to lesions of peripheral

Box 2.7 Neurological causes of acute pain in the arm

Peripheral nerve
    Carpal tunnel syndrome
    Peripheral neuropathy – diabetic, amyloid,
        paraneoplastic, ischaemic, drug-induced, e.g.
        metronidazole
Brachial plexus
    Trauma
    Cervical rib
    Inflammatory – neuralgic amyotrophy
    Malignant infiltration
    Irradiation
Cervical roots
    Trauma – avulsion
    Compression – disc, bony spur, malignancy
    Post-herpetic
Cervical cord
    Intramedullary tumour
    Syrinx
Central causes
    Thalamic lesion
    Extrapyramidal disorder

nerves, plexus or spinal roots, however, often does not follow an exact anatomical distribution. For example, pain due to compression of the median nerve at the wrist (carpal tunnel syndrome (CTS)) often spreads up the arm to the elbow or even to the shoulder. The pain due to damage to a spinal root is felt in the myotome and not in the dermatome, e.g. a lesion of C7 causes pain in the triceps, forearm extensors and pectoralis, while paraesthesiae occur in the middle finger. Pain in the arm also may be felt occasionally by patients with cerebral disease: for example, pain and clumsiness in one arm may be the first signs of Parkinson's disease.

Paraesthesiae, which describes positive sensory symptoms such as pins and needles or tingling, may be due to damage to peripheral sensory neurones from the peripheral nerve itself, to the spinal root, or due to lesions of the central sensory pathways or spinal cord, brainstem or internal capsule.

Cortical lesions generally do produce positive paraesthesiae, except in focal seizures arising in sensory cortex. Sensory disturbances, whether par-aesthesiae or sensory loss, are often difficult to put into words, and terms such as pins and needles, tingling, numbness, stiffness, constriction, wrapped in tight bandages, or like going to the dentist, all may be used to describe sensory deficit.

Weakness of the arm may be due to primary muscle disease (rare), lesions of peripheral nerves, brachial plexus or cervical roots, or to damage to central motor pathways.

The latter causes signs typical of upper motor neuron (UMN) lesions (weakness without wasting, spasticity, and enhanced reflexes). Lesions of peripheral nerves, plexus or roots cause the signs of a lower motor neuron (LMN) lesion (weakness with wasting, normal or diminished tone, reduced or absent tendon reflexes).

Acute pain in the arm

Acute disease of the shoulder joints or adjacent structures is a common cause of pain in the arm. A variety of conditions are responsible for the clinical syndrome of '**frozen shoulder**', which causes severe pain, restriction of movement and, later, wasting of the surrounding muscles. The frozen shoulder may be accompanied by a curious sympathetic disturbance of the hand which becomes swollen, painful, shiny and weak, for reasons that are not well understood. The shoulder-hand syndrome occurs in some patients with a hemiplegia due to a stroke if poorly managed and occasionally after myocardial infarction.

Primary muscle disease confined to the arm is very unusual, but giant cell arteritis may affect the muscles around the shoulder girdles to cause the syndrome of **polymyalgia rheumatica**. This causes increasing pain and stiffness of the shoulder girdle muscles.

Brachial neuritis (neuralgic amyotrophy) is another condition of unknown cause, probably arising from inflammatory plexopathy. This presents with very severe pain affecting one arm and shoulder girdle followed by rapid wasting of the arm muscles, usually around the shoulder, with winging of the scapula. Sensory disturbance may be minimal, although there may be a patch of altered sensation over the deltoid in the distribution of the circumflex nerve.

This may be hard to differentiate from a **cervical disc prolapse compressing a root**, usually C5, 6 or 7. Again there may be acute severe pain with paraesthesiae and weakness in the arm in the distribution of the affected nerve root. The neck is often 'fixed' and painful to move, and coughing or sneezing may provoke a surge of pain referred down the arm. When lateral flexion or rotation of the neck aggravates the pain on the same side (ipsilateral), this also points to nerve root irritation.

Herpes zoster may cause acute pain in the arm before the appearance of the characteristic skin rash, if cervical roots are affected.

The acute pain of neuralgic amyotrophy or a cervical disc prolapse usually resolves in a matter of weeks or months.

Chronic pain in the arm

A number of entrapment neuropathies affecting peripheral nerves in the arm are common causes of more chronic pain.

> **Carpal tunnel syndrome** is the most common cause of chronic arm pain, particularly in women. Often there is the complaint of unpleasant night pain accompanied by tingling in the fingers, particularly the thumb, index and middle fingers, relieved by moving the hands about or hanging them out of bed. Signs are often minimal.

In men, it is usually the **ulnar nerve** that is affected, particularly at the elbow. There may be pain and paraesthesiae in the ring and little fingers with weakness and wasting of the small muscles of the hand.

The **lower cord of the brachial plexus** may be compressed by a cervical rib, infiltrated by malignant disease from an apical lung carcinoma (Pancoast's syndrome) or local spread from a breast carcinoma. Unpleasant pain radiating down the inner aspect of the forearm with paraesthesiae and weakness of the small hand muscles often accompanies this. Cervical ribs and muscular bands may also compress the subclavian artery producing vascular symptoms in the arm.

Cervical spondylosis, degenerative disease of the cervical spine, is very common with increasing age. It may produce chronic pain accompanied by weakness and paraesthesiae in the distribution of the affected root or roots. Although sometimes this may follow an acute disc prolapse, more often it results from root compression by osteophytes narrowing the spinal exit foramina (C5, 6 and 7 are most often involved).

Spinal tumours may present with arm pain. Malignant disease of the cervical vertebrae may lead to spinal involvement and compression of cervical roots with sometimes spinal cord involvement. Benign neurofibromas and rarely intrinsic cord tumours, as gliomas, may present with chronic arm pain. **Syringomyelia** causes pain with a characteristic dissociated sensory loss, absent tendon jerks and wasting of the hand muscles.

The wasted hand

> Wasting of the small hand muscles with or without pain is a common clinical problem. These muscles are innervated predominantly by the **ulnar nerve** (the median nerve only supplies the thenar pad), **the inner cord of the brachial plexus, the T1 spinal root**, or the equivalent group of anterior horn cells. Lesions at these sites will give a wasted hand (Box 2.8).

However, wasting of the hand is also one of the common presenting features of **motor neurone disease**: here there will be fasciculation, usually signs of upper motor neurone damage and no sensory loss.

Wasting of the muscles around the shoulder occurs with a frozen shoulder, neuralgic amyotrophy, cervical spondylosis affecting the C5 roots, and in motor neurone disease. Symmetrical wasting around the shoulder may also be a sign of primary muscle disease, including thyrotoxicosis.

BACK PAIN

Low back pain is very common, affecting 60–70 per cent of the population at some time in their life. Most episodes are of short duration but they often recur. There appears to be a link with the physical demands of work and a previous history of back problems is an adverse risk factor.

Box 2.8 Neurological causes of wasted small hand muscles

Peripheral nerve
    Ulnar, median (thenar pad)
    Peripheral neuropathy
        Diabetic, amyloid, paraneoplastic, CMT, CIDP,
            ischaemic, toxic, e.g. alcohol
Brachial plexus
    Lower cord compression
        Cervical rib, fibrous band
        Malignancy
        Irradiation fibrosis
        Neuralgic amyotrophy
Cervical root C8/T1
    Spondylotic degenerative changes, disc prolapse
    Compression by tumour
    Trauma
Cervical cord
    Intramedullary tumour
    Motor neurone disease
    Poliomyelitis
    Syrinx
Disuse associated with arthritis
    Rheumatoid
    Osteoarthritis
    Ageing
Muscle
    Inclusion body myositis (finger flexors particularly)

CIDP, chronic inflammatory demyelinating polyneuropathy; CMT, Charcot-Marie-Tooth disease (peroneal muscular atrophy).

Simple back pain centred on the lumbosacral region and upper buttocks is probably mechanical in origin and carries a good outlook with most patients recovering within 6 weeks. The pain may be severe and the back 'locked'. It is best managed by physiotherapy.

If there is associated nerve root pain referred down the leg, most often the back of the leg and into the foot, sometimes with accompanying sensory symptoms, the outlook is less good with only some 50 per cent recovering by 6 weeks. If the pain appears more severe, progressive, and is not helped by rest and accompanied by more widespread neurological signs or features of systemic upset, these are considered 'red flags', marking the need for early investigation.

PAIN IN THE LEG

The painful, tingling or weak leg

As in the arm, the most common cause of leg pain is local bone or joint disease. The speed with which the quadriceps muscle wastes after a knee injury may amaze the young sportsman, while the most common cause of pain in the thigh with quadriceps wasting in later life is osteoarthritis of the knee. The most common cause of acute leg pain is sciatica, but a number of conditions may cause chronic leg pain.

Acute sciatica

Traditional terms, such as lumbago and sciatica, describe symptoms of acute pain in the back with radiation into the leg respectively.

Acute back pain (lumbago) probably has many causes including tears of the paraspinal muscles, or spinal ligaments, acute damage to hypophyseal joints of the spine, and acute ruptures of lumbar discs. Radiation of pain into the leg may follow from hip disease; however, when it is **unilateral and extends below the knee it is most usually due to irritation of the corresponding lumbosacral nerve root by a lateral disc protrusion**. Musculoskeletal pain of lumbar origin may radiate widely and into both legs. Sciatica is commonly accompanied by back pain, but each may occur on its own. Typically, the onset is sudden during physical activity, e.g. lifting a weight with the back flexed. The pain may be very severe and accompanied by spasm of the muscles so that the spine 'locks', and any slight movement is agonizing. Coughing, sneezing or straining to defaecate all aggravate the pain. The sciatica is in the distribution of the nerve root involved, down the back of the leg to the heel with S1, or down the lateral side of the leg to the instep with L5. **These two roots are those most often affected by disc degeneration at the L4/5 (L5 root) and L5/S1 (S1 root) disc spaces, respectively**. Root compression also gives rise to typical sensory symptoms of numbness or paraesthesiae and motor weakness in the appropriate distribution. When the onset is acute in the setting of physical exercise, the diagnosis of acute sciatica is rarely in doubt. However, disc protrusions not uncommonly may cause a more gradual onset of pain without any obvious precipitating cause. In this situation, alternative diagnoses have to be considered (Box 2.9).

Chronic leg pain

Pain referred into the leg may be due to pelvic malignancy spreading from the uterus, cervix, prostate or rectum to infiltrate the lumbar or sacral plexus. Such pain may have an insidious onset but usually becomes more severe and constant. A rectal examination, which is essential in all patients with unexplained persistent leg pain, may reveal the cause.

Meralgia paraesthetica is due to an entrapment neuropathy of the lateral cutaneous nerve of the thigh as it passes through the lateral end of the inguinal ligament. This may give pain, often with a burning quality, with tingling and numbness on the anterolateral aspect of the thigh within the distribution of the nerve, down to but not below the knee.

Diabetic amyotrophy or plexopathy is another common cause of leg pain. This diabetic complication presents with a subacute severe pain in the thigh accompanied by wasting of the quadriceps and minor sensory changes in the distribution of the femoral nerve. It is usually due to an acute vascular lesion affecting the vasa nervorum. The femoral nerve may also be compressed acutely after a haemorrhage into the iliopsoas muscle in those

Box 2.9 Neurological causes of acute leg pain

Peripheral nerve
   Peripheral neuropathy
      Diabetic, ischaemic, paraneoplastic, amyloid
   Tarsal tunnel, interdigital neuroma
Lumbosacral plexus
   Diabetic plexopathy
   Malignancy
   Haematoma - excess anticoagulants
Roots
   Prolapsed disc
   Malignancy
   Arachnoiditis
Lumbosacral cord (often bilateral leg symptoms)
   Tumour - include metastases
   Myelitis
   Infection - epidural abscess, meningomyelitis

with a bleeding diathesis or on excess anticoagulant therapy.

Foot drop

Foot drop
Paralysis of the dorsiflexors of the ankle may be due to lesions of the common peroneal nerve, the sciatic nerve, the L5 root, or occasionally the motor cortex.

The common peroneal nerve is extremely vulnerable in its course around the neck of the fibula, where it may be compressed by external pressure or stretched by prolonged bending or sitting with the knees fully flexed. Apart from the foot drop, such patients also have sensory loss on the dorsum of the foot, but the ankle jerk is preserved. The sciatic nerve is at risk from misplaced injections into the buttocks or thigh, which leave not only a foot drop, but also weakness of plantar flexion of the foot, sensory loss extending onto the sole of the foot, and the loss of the ankle jerk. L5 root lesions are difficult to distinguish from common peroneal nerve palsies, but the presence of back pain with sciatic radiation and extension weakness to involve the knee flexors will point to this proximal lesion. Extensor hallucis longus has an almost pure L5 innervation. Motor cortex lesions affecting the foot area may present with a foot drop but the plantar response will be extensor and there may be other UMN signs.

Cramps in the legs

Many patients use the word cramp to describe pain in the legs due to vascular insufficiency, or nerve damage. However, genuine cramp consists not only of pain but also intense and involuntary muscle contraction affecting particularly the calf muscles. Such cramps are common in the untrained athlete, the elderly and are well-known to occur in hot climates due to salt depletion. Muscle cramps occur in those recovering from sciatica and in motor neurone disease, but other findings will point to these diagnoses. Occasionally, isolated muscle cramps may be found to be due to primary metabolic muscle disease, but in the majority of such patients no obvious cause can be discovered and they can be difficult to treat.

True muscle cramps are electrically silent on EMG study. In contrast, flexor spasms of leg muscles that occur in those with damage to corticospinal pathways are associated with intense EMG activity and with signs of an UMN lesion (weakness without wasting, spasticity and exaggerated tendon reflexes).

Restless legs

Some patients will complain of discomfort in the legs that is not due to pain, cramp or paraesthesiae. They will find it impossible to put into words the quality of the intense discomfort they feel, but describe relief from movement. Such patients cannot sit still because of the discomfort and may be forced to get out of bed at night to walk around to gain relief from this distressing complaint. This common symptom, known as Ekbom's syndrome, is usually inherited and may be a minor form of dystonia. Some patients are found to have iron deficient anaemia or uraemic neuropathy and there is an overlap with periodic limb movements of sleep where jerky flexion movements occur in the legs during non-REM sleep.

Intermittent claudication

Pain in the calves or buttocks on exercise, relieved rapidly by rest, is the characteristic feature of arterial insufficiency in the legs.

However, this syndrome of intermittent claudication may occasionally be mimicked by disease of the lumbar spine, particularly in those with a narrowed spinal canal from congenital lumbar stenosis or more often from degenerative lumbar spondylosis. Such patients complain of pain in the legs on exercise, but the pain is often in the distribution of one of the spinal roots, and is accompanied by neurological symptoms including foot drop and paraesthesiae. Rest relieves the pain, but usually after a longer period of time than is required in the case of vascular intermittent claudication.

The neurological syndrome, because it mimics vascular claudication, has been called intermittent **claudication of the cauda equina**.

DIFFICULTY WALKING

This is one of the most common neurological complaints and it is necessary to distinguish the different anatomical causes. When considering gait disturbance it is logical to work mentally from muscles to cerebral cortex or vice versa (see Table 2.2).

Difficulty walking with wasted legs

Primary muscle disease (myopathy) often presents with an abnormality of gait, because it affects proximal muscles of the hip girdle symmetrically at an early stage. Similar symmetrical proximal muscle weakness around the shoulder girdle usually occurs later. Characteristically, the gait is waddling due to failure to stabilize the pelvis on the femur when the opposite leg is lifted from the ground. In addition, patients with primary muscle disease frequently complain of difficulty getting out of a low chair, and of climbing stairs, because of weakness around the hips. When the arms are affected, an early symptom is often difficulty raising the hand above the head to brush the hair or reach up into a high cupboard.

Other characteristics of primary muscle disease are that sensation is normal and sphincter function is not affected.

There are many causes for myopathy including hereditary muscular dystrophy, inflammatory myositis, thyrotoxicosis, steroid therapy and metabolic myopathies. A family history suggests muscular dystrophy, which causes painless progressive wasting of muscles in characteristic distribution. Pain and systemic disturbance suggest polymyositis. Many endocrine and electrolyte disturbances may cause metabolic myopathies.

The physical signs of primary muscle disease are muscle wasting and weakness, symmetrical and proximal, with normal or reduced tendon jerks, and no evidence of sensory deficit.

Defects of neurotransmission due to **myasthenia gravis**, or to the much rarer **Lambert–Eaton**

Table 2.2 Causes of difficulty walking

Muscle	Myopathy (proximal)
Neuromuscular junction	Myasthenia gravis (fatigue)
Peripheral nerve (LMN)	Neuropathy (distal)
Roots (LMN)	Disc protrusion, compressive, cauda equina (+ sphincters)
Spinal cord	Compression (tumours, discs)
	Demyelination, inflammatory
	Vascular, degenerative (MND), intrinsic damage (syrinx, tumour)
Brain, brainstem (UMN)	Vascular, demyelination, tumours (intrinsic, extrinsic), Abscesses, degenerative
Cerebellar (ataxic)	Vascular (acute), tumour, degenerative
Extrapyramidal	Parkinsonian
Sensory loss (JPS loss)	Locomotor ataxia
Psychogenic	Functional, chronic fatigue states
Joint disease	Painful arthritis, Charcot joints
Weakness (general)	Systemic disease, cachexia, hypotensive, malnutrition

JPS, joint position sense; LMN, lower motor neurone; MND, motor neurone disease; UMN, upper motor neurone.

myasthenic syndrome (**LEMS**) usually associated with carcinoma, may also present with difficulty in walking due to proximal leg weakness. However, the legs are not wasted in myasthenia. As in primary muscles disease, sensation is not affected. **The characteristic feature of myasthenia is muscle fatigue and fluctuation in strength**. The patient may not complain of feeling tired, but of weakness of muscle action on exercise. Thus, they may start the day walking strongly, but as time goes on and as exercise continues, they become weaker and weaker. Rest restores strength, but further exercise leads to further weakness.

Peripheral nerve disease may also cause difficulty walking. This may arise either as a result of damage to an isolated peripheral nerve (mononeuropathy) such as a peroneal or femoral nerve palsy, or to generalized peripheral nerve disease (peripheral neuropathy). In all such conditions, the signs will be those of a LMN lesion (wasting with weakness, normal or reduced tone, and normal or depressed tendon reflexes). In addition, there will be appropriate sensory disturbance in the distribution of the affected peripheral nerves. In the case of a generalized length dependent peripheral neuropathy, symptoms commence in the feet symmetrically, with paraesthesiae and numbness which spread upwards into the legs accompanied by a bilateral

foot drop from distal weakness. **Generalized peripheral neuropathies usually affect the legs before the arms, because long axons are affected first**. Sphincter function, however, is normal. An acute neuropathy with onset and progression over a few days or 2–4 weeks is most often due to an acute idiopathic inflammatory polyneuropathy known as the Guillain–Barré syndrome. More rarely, a subacute generalized neuropathy may occur with glandular fever, HIV infection, acute intermittent porphyria, or from toxic heavy metals and industrial agents. Diphtheria is now exceedingly rare, but the early palatal palsy and paralysis of accommodation is characteristic. There are many causes of a chronic peripheral neuropathy but the most common in the UK is diabetes, with alcohol and malignancy seen fairly often. In the world, the most common cause was leprosy but may by now have been overtaken by HIV-related neuropathies.

Proximal lesions of the lumbosacral roots (cauda equina lesions) may present with difficulty walking due to weakness of the legs associated with sensory disturbance which characteristically is focused around the perineum (the patient 'sits on their signs'), and early disturbances of sphincter function.

Motor neurone disease, too, may present with painless wasting, weakness and fasciculation of leg muscles, usually asymmetrically, and without sensory or sphincter disturbance.

Difficulty in walking with spastic legs

Lesions of the corticomotorneurone pathways bilaterally will cause a **spastic paraplegia**, which manifests as a characteristic disturbance of gait. **Patients walk with stiff straight legs, scuffing the toes and outer border of the feet along the ground.** They often trip. Physical examination will show UMN signs (weakness without wasting, spasticity, exaggerated tendon reflexes and extensor plantar responses). The next stage is to decide on the anatomical level and the cause (Table 2.2).

Acute paraplegia

Acute damage to the spinal cord from trauma, inflammatory disease (acute transverse myelitis) or a vascular lesion all produce an acute paraplegia. Initially, the signs are not those characteristic of spasticity. Sometimes acute cord compression may present with an acute paraplegia. Immediately after such an acute insult the segment of spinal cord below the lesion is in a state of shock, when it is unresponsive to peripheral input.

Acute spinal cord lesion

Immediately after an acute spinal cord lesion the legs are flaccid, the tendon reflexes absent and the plantar responses unobtainable. Spasticity, exaggerated reflexes and extensor plantar responses gradually emerge over a matter of some weeks following the acute insult.

An acute flaccid paraplegia, or quadriplegia if the arms are also affected, may be difficult to distinguish from a subacute peripheral neuropathy or even from severe acute metabolic myopathies such as that due to hypokalaemia, at least in the early stages.

The presence of sensory loss obviously will exclude primary muscle disease, and urinary retention points to spinal cord damage rather than a peripheral neuropathy. **In those with an acute paraplegia thought to be due to spinal cord damage, it is crucial to exclude spinal cord compression,**

e.g. by dorsal disc protrusion or extradural abscess (Box 2.10), for the longer the delay before surgery the less the chance of useful recovery. All such patients need immediate neurological assessment and imaging of the spinal cord if a compressive

Box 2.10 Causes of spinal cord damage

Trauma
  Fracture dislocations, burst fractures of vertebral body
Infection
  Epidural abscess – staphylococcal, tuberculosis
  Tuberculoma; gumma, tabes dorsalis (syphilis)
  Lyme disease
  Viral – HIV infection, CMV infection, HTLV-1, varicella-zoster, poliomyelitis, EBV
  Parasitosis – schistosomiasis
Inflammatory
  Demyelination (MS), neuromyelitis optica, Sarcoidosis, systemic lupus erythematosus
  Transverse myelitis (may be associated with infections)
Vascular
  Ischaemia, infarction
  Arteriovenous malformations, dural fistulae
  Epidural haemorrhage – bleeding diathesis, anticoagulant excess
Tumour
  Primary – intramedullary – glioma, ependymoma; extramedullary – meningioma, neurofibroma
  Metastatic deposits
Degenerative
  Disc prolapse, spondylotic changes
  Osteoporotic collapse, Paget's disease
  Atlanto-axial subluxation (congenital, rheumatoid arthritis)
  Motor neurone disease, spinal muscular atrophies
  Heredo-familial spastic paraplegias
  Syringomyelia
Others
  Arachnoiditis
  Subacute combined degeneration – vitamin B12 deficiency
  Radiation myelopathy
  Heroin abuse

CMV, cytomegalovirus; EBV, Epstein–Barr virus; HIV, human immunodeficiency virus; HTLV-1, human T lymphotropic virus type 1; MS, multiple sclerosis.

---

lesion is to be excluded. This is best undertaken by MRI, or when contraindicated by CT myelography.

Acute quadriplegia

> Sudden or rapid paralysis of all four limbs becomes a medical emergency if breathing is threatened.

Respiratory failure occurs when arterial oxygen tension falls below 8.0 kPa (60 mmHg), or if arterial carbon dioxide tension rises above 6.6 kPa (50 mmHg). However, patients with neurological disease causing weakness of the respiratory muscles may be on the brink of catastrophic respiratory failure long before the blood gases are compromised.

A rising respiratory rate and breathlessness indicate impending respiratory failure, which may require assisted respiration. The best index of respiratory reserve is the vital capacity (VC), which is the volume of maximal expiration following a maximal inspiration.

In an adult, a falling VC with a value of less than 50 per cent of the predicted normal is a warning of impending crisis, and action is undoubtedly required if the VC falls to 1.0 L or less. Peak expiratory flow rate (PEFR) is a measure of obstructive respiratory defects and is an inappropriate and dangerously misleading measure of respiratory function in patients with neuromuscular disease. **The combination of respiratory muscle weakness and bulbar failure is particularly dangerous**.

Causes of acute quadriplegia

The common causes of acute or subacute (with onset over days) quadriplegia are polymyositis, myasthenia gravis, acute inflammatory polyneuropathy (Guillain–Barré syndrome), and high cervical cord lesions due to trauma, inflammation or vascular damage. Rarer conditions include hypokalaemic paralysis, acute porphyria, poliomyelitis, tetanus, and other causes of high cervical cord damage, such as subluxation of the odontoid peg (as may occur in rheumatoid arthritis) or cord tumours. Brainstem lesions may also cause a quadriplegia, and bulbar muscles are involved to cause diplopia, dysphagia and dysarthria.

Chronic spastic paraparesis

> The most common cause of a chronic spastic paraparesis in the young adult is MS, and in the elderly individual it is cervical spondylosis. However, it is crucial to exclude other treatable causes of spinal cord disease in both age groups before accepting either diagnosis.

In particular, any patient with a chronic progressive spastic paraparesis requires imaging of the spinal cord to exclude a spinal tumour or other causes of cord compression, unless there are obvious signs or symptoms of MS elsewhere, or some other clear evidence to establish an alternative diagnosis. To carry out negative non-invasive imaging studies is much better than to miss treatable benign spinal tumours, such as neurofibromas or meningiomas, until the damage is severe and irreversible with surgical treatment. Unfortunately, in the older age group metastatic cancer deposits in the spine, most often from breast, lung or prostate, are more often the cause of spinal cord compression. Rarer causes include dorsal disc prolapse, arachnoiditis, intramedullary cord tumours and syringomyelia. It is also essential to exclude subacute combined degeneration due to vitamin B12 deficiency, neurosyphilis, and in patients particularly from abroad, infection with the human T lymphotropic virus type 1 (HTLV-1), as causes of chronic spastic paraparesis. Subacute combined degeneration nearly always presents with paraesthesiae first in the feet, due to the associated peripheral neuropathy, and the ankle jerks will be lost. The picture of a spastic paraplegia but with absent ankle jerks also may be seen in patients with hereditary spinocerebellar degenerations, and as a remote, non-metastatic complication of a primary neoplasm. Motor neurone disease also may present as a spastic paraparesis before evidence of LMN damage with wasting and fasciculation is evident.

Spastic weakness of one leg

Stiffness and dragging of one leg is a common presenting complaint in neurology.

The difficulty is always to decide whether the lesion lies in the spinal cord or in the brain.

Full investigation includes MR imaging of the

spine and brain. CSF examination may be helpful to support or refute a diagnosis of MS. Progression to involve the arm does not necessarily help to decide between spinal cord and brain, while spread to the opposite leg does not always indicate that the lesion is in the cord. The notorious but uncommon parasagittal meningioma may produce UMN signs in both legs.

Unsteadiness of gait

> **Ataxia of gait**
> An unsteady, uncertain gait may be caused by sensory loss (sensory ataxia), cerebellar disease (cerebellar ataxia), hydrocephalus, extrapyramidal disease (e.g. Parkinson's disease, chorea), or diffuse cerebral damage.

In **sensory ataxia**, the patient characteristically walks unsteadily with feet wide apart and lifted high off the ground to slap into the floor. In addition, the unsteadiness is much worse in the dark when vision cannot be used to compensate (the basis of Romberg's sign). The patient with **cerebellar ataxia** again walks with feet wide apart and reels from side to side as if drunk. The patient with **Parkinson's disease** slowly shuffles with small steps and a flexed posture. The patient with chorea unexpectedly dances and lurches (crab-like gait) as the balance is disturbed by unpredictable involuntary movements.

Gait disturbance with small shuffling steps may arise from a number of disorders. In Parkinson's disease, there is a tendency to festination with a flexed posture and impaired balance. In patients with a frontal lobe disturbance (often a 'gait apraxia'), there may be no weakness and normal individual muscle movements on the bed. However, there may be difficulty turning over in bed. Examination may show a degree of leg spasticity without sensory loss but walking using short steps on a wide base. There may be perseveration in some actions. Often there is a degree of dementia and sometimes urinary urgency and even incontinence. One such cause is widespread vascular disease with multiple lacunar infarcts resulting in a marche à petit pas. In patients with normal pressure hydrocephalus (NPH), again there may be a gait with short shuffling steps and a wide base (Figure 2.5). Commonly, there is an

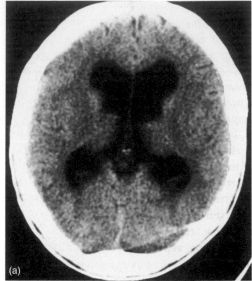

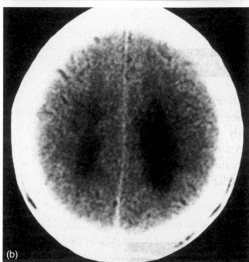

Figure 2.5 (a) Axial view CT brain scan to show triventricular enlargement and (b) absence of cortical sulci in a patient with normal pressure hydrocephalus. The patient presented with dementia, a gait with short shuffling steps and incontinence.

associated dementia and urinary incontinence. **Gait apraxia is a very common cause of gait disturbance in elderly hospitalized patients.**

Extensive sensory loss in the legs may be due to a sensory peripheral neuropathy or to degeneration of the posterior columns as in tabes dorsalis. In both conditions, the tendon jerks are absent: in peripheral neuropathy there will be distal motor signs, while in tabes dorsalis there is likely to be urinary retention with overflow and abnormal pupils.

Progressive cerebellar ataxia occurs in diffuse diseases of the central nervous system, e.g. in MS, when it is accompanied by a spastic paraparesis to produce a typical spastic-ataxic gait. Isolated progressive cerebellar ataxia may be due to a cerebellar tumour, hereditary spinocerebellar degeneration (Figure 2.6), alcohol, endocrine disturbance such as myxoedema, or as a remote effect of a primary neoplasm elsewhere. Patients who are ataxic sitting and standing are likely to have a mid-line cerebellar lesion. A cerebellar syndrome in childhood most frequently is due to a posterior fossa tumour, which may present without symptoms of raised ICP. In adults, this is seldom so, and most isolated slowly progressive cerebellar ataxias without headache and vomiting are found to have a degenerative origin.

Extrapyramidal diseases are discussed in the next section.

MOVEMENT DISORDERS

The term 'movement disorders' has come to be applied to those diseases of the nervous system, mostly of the basal ganglia, which cause disturbances of movement which cannot be attributed to sensory loss, weakness or spasticity, or obvious cerebellar ataxia.

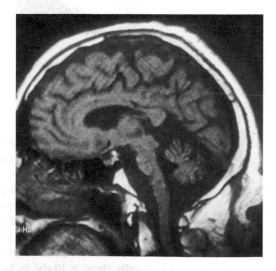

Figure 2.6 Sagittal view MRI scan (T1-weighted) to show cerebellar and brainstem atrophy in a patient with progressive unsteadiness.

> **Movement disorders fall into two main categories:**
> 1 Those characterized by a poverty (hypokinesia) and slowness of movement, the so-called akinetic-rigid or parkinsonian syndrome.
> 2 Those characterized by excess abnormal uncontrollable involuntary movements, otherwise known as dyskinesias.

Idiopathic Parkinson's disease, associated with characteristic pathology including the presence of Lewy bodies in affected pigmented nerve cells and loss of nigro-striatal neurones, is the most common cause of an akinetic syndrome in middle or late life. A similar condition could be produced as an aftermath of encephalitis lethargica (post-encephalitic parkinsonism), and occurs commonly nowadays as a result of neuroleptic drugs, such as phenothiazines or butyrophenones (**drug-induced parkinsonism**). Rarer causes include **multiple system atrophy** and **progressive supranuclear palsy** in the older age group, while in juveniles or young adults, **Wilson's disease** and the rigid form of **Huntington's disease** have to be considered. An important distinction is between Parkinson's disease, or the other conditions mentioned which may cause parkinsonism, and the akinetic-rigid features that occur in patients with many diffuse cerebral degenerations. In the latter conditions, which include diffuse cerebrovascular disease and Alzheimer's disease, the akinetic-rigid features are only part of a much greater disorder of higher mental function which produces profound disturbances of memory, intellect and cognitive function.

> **Abnormal involuntary movements**
> Abnormal involuntary movements (dyskinesias) are a feature of many diseases of the nervous system, but most can be included within five main categories – tremor, chorea, myoclonus, tics and torsion dystonia. These are not diseases, but present as clinically identifiable single symptoms or symptom complexes with many causes. In some patients, such dyskinesias are accompanied by other neurological deficits, but in others the involuntary movements occur in isolation and constitute the illness.

Tremor is a rhythmic sinusoidal movement which may occur at rest (rest tremor), or on action (action tremor), when it may be present while maintaining a posture (static or postural tremor), or executing a movement (kinetic or intention tremor). Rest tremor is characteristic of Parkinson's disease. Postural tremor often is no more than an exaggeration of physiological tremor by anxiety, drugs, alcohol or thyrotoxicosis. Intention tremor is a distinctive sign of cerebellar disease.

Chorea is characterized by continuous randomly distributed and irregular timed muscle jerks. Patients appear restless and fidgety. The limbs, face and trunk are continually disturbed by brief, unpredictable movements. Walking is interrupted by lurches, stops and starts (the 'dancing' gait); hand movements and fine manipulations are distorted by similar unpredictable jerks and twitches, while speech and respiration also are affected. Strength is usually normal, but the patient is unable to maintain their grip which waxes and wanes (milkmaid's grip), and the protruded tongue pops in and out (fly-catcher's tongue). The limbs are hypotonic and tendon jerks brisk. Sydenham's chorea and Huntington's disease are the most common causes of generalized chorea, but this may be the presenting feature of a number of general medical illnesses or may occur as a side-effect of drug therapy.

Hemichorea or hemiballism describe unilateral chorea most apparent in proximal muscles, so that the arm and leg are thrown widely in all directions.

Myoclonus consists of brief, shock-like muscle jerks, similar to those provoked by stimulating the nerve to the muscle. Myoclonic jerks may occur irregularly or rhythmically, and they often appear repetitively in the same muscles. In this respect, myoclonus differs from chorea, which is random in time and distribution.

Tics are brief stereotyped repetitive involuntary muscle contractions. They can be mimicked by the observer, and usually can be controlled through an effort of will by the patient, often at the expense of inner mounting tension. Typically they involve the face, e.g. with blinking, sniffing, lip smacking or pouting; and in the upper arms, e.g. with shoulder shrugging. Some may be associated with vocalizations. Tics may occur in at least one-quarter of children, but disappear with maturity. A number of normal adults also display persistent motor tics as part of their personality.

Torsion dystonia differs from other movements that are mentioned in that it is caused by sustained spasms of muscle contraction which distort the body into characteristic postures for prolonged periods of time. The neck may be twisted to one side, torticollis, or extended, retrocollis: the trunk may be forced into excessive lordosis or scoliosis; the arm may be extended and hyperpronated with the wrist flexed and the fingers extended; the leg may be extended with the foot in plantar flexion and in-turned. Initially, these muscle spasms may occur only on certain actions (action dystonia), so that patients walk on their toes or develop the characteristic arm posture on writing. Tremor often occurs with the dystonia affecting the same body part. In progressive dystonia, abnormal spasms and postures appear at rest causing increasing dystonic movements and deformity. The term 'athetosis' is also used to describe similar dystonic movements, although originally it was employed to describe slow writhing and wavering movements of the fingers and toes.

DECLINE OF MEMORY, INTELLECT AND BEHAVIOUR

A global loss of all higher intellectual function, memory and cognitive function, accompanied by disintegration of personality and behaviour, forms the clinical syndrome known as dementia, which is most frequently due to diffuse cerebral cortical disease.

Usually, there is a progressive impairment of memory plus loss of one other cognitive domain, such as language, praxis, perception, executive function, personality and social behaviour.

The syndrome of dementia may arise acutely, as after head injury or cerebral anoxia due to cardiac arrest, or may commence insidiously and be progressive, as in the various neurodegenerative illnesses of which **Alzheimer's disease** is the most common. A mixture of Alzheimer's disease and cerebrovascular disease is also common, and dementia with Lewy bodies is increasingly recognized. Vascular dementia is the second most common cause in white populations and is very common in the Far East. However, there are other causes of a progressive dementia, and some are reversible, including certain treatable brain tumours, metabolic diseases such as myxoedema or vitamin B12 deficiency (Box 2.11).

Box 2.11 Causes of dementia

Primary degenerative
  Alzheimer's disease (55%), dementia with Lewy
    bodies (15%), frontotemporal dementia (5%),
    Huntington's disease, Parkinson's disease,
    corticobasal degeneration
Vascular
  Multi-infarct (sometimes mixed with Alzheimer's)
    (20%), (Binswanger's subcortical leukoaraiosis
    – a radiological description)
  CADASIL
Prion disease
  Creutzfeldt–Jakob's disease – sporadic and new
    variant
Infective
  Chronic meningitis, neurosyphilis
  AIDS dementia complex
  Progressive multifocal leukoencephalopathy
  Post-meningo-encephalitis
Metabolic, endocrine
  Uraemia, hepatic encephalopathy, myxoedema
  Hashimoto's encephalopathy
  Hypopituitarism, hypoglycaemia
  Hypercalcaemia, hypocalcaemia
Deficiencies
  Thiamine, vitamin B12, multiple nutritional
Drugs
  Alcohol
  Barbiturates
Trauma
  Head injury, 'punch-drunk' boxers
  Subdural haematoma
Tumours
  Primary – glioma, meningioma
  Secondary – metastatic
  Paraneoplastic syndromes
  Obstructive hydrocephalus
Normal pressure hydrocephalus
Depression – pseudodementia

AIDS, acquired immunodeficiency syndrome; CADASIL, cerebral
autosomal dominant arteriopathy with subcortical infarcts and
leukoencephalopathy.

Percentages in brackets reflect the most common causes.

Diagnosing dementia

When faced with a patient, or their relatives, complaining of memory difficulty, intellectual decline, or changes in personality, three questions have to be answered:

1 Is this really due to a true dementia as a result of organic brain disease, or are these symptoms due to those of a 'pseudodementia' due to psychiatric illnesses such as depression?
2 Are these symptoms those of a true global dementing illness, or are they due to a focal cortical syndrome as the result of damage to one part of the cerebral cortex, rather than diffuse disease?
3 If they are due to a true global dementia, then is there any treatable cause for the condition?

Pseudodementia

Impairment of memory with change in personality and behaviour are, of course, typical symptoms of **depression**, which also produces sleep disturbance, diurnal mood swing, loss of libido, anorexia and weight loss and social withdrawal. Difficulty arises because a considerable proportion of patients with true organic dementing illnesses experience a reactive depression in the early stages of their illness. Accordingly, in a patient who exhibits a decline of memory and intellect with alteration of personality and behaviour accompanied by depression, it can be exceedingly difficult to distinguish primary depressive illness from a dementing process with depression. Careful assessment by experienced psychologists may assist, but often does not resolve the matter. If in doubt, it is prudent to treat depression and await events. Abnormal beliefs and perceptions may also arise in dementia raising the question of a psychotic illness. Other psychiatric conditions that may produce pseudodementia include conversion disorders and malingering, but these are relatively rare.

Focal cortical syndromes

Bilateral damage to the temporal lobes, particularly to their medial structures including the hippocampus, or to the hypothalamus, may produce a pure **amnesic syndrome**, consisting of dense loss of memory for recent events, with inability to retain new information, but with preserved intelligence and personality. Such amnesic syndromes are seen most commonly in Wernicke–Korsakoff syndrome as a result of thiamine deficiency in alcohol-dependent patients, but occasionally as a result of parapituitary tumours, or bilateral temporal lobe damage secondary to head injury or encephalitis. A **transient global amnesia** also occurs as a benign syndrome in which patients usually show a marked short-term memory loss extending for some hours during which they may repeatedly ask the same questions. This syndrome can be precipitated by emotion and straining. A similar syndrome may also arise with migraine and even as part of a complex partial seizure. An amnesic/confusional syndrome may persist for some time after head injury (post-traumatic amnesia), or after an epileptic seizure (post-epileptic amnesia).

Dysphasia may be mistaken for dementia. The severe disturbance of the content of spoken speech that occurs in Wernicke's/receptive dysphasia due to damage to the posterior temporal region of the dominant hemisphere may consist of such nonsensical language and jargon that the inexperienced observer may mistake this for dementia.

Damage to the frontal lobes by tumour, most often a slowly enlarging benign meningioma, or in myxoedema, may produce a remarkable change in personality and behaviour, without deterioration of intellect or memory.

Causes of dementia

If the conclusion is that the patient's symptoms are those of a diffuse global dementing illness, the next stage is to decide the cause (Box 2.11).

> In some 10 per cent of patients, some potentially treatable condition will be discovered on careful examination and full investigation, the yield being greatest in those under the age of 70.

The most common cause of dementia is Alzheimer's disease, which becomes increasingly frequent with age. Previously the term 'presenile dementia' was used for the syndrome with onset prior to the age of 65, while 'senile dementia' was applied when the illness commenced after the

Potentially reversible causes of dementia
Reversible causes of dementia include not only unexpected cerebral tumours (particularly frontal and non-dominant temporal lobes in site) and other mass lesions such as giant aneurysms, but also obstructive or communicating hydrocephalus, paraneoplastic syndromes, neurosyphilis and various metabolic conditions, vitamin B12 deficiency, chronic drug intoxication, myxoedema, Hashimoto's encephalopathy and disturbances of calcium metabolism. Full investigation is required to exclude such treatable causes and should be undertaken in every patient under the age of 75, and in all those over that age in whom the cause of dementia is not established.

age of 65. Senile dementia became equated with Alzheimer's disease which, in fact, can occur at any age and accounts for over 80 per cent of those dementing in later life. Cerebrovascular disease is also a common cause of dementia and usually is suggested by the presence of established hypertension and a history of repeated stroke-like episodes (**multi-infarct dementia**) often with diffuse small vessel damage (Figure 2.7). Other causes include

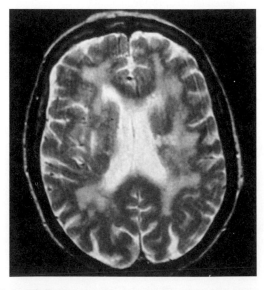

Figure 2.7 Axial view T2-weighted MRI scan of a patient with widespread small vessel disease and multi-infarct dementia.

dementia with Lewy bodies, frontotemporal dementias, Huntington's disease (which is suggested by typical chorea and family history), and Creutzfeldt-Jakob disease (CJD) which is a prion encephalopathy producing a subacute rapidly progressive dementia often with characteristic myoclonus, sometimes marked cerebellar signs, and EEG findings. In younger patients, variant CJD should be considered and the **HIV-associated** dementia complex is also seen regularly.

REFERENCES AND FURTHER READING

Bhidayasiri R, Waters MF, Giza CC (2005) *Neurological Differential Diagnosis – a Prioritized Approach.* Oxford: Blackwell Publishing.

Bradley WG, Daroff RB, Fenichel GM, Jankovic J (2007) *Neurology in Clinical Practice*, 5th edn. Boston: Butterworth-Heinemann.

Brazis PW, Masdeu JG, Biller J (2007) *Localisation in Clinical Neurology*, 5th edn. Philadelphia: Lippincott Williams and Wilkins.

Bronstein AM, Lempert T (2007) *Dizziness – A Practical Approach to Diagnosis and Management.* Cambridge: Cambridge University Press.

Marshall RS, Mayer SA (2007) *On Call Neurology*, 3rd edn. Philadelphia: Saunders.

Pendlebury ST, Giles MF, Rothwell PM (2009) *Transient Ischaemic Attack and Stroke.* Cambridge: Cambridge University Press.

Ropper AH, Samuels MA (2009) *Adams and Victor's Principles of Neurology*, 9th edn. New York: McGraw-Hill Medical.

Silberstein SD, Lipton RB, Dodick (2008) *Wolff's Headache and Other Head Pain*, 8th edn. New York: Oxford University Press.

CHAPTER 3

EXAMINATION OF THE NERVOUS SYSTEM

Tim Fowler, John Scadding and Nick Losseff

NEUROLOGICAL EXAMINATION

The neurological examination is often seen as difficult and time-consuming. However, in many patients, the diagnosis will become clear as the history is taken. Indeed, in most patients presenting with headache or blackouts, and in many patients with episodic dizziness (the three most common presenting symptoms in outpatient neurology), there will be no abnormal physical signs and the diagnosis will be based on the history alone.

As outlined in Chapter 2, the history provides the answer to the two crucial questions in diagnosis: *where* is the lesion (anatomy)? And *what* is the lesion (pathology)? Armed with this information, the examination can be focused, but at the same time it is essential to conduct an examination that effectively screens all the major parts and functions of the nervous system.

It is helpful to have in one's mind two simple plans:

1 The routine basic scheme of examination that is to be conducted in every neurological patient – the screening examination.
2 The parts of the examination requiring particular attention, based on the history.

This plan will be followed in this chapter. First, the basic routine examination will be described. Details of individual tests will not be elaborated, because they are best learned at the bedside. Second, more specific detailed examinations required in patients with certain problems will be discussed.

The basic scheme of neurological examination

This consists of:

1 Assess higher mental function:
   a. Intellect, memory, personality and mood
   b. Speech and cognitive function.
2 Observe gait and station.
3 Test the cranial nerves.
4 Test motor functions.
5 Test sensory functions.
6 Test autonomic function.
7 Examine related structures.

Higher mental function

Intellect, memory, personality and mood

The clarity with which a patient presents their story and answers questions, and their cooperation during examination, will convey a picture of their intellectual capacity and of their personality and mood. Compare your own estimate with what might be expected from the patient's type of work and scholastic record. A patient's mood and insight may be further demonstrated by their reaction to the illness; while their power of memory may be indicated by the coherence and ease with which symptoms and past history are recalled and dated. Whenever there is doubt about a patient's higher mental function, it is crucial to obtain the story and observations of an independent witness who can testify to the patient's intellectual competence.

If history taking does not suggest any defect of higher cerebral function, then no further testing is required. However, if impairment of higher mental function is suspected, more extensive examination is necessary (see later).

Speech and cognitive function

The content and articulation of speech will be evident while taking the history. Always note whether the patient is right-handed or left-handed and, if speech difficulty is apparent, it is also worth checking which eye and which leg are dominant. Abnormalities of speech may include the following:

1 **Dysphonia**, in which the content of speech is normal and articulation preserved but basic voice production is disturbed by mechanical abnormality of the organs of speech, including the vocal cords and resonating sound boxes. The hoarse voice of laryngitis and the nasal speech of the common cold are frequent non-neurological causes of dysphonia.

2 **Dysarthria**, which describes abnormal articulation resulting from damage to the nervous pathways or muscles responsible for speech production, with intact language content. Lower motor neurone paralysis of the soft palate produces nasal escape of air and the characteristic nasal speech of a paralytic dysarthria. Spasticity of the tongue, palate and mouth produces a monotonous, stiff, slurred type of speech known as a spastic dysarthria, which sounds as if the patient is talking with a plum in the mouth. Incoordination of muscular action responsible for speech because of cerebellar disease results in irregular, staccato and explosive speech known as scanning or cerebellar dysarthria. The akinetic-rigid syndrome of parkinsonism produces a characteristic slow, soft, monotonous speech known as an extrapyramidal or hyphonic dysarthria, a combination of dysphonia and dysarthria. Edentulous patients show a degree of dysarthria.

3 **Dysphasia**, which describes impairment of language, is either difficulty of understanding the spoken or written word, or of speaking or writing itself. The various types of dysphasia that may be encountered with lesions affecting the dominant hemisphere are described later.

Cognition refers to the capacity to know and perceive one's surroundings and one's self in relationship to those surroundings. The inability to recognize objects in space, colours, faces or even one's own body parts is known as **agnosia**. Inability to undertake a skilled motor act despite intact power, sensation and coordination is known as **apraxia** (different types of agnosia and apraxia will be described later).

Gait and station

It is traditional to examine the patient's gait at this stage of the examination. However, in the outpatient clinic setting, the opportunity to watch the patient's gait should not be lost as the patient walks into the clinic room.

The ability to stand and walk depends on the integration of several neurological functions, including:

- motor functions – cortex, upper and lower motor neurones, the basal ganglia and cerebellum, muscles and joints;
- position sensation from muscles and joints in the limbs and also in the trunk and neck;
- sensory input from vision and the labyrinths in the inner ear;
- intact autonomic control of blood pressure.

These functions will be examined in detail during the neurological examination, and it is often helpful to re-examine the gait at the end of the examination, when interpretation of any impairment will be easier in the light of the knowledge of the various individual deficits found on detailed examination.

Station refers to the ability of the patient to stand, and the posture of the stance. Examples of common abnormalities include the stooped stance in Parkinson's disease and the wide-based stance of a patient with cerebellar disease. It is important to observe how easily the patient is able to stand up and whether or not assistance is required. The ability to walk is then assessed. In a patient whose gait appears normal or only mildy abnormal, two further tests should be performed.

1 **Tandem gait**. The patient is asked to walk heel-to-toe along a straight line. This is a stringent test of balance and coordination, and in the presence of normal power, usually indicates impairment of cerebellar or vestibular function, or of postural sensation (sensory ataxia).

2 **Romberg's test**. If the tandem gait is normal, the patient is asked to stand with the feet together and then to close the eyes. An inability to maintain balance indicates impairment of either postural sensation or vestibular function.

In patients whose gait is already obviously impaired and unsteady, tandem gait and Romberg's test will not add anything of diagnostic value and are potentially dangerous to the patient, who may fall. They should not be performed under this circumstance.

Certain gait disorders are readily recognized:

- In a **spastic gait**, the patient walks slowly, with stiffness in the legs and sometimes scissoring due to thigh adductor spasm. The feet are plantar flexed and inverted and the toes scuff the ground. A hemiplegic gait is characterized by dragging, weakness and spasticity of one leg.

- The patient with an **ataxic gait** is unsteady and adopts a wide-based stance, and tends to lurch from side to side on walking.

- The **Parkinsonian gait** is typified by a stooped posture, difficulty in initiating walking (start hesitation), small shuffling steps with a tendency to gain pace (festinant gait).

- A **waddling gait** is produced by proximal weakness at the hip girdle. There is an inability to tilt the pelvis normally when swinging each leg through to take the next step, and this is compensated by exaggerated lateral movements of the trunk, producing a waddling motion.

- A **steppage gait** results from severe weakness of dorsiflexion of the feet, combined with impairment of position sensation. In order to clear the ground with each step, there is exaggerated flexion at the hip. There may also be associated stamping of each foot on the ground, particularly when weakness is associated with severe postural sensory loss.

- In an **apraxic gait**, the patient is able to stand, but unable to perform the planned sequence of motor function necessary for walking. The gait most often appears small-paced and shuffling.

- A **limping gait** is a very common observation, and usually not the result of any neurological deficit, but rather, a painful musculoskeletal condition affecting the leg or lumbar spine. The gait appears protective and when associated with pain, is also sometimes called an **antalgic gait**.

CRANIAL NERVES

I Olfactory nerve

The sense of smell should always be tested if there are complaints of disturbance of taste or smell. The most common cause of a complete loss of smell, **anosmia**, is damage to one or both olfactory nerves resulting from head injury. Smell should be tested if there is suspicion of a lesion involving the anterior fossa or of dementia. It is important to realize that patients complaining of loss of taste are usually describing the effects of damage to the olfactory nerve, which results in loss of appreciation of subtleties of good food or wine. Such patients can still recognize the elementary four tastes – sweet, sour, salt and acid – but cannot appreciate flavour. The sense of smell may be tested by the ability to identify and distinguish the odours of common objects, such as coffee, peppermint or orange peel, with each nostril in turn. Unilateral hyposmia or anosmia suggests a lesion of the olfactory nerve. Bilateral hyposmia is usually the result of local nasal disease, such as a common cold or sinusitis.

II Optic nerve

The function of the optic nerve can be tested by examining visual acuity, the visual fields and the optic fundus. This requires a Snellen visual acuity chart, a large red-headed (5 mm) hatpin and a grid card, and an ophthalmoscope.

The visual acuity (VA) is a measure of the integrity of central macular vision. The distance VA should be measured in each eye using the

Snellen chart at 6 m with the patient wearing spectacles to correct any refractive error. If the patient's spectacles are not available, or if VA is worse than 6/6 in a patient who does not normally wear glasses, VA should be remeasured by asking the patient to look through a pinhole aperture. Impaired VA that cannot be corrected with the patient's spectacles or a pinhole suggests a neurological or retinal lesion.

The normal distance acuity is 6/6, the numerator representing the distance of the patient from the chart (6 m) and the denominator the distance in metres at which a normal person is able to read that line (Figure 3.1). Decreasing acuity is recorded as 6/9, 6/12, 6/18, 6/24, 6/36, 6/60, and then as the ability to count fingers, perceive hand movements or, finally, perceive light. Near acuity is tested by asking the patient to read standardized test type, again correcting any refractive error. Near vision is a less accurate assessment of acuity. Most patients with a VA of 6/18 for distance can read N5 or N6 size test type. For driving in the UK, it is necessary to read a number plate at 75 feet (22.9 m), which is a VA between 6/9 and 6/12.

Colour vision may be affected by optic nerve damage and is tested with standard Ishihara plates. Some 8 per cent of the male population may be colour-blind, most often with red–green impairment.

The visual fields may be tested at the bedside by the confrontation technique, where the patient's field is compared with that of the tester.

Lesions of the posterior visual pathways cause defects in the opposite half of the peripheral fields (hemianopias).

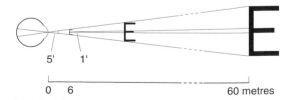

Figure 3.1 Distance visual acuity – the angles subtended by test type on a standard Snellen chart at 6 m.

With one eye covered, the patient faces the examiner and is asked to fix his gaze on that of the examiner. Using a 5 mm red pin, the target is brought from outside the peripheral extent of the field into each of the four quadrants to detect any impairment. First the patient is asked to say when they first see the pin (often described as dark) and after this to repeat the test asking them to say when they first perceive the pin as red. Each eye is tested separately and any peripheral defect is often matched in the initial peripheral field (dark) and that of the smaller field to red. Peripheral defects as hemianopias, quadrantanopias and altitudinal defects should be detectable using this technique. Visual fields should be recorded in the notes with the right-eye field on the right and the left-eye field on the left (Figure 3.2). More accurate visual field testing is now carried out using automated perimeters with a computer printout, for example, the Humphrey visual field analyser. In a subsequent examination, both eyes should be tested together to look for any visual inattention or neglect (see later). Here, small finger movements can be used as targets.

Central field loss occurs most often with lesions of the anterior visual pathways, particularly the macular area of the retina and the optic nerve.

Patients commonly show a depressed acuity and may complain of blurred vision or a central impairment (central scotoma). This can be confirmed using a 5 mm red hatpin or by checking central macular vision using an Amsler chart (Figure 3.3). This is a 'grid' printed on paper and the patient is asked to look at the central spot and point out any fault. It tests the central 10 degrees of the visual field. It is also often useful to look for colour desaturation in the central part of the field comparing the intensity of the red colour of the target between the two sides at the centre of the field.

Optic fundus examination
It is helpful to pursue a routine in fundus examination, concentrating initially on the optic disc, looking for swelling (papilloedema) or pallor (optic atrophy), then exploring the four quadrants of the retina looking for haemorrhages or exudates and examining the retinal arteries, which should be about two-thirds of the diameter of veins, the latter often being pulsatile at least as they converge near the optic disc.

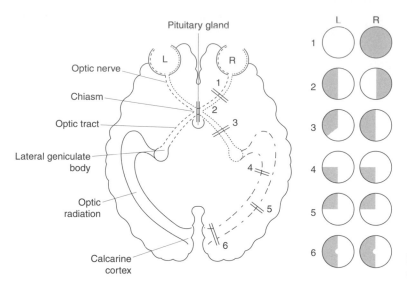

Figure 3.2 Common visual field defects.

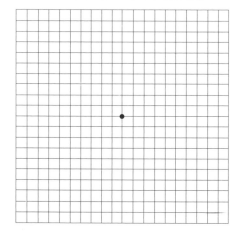

Amsler recording chart
A replica of Chart No. 1, printed black on white for convenience of recording

Figure 3.3 Amsler grid for recording central field of vision. When held at a reading distance of 14 in, 1/3 m, the full-size grid tests the central 10 degrees of the visual field, that is 10 degrees in all directions from the fixation point.

Examination of the optic fundi with an ophthalmoscope is a skill that can only be learnt by practice. Low ambient light and good ophthalmoscopic illumination is essential (Plate 1a).

Visible venous pulsations in the vessels entering the optic cup in the disc indicate there is no papilloedema. Venous pulsation is best seen if the patient is standing or sitting. It is important to distinguish between swelling of the optic nerve from local disease (optic neuritis) and papilloedema resulting from raised intracranial pressure.

Optic neuritis versus papilloedema
In optic neuritis, there will be an obvious and often profound drop in visual acuity accompanied by a central scotoma, while in papilloedema as a result of raised intracranial pressure the visual acuity remains normal, and the only field defect initially is an enlarged blind spot. Later effects of damage to the optic nerve or chiasm lead to a pale, clearly demarcated disc – optic atrophy (Plate 1b).

III, IV and VI Oculomotor, trochlear and abducens nerves

Examination of the three nerves innervating the muscles of the eyes involves assessment of pupillary function and of eye movement.

The size, shape and equality of the pupils should be recorded. Their reaction to a bright light should be tested both directly, by shining the light into the eye under observation, and consensually, by shining the light into the opposite eye, both of which should produce brisk and equal pupillary constriction. The light should be shone into each eye from a slight lateral angle, to avoid the patient focusing gaze on the light source, thereby leading to a convergence papillary constriction (see below). The **'swinging light'** test is a particularly sensitive method of detecting optic nerve lesions. The light is alternately focused on one pupil then the opposite. The pupil of the affected side will dilate slightly when the light is directed onto it because the optic nerve lesion reduces the direct light response, while the consensual response from the opposite eye is preserved. The pupillary response to accommodation or near-vision should be tested by asking the subject to focus upon a finger or object, which is carried towards the nose: again, the pupils will constrict on convergence. The position of the upper eyelid should be noted, looking particularly for the presence of drooping (ptosis). Defects of pupillary function are described later in this chapter.

Eye movements should be tested in two ways. The **saccadic system** is examined by asking the patient to look voluntarily to right and left, and up and down. The **pursuit system** is examined by asking the patient to follow an object moved to right and left, and up and down. Note the range of movement of each eye in all directions, and whether the movements of the two eyes are yoked together (conjugate eye movements). Note whether saccadic movements are carried out rapidly to the extremes of gaze in each direction, and whether pursuit movements are carried out smoothly without interruption. The significance of impaired saccadic and pursuit eye movements is discussed later in this chapter.

Ask whether the patient sees double at any point (diplopia); this is the most sensitive index

---

Assessment of diplopia

1 Is it constant, intermittent or variable?
2 Note the direction of separation of images – horizontal, vertical or tilted/oblique.
3 Note the direction of gaze in which there is maximal separation.
4 By 'cover' testing, check which is the most peripheral image. The weak muscle leads to the more peripheral image.
5 Note the presence of any head tilt, and whether this improves or worsens the diplopia
6 Any associated features:
   a. pupillary size and reactions
   b. ptosis
   c. weakness of eye closure
   d. proptosis
   e. peri-orbital changes

---

of defective ocular movement and may be evident to the patient even when the examiner can see no abnormality of gaze.

Look for any **nystagmus**, which is a repetitive drift of the eyeball away from the point of fixation, followed by a fast corrective movement towards it.

Nystagmus – peripheral versus central
Peripheral vestibular lesions cause horizontal nystagmus away from the side of the lesion, which enhances if fixation is lost. Central lesions causing nystagmus tend to produce a more coarse nystagmus towards the side of the lesion. Central nystagmus may also be multidirectional, vertical and rotatory, and may change direction with gaze.

V Trigeminal nerve

Both the motor and sensory divisions of the trigeminal nerve should be examined.

The motor functions of the trigeminal nerve are examined by comparing the size of the masseter and temporalis muscles on each side by palpation while the teeth are clenched. Look for unilateral wasting of these muscles on the side of a trigeminal nerve lesion. Then ask the patient to open their mouth; normally the jaw does not deviate from the midline on mouth opening. In a unilateral trigeminal nerve lesion, the jaw will deviate towards the side of damage, because of weakness of the pterygoid muscles, which normally protrude the jaw. However, a common cause of jaw deviation is subluxation of one temporomandibular joint, so before diagnosing a trigeminal nerve lesion, always check by palpation that the mandibular condyle has not flipped out of its socket. Finally, test the jaw jerk by a brisk tap applied to a finger placed on the point of the half open jaw.

The most sensitive index of impairment of the sensation in the trigeminal nerve is usually loss of the corneal reflex.

The reflex is elicited by touching the cornea with a wisp of cotton wool, introduced from laterally, out of the sight of the patient, to avoid a visually cued blink response. The stimulus evokes an afferent volley in the ophthalmic division of the trigeminal nerve to cause a bilateral blink, which is mediated by motor impulses in the facial nerve. Sensation in all three divisions of the trigeminal nerve should be examined with pin and cotton wool to test pain and light touch, respectively. Remember the anatomical confines of the trigeminal territory, which extends back to meet the zone innervated by the C2 sensory division well past the crown of the head behind the ears (Figure 3.4). Also the mandibular division of the trigeminal nerve supplies the skin over the jaw, but spares that portion over the angle of the jaw, which again is supplied by C2. These landmarks are of value in distinguishing true trigeminal sensory loss from elaborated claims of facial numbness. Another useful point is that fibres of the trigeminal nerve supplying the cornea travel with the nasociliary branch of the ophthalmic division, so that depression of the corneal reflex is almost always accompanied by impairment of pinprick sensation at the root of the nose next to the eye. The lining of the inner nostril is also supplied by the ophthalmic division of the trigeminal nerve.

VII Facial nerve

Test facial movements by asking the patient to wrinkle the forehead, screw up the eyes, show the teeth and whistle. Asking a patient to whistle often makes them laugh, which will give you the opportunity to assess facial weakness around the mouth.

> **Facial nerve lesions – upper motor neurone versus lower motor neurone**
> Lesions of the facial nerve, or of its nucleus, produce weakness of the whole side of the face, including the forehead. In contrast, a unilateral lesion of the supranuclear corticobulbar pathway for facial movement (an upper motor neurone (UMN) lesion) only affects the lower half of the face, sparing the forehead. The facial nerve also supplies a small branch to the stapedius muscle.

The facial nerve itself has no important sensory component. However, fibres originating in the lingual nerve, which carry the sensation of taste from the anterior two-thirds of the tongue, join the facial nerve via the chorda tympani branch in the petrous temporal bone. Rarely, it is necessary to test the sensation of taste. To do so, ask the subject to protrude the tongue, and keep it out, while a test

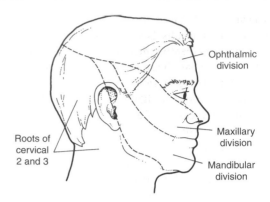

Figure 3.4 Trigeminal sensory innervation.

substance is applied to one side of the tongue tip. There are four tastes – salt, sweet, bitter (quinine) and acid or sour (lemon). The facial nerve also supplies the lacrimal gland.

VIII Auditory or vestibulocochlear nerve

> The auditory nerve has two divisions, one conveying impulses from the cochlea subserving hearing, and the other conveying impulses from the labyrinth responsible for vestibular function.

Hearing can be tested quickly by asking the patient to repeat whispered words or numbers with the eyes shut and one ear occluded by the examiner's forefinger. Alternatively, a wristwatch may be brought towards the ear and the distance at which the subject hears the ticking is noted for each side. A watch ticking is a high frequency sound and useful for detecting nerve deafness. If deafness is detected, define whether it is as a result of middle ear disease (**conductive deafness**) or a nerve lesion (**sensorineural or perceptive deafness**). To do this, compare the sound of a tuning fork (256 Hz or, better, 512 Hz) held close to the ear (air conduction) with that when the fork is placed on the mastoid (bone conduction): this is called Rinne's test. In normal subjects, and in those with sensorineural deafness, air conduction is better than bone conduction. In patients with conductive deafness, the reverse is true. Weber's test also may help to distinguish between unilateral conductive and sensorineural deafness. A tuning fork is placed on the centre of the forehead; in the normal subject this is heard equally well in both ears. In conductive deafness it is usually heard loudest in the deaf ear, whereas in perceptive deafness it is heard loudest in the normal ear. These bedside tests, however, are crude: deafness is more accurately assessed by formal audiometric investigation, which will provide a quantitative measure of auditory acuity at different frequencies of sound.

The vestibular nerve carries impulses from the semicircular canals: these sense head rotation (angular acceleration). It also carries impulses from the utricle and saccule, which are the sensors of linear motion (acceleration) and static tilt of the head. Apart from examining for nystagmus, it is not necessary to test vestibular function routinely. In patients with vertigo or imbalance, special tests are required that will be described later.

IX and X Glossopharyngeal and vagus nerves

The glossopharyngeal nerve supplies sensation to the posterior pharyngeal wall and tonsillar regions. The vagus nerve, apart from supplying autonomic fibres to thoracic and abdominal contents, supplies motor fibres to the muscles of the soft palate. Interference with glossopharyngeal and vagus nerve function causes difficulty with talking and swallowing.

Vagus function can be examined easily by watching the uvula rise in the midline when the patient says 'Aah'. A unilateral palatal palsy causes drooping of the affected side and, on phonation, the palate deviates to the opposite side, pulled in that direction by the intact muscles. A unilateral vagal lesion will also paralyse the ipsilateral vocal cord to cause a typical hoarse voice and 'bovine' cough. Watch and listen while a patient drinks sips of water.

It is not necessary to test glossopharyngeal sensation routinely, because this involves eliciting the 'gag' reflex, which is unpleasant. When required, the 'gag' reflex is obtained by touching the posterior wall of the pharynx with an orange stick, which causes the patient to 'gag'; both sides of the pharynx should be tested.

XI Accessory nerve

The accessory nerve innervates the sternomastoid and trapezius muscles. Its fibres are derived from the lower brainstem and the upper cervical cord segments. The sternomastoid turns the head to the opposite side, while the trapezius is activated by shrugging the shoulders. Bilateral weakness raises the possibility of muscle disease.

In a patient with a hemispheric stroke, it is the sternomastoid muscle contralateral to the hemiparesis that is affected (i.e. ipsilateral to the cerebral lesion). This will result in weakness of head-turning towards the side of the hemiparesis.

XII Hypoglossal nerve

The hypoglossal nerve innervates the muscles of the tongue. Normally the tongue is held in the floor of the mouth by activity in the tongue retractors. A unilateral hypoglossal lesion therefore will cause the tip of the tongue to deviate away from the affected side when lying in the floor of the mouth. On protrusion, the tip of the tongue will deviate towards the affected side. Wasting of the tongue results from lower motor neurone lesions, and is often accompanied by fasciculation. In bilateral upper motor neurone lesions, the tongue may be small and spastic. Spasticity is elicited by asking the subject to attempt rapidly to protrude the tongue in and out, or move it from side to side.

MOTOR FUNCTION

The standard order of the examination of the motor system is as follows:
- posture;
- muscle bulk; distribution of any wasting present; presence of fasciculation;
- muscle tone;
- power;
- coordination;
- reflexes.

In any patient whose history indicates the likelihood of finding a neurological deficit, it is always best to adhere to this order of examination.

However, in patients in whom the presence of a deficit in the limbs is considered unlikely, it is convenient to screen for motor deficits by examining coordination first. Any type of motor abnormality will impair the capacity to execute rapid fine arm and finger movements, or the ability to walk normally.

Motor function screen

- Hold arms outstretched
- Rapid finger movements, finger/nose testing
- Stance, observe balance
- Gait, observe walking and on tiptoe and heels

Screen of muscle strength

C5	deltoid	shoulder abduction
C6	biceps	elbow flexion
C7	triceps	elbow extension
C8	finger flexors	grip
T1	dorsal interossei	finger abduction
L1	ilio-psoas	hip flexion
L2	adductors	hip adduction
L3	quadriceps	knee extension
L4	tibialis anterior	foot dorsiflexion
L5	ext. hallucis longus	big toe dorsiflexion
S1	tibialis posterior	foot plantar flexion

Ask the patient to hold the arms outstretched, with fingers spread and with the eyes shut. Look for a tendency: for the arm to drop, which suggests weakness of the shoulder; for the forearm to pronate, which suggests mild upper motor neurone deficit or dystonia; for the fingers to waver uncertainly (pseudoathetosis), which suggests sensory loss; or for abnormal movements, such as tremor, to develop. Then ask the patient to touch their nose rapidly with the point of the forefinger and then the examiner's finger, going to and fro as accurately as possible. Such 'finger–nose testing' examines the skill of large proximal arm movements. Look particularly for kinetic or intention tremor, an oscillation that appears during movement and becomes worse as the point of aim is reached. Also note if the finger overshoots or undershoots its target (dysmetria). Then test the capacity for rapid finger movement by asking the patient to approximate the pulp of the thumb to the pad of each finger in turn rapidly and accurately. This 'five finger exercise' directly tests the integrity of the 'true pyramidal' pathway, which controls fine manual skills, and also detects parkinsonism, which causes slowness, reduced amplitude and fade of such repetitive movements. Finally, ask the patient to pronate and supinate the outstretched arms rapidly. Such

alternating movements are impaired in cerebellar disease (dysdiadochokinesis) and in parkinsonism.

During the examination for coordination of the arms and legs, look out for the presence of **wasting and involuntary movements**. Muscle wasting implies either primary muscle disease (myopathy) or a lower motor neurone lesion. It can be difficult, particularly in the elderly or in those with joint disease, to decide whether apparent thinning of muscle bulk is merely a result of disuse or whether it indicates neurological deficit.

> Muscle wasting is only of significance if it is accompanied by definite muscle weakness.

The characteristics of the typical abnormal movements of tremor, chorea, myoclonus, tics and dystonia have been described in Chapter 2. Other abnormal movements that may be observed include fasciculation, which is a random involuntary twitching of large motor units that occurs as a result of denervation and reinnervation. The characteristic of pathological fasciculation is that twitches of muscle fascicles occur randomly in time and site.

Rapidly test **muscle tone** by noting the resistance of the limbs to passive movement. In the arms, this can be studied by shaking the shoulders with the subject standing, looking for the ease with which the limp arms swing from side to side, or by pronation/supination movements of the forearm. In the legs, proximal tone can be assessed by rolling the thigh to and fro, or by passive flexion of the leg onto the abdomen. Tone distally at the ankle is tested by rapid passive dorsiflexion of the foot. Increased tone can be detected, and the manoeuvre

---

Muscle tone

Spasticity is a resistance to attempted stretch of the muscle that increases with applied force until there is a sudden give at a certain tension, the 'clasp-knife' or 'lengthening' reaction. Rigidity is a resistance to passive movement that continues unaltered throughout the range of movements, and so has a plastic or 'lead pipe' quality. Gegenhalten describes a curious intermittent resistance to movement in which the patient seems to be unknowingly attempting to oppose efforts to displace the limb.

will elicit clonus, if present. The optimal posture to undertake this examination is with the thigh slightly abducted and externally rotated and the knee flexed to greater than 45 degrees, supported in this posture by the examiner. This ensures good relaxation and thus a more reliable assessment of muscle tone. An increase in muscle tone may take one of three forms.

Muscle power is tested by asking the patient to exert force against resistance imposed by the examiner, with attention to the segmental innervation of the muscles being tested. Table 3.1 indicates those muscle groups that are routinely tested, in anatomical order. Assessment of normal strength needs to take account of the age and physique of the patient.

It is useful to grade power in each group tested, and the most commonly used scale is the Medical Research Council (MRC) scale:

Grade 0 – no movement at all
Grade 1 – flicker of movement
Grade 2 – movement with gravity eliminated
Grade 3 – movement against gravity
Grade 4 – movement against resistance. This includes a wide range of power and is often subdivided into grades 4–, 4 and 4+
Grade 5 – normal power

However, in patients in whom there is no reason from the history to suspect that there will be weakness, it is reasonable to undertake an abbreviated screening examination of strength, testing the power of two critical muscles, one proximal and one distal, in both arms and legs. The reason for choosing a proximal and distal muscle to examine is that primary muscle disease will be detected by proximal muscle weakness, while the impact of peripheral nerve disease will be apparent in distal muscle weakness.

The proximal and distal muscles chosen to test can be selected also to detect weakness resulting from an upper motor neurone lesion. The latter has a quite distinctive distribution, which can be remembered by recalling the posture of a patient rendered hemiplegic by a stroke. The stroke victim carries the arm held to the side, the elbow flexed and the wrist and fingers flexed onto the chest. The leg is held extended at both hip and knee, with the

Table 3.1 Innervation and examination of muscle groups[a]

Muscle/muscle group	Segmental/nerve innervation	
Diaphragm	C3, 4, 5	
Rhomboid	C4, 5	
Serratus anterior	C4, 5, 6	
Supraspinatus	C4, 5, 6	
Infraspinatus	C4, 5, 6	
Pectoralis major	C5, 6, 7, 8, T1	
Deltoid	C5, 6	
Biceps/brachialis	C5, 6	
Triceps	C6, 7, 8	Radial
Brachioradialis	C5, 6	Radial
Wrist extensors	C5, 6, 7, 8	Radial
Wrist flexors – carpi radialis	C6, 7	Median
carpi ulnaris	C7, 8, T1	Ulnar
Finger extensors	C6, 7, 8	Radial
Finger flexors	C7, 8, T1	Median
Abductor pollicis brevis	C8, T1	Median
Abductor pollicis longus	C7, 8	Radial
Interossei	C7, 8	Ulnar
Upper abdominal	T6-T9	
Lower abdominal	T10-L1	
Hip flexors – iliopsoas	L1, 2, 3	
Adductors of hip	L2, 3, 4	
Abductors of hip	L4, 5, S1	
Extensors of hip	L5, S1, 2	
Knee flexors – hamstrings	L4, 5, S1, 2	
Knee extensors – quadriceps	L2, 3, 4	
Dorsiflexion of foot	L4, 5	
Plantarflexion of foot	S1, 2	
Inversion of foot	L4, 5	
Eversion of foot	L5, S1	
Toe extension	L5, S1	
Extensor hallucis longus	L5	
Extensor digitorum brevis	S1	
Toe flexion	S1, 2	

[a]Those in bold type are the muscles/groups tested routinely.

foot plantar flexed and inverted. This characteristic posture is the result of a selective distribution of spasticity working against a selective distribution of weakness. **Hemiplegic weakness in the arm** affects the shoulder abductors, elbow extensors, wrist and finger extensors, and small hand muscles. **Hemiplegic weakness in the leg** affects hip flexors, knee flexors, and dorsiflexors and evertors of the foot. Accordingly, the critical muscles to test in a screening motor examination are: (1) in the arm, proximally the shoulder abductors and distally the small muscles of the hand, which spread the fingers; and (2) in the leg, proximally the hip flexors and distally the dorsiflexors and evertors of the ankle.

The reflexes

Elicit the following reflexes

The deep tendon reflexes of the biceps, triceps, supinator, and finger flexors in the arms, and of the knee and ankle in the legs (Table 3.2). When eliciting such 'tendon jerks' always compare the two sides, taking care to have the limbs in comparable positions. When hyper-reflexia is present, try to elicit **clonus** (a repetitive self-sustaining reflex contraction) by rapid passive dorsiflexion of the ankle, and by downward thrust of the patella. Also routinely elicit the superficial reflexes known as the **plantar responses** by firmly stroking the outer border of the sole of each foot upwards. This normally produces plantar flexion of the big toe (a flexor plantar response). The abnormal response consists of upwards movement of the big toe, often accompanied by fanning of the toes; this is known as an extensor plantar response or Babinski's sign. If there is doubt as to the presence of hyper-reflexia

Table 3.2 Reflexes

Arm	Biceps	C5/6
	Supinator	C5/6
	Triceps	C7
	Finger flexors	C8
Abdominal	Upper	T8–10
	Lower	T10–12
	Cremasteric	L1/2
	Anal	S4/5
Leg	Knee	L3/4
	Ankle	S1

or Babinski's sign, elicit the abdominal reflexes by gently stroking the skin of the abdomen in each quadrant in turn. This normally causes a twitch contraction of the appropriate quadrant of the underlying muscles, tending to pull the umbilicus in that direction. The abdominal reflexes are lost in an upper motor neurone lesion. They may also be absent after extensive abdominal surgery or with very lax stretched muscles.

Sensory functions

The student will soon learn that testing sensation can be difficult and frustrating. It is crucial to have some clear idea of what is being looked for before embarking on this part of the neurological examination. The sensory examination is performed at this stage of the overall examination because by now, the examiner should have ascertained whether or not sensory loss is likely to be present, and if so, of what type and distribution. In a routine screening of the nervous system, sensory examination may be brief, providing the patient has no sensory complaint and there is no other good reason for extensive sensory testing.

Spinal cord sensory pathways

The three main sensory systems entering the spinal cord are:
- Pain and temperature travelling via the spinothalamic tracts
- Vibration and position sense travelling via the posterior columns
- Light touch, which travels through both these other pathways

---

The anatomical pathways are outlined in Figure 3.5, where it is shown that all the sensory modalities pass via the dorsal root ganglion into the spinal cord. **Pain and temperature sense** cross to the other side of the spinal cord within one or two segments of entry and then ascend in the spinothalamic tracts to reach the thalamus, while **vibration and position sense** after entry, ascend in the posterior columns (fasciculus gracilis and cuneatus) of the same side of the spinal cord to reach the lower brainstem where the pathway crosses to ascend on the opposite side in the medial lemniscus to reach the thalamus and to relay to the cortex.

Test appreciation of light touch and pinprick on

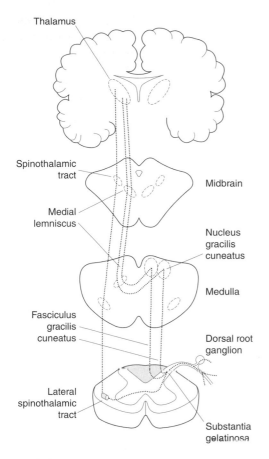

Figure 3.5 Ascending sensory pathways. Posterior columns – position sense, vibration, tactile sense, discrimination. Lateral spinothalamic tract – pain, temperature, tactile sense, tickle, itch.

the tips of the fingers and the dorsum of the toes. Pinprick should always be tested with a disposable pin; syringe needles are too sharp, may draw blood and thus should not be used. Also examine the ability to appreciate joint movement in the distal interphalangeal joints of a finger and the big toe. Remember joint position sense is extremely sensitive, such that small movements of only a few degrees may be perceived accurately. Finally, examine vibration by applying a standard tuning fork (128 Hz) to the pulps of the fingers and the dorsum of the big toes. Always set the tuning fork vibrating by 'tweaking' the ends together and rapidly releasing. This produces a fairly standardized degree of vibration and avoids the obvious auditory cue produced by hitting the tuning fork on a hard surface. Some estimate of quantitative sensory appreciation of vibration may be obtained

by checking whether the patient has ceased to recognize vibration after a standard 'tweak' when compared to the application of the same stimulus to the examiner.

The various patterns of sensory deficit typically found in different neurological conditions are described in the later chapters in this book.

Autonomic functions

The autonomic nerves innervate the viscera, bowel, bladder and sexual organs and are responsible for control of circulatory reflexes, sweating and pupillary reactions (Figure 3.6). Symptoms of autonomic failure may include constipation with impaired bowel motility, incomplete bladder emptying from a hypotonic bladder, which may lead to urinary incontinence, and impotence in the male. Failure of the circulatory reflexes may cause postural hypotension with feelings of faintness or dizziness on standing, sometimes syncope, and often a fixed relatively rapid heart rate. There may be impaired sweating with difficulties in temperature regulation, occasionally patchy hyperhidrosis, dry eyes and oral mucous membranes. The pupils may become non-reactive.

The easiest simple tests of autonomic function include measurement of the blood pressure (BP), when the patient is lying and after standing for 1 minute, and the measurement of the pulse rate at rest, during the Valsalva manoeuvre, when deep breathing and on standing.

With autonomic failure the BP will fall by more than 30 mmHg on standing. Orthostatic hypotension is defined as a fall in systolic BP of >20 mmHg and a fall in the diastolic BP of 10 mmHg on standing upright. The pulse rate normally rises on standing: in autonomic failure this may not occur. With a Valsalva manoeuvre, during the strain the BP normally falls and the pulse rate rises. With release, the BP rises and the pulse rate falls. With autonomic failure there is no change in pulse rate. Normally the pulse rate varies with deep breathing, but again with autonomic failure this may not occur. Measuring the R-R interval on an electrocardiogram during such tests is a useful way of measuring such heart rate changes. More detailed tests of urodynamic function, penile plethysmography and pharmacological tests for sweating and pupil-

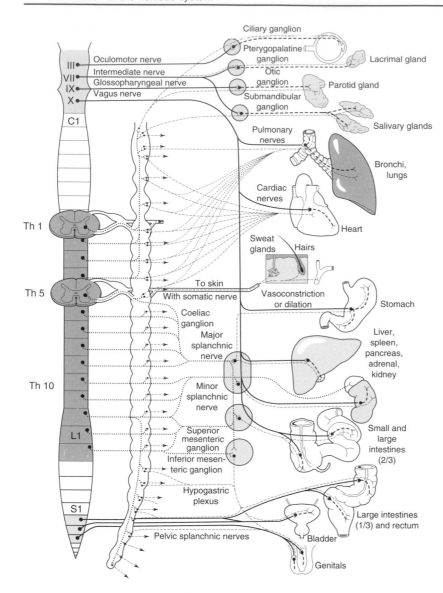

Figure 3.6 The autonomic nervous system and the organs supplied by this. Sympathetic pathways are shown in black. Parasympathetic pathways in grey. Only the left trunk is shown. (Reproduced with permission from P Duus (1988) *Topical Diagnosis in Neurology*. Stuttgart: Georg Thieme Verlag.)

lary reactions may also be used for further testing in appropriate patients.

Examination of related structures

> **The neurological examination is completed by looking at:**
> - the skeletal structures enclosing the central nervous system;
> - the extracranial blood vessels;
> - the skin;
> - a general physical examination.

Check the size and shape of the skull, noticing any palpable lumps. Bruits over the skull and neck may indicate arterial narrowing or the presence of an arteriovenous malformation. Check the skin for any birth marks or stigmata of cutaneous disease, for example neurofibromatosis (Plate 2a).

Look for **meningism** by flexing the head and neck onto the chest. Normally the chin will reach the chest but if the meninges are irritated by blood or infection, such movement is limited by painful spasm of the neck extensors. In severe instances, there may be actual head retraction.

In the case of spinal lesions, examine the spine for any local tenderness or deformity and test spi-

Meningeal irritation can also be found in the lumbar region, where spasm of the hamstrings causes limitation of leg movement so that when the thigh is at 90 degrees to the trunk, the knee cannot be straightened (Kernig's sign).

nal movements. Straight-leg raising, by flexing the thigh at the hip with the knee extended, will cause stretching of the sciatic nerve and if the contributing nerve roots are compressed or irritated, results in limitation of the movement with accompanying pain. The pain may be in the back or territory of the sciatic nerve and may be accentuated by dorsiflexing the foot while the leg is raised in the test.

Add a general physical examination for all patients. In particular the pulse rate and rhythm and the BP should be recorded. Check for any signs of heart disease, especially valvular damage. Any enlargement of lymph glands, liver or spleen should be noted and the presence of any other abdominal mass. This examination is to screen for possible sources of clues to neurological complications of systemic diseases.

Interpretation of abnormal findings

Anatomical site
As discussed in Chapter 2, the first object of history taking and clinical examination is to find the anatomical site of damage to the nervous system. Every abnormality discovered on physical examination suggests that a particular group of neurones is damaged. By defining the pathways involved, the likely site or sites of the disease may be deduced.

This exercise in applied neuroanatomy is hampered by the ease with which minor insignificant abnormalities may be discovered on examination. Even normal findings sometimes may be misinterpreted as indicating a disease process; for instance, the over-helpful patient may manufacture sensory abnormalities as fast as the examiner suggests that they might be present!

To overcome this problem, it is a useful exercise to classify each abnormality discovered as a 'hard' or 'soft' sign.

'Hard' signs are unequivocally abnormal – an absent ankle jerk, even on reinforcement; a clear-cut extensor plantar response; definite wasting of the small hand muscles. Any final anatomical diagnosis must provide an explanation for such 'hard' signs. 'Soft' signs are frequently found in the absence of any definite abnormality and are, therefore, unreliable. Examples of such 'soft' signs are a slight asymmetry of the tendon reflexes, slightly less facility of repetitive movements of the left hand in a right-handed person, and a few jerks of nystagmus of the eyes on extreme lateral gaze. When in doubt, it is best to ignore such findings in the initial assessment.

The importance of 'hard' signs
Base your first attempt at diagnosis on the 'hard' signs only. Having taken each of these into account in your final conclusion, then review the 'soft' signs that you discovered on the way, and just make certain that none of them raises doubts about your conclusion.

Another point of neurological examination must be emphasized. The speed and precision with which the site of the lesion may be established depends upon continual deduction throughout the process of history taking and examination. In these first few chapters, emphasis has been laid on the way the findings at one stage in the diagnostic process determine the pattern of the succeeding phases of history taking and examination. Whenever an abnormality has been detected, either in the history or on physical examination, its implications must be followed up to the full; for example, the discovery of a bitemporal hemianopia demands a careful search for evidence of pituitary dysfunction. If a patient with headache is discovered to have such a physical sign, then the examiner may immediately return to ask more questions on this history, such as whether a man still shaves regularly or whether a woman's menstrual periods remain regular. This is the true art and skill of neurology. Each clue that emerges during history taking or examination should prompt new thought. Previous provisional conclusions should be re-examined and new questions or physical tests considered. In other words, to arrive at the correct final conclusion requires a constant alert mental processing of every scrap of information that is available.

SPECIFIC ABNORMALITIES

Having described briefly a basic scheme for examination of the nervous system, one to be undertaken in every neurological patient, we will now turn to the more detailed examinations that may be required when certain abnormalities are discovered. The topics chosen by no means cover all the abnormalities that may be found on clinical examination, but they represent the most common problems, which will require further exploration.

Dementia

If the patient's complaint is one of memory difficulty or impairment of intellectual processes, or if a relative or acquaintance suggests that this may be the case, then extensive investigation of higher mental function will be required. Likewise, a detailed examination of the mental state is necessary if, in the course of history-taking and physical testing, the patient's intellectual processes seem impaired. Detailed analysis of intellect, reasoning and powers of memory can be a very time-consuming business, requiring the expertise of trained clinical psychologists. They will undertake a formal psychometric assessment of the patient's current level of intellectual performance, using tools such as the Wechsler Adult Intelligence Scale (WAIS), Raven's progressive matrices and other standardized test batteries. The WAIS test is used most widely, and consists of a number of subtests which assess both 'verbal' and 'performance' abilities. Details of such complex investigations are beyond the scope of this book. Here we are concerned with simple bedside testing of mental powers. However, once the need for formal examination of the mental state has been decided upon, it is best to proceed to gather information in a standard fashion.

An appropriate, standardized, practical and widely used bedside screening tool for evaluating higher mental function is the Mini-Mental State Examination (MMSE; Table 3.3). This provides a numeric score, helpful for serial examinations over time. The tests included in the MMSE have been devised to examine most aspects of mental activity briefly but reproducibly. The whole test takes no longer than 5 minutes to complete, and is a reliable index of intellectual function. In younger patients, a score of 28–30 is expected: this may fall to 24

in older patients. Its weakness is perhaps too much emphasis on language functions and too little on recent memory.

Aphasia

Once a defect of the use of language has been detected, either on history-taking or examination, a more extensive evaluation of speech function is required. A great deal of detailed information is available on the way in which human speech and the use of language can break down in neurological disease, but much of this is irrelevant to routine neurological practice.

> Disorders of language with faulty speech may arise from damage to the dominant hemisphere and are important localizing signs. The left hemisphere is dominant in right-handed subjects, but also in some 70 per cent of left-handers.

Much of our understanding of language disorders results from the study of patients who have sustained dominant hemisphere damage. More recently, positron emission tomography (PET) and functional magnetic resonance imaging (MRI) have added to our understanding of the anatomical localization of certain faults and in the production of 'normal' speech. Strictly, aphasia implies a severe or total loss of speech; dysphasia being a milder deficit.

A **global aphasia** describes the impairment of all functions – comprehension, expression, problems in naming, reading, writing and in repetition. These should all be tested. A global aphasia arises from extensive damage.

Two particular speech areas are recognized. Broca's area lies in the posterior frontal region (Figure 3.7), which is close to the motor regions concerned with articulation. **Broca's (expressive) aphasia** causes expressive difficulties with non-fluent speech with telegrammatic utterances. Short connecting words may be missing (agrammatic speech) and there may be difficulty with 'ifs, ands or buts'. Sometimes there is perseveration and there may be writing difficulties. Comprehension is good.

The second area lies in the posterior part of the superior temporal gyrus, Wernicke's area, which is close to the region of the brain concerned with auditory input. In **Wernicke's (receptive) aphasia**

Table 3.3 The mini-mental state examination

Assessing	Questions	Points (max.)
1 Orientation	Ask the date, the day, the month, the year and the time: score one point for each correct answer	(5)
	Ask the name of the ward, the hospital, the district, the town, the country: again score one point each	(5)
2 Registration and calculation	Name three objects and ask the patient to repeat these: score three for all correct, two if only two	(3)
	Ask the patient to subtract seven from 100 and repeat this five times (93,86,79,72,65)	(5)
	Recall: ask for the three objects to be named again	(3)
3 Language	Name two objects shown to the patient (e.g. pen, watch)	(2)
	Score one point if they can repeat 'No, ifs, ands or buts'	(1)
	Ask the patient to carry out a three-stage command, e.g. 'Take a piece of paper in your right hand, fold it in half and put it on the table'	(3)
	Reading: write in large letters 'Close your eyes' and ask the patient to read and follow this	(1)
	Write: ask the patient to write a short sentence: it should contain a subject, a verb and make sense	(1)
4 Visuo-spatial	Copying: draw two intersecting pentagons, each side about one inch and ask the patient to copy this	(1)
Total		(30)

there are comprehension difficulties with fluent speech, which exhibits many errors of content. Words and phrases may be incorrect and often repeated – paraphasia. Writing is abnormal and commonly there is difficulty understanding the written word, dyslexia.

The speech areas are connected by the arcuate fasciculus (Figure 3.7). A lesion in this pathway may separate the two sites, allowing fluent paraphasic speech with preserved comprehension,

so-called **conduction aphasia**. In such patients, repetition is highly abnormal. In some aphasic patients the deficit appears to be one of naming, word finding, anomic aphasia. This may occur with lesions in the left temporo-parietal region, including the angular gyrus, when it may be associated with alexia and agraphia. A rare symptom complex also arising from lesions in the region of the angular gyrus is Gerstmann's syndrome. This combines agraphia, acalculia, right–left disorientation and finger agnosia. In general, cortical lesions in the dominant hemisphere disrupt spontaneous speech and repetition. Subcortical lesions (**transcortical**

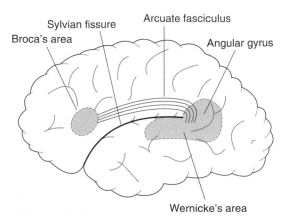

Figure 3.7 Speech areas of the brain.

Labels: Sylvian fissure, Arcuate fasciculus, Broca's area, Angular gyrus, Wernicke's area

---

Examination of language functions can be tested by observing six basic abilities:

1 Spontaneous speech (fluent versus non-fluent, errors of content)
2 Naming of objects
3 Repetition
4 Comprehension
5 Reading
6 Writing

aphasia) leave repetition intact, although understanding may be impaired (Table 3.4).

Agnosia

Agnosia is the failure to recognize objects when the pathways of sensory input from touch, sight and sound are intact. This sensory input cannot be combined with the ability to recall a similar object from the memory areas of the brain, a sort of 'mind-blindness'. Such deficits can be tested by asking patients to feel, name and describe the use of certain objects.

Tactile agnosia, astereognosis, is the inability to recognize objects placed in the hands. There must be no sensory loss in the fingers and sufficient motor function and coordination for the patient's fingers to explore the object. Such defects reflect parietal lobe damage.

Visual agnosia is the inability to recognize what is seen when the eye, optic nerve and main visual pathway to the occipital cortex are preserved. Affected patients can often describe the shape, colour or size of an object without recognizing it. Prosopagnosia is the inability to recognize a familiar face. Parieto-occipital lesions are responsible.

Anosognosia is a term used to describe the lack of awareness or realization that the limbs on one side are paralysed, weak or have impaired sensation. It is most often seen in patients with right-sided parietal damage who may seem to be unaware of their faulty left limbs.

Topographagnosia is the inability to find one's way in familiar surroundings. It is most frequently due to lesions in the non-dominant parietal lobe.

Apraxia

Apraxia is the inability to perform purposeful willed movements in the absence of motor paralysis, severe incoordination or sensory loss. It is the motor equivalent of agnosia. Patients should also be able to understand the command, although it is quite common for some dysphasia to be present. To test for apraxia, patients should be asked to perform a number of tasks, such as to make a fist, to pretend to comb their hair, lick their lips, or to construct a square with four matches. In ideomotor apraxia patients cannot perform a movement to command, although they may do this automatically, for example, lick their lips. In ideational apraxias there is difficulty in carrying out a complex series of movements, like squeezing toothpaste onto a toothbrush.

Gait apraxia describes problems walking. In dressing apraxias, patients cannot put their clothes on correctly. Constructional apraxias produce problems in copying designs or arranging patterns on blocks.

In most instances, apraxias are caused by dominant parietal lobe damage with breakdown in the connections via callosal fibres with the opposite hemisphere, and in the links between the parietal lobes and the motor cortex.

Visual field defects

Light from an object on the left-hand side of the body falls on the right-hand half of each retina after passing through the narrow pupillary aperture. The temporal or outer half of each retina eventu-

Table 3.4 Aphasia

Broca's aphasia	Wernicke's aphasia	Conduction aphasia	Anomic aphasia
Speech non-fluent telegrammatic	Fluent speech poor content, paraphasic errors	Fluent speech, paraphasic errors	Fluent speech
Comprehension good	Comprehension poor, both verbal and written	Comprehension good	Comprehension good
Repetition good	Repetition poor	Repetition very poor	Repetition normal
Object naming poor	Object naming poor	Object naming poor	Object naming poor
Often hemiparesis arm > leg	Absent or mild hemiparesis, ± hemianopia	Cortical sensory loss	Usually no hemiparesis
Global aphasia - large lesions affect all functions			
Although strict divisions are made, in nearly 60 per cent of aphasic patients there appears to be a mixture of problems.			

ally is connected to the cerebral cortex on that side by nerve fibres, which never cross the midline. The inner, or nasal, half of the retina is connected to the cortex on the opposite side by fibres which cross the midline of the optic chiasm. It follows that the right-hand halves of both retinae are connected to the right occipital cortex, which views objects on the left side of the body. Analysis of visual field defects follows from these simple anatomical arrangements.

Visual field defects may be caused by a lesion affecting the eye, the optic nerve, the optic chiasm, the optic tract between the chiasm and lateral geniculate bodies, the optic radiation, or the occipital cortex. The resulting patterns of visual field defect are illustrated in Figure 3.2.

Optic nerve lesions

In the case of optic nerve lesions, the macular fibres are often damaged first, as these are most sensitive to pressure or ischaemia. Accordingly, the initial symptoms of an optic nerve lesion are a loss of visual acuity accompanying a central visual field defect (a central scotoma). Degeneration of optic nerve fibres can be seen with the ophthalmoscope as optic atrophy, in which the disc becomes unnaturally white and flattened, with loss of the normal optic cup. This leads to the appearance of a particularly sharp edge to the optic disc. As an optic nerve lesion progresses, visual acuity falls further and the size of the central scotoma enlarges. Eventually, a complete optic nerve lesion will lead to blindness in that eye (Figure 3.2). However, the patient will still be able to see clearly and to either side with the remaining opposite intact eye. The pupil of the blind eye will not react to light shone directly into it, but will react briskly when the light is shone in the opposite eye to evoke the consensual reaction (afferent papillary defect).

Afferent pupillary defect

The 'swinging light test' employs the principle that there is a difference in the direct and consensual pupillary reactions to light when there is a fault in the afferent visual pathway, the optic nerve or a severe degree of retinal damage. If a light is flashed from one eye to the other, the direct response on the side of the affected optic nerve will be less powerful than the consensual response evoked from the normal eye. As a result, when the light is shone in the affected eye, the pupil will dilate. In normal subjects, the response is symmetrical. When there is an asymmetry in the response this is called the afferent pupillary defect or Marcus Gunn phenomenon.

Chiasmal lesions

The optic chiasm contains both non-crossing fibres from the outer halves of the retina, which lie laterally, and decussating fibres from the inner halves of the retina. The decussating fibres are arranged with those from the upper part of the retina above and posteriorly, and those from the lower part below and anteriorly. Macular fibres also lie in the posterior part of the chiasm.

Another anatomical peculiarity is that fibres from the lower part of the nasal retina, having passed in the chiasm, may loop anteriorly into the optic nerve before passing posteriorly into the optic tract. Accordingly, a posteriorly placed lesion of the optic nerve will cause not only a central scotoma on that side, but also an upper temporal quadrantic defect in the visual field of the opposite eye, the so-called 'junctional scotoma'.

A lesion dividing the optic chiasm in the midline interrupts fibres from the inner half of each retina and results in the loss of the temporal field of vision in each eye, the bitemporal hemianopia (Figure 3.2).

It is important to realize that the visual fields of the two eyes overlap binocularly when they are both open. The extent of overlap is almost complete except for a few degrees at each temporal crescent. Accordingly, it is possible to miss entirely a total bitemporal hemianopia when examining the visual fields to confrontation, unless each eye is tested separately. The details of the anatomical arrangement within the optic chiasm dictate the pattern of visual defects caused by different lesions in this region.

Pressure on the chiasm from behind and below, such as by a pituitary tumour, often affects the decussating macular fibres first to produce bitemporal paracentral scotomas.

As such a tumour enlarges, the scotomas extend out to the periphery to cause the characteristic bitemporal hemianopia. Pressure on the chiasm from one side first affects the non-crossing fibres from the outer half of the retina, to cause a unilateral nasal hemianopia.

Posterior lesion

Lesions of the optic tract

Lesions in the optic tract will damage all fibres conveying vision from the opposite side of the patient to cause a homonymous hemianopia, in which the field defects of the left and right eyes will be the same (Figure 3.2).

However, such lesions also often impinge upon the posterior part of the chiasm, thereby damaging fibres from the upper inner quadrant of the ipsilateral retina before they cross to the opposite side. This results in the addition of an ipsilateral lower temporal field defect to the contralateral hemianopia, so that optic tract lesions commonly are incongruous.

Lesions in the region of the optic nerve, optic chiasm and optic tract lie close to, and may arise from, the pituitary, and to the adjacent hypothalamus above. Accordingly, such parapituitary lesions often produce disturbances other than visual field defects, including abnormalities of eye movement, hypopituitarism and diabetes insipidus. The effect of damage to the optic nerve on the pupillary reaction to light was described earlier, and any lesion in this region causing damage to central vision may produce an afferent pupillary defect. However, if the field defect is a hemianopia, sufficient vision remains in the intact half of the macular region to preserve visual acuity as normal, and the pupillary reaction likewise will be normal.

Lesions of the optic radiation

The fibres of the optic radiation leave the lateral geniculate body to pass via the posterior limb of the internal capsule to the visual cortex. In their course, fibres carrying impulses from the homonymous upper portions of the retinae pass via the parietal lobe to the supracalcarine cortex. Fibres representing the lower portions of the retinae pass over the temporal horn of the lateral ventricle, where they lie in the posterior portion of the temporal lobe before reaching the infracalcarine cortex.

Optic radiation damage

Destruction of the whole optic radiation produces a contralateral homonymous hemianopia (see Figures 1.1 and 3.2) without loss of visual acuity, without optic atrophy (because optic nerve fibres have synapsed in the lateral geniculate body), and without alteration in the pupillary light reflex. Partial lesions of the radiation are common. Parietal lobe lesions will produce predominantly inferior homonymous quadrantic field defects, while temporal lobe lesions produce superior homonymous quadrantic defects.

When dealing with hemianopic field defects, it is important to test both eyes simultaneously to confrontation.

The earliest sign of a hemianopia may be the inability to perceive an object in the affected field of vision when the corresponding portion of the normal field is tested at the same time; this is called an **inattention hemianopia**.

Lesions of the occipital cortex

The characteristic field defect resulting from a lesion of the occipital cortex is a contralateral homonymous hemianopia (Figure 3.2) without loss of visual acuity and with preserved pupillary responses. However, local anatomical arrangements of visual representation in the occipital cortex and of blood supply to this area may cause a variety of other field defects. The macula is extensively represented in the cortex of the tip of the occipital pole, an area sometimes supplied by the middle cerebral artery. Compressive lesions at this site, or middle cerebral arterial insufficiency, may produce **contralateral homonymous paracentral scotomas** (Figure 3.2). The remainder of the occipital cortex is supplied by the posterior cerebral arteries, which, because they derived from a common stem, the basilar artery, often are occluded simultaneously. If the occipital tip is supplied by the middle cerebral artery in such patients, then bilateral occlusion of posterior cerebral artery flow will cause **grossly constricted visual fields with preservation of small tunnels of central vision**. These central 'pinholes', the size of which will depend upon the extent of the middle cerebral supply to the occipital cortex, may be sufficient to preserve normal visual acuity. It is important to distinguish such constrictive visual fields from those seen in some patients with hysterical visual loss. It is a physical fact that the size of the central pinhole must increase, the further away from the patient one moves. In contrast, hysterical 'tunnel' vision commonly takes the form of preservation of a central area of vision, the size of which remains the same whether one is 1 foot (0.31 m) or 10 feet (3.1 m) from the patient's face – this is physically impossible. Finally, if the whole of the occipital cortex is supplied by the posterior cerebral arteries, and both are occluded, then the patient will develop **cortical blindness**, in which the patient can perceive nothing yet pupillary responses are preserved and the optic discs appear normal. Because damage often also involves adjacent areas of cortex in some patients, many of them may exhibit other cognitive deficits, including even **denial of blindness – Anton's syndrome**.

Pupillary abnormalities

The size of the pupil is controlled by the influence of the two divisions of the autonomic nervous system, which act in response to the level of illumination and the distance of focus. The sphincter muscle makes the pupil smaller (miosis), and is innervated by cholinergic parasympathetic nerves; the dilator makes it larger (mydriasis), and is innervated by noradrenergic sympathetic fibres.

The parasympathetic fibres, which control both pupillary constriction and contraction of the ciliary muscle to produce accommodation, arise from the Edinger–Westphal nucleus. They travel by the IIIrd nerve to the ciliary ganglion in the orbit; post-ganglionic fibres from the ciliary ganglion are distributed by the ciliary nerve. A lesion of the parasympathetic nerves produces a dilated pupil, which is unreactive to light or accommodation. The parasympathetic fibres to the eye are nearly always damaged by lesions affecting the IIIrd nerve, which also produce ptosis and a characteristic loss of ipsilateral eye movement (see later).

Adie's tonic pupil

Adie's tonic pupil is a rare cause of damage to the parasympathetic fibres within the ciliary ganglion, presenting usually with a large pupil (Figure 3.8).

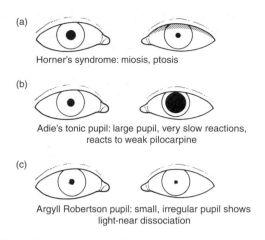

(a) Horner's syndrome: miosis, ptosis

(b) Adie's tonic pupil: large pupil, very slow reactions, reacts to weak pilocarpine

(c) Argyll Robertson pupil: small, irregular pupil shows light-near dissociation

Figure 3.8 Abnormal pupils.

The condition commonly presents in young women with the sudden appreciation that one pupil is much larger than the other. The dilated pupil does not react immediately to light, but prolonged exposure in a dark room may cause slow and irregular contraction of the iris. Likewise, accommodation on convergence is very slow to take place. With time, the dilated tonic pupil gradually constricts and may end up eventually smaller than the other. Inspection of the affected pupil with a slit-lamp may show irregular wormlike movements of the iris border. Pharmacological testing will confirm the label by showing denervation hypersensitivity to weak pilocarpine (0.125 per cent) or methacholine (2.5 per cent) eye drops. These drugs will cause a tonic pupil to constrict but have no effect on the normal pupil. Some patients with a tonic pupil, or tonic pupils, also lose their tendon jerks in the so-called **Holmes–Adie syndrome**.

Argyll Robertson pupils

The pupillary response to light depends on the integrity of the afferent pathways. As already described, the direct light response is impaired, with damage to the retina or optic nerve, and this can be shown by the presence of an afferent pupillary defect. The relevant optic nerve fibres responsible for the light reaction leave those responsible for the perception of light to terminate in the pretectal region of the midbrain, from whence a further relay passes to the Edinger–Westphal nucleus. Damage to this pretectal region is believed to be responsible for the Argyll Robertson pupil classically seen in neurosyphilis. The characteristics of these pupils are that they are small, irregular and unequal, and exhibit **light–near dissociation** (Figure 3.8). Light–near dissociation refers to the loss of pupillary reaction to light, with preservation of that to accommodation. Pupils resembling those of Argyll Robertson also occur occasionally in diabetes and in other conditions with autonomic neuropathy. Large pupils exhibiting light–near dissociation are characteristic of damage in the region of the superior colliculi, as may be produced by tumours of the pineal gland. These cause **Parinaud's syndrome** in which there is pupillary light–near dissociation, with paralysis of upgaze and convergence.

Horner's syndrome

The sympathetic fibres supplying the eye arise from the eighth cervical and the first two thoracic segments of the spinal cord. They synapse in the cervical ganglia and pass via the carotid plexus to the orbit. The activity of these fibres is controlled by hypothalamic centres, from which central sympathetic pathways pass to the spinal cord (Figure 3.9b). A lesion of the ocular sympathetic pathways anywhere along this route will produce a Horner's syndrome (Figure 3.8).

Horner's syndrome (Figure 3.9a,b)
The pupil on the affected side is constricted. It reacts to light and accommodation, but does not dilate normally in response to shade or pain. In addition, denervation of the smooth muscle of the upper eyelid leads to ptosis, which can be overcome by voluntary upgaze, enophthalmos and denervation of the facial sweat glands causes loss of sweating on the affected side of the face.

As indicated, a Horner's syndrome may appear as a result of lesions affecting the hypothalamus, brainstem or spinal cord, or as a result of damage to the emergent T1 root and cervical ganglion containing sympathetic nerve output, or to the sympathetic plexus on the carotid artery anywhere from the neck to the head. Pharmacological testing may help to establish the anatomical level of the sympathetic damage. Nearly all post-ganglionic lesions are 'benign': preganglionic or central lesions may affect the brainstem, cervical cord and particularly

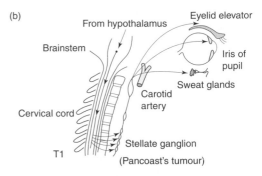

Figure 3.9 Horner's syndrome. (a) Pharmacological testing of the pupil with 4 per cent cocaine and 1 per cent pholedrine (*N*-methyl hydroxyamphetamine) to show the site of the lesion. (b) Anatomical pathways of sympathetic innervation of the eye and pupil.

lesions at the lung apex or lower neck. With preganglionic and central lesions, application of 4 per cent cocaine eye drops will cause slight dilatation of the affected pupil. With post-ganglionic lesions, 1 per cent hydroxyamphetamine or 1 per cent pholedrine eye drops will cause no reaction, while preganglionic and central lesions show dilatation. Phenylephrine (1 per cent) will also cause dilatation of the affected pupil in post-ganglionic but not in preganglionic or central lesions (Figure 3.9a).

Defects of ocular movement and diplopia

Abnormalities of eye movement may arise at one of three levels in the nervous system: in the muscles, in the brainstem and more centrally.

Primary muscle disease may impair ocular motility (ocular myopathy), when eye movements usually remain conjugate, or in myasthenia gravis, in which fatigue is typical. Lesions of individual muscles or their nerve supply, caused by damage of the IIIrd, IVth or Vth cranial nerves or their nuclei, will impair specific individual movements of the eye. This will result in a breakdown of conjugate gaze to cause double vision (diplopia). Within the brainstem, complex pathways link together centres for conjugate gaze to the individual ocular motor nuclei; for example, horizontal gaze to one side demands conjugate activation of one VIth nerve nucleus and the portion of the opposite IIIrd nerve nucleus innervating the medial rectus. These two nuclear regions are linked by fibres passing in the medial longitudinal bundle (Figure 3.10). Damage to such pathways produces dysconjugate gaze known as an internuclear ophthalmoplegia. Finally, conjugate gaze to either side and up and down is controlled by pathways from the cerebral hemispheres arising in frontal and occipital eyefields. Damage to these pathways will cause defects of conjugate eye movements known as supranuclear gaze palsies.

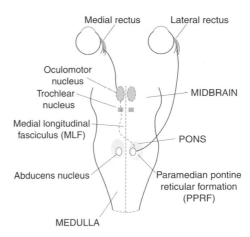

Figure 3.10 Pathway of medial longitudinal fasciculus yoking the abducens and oculomotor nuclei for conjugate horizontal eye movements.

Infranuclear lesions

Each eye is moved by three pairs of muscles. The precise action of these depends upon the position of the eye, but their main actions are as follows:

1 The lateral and medial recti, respectively, abduct and adduct the eye.
2 The superior and inferior recti, respectively, elevate and depress the abducted eye.
3 The superior and inferior obliques, respectively, depress and elevate the adducted eye.
4 The superior oblique also internally rotates, and the inferior oblique externally rotates the eye.

Weakness of an individual muscle will cause limitation of movement of one eye in a characteristic direction, and diplopia will occur as a result of misrepresentation of the object on the retina. The term **squint** (also called strabismus) describes a misalignment of ocular axes, but is sufficiently great as to be obvious to the observer. When the misalignment is present at rest and equal for all directions of gaze (concomitant squint), it is not caused by a local weakness of the ocular muscles.

Concomitant squint develops during childhood because of failure to establish binocular vision. The abnormal image from the squinting eye is suppressed, so there is no diplopia. In contrast, a misalignment of the eye that is more apparent when gazing in a particular direction indicates weakness of the muscle acting in that direction (paralytic squint), and diplopia. It should be noted that slight muscle weakness will produce diplopia before any defect of movement can be observed by the examiner.

Although these rules sound simple, in practice it can often be difficult to analyse complex diplopia at the bedside. The use of red and green spectacles to identify two images, and the use of Hess charts to plot their position, may sometimes be required to make analysis easier and to follow progress.

Disorders of function of individual eye muscles, and the diplopia so produced, may be caused by disorder of the eye muscles themselves, or by lesions of the nerves controlling them. Lesions of the eye muscles occur in two situations. **Primary ocular myopathy** occurs in the group of disorders known as chronic progressive ophthalmoplegia (CPEO; see Chapter 18). Such patients have profound defects of all forms of eye movement, but the ocular axes remain parallel so that diplopia does not develop. In contrast, **myasthenia gravis**, which commonly affects the eyes, causes loss of conjugate gaze and inevitable diplopia.

Diplopia assessment

A scheme to examine the eyes in patients complaining of diplopia has been outlined above under Assessment of diplopia. Three cardinal points should be emphasized:

1 The diplopia may consist of images that are side by side (horizontal), or one above the other (vertical), or both. Horizontal diplopia must be a result of weakness of a lateral or medial rectus muscle. Vertical diplopia, or diplopia in which the two images are at angles to one another, can result from weakness in any of the other muscles.

2 Separation of the images is maximal when the gaze is turned in the direction of action of the weak muscle; for example, maximal separation of images on looking to the right, with horizontal diplopia, indicates weakness of the left medial or right lateral rectus.

3 When the gaze is directed to cause maximal separation of the images, the abnormal image from the lagging eye is displaced further in the direction of gaze; for example, if horizontal diplopia is maximal on looking to the right, and the image furthest to the right comes from the right eye (tested by covering each eye separately), the right lateral rectus is weak. Conversely, diplopia is minimal when the gaze is directed in such a way as to avoid the use of the weak muscle. Patients sometimes make use of this fact to prevent double vision, by adopting a convenient head posture. Thus the patient with a right lateral rectus palsy will maintain the head deviated to the right so as to be gazing slightly to the left, when the image will be single.

Characteristic of myasthenia is fatigue of eye muscle contraction with exercise, so that diplopia occurs towards the end of the day, or on sustained gaze in a particular direction. Ptosis is also often present and there may be weakness of eye closure (orbicularis oculi).

Lesions of the nerves to the ocular muscles may result from disorders affecting the nuclei in the brainstem, or from damage to the nerves themselves in their course to the orbit. Such lesions inevitably produce diplopia (unless the patient is blind in one eye), for conjugate gaze is destroyed.

Oculomotor (IIIrd nerve) lesions produce ptosis because the levator palpebrae is paralysed. On lifting the lid, it will be apparent that the eye is deviated outwards and downwards, because of the respective actions of the intact lateral rectus and superior oblique (which are supplied by the VIth and IVth nerves) (Figure 3.11). The pupillomotor fibres lie towards the outside of the nerve so compressive lesions cause the pupil to be dilated and unresponsive to light, and accommodation may be paralysed. Partial lesions of the IIIrd nerve are common, however, and in these the parasympathetic fibres to the pupil may either be spared or selectively involved.

Trochlear (IVth nerve) lesions paralyse the superior oblique muscle, producing inability to look downwards and inwards. Such patients commonly present with a complaint of diplopia when walking downstairs. The presence of intact IVth nerve function can be demonstrated by showing the eye intorts, that is, it rolls inwards about an anterior-posterior axis, when the patient is asked to look at the root of their nose (Figure 3.12). Many patients may show a head tilt to the side opposite to that of the defective eye.

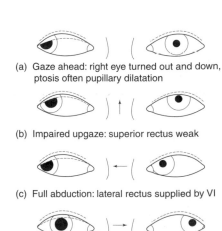

(a) Gaze ahead: right eye turned out and down, ptosis often pupillary dilatation

(b) Impaired upgaze: superior rectus weak

(c) Full abduction: lateral rectus supplied by VI

(d) Impaired adduction: medial rectus weak

(e) Impaired downgaze: inferior rectus weak

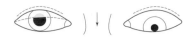

Figure 3.11 Right oculomotor palsy.

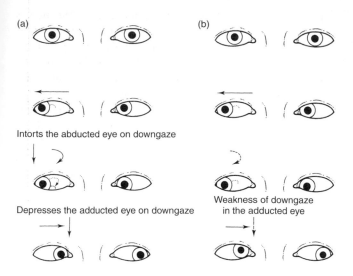

(a)

(b)

Intorts the abducted eye on downgaze

Depresses the adducted eye on downgaze

Weakness of downgaze in the adducted eye

Figure 3.12 (a) Actions of normal superior oblique muscle. (b) Right superior oblique palsy.

Abducens (VIth nerve) lesions paralyse the external rectus, producing inability to abduct the eye (Figure 3.13).

Internuclear lesions

The complex details of interconnection between ocular motor nuclei and pontine gaze centres (see below and Figure 3.10) are beyond the scope of

> A unilateral lesion of the medial longitudinal bundle causes the characteristic features of an internuclear gaze palsy (internuclear ophthalmoplegia (INO)). These consist of difficulty in adducting the ipsilateral eye on horizontal gaze, with the development of coarse jerk nystagmus in the contralateral abducting eye (Figure 3.14).

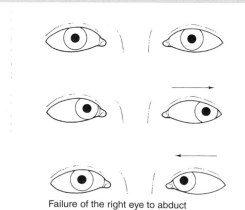

Failure of the right eye to abduct

Figure 3.13 Right abducens palsy.

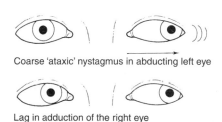

Coarse 'ataxic' nystagmus in abducting left eye

Lag in adduction of the right eye

Figure 3.14 Right internuclear ophthalmoplegia. Lesion of the medial longitudinal fasciculus.

this book. The important point is the critical role played by the medial longitudinal bundle linking the VIth nerve nucleus in the pons with the IIIrd nerve nucleus in the midbrain.

The syndrome is sometimes called ataxic nystagmus of the eyes. Lesser degrees of INO may be evident simply as a relative slowness of adduction compared with abduction on horizontal gaze. The adducting eye is seen to lag behind the abducting eye. Diplopia is unusual in an INO, but oscillopsia, that is, a tendency for the outside world to bob up and down, often occurs with brainstem lesions. Bilateral INO is almost always due to multiple sclerosis, although vascular disease and brainstem tumours occasionally may produce unilateral internuclear lesions.

Supranuclear lesions

These systems for controlling conjugate gaze may be interrupted in many different ways. Lesions

Supranuclear lesions

Four separate mechanisms exist for eliciting conjugate ocular gaze in any direction:

1 The saccadic system allows the subject voluntarily to direct gaze at will, even with the eyes shut. The pathways responsible for saccadic gaze arise in the frontal lobe and pass to the pontine gaze centres.

2 The pursuit system allows the subject to follow a moving object. The pathways responsible for pursuit gaze arise in the parieto-occipital region and pass to the pontine gaze centres.

3 The optokinetic system restores gaze, despite movements of the outside world. The operation of the optokinetic system is seen in the railway train, where the eyes of the subject gazing out of the window are seen to veer slowly as the train moves, to be followed by rapid corrections back to the primary position of gaze.

4 The **vestibulo–ocular reflex (VOR)** system corrects for movements of the head to preserve the stable visual world. Inputs from the labyrinths and from neck proprioceptors are directed to the brainstem ocular mechanisms to achieve stabilization of the visual image, despite head movements.

of the frontal lobes commonly disrupt voluntary saccadic gaze, while pursuit, optokinetic and vestibulo-ocular mechanisms remain intact. Diffuse cerebral disease, of whatever cause, may interfere with both saccadic and pursuit systems. Saccadic movements become slowed and hypometric, while smooth pursuit is broken up into small jerky steps. Optokinetic nystagmus, as tested with a hand-held drum bearing vertical black and white stripes, is also disrupted in such patients. In fact, optokinetic nystagmus tested in this way is frequently disturbed before evidence of interruption of the pursuit system is apparent. Patients with such supranuclear gaze palsies for saccadic and pursuit movements, often have preserved VOR movement. This is tested by the doll's head manoeuvre, the **oculocephalic reflex**. The patient is asked to fixate on the examiner's face, and the head is briskly rotated from side to side or up and down. Patients unable voluntarily to direct their gaze to either side, and unable

to follow a moving object in the same direction, may exhibit a full range of ocular movement to the doll's head manoeuvre. It is this preservation of VOR eye movement in the absence of voluntary saccadic or pursuit movements that is diagnostic of a supranuclear gaze palsy. Caloric tests may also demonstrate preserved VOR function in the brainstem. The VOR may also be assessed at the bedside by the **head impulse** test. The patient is asked to fixate on a nearby target and then the head is turned briskly by the examiner's hands, first to one side and then to the other, rotating the head by about 30 degrees. The test is abnormal if the eyes have to make a few saccadic jerks before refixing on the target. With an intact VOR, the patient can maintain fixation despite the head movements. This test is sensitive in detecting a unilateral peripheral vestibular fault.

Despite defects in gaze, the eyes remain conjugate in supranuclear palsies, so diplopia does not occur.

The centres in the cerebral hemispheres responsible for saccadic and pursuit movement control deviation of the eyes conjugately towards the opposite side of the body.

Thus, a unilateral hemisphere lesion will cause weakness of conjugate deviation of the eyes away from the side of the lesion. As they descend towards the brainstem, these pathways cross before they reach the pons. Accordingly, damage to the region of the pontine gaze centres will cause weakness of deviation of the eyes towards the side of the lesion.

The combination of damage to the pontine paramedian horizontal gaze centre with involvement of the ipsilateral medial longitudinal bundle (internuclear ophthalmoplegia) may produce the **one-and-a-half-syndrome** (Figure 3.15).

The centres for conjugate vertical gaze in the brainstem lie in the midbrain. Lesions at that site cause difficulty in conjugate upgaze. The centres responsible for downgaze are less well localized, and lesions both in the midbrain and at the level of the foramen magnum can produce defects of voluntary downgaze. **Downbeat nystagmus strongly suggests a lesion at the craniocervical junction or in the cerebellum** (Figure 3.16).

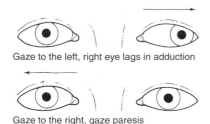

Gaze to the left, right eye lags in adduction

Gaze to the right, gaze paresis

Figure 3.15 Right 'one-and-a-half' syndrome. This is a combination of an internuclear ophthalmoplegia and an ipsilateral gaze paresis on the same side.

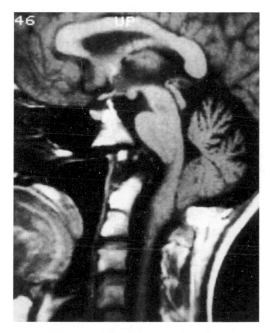

Figure 3.16 MRI sagittal view of craniocervical junction to show basilar impression in a patient who presented with slight ataxia and showed downbeat nystagmus.

Defects of vestibular function and nystagmus

The **vestibular system** is responsible for maintaining balance, and the direction of gaze, despite changes in head and body positions. Its components provide information on the static position of the head in space (from the otolith organs in the utricle and saccule), and on the character of dynamic changes in head position (from the semicircular canals). The information is correlated from that arising in neck proprioceptors, which provide data on the relationship of the head to the body.

The integration of these various data on posture occurs in the brainstem and cerebellum. The information is used to adjust postural muscle activity to maintain balance, and eye position to maintain gaze. Damage to the vestibular system, whether it be in the labyrinth or in the brainstem/cerebellum, inevitably leads to imbalance and defects of eye movement control.

> Each labyrinth at rest exerts tonic influence tending to deviate the eyes to the opposite side.

The effects from the two sides counterbalance each other, thereby maintaining a forward gaze. Sudden destruction of one labyrinth produces a forced drift of the gaze to the affected side because of the unopposed action of the normal labyrinth, followed by a rapid correction in an attempt to restore visual fixation.

> The jerk nystagmus provoked by such unilateral labyrinthine destruction (**'canal' vestibular nystagmus**) has the following characteristics:
> - the slow phase is always directed to the abnormal ear;
> - it is most marked when the gaze is directed away from the abnormal ear;
> - it is predominantly horizontal or rotator;
> - it is independent of vision, for it persists or is enhanced when the eyes are shut or defocused using strong plus lenses (Frenzel's lenses);
> - it is frequently accompanied by vertigo and evidence of damage to the cochlear portion of the middle ear in the form of deafness or tinnitus.

Peripheral vestibular damage causes intense vertigo, accompanied by all the other symptoms associated with 'sea-sickness' including nausea, sweating and vomiting. These symptoms are accompanied by fear. In addition, the patient is severely ataxic, and often can only move around by crawling on the floor.

Compensation rapidly occurs after loss of one vestibular apparatus. The remaining intact labyrinth adapts to the new conditions so that balance is restored and vertigo disappears over a matter of a few weeks. Indeed, even when both labyrinths are destroyed, the patient soon can walk and even dance, provided the floor is even, because visual, cutaneous and proprioceptive sensations provide the necessary alternative information.

> In contrast to the dramatic and explosive symptoms caused by peripheral vestibular damage, lesions of the vestibular nerve or its brainstem connections produce fewer symptoms.

Vertigo and ataxia may be evident, but dramatic nausea and vomiting are unusual. Such brainstem damage causes **'central' vestibular nystagmus** (Table 3.5), which differs from 'canal' vestibular nystagmus in certain important characteristics: frequently it is vertical as well as horizontal; its direction changes with the direction of gaze, such that the jerk is to the right on right lateral gaze and to the left on left lateral gaze; compensation occurs but slowly; and it is improved or abolished by eye closure.

Lesions of the brainstem may cause nystagmus, not only by compromising vestibular connections, but also by interfering with the mechanisms responsible for gaze. Gaze nystagmus, which is analogous to the oscillatory movement that may occur in a weak limb when the patient attempts to maintain it in a given position against gravity, occurs when the eyes are deviated in the direction of weakness of gaze. Because the pontine gaze centres are responsible for drawing the eyes towards that side, damage to this region will cause nystagmus on looking towards the lesion. In contrast, as noted above, damage to the vestibular system causes nystagmus, which is maximal on looking away from the side of the lesion. As a consequence, a lesion in the cerebellopontine angle, such as an acoustic neuroma, may initially cause nystagmus

Table 3.5 Characteristics of nystagmus

Peripheral	Central
Unidirectional	Directional
Fast phase away from side of lesion	Fast phase towards the site of lesion
	May include vertical, rotatory
Fixation inhibits	No change with fixation
Darkness, defocus enhances	Darkness, defocus may reduce

on gaze away from the affected side because of damage of vestibular fibres in the VIIIth nerve, but subsequently the nystagmus changes and becomes maximal on looking towards the side of the lesion when it has grown large enough to impinge upon the brainstem.

The semicircular canals are the sensors of dynamic changes (angular acceleration) of head position, while the otolith organs, the utricle and saccule, are the sensors of linear acceleration and gravity changes (including head tilt). The hair cell is the basic sensory cell. In each semicircular canal, there is a mound of hair cells, the ampulla, with a divider, the cupula. These hair cells either increase or decrease their firing rate depending on the direction of fluid displacement. In the otolith organs, the hair cells are situated in the maculae and are covered by a crystal-laden gelatinous membrane. These crystals are particles of calcium carbonate, the otoconia. Movements of the head by tilting or by linear acceleration may displace the otoconia and stimulate the otolith hair cells.

Benign paroxysmal positional vertigo is the most common cause of vertigo and reflects dislocation of otoconia from the utricle that have migrated into the posterior semicircular canal causing abnormal stimulation. The Dix–Hallpike manoeuvre is the diagnostic test to show whether this is so. With the patient sitting on the couch, their head is turned slightly to one side and the neck extended. The eyes of the patient should be fixed on the examiner's eyes. The patient is then lain supine quickly, the head still being supported by the examiner's hands and their eyes still fixed on those of the examiner (Figure 3.17). In a normal patient, there is no nystagmus or distress. In patients suffering with positional vertigo, there is a brief latent period of 2–6 seconds, then usually a torsional upbeating nystagmus lasting 20–30 seconds which is accompanied by intense vertigo. The rotatory nystagmus is directed to the undermost ear. The signs and symptoms settle only to reappear, but to a lesser degree, on sitting up again. If the test is then repeated it fatigues – that is, it is much less or has largely disappeared.

A similar complaint, but usually less severe, may occur in patients with brainstem lesions causing vertigo, **central positional vertigo**. This is accompanied by persistent positional nystagmus without any latent period and which does not show fatigue.

(a)

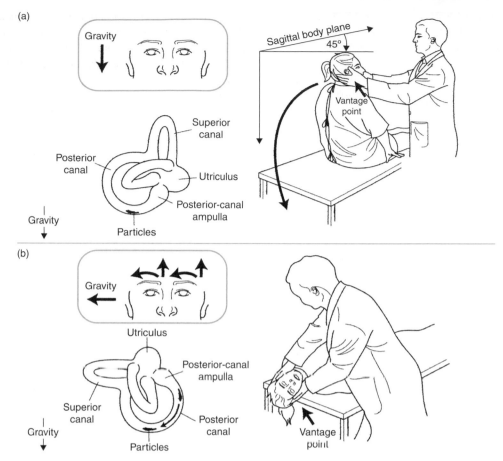

Figure 3.17 Dix–Hallpike manoeuvre to test for paroxysmal positional vertigo arising from the right posterior semicircular canal. (a) The patient's head is held in the examiner's hands and turned some 45 degrees to the right with the neck slightly extended. The patient is then lain supine with the instructions that they should fix their eyes on the eyes of the examiner. (b) If the test is positive, the patient will notice brief intense vertigo accompanied by nystagmus. The latency, direction and duration of that nystagmus should be noted. The arrows in the inset show the direction of that nystagmus in a fault arising from the right posterior semicircular canal. The presumed location of the free-floating debris in the canal is also shown. If the patient then sits up, there may be a further brief spell of vertigo and nystagmus, although to a lesser degree. (Redrawn, with permission, from Furman J, Cass S. (1999) *New England Medical Journal* **341**:1590–1596. Copyright © 2003 Massachusetts Medical Society.)

Many of the vestibular defects described here may be deduced from careful clinical examination at the bedside. However, full assessment of vestibular function requires specialized neuro-otological investigation. This would include caloric testing, in which air 7°C above and below body temperature is blown into the external auditory canal. With the patient lying supine and the head flexed to 30 degrees from the horizontal, this stimulates the horizontal semicircular canals to produce nystagmus, often with vertigo. Damage to the semicircular canals or to the vestibular nerve may abolish caloric-induced nystagmus, **canal paresis**. Damage

to the vestibular apparatus in the brainstem often produces a lesser degree of abnormality on caloric testing, in which the response to one direction is reduced to produce a directional preponderance. Other more detailed tests of vestibular function are available, such as posturography.

Muscle weakness

Muscle wasting

The integrity of muscle fibres depends not only on their own health, but also on an intact nerve sup-

Muscle weakness

Weakness of muscles may be from disease of the muscle itself (myopathy), defects in the transmission of the neuromuscular impulse at the muscle end-plate (myasthenia), damage to the motor nerve or anterior horn cell that gives rise to it (lower motor neurone (LMN) lesion), or damage to the corticomotor neurone pathway (UMN) lesion. The characteristic findings that enable these different lesions to be distinguished are shown in Table 3.6. The critical differences are in the presence or absence of muscle wasting, changes in muscle tone and stretch reflexes, and in the distribution of weakness.

ply. Muscles waste either because they themselves are damaged (myopathy), or because of lesions of the LMN. The more proximal the damage to the LMN, the greater is the opportunity for collateral reinnervation from adjacent nerve fibres, in an attempt to overcome the consequences of denervation. Such collateral reinnervation produces abnormally large motor units, which are responsible for the involuntary twitching (**fasciculation**) that occurs in denervated muscles.

Muscle tone and the stretch reflex

Our understanding of the functions of the nervous system were built upon Sherrington's discovery of the stretch reflex. Muscle tone and the tendon jerks are believed to represent operation of stretch reflex mechanisms, but still there is considerable ignorance about their exact relationship.

Delivery of a tendon tap produces a transient sudden stretch of muscle, which excites primary endings wrapped around the central portion of the muscle spindles. The resulting afferent volley is rapidly conducted to the spinal cord via large group IA fibres, which synapse with anterior horn cells of both the same muscle and of synergistic muscles. The number of anterior horn cells discharged by this synchronous afferent volley depends upon excitability of the anterior horn cell pool and the size of the afferent volley. The sensitivity of the muscle spindle endings is controlled by the pre-existing tension exerted on the central portion of the spindle muscle fibres by the contractile pull of the intrafusal fibres. Contraction of the intrafusal fibres increases the tension exerted on the central receptor and, hence, increases its sensitivity to stretch. The intrafusal fibres are innervated by fusimotor nerves originating in small anterior horn cells (gamma motor neurones). Alteration of fusimotor activity therefore will change the 'bias' of the muscle spindles. It follows that the amplitude of a response to a tendon tap depends on:

- the integrity of the spinal reflex;
- the sensitivity of the muscle spindles as determined by pre-existing activity of fusimotor neurones;
- the excitability of the appropriate alpha motor neurone pool.

Peripheral nerve lesions decrease the size of the tendon jerk. This is much more evident with sensory lesions than with pure motor abnormalities.

Damage to sensory nerve fibres, which desynchronizes the afferent volley, soon abolishes tendon jerks. In contrast, quite extensive muscle wasting by itself may be insufficient to remove the response to a tendon tap. The tendon jerks are exaggerated (hyper-reflexia) in damage to the UMN pathway, as a result of enhanced anterior horn cell excitability. The latency of the tendon jerk is more difficult to judge at the bedside, but slow muscle relaxation may be evident in patients with myxoedema, and certain other metabolic disorders that delay muscle relaxation time.

Although Sherrington considered the tendon jerk to be a fractional manifestation of the stretch reflex, the basis of muscle tone as appreciated by the clinician at the bedside is unclear. Muscle tone is defined as the resistance to passive movement

Table 3.6 Differences between upper and lower motor neurone lesions (UMN and LMN)

UMN	LMN
Weak	Weak
	Wasted
	Fasciculation
Hypertonic, spastic	Hypotonic, flaccid
Clonus	
Reflexes exaggerated	Reflexes depressed or absent
Plantar responses	Plantar responses flexor extensor

imposed by the examiner. Such resistance must comprise both passive elements of viscosity and elasticity arising in muscle, tendons and joints, as well as the active response of the muscle itself. Probably, muscle tone involves the combined effect of activation of both primary and secondary muscle spindle endings, both of which cause reflex muscle contraction.

Decreased muscle tone and depression of tendon jerks occur physiologically during sleep, including rapid eye movement sleep, and in anaesthesia or deep coma. In all these situations, fusimotor activity and anterior horn cell excitability are likely to be decreased. Muscle tone is also diminished in cerebellar disease, perhaps as a result of decreased fusimotor spindle drive.

> Increased muscle tone is characteristic of lesions of the descending motor pathways from the brain to the spinal cord.

Spasticity is a resistance to attempted stretch of the muscle that increases with the applied force, until there is a sudden give at a certain tension, the 'clasp knife' or 'lengthening' reaction. **Rigidity** is a resistance to passive movement that continues unaltered throughout the range of movement, and so has a plastic or 'lead-pipe' quality. Both types of hypertonia are the result of excessive alpha-motor neurone discharge in response to muscle stretch. In spasticity, the tendon jerks are also exaggerated (hyper-reflexia), but in rigidity the tendon jerks are usually of normal amplitude and threshold.

The distribution of spasticity and rigidity differs. The spastic posture of the patient after a stroke, with flexed arm and extended leg, indicates that tone is increased mainly in the adductors of the shoulder, the flexors of the elbow, the flexors of the wrist and fingers, the extensors of the hip and knee, and the plantar flexors and invertors of the foot. By contrast, the posture of generalized flexion in Parkinson's disease illustrates that rigidity is maximal in all flexor muscles in the body, although it is appreciated in extensors as well.

The complete picture of damage to UMN pathways includes not only spasticity and hyper-reflexia, but also absence of the abdominal reflexes and an extensor–plantar response. However, different corticoneurone pathways may be involved in the expression of these various manifestations of a UMN lesion. A lesion restricted to the 'pyramidal' pathway in the medulla, thereby sparing all other corticomotor neurone systems, only causes loss of abdominal reflexes and an extensor plantar response. Spasticity and hyper-reflexia appear when the alternative non-pyramidal corticomotor neurone pathways are interrupted. Such damage liberates overactive stretch reflex mechanisms to produce the increased muscle tone and exaggerated reflexes.

Distribution of muscle weakness

Careful analysis of the distribution of muscle weakness in a patient discovered to have motor signs may be invaluable. It is much easier to examine the motor than the sensory system, and deductions based upon motor deficit may dictate the pattern of subsequent sensory examination.

> **The distribution of UMN weakness**
> The distribution of weakness resulting from a UMN lesion can be recalled. The hemiplegic patient has the arm flexed across the chest and the leg extended with the toes scraping the ground. Accordingly, UMN weakness selectively involves shoulder abduction, elbow extension, wrist and finger extension, and the small muscles of the hand, and in the leg, hip flexion, knee flexion, dorsiflexion and eversion of the foot.

Damage to the **motor roots or anterior horn cells** also causes distinctive patterns of weakness, depending upon the level involved (see Figures 1.3 and 3.18). Likewise, lesions of a peripheral nerve containing motor fibres also produce a distinctive pattern of weakness. Careful attention to detail allows the examiner to distinguish weakness resulting from a UMN lesion from that caused by root or peripheral nerve damage. The following examples will illustrate the point.

Weakness of shoulder abduction may be the result of a UMN lesion, a C5 root lesion, or from damage to the circumflex nerve. In a UMN lesion, elbow extension and wrist and finger extension will also be weak; in a C5 root lesion, the biceps will be weak and the biceps jerk will be lost; in a circumflex nerve lesion, weakness will be restricted to shoulder abduction and the biceps jerk will be normal.

Elbow extension may be weak because of a UMN lesion or because of damage to the radial nerve. In a UMN lesion, shoulder abduction will also be weak.

Weakness of one hand may result from a UMN lesion, from damage to the T1 motor root or anterior horn cells, or to an ulnar nerve lesion. If a UMN lesion is responsible, there will also be weakness of wrist and finger extension, and elbow extension, and of shoulder abduction. If the ulnar nerve is involved, the thenar eminence is not wasted and the abductor pollicis brevis is strong because these are innervated by the median nerve. If the ulnar nerve is involved at the wrist, only the hand muscles will be weak. If the ulnar nerve is

involved at the elbow, there will be weakness of the long finger flexors (flexor digitorum profundus) of the ulnar two digits, which flex the top joints of the fingers.

Weakness of hip flexion may be from a UMN lesion, damage to the L1/2 motor roots, or result from a femoral nerve lesion. If a UMN lesion is responsible, then knee flexion and dorsiflexion and eversion of the foot will be weak. If the L1/2 roots are involved, then hip adduction will also be weak, but knee flexion and dorsiflexion of the foot will be normal.

A **foot drop** may be caused by a lesion of the UMN, of the L4/5 root or the peroneal nerve. If a UMN lesion is responsible, hip flexion and knee

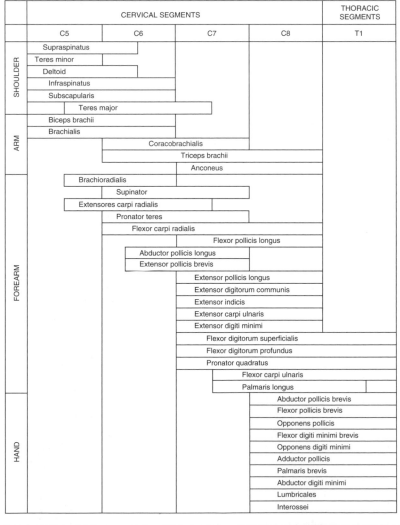

(a)

Figure 3.18 Segmental innervation of (a) arm muscles; (b) leg muscles. (Courtesy of Lord Walton of Detchant and Oxford University Press, *Brain's Diseases of the Nervous System*, 8th edn. Reproduced with permission.)

flexion will also be weak. If the L4/5 roots are involved, then hip extension and knee flexion will be weak. If the peroneal nerve lesion is responsible, then hip movements and knee flexion will be normal.

In addition to the very distinctive patterns of weakness caused by UMN lesions, root lesions and peripheral nerve lesions, diffuse generalized peripheral neuropathies and primary muscle disease (myopathy) also produce characteristic patterns of muscle weakness. A **generalized peripheral neuropathy** usually affects the longest nerve fibres first, so that the distal parts of the limbs are most affected, and the legs before the arms. Accordingly, weakness around the feet in dorsiflexion and plantar flexion with wasting of the lower limb are

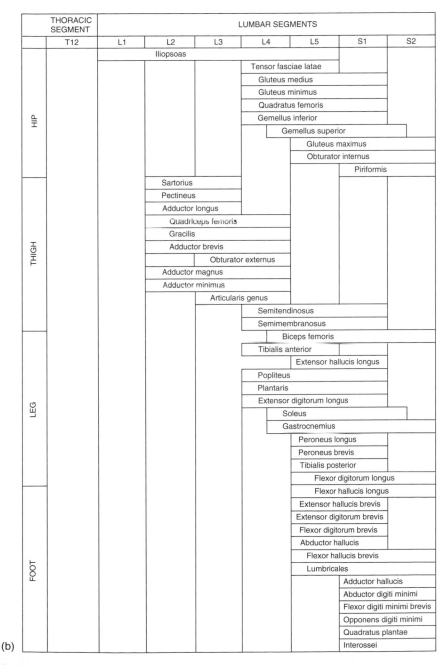

(b)

Figure 3.18 (*Continued*)

the most common earliest signs of a peripheral neuropathy, to be followed by wasting and weakness of the small muscles of the hand.

In contrast, **primary muscle disease** usually selectively involves the more proximal muscles, to cause weakness and wasting around the hip and shoulder girdle.

In both peripheral neuropathy and primary muscle disease, flexors and extensors are involved more or less equally. UMN lesions, root lesions and peripheral nerve lesions usually preferentially affect flexors or extensors, with relative sparing of antagonists.

Bulbar and pseudobulbar palsy

Bilateral LMN lesions affecting the nerves supplying the bulbar muscles of the jaw, face, palate, pharynx and larynx cause **a bulbar palsy**. Speech and swallowing will be impaired. In particular, speech develops a nasal quality caused by escape of air through the nose. The paralysed soft palate no longer can occlude the nasopharynx. Swallowing of liquids is badly impaired, with a tendency to regurgitate fluids back through the nose and to cough because fluids spill over into the trachea. Paralysis of affected muscles will be evident, and the tongue appears wasted.

A **pseudobulbar palsy** results from bilateral damage to corticomotorneurone pathways inner-vating the bulbar musculature. In other words, a pseudobulbar palsy is the result of a UMN lesion affecting corticobulbar systems. A unilateral UMN lesion produces only transient weakness of many of the muscles supplied by the cranial nerves. Thus after a stroke, there is no loss of power in the upper part of the face, and weakness of the muscles of the jaw, palate, neck and tongue is transient.

Bilateral damage to the corticobulbar tracts causes persistent weakness and spasticity of the muscles supplied by the bulbar nuclei. As a result, there is slurring of speech, known as a spastic dysarthria, and difficulty in swallowing (dysphagia). The jaw jerk is abnormally brisk, and movements of the tongue are reduced in velocity and amplitude as a result of spasticity. In addition, patients with a pseudobulbar palsy exhibit emotional incontinence. This describes a loss of voluntary control of emotional expression such that the patient may laugh or cry without apparent provocation.

The distinguishing features of bulbar and pseudobulbar palsies are shown in Table 3.7.

Sensory defects

The assessment of sensory function starts with the history, because symptoms may precede any demonstrable abnormality of simple sensation as tested by standard bedside techniques.

Table 3.7 Differentiation between bulbar and pseudobulbar palsies

Bulbar	Pseudobulbar
Weakness of muscles (LMN) from motor brainstem nuclei V–XII	Bilateral corticobulbar (UMN) lesions
Tongue: atrophic, fasciculating	Tongue, small, spastic, difficulty with rapid movements, protrusion
Speech: monotonous, hoarse, nasal	Speech: spastic slurring dysarthria
	Exaggerated reflexes: jaw jerk, snout, pout
Gag may be depressed	Brisk gag reflex
Lips, facial muscles may be weak	Stiff, spastic facial muscles
Saliva may pool and dribble out	Trouble chewing, food may stay in mouth or spill
Spill-over of fluids, occasional nasal regurgitation	May choke
Weak cough	Emotional incontinence
	Often bilateral corticospinal tract signs in limbs

LMN, lower motor neurone; UMN, upper motor neurone.
Motor neurone disease, which is the commonest cause of a bilateral wasted tongue, may also show UMN signs.

The patient's symptoms will suggest which area of the body, or which type of sensory function, needs the most detailed attention. The preceding examination of the motor system will also direct attention to the appropriate sensory testing.

Sensory symptoms are of two types.

Defects of sensation

If there is impairment of all forms of cutaneous sensation, the patient may complain of numbness, deadness or freezing feelings, or even weakness. Many liken it to the sensation that follows dental treatment under local anaesthesia. If there is more specific sensory loss, it may only come to attention indirectly. Thus, inability to perceive pain usually is detected because unexpected painless injuries occur, such as burns of the fingers on cooking utensils or by cigarettes. Loss of temperature appreciation may be recognized by inability to perceive the heat of bath water.

Abnormal sensations

Abnormal sensations may be qualitative changes in an existing sensation (dysaesthesiae), or spontaneous sensations (paraesthesiae). Paraesthesiae may take the form of burning, coldness, wetness or itching (all of which suggest a lesion of pain pathways), or they may consist of feelings of pins and needles, vibration, electric shock or tightness as if wrapped in bandages (all of which suggest a lesion of the posterior column sensory pathways). Two other types of distorted sensation may occur: hyperpathia refers to exaggeration of pain to a painful stimulus; allodynia refers to pain evoked by a non-painful stimulus.

The anatomical arrangements of sensory pathways are such that the signs on physical examination usually make it possible to distinguish between lesions at the following sites; a peripheral nerve or trunk of a nerve plexus, a spinal root, the spinal cord, the brainstem, the thalamus, and the cerebral cortex (see Figure 1.5). The distribution of the resulting sensory signs is illustrated in Figures 3.19, 3.20, 3.21 and 3.22.

A lesion of the peripheral nerve or of one trunk of a plexus usually causes both sensory and motor loss in its area of distribution, although one may strikingly precede the other. The sensory loss involves all sensory functions, and its site roughly corresponds with the anatomical distribution of the nerve (Figure 3.19). There is, however, considerable overlap in the area of supply of individual peripheral nerves, so that the extent of sensory loss after damage to a given nerve varies considerably from one subject to another. Partial lesions of peripheral nerves tend to affect the appreciation of touch more than that of pain.

Peripheral neuropathies tend to affect the longest fibres first, so symmetrical sensory loss starts in the legs before the arms, and begins in the feet and then in the hands. The result is the classical 'glove-stocking' pattern of sensory disturbance (Figure 3.20).

Lesions of the **posterior spinal root** cause sensory loss without motor deficit, although the appropriate tendon jerk is depressed or absent. The sensory loss will correspond roughly with the anatomical area of root supply (the dermatome) (Figure 3.19). However, there is considerable overlap of dermatomes, so that the extent of a sensory deficit after individual root damage is much less than that predicted from its known distribution. Indeed, loss of a single posterior root may produce no sensory deficit that can be detected. Root damage commonly impairs appreciation of pain more than that of touch.

Complete **lesions of the spinal cord** cause loss of all forms of sensation, and of motor activity, in those areas supplied by the cord below the lesion (Figure 3.21). Also, there will be a fairly well defined 'upper level' for the loss of both sensory and motor function. Partial lesions may cause a sensory loss unaccompanied by motor loss, and also may cause selective loss of one or more types of sensation. Such dissociated sensory loss occurs because the different sensory pathways follow different anatomical routes in the spinal cord (Figure 3.20).

The **lateral spinothalamic** tract contains the second sensory neurone conveying the sensations of pain, temperature, tickle and itch, and to some extent those responsible for appreciation of touch, from the contralateral side of the body (Figure 3.5). The **posterior columns** contain the central processes of the primary sensory neurones conveying the sensations of joint position, vibration and, to some extent, those of touch for the ipsilateral half of the body. The posterior (dorsal) columns also carry the sensory fibres responsible for judgement of location of the site of the stimulus, its weight, texture and the capacity to distinguish between two separated points.

Lesions that cause dissociated sensory loss include damage to one half of the spinal cord (**Brown–Séquard syndrome**), damage to the anterior half of the cord, and expanding intramedullary lesions. Each of these disorders will produce a particular pattern of dissociated sensory loss in combination with distinctive motor signs below

the lesion. In the Brown–Séquard syndrome, there is ipsilateral loss of vibration and position sense, and impairment of tactile discrimination, with contralateral loss of pain and temperature sensation (Figure 3.20). Voluntary motor activity is lost on the side of the lesion. With damage to the anterior half of the spinal cord, there is bilateral loss of pain and temperature sensation and of voluntary motor activity, but preservation of touch, vibration and position sense. An **intramedullary lesion** that interrupts the decussating fibres from the dorsal grey column to the lateral spinothalamic tract often causes preferential loss of pain and temperature appreciation in a segmental distribution corresponding to the site of cord involvement.

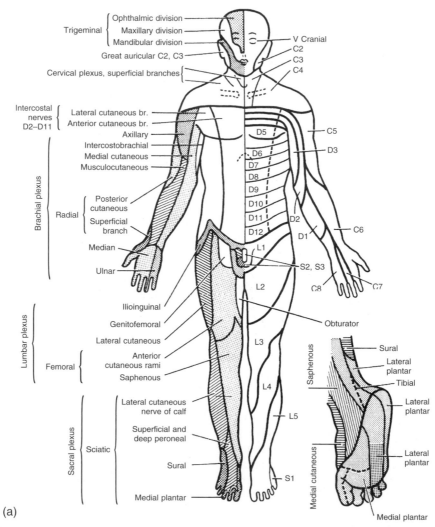

(a)

Figure 3.19 Cutaneous areas of distribution of spinal segments and peripheral nerves: (a) anterior aspect; (b) posterior aspect. (Courtesy of Lord Walton of Detchant and Oxford University Press, *Brain's Diseases of the Nervous System*, 8th edn. Reproduced with permission.)

The **anatomical level of sensory loss** that accompanies spinal cord lesions is affected by a number of factors, and may be misleading; for example, in spinal cord lesions, the upper level of loss of pain and temperature is often two or three segments below the site of the lesion. This is because the fibres conveying pain and temperature cross the cord obliquely, and may ascend for a few segments before decussation. A lesion compressing the spinal cord from the outside tends to affect the most superficial fibres first. In the lateral spinothalamic tract, these are from the legs. Thus, extramedullary cord compression initially produces sensory distur-bance in the legs, which then ascends as the lesion progresses. In contrast, intramedullary lesions of the cervical cord produce loss of pain and temperature sensation in the arms, before the legs or sacral regions show any sensory deficit (suspended sensory loss) (Figure 3.22).

Within the **brainstem**, the arrangement of sensory tracts changes. The first neurones of the posterior column synapse in the gracile and cuneate nuclei, and then decussate to enter the medial lemniscus, now lying in close relation to the lateral lemniscus carrying fibres from the auditory pathway (Figures 3.5 and 3.21). In addition, sensory fibres from the

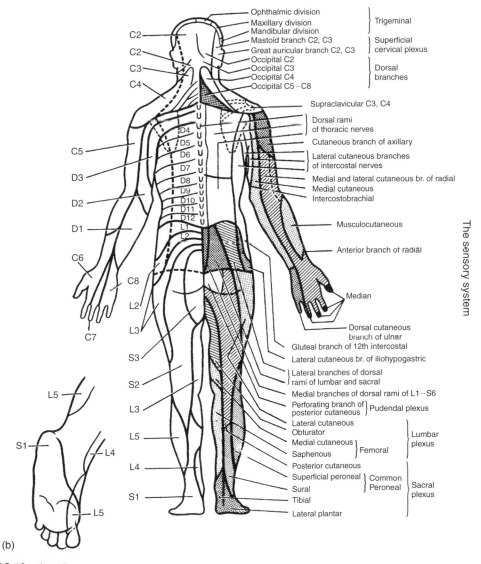

(b)

Figure 3.19 (Continued)

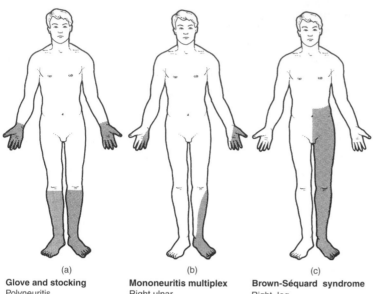

Glove and stocking
Polyneuritis
Hysteria

Mononeuritis multiplex
Right ulnar
Left median
Left lateral popliteal

Brown-Séquard syndrome
Right leg
  Pyramidal weakness
  Posterior column loss
Left leg
  Spinothalamic sensory loss

Figure 3.20 Patterns of sensory loss: glove-stocking; mononeuritis multiplex; and Brown–Séquard.

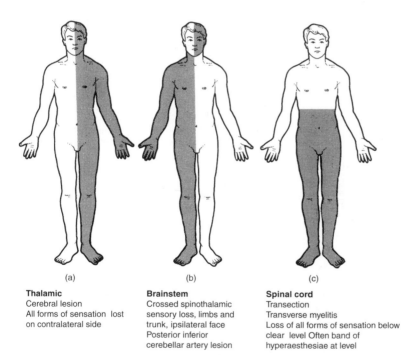

Thalamic
Cerebral lesion
All forms of sensation lost on contralateral side

Brainstem
Crossed spinothalamic sensory loss, limbs and trunk, ipsilateral face
Posterior inferior cerebellar artery lesion

Spinal cord
Transection
Transverse myelitis
Loss of all forms of sensation below clear level Often band of hyperaesthesiae at level

Figure 3.21 Patterns of sensory loss: thalamic; brainstem; and spinal cord.

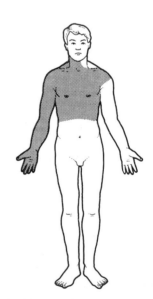

Figure 3.22 Sensory loss in an intramedullary spinal cord lesion. Spinothalamic sensory loss in the right arm and 'cuirasse' distribution over the chest. Lost arm reflexes. Pyramidal signs and posterior column sensory loss in the legs, that is dissociated sensory loss.

fifth nerve join the lemniscal system so that a uni-lateral lesion in the pons tends to cause loss of all varieties of sensation from the opposite half of the body. However, a lesion of the medulla may cause crossed sensory loss. This consists of contralateral loss of all sensation and ipsilateral loss of pain and temperature over the face. Such a pattern arises because fibres of the fifth nerve subserving pain and temperature descend in the spinal tract of the fifth nerve into the medulla, before synapsing in the nucleus of that tract, crossing and then ascending in the trigeminal lemniscus.

The second sensory neurones from the opposite side of the body all terminate in the thalamus, from which the third sensory neurone fibres pass to the cortex on the same side. **Thalamic lesions** thus cause loss of all modalities of sensation on the opposite half of the body (Figure 3.21). In addition, for reasons that are not understood, thalamic dam-age may cause an abnormally heightened affective response to sensory stimuli. Thus, the single pin-prick produces a perverted sensation of pain, which is poorly localized, protracted and intensely disa-greeable, hyperpathia. In addition, thalamic lesions may produce spontaneous thalamic or central pains (see Chapter 30).

Lesions of the **cerebral cortex** characteristically affect the ability to integrate sensory information, and to make judgements based upon crude sensory appreciation from the opposite half of the body. Cortical damage does not impair the ability to be able to appreciate simple touch, pain, temperature or vibration. However, the patient cannot utilize such information to make sensory judgements. Thus, appreciation of joint position and two-point discrimination is impaired. The ability to identify familiar objects placed in the hand (stereognosis), and the ability to judge the comparative size and weight of different objects placed in the hand, are compromised by cortical lesions. Another useful test of cortical sensory function is the ability to perceive two simultaneous sensory stimuli applied with equal intensity to corresponding sites on opposite sides of the body. A unilateral cortical lesion may lead to failure to perceive the contralat-eral stimulus, even though it is easily detected when administered by itself. Such sensory inattention or neglect, when severe, may extend to an apparent unawareness of the contralateral limb or even one whole half of the body, a form of agnosia.

Coma

Impairment of cerebral function may cause depres-sion or clouding of consciousness leading to coma. Consciousness, or the maintenance of the alert state, relies on an intact ascending reticular acti-vating system. This starts in the brainstem in the pons, ascending through the midbrain to end in the hypothalamus and thalamic reticular formation (Figure 3.23). Any structural damage in this path-way will cause a depressed conscious level so that infarcts, haematomas or mass lesions at this site may be responsible. These may be relatively small in size. In the supratentorial compartments, bihemi-sphere lesions, bilateral thalamic infarcts or a mas-sive unilateral lesion causing significant shifts or distortion may also cause a depressed conscious level. Other important causes include:

- metabolic upsets – such as, uraemia, hepatic failure, hypoglycaemia or hyperglycaemia;
- infective processes – meningitis, encephalitis;
- hypoxic/ischaemic disturbances – cardiac/respi-ratory arrests;
- poisoning – from drugs or alcohol overdosage.

Many terms are used to describe various levels of depression of consciousness. **Comatose** patients are unconscious and unable to respond to ver-bal command, although they may show motor responses to painful stimuli. **Stuporose** patients are unconscious but can be roused by verbal command

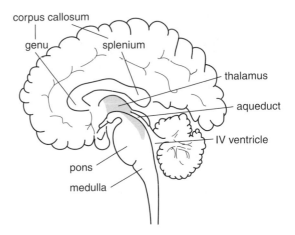

Figure 3.23 Sagittal section to show ascending reticular activating system in the brainstem and diencephalon (shaded).

or painful stimuli for short periods to produce a verbal response. When stimulation ceases, they lapse back into coma. **Confused patients** are alert, but disorientated for time, place, and even person. In **delirium**, patients are confused, but also restless and overactive. Another term to describe delirium is **toxic confusional state**.

Such grades of depression of consciousness are difficult to define and a valuable method of recording data is the international **Glasgow Coma Scale** (Table 3.8), which has proved easy to administer by doctors and nurses. The scale describes the best verbal, motor and eye responses to stimulation, either by verbal command or pain. Each of the three categories of response is graded on a scale ranging from normal (the patient is orientated, obeys command and shows spontaneous eye opening – a score of 15) to deep coma (the patient exhibits no verbal response to stimulation, no motor response to pain and never spontaneously opens the eyes – a score of 3). In addition, it is essential to record the pupillary responses to light, the reflex eye movements in both vertical and horizontal plane to oculocephalic (doll's head manoeuvre) and/or caloric stimulation, the blood pressure, respiration, pulse and temperature in every unconscious patient.

Other terms are used to describe the level of consciousness and physical state of patients surviving coma. A **vegetative state (VS)** is defined as a 'clinical condition of unawareness of self and environment in which the patient breathes spontaneously, has a stable circulation and shows cycles of eye closure and eye opening, which may simulate sleep and waking'. Such patients survive coma, but do not speak or exhibit any purposeful response to the outside world. They may show periods of wakefulness, groan and grunt, and exhibit stereotyped primitive movements in response to external stimuli, but they have no intelligent communication. This state has also been called the apallic syndrome. The term continuing vegetative state is applied when the state continues for more than 4 weeks and the term **persistent (permanent) vegetative state** is best used when the diagnosis of an irreversible state can be made with a high degree of clinical certainty. No absolute timescale has been established, although the term persistent VS may reasonably be made in patients stable some 12 months after a head injury or six months after other causes of brain damage. Akinetic mutism may also refer to a patient with a continuing vegetative state, although not all such patients are akinetic.

The **'locked–in' syndrome** refers to patients who have sustained extensive damage to the pons, causing complete loss of speech and a quadriplegia. However, because the midbrain is intact such patients are alert and give normal results on electroencephalography (EEG). Their only means

Table 3.8 Glasgow coma scale (adults and children). Reprinted from The Lancet, 338, Teasdale G., Jennett B., An assessment of coma and impaired consciousness: a practical scale, 81–4, 1974, with permission from Elsevier.

Assessment of conscious level	Adults	Children	Score
Eye opening	Spontaneous	Spontaneous	4
	To speech	To sound	3
	To pain	To pain	2
	None	None	1
Best motor response	Obeys command	Appropriate for age	6
	Localizes to pain	Localizes to pain	5
	Flexion to pain	Flexion to pain	4
	Spastic flexion	Spastic flexion	3
	Abnormal extension	Abnormal extension	2
	None	None	1
Best verbal response	Orientated	Appropriate for age	5
	Confused	Cries	4
	Monosyllabic	Irritable	3
	Incomprehensible sounds	Lethargic	2
	None	None	1

of communication is by eye movements. The pontine damage paralyses horizontal gaze, but eyelid movements and vertical gaze are preserved. These patients can see, hear and think normally.

Causes of coma

The causes of coma are shown in Box 3.1 and Table 3.9. Loss of consciousness is caused by diffuse brain disease affecting both cerebral hemispheres, large space-occupying supratentorial lesions causing considerable shifts or distortions, or by rela-

Box 3.1 Causes of coma

Diffuse
  Self-poisoning
    Drugs, alcohol
    Accidental – children
  Metabolic
    Diabetic, hypoglycaemic
    Hepatic
    Uraemic
    Electrolyte disturbance, commonly
      hyponatraemic
    Wernicke's encephalopathy, carbon dioxide
      narcosis
    Endocrine (rare) – myxoedema, pituitary
      apoplexy
  Hypoxic/ischaemic – cardiorespiratory arrest,
    carbon monoxide poisoning
  Infective – meningitis, encephalitis, cerebral
    malaria, septicaemia
  Vascular
    Subarachnoid haemorrhage, vasculitis,
    Hypertensive encephalopathy
  Trauma – head injuries
  Epilepsy – post-ictal state
Focal
  Supratentorial
  Haemorrhage
    Infarct
    Subdural, extradural haematoma
    Tumour
    Abscess
  Infratentorial
    Haemorrhage
    Infarct
    Tumour
    Abscess
  Psychogenic

Table 3.9 Frequency of causes of coma in 386 patients admitted to an emergency department (%)

Diffuse – metabolic/toxic	261 (68)
Overdoses	99 (26)
Metabolic/endocrine	81 (21)
Hypoxic/ischaemic	51 (13)
Infection	11 (3)
Subarachnoid haemorrhage	10
Focal lesions	
Supratentorial	69 (18)
Haematoma, intracerebral	33 (9)
Haematoma, subdural, epidural	25 (6)
Infarct	5
Tumour	5
Abscess	3
Infratentorial	52 (13)
Infarct	37 (10)
Haemorrhage, brainstem cerebellar	11 (3)
Tumour	2
Abscess	2
Psychiatric	4

After Plum and Posner (1972) with permission of Dr F Plum and Oxford University Press.

tively focal upper brainstem lesions. Diffuse brain disease may be the result of some generalized extrinsic condition, whose primary cause lies outside the brain, or of diffuse intrinsic disease of the brain itself. Extrinsic conditions include metabolic disturbances and poisoning with drugs or alcohol; intrinsic causes include meningitis and encephalitis. Focal lesions causing coma are most commonly abscesses, traumatic extradural or subdural haematomas, primary intracerebral haemorrhage or post-infarct swelling, or tumours.

The pathophysiology of coma

Diffuse brain disease usually causes coma by interfering with cerebral metabolism. The energy requirements of the brain are normally supplied by the oxidation of glucose. Each 100 g of human brain utilizes 5 mg of glucose/min, and the brain as a whole consumes 15–20 per cent of the total oxygen consumption of the body at rest, which amounts to 3.3 mL O_2/100 g brain/h. The carbohydrate reserves of the brain are only 2 g, and there are almost no reserves of oxygen. The brain is therefore critically dependent on its blood supply for its large requirements of both glucose and oxygen. The resting cerebral blood flow is about 50 mL/100 g of brain/min, which amounts to nearly one-fifth of the cardiac output.

> When the brain is deprived of its supply of oxygen or glucose, function declines almost immediately and consciousness is rapidly lost.

The higher cortical functions and awareness are affected first. Focal brain lesions cause coma in one of two ways.

Coma caused by focal lesions

Focal damage to the upper brainstem destroys the ascending reticular activating systems responsible for consciousness. Focal space-occupying lesions supratentorially, or in the posterior fossa, cause coma by impairing brainstem function as a result of pressure and distortion. Small lesions of the cerebral hemispheres usually do not produce coma, but as a tumour grows or a blood clot or abscess expands inside the skull, they begin to displace the intracranial contents.

Because the skull and spinal canal have very rigid walls, a mass lesion can only be accommodated by displacement of other intracranial materials. A little blood can be displaced by the collapsible veins (but not from the major sinuses which are well protected by tough dural and bony walls), and the total cerebrospinal fluid (CSF) pool can be reduced. However, once these compensatory mechanisms have taken place, further growth of a mass will cause a rise of pressure within the skull and displacement of brain away from the lesion. The latter may lead to blockage of the major drainage routes of CSF, which may further increase the intracranial pressure.

The tentorium cerebelli and the falx cerebri act as relatively immobile partitions within the skull. An enlarging mass lesion thus causes severe distortion of the displaced brain in the neighbourhood of the dural folds. A supratentorial mass lesion pushes the brain towards the opposite side, and some of it is squeezed under the falx. The midbrain and diencephalon are squeezed through the tentorial notch into the infratentorial compartment (see Figure 9.1). The upper brainstem thus is distorted by stretch and by compression against the unyielding edge of the tentorium. In addition, the inferomedial portion of the temporal lobe, the uncus, may be squeezed through the tentorial notch to compress and distort the midbrain, together with the adjacent IIIrd cranial nerve. As this process of **transtentorial herniation** occurs, not only is the brainstem distorted and stretched, but the blood vessels supplying it, which are relatively tethered, are also torn and stretched. As a result, haemorrhage occurs in the upper brainstem as transtentorial herniation occurs and consciousness is lost.

Infratentorial posterior fossa mass lesions also cause shifts of intracranial content. They force the brainstem upwards through the tentorial notch, causing midbrain distortion, and force the medulla and tonsils down through the foramen magnum, leading to **medullary herniation**. The shift of intracranial contents through the tentorial notch or through the foramen magnum generally is referred to as 'coning'.

It is obvious that both large supratentorial and infratentorial mass lesions may result in compression, distortion and ischaemia of the brainstem as a result of coning. However, in addition to the mass itself, other important factors also may contribute to impairment of brain function in these circumstances. The volume and pressure of blood in capillaries is controlled in part, by the tone of the cerebral arterioles and these will dilate in response to a rise in local PCO_2, or a fall of PaO_2.

> Consequently, hypoventilation can result in a further increase in intracranial pressure.

The rise in PCO_2 and fall in PaO_2 that follows respiratory failure leads to cerebral arteriolar dilatation and an increased volume of blood in the skull, which must cause further coning.

> A period of respiratory depression can thus be disastrous for a patient with an intracranial mass lesion.

Indeed, when an intracranial mass produces coma by brainstem compression, matters are delicately poised. Once the compression begins to cause impairment of function in the respiratory centre in the medulla, a 'vicious circle' may be initiated, which can rapidly lead to death. Fortunately, the development of a pressure cone is accompanied by a sequence of physical signs resulting from progressive impairment of brain function. These should give sufficient warning of the impending disaster, provided the patient is examined frequently. As will be described later, the process of coning causes an orderly and predictable sequence of loss of neuronal function, which can point clearly to what is happening.

> Patients at risk of coning, or in the process of coning as a result of large intracranial mass lesions may be treated as an emergency by shrinking the intracranial contents.

Acute medical treatment of raised intracranial pressure

Assisted ventilation will reduce cerebral blood volume to give more space, and cerebral oedema around infarcts, haemorrhages or tumours may be reduced by the use of intravenous mannitol. Critically ill patients may be intubated and hyperventilated. The head of the bed should be elevated to 30–45 degrees. Mannitol, a hyperosmolar agent, withdraws oedema fluid from the brain and causes a brisk diuresis. Intravenous infusion of 100–200 mL of 20 per cent mannitol will rapidly reduce intracranial pressure and may stop or reverse the process of coning long enough to allow further investigation and definitive treatment to be undertaken. Patients with a depressed conscious level should have a urinary catheter inserted. Corticosteroids also reduce cerebral oedema, but their effect is slower in onset. Dexamethasone 5–10 mg intravenously followed by 4 mg 6-hourly may help to control cerebral oedema around tumours. If a mass lesion is present, a neurosurgical consultation should be sought.

Examination of the unconscious patient

Because the unconscious patient cannot cooperate, a different system of examination must be employed to assess coma. A suitable sequence (Box 3.2) should include the investigations detailed in the following paragraphs.

Respiration and circulation: the first and most urgent need is to make sure that the airway, breathing and circulation (ABC) are adequate to sustain life. If these are compromised, emergency action should be taken to ensure an airway with assisted ventilation, and an adequate cardiac output. Once emergency resuscitation has been completed, further examination can continue.

Blood pressure, the pulse rate and rhythm, and temperature are recorded. The character of respiration is noted.

Damage to the respiratory neurones produces a variety of abnormalities of breathing. **Cheyne–Stokes breathing** refers to periodic cycles of

Box 3.2 Examination of the unconscious patient

> **A** Airway
> **B** Breathing – respiratory rate, rhythm
> **C** Circulation – pulse rate, rhythm, blood pressure, cardiac output
> Temperature
> Meningism
> Conscious level – Glasgow Coma Scale
>   Best verbal response
>   Best motor response
>   Eye opening
> Appearance – jaundice, rashes, fetor (ketotic, ethanol), bruising, needle marks (addicts), blood from nose, ears, bitten tongue
> Pupils – size, symmetry, reactions
> Fundi
> Eye movements
>   Spontaneous, conjugate, dysconjugate, abnormal
>   Doll's head
>   Cold calorics
> Corneal, lash reflexes
> Facial movements – grimaces
> 'Gag', cough reflexes
> Spontaneous limb movements
> Abnormal movements – myoclonus
> Response to pain
>   Decorticate rigidity
>   Decerebrate rigidity
> Reflexes, plantar responses
> General examination

hyperventilation alternating with apnoea in a waxing and waning pattern. Each cycle lasts about a minute. The patient ceases respiration, then begins to breathe again, the rate and depth increasing to a peak, and then dying away again. This respiratory drive is linked to the carbon dioxide level: when this is high, it stimulates the medullary respiratory centre and a number of deep breaths follow, the level then falls and the drive is lowered and the breaths diminish. The most common cause is circulatory failure but it may also arise with metabolic disturbances, such as with uraemia, and with bihemisphere cortical lesions and supratentorial herniation. A similar pattern with a shorter cycle length of about half a minute, occurs in some patients with midbrain and internal capsule lesions. **Central neurogenic hyperventilation** is associated with destruction of the reticular formation in the pons and midbrain. It causes respiratory alkalosis. **Apneustic breathing** describes a prolonged pause after each inspiration and before the next expiration occurs. It results from damage to the lower half of the pons. **Ataxic breathing** is completely irregular in amplitude and frequency. It indicates damage to the medullary respiratory neurones. **Gasping respiration** is characterized by an abrupt inspiration followed by expiration, then a long pause before the next breath. It occurs shortly before death.

Progressive transtentorial herniation of the brainstem thus may produce an orderly sequence of changes in respiration. As coning occurs, central neurogenic hyperventilation may give way to apneustic breathing, followed by ataxic breathing, gasping respiration and then death.

Assess the level of consciousness: take note of the patient's spontaneous verbal, motor and ocular responses, and observe how they react to external circumstances and your commands.

> The aim will be to place the patient in the appropriate category on the Glasgow Coma Scale in due course.

Suitable graded stimuli are spoken commands, shouted commands, pinprick, pressing on the sternum or supraorbital notch, which causes pain. While watching the response of the patient to stimuli, always look for asymmetric motor reactions, or apparent neglect of such stimuli on one half of the body.

Examine the head and skull: palpate the skull for signs of fracture and for bruising. Note any bruising or discharge of blood or CSF from the ears, nose or mouth. This might suggest a basal skull fracture. Check the skin for any rash, such as the purpuric changes of a meningococcal septicaemia, or for jaundice or extensive bruising, the last suggesting a haemorrhagic state.

The neck: flex the neck on the head and note any resistance to movement suggesting meningeal irritation from either blood or infection. However, the absence of meningism in a deeply unconscious patient does not exclude the possibility of meningitis or subarachnoid haemorrhage. Obviously movement of the neck should not be attempted if there is a suspicion that cervical vertebrae may have been fractured.

The eyes: the visual fields may be examined in such patients either by advancing a bright light in each quadrant, or by making threatening movements of the hand towards the eye. Patients whose level of consciousness allows reaction to such stimuli, will turn the head and eyes away, or blink.

Examine the optic fundi to check for disc swelling, retinal haemorrhages or other retinal changes.

Note the size of **the pupils and their response to light**. The midbrain contains the IIIrd nerve, parasympathetic and pretectal nuclei, so that midbrain lesions produce obvious pupillary abnormalities.

> The pupils, therefore, are invaluable in indicating the presence of a focal brain lesion responsible for coma. In a comatose patient, mydriatics should not be used in order to obtain a better view of the optic fundi. Serial observations of pupillary size and reactions can be invaluable in assessing progression or recovery in coma, and outweigh the information gained from fundoscopic examination, particularly when there is easy access to brain imaging with CT or MRI.

Some specific poisons also affect the pupillary responses, e.g. atropine and gluthemide cause dilatation, opiates cause constriction.

> The pupillary responses are, perhaps, the single most important guide to the cause of coma.

COLOUR PLATES

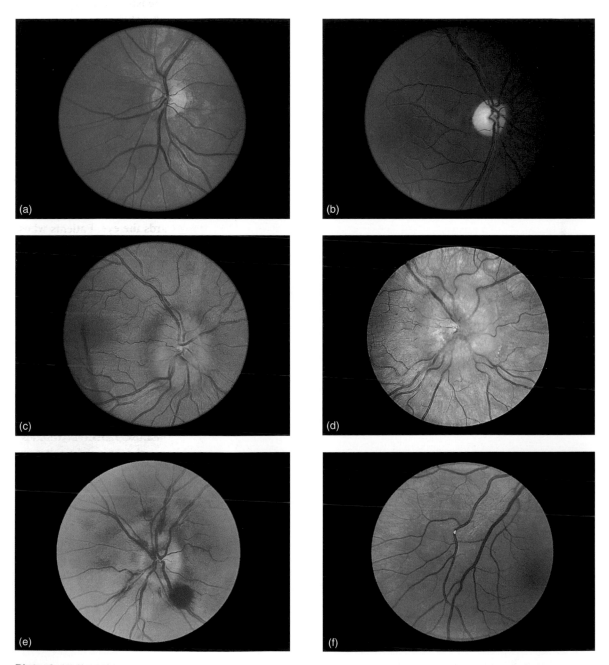

Plate 1 (a) Normal optic disk; (b) Optic atrophy – the pallor of the disc appears accentuated because the patient was pigmented (Indian); (c) Acute papilloedema; (d) More chronic and more severe papilloedema; (e) Haemorrhagic lesions in a patient with acute leukaemia; (f) Cholesterol embolus in a retinal artery branch.

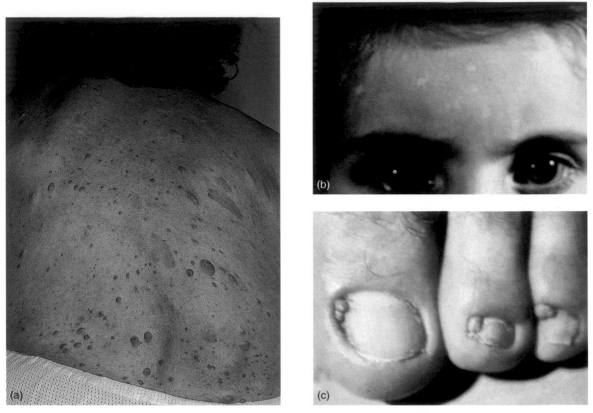

Plate 2 (a) Typical widespread skin changes in a patient with type I neurofibromatosis. Note there is also a scoliosis; (b) Depigmented skin lesions on a child's face with tuberous sclerosis; (c) Subungual fibroma in patients with tuberous sclerosis.

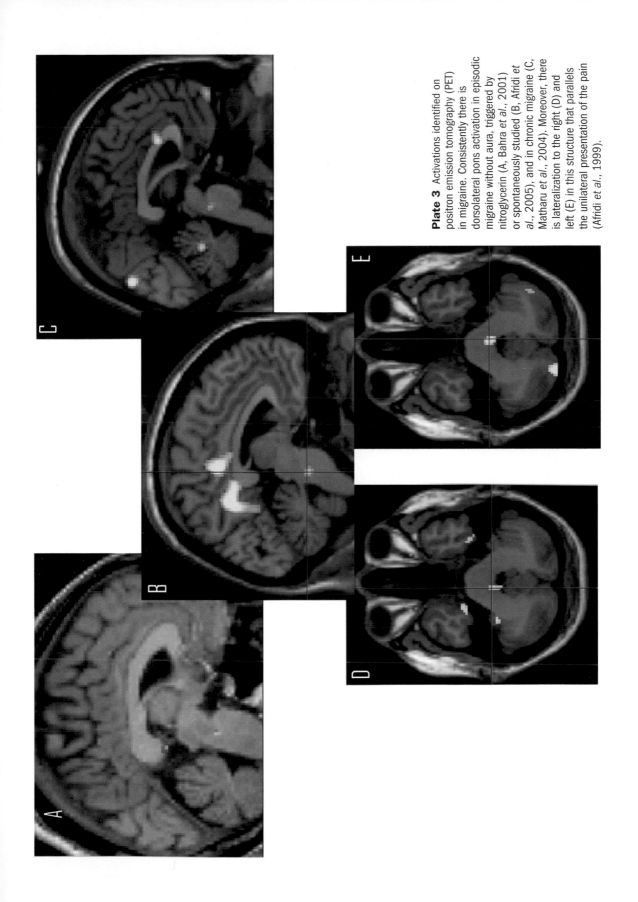

Plate 3 Activations identified on positron emission tomography (PET) in migraine. Consistently there is dorsolateral pons activation in episodic migraine without aura, triggered by nitroglycerin (A, Bahra et al., 2001) or spontaneously studied (B, Afridi et al., 2005), and in chronic migraine (C, Matharu et al., 2004). Moreover, there is lateralization to the right (D) and left (E) in this structure that parallels the unilateral presentation of the pain (Afridi et al., 1999).

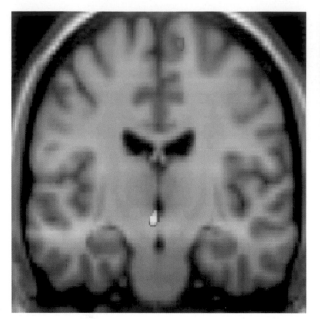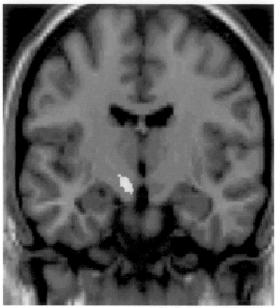

Plate 4 Activation on positron emission tomography (PET) in the posterior hypothalamic grey matter in patients with acute cluster headache (A). The activation demonstrated is lateralized to the side of the pain (May *et al.*, 1998). When comparing the brains of patients with cluster headache with a control population using an automatic anatomical technique known as voxel-based morphometry (VBM) that employs high-resolution T1 weighted MRI, a similar region is demonstrated (B) and has increased grey matter (May *et al.*, 1999).

Pupillary changes in coning

A unilateral supratentorial mass lesion causing transtentorial coning leads to a IIIrd nerve palsy as the process evolves. The pupil on the side of the lesion dilates, becomes unreactive to light and accommodation, ptosis develops and the eye turns down and out. Bilateral supratentorial mass lesions, or diffuse brain swelling, which produces a central transtentorial herniation, tend to affect pupillary pathways in the diencephalon and brainstem in an orderly sequence. At first, damage to the sympathetic fibres causes the pupils to become small but reactive. Then, as the process evolves, the pupils begin to dilate and eventually become dilated and unreactive to light. Primary pontine lesions spare the parasympathetic pupillary systems causing disruption only of the sympathetic mechanisms. As a result, the pupils are constricted and may become very small ('pinpoint pupils'). Lesions of the lateral part of the medulla affect the descending sympathetic fibres to produce a unilateral Horner's syndrome.

'Metabolic coma'

It can be stated that an unconscious patient showing no focal motor deficit, who has equal, normal-sized and reactive pupils, is in coma because of diffuse brain disease. The absence of a history or signs of cerebral trauma, and a normal CT brain scan and CSF examination in such patients will exclude intrinsic causes of diffuse brain disease. In such circumstances, a confident diagnosis of extrinsic diffuse brain disease or 'metabolic' coma can be made.

Examine the eye movements: provided the patient is capable of some response to command, the range of eye movements can be assessed simply. However, many stuporose and/or comatose patients will not obey verbal commands, so eye movements must be tested in other ways. Two techniques can be used. Eye movement may be provoked by the **oculocephalic reflexes** elicited by the **doll's head manoeuvre**. Brisk rotation of the head from side to side, or flexion and extension of the neck, will produce conjugate eye movements in the opposite direction to the head movement. This gives the impression that the patient's gaze is focused on an object straight in front. Such oculocephalic responses are attributed to the effect of vestibular input combined with proprioceptive impulses from the neck. This information eventually ascends via the medial longitudinal bundle in the brainstem to the ocular motor nuclei.

> Preservation of horizontal and vertical eye movement in response to the doll's head manoeuvre implies that the brainstem is intact.

Loss of reflex conjugate upgaze indicates damage to the midbrain. Loss of reflex conjugate horizontal gaze indicates damage to the pons. Dysconjugate eye movements may be provoked by the doll's head manoeuvre, or may occur spontaneously in the comatose patient. Failure of lateral deviation of one eye when gaze is reflexively provoked in that direction indicates a VIth nerve palsy. Failure of adduction of the eye with normal abduction suggests an internuclear ophthalmoplegia. If the doll's head manoeuvre is insufficient to provoke eye movement, then caloric responses may be employed to elicit VOR, which again depend upon an intact brainstem. Ice-cold water is syringed into each ear in turn, making sure that the ear drum is normal before doing so. If brainstem function is intact, there will either be nystagmus in the direction away from the irrigated ear, or conjugate deviation of the eyes to the irrigated side. Again, patients with specific ocular motor palsies may show a dysconjugate response to caloric stimulation. In addition to examination of voluntary or reflex eye movements, spontaneous eye movements should be carefully recorded in the unconscious patient.

Tonic ocular deviation

Tonic deviation of the eyes conjugately to one side suggests a focal lesion, either of the cerebral hemisphere or of the brainstem. With a hemisphere lesion, the opposite limbs will be paralysed and the eyes look away from them towards the side of the lesion. In a brainstem pontine lesion, the opposite limbs will be paralysed, but the eyes will look towards them, that is, away from the side of the lesion.

Other abnormalities of spontaneous eye movements are described in coma; these include ocular bobbing, repetitive divergence and nystagmoid jerking of one eye.

The face: look for signs of a unilateral facial paralysis (drooping of one side of the mouth which is puffed out with each breath). Test the corneal and lash reflexes with a wisp of cotton wool, and the facial response to pinprick or supraorbital pressure. Both of these stimuli should cause screwing up of the same side of the face.

The ears: examine the ear drums with an auroscope, looking for evidence of middle ear infection, such as an opaque, bulging drum or a ruptured drum with purulent discharge. With trauma, there may be blood behind the drum or in the external auditory meatus.

The mouth: smell the breath for alcohol, ketones or other distinctive odours. Look for lacerations of the tongue, which suggest a recent epileptic fit. Check for the presence of a gag reflex.

Examine the limbs: establish whether all four limbs move, either spontaneously or in response to painful stimuli. Squeezing the Achilles tendon or a finger nail, or rubbing the sternum are useful means of provoking reflex movement. Such stimuli should always be applied at various sites to allow for local anaesthesia. Failure to move an arm or leg on one side in response to stimuli to each side indicates a hemiplegia. Absence of any limb movement in response to strong stimuli occurs with bilateral severe damage to the brainstem, as in the 'locked-in' syndrome, but also occurs in very deep coma without any focal brain damage.

Provided the limbs are not paralysed, stimuli may provoke appropriate or inappropriate reflex responses. When there is no motor deficit, painful stimuli will cause withdrawal of the limb, attempts to remove the source of pain with the opposite limb, screwing up of the face, and even verbal responses. An early motor sign of severe focal cerebral damage is the appearance of stereotyped limb movements in response to painful stimuli. Destructive lesions involving the internal capsule cause **decorticate rigidity**. A painful stimulus provokes flexion and adduction of the arm with extension of the leg on the affected side. Damage to the upper brainstem causes **decerebrate rigidity** in response to a painful stimulus. The neck retracts and the teeth clench. The affected arm extends, adducts and the forearm pronates. The affected leg extends and the foot plantar flexes. Spontaneous spasms of decerebrate rigidity may occur with severe brainstem lesions, often accompanied by shivering, hypertension and hyperpyrexia.

Muscle tone can be assessed in the unconscious patient by passive manipulation of the limbs, or by noting the response to dropping the limb to the bed. Lift the arms and legs, individually or together, and note the speed with which they fall to the bed when dropped. Hemiplegic limbs, which are flaccid in the acute stage, fall harder and faster than normal limbs.

Examine the tendon jerks and plantar responses. However, remember that it may take some days for hyper-reflexia and Babinski's sign to appear after an acute lesion of corticomotorneurone pathways. In the stage of shock following an acute hemiplegia, the limbs are flaccid, the tendon jerks are normal or absent, and the plantar response may be unresponsive.

General examination: examine the heart, lungs and abdomen.

Always test the urine for protein, glucose and ketones, and examine it with a microscope for pus cells and casts.

Measure the glucose in all unconscious patients

If the cause of coma is not apparent at this stage, **always measure the blood glucose** concentration and administer glucose intravenously. Most accident and emergency departments have an absolute rule that blood glucose must be measured in all unconscious patients. In addition, it is essential to give thiamine by injection. Many unconscious patients admitted to accident and emergency departments are victims of chronic alcoholic abuse, and may have Wernicke's encephalopathy. Administration of glucose to patients with Wernicke's encephalopathy increases metabolic demand and this may intensify or precipitate the encephalopathy (see Chapter 27).

The differential diagnosis of coma

The important features distinguishing diffuse brain disease and focal brain lesions causing coma are shown in Box 3.3. The important features distin-

Box 3.3 Differentiation of diffuse and focal brain lesions leading to coma

Diffuse
  Absence of focal or lateralizing signs: motor or sensory
  May be bilateral changes in tone, reflexes and extensor plantar responses
  Brainstem functions often preserved initially, especially ocular movements and papillary responses
  Often self-poisoning, metabolic causes, infection, bleeding or epilepsy, so CT brain scan often negative
Focal
  Focal or lateralizing signs usually present to suggest hemisphere or brainstem damage
  Include flaccid weakness and loss of response to pain on one side
  Reflex asymmetry, including plantar response
  Tonic deviation of eyes to one side
  Derangements in ocular motility and papillary responses
  Often supratentorial mass (abscess, tumour, haematoma) or infratentorial mass (haematoma, infarct, tumour), so CT brain scan positive

Box 3.4 Differentiation of supratentorial focal from infratentorial lesion in patients with a depressed conscious level

Supratentorial
  Focal mass has to expand to compress the other hemisphere and cause brainstem compression to cause coma
  May be clear unilateral focal signs
  Often brainstem reflexes initially preserved: pupillary responses, ocular movements, gag, corneal, etc.
  Eyes may be tonically deviated to side of lesion away from hemiplegia
  May be focal epileptic seizures
  Sometimes decorticate rigidity
  Late: unilateral oculomotor palsy with uncal cone
Infratentorial
  Small lesions damaging the reticular formation may cause early coma often with signs of midbrain or even foramen magnum coning
  Brainstem reflexes impaired: abnormal pupils (e.g. bilateral pinpoint), impaired ocular motility, lost corneal, gag, etc.
  Impaired doll's head and cold caloric reflexes
  Eyes may be tonically deviated away from the side of the pontine lesion towards hemiplegia
  Hyperventilation, irregular breathing patterns: apnoea
  Decerebrate rigidity

guishing a supratentorial focal brain lesion from an infratentorial focal lesion causing coma are shown in Box 3.4.

The initial clinical assessment and examination may have revealed the obvious cause of coma. If not, blood glucose is measured, and glucose and thiamine administered.

Now is the time to obtain as much information as possible on the background of the patient.

Witnesses to the circumstances in which the individual was found must be questioned. These will include policemen, ambulance attendants, relatives and friends. The patient's clothing must be searched, for evidence such as a diabetic or steroid card, or an empty bottle for sleeping tablets. If known, the patient's general practitioner can be approached for further information and other relatives contacted. Any containers brought in by relatives or witnesses should be kept for analysis in patients suspected of self-poisoning.

If the cause for coma is still not apparent, then a series of investigations should now be set in train (see later), and the patient kept under close observation. Subsequent events may clarify the situation so it is particularly important to repeat parts of the initial examination at intervals to assess progress.

The most sensitive index of change is the state of consciousness, but heart rate, blood pressure, temperature, limb movements, pupillary size and reaction to light, and respiratory pattern, should all be regularly observed and recorded.

Investigations in coma

In those in whom the cause of coma is not evident, the direction of investigation is determined by whether examination suggests that it is a result of diffuse brain disease or a focal brain lesion (Box 3.3).

> If a focal lesion is suspected, investigations should be directed to imaging of the head.

This is usually undertaken by a CT brain scan, although occasionally an MRI brain scan may be possible. An EEG may sometimes prove helpful; for example in some forms of status epilepticus or an encephalopathy. It also may help in prognosis. Somatosensory evoked potentials may be useful in prognosis of coma, although this is very dependent on the cause. With median nerve stimulation 5 days or more after the onset of hypoxic-ischaemic coma, the absence of a cortical response implies a bad prognosis, with the possibility of a persistent VS. Examination of the CSF in the presence of a focal mass lesion may prove dangerous because this may precipitate coning and death. However, if a mass lesion has been excluded by scanning or there are clear pointers to a meningitic or encephalitic process, CSF examination is required to detect the presence of pus, blood or inflammatory changes.

> When diffuse brain disease is suspected as the cause for coma, and there are no signs of a focal mass lesion, then lumbar puncture is necessary to exclude meningitis, encephalitis or a subarachnoid haemorrhage.

This is particularly so in any drowsy patient with meningism. Blood cultures should also be set up.

> If diffuse brain disease is suspected and there is no meningism and the CSF is normal, then the following metabolic and other investigations should be undertaken:
> - full blood count, ESR;
> - blood glucose, urea and electrolytes;
> - liver function tests, blood alcohol and ammonia levels;
> - arterial blood gases;
> - a screen for drug levels that might be responsible for self-poisoning.

If the patient has a raised temperature, or there are other clues to suggest an infection, blood and urine cultures should be set up. A urine sample should be sent for routine analysis, also for estimation of drug levels, osmolality and even porphyrins. The EEG is a valuable test in suspected 'metabolic' coma. The finding of a local abnormality may suggest the presence of a focal lesion. Generalized abnormalities may be found in any metabolic disorder, or in meningitis and encephalitis. Epileptic discharges may be detected and occasionally forms of minor status. Certain rare encephalitic diseases may show diagnostic changes with periodic widespread discharges.

> While awaiting these results, the patient should be continuously monitored, as described earlier. An adequate airway and ventilation should be maintained.

This may require an oropharyngeal airway, an endotracheal tube or even assisted respiration. Fluid and caloric supplements should be given with added vitamins, particularly thiamine. Initially, this may require intravenous infusion, but a nasogastric tube may be used subsequently. The bladder should be catheterized and regular fluid balance charts instituted. The patient should be regularly turned every 2 hours to prevent bedsores.

Cerebral death

Rapid and efficient resuscitation is now widely available and saves lives. However, it also reclaims some individuals in whom the brain is so severely damaged that they will never recover an intelligent existence. For all intents and purposes, their brain is dead, but the heart continues to beat. Eventually, even the heart will cease beating. Such patients may be said to have suffered cerebral death.

The importance of defining cerebral death is two-fold. First, once it can be established with certainty that cerebral death has occurred, the patient's relatives may be informed that there is no point in continuing resuscitation and life support. After discussion, it may be deemed appropriate to cease artificial ventilation. Second, once the diagnosis of cerebral death has been established beyond doubt, the possibility of using that patient's organs for transplantation arises.

The criteria for cerebral death must be fool-proof. If there is any doubt, the diagnosis should not be made. Irreversible brainstem damage from a known cause is synonymous with cerebral death.

To diagnose cerebral death, the **cause** of the brain damage must be known. Often this is obvious, as after major trauma or a subarachnoid haemorrhage. Such a cause must be **irreversible**: this will exclude patients who are hypothermic, have received doses of neuromuscular blocking drugs, depressant drugs or who have a possible metabolic or endocrine defect causing coma.

The affected patient will be on a ventilator as spontaneous breathing has failed and will not be 'fighting' the machine. There must be no signs of any residual brainstem function.

Brain death criteria

1 The pupils are fixed, dilated and unreactive.
2 There are absent corneal reflexes.
3 There are absent oculocephalic (doll's head) and oculovestibular (cold caloric) reflexes.
4 There is an absent 'gag' reflex or no response to a suction catheter in the trachea.
5 No purposeful movements should be elicited, nor facial grimaces to painful stimuli applied to the limbs, trunk or face.
6 The patient's medullary respiratory centre will not respond to a rise in arterial carbon dioxide ($PaCO_2$) of greater than 6.65 kPa (50 mmHg) if the patient is disconnected from the ventilator, that is, to an adequate chemical stimulus for that centre.

Such tests should be repeated after an interval to ensure that the signs remain absent.

REFERENCES AND FURTHER READING

Acheson JF, Sanders MD (1997) Common problems in neuro-ophthalmology. In: *Major Problems in Neurology*. Philadelphia: WB Saunders.

Brandt T (1999) *Vertigo, its Multisensory Syndromes*, 2nd edn. Berlin: Springer Verlag.

Devinsky O (1992) *Behavioural Neurology: 100 Maxims*. (100 Maxims in Neurology Series). London: Arnold.

Duus P (1998) *Topical Diagnosis in Neurology*, 3rd revised edn. Stuttgart: Georg Thieme.

Folstein MF, Folstein SE, McHugh PR (1975) Mini-mental state – a practical method for grading the cognitive state of patients for the clinician. *Journal of Psychiatric Research*, 12:189–198.

Gilman S (2000) *Clinical Examination of the Nervous System*. New York: McGraw-Hill.

Goebel JA (2001) *Practical Management of the Dizzy Patient*. Philadelphia: Lippincott, Williams and Wilkins.

Haerer AF (1992) *De Jong's the Neurological Examination*, 5th edn. Philadelphia: JP Lippincott.

Hodges JR (1994) *Cognitive Assessment for Clinicians*. Oxford: Oxford University Press.

McCarthy RA, Warrington EK (1990) *Cognitive Neuropsychology – a Clinical Introduction*. San Diego: Academic Press.

Plum F, Posner JB (1980) *Diagnosis of Stupor and Coma*, 3rd edn. Philadelphia: FA Davis Coy.

Teasdale G, Jennett B (1974) Assessment of coma and impaired consciousness: a practical scale. *Lancet*, ii:81–84.

Working Party of the Royal College of Physicians (2003) The Vegetative State: guidance on diagnosis and management. *Clinical Medicine*, 3:249–254.

NEUROIMAGING

Philip Rich

INTRODUCTION

Diagnostic neuroimaging is central to modern neurology practice. Magnetic resonance imaging (MRI) is the investigation of choice in most circumstances and in routine clinical use produces images that resemble gross pathology. MRI also offers physiological information beyond anatomical imaging. Diffusion weighted imaging has rapidly become established in clinical use, whereas other advanced applications such as spectroscopy and functional magnetic resonance imaging (fMRI) still have only limited usefulness outside research. Computed tomography (CT) remains the workhorse of emergency imaging. Most vascular imaging is now performed non-invasively although catheter angiography still has a role in selected patients, mainly following intracranial haemorrhage.

TECHNIQUES

Plain radiography

In neuroradiology, plain x-rays are now only used for assessing integrity of ventricular shunt tubing, screening after spinal trauma and occasionally to locate a foreign body. **The practice of obtaining skull films after most head injuries, as a fracture increases the likelihood of intracranial complications, has been rendered obsolete by recent trauma management guidelines.** Now, in any head injury warranting imaging, CT is used for direct visualization of the intracranial contents. The only routine exception to this is non-accidental head injury in infants when skull films are required for forensic purposes. Tumours of the skull vault are usually better shown on CT.

Plain x-rays are still used for initial screening after spinal trauma. However, a single lateral x-ray of the cervical spine will only show around 75 per cent of acute fractures and failure to adequately show the C7/T1 disc space risks missing a dislocation of the cervicothoracic junction. The images should be scrutinized for alignment and spacing between vertebrae. Increased width of prevertebral soft tissues may be seen after a cervical spine fracture but this sign is not always present. Spinal fractures are far more easily diagnosed on CT, particularly now that high quality sagittal and coronal reformat images are routinely produced.

Cross-sectional imaging

Normal radiologic anatomy is demonstrated in Figures 4.1, 4.2 and 4.3 using MRI.

MRI techniques and applications

MRI is the pre-eminent neuroimaging modality offering the highest sensitivity and diagnostic specificity in most clinical circumstances. The

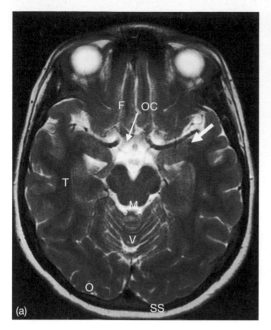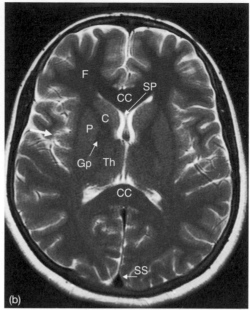

Figure 4.1 Normal radiological neuroanatomy. Axial T2-weighted scans. Frontal (F), temporal (T), occipital (O) lobes. Sylvian fissure (thick arrows) with middle cerebral arteries (left image). Optic chiasm (OC, arrowed) with pituitary stalk behind. Midbrain (M). Cerebellar vermis (V) with superior surface of hemispheres either side. Superior sagittal sinus (SS, arrowed). Caudate (C), putamen (P), globus pallidus (Gp, arrowed), thalamus (Th). In the axial plane the internal capsule is bounded laterally by the putamen and globus pallidus, and medially by the caudate nucleus and thalamus. The third ventricle lies in the midline between the thalami. Corpus callosum (CC). Septum pellucidum (SP, arrowed) separating frontal horns of lateral ventricles.

scanner creates a very strong magnetic field that causes parallel alignment in direction of spin of mobile protons, mainly in water molecules.

Transient changes in spin alignment are induced by pulsed radiofrequency gradients. Subsequent proton spin realignment to the background scanner field results in release of energy as signal from which MR images are formed. The various MRI sequences such as T1-, T2-weighted and so on depend on the different processes and times taken for protons to return to their resting state within the scanner field, known as 'relaxation'.

On T1-weighted sequences cerebrospinal fluid (CSF) is dark, and myelinated white matter is lighter than grey matter (Figure 4.4). Oedema makes brain tissue appear darker than normal and most pathological soft tissue is low signal (Box 4.1).

On T2-weighted sequences CSF or other fluid is bright, and myelinated white matter is darker than grey matter. Most abnormal tissue returns high signal. Fluid attenuated inversion recovery (FLAIR) imaging nulls the signal from water which renders CSF black, thereby increasing conspicuity of periventricular and cortical lesions. Abnormal tissue or fluid accumulation such as oedema, pus or haemorrhage remains bright on FLAIR images.

Box 4.1 High signal on T1-weighted MRI

Fat
Posterior pituitary lobe
Contrast enhancement
Methaemoglobin
Manganese (deposited in basal ganglia in liver disease)
Microcalcification
Proteinaceous/mucinous material
Melanin

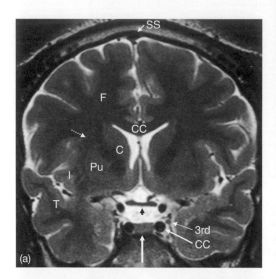

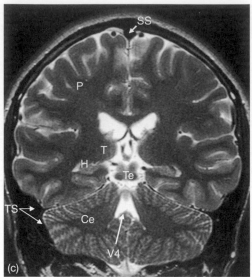

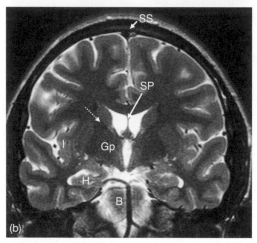

Figure 4.2 Normal radiological neuroanatomy. Coronal T2-weighted scans. Frontal (F), temporal (T), parietal (P) lobes, corpus callosum (CC), caudate (C) lateral to frontal horn of lateral ventricle, putamen (Pu), globus pallidus (GP). Internal capsule (dotted arrow). Insula and Sylvian fissure (I). Optic chiasm (short arrow) and pituitary gland (long arrow). Note adjacent round signal voids of supraclinoid and cavernous portions of internal carotid arteries, respectively. Cavernous sinuses (CC, arrowed), with oculomotor nerve visible in its lateral dural wall (3rd, arrowed). Septum pellucidum (SP) separating lateral ventricles, with fornices in its lower margin and third ventricle below. Hippocampus (H), thalamus (T), basilar artery (B) in front of pons, tectal plate (Te), cerebellar hemispheres (Ce) around fourth ventricle (V4), superior sagittal sinus (SS, arrowed), transverse/sigmoid sinus (TS, arrowed).

Gradient echo or susceptibility weighted imaging depend on local field inhomogeneities from paramagnetic substances, such as iron or gadolinium contrast media, and the signal loss they cause. These sequences show blood products not readily visible on other sequences and are particularly important in acute stroke imaging. Susceptibility effects induced by an infused bolus of gadolinium contrast medium form the basis of perfusion weighted imaging. Arterial spin labelling is a perfusion imaging technique that does not require injected contrast medium. Moving protons in arterial blood are 'labelled' and a territorial map of brain perfusion can be made by labelling individual arteries.

Diffusion weighted imaging (DWI) exploits variations in water diffusivity induced by cell swelling and changes in extracellular fluid space volume. Additionally, in the normal state, water diffuses more readily parallel to major white matter fibre bundles than perpendicular. Thus clinical DWI is acquired in three orthogonal planes, with signal summated to correct for anisotropy produced by white matter tracts. Most DWI sequences in clinical use have some inherent T2 weighting which may cause 'shine through' of bright signal on the diffusion weighted image from chronic lesions. To avoid misdiagnosis as acute restricted diffusion it is necessary to correlate the DW image with an apparent diffusion coefficient (ADC) map, automatically calculated from the DWI data and not susceptible to such artefacts. Rapid diffusion of water molecules dissipates signal, producing a dark

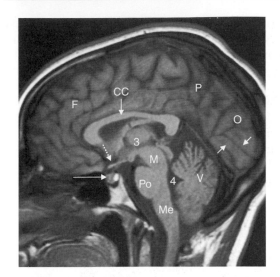

Figure 4.3 Normal radiological neuroanatomy. Mid-sagittal T1-weighted scan. Frontal (F), parietal (P), occipital (O) lobes. Calcarine fissure lined by primary visual cortex (short arrows), corpus callosum (CC, arrowed), optic chiasm (dotted arrow), with pituitary stalk beneath. Pituitary gland and fossa (long arrow), with high signal posterior pituitary lobe. Third ventricle (3), midbrain (M), pons (Po), medulla (Me), Fourth ventricle (4), cerebellar vermis (V).

imaging but has wider applications such as prion disease, encephalitis, some metabolic disorders, grading tumour malignancy and differentiating between necrotic tumours and pyogenic abscesses.

An extrapolation of DWI is diffusion tensor imaging or tractography, which involves data acquisition in many more planes to produce detailed statistical maps of diffusivity, effectively predicting white matter tract organization in some detail. This remains work in progress, but it is already possible to produce quite spectacular 3D colour images of fibre tracts. This may be useful in guiding surgery, showing damage from acquired lesions such as infarcts, tumour invasion and brain connectivity in developmental and cognitive disorders.

Magnetic resonance spectroscopy (MRS) measures metabolite concentrations either as a linear trace or brain map. Although intuitively useful, in most clinical circumstances MRS adds little to careful analysis of structural imaging. fMRI exploits very slight alterations in local tissue blood flow that occurs with neuronal activity. This may help to localize brain functions prior to surgery but rather like MRS, fMRI is used more in research than clinical practice at the moment.

area on DWI, and as diffusion is increased this is bright on an ADC map. A normal example of this is the appearance of ventricular CSF. Restricted water diffusion results in a relatively strong and coherent signal that appears bright on DWI and dark on an ADC map. **DWI is extremely useful in acute stroke**

MR angiography and venography are widely used clinical sequences. Contrast enhancement improves the quality of neck vessel imaging but is not necessary for intracranial studies.

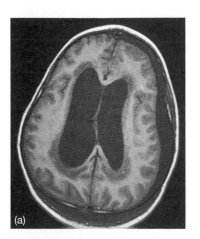
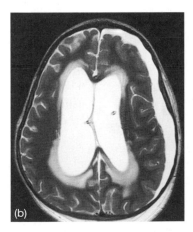
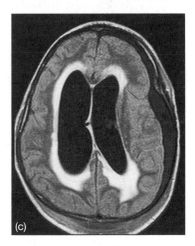

Figure 4.4 Comparison of different MRI sequences. Axial T1 weighted, T2-weighted and fluid attenuated inversion recovery (FLAIR) images. There is hydrocephalus with a shunt tube in the left lateral ventricle and increased transependymal CSF flux causing a rim of signal abnormality around the ventricles. On the left there is a subdural collection with similar signal characteristic to CSF. Note on T1 white matter is lighter than grey matter (cortex) whereas the reverse is the case on T2 and FLAIR. On T1 fluid such as CSF and periventricular oedema is dark. On T2 fluid is bright. On FLAIR signal from normal fluid such as CSF is nulled (dark) rendering more conspicuous signal from abnormal fluid such as oedema around the ventricles.

There are safety considerations in MRI that do not apply to CT. The MRI magnet is 'always on'. The field affects anyone in the scanning room, not just the patient in the bore of the magnet. MR radiographers apply safety procedures to ensure that no-one is allowed into the vicinity of the scanner if they have an implant that may be affected by the magnetic field. This includes medical devices such as pacemakers, spring-loaded aneurysm clips, cochlear implants, some recently inserted stents or plates, and foreign bodies such as shrapnel or occupationally acquired orbital metal fragments. However, some other implants and clips are safe and in all cases local staff will be able to advise.

Strict rules must also apply to the design and use of other equipment, such as trolleys or wheelchairs, and even small mundane objects such as scissors or pens can become high velocity projectiles if inadvertently carried into the magnetic field. Medical equipment such as ventilators and monitors must be modified or kept out of the scanner room.

CT techniques and applications

> CT scanning remains of great value in clinical neuroradiology practice, despite not offering the image clarity of MRI. Its ease of use and reliability for detecting acute haemorrhage, hydrocephalus and mass effect ensure it is still the technique of first choice for most emergency cranial imaging. A diagnostic brain scan can be acquired in 10 seconds scanning time and less than 5 minutes table time on a modern CT scanner.

Modern CT scanners consist of an x-ray tube and multiple detector arrays arranged in rings that rotate as the patient is moved through the scanner gantry on a mobile table ('multislice CT'). High resolution reformatted images can be made in different planes and a bolus of contrast medium can be 'chased' through different circulatory phases in CT angiography or venography.

Tissue density is expressed in Hounsfield units (HU), by convention ranging from −1000 to +1000 with water (including normal CSF) having a Hounsfield value of zero. Any substance denser than water will have a higher HU value and appear brighter than CSF on a brain scan and anything less

dense, such as fat or air, will appear darker. Oedema and the centre of cavitated lesions appear darker than normal brain parenchyma. Acute thrombus is denser than brain tissue or flowing blood, and therefore recent haemorrhage and thrombosed vessels appear bright on CT.

Once a scan has been acquired, the images can be manipulated to show different tissues, with window settings varied accordingly. Brain window settings are best centred on 40 HU with a width of around 80 HU for the cerebrum and slightly wider for the posterior fossa. Narrowing the width to around 40 HU exaggerates different tissue densities, which increases the conspicuity of early infarcts and is therefore useful in acute stroke imaging. However, it also produces much coarser images that are less sensitive for some smaller lesions. Window settings are changed at the touch of a button on the viewer keyboard, and it is routine practice to review the same image at more than one setting. Unlike CT, which uses set window values, in MRI, brightness can be altered by the observer to highlight any features of interest variably between scans.

Angiography

MR and computed tomography angiography (CTA) have greatly reduced the need for invasive digital subtraction catheter angiography (DSA). DSA requires an arterial puncture, bed rest for several hours afterwards and carries up to 5 per cent risk of groin haematoma and occasionally arterial damage at the puncture site. **The risk stroke from DSA is at least 1 per cent in patients with ischaemic cerebrovascular disease or atheroma in the great vessels.** After subarachnoid haemorrhage (SAH), the risk of permanent stroke is smaller (nearer 1:1000 in one large series), but there is still an approximately 1 per cent incidence of transient neurological symptoms.

> CTA should now be the first investigation after SAH, with DSA reserved for clarifying aneurysm anatomy in selected cases or after a negative CTA. Coiled cerebral aneurysms can be satisfactorily followed on unenhanced magnetic resonance angiography (MRA).

Currently, only DSA provides the spatial and temporal resolution necessary for detailed assessment of arteriovenous malformations (AVM). In due course, CT and MRI will contribute more in this area. It should always be possible to diagnose intracranial venous thrombosis and cervical arterial dissection using non-invasive techniques without recourse to DSA. Occasionally, DSA is used to plan embolization of tumours.

Myelography and cisternography

Myelography is still occasionally required when a patient has a pacemaker or there is another contraindication to MRI. Cisternography is used to investigate a CSF leak if the source is not apparent on MRI or high resolution skull base CT. For either procedure, a fluoroscopically guided lumbar or lateral cervical puncture allows introduction of contrast medium into the subarachnoid space, followed by a CT scan of the relevant part. Cisternography should only be performed if there is a persistent CSF leak at the time of the procedure.

Contrast media

CT contrast media contain iodinated compounds that are relatively radiodense. In central nervous system (CNS) imaging, MR contrast media are chelates of gadolinium. There is normal enhancement of flowing blood and structures normally lacking a blood–brain barrier (BBB). Diseases that cause disruption of the BBB allow contrast media to enter the extracellular space, producing tissue enhancement on imaging (Box 4.2).

Life-threatening allergic reactions to injected contrast media are now very rare. The risk of exacerbating renal impairment with injudicious use of iodinated contrast media has long been recognized. However, an association has recently been recognized between nephrogenic systemic fibrosis and previous administration of gadolinium-based contrast media to patients in severe renal failure. The need for contrast media of any sort should be carefully considered in patients with renal impairment.

Radiation exposure

X-ray based imaging modalities should be avoided when not strictly necessary. Sometimes the information required can be obtained by other means, namely MRI, ultrasound, or in some circumstances a more experienced clinical opinion. This particularly applies in children, young adults and women of reproductive age. In practice, the benefits of imaging almost always outweigh dose considerations in neuroimaging, particularly in emergency situations.

CLINICAL APPLICATIONS

Head injury

Acute extradural or subdural haemorrhages are readily shown on CT, the latter often associated with severe underlying brain injury. Extradural haemorrhages are constrained by the dural attachment at skull sutures and therefore biconvex. Subdural collections are not so limited and can extend over the whole cerebral surface. Both types appear bright when acute. Chronic subdural collections are frequently a mixture of recent haemorrhage and older fluid that is dark, often within thick, vascularized membranes. If they are bilateral, there may be symmetrical brain compression and no midline shift.

Severe brain swelling or midline shift may obliterate basal cisterns and cause coning at the tentorial hiatus or foramen magnum as the brain herniates downwards (Figures 4.5, 4.6 and 4.7). Patients who recover are often left with occipital infarcts from vascular compression.

In diffuse axonal injury, there may be little to see acutely on CT scans, other than mild brain swelling and generally diminished grey-white differentiation. Small areas of white matter haemorrhage may be seen close to the corticomedullary junction and in the corpus callosum. In more severe cases, there may be lesions in the basal ganglia and brainstem.

Box 4.2 Normal structures on brain MRI that show contrast enhancement

Blood vessels
Meninges
Pituitary gland and stalk
Pineal body
Choroid plexus
Paranasal sinus mucosa
Extraocular muscles and optic sheath

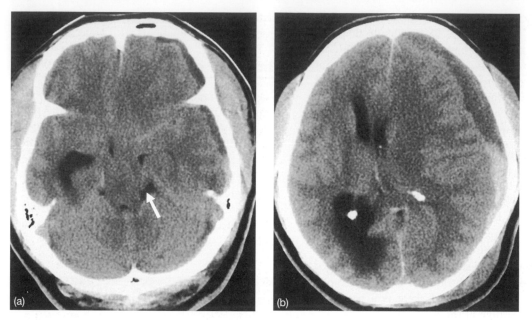

Figure 4.5 Subdural haematoma with midline shift and tentorial pressure cone. Unenhanced axial CT brain scans on a 30-year-old man with a 3-week history of progressive headache and reduced conscious level on the day of presentation. There is a subacute subdural haematoma over the left cerebral hemisphere that contains a mixture of bright thrombus posteriorly and lower density, darker fluid anteriorly. There is compression of the left cerebral hemisphere with shift of midline structures to the right and right-sided hydrocephalus due to obstruction at foramen of Munro. The left uncus has herniated over the tentorial edge and is compressing the left side of the brainstem (arrow). The basal cisterns around the brainstem are obliterated (compare with **Figure 4.1**).

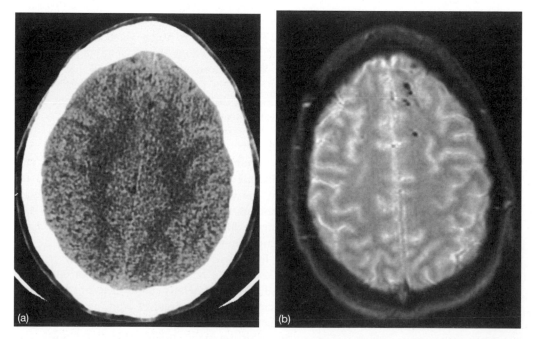

Figure 4.6 Head injury. (a) Axial CT and (b) T2 gradient echo MRI. The brain appears unremarkable on CT. This MRI sequence is very sensitive to haemorrhage which appears low signal. There are foci of haemorrhagic shearing injury in the left superior frontal gyrus.

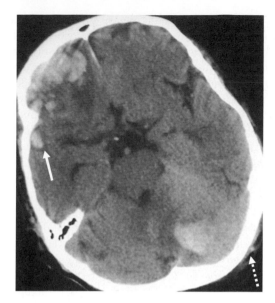

Figure 4.7 Unenhanced axial CT brain scan showing the typical appearance of contracoup haemorrhagic contusions on the orbital surface of the right frontal lobe and at the right temporal pole (arrow). The patient suffered an impact injury to the back of the head on the left and there is haemorrhage in the left cerebellar hemisphere with overlying scalp swelling (dotted arrow).

Fractures of the skull vault or base may also be apparent. Images should be inspected for intracranial air indicating a compound fracture, usually through a paranasal sinus or mastoid air space.

The late effects of head injury include focal and generalized cerebral atrophy, areas of superficial cortical scarring and white matter lesions. Other than global atrophy, these are generally easier to see on MRI.

Cerebrovascular disease

Intracranial haemorrhage

Acute haemorrhage appears brighter than normal brain on CT and is usually readily diagnosed, although a small volume subarachnoid haemorrhage may produce only subtle changes (Figure 4.8). As blood clot is broken down, its density reduces. After a week or so, it becomes isodense with surrounding brain tissue and lower density after about 3 weeks, although high density persists for longer at the centre of a large clot. A small haemorrhage may be indistinguishable from a cerebral infarct after 7–10 days.

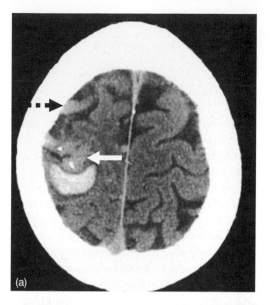

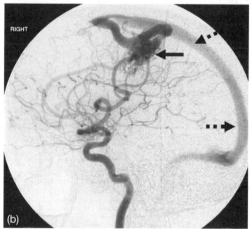

Figure 4.8 Haemorrhage from an arteriovenous malformation. (a) Unenhanced axial CT brain scan shows a small, crescent-shaped acute haematoma in the right parietal lobe immediately behind an AVM nidus (arrow) which contains two dense foci of calcification. The nidus is slightly denser than normal brain tissue. The draining vein is also visible (dotted arrow). (b) DSA via injection into the right internal carotid artery shows the nidus (arrow) supplied from below by hypertrophied branches of the right middle cerebral artery and draining via a single enlarged vein upwards to opacify the superior sagittal sinus (dotted arrows).

The appearance and evolution of haemorrhage on MRI is more complex, and routine sequences are less sensitive than CT acutely. After 3 days, conversion to methaemoglobin begins and the clot becomes bright on T1-weighted scans. The chronic state is haemosiderin, which is dark on all MRI sequences. Susceptibility weighted sequences have high sensitivity for blood products.

On CT, an acute parenchymal haematoma is usually uniformly dense, although a hyperacute haemorrhage may contain areas of lower density unclotted blood. Fluid levels are seen in coagulopathies and after haemorrhage into a pre-existing cavity. There is normally only a thin halo of low density around an acute haemorrhage due to clot retraction and brain injury. Surrounding vasogenic oedema develops over subsequent days with increasing mass effect, but extensive oedema on the day of haemorrhage is suggestive of an underlying tumour. Blood products of different densities may be seen in haemorrhage from a tumour or vascular malformation. Both entities may be associated with calcification, the latter in serpiginous or curvilinear form when in the walls of vessels, which will also enhance if contrast is given. However, contrast enhancement is usually unnecessary initially and for several weeks afterwards there is normally enhancement of the haematoma cavity rim regardless of the cause, due to BBB disruption. If follow-up imaging is required, MRI a few weeks later is preferable, once mass effect has subsided, in order to assess residual brain injury, and to look for microbleeds or other haemorrhagic lesions and associated ischaemic changes.

In hypertensive patients, haemorrhages commonly occur in the basal ganglia/external capsule, thalamus, pons and cerebellum. Peripheral haemorrhages are associated with amyloid angiopathy.

This mirrors the distribution of microbleeds shown on gradient echo MRI. MRA or CTA may be used to diagnose an AVM and show its gross architecture, but currently, DSA is still required for treatment planning, and also to confidently exclude a small AVM or fistula in younger patients. The characteristics of an AVM are one or more enlarged feeding arteries and draining veins, with a nidus of variable definition. On DSA, draining veins opacify early, as shunting through an AVM bypasses the capillary circulation. Arterial or venous aneurysms are commonly associated abnormailities.

Cavernous haemangiomas (cavernomas) are capillary malformations arising anywhere in the CNS. They may be single or less commonly multiple, the latter sometimes familial. They can be found incidentally or present with haemorrhage or seizures. Typically, they are round with heterogeneous signal characteristics on MRI and a surrounding dark rim due to chronic leakage of haemosiderin. CT often shows calcification. Occasionally, following repeated haemorrhages, they enlarge with multiple cavities containing blood-fluid levels and may be confused with neoplasms.

Cavernomas are angiographically occult. They are often colocated with a developmental venous anomaly (DVA or 'venous angioma'). This variant in venous anatomy consists of a caput of vessels that converge on a single vein draining towards a normal venous sinus. They are not a pathological malformation in their own right. Although an associated cavernoma could cause symptoms, the DVA itself is asymptomatic and ligation would cause a venous infarct. A DVA can usually be diagnosed on routine MRI but, if in doubt, the characteristic arrangement of veins is clearly seen following contrast enhancement. DSA is not required to make this diagnosis.

Subarachnoid haemorrhage

Acute subarachnoid haemorrhage (SAH) is due to an aneurysm in around 75 per cent of cases, a vascular malformation in 5–10 per cent and in 15-20 per cent angiography does not show a cause.

In aneurysmal SAH, blood is visible in the basal cisterns, which become bright on CT (Figures 4.9, 4.10 and 4.11). Asymmetrical blood distribution or a sentinel clot sometimes indicates the likely site of origin, although in many cases haemorrhage extends diffusely in the fissures and cerebral sulci. In larger volume haemorrhages, there is usually intraventricular blood and hydrocephalus. **The sensitivity of CT for detecting SAH is around 95 per cent at 12 hours after the ictus, but this falls rapidly as the blood is broken down and diluted by CSF, to only 75 per cent by the third day.** In patients with a suggestive history but normal CT scan, lumbar puncture can be used to examine

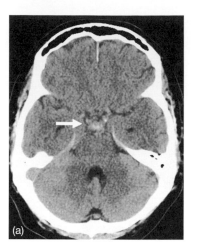
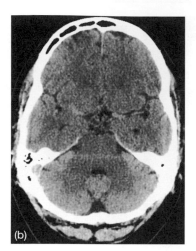
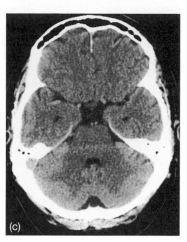

Figure 4.9 Perimesencephalic subarachnoid haemorrhage. Unenhanced axial CT brain scans on days 1, 2 and 4 (a, b and c, respectively) after a sudden onset, persisting meningitic headache. The patient was neurologically intact. The first scan shows a small volume of high density blood around the upper basilar artery in the typical distribution of the 'perimesencephalic syndrome' (arrow). Note that 24 hours later the blood is no longer clearly visible and there is only subtle loss of clarity of the basal cisterns that could easily be overlooked. By day 4, the scan is normal with uniformly dark CSF in the basal cisterns. Subsequent angiography was normal. A larger subarachnoid haemorrhage would remain visible on CT for longer but this small volume haemorrhage demonstrates the rapidly decline in sensitivity of CT within a few days in some cases.

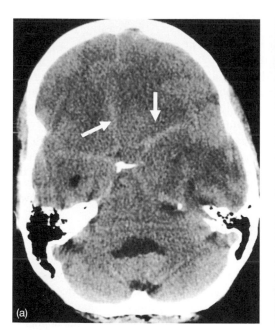
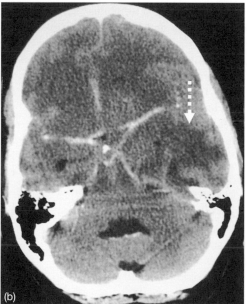

Figure 4.10 (a) Axial CT before and after contrast medium shows 'pseudosubarachnoid haemorrhage' due to severe brain swelling. There is increased density in the Sylvian fissures and interhemispheric fissure that could be mistaken for SAH (arrows). (b) Following contrast, there is enhancement confirming these are vessels surrounded by swollen brain. There is also oedema in the left temporal lobe (dark area; dotted arrow). This was due to a tumour (on higher slices; not shown).

the CSF for blood, though sometimes, when clinically appropriate, MRI is preferable in the first instance (e.g. if venous thrombosis is suspected). Unfortunately, a traumatic tap with inadequate

examination of the CSF for xanthochromia is a commonly encountered scenario, and the three tube test is unreliable. The lack of a definitive negative result sometimes commits the patient to vascular

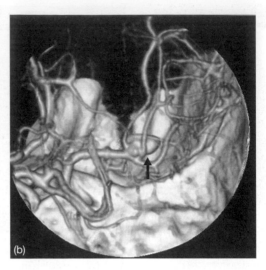

Figure 4.11 Ruptured middle cerebral artery aneurysm. Unenhanced axial CT brain and intracranial CT angiogram. (a) There is a haematoma in the right temporal lobe and diffuse subarachnoid haemorrhage (arrows). (b) The CTA shows a lobulated aneurysm at the main trifurcation of the right middle cerebral artery, viewed from behind (arrow).

imaging, which is particularly regrettable, as in this situation angiography is usually negative. Careful attention to lumbar puncture technique avoids unnecessary investigations and the risk of iatrogenic stroke from catheter angiography.

A high sensitivity for SAH is claimed for MRI. It may show haemorrhage days or weeks after it becomes occult on CT but there are persisting issues with artefacts that hamper confident interpretation, particularly related to physiological CSF movement around the brainstem.

> CTA is now preferred to DSA as the first investigation after SAH. Despite persisting scepticism, it has rapidly gained widespread acceptance for its ease of use, high sensitivity in expert hands, and absence of stroke risk. CTA is usually sufficient to triage aneurysms between clipping and coiling with DSA available to clarify anatomy in selected cases.

It is possible to achieve sensitivities higher than 95 per cent for ruptured aneurysms, but occasionally lesions are missed, so it remains routine practice in most centres to confirm a negative CTA result with DSA. Aneurysms sited peripherally or close to the skull base are more likely to be missed on CTA. Even DSA has less than perfect sensitivity, due to vasospasm or perception errors, so it is

common practice to repeat a negative study if the distribution of haemorrhage on CT is suggestive of a ruptured aneurysm. The sensitivity of CTA is observer-dependent and lower outside specialist centres.

The 'perimesencephalic syndrome' comprises a small blood load limited to the region around the basilar artery and upper brainstem in a patient who is neurologically intact. Angiography is typically negative and the risk of further haemorrhage no higher than the general population. Evidence is accumulating that an aneurysm can reliably be excluded in this group on CTA alone.

Ischaemic stroke

There has been a revolution in stroke imaging, alongside the introduction of thrombolysis and acute stroke units (Figures 4.12, 4.13 and 4.14). CT is still widely used for early stroke imaging, primarily to rule out acute haemorrhage or other common stroke mimics, but large infarcts are often visible even within an hour or two of onset. Advanced techniques may help to refine patient selection for thrombolysis, but availability is limited and increasing imaging time delays treatment.

Non-lacunar middle cerebral artery territory infarcts within 3 hours of onset can be detected on CT with sensitivity up to 80 per cent. CT is much less useful for detecting a new lacunar infarct in

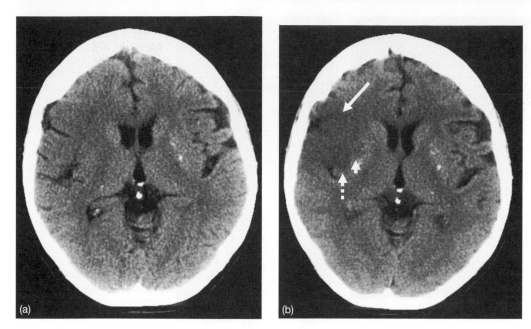

Figure 4.12 Acute infarct. Unenhanced axial CT brain scans show an acute infarct at 2 and 22 hours after symptom onset (a and b, respectively). There is reduced density in right frontal lobe (solid arrow) and insula cortex (dotted arrow) causing loss of normal grey-white differentiation compared with the left. The putamen is also affected (short arrow). The changes are barely visible on the presenting scan but much more obvious the following day due to increased oedema. This has also caused mild swelling with effacement of sulci in the affected area. Note punctuate bright areas in the basal ganglia on both scans are incidental calcification.

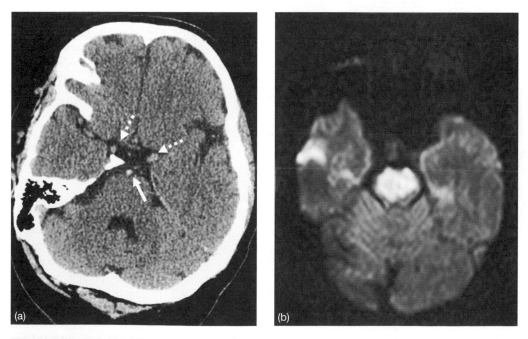

Figure 4.13 Basilar thrombosis. (a) Unenhanced axial CT brain scan shows the basilar artery is abnormally dense due to acute thrombus (arrow) compared with the normal internal carotid arteries (dotted arrows). No ischaemic change is visible on CT but diffusion weighted MRI (b) shows high signal in the pons due to a large infarct.

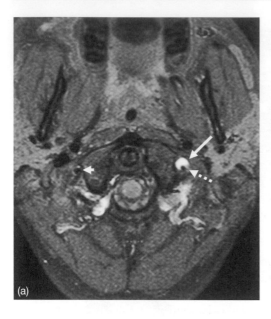

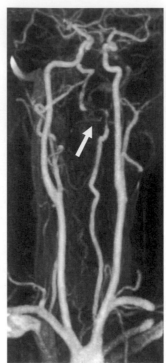

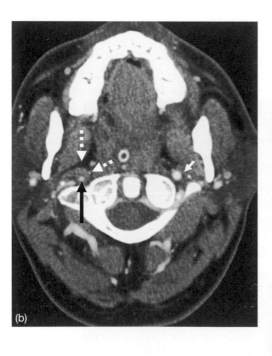

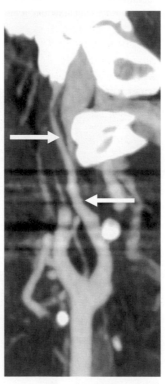

Figure 4.14 (a) Acute vertebral artery dissection. Axial T1-weighted scan with fat suppression at C1 level. Fat signal is nulled making the background dark. This increases conspicuity of bright mural thrombus in the left vertebral artery within its foramen transversarium (arrow). The eccentric patent lumen is dark (dotted arrow). This appearance is diagnostic of dissection. The normal right vertebral artery returns black flow void (short arrow) and there is no mural thickening. The corresponding contrast enhanced MR angiogram shows the great vessels from the aortic arch to the circle of Willis. There is focal narrowing of the left vertebral artery at C1 (arrow). (b) Acute internal carotid artery dissection. CT angiogram; axial source image at C1 shows eccentric enhancing lumen (long arrow) surrounded by a crescent of non-enhancing mural thrombus (dotted arrows), analogous to the appearance on MRI and diagnostic of acute right internal carotid artery dissection. The left internal carotid artery is normal calibre without mural thickening (short arrow). Sagittal maximum intensity projection of the right carotid bifurcation shows a tapered 'rat tail' stenosis from slightly above the bifurcation to the skull base (arrows).

the presence of pre-existing subcortical ischaemic changes, and infarcts at any stage are poorly shown in the brainstem. Thus, CT has very low sensitivity for acute stroke when all subtypes are included.

Diffusion-weighted MRI is by far the most sensitive imaging technique for the detection of acute infarction, whereas routine structural MRI sequences add little to CT acutely.

Occlusive thrombus may be appreciable on CT from the time of onset as a 'hyperdense artery sign'. The early autoregulatory response to reduced cerebral perfusion causes expansion of the vascular bed and an increase in cerebral blood volume (CBV) that is measurable on MR or CT perfusion imaging. With progression towards infarction, CBV falls and cells begin to swell, the latter causing a reduction in volume of the extracellular space. This restricts water diffusion and is visible within minutes as high signal on DWI and dark on a corresponding ADC map. This is almost always irreversible. As oedema develops, grey matter becomes darker on CT with loss of grey–white differentiation and effacement of sulci. On T2-weighted MRI, acute infarcts return high signal. Early ischaemic changes on CT or MRI other than DWI are very subtle, and the clinical localization of an infarct is a useful guide when interpreting the scan.

The concept of mismatch is useful when triaging patients for thrombolysis. Mismatch is the difference between the irretrievable core infarct and surrounding ischaemic penumbra. The aim of thrombolysis is reperfusion of the penumbra before it also infarcts. Tissue already infarcted is shown on DWI, but as CBV is also diminished, CT perfusion data provide a practical surrogate for diffusion-weighted MRI. The wider perfusion deficit on a mean transit time map or equivalent indicates the penumbra, and this predicts the potential final infarct size without spontaneous or therapeutic reperfusion. Matched defects are said to exist when core and penumbra are congruent, and apart from rare anecdotal exceptions indicate no residual salvageable ischaemic tissue.

Around half of transient ischaemic attacks (TIAs) will show an abnormality on DWI, which if positive confirms the ischaemic basis of the clinical event. It also demonstrates that radiologically, stroke and TIA are part of the same spectrum. Haemorrhage is not reliably detected on DWI, so if MRI is used for acute stroke imaging, a T2-weighted gradient echo sequence providing equivalent sensitivity to CT must be acquired.

However, it is also possible to use non-contrast CT without advanced techniques for brain imaging prior to thrombolysis. For cortical strokes clinical assessment and stroke scores indicate the likely penumbra. Most patients with a significant clinical deficit due to middle cerebral artery territory ischaemia will only have a small completed infarct at the time of imaging if the presenting CT scan is normal. Lacunar or brainstem infarcts can cause a major clinical deficit without being visible on CT, but these lesions are much smaller in volume and there is less risk of bleeding after thrombolysis.

As the infarcted tissue loses its structural integrity, water diffusivity increases, and at around 4–10 days the diffusion imaging characteristics reverse, becoming low signal on DWI and bright on the ADC map. There is a transient intervening period of 'pseudonormalization' which can render small lesions undetectable on DWI, although large infarcts tend to change non-uniformly and will still be appreciable.

The BBB is disrupted after an infarct and it is normal for contrast medium to cause enhancement within a few days of onset that persists for 2–3 months. Cortical infarcts usually show a gyriform pattern of enhancement and this is also appreciable on CT. Swelling of large infarcts should be maximal at around a week with atrophy developing by 3–4 weeks. Persisting mass effect after this time should prompt reassessment of the diagnosis.

Vascular imaging is normally required after stroke or TIA, although only a minority are associated with >50 per cent stenoses in the neck vessel, around 11 per cent for anterior circulation strokes and 25 per cent in the posterior circulation. Doppler ultrasound is a convenient means of examining the carotid bifurcations but offers limited views of the neck vessels more generally and has very low sensitivity for vertebral artery stenosis. Contrast enhanced MRA or CTA show the great vessels from the aortic arch to the circle of Willis and are less operator dependent than ultrasound.

The choice partly depends on local resources, with all three modalities having similar sensitivity in experienced hands for diagnosing clinically significant carotid bifurcation disease. Contrast enhanced MRA, and to a slightly lesser degree CTA, have much higher sensitivity for detecting stenoses at other sites, particularly in the vertebral arteries and intracranial vessels. Thus ultrasound is often first choice for carotid disease, and MRA or CTA for posterior circulation strokes.

In many centres, a positive finding of stenosis is confirmed on another modality prior to intervention. Carotid plaque imaging to stratify stroke risk is a current area of research. Intraplaque haemorrhage and lipid accumulation appear to be adverse risk factors.

The historical 'gold standard' for neck vessel imaging is DSA but this carries a stroke risk of at least 1 per cent when performed for investigation of stroke or TIA and it should not be used for first-line screening of stroke patients. DSA is still occasionally necessary for clarification, more commonly now at the vertebral origins than the carotid bifurcation.

The cardinal sign on cross-sectional imaging of acute arterial dissection is vessel expansion with a crescent of mural thrombus and an eccentrically placed lumen. In internal carotid dissection that extends to the skull base, this is readily visible on the lowermost slice of routine T2-weighted axial brain scans without recourse to special sequences. If in doubt, fat suppressed axial scans through the neck are often diagnostic. The classical angiographic sign of a 'rat's tail' tapered occlusion is often appreciable on CTA or MRA, however in some cases dissection causes little if any luminal narrowing, hence the importance of imaging the vessel wall. Follow up imaging often shows resolution, although some vessel irregularity can persist and false aneurysms may develop. Vertebral artery dissection produces similar signs but can be more difficult to diagnose as the vessels are smaller. The appearance on CTA is analogous, with vessel expansion and a patent eccentric lumen surrounded by non-enhancing mural thrombus.

Venous thrombosis

Acute thrombosed venous sinuses appear dense on non-contrast CT and are often expanded. A confident diagnosis can be made when these signs are present. However, CT is less sensitive for excluding venous thrombosis, particularly when subacute, as the density of thrombus falls within days. Following contrast medium the sinus lumen will not enhance but the surrounding dura does. On MRI, the normal black signal void from flowing blood is lost in a thrombosed sinus.

MR or CT venography are definitive and are useful for a full assessment of the intracranial veins and as a baseline for follow up imaging. Venous oedema or infarction conforms to venous rather than arterial territories: parafalcine for the superior sagittal sinus, lateral temporal for the transverse sinus and thalamic for the deep veins. Areas of restricted diffusion may resolve in venous ischaemia, which in practice very rarely happens after arterial occlusion. Venous infarcts are commonly haemorrhagic.

DSA is no longer required to diagnose either arterial dissection or venous thrombosis.

Small vessel disease

Small vessel disease causes a mixture of ischaemic demyelination, gliosis, lacunar infarcts and microbleeds in cerebral white matter, deep nuclei and pons (Figure 4.15). It is best shown on T2-weighted or FLAIR sequences as small dots or larger irregular patches of high signal. Lacunar cavities are dark centrally on FLAIR imaging. Microbleeds are shown on T2-weighted gradient echo scans as small dots of signal void in 5–6 per cent of all older people and a quarter of those with extensive small vessel disease. Acute lacunar infarcts are usually only distinguishable from background changes on DWI and occasionally asymptomatic acute lesions are found coincidentally.

Age is the strongest risk factor and hypertension is also an associated factor. **Less than 5 per cent of those over 65 years have no ischaemic lesions on MRI.** A third of over 65s without a history of stroke or TIA will have at least one asymptomatic infarct or haemorrhage. Most people have relatively mild disease, and ischaemic change on a scan done for cognitive impairment is not in itself proof positive of 'vascular dementia'. However, very extensive changes are associated with cognitive decline, depression and rarer vasculopathies such as CADASIL (Chapter 23) are strongly associated with dementia.

Small vessel vasculitis can be indistinguishable on MRI from age-related ischaemic change. Imaging evidence of activity, such as excessive meningeal enhancement or repeated acute events, is helpful in differentiating when present. Vasculitis may produce multiple stenoses and vessel beading, which are sometimes visible on MRA or CTA. DSA is more sensitive but frequently negative and even if stenoses are shown the appearance is often non-specific. In practice, DSA is not helpful as a diagnostic test for vasculitis as it is neither specific or sensitive.

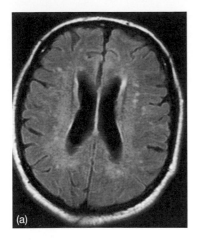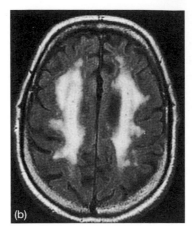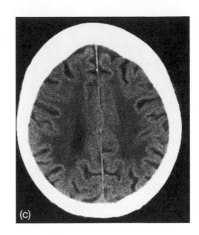

Figure 4.15 Ischaemic white matter lesions in two different patients. FLAIR axial image (a) shows only a few small bright dots due to mild ischaemic white matter disease. (b) and (c) Severe white matter involvement that causes diffuse high signal on FLAIR MRI and low density on non-contrast CT.

A few small dots of high signal in cerebral white matter on T2-weighted MRI are common findings in young adults and even children. These are non-specific and usually incidental. It is not helpful, or in most cases accurate, to dismiss them as 'small vessel disease', which in the young requires further investigation.

Demyelination, infection, inflammatory conditions

For all these conditions, MRI is far superior to CT (Figures 4.16, 4.17 and 4.18). Diffusion weighted imaging should be acquired and may show changes earlier than structural sequences. Contrast enhanced imaging may contribute but other than in conditions such as sarcoidosis that thicken the meninges it is of little value if the unenhanced scans are normal.

Multiple sclerosis is one of the most common neurological diseases investigated on imaging and it produces multiple CNS lesions, mainly in white matter. However, incidental white matter lesions are common on MRI. Therefore, specific diagnostic criteria must be satisfied, based on the clinical context, the number of lesions and location, particularly juxtacortical, periventricular, infratentorial or in the spinal cord.

Dissemination in time can be confirmed by an enhancing MRI lesion at least three months after a first clinical event, or a new T2 lesion on follow up imaging.

Acute lesions are often ovoid with a T2 hyperintense centre and a halo of milder signal change. Any enhancement only persists for a few weeks. Over time they regress leaving smaller, well-defined scars. Disability is more strongly associated with residual 'black holes' on T1-weighted scans than the extent of T2 abnormality. The disease process is not confined to visible focal lesions. Diffuse white matter atrophy also occurs, and advanced techniques such as diffusion tensor imaging and spectroscopy confirm abnormality of the normal appearing white matter.

Optic nerve signal change, swelling and sometimes enhancement are features of optic neuritis. The risk of developing multiple sclerosis correlates with the number of associated brain lesions. Occasionally, demyelination produces tumour-like lesions, although sequential imaging will show regression over several weeks.

Vasculitides, such as SLE, produce focal lesions that are sometimes indistinguishable from demyelination, although cord involvement is less common and there may be multiple infarcts that indicate the likely diagnosis. In neurosarcoidosis, white matter lesions are usually more suggestive of ischaemia and occasionally multiple acute infarcts are seen. Contrast enhanced scans should be acquired, as enhancing granulomas and meningeal thicken-

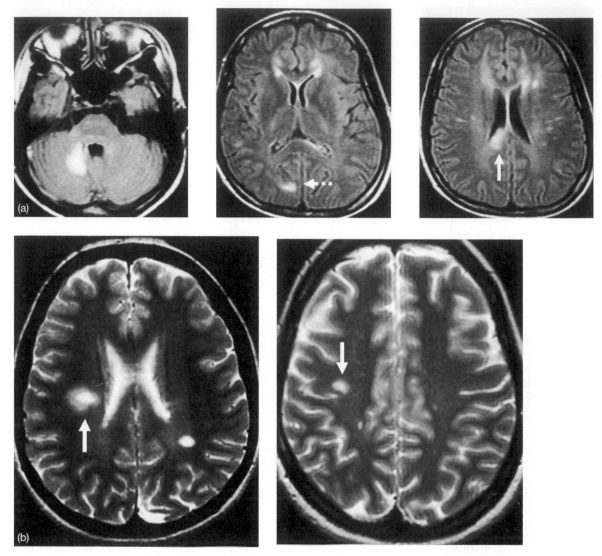

Figure 4.16 (a) SLE. Axial FLAIR images show widespread high signal lesions in cerebral white matter including corpus callosum (arrow), juxtacortical white matter (dotted arrow) and cerebellum. (b) Multiple sclerosis. Axial T2-weighted scans in two different patients. On the left, there are bilateral white matter lesions and an acute plaque with inflammatory halo creating a 'target' lesion (arrow). The right hand image shows a juxtacortical plaque (arrow) and a few smaller dots elsewhere. Note the similarity between the two sets of scans.

ing are typical features. There may be associated hydrocephalus.

A pyogenic cerebral abscess appears on CT or MRI as a cavitated ring-enhancing lesion surrounded by white matter oedema. Abscesses are usually thin-walled and may have adjacent 'daughter' lesions. Other infections can produce a similar appearance including toxoplasmosis or fungal infections in immunocompromised patients. Haemorrhage may occur in either type of lesion, leading to infarction. Tuberculosis also produces

ring lesions. However, the caseous material in tuberculomas is usually dark on T2-weighted MRI, unlike pus in an abscess which returns high signal. In tuberculous meningitis there is often a thick layer of enhancing material in the basal cisterns, causing hydrocephalus and infarcts. The affected cisterns often appear dense on unenhanced CT. The spinal cord may also be affected.

CT is relatively insensitive for early diagnosis of viral encephalitis and less specific than MRI, which is the investigation of choice. Grey matter involve-

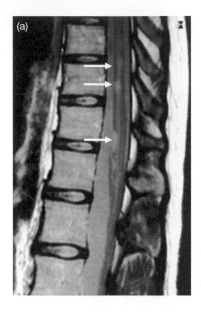

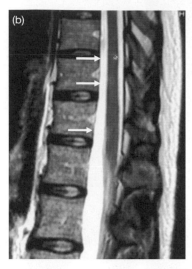

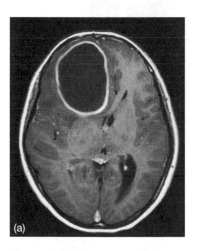

Figure 4.17 Spinal cord imaging in multiple sclerosis. Proton density and T2-weighted sagittal images. High signal plaques in the lower spinal cord are more conspicuous on the proton density scan (arrows).

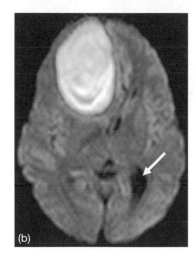

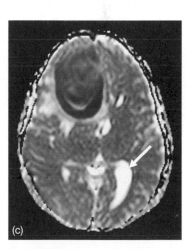

Figure 4.18 Abscess on diffusion weighted imaging. (a) Axial MRI T1-weighted post-contrast, (b) DWI and (c) ADC map. There is a large right frontal cavitated lesion with a thin rim of enhancement. The contents are very high signal on DWI and dark on the ADC map indicating restricted diffusion which is typical of a pyogenic abscess. The diagnosis was confirmed at surgery. Free diffusion, for example within the left lateral ventricle, produces low signal on DWI and is bright on ADC (arrow).

ment is usually more conspicuous initially. There may be restricted diffusion, enhancement and, in severe cases, haemorrhagic necrosis. Although no radiological appearance is pathognomonic for a particular organism, herpes simplex encephalitis is typically bilateral but asymmetrical, affecting temporal, frontal and insular cortex. Enteroviruses may involve the brainstem. Changes restricted to the mesial temporal structures may be due to paraneoplastic or autoimmune limbic encephalitis.

Sporadic Creutzfeldt–Jakob disease (CJD) involves the basal ganglia, sometimes accompanied by milder signal abnormality in the thalami and cortex. Diffusion weighted imaging is more sensitive than other MRI sequences. Contrast enhancement is of no value. The variant form of CJD principally affects the pulvinar nuclei of the thalami.

Tumours

Metastases and gliomas are the most common adult intrinsic brain tumours (Figures 4.19, 4.20

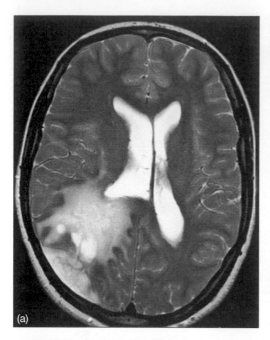
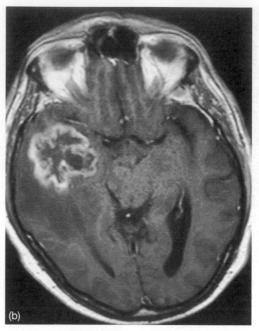

Figure 4.19 Gliomas in two different patients. On the left, an axial T2-weighted scan shows a diffusely infiltrating WHO grade 2 astrocytoma in the right parietal lobe that crosses the corpus callosum. There is some cystic degeneration within the tumour but no enhancement was shown on other sequences. On the right, axial T1-weighted post contrast medium shows a glioblastoma multiforme in the right temporal lobe with irregular peripheral enhancement and surrounding oedema which appears dark on T1 imaging. Typically in gliomas the tumour infiltrates beyond the area of enhancement.

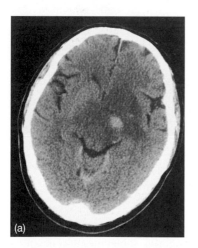
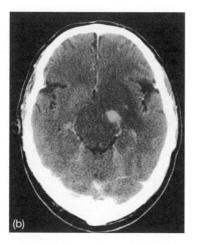
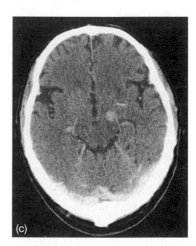

Figure 4.20 Primary cerebral lymphoma. CT scans before and after contrast medium (left and middle) show a hyperdense subthalamic mass that uniformly enhances, surrounded by low density due to oedema. The contrast enhanced CT scan on the right was obtained 6 days later after steroid therapy. There has been shrinkage of enhancing tumour and resolution of oedema and mass effect. The appearance is typical of lymphoma and this dramatic response to steroids is not seen in other tumours.

and 4.21). Glioblastoma multiforme (GBM) occurs at any age but more frequently in older adults. It is highly malignant, often large with an irregular enhancing rim and central necrosis. There is usually surrounding oedema and frequently haemorrhage.

Occasionally, GBM may be confused with an infarct if presenting early with seizures when not yet necrotic. History and rapid progression on follow-up imaging are diagnostic. A round GBM may be indistinguishable from a solitary metastasis.

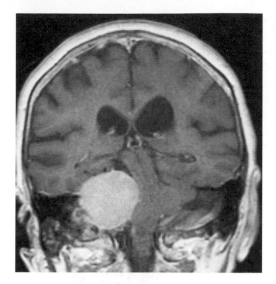

Figure 4.21 Meningioma. Coronal T1-weighted following intravenous contrast shows a large extra-axial mass in the right side of the posterior cranial fossa that displaces the brainstem to the left. The appearance is typical of a meningioma.

Multiple brain tumours are usually metastases. A glioma sometimes appears 'multifocal', although in reality it is a diffuse lesion. By far the most common cerebellar tumour in adults is a metastasis. Metastases are typically round with solid or ring enhancement and white matter oedema. They are frequently haemorrhagic. Small cortical lesions may be missed without contrast enhanced scans. Common primary tumours include lung, breast, gastrointestinal tract and melanoma.

Low grade gliomas occur in younger adults, usually frontal or temporal, and are predominantly astrocytomas, which have a rather bland appearance without necrosis or oedema. Oligodendrogliomas are rarer, usually cortical and often quite heterogeneous, with haemorrhage and calcification.

Infratentorial gliomas and brainstem tumours of any sort are much rarer in adults than children. The most common cerebellar primary tumour in adults is a haemangioblastoma, which is typically cystic with an enhancing nodule and enlarged adjacent vessels.

Primary CNS lymphoma is typically a disease of older adults, producing solid periventricular lesions that appear hyperdense on non-contrast CT, enhance strongly and frequently show dra-matic radiological regression within a few days of commencing steroid therapy.

Secondary spread of lymphoma from outside the CNS usually affects the meninges rather than brain parenchyma. Immunosuppressed patients develop lymphoma at a younger age with cavitated lesions that may be indistinguishable from infections such as toxoplasmosis, necessitating biopsy for definitive diagnosis.

Rarely, lymphoma can produce extensive oedema due to perivascular tumour infiltration without a focal mass. Perivascular space enhancement is seen on MRI but is not visible on CT. The differential diagnosis is sarcoidosis.

The most common extra-axial tumour is a meningioma, which may occur anywhere over the brain or spinal cord and rarely in a ventricle. Meningiomas are usually solid and enhancing and may be calcified.

Most sellar region masses are pituitary adenomas which may become large enough to compress the optic chiasm, invade the skull base or occasionally deeply indent the brain and present with epilepsy. Adenomas can invade the cavernous sinuses, although in contrast to meningiomas they do not narrow the internal carotid arteries and cranial nerve palsies are relatively unusual, other than in pituitary apoplexy. MRI is the investigation of choice, although a pituitary adenoma large enough to compress the optic chiasm will be visible on CT. Pituitary tumours may contain haemorrhage or cystic areas. Contrast enhancement is often helpful to identify a microadenoma in Cushing's disease or acromegaly but is not necessary in prolactinomas which are managed medically. Sarcoidosis and histiocytosis can also cause enhancing lesions involving the hypothalamus.

The differential diagnosis for suprasellar masses includes optic pathway glioma and germinoma in younger patients and craniopharyngioma at any age. The latter classically produces a complex lesion with cysts, calcification and enhancing solid tissue.

Conditions that can mimic tumours include infarcts, demyelination, abscesses and cerebral malformations. The gyriform enhancement pattern that develops within a few days of an infarct is usually diagnostic if there is clinical uncertainty and mass effect should regress after a week or two. Demyelination often produces a characteristic, incomplete ring of faint enhancement and there may be other, smaller plaques. Abscesses are not always associated with a history of infection or constitutional disturbance. However, DWI reliably differentiates restricted diffusion of pus from free diffusion of a necrotic tumour. Malformations consist of disordered grey and white matter, usually with appropriate signal characteristics and no enhancement. Occasionally they present in adulthood, although there is usually a history of seizures.

Supratentorial brain tumours are often adequately shown on CT. MRI adds little if CT shows multiple metastases, a typical convexity meningioma or a large GBM in an appropriate clinical setting. However, MRI is indicated when infection is a possibility or for infiltrative tumours that can be rather non-specific in appearance on CT. It is also used for surgical planning in selected cases if anatomy is unclear, for example, when a meningioma lies in proximity to a venous sinus and invasion is a possibility.

Neurodegenerative conditions

The radiological signs of neurodegenerative conditions generally become more obvious and specific with disease progression (Figures 4.22 and 4.23). Traditionally, brain scans were carried out in patients with dementia to rule out 'surgical' conditions such as tumour, subdural collections or hydrocephalus. CT is sufficient and contrast is not required unless a tumour is shown. Positive findings are rare. However, an assessment of atrophy and vascular damage contributes to diagnosis in many more cases. Unenhanced CT remains adequate in most routine clinical circumstances, particularly now that high quality coronal reformat images are possible.

MRI is helpful when the presentation is atypical or the differential diagnosis includes prion disease, which cannot be diagnosed on CT. Small, strategic infarcts are more easily detected on MRI but generalized ischaemic change sufficient to contribute to a global dementing illness is adequately demonstrated on CT. In research, MRI allows automated comparison between scans to detect progression of brain atrophy beyond the limits of visual inspection.

Normal ageing causes minimal cerebral atrophy before around 50 years of age, and only 0.3–0.5 per cent per annum volume loss thereafter. Accurate discrimination between 'normal involution' and excessive atrophy on a single scan is highly subjective. Mild loss of volume in mesial temporal structures may occur, but conspicuous atrophy is not a normal feature. In Alzheimer's disease, whole brain volume reduces at approximately 2 per cent per annum, which may be appreciable on scans a year or two apart, whereas the normal rate of volume loss is only 0.2 per cent per annum and is not detectable on visual inspection over a similar time period.

The pattern of atrophy is important. Alzheimer's disease causes diffuse, symmetrical mesial temporal atrophy which may be visible before dementia is diagnosed and predicts progression from mild cognitive impairment. The rarer posterior cortical variant causes early parieto-occipital atrophy which may be lateralized. Asymmetrical frontotemporal atrophy that is more severe anteriorly is a feature of frontotemporal dementias. Dementia with Lewy bodies typically causes generalized atrophy without conspicuous hippocampal volume loss.

Ventricular enlargement due to cerebral atrophy is sometimes confused with hydrocephalus. Various measurements and advanced imaging tests have been devised to diagnose 'normal pressure hydrocephalus'. None have gained universal acceptance and in many centres patients are selected for ventricular shunt placement if they exhibit the triad of gait disturbance, urinary incontinence and cognitive impairment and their scan shows ventriculomegaly out of proportion to sulcal enlargement.

Atypical Parkinsonian disorders, spinocerebellar atrophies and Huntington's disease cause atrophy patterns and signal changes of differing specificity and sensitivity that are best diagnosed on MRI, with CT being of little value. Huntington's causes characteristic atrophy of the caudate nuclei. Corticobasal degeneration may cause asymmetrical parietal cortical atrophy, appropriately lateralized for the clinical signs. Progressive supranuclear palsy causes disproportionate atrophy of the midbrain. In multiple system atrophy, there is signal change and atrophy of the basal ganglia, brainstem and cerebellum with a cruciate pattern of signal change in the pons which has been likened to a

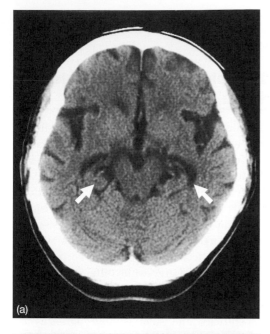

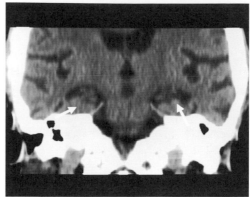

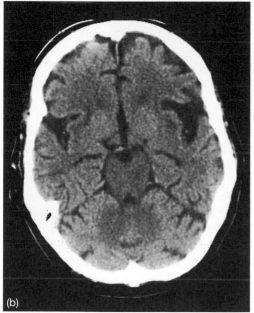

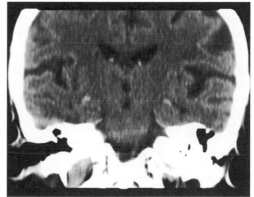

Figure 4.22 Alzheimer's disease. Axial CT with coronal reformat images in two different patients. The top row shows a 79-year-old with a clinical diagnosis of Alzheimer's disease. There is mild generalized cerebral volume loss with disproportionate, symmetrical hippocampal atrophy (arrows). The bottom row shows a cognitively normal 88-year-old. There is less cerebral atrophy and hippocampal volumes are preserved.

'hot cross bun', due to atrophy of pontine nuclei and transverse fibres.

Cranial nerve imaging

Imaging of the internal auditory canals to exclude a vestibular schwannoma is one of the most common indications for cranial MRI, and requires only a short T2-weighted scan without contrast medium.

Similar sequences are often requested in trigeminal neuralgia to show impingement by blood vessels on trigeminal nerves, although this is also a very common asymptomatic finding. Investigation of other cranial neuropathies usually requires detailed views tailored to the clinical indication. Contrast enhancement is often helpful to look for inflammatory changes or infiltration of the nerves and overlying meninges not easily appreciated on

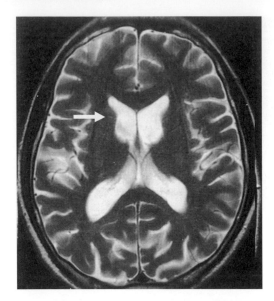

Figure 4.23 Huntington's disease. Axial T2-weighted scan through the basal ganglia in a 40-year-old male with Huntingdon's disease. The brain appears atrophied. There is disproportionate basal ganglia atrophy including the heads of caudate nuclei (arrow; compare with normal scans in **Figure 4.1**).

unenhanced images. Imaging the optic nerves for visual failure can be performed with MRI or CT, the former required to investigate suspected optic neuritis and the latter often preferred for investigation of orbital masses.

Epilepsy

According to the UK National Institute of Health and Clinical Excellence (NICE), all patients after a first seizure should have brain imaging, ideally MRI. More complex imaging protocols are required for epilepsy surgical assessment than for a routine diagnostic screen (Figures 13.1-13.11 in Chapter 13). The most common specific abnormality in adults with intractable epilepsy is hippocampal sclerosis. The affected hippocampus is smaller and brighter than its contralateral fellow on thin slice coronal T2-weighted scans. Adjacent white matter and the amygdala may also be affected. Bilateral sclerosis may be more difficult to detect if the changes are mild and symmetrical. Less commonly, tumours or vascular malformations are shown. Unsurprisingly, there is a higher yield of malformations and subtle cortical dysplasias using higher resolution imaging in specialist centres. Contrast enhanced imaging is not usually required, even

in focal epilepsies, unless a neoplasm is shown on unenhanced scans, or the patient has Sturge-Weber syndrome.

Hydrocephalus and intracranial pressure

The diagnosis of raised intracranial pressure is obvious when a large mass or collection causes shift of midline structures, brain herniation and obliteration of basal cisterns (Figures 4.4 and 4.24). Occasionally on CT in a comatose patient, the vessels and meninges in the basal cisterns appear bright compared with surrounding swollen, oedematous brain, causing a 'pseudosubarachnoid haemorrhage' effect. The clues to the correct diagnosis are diminished grey-white differentiation and the relatively small volume of 'haemorrhage' which would not usually be associated with deep coma. Small ventricles and sulci without parenchymal changes are an unreliable guide to intracranial pressure or cerebral swelling, particularly in younger patients with preserved brain volume.

Acute hydrocephalus causes ventricular enlargement, often with a broad rim of periventricular signal change due to increased transependymal flux of CSF. This can be seen whether it is obstructive or communicating and, in the latter, when no mass is visible, contrast may help to identify and delineate meningeal disease. The relationship between ventricular size and pressure is non-linear, due to the influence of premorbid dimensions and brain compliance. Obstructive hydrocephalus is commonly due to tumour, occasionally a small lesion at the level of the aqueduct, but more frequently a posterior fossa mass. Large cerebellar infarcts may also result in hydrocephalus and haemorrhage is another common cause, either intraventricular or subarachnoid. Occasionally, aqueduct stenosis presents in adult life. Communicating hydrocephalus is a late complication of subarachnoid haemorrhage or meningitis and is frequently seen in other conditions that affect the basal meninges such as tuberculosis or sarcoidosis.

Idiopathic intracranial hypertension often causes a deep sella and flattened or concave pituitary gland. The optic sheaths may be patulous. These are non-specific signs of chronic raised pressure. The main differential is a missed venous thrombosis. Very rarely, venous obstruction may be due to an unsuspected tumour such as a jugular

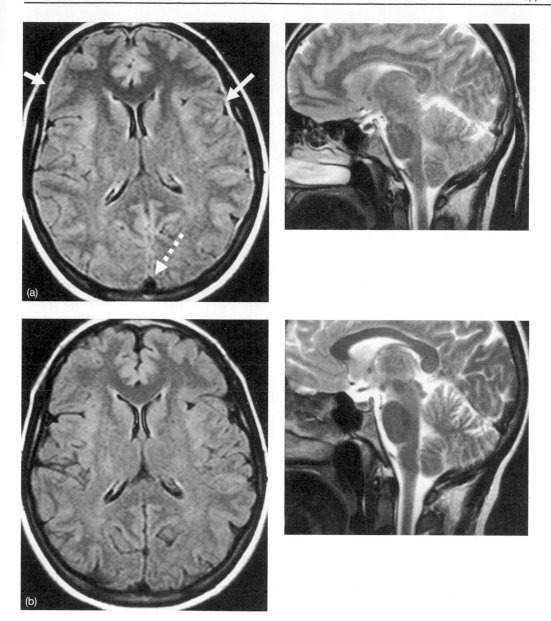

Figure 4.24 Low CSF volume syndrome. Axial FLAIR and sagittal T2 images. The upper scans were obtained while the patient was symptomatic and show a bright layer around the brain due to diffuse dural thickening (solid arrows), expansion of the superior sagittal sinus (dotted arrow) and the hindbrain lying low in the posterior fossa. The lower scans acquired after the symptoms had resolved show resolution of radiological signs.

fossa meningioma or paraganglioma obstructing sinus outflow.

The characteristic radiological features of the low CSF volume syndrome are diffuse dural thickening, shallow subdural hygromas above or below the tentorium and downward displacement of the hindbrain. Venous engorgement also occurs with increase in size of the venous sinuses and upward bulging of the pituitary gland. The meningeal changes and subdural effusions are often also appreciable on spinal imaging, although the site of the leak is usually not shown. The appearances reverse after treatment. Traditionally, contrast enhanced MRI is requested as dural thickening is easier to see when enhanced but in most cases it is also visible as a thin high signal layer on FLAIR.

Spinal imaging

Imaging of the spinal cord with MRI is far superior to CT, although cervical cord compression is often appreciable on CT (Figure 4.25). T2-weighted scans are used to assess spinal cord parenchyma. High signal due to demyelination or other inflammatory conditions is usually readily apparent. In multiple sclerosis, smaller cord plaques are more easily seen on proton density images. Marrow texture and bony infiltration or oedema is best assessed using T1-weighted scans or fat suppressed T2-weighted sequences on which abnormal signal from oedema or tumour is more conspicuous. Contrast enhancement contributes little to diagnosis in most inflammatory cord lesions, although it provides an additional radiological marker to follow.

Spinal cord infarcts tend to be rather indistinct on scans carried out within hours of clinical onset, becoming more conspicuous over a few days. This is in contrast to inflammatory myelopathies which are usually obvious on imaging at clinical presentation. Spinal vascular malformations are uncommon. They are most commonly arteriovenous fistulae on a dural root sheath which cause venous hypertension and cord oedema. The radiological findings are diffuse cord T2 high signal and swelling, sometimes with enhancement due to disrupted blood–cord barrier. Enlarged veins are visible on the surface of the spinal cord as flow voids which may be dots or serpiginous. These should not be confused with almost ubiquitous ill-defined patches of signal loss within the CSF dorsal to the cord due to normal fluid motion. Definitive diagnosis or exclusion still requires catheter angiography which is a prolonged procedure, carrying a risk of neurological deterioration and normally performed under general anaesthetic. CTA and MRA can shorten the catheter angiogram by indicating the likely level of fistula.

Spinal cord compression is usually due to tumour or degenerative disease of the spine. Contrast enhanced images are required if the preliminary scans suggest spinal epidural abscess or other infection.

CT is important after trauma to demonstrate fractures. It is used to assess bone texture in some tumours and is sometimes required for surgical planning. CT myelography still has a role when MRI is contraindicated, or occasionally in patients with persistent symptoms after surgery for degenerative change that are not explained on MRI.

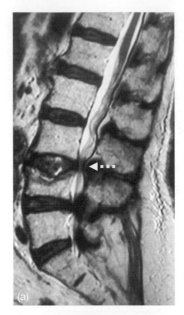

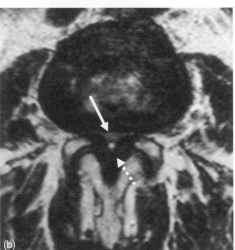

Figure 4.25 Lumbar canal stenosis. Sagittal and axial T2-weighted scans of the lumbar spine The spinal canal is severely narrowed at L3/4 (arrow) by disc in front and thickened ligamentum flavum behind (dotted arrows) obliterating all space between the roots of the cauda equina. The sagittal scan shows coiling of redundant intrathecal roots above the level of stenosis. These are features of a severe stenosis and correlate better with symptoms than milder canal narrowing.

Degenerative disease is the most common indication for all spinal imaging. There is an uncertain relationship between symptoms and imaging and careful correlation with clinical findings is essential.

It is common for asymptomatic root compression to be found, and the degree of spinal cord impingement correlates poorly with symptoms and signs, unless there is also signal change within the cord substance. CT and MRI both show lumbar disc protrusions and canal stenosis, but MRI is preferred to avoid excessive radiation dose. MRI should be used in the cervical spine.

SCANNING FOR REASSURANCE, 'INCIDENTALOMAS' AND CONCLUDING REMARKS

Medical imaging, in particular MRI, has given us unprecedented views inside the living body to the great benefit of our patients. However, it has also created a new dilemma by revealing occult pathology or previously unanticipated variants of normal, frequently of uncertain immediate significance or future prognosis.

Scans 'for reassurance' do not usually show anything of direct clinical relevance but in around 2.5 per cent of patients reveal asymptomatic lesions such as vascular changes, demyelination, small meningiomas, pituitary gland abnormalities and unruptured cerebral aneurysms. Sometimes this is fortuitous, but the prognosis of chance findings is often uncertain and further interventions may result. This may expose the patient to the physical risks and psychological burden of a prolonged investigation trail and follow up imaging, or merely from knowing there is 'something in their head'. While not disputing the benefits of a normal scan report, the small risk of an unexpected abnormal result should also be considered. This is also a significant ethical issue in research imaging as the subjects are often asymptomatic volunteers. The higher resolution MRI sequences frequently used in these circumstances are even more likely to show unexpected findings, in over 4 per cent of cases according to one recent meta-analysis.

In conclusion, the current state and future potential of neuroimaging represent an exceedingly powerful weapon in the medical armamentarium. However, clinical scans are assessed by subjective means, not objective measurements, and findings are often non-specific. Accurate interpretation is always dependent upon the context provided by a thorough clinical assessment of the patient prior to imaging.

REFERENCES AND FURTHER READING

Adam A, Dixon AK, Grainger RG, Allison DJ (eds) (2008) Neuroradiology, including the head and neck. In: *Grainger and Allison's Diagnostic Radiology*, 5th edn. Oxford: Elsevier.

Atlas SW (ed.). (2008) *Magnetic Resonance Imaging of the Brain and Spine*, 4th edn. Philadelphia: Lippincott-Raven.

Barber PA, Hill MD, Eliasziw M *et al.* for the ASPEC study group (2005) Imaging of the brain in acute ischaemic stroke: comparison of computed tomography and magnetic resonance imaging. *Journal of Neurology, Neurosurgery and Psychiatry*, **76**:15228–15233.

Chalela JA, Kidwell CS, Nentwich LM *et al.* (2007) Magnetic resonance imaging and computed tomography in emergency assessment of patients with suspected acute stroke: a prospective comparison. Lancet, **369**:293–298.

Hayward R (2003) VOMIT (victims of modern imaging technology)-an acronym for our times. *British Medical Journal*, **326**:1273.

Kaufmann TJ, Huston J, Mandrekar JN *et al.* (2007) Complications of diagnostic cerebral angiography: evaluation of 19826 consecutive patients. *Radiology*, **243**:812–819.

Lin K, Rapalino O, Law M *et al.* (2008) Accuracy of the Alberta Stroke Program Early CT Score during the first 3 hours of middle cerebral artery stroke: comparison of noncontrast CT, CT angiography source images and CT perfusion. *American Journal of Neuroradiology*, **29**:931–936.

Longstreth WT, Manolio TA, Arnold A *et al.* (1996) Clinical correlates of white matter findings on cranial magnetic resonance imaging of 3301 elderly people. The Cardiovascular Health Study. *Stroke*, **27**:1274–1282.

Marquardt L, Kuker W, Chandratheva A *et al.* (2009) Incidence and prognosis of ≥50% symptomatic vertebral or basilar artery stenosis: prospective population-based study. *Brain*, **132**:982–988.

Morris Z, Whiteley WN, Longstreth WT *et al.* (2009) Incidental findings on brain magnetic resonance imaging: systematic review and metaanalysis. *British Medical Journal*, **339**:b3016.

National Institute for Health and Clinical Excellence Guidelines (Epilepsy 2004, Head Injury 2003; updated 2007).

Polman CH, Reingold SC, Edan G *et al.* (2005) Diagnostic Criteria for multiple sclerosis: 2005 Revisions to the 'McDonald Criteria'. *Annals of Neurology*, **58**:840–846.

CHAPTER 5

CLINICAL NEUROPHYSIOLOGY

Veronica Tan

INTRODUCTION

Neurophysiological studies extend the neurological examination by providing additional information which, when interpreted in the context of the clinical picture, can improve diagnostic accuracy. When performed in the appropriate setting, these studies can also provide useful prognostic information. **It is important for clinicians to have an understanding of these techniques and their limitations in order to optimize the use of these investigations.**

This chapter will concentrate on peripheral neurophysiology and electroencephalography, with a brief overview of other techniques currently in use in adults.

PERIPHERAL NEUROPHYSIOLOGY

Routine nerve conduction studies (NCS) and electromyography (EMG) are used to assess the function of sensory and motor nerves, the neuromuscular junction, and skeletal muscles.

The type of test performed, the choice of nerves and muscles to be studied, and the extent of the examination, must be individually tailored to the patient depending on the presenting symptoms and signs and the main differential diagnoses. The study will often need to be modified depending on the results as they emerge. It is important to recognize that an apparently similar set of results may indicate different pathologies in alternative clinical situations, and it is therefore critical that the person performing the study has all the relevant clinical data to facilitate correct interpretation of the results.

NERVE CONDUCTION STUDIES

Sensory studies

Sensory nerve conduction studies assess the function of the large diameter sensory nerve axons distal to the dorsal root ganglion. Because the connection between the cell body and peripheral axons is unaffected by lesions proximal to the dorsal root ganglion (e.g. in the root or cord), such proximal lesions do not result in any abnormality being found on routine sensory studies.

Sensory axons are stimulated with surface electrodes and the sensory nerve action potential (SNAP) recorded with surface electrodes several centimetres along the nerve. An example of electrode placements for median sensory studies is illustrated in Figure 5.1.

Sensory studies may be orthodromic (i.e. recorded in the direction of physiological sensory nerve conduction) or antidromic (in the opposite direction). Amplitudes are greater with antidromic stimulation, an important point to bear in mind when comparing SNAP results recorded from different centres. The amplitude of the recorded SNAP provides an indication of the number of conducting large diameter sensory axons, and the conduction velocity reflects the function of the myelin sheath between the stimulating and recording electrodes (Figure 5.2). In addition to pathological factors, the SNAP amplitude and conduction velocities may be influenced by technical and physiological factors (Table 5.1). Normal ranges vary slightly in different centres, but a rough guide is ≥50 m/s in the upper limb, and ≥40 m/s in the lower limb for a surface temperature of 32°C.

Technical difficulties related to electrical noise can be a problem in the intensive care setting, and creams and ointments on the skin can cause particular difficulties if they cannot be removed (as in some dermatological conditions).

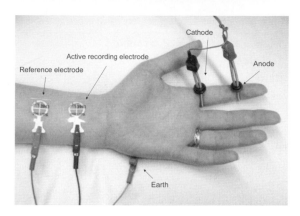

Figure 5.1 Electrode placement for orthodromic median sensory nerve conduction studies. Stimulation is of the sensory digital nerves on the index finger, recording is made over the median nerve at the wrist.

Motor studies

In motor nerve conduction studies, stimulation is performed over various segments of the main trunk of the nerve, and the recording electrodes are placed over the relevant muscle to selectively record the motor component (Figure 5.3). A compound muscle action potential (CMAP) is recorded, which represents the summation of the individual muscle fibre action potentials. The latency, amplitude, duration and area for the responses from each stimulation site are measured (Figure 5.4). Motor conduction velocities are calculated for each segment as illustrated. Because the distal motor latency reflects a combination of the time for motor

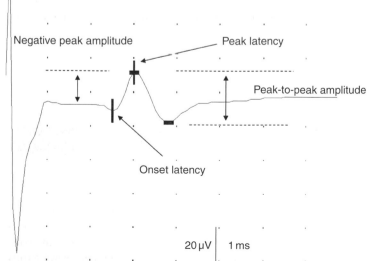

Figure 5.2 Measured parameters of a sensory nerve action potential.

Table 5.1 Factors affecting sensory nerve action potential amplitudes and conduction velocities

Factors affecting SNAP recordings	Amplitude	Velocity
Technical		
Noise		
Environmental electrical noise	↓	↔
Failure to ensure the patient is relaxed		
High skin impedance (e.g. use of moisturising creams)	↓	↔
Physiological		
Temperature		
Cold	↑	↓
Habitus		
Increased subcutaneous tissue (particularly over recording sites)	↓	↔
Age		
Variable effect, but may need to be considered in individuals >65 years	↓	↓ or ↔
Height		
Variable effect, consider in very tall (>6′3″) individuals	(↓)	(↓ or ↔)
Pathological		
Loss of sensory axons (e.g. axonal neuropathy)	↓	↔ , or mild ↓ due to loss of the fastest conducting fibres
Demyelination (primary or secondary)	↓ Due to dispersion and phase cancellation	↓
Lesion proximal to the dorsal root ganglion (pre-ganglionic lesions)	No effect	No effect

↓ decreased; ↑ increased; ↔ no change.

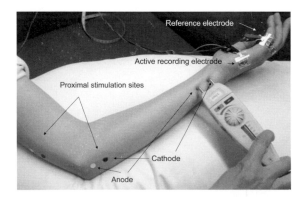

Figure 5.3 Electrode placement for ulnar motor conduction studies, with surface recording electrodes on abductor digiti minimi. The stimulator is shown at the distal stimulation site at the wrist; proximal stimulation sites below and above the elbow are shown with skin markers.

conduction along the nerve to the neuromuscular junction, the neuromuscular transmission time, and the time for muscle depolarization, unlike sensory studies, motor studies require stimulation at two sites to allow subtraction of the conduction time between the distal stimulation site and the muscle. Normal ranges for motor conduction velocities in the upper and lower limbs are similar to those quoted for sensory studies above.

Factors that may affect the amplitude of the CMAP and the motor conduction velocity are shown in Table 5.2. It is worth noting that 'normal' conduction velocities are based on the measurements of the fastest conducting large diameter fibres, and loss of these fibres as part of a general loss of axons may lead to slowing of the measured conduction velocity. In addition, in regenerating axons, the nodes of Ranvier are more closely

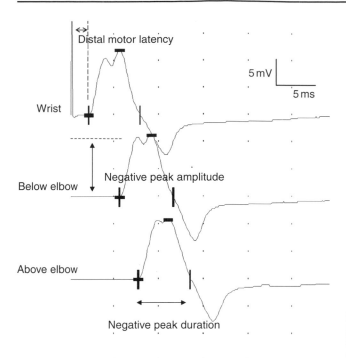

Figure 5.4 Ulnar compound muscle action potential (CMAPs) obtained with stimulation at the wrist, and below- and above-elbow positions, marked to illustrate routinely measured parameters.

> The amplitude of the CMAP provides an indirect measure of the number of conducting motor axons, since the survival of muscle fibres is dependent on the trophic effect of the associated motor nerve. As with sensory studies, the motor conduction velocity reflects the integrity of the myelin sheath along the segment of nerve under study.

spaced; saltatory conduction is therefore slower. Thus slowing of motor conduction is not limited to demyelinating lesions (demyelinating neuropathies) and can occur in conditions primarily affecting axons (axonal neuropathies). Interpretation depends on the clinical scenario and timing of the study in relation to the nerve damage.

Mixed nerve studies

The main trunk of the nerve is stimulated with surface electrodes and the response from the nerve recorded using surface electrodes placed more proximally along the nerve. The response recorded is from both motor and sensory fibres but a large contribution is from the fastest conducting fibres in the nerve trunk, i.e. the large myelinated Ia muscle spindle sensory afferents.

Mixed nerve studies are helpful in mild compressive lesions of the main trunk of a nerve which affect the largest myelinated fibres early, resulting in a reduced nerve action potential (NAP) across the affected segment. In very mild lesions, this may be the only demonstrable abnormality, although in most cases focal motor slowing is also demonstrable over the same segment.

In inflammatory neuropathies with motor conduction block, a normal NAP over the same segment suggests relative sparing of sensory fibres and helps to differentiate conditions selectively affecting motor nerves (such as multifocal motor neuropathy with conduction block (MMNCB)) from other inflammatory neuropathies associated with patchy demyelination with conduction block affecting both sensory and motor fibres (e.g. the Lewis Sumner variant of chronic inflammatory demyelinating neuropathy/multifocal acquired demyelinating sensory and motor neuropathy (MADSAM)).

Late responses

F wave responses

The F wave (first recorded from intrinsic Foot muscles) is a late motor response which arises as a result of antidromic conduction of the stimulus to the anterior horn cells, causing activation of a small

Table 5.2. Factors affecting compound muscle action potential amplitudes and conduction velocities

Factors affecting CMAP recordings to distal stimulation	Amplitude	Velocity
Technical		
Position of the recording electrodes		
Precision of the placement of the active recording electrode over the motor point is particularly important in certain muscles (e.g. abductor pollicis brevis)	↓	↔
Area of recording electrodes		
Larger recording electrodes	↓	↔
Physiological		
Temperature		
Cold	(↑)	↓
Age		
Variable effect, but may need to be considered in distal muscles in individuals >65 years	↓	↓ or ↔
Pathological		
Loss of anterior horn cells	↓	↔
Loss of motor axons	↓	↔, or ↓ if CMAP very small, because of loss of fastest conducting fibres, or ↓ in regenerating motor nerves due to short internodes
Distal conduction block (between the distal stimulating electrode and the neuromuscular junction)	↓	↓ or ↔
Demyelination	↓, dispersion	↓
Disorder of neuromuscular transmission (LEMS, severe myasthenia gravis, neuromuscular blockade)	↓	↔
Severe myopathy	↓	↔

proportion (about 1–5 per cent of muscle fibres) of motor axons which travels back down the axon to elicit a small late CMAP (Figure 5.5). The normal range for minimum F wave latencies depends on the arm and leg length, which typically correlates with the patient's height, although in individuals with disproportionately long limbs, calculation of F wave conduction velocities may be a more accurate indicator of the presence of absence of pathology.

F wave persistence (percentage of stimuli associated with an accompanying F wave response) is normally >50 per cent in most motor nerves, with the exception of the common peroneal nerve where F waves may be difficult to elicit in normal subjects. The F wave may be absent in normal sedated patients, which is of particular relevance in ITU patients.

F wave chronodispersion is the difference between the fastest and slowest F wave responses and is normally up to 4 ms in the upper limbs, and 6 ms in the lower limbs.

Prolongation of minimum F wave latencies beyond what may be accounted for by peripheral conduction velocities is suggestive of proximal slowing, and may be the only abnormality seen in the early stages of acute inflammatory demyelinating polyradiculoneuropathies.

H responses

The H (Hoffman) response is the electrophysiological equivalent of the ankle jerk and is of limited clinical value if the ankle jerk is present. A prolonged H reflex may be seen in any condition that depresses the ankle jerk, including peripheral neuropathies or S1 radiculopathies.

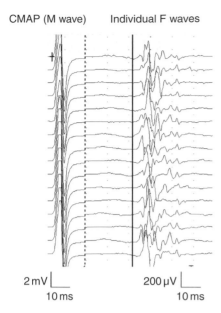

CMAP (M wave)   Individual F waves

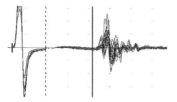

Superimposed F waves

2 mV |
10 ms

200 µV |
10 ms

Figure 5.5 F wave recordings obtained on stimulation of the tibial nerve.

A comment on terminology

Pre- and post-ganglionic lesions

These terms are relatively well established in clinical neurophysiology usage, but are potentially confusing. The terms are based on the location of a lesion as might be described in an anatomical drawing of nerve roots arising from the spinal cord, and not in terms of the direction of physiological conduction in a sensory nerve. Thus, 'pre-ganglionic' refers to a lesion proximal to the sensory dorsal root ganglion and includes lesions in the root or the spinal cord, and 'post-ganglionic' refers to a lesion in the peripheral sensory nerve distal to the sensory ganglion.

'Motor radiculopathies'

In radicular lesions involving both sensory and motor fibres, the damage to the proximal sensory fibres is not demonstrable on routine neurophysiology because lesions proximal to the sensory root ganglion do not result in loss of peripheral sensory fibres. Because the only abnormality detectable on routine neurophysiology is neurogenic change on EMG, with or without a reduced CMAP in the affected myotome, the abnormalities are reported either as 'consistent with a [root level] motor radiculopathy' or as suggestive of a 'pre-ganglionic' lesion in the affected myotome. Very localized lesions affecting only the sensory root will not be detectable on routine neurophysiology. This also applies to sensory radiculopathies of inflammatory origin. In such cases, dermatomal evoked potentials may be helpful, but these studies are generally only available in specialist centres.

ELECTROMYOGRAPHY

Changes in motor unit action potential morphology in needle electromyography (Table 5.3) are helpful for differentiating neurogenic (Figure 5.6) from myopathic (Figure 5.7) processes.

Spontaneous activity in the form of fibrillations and positive sharp waves (Figure 5.8) is an indication of muscle fibre membrane instability and occurs both in primary disorders of muscle and as a result of denervation.

Some forms of spontaneous activity are more specific; for example, fasciculations (Figure 5.9), doublets and triplets (Figure 5.10) and myokymic and neuromyotonic discharges, and are indicative of a neural origin, whereas myotonic discharges (Figure 5.11) arise from the muscle fibre. However, pseudomyotonic or complex repetitive discharges may occur both in neurogenic and myopathic disorders.

Recruitment patterns (normally the first units that start firing are the small units and they follow

Table 5.3 Typical characteristics of neurogenic and myopathic motor unit action potentials (MUAPs)

	Normal	Myopathic	Neurogenic
Duration (ms)	5–16	<5	>16
Amplitude (mean, μV)	200–400	<200	>400
Configuration	Triphasic	Polyphasic	Polyphasic
Recruitment	According to size principle as force increases	Rapid recruitment of many small units with weak contraction	Large units recruiting early
Interference pattern	Full	Full	Reduced

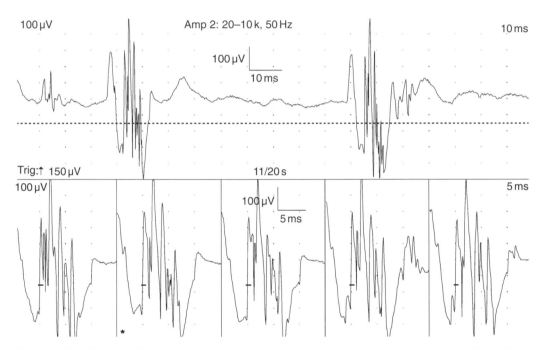

Figure 5.6 EMG changes following a neurogenic lesion. Large amplitude, long duration polyphasic units are illustrated.

an orderly size principle with increasing force), the firing rate of the units (i.e. whether the number of different motor units firing is appropriate for the rate of the fastest firing unit: normally the ratio of firing frequency to the number of units firing is 5:1), and changes in the interference pattern (formed by the overlapping of motor units, which reflects the number of units firing) are also helpful for differentiating neurogenic from myopathic conditions. Rapid recruitment of many small motor units with weak contraction (i.e. increased force requires rapidly increasing the number of motor units firing) is suggestive of a myopathic disorder, whereas larger units recruiting early and firing at high rates with a reduced interference pattern (increased force is generated by a higher rate of firing of the few motor units available) is suggestive of a neurogenic disorder.

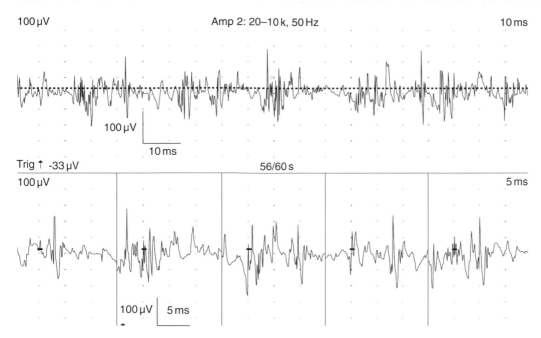

100 µV   Amp 2: 20–10 k, 50 Hz   10 ms

100 µV

10 ms

Trig ↑ -33 µV   56/60 s

100 µV   5 ms

100 µV   5 ms

Figure 5.7 EMG changes in a myopathy. Small spiky short duration polyphasic units are illustrated.

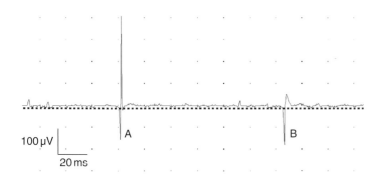

100 µV

20 ms

A   B

Figure 5.8 Fibrillation potential (A) and positive sharp wave (B).

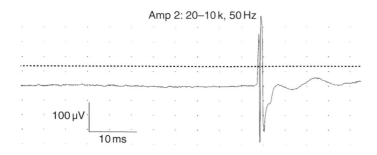

Amp 2: 20–10 k, 50 Hz

100 µV

10 ms

Figure 5.9 Fasciculation potential.

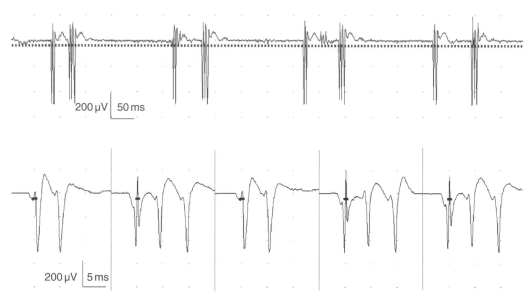

200 µV | 50 ms

200 µV | 5 ms

Figure 5.10 Spontaneous motor unit action potentials firing in groups of two (doublets) and three (triplets).

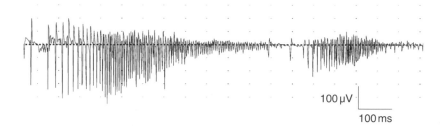

100 µV

100 ms

Figure 5.11 Myotonic discharge. Note the waxing and waning in both amplitude and frequency.

IMPORTANT CONCEPTS IN THE INTERPRETATION OF NCS AND EMG

Estimating the degree of traumatic nerve injury

Provided the studies are performed at the appropriate time after injury, neurophysiology can help classify lesions into the following broad categories, and thus inform decisions regarding the need for surgical intervention.

(a) Lesions with little or no axonal loss (**neurapraxia**/first-degree injuries) where the clinical deficit is due to conduction block at the site of the injury (due to ischaemia or focal demyelination). The prognosis is good, with recovery occurring any time from hours to up to about three months.

(b) Lesions with axonal loss (**axonotmesis**) where recovery depends on axonal regrowth, which in turn depends on the degree of associated disorganization of the surrounding stroma and the distance from the end organ. Neurophysiology can broadly quantify the degree of axonal damage provided sufficient time has elapsed for complete Wallerian degeneration to occur (typically about 9–11 days post-injury).

(c) Severe lesions with complete disruption of all axons, where surgical intervention is likely to be required. Where there is complete disruption of axons, lesions without loss of the endoneurial tubes (**axonotmesis**) carry a much better prognosis than where there is complete disruption (**neurotmesis**); however, neurophysiology is unable to categorically distinguish between the groups. Where axons remain in continuity, although neurophysiology can estimate the number of axons remaining, it cannot directly estimate the degree of associated endoneurial damage at the site of injury. In both situations, the nature of the injury is probably the best indicator of the likely degree of associated stromal disruption; the likelihood being higher in injuries associated with a high degree of force, or with traction injuries, than with compression injuries.

(d) A combination of conduction block and axonal loss can occur, which together determine the degree of clinical deficit during the first few months. The contribution of each can also be estimated by comparing side to side distal CMAP differences, and by comparing the size of the CMAPs obtained on stimulation proximal and distal to the site of the injury. Clinical recovery in such lesions is usually biphasic, with more rapid initial recovery due to reversal of block, and a slower second phase as axons regenerate.

Timing of pathological changes in peripheral nerve injuries

An understanding of the timing of the changes that occur after nerve injury is necessary for the interpretation of the neurophysiological findings after traumatic peripheral nerve injury. Studies performed too early will underestimate the degree of damage because there has been insufficient time for complete Wallerian degeneration to occur, and those performed late (>2–3 months after the injury) will underestimate the degree of axonal loss from the original injury because of reinnervation.

In motor nerves, changes in the distal CMAP may start to occur at 3–5 days post injury, although this is dependent on the length of the remaining distal segment; shorter segments degenerate more rapidly. The initial fall in CMAP is due to failure of neuromuscular transmission, followed by loss of conduction along the nerve. This is usually complete by day 9 post injury. Wallerian

degeneration in sensory nerves is estimated to take about 11 days.

Timing of neurophysiological changes and limitations of NCS and EMG

Immediately after nerve transection, there will be failure of conduction across the site of the lesion but the distal segment will conduct normally. The following points are worth noting.

- Studies performed before there has been sufficient time for Wallerian degeneration to occur will underestimate the degree of axonal loss. Within the first few days after injury, the nerve conduction studies will be indistinguishable from neurapraxic lesions with conduction block. Similarly, a 'pseudoconduction block' may be seen in the first few days of a vasculitic neuropathy. The clinical history and presentation are therefore critical for correct interpretation of the findings.

- If the lesion is too proximal to allow stimulation of the nerve proximal to the lesion, it may not be possible to demonstrate any abnormality until failure of neuromuscular transmission and subsequent Wallerian degeneration cause a drop in the CMAP to distal stimulation. In trunkal or proximal leg muscles where CMAPs cannot be easily obtained for technical reasons, evidence of axonal loss may not be apparent until the development of neurogenic changes on EMG.

Neurogenic fibrillations and positive sharp waves generally appear only after Wallerian degeneration has occurred. As noted above, the time taken varies depending on the length of the distal nerve fragment and is estimated at 10–14 days for a distal lesion and up to 3–4 weeks for proximal lesions when sampling a distal muscle.

Muscle fibres continue to fibrillate until they are either reinnervated or replaced by fibrotic tissue. Muscle fibres which are not reinnervated generally survive for up to 18–24 months, although individual cases vary. The importance of this point is that nerve repair may fail to improve outcome even if the surgery is technically successful if it is performed too late for the muscle to be reinnervated in time. Axonal growth is estimated at about

1–5 mm per day, so surgical repair for proximal nerve lesions must be performed at the earliest opportunity for optimal outcome.

It should be noted that in cases of trauma, fibrillations and positive sharp waves may also arise as a result of direct muscle injury, which may cause difficulties when trying to localize the site or degree of nerve injury neurophysiologically.

In cases where there is a combination of axonal loss and conduction block in the remaining axons, the presence of fibrillations and the absence of voluntary units may mimic complete loss of axons. If the lesion is very proximal and CMAPs cannot be measured, it may not be possible to distinguish the two conditions electrophysiologically.

EMG changes of reinnervation from collateral sprouting are typically seen 3–6 weeks after a partial nerve injury. These take the form of larger longer duration polyphasic units. In complete nerve lesions, reinnervation depends on regrowth of the axons and the generation of new neuromuscular junctions; these reinnervating motor units are small, polyphasic and typically unstable (i.e. tend to change in amplitude and number of phases each time it fires).

TIMING PERIPHERAL NEUROPHYSIOLOGY REQUESTS

Since accurate neurophysiological estimation of the severity of a nerve lesion cannot be made before 9–14 days, there will be situations where such a delay is not in the best interests of the patient. The following recommendations assume access to specialist neurosurgical expertise.

When surgical exploration should not be delayed
In trauma cases where the force of the impact is likely to have been sufficient to cause neurotmesis or avulsion, or where there has been a traction injury to a nerve which is relatively fixed at certain points (e.g. the common peroneal nerve), patients with complete loss of function due to nerve injury should be referred directly to a specialist peripheral nerve unit for surgical exploration.

Any associated orthopaedic injuries could be attended to simultaneously. As already outlined above, the potential cost to the patient of delaying referral if nerve repair is required is high, whereas there is little to be lost if exploration finds an intact nerve that does not require any surgical intervention.

In acute penetrating or laceration injuries where the neurological deficit is highly likely to be due to axonal damage, immediate surgical exploration and repair is usually required.

Severe neuropathic pain (see Chapter 30), with or without associated neurological deficit, occurring immediately following elective surgery (e.g. total hip replacement), usually indicates acute nerve injury or ischaemia. Imaging to exclude a surgically treatable cause of nerve compression (e.g. haematoma) followed by exploratory surgery to exclude any potentially remediable cause (e.g. a stitch through the nerve) is usually indicated.

When it is reasonable to wait until neurophysiology can provide meaningful data
In compressive lesions (e.g. 'Saturday night palsy'), especially when there is partial preservation of nerve function (i.e. the lesion is clinically incomplete), and the main clinical question is one of prognosis in order to aid rehabilitation planning, delaying neurophysiological studies for 2 weeks enables a more accurate assessment of the degree of injury.

When follow-up studies are likely to be required before a clear diagnosis can be made

In cases of suspected acute inflammatory demyelinating polyradiculoneuropathy (AIDP), neurophysiology is usually requested early if the patient is severely weak. In such cases, the main purpose of the neurophysiology is to exclude alternative diagnoses. In the very early stages of AIDP, a patient may be profoundly weak from proximal demyelination of the roots, but investigations in the first week may be normal, or show only F wave abnormalities. In such cases, a follow-up study in the second or third week of illness is usually required. In mild cases, especially where the deficit is predominantly sensory, it is usually reasonable to delay the initial nerve conduction studies to the second week.

PATTERNS OF CHANGE AND INTERPRETATION OF PERIPHERAL NEUROPHYSIOLOGICAL STUDIES

Sensory, motor or sensory-motor neuropathies

Nerve conduction studies aid in the differential diagnosis of a neuropathy by classifying the abnormalities as affecting only sensory or motor nerves, or both types of nerves (see Chapter 16).

Length-dependent or patchy changes

Toxic, metabolic or degenerative neuropathies are typically length-dependent, i.e. the pathology is seen earliest and most severely in the longest nerves, because these are the most vulnerable to compromise of neuronal metabolism or axonal transport. Patchy changes and multiple mononeuropathies are typically due to inflammatory processes, such as demyelination or vasculitis. Patchy changes may also be seen with multiple compressive neuropathies in hereditary neuropathy with pressure palsies (HNPP), or other conditions predisposing to multiple superadded pressure palsies (e.g. diabetes).

Axonal or demyelinating

Slowing of conduction

As mentioned previously, loss of the fastest conducting axons as part of an axonal neuropathy will result in a reduction of measured velocities. **When interpreting conduction velocities, a judgement must therefore be made as to whether the degree of slowing is more than could be accounted for by axonal loss alone.** Because of the distribution of velocities in the upper and lower limb axons, it been suggested that velocities of <75 per cent of the lower limit of normal (i.e. <37 m/s in the upper

limb (UL) and <30 m/s in the lower limb (LL)) would suggest a demyelinating process.

Accordingly, the genetic neuropathies (e.g. Charcot–Marie–Tooth (CMT), see Chapter 16) are classified based on motor conduction velocities: CMT1 (UL velocities of <38 m/s), CMT2 (UL velocities >38 m/s) or CMT intermediate (UL velocities 25–45 m/s).

These ranges provide a useful guide, although in acquired neuropathies, depending on the clinical setting, the possibility of slowing due to shortened internodes in regenerating axons also needs to be considered. This, coupled with a reduction of temperature in wasted limbs, may result in some axonal neuropathies mimicking a demyelinating process, especially when the initial study is performed several months after the onset. The clinical context is therefore critical for interpretation.

Homogeneous or variable slowing

Conduction velocities in hereditary demyelinating neuropathies (such as CMT1) are typically uniform, being very similar for all the nerves in the upper and lower limbs, whereas in acquired demyelinating neuropathies, the velocities tend to vary from nerve to nerve and along different segments of the nerve. Notable exceptions exist, in particular CMTX (X-linked CMT), where the neurophysiology may mimic an acquired demyelinating neuropathy.

Conduction block and dispersion

Both conduction block (Figure 5.12) and dispersion (Figure 5.13) of the CMAP are features of a demyelinating process. Non-uniform slowing of conduction leads to dispersion and an increased duration of the CMAP with a reduction in amplitude, often with an irregular CMAP outline. The definition of conduction block varies in the literature and is variously quoted as a reduction in the CMAP of >20–50 per cent without significant increase in CMAP duration.

CMAP duration may also be increased in some forms of primary muscle disease (e.g. critical illness myopathy (Figure 5.14)) because of slowing of muscle fibre conduction. In this case, the CMAPs are small and of long duration but the outline remains smooth, unlike neurogenic dispersion.

Slowing of conduction alone does not cause significant clinical weakness. In the absence of axonal loss, clear weakness is suggestive of con-

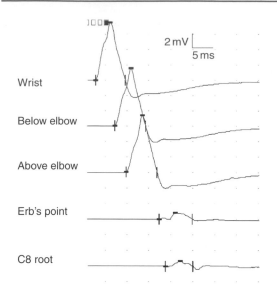

Wrist

Below elbow

Above elbow

Erb's point

C8 root

Figure 5.12 Ulnar nerve motor studies showing conduction block in the segment of nerve between Erb's point and the stimulation point above the elbow. Note the drop in amplitude without increase in duration of the compound muscle action potential.

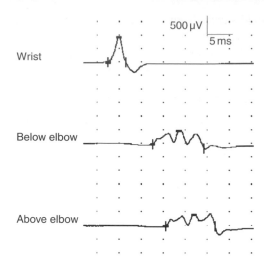

Wrist

Below elbow

Above elbow

Figure 5.13 Ulnar nerve motor studies showing dispersion of compound muscle action potential (CMAP) following stimulation of the nerve proximal to the wrist. Note the increase in the CMAP duration and the irregular complex shape of the dispersed CMAP.

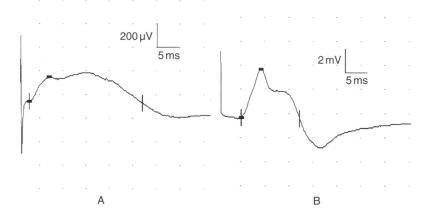

A   B

Figure 5.14 Increased duration and small amplitude common peroneal compound muscle action potential (CMAP) (surface electrodes on tibialis anterior) in critical illness myopathy (A). Note the regular CMAP outline despite the increased duration. Normal CMAP for comparison (B). Note the difference in the amplitude scale between (A) and (B).

duction block. EMG may also be helpful in cases where proximal conduction block cannot be easily demonstrated on nerve conduction studies, either because proximal stimulation of the nerve is not technically possible, or when proximal stimulation results in co-stimulation of other nerves making the CMAP amplitude unreliable for indicating conduction block (such as in the median or radial nerves when stimulating at Erb's point). A markedly reduced interference pattern with rapidly firing units in the context of clinical weakness and a large CMAP to distal stimulation (typically without

muscle wasting) supports the presence of proximal conduction block.

Conduction block and dispersion are more commonly seen in acquired neuropathies, but may also occur in CMTX.

Localization

Pre- or post-ganglionic localization
In a patient with sensory loss and neurogenic change in a particular myotome on EMG, the presence of a normal SNAP in the relevant dermatome

would suggest that the lesion is pre-ganglionic. If there is a pre-existing sensory neuropathy, however, it may not be possible to distinguish between pre- and post-ganglionic lesions.

Simultaneous multiple injuries

Multiple peripheral nerve lesions may be indistinguishable from a plexus injury and post-ganglionic lesions will mask the presence of concomitant pre-ganglionic lesions. In such cases, the results of neurophysiological studies will need to be interpreted with regard to the clinical presentation, and supported by imaging and occasionally, neurosurgical findings.

Myopathic or neurogenic disorders

Inflammatory myopathies may be associated with mixed changes, with some myopathic and some 'neurogenic' units, because of axonal sprouting and reinnervation of functionally denervated muscle fibres. Active disease is often associated with fibrillations and positive sharp waves. In cases where there are many longer duration units, the findings may rarely be mistaken for early anterior horn cell disease. In the latter, the presence of fasciculations is helpful for suggesting a primary neurogenic process.

The combination of myopathic units and spontaneous activity is not specific to inflammatory myopathies and may be seen in any myopathic condition in which the pathology results in instability of the sarcolemmal membrane, including some congenital myopathies and muscular dystrophies. Interpretation, as always, is dependent on the clinical context.

In severely wasted muscles due to chronic disease (chronic muscular dystrophies, spinal muscular atrophies, severe chronic inflammatory or necrotizing myopathies or neuropathies), the EMG may be non-diagnostic. This is because similar processes tend to occur in end-stage muscle, with muscle fibres being replaced by fibrosis, and axonal sprouting to innervate functionally denervated muscle fibres. In such cases, muscle biopsy of a less severely affected muscle or genetic testing may be more helpful.

EMG changes may be absent or minimal in metabolic and endocrine myopathies and cannot be used to exclude these conditions.

Myokymic discharges

In the context of a brachial or lumbosacral plexopathy appearing many years after radiotherapy to the region, the presence of myokymic discharges favours post-radiation changes over neoplastic infiltration. Myokymic discharges in the cranial nerve distribution may be seen in brain stem demyelination, although myokymia limited to orbicularis oculi may be seen in normal individuals. Generalized myokymic discharges are seen in Isaac's syndrome (Chapter 18), and in episodic ataxia type 1 (EA1) (Chapter 21).

Myotonic discharges

These are seen in the dystrophic and non-dystrophic myotonias (Figure 5.11). Occasional myotonic discharges may be seen in acid-maltase deficiency, typically in the paraspinal muscles.

REPETITIVE NERVE STIMULATION AND SINGLE FIBRE EMG

Repetitive nerve stimulation and single fibre EMG (SFEMG) studies are used in the investigation of disorders of neuromuscular transmission such as myasthenia gravis, Lambert–Eaton syndrome and botulism.

The congenital myasthenic syndromes (with the exception of slow channel syndrome) typically present in childhood and will not be discussed here.

In postsynaptic syndromes such as myasthenia gravis, the resting CMAP is typically normal (except in very severe disease).

In weak muscles, slow rates (2–5 Hz) of repetitive stimulation are associated with a decrement which is maximal with the 4th or 5th stimulus ('U' shaped decrement), due to progressive depletion of acetycholine quanta, which begin to be replenished from the secondary store by the 6th–10th stimuli (Figure 5.15).

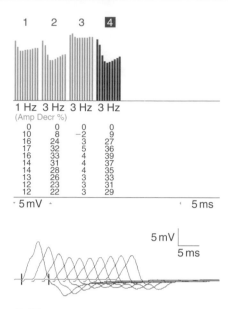

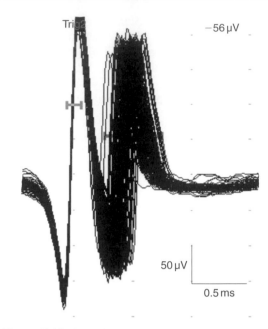

Figure 5.15 Repetitive stimulation in a patient with myasthenia gravis, stimulating the median nerve at the wrist and recording over abductor pollicis brevis. The figure illustrates the typical pattern of decrement which is maximal with the 4th or 5th stimulus ('U' shaped decrement), due to progressive depletion of acetycholine quanta, which begins to be replenished from the secondary store by the 6th–10th stimuli. The numbers beneath the histograms represent percentage decrement from baseline. The decrement is greater at 3 Hz (2) than at 1 Hz (1), there is repair of decrement following 15 s of exercise (3), and post-exercise exhaustion (4) when retested after 3 minutes of rest.

Figure 5.16 Single fibre electromyography showing increased jitter in a patient with myasthenia gravis. The trigger is on the first fibre of the pair, and the increased jitter (variation in the time interval between the firing of the two fibres belonging to the same motor unit) is shown on the superimposed images.

After more prolonged exercise (e.g. 1 minute), a larger decrement is typically seen following 2–4 minutes of rest ('post exercise exhaustion'). SFEMG in weak muscles shows increased jitter (Figure 5.16) with blocking.

In Lambert–Eaton myasthenic syndrome (LEMS), a presynaptic disorder, the resting CMAP is typically low in amplitude, due to the low quantal release of acetylcholine with a single stimulus. Low rates of repetitive stimulation are as associated with the typical 'U' shaped decrement, but high rates of repetitive stimulation (or brief maximal voluntary exercise) results in an increase in the CMAP amplitude due to calcium accumulation in the nerve ending causing increased quantal release (typically >200 per cent of the resting CMAP) (Figure 5.17) and may restore the CMAP to normal values. SFEMG shows increased jitter and blocking which is maximal at low rates (1–5 Hz) and which improves at higher firing/stimulation rates (e.g. 15–20 Hz).

In botulism, the electrophysiological findings vary depending on the time of examination and the severity of the disease. In mild disease, the resting CMAPs may be 'normal' or low-normal in amplitude, and show little or no decrement at low rates of repetitive stimulation, but demonstrate an increment of >40 per cent after exercise or after high rates of repetitive stimulation, consistent with the presynaptic nature of the pathology. Unlike LEMS and myasthenia gravis, there is no post-activation exhaustion and the increment usually persists for longer (4–20 minutes). In more severe disease, the resting CMAP is usually small, there may or may not be decrement at low rates of repetitive stimulation, and the incremental response to high rates of stimulation may be minimal or absent. Needle EMG may show fibrillation potentials and positive sharp waves in severely affected muscles, and small amplitude potentials resembling a myopathic pattern, mimicking and inflammatory myopathy. Both amplitude and interference pattern may increase with sustained effort. SFEMG is often abnormal early in the disease, with increased jitter and blocking in affected muscles. As in LEMS, the

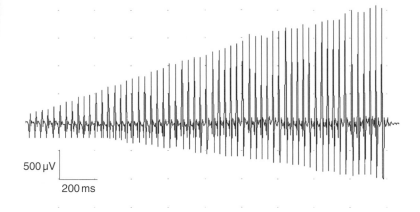

Figure 5.17 Tetanic stimulation (30 Hz for 2 s) of the ulnar nerve (surface electrodes on abductor digiti minimi) in a patient with Lambert-Eaton syndrome showing the marked increase in amplitude. Compound action muscle potential (CMAP) at rest was 0.1 mV. CMAP at the end of the titanic train was 3 mV.

500 µV

200 ms

amount of jitter decreases with an increase in the firing rate.

Abnormal single fibre EMG and mild decrements on repetitive stimulation are not specific for disorders of neuromuscular transmission; they may also be seen in neurogenic conditions, and in some inflammatory myopathies, due to the presence of axon sprouts with immature unstable neuromuscular junctions. Decrements on repetitive stimulation may also be seen in the chloride channel myotonias and in the myotonic dystrophies. It is therefore important that these studies should always be interpreted in the context of the clinical presentation and other nerve conduction and EMG findings.

SMALL FIBRE STUDIES

The very slowly conducting small sensory (C and Aδ) nerve fibres involved in pain and temperature sensation cannot be assessed using routine nerve conduction studies, and requires specialist equipment which tests the patient's ability to sense changes in temperature (thermal threshold testing). In most systems, a thermistor is applied to the skin and the initial temperature is set to the patient's skin temperature. The temperature is then gradually increased or decreased and the patient asked to press a button when he/she is first able to detect a sensation of cold or warmth. These studies involve the whole small fibre sensory pathway and therefore cannot distinguish between abnormalities

caused by central or peripheral lesions. As with all psychophysical studies, thermal threshold testing requires good patient cooperation for accuracy.

The Contact Heat-Evoked Potential Stimulator (CHEPS) is a newer, more objective method of assessing small fibres, in which cortical evoked potentials in response to thermal-related pain are recorded; it is only available in specialist centres.

The blink reflex

The blink reflex is analogous to the corneal reflex: the afferent impulses travel along the trigeminal nerve, and the efferent arc is via the facial nerve to both orbicularis oculi muscles; synapses occur in the pons and lateral medulla. The blink reflex may be abnormal in lesions of the trigeminal or facial nerves (including due to lesions of the cerebellopontine angle), and in brainstem lesions. Prior to the widespread availability of MRI, abnormal blink reflexes were helpful in demonstrating clinically silent lesions in multiple sclerosis.

Exercise testing in muscle channelopathies

Several distinct patterns of change in the CMAP amplitude and area have been described following repeated 10 s of isometric exercise (the short exercise test) at room temperature and after cooling, which help distinguish chloride from sodium channel myotonias, and paramyotonia congenita (Figure 5.18). These changes are helpful for guiding genetic analysis of patients with non-dystrophic myotonias (see Chapter 18).

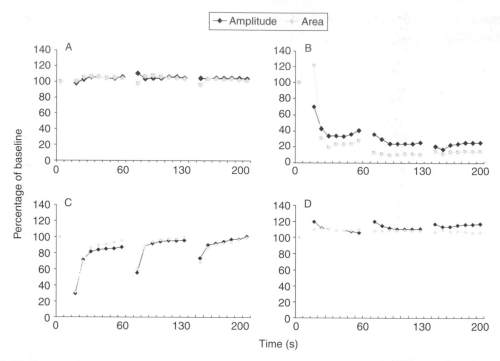

Figure 5.18 Short exercise test patterns at room temperature in patients with non-dystrophic myotonia. The ulnar nerve is stimulated at the wrist and the compound muscle action potential (CMAP) recorded with surface electrodes on abductor digiti minimi (ADM). Isometric exercise of ADM is performed for 10 seconds and the CMAPs recorded immediately after exercise and then at 10 s intervals for 60 seconds of rest. The exercise is then repeated for a total of three exercise trials. The amplitude and area change in the CMAP is plotted as a percentage of the baseline. A: Normal control; B: Paramyotonia congenita; C: Myotonia congenita; D: Sodium channel myotonia/Potassium-aggravated myotonia.

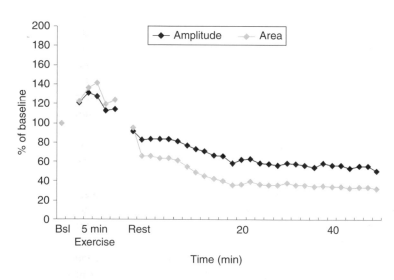

Figure 5.19 The long exercise test in a patient with familial periodic paralysis. The ulnar nerve is stimulated at the wrist with surface electrodes over the abductor digiti minimi (ADM). The ADM is exercised for 5 minutes and then rested. Compound muscle action potentials (CMAPs) are recorded at rest, each minute during the 5 minutes of exercise and then at 1–2 minute intervals for a total rest period of 50 minutes. Decrement is calculated as a percentage of the maximum CMAP obtained during the 5 minutes of exercise (upper limit of normal for amplitude change: 40 per cent) and as a percentage of the baseline CMAP (upper limit of normal for amplitude change: 30 per cent).

The long exercise test (CMAPs monitored for 40–50 minutes following 5 minutes of isometric exercise) is helpful in patients with suspected periodic paralysis (Figure 5.19). An abnormal result is helpful in suggesting that genetic analysis should be pursued, but a normal result does not exclude the possibility of periodic paralysis if the history is highly suggestive.

NEWER TECHNIQUES

Nerve excitability studies – threshold tracking techniques

In contrast to standard nerve conduction studies, where maximum amplitudes and velocities to supramaximal stimuli are measured in threshold tracking techniques, the response is set at a target level (usually 40–50 per cent of the maximum CMAP) and it is the stimulus current required to achieve this target response under varying conditions that is monitored.

Nerve excitability studies are now providing insights into the behaviour of neuronal ion-channels and the mechanisms underlying some acquired and genetic neuropathies (including renal failure and EA1).

Muscle excitability studies

There are now also methods for demonstrating changes in the muscle membrane potential by measuring changes in muscle fibre conduction velocities in response to conditioning stimuli at varying intervals from the test stimulus. These are now giving insights into changes that occur in ischaemia, critical illness myopathy and renal failure.

ELECTROENCEPHALOGRAPHY

Basic concepts

The electroencephalogram (EEG) comprises a recording of electric field potentials generated by summated cortical pyramidal cell inhibitory and excitatory postsynaptic potentials, together with some intrinsic currents generated by the thalamus. These are recorded as voltage differences between electrodes placed at various points on the scalp, which are then amplified and plotted against time to produce the EEG trace.

Routine recordings last approximately 20 minutes. When clinically indicated, longer recordings to include sleep, additional activation procedures, prolonged day case or ambulatory recordings, or telemetry can be performed. A standard recording in adults uses a minimum of 21 electrodes, placed on specific locations on the scalp using bony landmarks as a guide (known as the international 10–20 system) (Figure 5.20). The voltage from each electrode is recorded either with reference to a specified common reference potential which may or may not be electrically silent (referential or 'monopolar' recording), or with reference to another active electrode in an orderly sequence (bipolar recording). The results are then displayed in various arrangements of electrodes (montages). For clarity, all the EEG examples in this article are displayed in a bipolar montage, with the electrodes linked as illustrated in Figure 5.20.

In addition to the EEG, a single channel electrocardiogram (ECG) trace is routinely simultaneously recorded. The recording can be further augmented by simultaneous monitoring of respiration, eye movements, surface EMG and skin resistance (polygraphic recordings). Polygraphic recordings are tailored to the patient, depending on seizure type and preceding EEG findings.

This chapter will concentrate on the use of EEG in adult patients.

TYPES OF EEG RECORDINGS

EEG recordings in most centres now include a synchronized digital video recording and a single channel ECG recording. The main types of recording may be divided into the standard 'interictal' outpatient recordings, with or without sleep, and more prolonged recordings aimed at capturing an ictal event. The various types of EEG recordings, the methods used, the aim of the recording and the typical indications for requests are outlined in Table 5.4.

Additional procedures, generally only performed at centres for epilepsy surgery, include video telemetry using intracranial electrodes (foramen ovale, depth or subdural electrodes), electrocorticography (EEG recorded using grids of electrodes placed directly on the cortex) and magnetoencephalography (a digital recording of magnetic field values produced by neuronal intracellular currents).

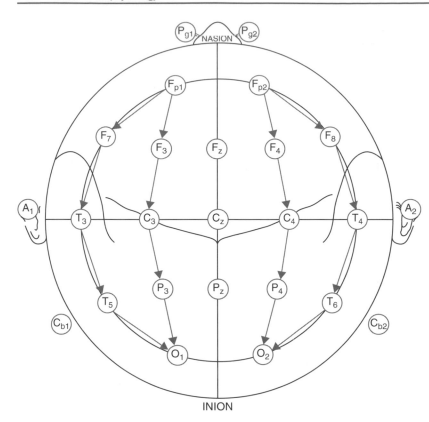

Figure 5.20 Diagrammatic representation of the International 10–20 system. The arrows represent how the channels are linked in a typical bipolar montage.

Basic EEG nomenclature

The typical EEG report comprises a factual description of the trace followed by a clinical comment or conclusion. The following are definitions for some of the common technical terms used:

Cortical rhythms are classified according to their frequency range:	
<4 Hz	Delta (or slow)
4 to <8 Hz	Theta
8–13 Hz	Alpha
14–15 Hz	Sigma (sleep spindles)
>15–40 Hz	Beta (or fast)
>40 Hz	Gamma

Spike: A suddenly appearing (paroxysmal) sharp component of ≤70 ms duration standing out from the background activity. Sharp wave: A broader sharp component lasting 70–200 ms.

The normal resting record (Figure 5.21) in the alert patient should contain well-formed alpha activity in the posterior leads. Low amplitude beta activity is usually present anteriorly.

Slow activity is abnormal in the alert waking adult recording, and suggests the presence of underlying cerebral dysfunction. Theta activity is a less specific finding and interpretation of its significance depends on the clinical context. It may be a normal finding in a drowsy patient. In patients with the appropriate clinical history (see Chapter 13), rhythmic bursts of slow or theta activity may represent ictal (seizure) activity (e.g. temporal intermittent rhythmic delta activity, or rhythmic theta discharges in mesial temporal lobe seizures due to hippocampal sclerosis).

Although spikes and sharp waves are often seen as part of epileptiform discharges, they need not always represent pathology, being part of normal sleep activity (vertex sharp waves), some benign variants (e.g. small sharp spikes in sleep), or variants of doubtful/uncertain association with epilepsy.

Table 5.4 Types of EEG recordings

Type of EEG	Method	Aim	Indications
Standard video EEG	EEG recording at rest and following various activation procedures including hyperventilation, photic stimulation, and where relevant, other suspected triggers such as pattern stimulation, video games, startle, listening to music, and reading	Record paroxysmal interictal or ictal epileptiform activity and document any associated clinical manifestations	Episodes of loss of consiousness, suspected seizures
			Syndromic classification of epilepsy
			Impaired responsiveness, suspected subclinical seizures
			Organic brain syndromes
			Suspected encephalitis or encephalopathy
Sleep recordings	The patient is either sleep-deprived or given a sedative. The patient is then woken from sleep and, when appropriate, activation procedures are performed immediately afterwards	Increase the likelihood of capturing epileptiform discharges	High clinical suspicion of epilepsy, but routine EEG either noral or nondiagnostic
Longer term recordings			
Outpatient ambulatory EEG (no video)	The patient presses an event button and keeps a diary	Capture habitual ictal events for diagnosis and presurgical evaluation	Multiple recurrent mild attacks/attacks with aura, of uncertain aetiology. However, limited number of channels (up to 16) limits accurate localization of discharges
Prolonged video EEG (day case recordings)	Prolonged recording which includes sleep and various activating procedures with physiologist in attendance and medical staff available for consultation		Diagnosis of seizure type and epilepsy syndrome
Inpatient EEG telemetry (surface electrodes)	Continuous EEG and video recording over days, with constant monitoring by nursing and medical staff; medication may be tapered		Localization of discharges as part of presurgical assessment
			Suspected non-epileptic attacks

It is important that the presence of sharp or rhythmic components in the factual report should not be taken as necessarily representing confirmation of an epileptic tendency. If there is uncertainty, the findings should always be discussed with the electrophysiologist.

Factors affecting the normal EEG

Age

The normal EEG alters with maturation until adulthood; this is of particular importance when studying premature babies and neonates, where correct

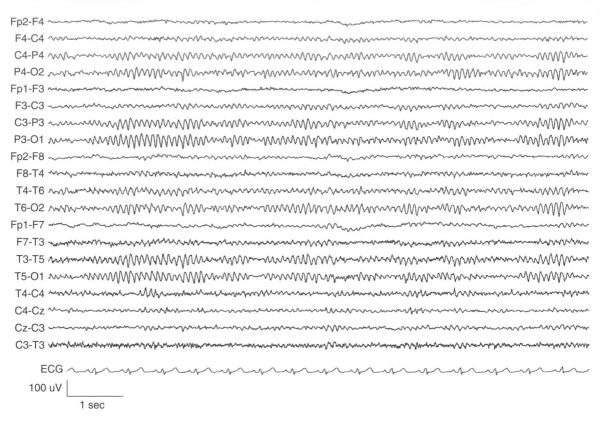

Figure 5.21 Normal waking adult EEG showing alpha rhythm posteriorly.

information regarding gestational age is important for accurate interpretation of the findings. In normal teenagers, some slow activity is often seen posteriorly (posterior slow waves of youth).

State of arousal

The normal posterior alpha rhythm of the relaxed alert state is replaced by theta in drowsiness (stage I sleep), and progression to the deeper stages of sleep is accompanied by various sleep phenomena (Positive Occipital Sharp Transients of Sleep or 'POSTS', sleep spindles, vertex sharp waves, and K complexes – stage II sleep), and deeper sleep (stages III and IV) are characterized by further symmetrical slowing of the background activities to 3 Hz or less.

Sedation produces similar background slowing and, in intensive care patients, the residual effects of intravenous sedation may interfere with interpretation of the EEG, if the record is taken too early after sedation is withdrawn.

Activation procedures

Hyperventilation, photic stimulation, sleep (drug-induced or natural sleep) and sleep deprivation are all used on occasion, in the appropriate clinical context, to bring out abnormalities not present in the resting record. These interictal epileptiform discharges or minor seizures provoked during the standard 'interictal' EEG are often sufficient to allow syndromic diagnosis, particularly in the idiopathic generalized epilepsies (IGEs) (see Chapter 13).

Hyperventilation

The subject is asked to breathe deeply and regularly at about 20 breaths per minute for about 3 minutes. The reduction in plasma CO_2 results in a mild degree of cerebral vasoconstriction. The changes are most marked in children and young adults in whom high voltage slow activity is induced, maximal anteriorly. In adults, the changes are usually less marked, the exception being in the presence of hypogly-caemia; the response may also be more marked in patients with migraine. The effect typically subsides after 60–90 s; prolonged slowing usually suggests areas of vascular compromise.

> Hyperventilation is used as an activation procedure to induce the appearance of epileptiform activity, particularly in patients with suspected IGE such as typical absence seizures. Combining overbreathing with breath-counting allows the detection of mild impairment of consciousness which may not otherwise be noticed with routine video recording. This is of particular importance if phantom absences are suspected (see Chapter 13).

Focal interictal spike wave activity can, however, be activated by hyperventilation in both IGE as well as some focal epilepsies, and syndromic diagnosis must, as always, depend on the combination of the EEG and the clinical history and presentation.

Photic stimulation

Photic stimulation is performed at various frequencies using a stroboscopic light. Generalized photoparoxysmal responses are typically seen in IGE, most commonly at frequencies between 12 and 20 Hz. Photoparoxysmal responses, particularly those limited to the posterior head regions, may sometimes be seen in patients with no history of seizures, and care should be taken to distinguish isolated photosensitivity from photosensitive epilepsy.

Sleep

Discharges in both focal epilepsies and in IGEs are activated during drowsiness and light sleep (drug-induced or natural sleep). During sleep, the discharges in IGE are particularly associated with phase A (greater arousal level) of the cyclic alternating pattern.

Sleep deprivation

Sleep deprivation and forced awakening are activating factors in the IGEs. Practice varies between centres and depending on the indication; all night deprivation may be used to induce a seizure in sleep, however most out-patient recordings are performed after only partial sleep deprivation. **There is an important benefit risk issue to be considered when sleep depriving a patient as seizures are dangerous, carry significant morbidity and sometimes mortality. The decision to sleep deprive must be justified in terms of a significant management outcome.**

CLINICAL INDICATIONS FOR AN EEG

Patients with suspected epileptic attacks

The EEG is not a 'test' for epilepsy but an interictal EEG is often helpful in providing support in patients with a highly suggestive clinical history, and principally is used in syndromic classification of patients with recurrent seizures.

The electrographic hallmark of the IGEs is the 3 per second (or faster) generalized spike-wave discharge which shows an abrupt bilateral and synchronous onset (Figure 5.22). These are the typical discharges seen in childhood absence, juvenile absence epilepsy and phantom absences. The background activity is normal.

In IGE syndromes predominantly manifesting with myoclonic seizures, such as juvenile myoclonic epilepsy, the interictal and ictal discharges are typically associated with irregular polyspike-and-wave activity, starting at >3 Hz but with unstable intradischarge frequencies. Interictal focal abnormalities are frequently seen, and there is often reflex seizure activation (most commonly in response to photic stimulation, but less frequent triggers include reading, some cognitive processes and praxis induction). In eyelid myoclonia with absences, eye closure may induce EEG paroxysms or seizures.

Temporal lobe epilepsy (TLE) is classified as mesial or lateral depending on the site of seizure onset. In mesial temporal epilepsy (as in hippocampal sclerosis), interictal anterior- to mid-temporal spikes may be seen, with the ictal discharge often taking the form of a rhythmic theta or delta discharge maximal over the anterior temporal region. In lateral temporal lobe epilepsy, the spikes are localized to more posterior/lateral temporal regions. Where bilateral onset is consistently seen on scalp,

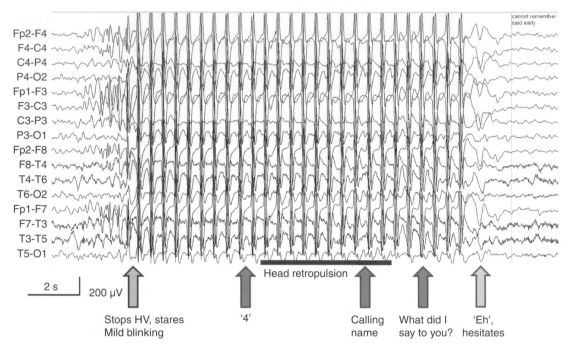

Fp2-F4
F4-C4
C4-P4
P4-O2
Fp1-F3
F3-C3
C3-P3
P3-O1
Fp2-F8
F8-T4
T4-T6
T6-O2
Fp1-F7
F7-T3
T3-T5
T5-O1

cannot remember
said early

Head retropulsion

2 s   200 μV

Stops HV, stares   '4'   Calling   What did I   'Eh',
Mild blinking   name   say to you?   hesitates

Figure 5.22 Typical absence seizure induced by hyperventilation in a patient with childhood absence epilepsy. Motor manifestations are minimal and consist of mild blinking (arrowed) and head retropulsion (black horizontal bar). Auditory stimulation delivered by the physiologist during the absence is marked on the trace. He showed no response or any behavioural change to the stimuli given and had no recollection of them after the absence. Note that motor arrest (stopping hyperventilation) and staring coincide with the first generalized spike wave oscillation of the discharge.

EEG and positron emission tomography (PET) scanning shows bilateral temporal hypometabolism, intracranial recordings using cortical subdural electrodes or stereotactic depth electrodes are required in patients being considered for epilepsy surgery.

In occipital epilepsies, the interictal scalp EEG may show unilateral occipital spikes, fast multiple spikes or occipital paroxysms. Fixation-off sensitivity (see Chapter 13) is characteristically seen in idiopathic occipital epilepsies, but may occasionally be seen in symptomatic occipital epilepsies (Figure 5.23).

In frontal lobe seizures, the interictal and ictal scalp EEG may be normal, and therefore most patients being considered for epilepsy surgery require intracranial EEG recordings. Simple partial seizures and epilepsy partialis continua are also frequently associated with normal surface EEG recordings.

It is important to note that the interictal EEG on its own cannot diagnose or exclude epilepsy, and cannot predict the likelihood for seizure relapse after discontinuation of antiepileptic drugs (AEDs).

In patients with frequent non-epileptic attacks (previously also known as pseudo-seizures or psychogenic seizures), recording a habitual attack can be very helpful in establishing the nature of the episodes. It should be remembered, however, that it is not uncommon for non-epileptic attacks and genuine seizures to coexist.

Patients with altered mental status

The EEG is helpful in differentiating altered mental status arising from an acute psychosis, in which the EEG does not show any gross abnormalities, from that due to an encephalopathy/encephalitis which is typically associated with diffuse slowing of cortical rhythms, with or without focal abnormalities. It is also helpful in identifying cases where impairment of consciousness is due to non-convulsive status epilepticus (Figure 5.24). Normal alpha activ-

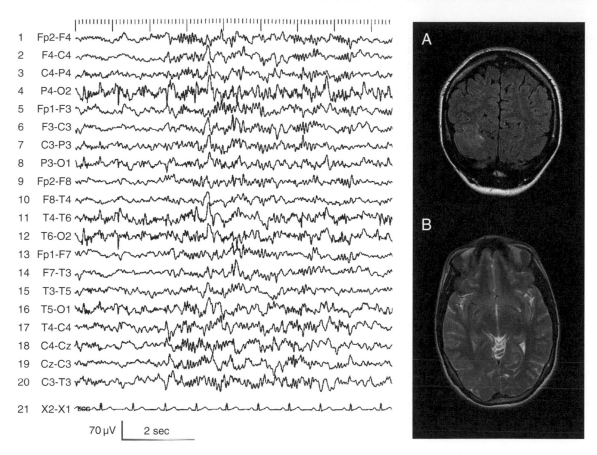

Figure 5.23 Left panel: Right occipital spiking during sleep. Right panel: Brain MRI of the same patient. Coronal FLAIR (A) and axial TW2 sequences (B) show a sizeable dysplastic area with cortical thickening, a blurred grey-white matter junction and faint cortical and subcortical T2 high signal in the right lateral occipital gyri.

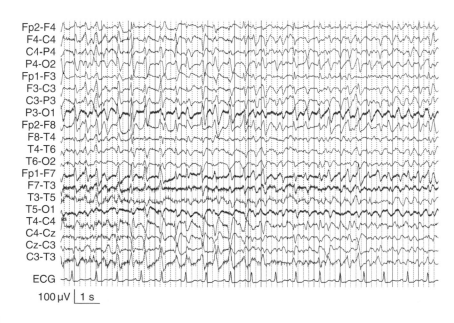

Figure 5.24 Complex partial status epilepticus. The discharges are generalized but phase-reverse over the midline.

ity during an attack of apparent unresponsiveness would suggest a non-epileptic/psychogenic cause (in the absence of paralysis due to neuromuscular disease, or a brainstem stroke, as in locked-in syndrome). An EEG containing an unusual amount of generalized fast activity in a poorly responsive or comatose patient would raise the possibility of benzodiazepine or barbiturate poisoning. Focal slowing would suggest a localized area of cerebral dysfunction.

Because the EEG reflects neuronal activity, it is helpful in providing some indication of the severity of cerebral dysfunction. However, it is not helpful in determining aetiology, since there are only a limited number of ways brain activity can alter in response to injury; thus similar electrographic changes can arise as a result of insults of various causes.

Nevertheless, some patterns, when present, are helpful in pointing towards a broad aetiological category. Triphasic waves are frequently associated with metabolic encephalopathies such as hepatic encephalopathy (Figure 5.25), uraemia, electrolyte abnormalities, anoxia and lithium intoxication. Generalized periodic complexes are seen in Creutzfeldt–Jacob disease (CJD) (Figure 5.26), subacute spongiform panencephalitis (SSPE) and severe anoxia. Bitemporal periodic lateralized epileptiform discharges (PLEDs) in the appropriated clinical context would raise the possibility of herpes simplex encephalitis (HSVE) (Figure 5.27). However, if the patient has received early treatment with acyclovir,

the EEG may show less specific temporal, frontal or generalized slowing. PLEDs are not specific for aetiology, and may also be seen in association with other acute or subacute destructive lesions (including cerebral infarcts) (Figure 5.28), again emphasizing the importance of the clinical context when interpreting EEG findings. Frontal intermittent rhythmic delta activity (FIRDA) was initially described in association with deep midline lesions, raised intracranial pressure, or subcortical dysfunction, but is now recognized as being much less specific and is more often found as a non-specific finding in diffuse encephalopathies.

In patients with psychiatric disorders, it is important to note that a variety of medications can alter the EEG. Sedative or recreational drugs, and some anti-psychotic drugs, particularly lithium and clozapine, may give rise to slowing and epileptiform changes. It is therefore important that full and accurate information on medication should always be provided with the EEG request.

Unresponsive patients on the intensive care unit

The EEG can provide helpful prognostication in patients who have suffered a severe cerebral anoxic insult. Provided all other factors likely to be contributing the EEG pattern (such as metabolic abnor-

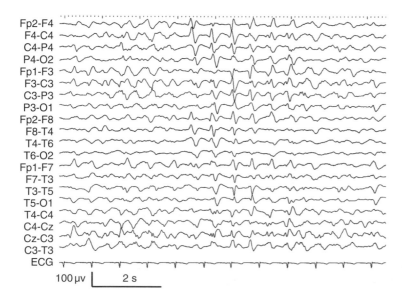

Figure 5.25 Triphasic sharp waves in a patient with hepatic encephalopathy.

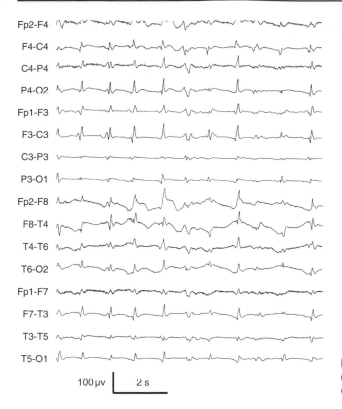

Fp2-F4
F4-C4
C4-P4
P4-O2
Fp1-F3
F3-C3
C3-P3
P3-O1
Fp2-F8
F8-T4
T4-T6
T6-O2
Fp1-F7
F7-T3
T3-T5
T5-O1

100 µv   2 s

Figure 5.26 Generalized, one per second, periodic complexes in a patient with sporadic Creutzfeldt-Jacob disease.

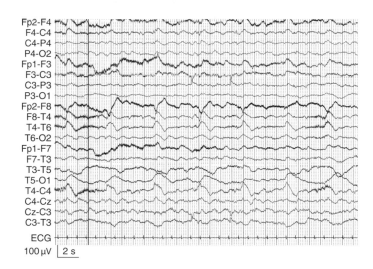

Fp2-F4
F4-C4
C4-P4
P4-O2
Fp1-F3
F3-C3
C3-P3
P3-O1
Fp2-F8
F8-T4
T4-T6
T6-O2
Fp1-F7
F7-T3
T3-T5
T5-O1
T4-C4
C4-Cz
Cz-C3
C3-T3
ECG
100 µV   2 s

Figure 5.27 Generalized slowing and periodic lateralized epileptiform discharges (PLEDs) over the right temporal region in a patient with acute herpes simplex encephalitis.

malities, sedation, hypothermia, sepsis) have been excluded, certain patterns are generally accepted as associated with a poor outcome. These include an unresponsive very low amplitude (<20 uV) trace, pseudoperiodic patterns (burst suppression, pseudoperiodic generalized epileptiform discharges (Figure 5.29), post-anoxic myoclonus status epilepticus, or continuous widespread unresponsive alpha or theta activity. Spontaneous fluctuation in cerebral activity, or evidence of responsiveness of the cerebral activity to external stimuli is a favourable prognostic indicator.

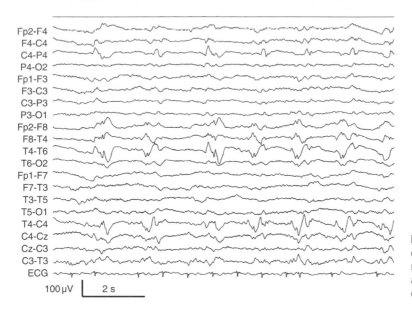

Figure 5.28 Periodic lateralized epileptiform discharges (PLEDs) over the right centrotemporal region following an acute cerebral infarct in the right middle cerebral artery territory.

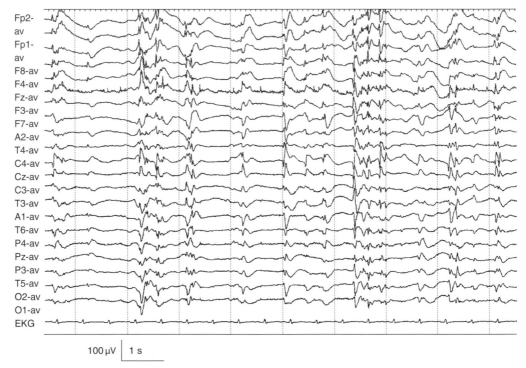

Figure 5.29 Pseudoperiodic generalized epileptiform discharges (PGED) alternating with periods of suppression lasting up to 2 seconds in a comatose patient following an out-of-hospital cardiac arrest. This EEG pattern was recorded 4 days after the event and indicates severe hypoxic brain damage and a grave neurological prognosis.

The EEG is also useful for monitoring seizure control in patients admitted in status epilepticus, and to assess progress in patients with drug intoxication or acute encephalitis.

It cannot be overemphasized that interpretation of the EEG findings is dependent on the clinical context. For example, a burst-suppression pattern carries a different prognosis following an episode

In patients in whom paroxysmal movements, autonomic fluctuations or sudden changes in conscious level raise the possibility of seizure activity, a video-EEG, with appropriate monitoring (EMG, oximetry, ECG, blood pressure (BP), skin impedence) is useful for differentiating ictal from non-ictal events.

of prolonged cerebral anoxia, compared to this pattern seen in the context of a drug overdose, severe hypothermia or use of anaesthetic agents.

Dementia

The EEG is of only limited diagnostic usefulness in dementia. It is helpful when sporadic CJD is suspected, when profound slowing and generalized 1 Hz periodic triphasic complexes may be seen (Figure 5.26); repeated recordings are often required. This finding is not specific to sporadic CJD, but is helpful if the history and clinical findings are highly suggestive. Periodic complexes and severe slowing may sometimes be seen in Lewy body dementia. In Alzheimer's disease, the record shows progressive slowing of waveforms; initially with loss of the posterior alpha activity, followed in the later stages by more widespread slowing. In fronto-temporal dementia, the EEG may be normal despite clear atrophy on imaging. The EEG has been superseded by imaging for the diagnosis of vascular dementia.

Brain death

An EEG is not required for the diagnosis of brain death in the UK. However, in the United States, determination of brain death includes demonstrating enduring loss of cerebral electrical activity (electrocerebral inactivity) according to a special recording protocol (American EEG Society, 1994).

THE EEG REPORT

The 'normal' EEG

A record is reported as normal if EEG patterns recognized as associated with clinical pathology are not seen during the period of the recording. However, it is well recognized that certain types of seizure activity (e.g. frontal lobe seizures), may be associated with no recordable abnormality on the scalp EEG, and a 'normal' record must therefore always be interpreted in the context of the likely clinical differential diagnoses.

The 'abnormal' EEG

The EEG is reported as abnormal if specific features recognized as being associated with pathology are present. These include epileptiform activity, photo-paroxysmal activity (paroxysmal activity induced by photic stimulation), slow waves (generalized or focal), amplitude asymmetries or other specific abnormal patterns.

However, an abnormal EEG does not always indicate the presence of clinically relevant cerebral pathology. Epileptiform changes may be seen in 10 per cent of patients who have undergone intra-cranial surgery, and in about 3 per cent of individuals with psychiatric disorders who do not have epilepsy. They may also be seen with therapeutic levels of certain medications (e.g. clozapine). The presence of photoparoxysmal responses induced in a laboratory setting does not necessarily imply that the patient has photosensitive epilepsy, and may be an incidental finding if the patient has no history of photic induced seizures. In the ITU setting, if performed too soon after sedation has been withdrawn, slowing of the record may be due to the persisting effects of sedative medication rather than underlying cerebral pathology.

Performed in the appropriate clinical setting, the EEG remains a useful investigation, particularly where there is impairment of consciousness. The best results are obtained when the studies are tailored to each patient depending on the differential diagnoses raised by the clinical presentation.

EVOKED POTENTIALS

Sensory EPs

The visual, brain stem and somatosensory evoked potentials (EPs) are electrical signals generated at various points along the nervous system in response to specific sensory stimuli. The timing and locations of these signals are determined by the anatomy of the sensory system involved. As with nerve conduction studies and EEGs, EPs are tests of function, and are not aetiologically specific. Their use has declined with the widespread availability of high quality MRI, although specific indications remain relevant.

Visual evoked potentials

Visual evoked potentials (VEPs) are responses of the visual cortex recorded in response to a set of standard stimuli. In adults, pattern-reversal stimuli (checkerboard of black and white squares which reverse in colour) to full and hemi-fields are routinely used; flash VEPs provide only limited information about the integrity of the visual pathways and tend only to be used when the subject is unable to cooperate with pattern-reversal; they will not be discussed further here.

VEPs are used to assess the function of the visual pathways anterior and posterior to the optic chiasm. Although MRIs have largely replaced evoked potentials for identifying lesions in other parts of the visual pathway, VEPs continue to be useful for identifying evidence of recent or previous (silent) optic neuritis in patients suspected of having multiple sclerosis (see Chapter 22). Electroretinography (ERG) represents the composite responses of the retina. Concomitant pattern ERGs are vital for accurate interpretation of VEPs when acuity is impaired, or when there is reason to suspect the presence of retinal disease. Ideally, VEPs and pattern ERGs should be routinely performed and interpreted together; in practice, pattern ERGs are largely limited to specialist centres.

Interpretation of the VEP is based primarily on measurement of the latency of the P100 component (the major positive peak with a latency of around 100 ms in normal subjects) following monocular stimulation. In optic neuritis, the typical finding is a delayed, but well-formed, waveform of normal amplitude. However, variations occur: cortical responses may be absent during the acute phase, or if subsequent recovery is poor. There is also some controversy as to whether the P100 latency always remains abnormal; some authors reporting that gradual latency recovery means that about 20 per cent of cases are within normal limits after 1–2 years. As with other neurophysiological investigations, the clinical context is always important; the VEP may be delayed in a maculopathy, or if there is a reduction in luminance (unilateral or bilateral ptosis, or in a drowsy patient).

Brain stem auditory evoked responses

The auditory evoked potentials include short-, middle- and long-latency potentials. The waveforms of the short-latency auditory evoked potential (AEP) mostly originate in the brainstem and are therefore also known as brainstem AEPs. Middle- and long-latency AEPs are not in routine clinical use and will not be discussed here.

Brief auditory stimuli in the form of clicks are presented to one ear while the other is masked with white noise. The normal response comprises five peaks labelled waves I–V. Wave I corresponds to the auditory nerve action potential and arises in the distal portion of the nerve. Wave II is generated by the proximal eighth nerve and cochlear nucleus. Wave III arises from the region of the superior olive and trapezoid body, and waves IV and V arise from generators in the upper pons and midbrain and inferior colliculus.

The use of brain stem auditory evoked responses (BSAEPs) for identifying lesions in the brainstem has largely been superseded by MRI. However, BSAEPs probably remain the most sensitive screening test for acoustic neuromas/schwannomas. In multiple sclerosis, the BSAEP is estimated to be abnormal in approximately 20 per cent of patients with possible or probable multiple sclerosis, even in the absence of clinical signs of brainstem dysfunction.

Somatosensory evoked potentials

The commonly used somatosensory evoked potentials (SSEPs) are those from the median, ulnar and tibial nerves. Upper limb SSEP responses are recorded at Erb's point, the cervical spine and cortex. Lower limb SSEPs are recorded over the spine at about the T12/L1 level and cortex. SSEPs test the integrity of the sensory pathways from the stimulated nerve, the relevant root, the dorsal column pathways in the spinal cord and brainstem to the cortex.

As with BSAEPs, SSEPs have largely been superseded by MRI for the detection of lesions in the spinal cord, although they may be helpful for documenting a lesion in the occasional patient with sensory symptoms but negative imaging. The main application of SSEPs today is as part of intraoperative monitoring during spinal surgery.

Motor evoked potentials

Motor evoked potentials (MEPs) assess the integrity of descending motor pathways. The motor cortex is stimulated by an electrical or magnetic stimulus, and the evoked response is recorded from an appropriate muscle in the upper or lower limb. MEPs can be generated by electrical or magnetic stimulation. Electrical stimulation, which produces more stable responses, is painful and therefore reserved for intraoperative monitoring. Transcranial magnetic stimulation (TMS) is generally well tolerated and can be used to measure the central motor conduction time (CMCT), which is often increased in demyelinating lesions. However, prolonged central motor conduction times may also occur in a variety of other conditions including motor neurone disease, hereditary spastic paraparesis and vascular lesions. CMCT measurements are often requested to investigate the integrity of motor pathways in apparently paralysed patients in whom no other investigation has provided evidence of pathology, and are helpful in the diagnosis of functional weakness.

More recently, with the use of various stimulation paradigms, TMS has been employed as a research tool for assessing changes in neuronal excitability in a variety of neurological conditions. Cortical stimulation with TMS is also being explored as a treatment modality in psychiatry, movement disorders, treatment resistant epilepsy and stroke.

Intraoperative monitoring

Electrophysiological monitoring of the integrity of SSEPs and MEPs pathways during spinal cord surgery is now widely used. SSEP monitoring alone is insufficient as it will not detect lesions in the ventral portion of the cord where infarction may occur without changes in dorsal column function. Early detection of neurological compromise allows prompt corrective measures which may prevent permanent neurological injury.

Monitoring facial nerve function by recording nerve or muscle action potentials to direct stimulation of the intracranial portion of CN VII reduces the risk of permanent facial palsy following surgery for cerebellopontine angle tumours.

REFERENCES AND FURTHER READING

Bradley WG, Daroff RB, Fenichel GM, Marsden CD (2000) *Neurology in Clinical Practice. Principles of Diagnosis and Management*, 3rd edn. Oxford: Butterworth Heinemann.

Dumitru D, Amato AA, Zwarts MJ (2002) *Electrodiagnostic Medicine*, 2nd edn. Philadelphia: Hanley and Belfus.

Ebersole JS, Pedley TA (2003) *Current Practice of Clinical Encephalography*, 3rd edn. Oxford: Lippincott Williams and Wilkins.

Panayiotopoulos C (2007) *A Clinical Guide to Epileptic Syndromes and their Treatment*, 2nd edn. London: Springer.

Preston DC, Shapiro BE (2005) *Electromyography and Neuromuscular Disorders. Clinical-Electrophysiologic Correlations*, 2nd edn. Oxford: Elsevier.

Robinson LR (2000) Traumatic injury to peripheral nerves. *Muscle and Nerve* 23:863–873.

CHAPTER 6

CRANIAL NERVE SYNDROMES

Tim Fowler, John Scadding and Nick Losseff

CRANIAL NERVE I

Anosmia

The olfactory nerve arises from nerve fibres in the nasal mucosa at the top of the nose, which pass through the cribriform plate forming the olfactory tract lying on the orbital surface of the frontal lobe. In most instances, the sense of smell relies on the inhalation of very small particles (airborne chemicals) of the substance under test. **Although many patients refer to the taste of foods, in nearly all instances this involves smell, as taste only differentiates sweet, salt, bitter and sour (acid).**

Smell may be lost (anosmia), diminished (hyposmia), perverted (parosmia), distorted (dysosmia) or unpleasant (cacosmia). Olfactory hallucinations are most commonly reported as part of the aura of complex partial seizures. These are usually unpleasant, very brief and may arise in the uncinate lobe. Olfactory hallucinations may also occur in psychiatric disorders.

Causes of anosmia are given in Table 6.1. Hynosmia is found very frequently with the common cold, sinusitis or nasal polyps. Head injuries may cause anosmia, due to shearing of the delicate olfactory fibres. Such loss is usually permanent: it is commonly associated with fractures of the floor of the anterior fossa. Anosmia may also arise from subfrontal tumours. These may present with dementia or altered behaviour and the most impor-

Table 6.1 Causes of anosmia

Local nasal disease	Infections, e.g. common cold, allergic rhinitis, nasal polyps
Trauma	Head injuries
Tumours	Subfrontal, e.g. meningioma, frontal glioma, pituitary
Degenerative	Alzheimer's disease, Huntington's chorea, Parkinson's disease
Endocrine	Addison's disease, diabetes mellitus

tant localizing sign may be anosmia. If the tumour is very large, it may cause papilloedema and optic nerve damage leading to optic atrophy.

CRANIAL NERVE II

Optic disc swelling

Papilloedema
This describes swelling with elevation of the optic disc. By definition this is a pathological swelling caused by raised intracranial pressure (ICP). As the disc swells, the veins become engorged and venous pulsation is lost (venous pulsation is best seen with the patient sitting or standing). The margins of the disc become indistinct and then radial streak haemorrhages may appear around the edges (Plate 1c,d).

Causes are shown in Box 6.1.

Optic disc swelling can be asymptomatic but usually there are symptoms related to the cause – from raised ICP or the site of a mass lesion. Visual acuity is usually unaffected, but there is only slight enlargement of the blind spots. With persistent raised ICP, there may eventually be a drop in acuity and some concentric constriction of the visual fields. With very high ICP, there may be transient visual obscurations with complete loss of vision lasting a few seconds, provoked by bending, coughing or straining – measures that produce a transient rise in ICP. Causes of monocular visual loss are given in Table 6.2.

Papilloedema may develop very rapidly, for example, with a cerebral haemorrhage, but more commonly arises slowly over days or weeks, as with a tumour. It should be emphasized that only some 50 per cent of cerebral tumours cause papilloedema.

Optic neuritis

Optic neuritis is an acute inflammation of the optic nerve causing acute visual loss, usually in one eye. If the nerve head, the papilla, is involved causing it to swell; this is papillitis.

Papillitis

A papillitis describes local swelling of the nerve head with involvement of the optic nerve and is characterized by a fall in visual acuity, an afferent pupillary defect and a central scotoma.

If the inflammation lies behind the nerve head, the disc may appear normal – a **retrobulbar neuritis**. Commonly, optic neuritis affects younger patients, aged 15–40 years. In children, both eyes may be affected and this may follow an acute viral infection. Most patients with optic neuritis describe acute or subacute visual loss with a fall in acuity varying from mild (6/9–6/12) to severe with almost complete loss. The process may progress over hours or days, usually reaching its worst within 1 week. There may be tenderness of the globe with pain on movement in the affected eye. Most often there is a central or paracentral scotoma, sometimes very large. Colour vision is impaired and there is an afferent pupillary defect. Later, pallor, indicating atrophy, may follow both optic neuritis (papillitis) or retrobulbar neuritis.

Box 6.1 Causes of papilloedema

Raised intracranial pressure
Mass lesions – tumours, abscesses, haematomas
Cerebral oedema – trauma, infarcts
Infections – meningitis, encephalitis
Obstructive hydrocephalus
Venous sinus thrombosis – cavernous, sagittal
Idiopathic intracranial hypertension
Medical disorders
Severe anaemia, including B12 deficiency
Polycythaemia rubra vera
Accelerated hypertension
Lead poisoning
Carbon dioxide retention
Drugs – tetracycline, excess vitamin A, lithium, isoretinoin, ibuprofen, steroids (withdrawal)

Table 6.2 Causes of monocular visual loss (usually acute)

Optic neuritis	MS
	Viral (childhood)
	Epstein–Barr virus
	Post-infectious
	Sphenoid sinusitis
	Unknown
Ischaemic optic neuritis	GCA, atheroma (may be sequential)
Orbital tumour	
Chiasmal compression[a]	Usually slower
Leber's optic atrophy[a]	
Retinal vascular	Arterial (GCA), occlusion embolic, venous (dysproteinaemia)
Elevated ICP[a]	Late
Toxic[a]	Methyl alcohol

[a]May be bilateral.

GCA, giant cell arteritis; ICP, intracranial pressure; MS, multiple sclerosis.

Optic neuritis is the initial symptom of multiple sclerosis (MS) in about 25 per cent of patients. However, if patients with an episode of optic neuritis are followed up, 50–70 per cent develop MS. An abnormal MR brain scan increases the risk of developing MS.

In most instances, recovery of vision occurs over 6–8 weeks, and about 90 per cent of patients recover acuity to 6/9 or better. In many there will be a residual afferent pupillary defect, impaired colour vision and disc pallor. A few patients are left with severe visual loss. Recurrent attacks in the same eye occur in 20–30 per cent of patients. Visual evoked potentials will show a prolonged latency which persists. MRI shows abnormal signal in the affected optic nerve.

Steroid treatment may shorten symptoms, relieving pain and allowing more rapid recovery of acuity, but in most cases is not given.

The American optic neuritis trial

This found that the clinical diagnosis of optic neuritis was sufficient without the need for special investigations. The outcome in terms of recovery of visual acuity was not altered whether steroids were used or not. However, there was a more rapid return of acuity in patients treated with pulsed IV steroids.

Those patients treated showed a reduced risk of relapse at two years compared to those treated with placebo or oral steroids, although by four years the figures were not significantly different.

There was the suggestion that patients treated with pulsed IV steroids showed a reduced rate of the development of MS during the first two years of follow-up in those who had shown abnormal MR brain scans (more than two white matter lesions) at the time of the optic neuritis. An MR brain scan showing more than three white matter lesions of greater than 3 mm size predicted an increased risk of the development of MS. By three years, 43 per cent of those presenting with optic neuritis had developed MS.

The most common clinical practice now is to use high dose pulsed IV steroids in patients with:

- bilateral ON;
- poor vision in the fellow eye and in whom the good eye has been affected;
- severe loss of acuity and marked pain.

The CHAMPS (Controlled High Risk Subjects Avonex Multiple Sclerosis Prevention Study) study suggested that the use of beta interferon Ia in patients presenting with an acute optic neuritis and abnormal MR brain scan reduces the risk of developing clinically definite MS over a three-year period.

Ischaemic optic neuritis

Vascular optic nerve damage

In older people, infarction of the optic nerve may arise from vascular damage. This may follow giant cell arteritis (GCA) or be part of atherosclerotic arterial disease. If the posterior ciliary arteries or peripapillary choroidal vessels occlude, the anterior part of the optic nerve and its head may infarct.

Usually there is an acute, painless, severe loss of vision in one eye, occasionally less severe. There is an afferent pupillary defect, a swollen disc and often rather attenuated thin retinal arteries. **With GCA, there is permanent visual loss in up to 50 per cent of patients. Once infarction has occurred in one eye, there is a severe risk that the second eye may sequentially be affected, unless prompt treatment with steroids has been started.** With GCA there may be complaints of headache, scalp tenderness, jaw claudication, malaise, fever, myalgia and proximal muscle weakness – there is an overlap with polymyalgia rheumatica.

In such patients, this loss of vision is an emergency and the erythrocyte sedimentation rate (ESR) must be measured urgently. This is nearly always raised in GCA, but if the clinical suspicion is strong, prednisolone 60–80 mg daily should be started immediately. The dose is later adjusted according to the patient's response and the ESR level, although prolonged low-dose steroids are often needed for 1–2 years. A temporal artery biopsy should be carried out within 72 hours, although arteries may be patchily affected – 'skip' areas. Affected vessels may show luminal narrowing from intimal proliferation and cellular infiltration of the media by round cells and giant cells. More commonly, optic nerve infarction arises from atheroma; it is also found in diabetics.

Retinal vascular occlusion

The **central retinal artery** may occlude suddenly, most often from an embolus or thrombosis, in older patients. Typically, there is an acute painless loss of acuity with either complete blindness or an altitudinal field loss from a branch occlusion. The retina appears pale and swollen with thinned arteries. Cotton wool spots, small haemorrhages and a cherry red spot at the fovea may be seen in the retina. GCA should always be considered and excluded.

Venous occlusions arise from thrombosis and characteristically cause acute visual loss of varying degree. Dysproteinaemias may be a cause. The retina shows massive haemorrhages ('blood and thunder'). There may be a persistent defect, sometimes improvement, but conversely deterioration linked with neovascularization and the development of glaucoma.

Treatment of acute arterial occlusion involves attempts to lower the intraocular pressure by IV acetazolamide, anterior chamber aspiration and ocular massage.

Optic atrophy

Optic atrophy indicates that the optic nerve has been permanently damaged. The signs are those of impaired visual acuity with a field defect and pallor of the optic disc (Plate 1b). The causes are listed in Box 6.2.

Slowly progressive visual deterioration may also be caused by toxins and certain deficiencies. These are well illustrated by tobacco/alcohol amblyopia, which is found most commonly in older patients, often chronic alcoholics whose dietary calories are largely provided by alcohol, accompanied by malnutrition. It is also found in heavy smokers using strong tobacco to roll their own cigarettes. There is a progressive fall in acuity accompanied by bilateral centrocaecal scotomas.

The latter are often difficult to chart but are most easily found with red targets. Such field defects commonly cross the vertical meridian of the field. Electrophysiological studies on the visual pathways may help to confirm such damage. Abstention from alcohol, cessation of smoking, a good diet with added injections of thiamine and vitamin B12 may prevent deterioration and often allow a degree of recovery, although this may prove incomplete.

Box 6.2 Causes of optic atrophy

Raised intracranial pressure – consecutive
  Mass lesions – tumours
  Infections
    Meningo-encephalitis
    Tuberculosis, syphilis
Optic nerve
  Inflammatory – optic neuritis
  Vascular – infarction
  Compression – glioma, meningioma, orbital tumour
  Toxic – alcohol, isoniazid, hydroxyquinolines
  Inherited – Leber's
  Deficiencies – B12, thiamine
  Trauma
Chiasmal compression
  Pituitary and parapituitary tumours
  Aneurysms
Retinal and ocular causes
  Tapeto-retinal degenerations
  Glaucoma
  Severe myopia
  Metabolic storage diseases
  Anterior visual pathways
  Radiation

Investigation of visual loss
Record the visual acuity and chart the visual fields

- Blood tests – blood count, ESR, serum proteins and electrophoresis, serum B12 level, fasting glucose, liver function tests, *Treponema pallidum* haemagglutination test (TPHA) or equivalent, pituitary function (where appropriate)
- Electrophysiological tests – visual evoked potentials, electroretinograms
- Imaging – MR scanning to include the optic nerves, chiasm, brain
- MR angiography may be indicated. Computed tomography (CT) scanning with bone windows to look at the skull base
- Test cerebrospinal fluid (CSF) – for cells, protein, oligoclonal bands; cytology for malignant cells.

Ophthalmological referral to exclude ocular causes.

Slowly progressive visual loss always requires full investigation to exclude a local ocular cause, or compression of the optic nerve or chiasm.

Leber's hereditary optic atrophy

Leber's hereditary optic atrophy is a rare inherited condition presenting in the teens or early adult life, with males more commonly affected. There may be acute or subacute visual failure either in one eye or both eyes, progressing over weeks or months to an acuity of 6/36–6/60, accompanied by a dense central or centrocaecal scotoma. Colour vision is severely affected. The optic disc may appear swollen with abnormal blood vessels, and later pallor, but is sometimes normal. Often one eye is affected first and deterioration of the second follows within weeks.

Leber's hereditary optic atrophy is caused by a mitochondrial DNA defect resulting from a point mutation, most commonly at the 11778 location. About 50 per cent of patients have no positive family history. Mutations may arise at other sites – 3460 and 14484; these carry differing prognoses (14484 carries the best prognosis). However, 11778 and 3460 mutations are responsible for the condition in most patients of European origin.

Clinically, there appears to be some overlap with the optic neuropathies produced by tobacco/alcohol intake, B12 deficiency, the toxic effects of methanol or drugs such as ethambutol. The mechanism appears to be a block in oxidative phosphorylation.

There is no effective treatment but injections of hydroxocobalamin are usually added. Patients are advised to stop smoking and to avoid alcohol.

CRANIAL NERVES III, IV AND VI; OCULAR MOTOR PALSIES

Damage to cranial nerves III, IV and VI will cause weakness or paralysis of the ocular muscles they supply, producing diplopia if the two eyes are not in parallel. Table 6.3 indicates some of the causes and their frequency.

Diplopia may also arise from pathology of the ocular muscles, for example dysthyroid restrictive ophthalmopathy, or from diseases affecting the neuromuscular junction, for example myasthenia

Table 6.3 Causes of ocular motor palsies

	Cranial nerve		
	III	IV	VI
Trauma	13	28	11
Vascular	17	15	9
Neoplasm	18	10	31
Aneurysm	18		3
Undetermined	20	34	22
Other	14	13	24

Figures as percentages.

gravis. **If there is a very slow onset and progression, particularly if this occurs early in childhood, there may be suppression of the image from the weak eye, amblyopia. This is often accompanied by a visible squint, strabismus.** In a divergent squint, the eyes are deviated away from each other (wall-eyed), **exotropia**: in a convergent squint the eyes are turned towards each other (cross-eyed), **esotropia**. If one eye is obviously higher (above) the other, this is termed **hypertropia**, or below the other, **hypotropia**. A latent squint may be demonstrated by asking the patient to fix on an object and then covering each eye in turn. If the uncovered eye moves to fix on the target, a latent squint has been elicited.

The cover test will also distinguish between a concomitant squint (where the affected eye will show a full range of movement when its fellow is covered) and a true paralytic squint. The testing for diplopia has been described in Chapter 3.

Oculomotor palsy

Oculomotor palsy

In a complete oculomotor palsy, the eyelid droops to cover the eye and the globe is turned down and out as a result of the unopposed actions of the unparalysed lateral rectus and superior oblique muscles (see Figure 4.11). The pupil may be enlarged and unreactive if the pupillomotor fibres that lie around the periphery of the nerve are affected.

Thus a 'surgical' lesion such as an aneurysm (Figure 6.1) or tumour compressing the oculomo-

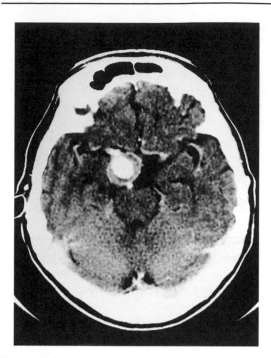

Figure 6.1 Computed tomography brain scan with enhancement showing a large aneurysm at the termination of the internal carotid artery. The patient presented with a painful partial oculomotor palsy with pupillary involvement.

tor nerve usually result in a large unreactive pupil. There will also be paralysis of the superior and inferior rectus, the medial rectus and inferior oblique muscles. Vascular lesions, which may infarct the nerve, for example as a result of diabetes mellitus or an arteritis, may produce a complete oculomotor palsy with pupillary sparing. Such lesions recover spontaneously over 3–4 months. Because of the anatomical arrangement of the various divisions of the oculomotor nuclei in the midbrain tegmentum, a nuclear lesion will cause bilateral ptosis and loss of upgaze in both eyes, with ipsilateral involvement of the medial and inferior rectus and inferior oblique muscles.

Trochlear palsy

The superior oblique depresses the adducted eye and intorts the abducted eye. This will cause **diplopia on downgaze with vertical separation of images**. There is often an associated **head tilt** to the opposite shoulder. Head injury is the most common cause.

Abducens palsy

The lateral rectus muscle abducts the eye, causing diplopia with horizontal separation of images maximal on gaze to the affected side. The sixth nerve has a relatively long course across the base of the skull, through the cavernous sinus and into the orbit via the superior orbital fissure. On this course, it may be affected by trauma, compression from masses, or inflamed or damaged as an effect of raised intracranial pressure.

Ocular motor palsies (Table 6.3) may arise centrally within the pons and midbrain from strokes, neoplasms, plaques of multiple sclerosis and thiamine deficiency (Wernicke's encephalopathy). Usually such lesions produce other signs, particularly involvement of other cranial nerves, a Horner's syndrome, cerebellar signs and sometimes long tract signs in the limbs. At the base of the brain, nerves may be damaged by meningitis or from basal neoplasms, for example nasopharyngeal carcinoma, or chordoma.

Cavernous sinus lesions

Cavernous sinus lesions cause involvement of the IIIrd, IVth and VIth cranial nerves and impaired sensation, most commonly in the territory of the ophthalmic division of the Vth (very occasionally the maxillary division if the lesion is inferior and posterior, see Figure 6.2). Sometimes the optic nerve may be involved. Most often the pathology

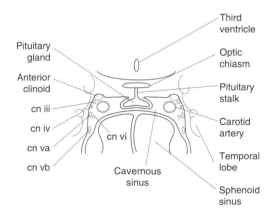

Figure 6.2 Diagram of coronal section in the parasellar region to include the cavernous sinus. cn iii, oculomotor nerve; cn iv, trochlear nerve; cn va, ophthalmic division of trigeminal nerve; cn vb, maxillary division of trigeminal nerve; cn vi, abducens nerve.

is from an aneurysm, caroticocavernous fistula or thrombosis (often secondary to infection), a tumour (pituitary, meningioma, nasopharyngeal carcinoma, metastasis) or from a granuloma (sarcoid, Tolosa–Hunt syndrome, Wegener's). More anteriorly, at the back of the orbit, mass lesions and granulomas may displace the globe producing diplopia and an axial proptosis.

Dysthyroid eye disease

An overactive thyroid (hyperthyroidism) may produce abnormal eye signs. **These include exophthalmos, a lid lag, conjunctival suffusion and diplopia**. The last is most often diplopia with vertical separation of images from restriction of upgaze, or less commonly from limitation of abduction. Dysthyroid eye disease is a restrictive ophthalmopathy where direct infiltration of the ocular muscles causes thickening and fibrosis, which results in tethering and restricted movements, most often found in the inferior and medial rectus muscles. This leads to impaired upgaze and abduction. The affected muscles appear swollen on orbital views of a CT or MRI scan. Blood tests will usually confirm the presence of thyrotoxicosis, but sometimes the evidence for thyroid disease is subtle and requires more specialized endocrine investigation.

Investigation of patients with ocular motor palsies and diplopia

Blood tests – full blood count, ESR, fasting glucose, thyroid function, TPHA or equivalent, autoantibodies including those for acetylcholine receptor

Edrophonium test

Electromyography – specialized tests of the neuromuscular junction

Imaging – MRI scanning of the orbits and brain, CT scanning of orbits or skull base, MR or CT angiography, chest x-ray – MRI of chest (to exclude thymoma)

Evoked potentials – visual and auditory (particularly combined with MRI of brain to support a diagnosis of MS)

CSF examination – to diagnose meningitis, a subarachnoid haemorrhage, to support MS

Myasthenia gravis

In any patient with variable diplopia, the diagnosis of myasthenia gravis should be considered. The condition may remain confined to an ocular distribution (ocular MG), but frequently later extends to involve facial and bulbar muscles, and may become generalized, with involvement of limb and trunk muscles. The diagnosis is confirmed by a raised titre of acetylcholine receptor antibodies, or by electrodiagnostic tests. An edrophonium test may be helpful (Chapter 18).

CRANIAL NERVE V

Trigeminal neuralgia, tic douloureux

Trigeminal neuralgia describes episodes of acute neuralgia, usually appearing as stabs, jabs or intense shoots of pain lasting seconds, and in the vast majority in the territory of the maxillary or mandibular divisions of the trigeminal nerve on one side. The pains are commonly triggered by touch, contact, for example washing, shaving, eating, cleaning the teeth, talking or a cold wind on the face.

Trigeminal neuralgia is considered further in Chapter 11.

Trigeminal sensory neuropathy

Trigeminal sensory neuropathy is a rare condition of unknown aetiology causing the slow progressive loss of sensation starting in one side of the face and becoming bilateral in 70 per cent of patients, usually asymmetrical in severity. The aetiology is unknown but there is an association with connective tissue disease, including systemic sclerosis, mixed connective tissue disease, systemic lupus erythematosus, Sjögren's syndrome and rheumatoid arthritis.

It usually starts with a patch of numbness, which increases in size, sometimes extending throughout the territory of the trigeminal nerve. In some patients pain or paraesthesiae may be the presenting symptoms, and progressive sensory loss then follows. Other causes of facial sensory loss are given in Table 6.4. The pathology for these may start in the pons, skull base or in the sinuses or face. Meningiomas, basal tumours, aneurysms or infiltration from a nasopharyngeal carcinoma or lymphoma are the most common symptomatic causes. Usually, such pathology involves the lower cranial nerves and sometimes the long tracts as well. In MS, facial numbness is common. Toxic damage may arise from substances such as trichlorethylene.

Investigations

In trigeminal sensory neuropathy, investigations should be negative. Brain scanning with MRI and CT scanning of the skull base are combined useful measures to exclude other pathology. A CSF examination may help to confirm the presence of a malignant or infective meningitis or MS. An ear, nose and throat (ENT) examination is important to look for sinus or nasopharyngeal lesions.

Numb chin syndrome

A small localized patch of sensory loss may be found on the chin in patients where the mental nerve has been involved by malignancy in the mandible. Such patients may have palpable submental lymph glands.

The finding of sensory loss within a mental nerve distribution is an important sign which should always prompt careful investigation.

CRANIAL NERVE VII

Bell's palsy

Bell's palsy is a common condition that presents with an acute onset of a lower motor neurone facial weakness affecting the muscles on one side of the face.

It has an annual incidence of 23 per 100 000 and all ages may be affected, including children, although the highest incidence is in patients aged 30–50 years. The causes of lower motor neurone facial palsy are listed in Table 6.5.

Pathogenesis

Electrophysiological studies in Bell's palsy suggest that there is segmental demyelination resulting in a local conduction block proximally. This allows a relatively rapid and complete recovery in about 85

Table 6.4 Causes of facial numbness

Inflammation	MS, connective tissue diseases
Infection	Herpes zoster, leprosy
Neoplastic	Trigeminal neuroma, meningioma, cerebellopontine angle tumours, gliomas, carcinomatous infiltration, metastases, nasopharyngeal carcinoma
Toxic	Trichlorethylene, cocaine abuse, allopurinol
Vascular	Pontine and medullary infarction, basilar aneurysms, AVMs, sickle-cell disease
Granuloma	Sarcoidosis
Trauma	Head injury, dental (extractions, anaesthesia)

AVMs, arteriovenous malformations; MS, multiple sclerosis.

Table 6.5 Causes of facial palsy

Idiopathic	Bell's
Infective	Viral – zoster, mumps, EBV, Borrelia[a], herpes
Vascular	Hypertension, diabetes, pontine infarction, vasculitis (collagen vascular disease)
Inflammatory	Guillain-Barré[a], MS (pontine plaque), otitis media
Tumour	Cerebellopontine angle tumour, cholesteatoma, meningeal carcinomatosis, pontine glioma, parotid
Trauma	Temporal or basal skull fractures
Granuloma	Sarcoidosis[a]

[a]May often be bilateral.
Muscular dystrophies and myasthenia may affect the facial muscles.
EBV, Epstein-Barr virus; MS, multiple sclerosis.

per cent of cases. In others, axonal degeneration occurs, which will produce a severe paralysis. Often this is then followed by incomplete recovery associated with aberrant reinnervation, that is, fibres to the periocular muscles may regenerate and supply the mouth, and vice versa. Such faulty reinnervation may lead to 'jaw-winking', and hemifacial spasm. Where axonal degeneration has occurred, electromyography of the facial muscles will show fibrillation and features of denervation, although these changes may not appear until some 10 days after the onset. In some instances the pathogenesis is a mixture of axonal degeneration and demyelination.

Symptoms and signs

> Patients may present with pain in or behind the ear preceding or appearing with the development of facial weakness. There is inability to close the eye or move the lower face and mouth.

The lack of blinking leads to tears spilling out of the eye, which waters to cause complaints of blurred vision. The cheek is flaccid and saliva and fluids may escape from the corner of the mouth. The weakness commonly progresses over 24–72 hours to reach a maximum. In many patients there are complaints of 'numbness' or 'deadness' in the affected side of the face, although trigeminal sensation is spared and there should be no weakness of jaw movement (supplied by the motor root of the trigeminal nerve).

About 40–50 per cent of patients are aware of disturbed taste on the ipsilateral anterior part of the tongue. This points to a lesion in the distal part of the facial nerve below the geniculate ganglion, but above the origin of the chorda tympani. Many patients also notice hyperacusis because the stapedius muscle is supplied by a branch of the facial nerve, which leaves the nerve in the facial canal proximal to the chorda tympani. **If herpes zoster infection is responsible, there will be herpetic vesicles on the pinna or in the external auditory canal on the affected side.** Ramsay Hunt described a herpetic infection of the geniculate ganglion with the development of an acute facial palsy (Hunt's syndrome). In some of these patients the eighth cranial nerve may also be infected, producing acute vertigo, deafness and tinnitus (see Chapter 11, Craniofacial pain). A few patients may show a bilateral facial palsy of lower motor neurone pattern; this may appear as part of a Guillain–Barré syndrome, from Lyme disease, from sarcoidosis or even carcinomatous meningitis.

Prognosis

About 85 per cent of patients show signs of improvement within 3–4 weeks of the onset. About 70 per cent of patients recover normal function in the face but approximately 16 per cent are left with asymmetry, signs of aberrant reinnervation and some weakness. An incomplete palsy at the onset or signs of recovery starting within 3–4 weeks are usually good prognostic features for recovery. This is mirrored in the electrophysiological findings. In the more severely affected, where axonal degeneration has taken place, recovery is slower and often incomplete. Recurrent facial palsies require more intensive investigation to exclude any compressive lesion in the middle ear or skull base, and to look for any systemic upset such as sarcoidosis, hypertension or diabetes.

Investigations

Blood tests – full blood count, ESR, fasting glucose, tests for Borrelia

Imaging – in selected patients MRI and/or CT scanning. Chest x-ray

EMG studies – these may assess the severity of damage and help in prognosis; they may also indicate a more widespread neuropathy

ENT examination

CSF examination – in selected patients

Treatment

There appears to be little difference in outcome between patients treated with corticosteroids and those who are not. There is evidence that a short intensive course of corticosteroids given within 5–7 days of the onset of the palsy may reduce the swelling of the facial nerve and so prevent axonal degeneration. Prednisolone 40 mg daily for 5 days and then tapered off over the next week is a typical regimen. It has been suggested that such a course should be given to all patients seen acutely with a complete palsy at the time of consultation or with impaired taste.

Because of the possible infective causation by the herpes virus, acyclovir has also been used in the treatment of an acute facial palsy. This certainly should be given if zoster infection (Ramsay Hunt syndrome, see Chapter 11) is suspected. The combination of acyclovir with steroids in those patients with complete facial palsies has also been used. Surgical decompression of the facial nerve has had its supporters over the years, although there has been no rigorous controlled trial to indicate benefit and, as over 70 per cent of patients will make a full recovery with no treatment, it is hard to justify the surgical risks.

Care of the eye is always important if there is incomplete lid closure but as the cornea is not anaesthetic, the patient will be aware of any intruding foreign body. Occasionally it may be necessary to suture the lids partially together, a tarsorrhaphy, to protect the eye.

In those patients left with marked residual weakness or asymmetry, a number of surgical measures may be used to try to improve their appearance. These include plastic surgery with implants of soft tissues to restore the contours. Such measures will improve the symmetry of the face at rest but are by no means a 'cure'.

Hemifacial spasm

Hemifacial spasm describes an involuntary twitching of the muscles on one side of the face. The muscles around the eye (blepharospasm), in the cheek or around the mouth are those usually affected. The twitches are irregular clonic movements, which may be mild and infrequent or very prominent and repetitive, even leading to closure of the eye. Often muscles appear to wink and the cheek and corner of the mouth to draw up. Many patients are aware of considerable variation in the movements; these are worse when tired or when physically or emotionally stressed. They may lead to great distress.

Electromyography studies show synchronous motor discharges in bursts firing rapidly. Rarely, such spasms may reflect irritation of the facial nerve by a cerebellopontine angle tumour or a basilar aneurysm. In a few instances, the spasm may follow a previous facial palsy. At operation, an increasing number of patients have been found to have a small blood vessel lying in contact with the facial nerve close to where it leaves the pons. By careful separation of this vessel from the nerve under the direct vision of an operating microscope, the spasms may be relieved. Medical treatment is disappointing; carbamazepine and clonazepam have been tried but usually with very limited benefit. The best treatment now, apart from surgical microdecompression, is by the injection of small doses of **botulinum toxin A** into the affected facial muscles. Such treatments need to be repeated, often at regular intervals – every 3–4 months.

Hemifacial spasm needs to be differentiated from facial **myokymia**. In the latter, there is a very fine involuntary movement in the facial muscles on one side, often in the cheek, like a fine rippling under the skin. Myokymia arises from intrinsic pontine lesions, most commonly from plaques of demyelination, but also from other pathology such as a pontine glioma.

Facial hemiatrophy

The soft tissues, fat and connective tissue on one side of the face, most often in the cheek, may gradually disappear and atrophy. This may lead to a curious indentation in the contour of the face. It usually progresses very slowly over many years and is of unknown aetiology. If asymmetry is very marked, plastic surgery may be helpful.

CRANIAL NERVE VIII

The eighth cranial nerve has two divisions, the cochlear and vestibular components. Disturbances may produce symptoms of deafness, tinnitus and vertigo.

In assessment of hearing loss, it is important to determine the onset: whether acute, fluctuating or slowly progressive, and also whether this affects one or both ears. Familial (hereditary) forms of deafness may occur and are sometimes associated with other neurological problems. A history of trauma, exposure to noise or certain drugs, for example aminoglycosides, may be of relevance. Examination should include particular attention to the cochlear and vestibular functions of the eighth nerve (see Chapter 3) and to the presence of nystagmus, trigeminal sensory loss or cerebellar disturbance.

Fluctuating deafness suggests Ménière's disease; while progressive unilateral deafness suggests a possible acoustic neuroma. Deafness may arise from lesions of the middle ear and is then conductive in type. This may arise from damage to the ossicles, from a blocked external canal, from otitis media, a perforated ear drum, otosclerosis or Eustachian tube blockage. Such pathology can be confirmed by careful examination of the ear. Deafness may also arise from damage to the cochlea or cochlear division of the eighth nerve, sensorineural deafness. This may be caused by trauma, drugs (e.g. quinine, aminoglycosides), Ménière's disease, cerebellopontine angle tumours, hypothyroidism and by presbyacusis. A watch-tick or a 512 or 1024 Hz tuning fork will test high tone frequency hearing loss: this is impaired in nerve deafness. Audiometry and auditory-evoked brainstem potentials allow very accurate and detailed assessment of hearing disorders.

Tinnitus, a hallucination of sound, may be described as ringing, buzzing, hissing or roaring. It is frequently associated with deafness. Occasionally it reflects a vascular flow murmur from an arteriovenous malformation or dural shunt and then is usually pulsatile.

Deafness is very common in old age: assessment of such patients may allow provision of a hearing aid or other measures for relief.

Ménière's disease, endolymphatic hydrops

Ménière's disease is a common disorder affecting the 30- to 50-year-old age group with an incidence of about 50–200 per 100 000 a year. Most patients present with unilateral involvement but about 30–50 per cent develop bilateral disturbance. It has been suggested that an excessive accumulation of fluid arises in the system because of a failure to reabsorb the endolymph. This in time leads to cochlear degeneration. **It causes recurrent episodes of severe vertigo associated with fluctuating deafness and tinnitus**. In about 40 per cent, the symptoms start with deafness, distorted sounds and sometimes a sensation of fullness or pressure in the affected ear. This may be associated with a low-pitched tinnitus. In about two-thirds of patients, episodes of rotational vertigo develop within six months of

onset, usually associated with nausea and vomiting. The vertigo lasts from 30 minutes to hours and during an attack the patient appears unsteady and will fall to the affected side. They prefer to lie down with the affected ear uppermost and during the episode there is obvious nystagmus with the fast phase away from the diseased ear. Afterwards, a sensation of imbalance may persist for several days.

Over many years, such patients will commonly experience repeated attacks and sometimes long periods of remission. A few patients may end up with positional vertigo, drop attacks or persistent ataxia. There is usually a slowly progressive deafness and bilateral disease may develop.

Hearing tests will confirm a sensorineural deafness. Initially, caloric tests may be normal but later a canal paresis or evidence of directional preponderance develops. Imaging tests are normal; a thin slice MR brain scan with gadolinium enhancement may be needed to exclude a small acoustic neuroma. It is important to check a TPHA or equivalent, as syphilis may cause deafness and vertigo.

Treatment

In the acute attack, most patients require bed rest accompanied by an injection or suppository to relieve the vomiting. In adults, a prochlorperazine suppository of 25 mg or an injection of 6.25–12.5 mg should be given. Frequent attacks may be treated with a vestibular sedative such as cinnarizine or betahistine, although there have been no proper trials of treatment in the acute phase. Most treatment regimens now use a graded approach, starting with dietary changes with the elimination of caffeine and a reduced sodium intake. These may be combined with the use of a diuretic and, in the acute phase, a vestibular sedative. Vestibular rehabilitation exercises may also be used. About 80 per cent of patients respond to such measures but in those that do not, surgery may be employed – either endolymphatic sac surgery or ablative therapy to destroy the affected labyrinth or its function. These procedures will produce deafness but can give relief in selected patients.

Episodic vertigo

Labyrinthine disease is the usual cause for episodic vertigo. The most common cause is travel (motion) sickness, which many people have experienced and such symptoms well illustrate those found in vertigo. These include hallucinations of movement, nausea and vomiting, fear and prostration.

Any insult to the vestibular system on one side may result in severe spinning vertigo with accompanying nausea, and often vomiting. As central compensation occurs, the spinning settles, to be replaced by feelings of imbalance. These may be described as light-headedness and are aggravated by rapid head movements. Gradually, improvement continues unless there are further fresh exacerbations. There is a significant correlation beween migraine and vestibular failure in adults.

The duration of the actual spinning vertigo (not the duration of the feelings of imbalance) is an important diagnostic aid: that of benign paroxysmal positional vertigo lasts seconds; that of vertebrobasilar ischaemia lasts minutes; that of Ménière's disease lasts hours; and that of vestibular neuronitis lasts days.

Ménière's disease has already been discussed. An acoustic neuroma (strictly a vestibular nerve schwannoma) is a relatively rare cause of vertigo but may cause ataxia (Figure 6.3). Middle ear disease, particularly infections, damage following ear surgery, a cholesteatoma or barotrauma may sometimes produce a **perilymph fistula**. This causes episodic vertigo, often with the sensation of tilting, fluctuating or progressive hearing loss, tinnitus and

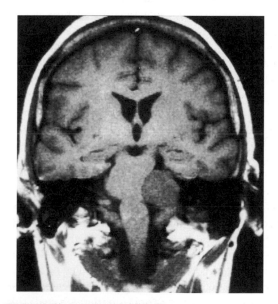

Figure 6.3 Magnetic resonance imaging brain scan, T1-weighted, coronal view, to show a large acoustic neuroma indenting the brainstem.

aural fullness. Patients may experience either auditory or vestibular symptoms or both. A history of vertigo worsened by straining, such as a Valsalva manoeuvre, is suggestive. A positive fistula test using a pneumatic otoscope to induce nystagmus supports the diagnosis and the need for ENT referral.

Other local causes of episodic vertigo include otitis media, drug-induced vertigo and acute alcoholic poisoning – the last described as 'pillow spin' provoked by the intoxicated patient lying down.

Positional vertigo

> **Positional vertigo**
> Here patients complain of acute episodes of vertigo provoked by changes of position, most usually lying down or sitting up quickly, or by turning over in bed. Vertigo may also be provoked by acute head turning or neck extension. Most frequently such positional vertigo is produced by damage to part of the labyrinth.

The hallmark of positional vertigo is the ability to elicit vertigo accompanied by nystagmus using the Dix–Hallpike manoeuvre (see Chapter 3).

Positional vertigo may follow a head injury, a vascular lesion or viral infection but the cause is often uncertain. It must be emphasized that many types of vertigo may be aggravated by positional changes or head turning. These include vertigo of both peripheral and central origin.

Benign paroxysmal positional vertigo

> Benign paroxysmal positional vertigo is the most common cause of episodic vertigo and is caused by a peripheral labyrinthine disturbance. It is characterized by spontaneous remissions and exacerbations with very short-lived but intense episodes of vertigo triggered by position change. It is common after trauma, ear infections and 'colds' but in many patients develops without obvious cause.

The duration of the intense spinning vertigo is usually less than 30 seconds and may be provoked by lying down or sitting up quickly or turning over onto the affected side. Although the actual vertigo is very brief, many patients feel off balance for long periods – hours or even days.

Testing with the Dix–Hallpike manoeuvre (see Figure 3.17) confirms the diagnosis. The patient is lain down supine with their head slightly turned to one side with the neck extended, while they are asked to fix their gaze on the examiner's nose. Normally there is no vertigo or nystagmus, but in affected patients with the faulty ear undermost there is a latent period of about 2–6 seconds then acute rotatory nystagmus appears beating towards the undermost affected ear and the patient feels acutely vertiginous and fearful. These symptoms rapidly settle, only to reappear as the patient is then sat upright quickly. This time the nystagmus reverses in direction. If the test is repeated, it shows fatigue – that is the symptoms and nystagmus are much less or have virtually disappeared.

Central lesions may also cause positional verti-

go but there is no latent period, the nystagmus usually lasts longer and may be variable and does not fatigue. The vertigo is not distressing. Commonly there are other signs of brainstem or cerebellar disease and conditions such as MS, cerebellar tumours or basilar territory disease may be responsible.

It is thought that in benign paroxysmal positional vertigo, otoconial debris from the utricle has migrated to the ampulla of the posterior semicircular canal (canalithiasis) and that this may then stimulate the hair cells there, which normally signal angular acceleration, as opposed to signalling linear acceleration/gravity, which arise from the utricle and saccule.

This is the basis for treatment, which relies on the so-called **Epley manoeuvre, which aims to reposition the otoconial debris out of the semicircular canal and back into the vestibule**. The provocative test is then followed by turning the patient's head slowly through 180 degrees and gradually sitting them up (Figure 6.4). Explanation and reassurance are also important measures because vertigo is frightening. Some patients require vestibular rehabilitation exercises and the Brandt–Daroff exercises based on repeated side-lying manoeuvres with the head turned to the same side have also proved useful.

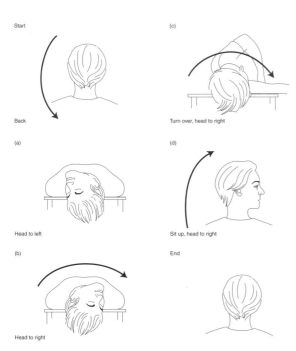

Figure 6.4 Epley repositioning manoeuvre. In this instance, the fault lies in the left posterior semicircular canal. (a) The patient is lain supine with their head turned to the left and the neck slightly extended (like a Dix–Hallpike test). (b) The head is then rotated some 45 degrees to the right (the opposite side). The neck is still extended. (c) The head and body are then turned so the patient is facing downwards. (d) The patient then sits up with the head still turned to the right and the neck slightly flexed.

Acute vestibular failure

In many instances of acute vertigo, the cause is uncertain, but there appears to have been an acute loss of labyrinthine function on one side. Some may arise from a vascular disturbance, perhaps from occlusion of the anterior vestibular artery, others perhaps from a viral infection where the term **vestibular neuronitis (viral labyrinthitis, acute vestibulopathy)** may be used. The last is sometimes seen in young adolescents and may follow an infection.

Patients present with acute prostrating vertigo accompanied by nausea and vomiting, but without hearing loss or tinnitus (cochlear symptoms). During the attack, patients lie with the affected ear uppermost. Nystagmus is present with the fast phase away from the affected ear and caloric tests will show a canal paresis on the affected side. Attempts at walking will produce ataxia. Usually the vertigo will settle within 2–3 weeks.

In the acute phase, bed rest, anti-emetics and vestibular sedatives are the mainstay of treatment. Steroids have been prescribed in the acute phase with little trial support. Later, compensatory balancing exercises help the patient to regain mobility and confidence. After vestibular damage, late fluctuations may occur in which recurrent vertigo occurs, not because of a new lesion, but because of a breakdown in central compensation secondary to intercurrent illness.

An **acute vestibular syndrome** may also arise from infarction of the inferior part of the cerebellum. Such patients may present with acute severe vertigo, nystagmus and ataxia. Such cerebellar infarction may arise from occlusion of the posterior or anterior inferior cerebellar artery. Many such patients have vascular risk factors such as hypertension, diabetes mellitus, a past history of myocardial infarction, smoking or atrial fibrillation. In many patients, there may also be other signs of acute brainstem disturbance such as diplopia, dysarthria, dysphagia and focal sensory or motor deficits. In most patients, the severity of their ataxia and the nature of their nystagmus points to a central fault. The nystagmus may be vertical, torsional, or change with the direction of gaze. Brain scanning with MRI is the investigation of choice to find evidence of infarction in the inferior cerebellum.

CRANIAL NERVES IX, X, XI AND XII

The glossopharyngeal and vagus nerves supply the bulbar muscles concerned with articulation and swallowing. Damage to the innervation of the soft palate will allow nasal regurgitation of fluids and if the laryngeal muscles are paralysed, the voice becomes hoarse and weak.

The common causes of an acute bulbar palsy, which are treatable, include:
- Guillain–Barré syndrome
- Myasthenia gravis
- Thyrotoxicosis
- Polymyositis

Acute bulbar problems also arise with cerebral infarcts and a slowly progressive bulbar palsy is most often seen with motor neurone disease. Rare neurological causes of dysphagia include diphtheria, tetanus and botulism. Carcinomatous invasion of the lower cranial nerves may also cause progressive loss of bulbar function and rare intrinsic brainstem infiltrating tumours may do the same. Wegener's granulomatosis may involve lower cranial nerves when there is a direct extension of the necrotizing granulomas from the nasal cavities and sinuses.

The jugular foramen syndrome

Features of jugular foramen syndrome
Cranial nerves IX, X and XI pass through the skull base in the jugular foramen. At this site they may be compromised by tumour compression, bony carcinomatous infiltration, granuloma, or chronic meningitis (e.g. Lyme disease). This results in a combination of lower cranial nerve palsies, which sometimes includes the hypoglossal nerve. Often there is local pain. Symptoms include diminished sensation in the ipsilateral soft palate, a depressed gag reflex, hoarse voice, difficulties swallowing, wasting and weakness of the ipsilateral sternomastoid and trapezius muscles and sometimes wasting of the ipsilateral tongue. If there is involvement of the brainstem, there may be a Horner's syndrome and eventually, long tract signs.

A **glomus jugulare tumour** is a rare, very vascular tumour that arises usually below the floor of the middle ear affecting lower cranial nerves on that side. Lower cranial nerve palsies are characteristically associated with ipsilateral conductive deafness and Horner's syndrome. Sometimes there is a visible vascular mass behind the tympanic membrane or in the external ear canal, with a bruit that is also audible to the patient. Commonly it produces bone erosion.

In patients presenting with a jugular foramen syndrome, imaging with MRI and CT with bone windows to demonstrate the skull base will usually show any mass lesion or bone erosion. Examination of the CSF may be necessary to show the presence of malignant cells (carcinomatous meningitis) or the presence of infection. The finding of antineutrophil cytoplasmic antibodies (ANCA) is relatively specific for Wegener's granulomatosis. Tumour treatment is by surgery, radiotherapy and sometimes chemotherapy. Glomus tumours may require a combination of embolization, surgery and radiotherapy.

Glossopharyngeal neuralgia

Glossopharyngeal neuralgia has many similarities to trigeminal neuralgia with brief intense stabs of pain experienced at the base of the tongue, at the angle of the jaw, in the throat, ear or side of the neck.

The condition is considered further in Chapter 11.

Polyneuritis cranialis

Multiple cranial nerve palsies may arise from the patchy involvement of a number of cranial nerves. Causes are given in Table 6.6. Carcinomatous invasion or cuffing of the cranial nerves by tumour cells or from those of a leukaemia or lymphoma are the common causes. Infective causes include tubercu-

Table 6.6 Causes of polyneuritis cranialis

Infective	Tuberculosis, listeria, borrelia, EBV, fungal
Granuloma	Sarcoidosis, Wegener's
Neoplastic	Carcinomatous meningitis – breast, bronchus
	Lymphoma, leukaemia
	Local spread – nasopharyngeal carcinoma. chordoma
Trauma	Basal skull fracture
Vascular	Vasculitis – PAN, collagen vascular disease
Inflammatory	Guillain–Barré, Miller Fisher
Always exclude	**Myasthenia gravis – ocular, facial and bulbar involvement**

EBV, Epstein-Barr virus; PAN, polyarteritis nodosa.

lous meningitis, fungal infections and glandular fever. Granulomatous infiltration may also occur, for example sarcoidosis, Wegener's granulomatosis. In a few patients, no cause is found.

Diagnosis rests on careful examination and identification of the neurological disturbance. The nasopharynx should be examined by an ENT surgeon, under anaesthetic if necessary. A search for any primary neoplasm is important, breast and bronchus being the most common sites. Extensive imaging studies may be necessary using MRI; gadolinium enhancement may show the presence of widespread meningeal involvement. CT scanning with bone windows is used to look at the skull base. Examination of the CSF is important. Cytology may allow identification of malignant cells and, in neoplastic meningitis, the CSF glucose is often very low. Staining and culture of the CSF may identify infective causes.

Treatment is that of the underlying cause. Intrathecal cytotoxic drugs, for example methotrexate, may be tried in malignant meningitis, although often with only limited benefit.

REFERENCES AND FURTHER READING

Acheson J, Riordan-Eva P (1999) *Neuro-ophthalmology: Fundamentals of Clinical Ophthalmology*. London: BMJ Books.

Balcer LJ (2001) Optic neuritis. *Current Treatment Options in Neurology*, 3:389–398.

Epley JM (1992) The canalith repositioning procedure: for treatment of benign paroxysmal positional vertigo. *Otolaryngological Head and Neck Surgery*, 107:399–404.

Furman JM, Cass SP (2003) *Vestibulae Disorders. A Case Study Approach*, 2nd edn. New York: Oxford University Press.

Goebel JA (2001) *Practical Management of the Dizzy Patient*. Philadelphia, PA: Lippincott, Williams and Wilkins.

Hickman SJ, Dalton CM, Miller DH, Plant GT (2002) Management of acute optic neuritis. *Lancet*, 360:1953–1961.

Trobe JD (1993) *Physicians Guide to Eye Care*. San Francisco, CA: American Academy of Ophthalmology.

CHAPTER 7

NERVE AND ROOT LESIONS

Tim Fowler, Nick Losseff and John Scadding

PRESSURE PALSIES

Compression of peripheral nerves may occur acutely or as part of a more chronic process. This may result in damage varying in severity. Mild compression is readily recognized and is experienced when sitting with the legs crossed, causing compression of the common peroneal nerve on the head of the fibula. With any duration of compression the blood supply to the nerve is compromised, **tingling develops and later numbness and weakness appear in the territory of the affected nerve**. With relief from the compression, there is usually rapid and complete recovery.

Moderate compression will produce damage to the insulating myelin sheath (segmental demyelination), producing a local conduction block or slowing of conduction with preservation of the continuity of the axon. This is called a **neurapraxia**. Usually the large, fast-conducting myelinated fibres are involved but small and unmyelinated fibres may be spared so that there is often preservation of some sensation. Repair is by remyelination and is usually complete with full recovery within a number of weeks or months.

More severe compression will damage the myelin sheath and the axon leading to axonal degeneration (Wallerian) distal to the site of injury. There will be conduction block in the distal part of the affected nerve.

The muscles supplied by the nerve become inexcitable, later showing signs of denervation with the development of fasciculation and wasting. The nerve trunk remains in continuity. Small and unmyelinated fibres are commonly involved. This type of damage is termed an **axonotmesis**. Repair is by regeneration over many months at the rate of 1–2 mm/day (consider the length of the average adult's leg) and may be incomplete.

If the nerve is severed or torn apart, causing the connective tissue framework to separate and disrupting the continuity of the axons and myelin sheaths, the ends of the nerve are free: this is termed a **neurotmesis**. In this situation, unless the two ends are sutured together or lie in close proximity, then repair by regeneration is likely to be poor.

Nerve conduction studies will usually give important information about the pathogenesis of such lesions and may demarcate the site of damage if there is a local conduction block. The electrical signs following axonal degeneration may take 5–7 days to appear in affected muscles after a severe injury so electrodiagnostic tests performed too early, within 2–3 days of injury, may prove misleading.

Many compressive nerve lesions are a mixture of axonal degeneration and demyelination.

Acute compression may arise in an unconscious patient as a result of direct pressure of the weight of an inert limb against a sharp edge or unyielding surface. Patients with a depressed conscious level from sedative drugs, excess alcohol or a general anaesthetic are particularly at risk. The 'Saturday night paralysis' of the intoxicated is the classic example, where the radial nerve in the upper arm is compressed against the humerus as the arm hangs over a chair back. Such damage may be of varying severity so that pressure palsies may take weeks or even months to repair.

Chronic compression or entrapment is likely to arise at certain sites where peripheral nerves travel in fibro-osseous tunnels or over bony surfaces so the nerve may be constricted, stretched or deformed (Box 7.1). The damage may be persistent or intermittent and the term entrapment is often used for lesions where surgical release of the compression may afford relief. In chronic entrapment, the affected nerve may appear thickened at the site and this may be palpable. It should be emphasized that nerves already diseased or damaged from some other neuropathic process are more liable to compression. Thus, patients with a diabetic neuropathy are particularly prone to develop carpal tunnel syndrome. A past history of other compressive neuropathic lesions always raises the possibility of an underlying hereditary neuropathy with a liability to pressure palsies. Occasionally, neoplastic or granulomatous infiltration of nerves may produce local compressive lesions, such as with leprosy or lymphoma.

Acute traction or stretch injuries can sometimes produce severe nerve damage, as when the brachial plexus is injured by a motor cyclist landing forcefully on the shoulder. In such injuries, the nerve roots may actually be torn out of the spinal cord with complete loss of continuity. Such severe injuries will produce signs of denervation in the affected arm muscles and there will be no recovery. Neurography with magnetic resonance imaging (MRI) is the investigation of choice to demonstrate the anatomy of such damage and electrodiagnostic studies may also be helpful.

Causalgia describes the severe pain produced by a partial injury to a peripheral nerve. Such pain is often intense and burning, with contact sensitivity, and may prove difficult to control. There may be accompanying sudomotor, vasomotor and trophic changes. This is complex regional pain syndrome (formerly known as reflex sympathetic dystrophy), considered further in Chapter 30. Usually there are complaints of troublesome pain, with impaired motor function and sensation, sometimes accompanied by abnormal sweating, temperature changes, swelling, often pallor or cyanosis, and later trophic changes, including osteoporosis.

Box 7.1 Entrapment neuropathies

> Common entrapment neuropathies
>   Median nerve in the carpal tunnel
>   Ulnar nerve at the elbow
>   Lateral cutaneous nerve of the thigh at the
>   inguinal ligament
>   Common peroneal nerve at the head of the fibula
> Rare entrapment neuropathies
>   Ulnar nerve at the wrist
>   Radial nerve
>   Posterior tibial nerve in the tarsal tunnel
>   Lower cord of the brachial plexus by cervical rib
>   or fibrous band

CARPAL TUNNEL SYNDROME

The median nerve may be compressed in the fibro-osseous carpal tunnel at the wrist. The nerve is supplied from the C6, C7, C8 and T1 roots. Certain features increase the risk of carpal tunnel compression (Box 7.2): women have narrower tunnels; the presence of rheumatoid arthritis; osteoarthritis or deformity from previous fractures, for example Colles', may encroach on the nerve. Diabetes mellitus, myxoedema, acromegaly, deposition of amyloid or even myeloma may compromise the nerve and there is an increased incidence in pregnancy. The symptoms are aggravated by use, particularly manual work.

Box 7.2 Carpal tunnel syndrome

Carpal tunnel syndrome may be associated with:
  Pregnancy
  Diabetes mellitus
  Myxoedema
  Acromegaly
  Rheumatoid arthritis
  Previous wrist trauma
  Myeloma
  Amyloid

Symptoms and signs

Symptoms of carpal tunnel syndrome
Symptoms include nocturnal painful tingling, usually described in all the fingers and hand, spreading up the forearm but not usually above the elbow. The symptoms may awaken the patient from sleep or appear on waking, or with lifting, carrying in certain positions, or with driving. They are usually eased by hanging the hand down, shaking it or changing position.

There are sometimes no abnormal signs, although with more severe lesions the thenar muscles are wasted and weak, particularly the *abductor pollicis brevis*, and some sensory changes may appear in the tips of the thumb, index, middle and ring fingers (Figure 7.1). A tourniquet test may be positive in patients with no signs, when inflation of the cuff around the upper arm rapidly produces similar sensory symptoms in the affected fingers within minutes. In Phalen's test, forced wrist flexion may provoke similar sensory symptoms.

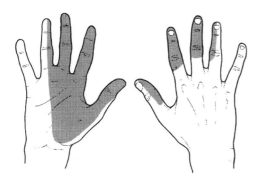

Figure 7.1 Area of sensory loss in the right median nerve lesion.

Investigation

Nerve conduction studies (described in detail in Chapter 5) in early compression will show diminution of the size of the sensory action potentials with delay seen first in the median palmar branches. Later there may be absence of the median sensory action potentials, prolonged distal motor latencies and signs of denervation in the *abductor pollicis brevis*. These studies have some predictive value in determining the outcome from decompression. Very severe damage (absent sensory action potentials and poor motor responses) may be followed by imperfect recovery. Moderate electrical damage is usually followed by a good surgical outcome.

Treatment

Treatment depends on the severity of the lesion and whether there are any added factors, such as diabetes or pregnancy. In mildly affected patients, a degree of rest and the use of a wrist splint at night may give relief. In some patients, local injection of steroids under the carpal ligament may also be of benefit, together with a reduction in the amount of manual work performed. In more severely affected patients, surgical decompression is necessary. This will usually relieve pain and sensory upset, although severe muscle wasting (in the thenar pad) may not recover, particularly in the elderly. Occasionally surgery may not relieve symptoms, raising the possibility of an incorrect diagnosis or inadequate decompression. Further conduction studies may be useful in such instances.

ULNAR NERVE LESIONS

The ulnar nerve arises from the roots of C8 and T1. The most common ulnar nerve lesion is compression of the nerve by the fibrous arch of *flexor carpi ulnaris* (the cubital tunnel), which arises as two heads from the medial epicondyle and the olecranon. Other ulnar nerve lesions at the elbow may reflect long-standing damage to the joint, often from an old fracture, causing deformity and angulation. This may result in a wide carrying angle with stretching of the nerve in its bony groove at the elbow, where it may be palpably thickened. Recurrent dislocation of the nerve from its groove is another mechanism and external pressure may arise, either from repeated trauma, or, more often, from patients confined to bed supporting their weight on their elbows. Ulnar nerve lesions may also arise after an anaesthetic, where presumably the nerve has been acutely compressed at the elbow while the patient was unconscious.

Symptoms and signs

> **Ulnar nerve symptoms and signs**
>
> Patients may complain of tingling or numbness involving the little finger, part of the ring finger and sometimes the ulnar side of the hand distal to the wrist. Sensory loss on the medial side of the forearm indicates a more proximal lesion (lower cord of brachial plexus or C8 root). Weakness may appear in the ulnar innervated small hand muscles causing difficulties in the use of the hand for fine manipulative tasks. In time, wasting of the first dorsal interspace muscles becomes evident, and later also in the dorsal interossei and hypothenar pad.

This will be associated with weakness of varying degree. With severe muscle wasting, the hand is deformed, 'clawed' with flexion of the little and ring fingers, associated with the inability fully to extend the tips, as the lumbricals of these two fingers are involved. The other fingers will appear slightly abducted from weakness of the interossei. Often the ulnar innervated long finger flexors, flexor digitorum profundus to the ring and little fingers, may be affected. Weakness usually involves the thumb adductors, the interossei – with difficulty abducting and adducting the outstretched fingers – and the hypothenar muscles. The area of sensory loss is shown in Figure 7.2.

At the elbow, the ulnar nerve may be thickened or unduly tender. There may be obvious deformity of the elbow, with restricted joint movements. If the forearm flexors are involved, the muscles of the medial side of the forearm will be wasted.

Investigation

Nerve conduction studies will usually show an absent or diminished ulnar sensory and ascending nerve action potential. There may be electrical signs

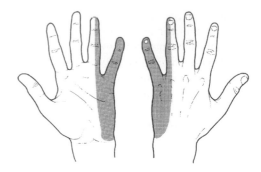

Figure 7.2 Area of sensory loss in the left ulnar nerve lesion.

of denervation in the first dorsal interosseous and *abductor digiti minimi.* Commonly, there is slowing of motor conduction across the elbow. In milder cases, there may be a significant decrement in the amplitude of the evoked muscle action potential from stimulation of the ulnar nerve above the elbow when compared with that below or at the wrist. MRI is also being increasingly used to delineate the anatomy of ulnar compression.

Treatment

In ulnar nerve lesions, treatment is less satisfactory. If there has been acute compression or repeated external pressure, then a period of rest and careful attention to avoiding any local pressure on the nerve at the elbow may be worth a trial. This includes towel splinting the elbow in extension at night to avoid repetitive or fixed flexion when sleeping. In more severe lesions, exploration of the nerve at the elbow allows decompression if such a lesion is exposed. If this is not found, the nerve may undergo anterior transposition, resiting it more anteriorly across the elbow. Medial epicondylectomy is an alternative decompressive operation that is sometimes successful. However, such measures seldom reverse any major wasting or weakness in the small hand muscles, although pain, paraesthesiae and discomfort may be eased. In milder lesions, recovery may take place but some lesions treated conservatively may do as well. Surgical treatment may sometimes prevent further progression of ulnar nerve damage.

Ulnar nerve lesions at the wrist

Ulnar nerve lesions at the wrist are far less common. The deep palmar branch of the ulnar nerve may be compressed in Guyon's canal, which runs between the pisiform and the hook of the hamate. The nerve may be compressed here by a ganglion, a neuroma or more commonly have an occupational link and be caused by, for example, the twist-grip of a motorbikes throttle or the 'proud' edged handle of a butcher's cleaver.

The deep palmar branch is purely motor and damage will cause wasting and weakness of the interossei, particularly the first dorsal and adductor pollicis, but sensation will be spared. The hypothenar muscles are usually spared, although the third and fourth lumbricals may be affected.

On electromyography (EMG) studies, the ulnar sensory action potential is present but there is a prolonged distal motor latency to the first dorsal interosseous with a normal latency to *abductor digiti minimi*, and normal motor conduction in the ulnar nerve in the forearm.

If there is no history of repeated trauma, MRI of the wrist and surgical exploration of the nerve may be necessary.

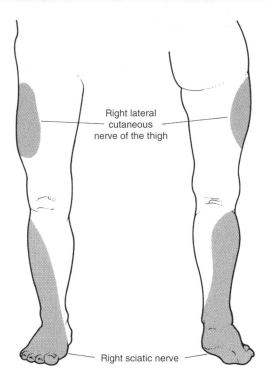

Right lateral cutaneous nerve of the thigh

Right sciatic nerve

Figure 7.3 Areas of sensory loss in lesions of the right lateral cutaneous nerve of the thigh and the right sciatic nerve.

LATERAL CUTANEOUS NERVE OF THE THIGH (MERALGIA PARAESTHETICA)

The sensory lateral cutaneous nerve of the thigh arises from L2 and L3 and emerges from the lateral border of the psoas and to the superior iliac spine. At this site, it may be compressed or stretched within its fascial tunnel. Sometimes this is provoked by obesity, pregnancy and certain physical activities particularly cycling and football. It may also be compressed by a neuroma. **Patients complain of tingling, numbness and sometimes pain in a patch about the size of a hand on the anterolateral aspect of the thigh above the knee (see Figure 7.3). There is no weakness or reflex change. Sensation is reduced within the territory of the nerve and light touch or stroking the skin may reveal unpleasant contact sensitivity (allodynia).**

In most patients, explanation, reassurance and sometimes weight loss are often all that are necessary. In a few patients where pain is troublesome, regional nerve block or surgical exploration may be required.

THE COMMON PERONEAL NERVE (LATERAL POPLITEAL NERVE)

The common peroneal (lateral popliteal) nerve divides into two branches. The superficial branch supplies the *peronei* (evertors) and the skin of the lateral side of the lower leg. The deep peroneal branch supplies the toe and ankle dorsiflexors and an area of skin on the dorsum of the foot between the first and second toes. The common peroneal nerve is very vulnerable at the head of the fibula, where it lies on a hard bony surface with only a covering of skin and connective tissue. External compression from a single prolonged exposure, such as from leaning on a sharp surface, continued squatting (strawberry-pickers foot), or repeated trauma (sitting cross-legged, wearing high stiff boots), may produce a lesion. It may also be compressed by a ganglion (which may arise from the superior tibiofibular joint) or even from the tendinous edge of *peroneus longus*.

Symptoms and signs

The presentation is usually with a painless foot drop, which may become more noticeable if the patient is tired or has walked any distance. This may cause the patient to trip. There is weakness of tibialis anterior and often the evertors, with a preserved ankle jerk. **The sensory loss is variable (Figure 7.4)**: if the deep peroneal branch is affected the area is small (Figure 7.4).

Investigation

Electromyography studies may show denervation in *tibialis anterior* and *extensor digitorum brevis*. There may be a local conduction block or slowing in the region of the head of the fibula. Usually the ascending common peroneal nerve action potential is lost. The sural nerve action potential is preserved and tibial conduction should be unaffected, which should help to localize the lesion.

Treatment

Physiotherapy, and an artificial foot orthosis, may be useful while waiting for recovery if an external

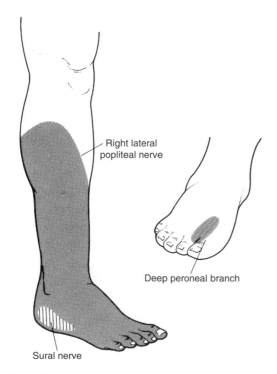

Figure 7.4 Areas of sensory loss in lesions of the right common peroneal and deep peroneal nerves.

Right lateral popliteal nerve

Deep peroneal branch

Sural nerve

compressive lesion, or acute trauma is causative. In a few instances, MR imaging of the common peroneal nerve or exploration is necessary to exclude a ganglion or compressive lesion.

LESS COMMON LESIONS

Radial nerve

The nerve is supplied by C7 and to a lesser extent C6 and C8. It supplies the *triceps, brachioradialis, supinator*, wrist and finger extensors and the long abductor of the thumb. Sensation may be impaired on the posterolateral aspect of the forearm or with more distal lesions over the dorsum of the web between the thumb and index finger. **An acute wrist drop is the major symptom and sign**. More proximal lesions cause additional weakness of triceps.

Most radial palsies reflect acute compression of the nerve either in the axilla or where it winds around the humerus (Saturday night palsy) or from direct trauma. The posterior interosseous nerve (a branch of the radial) may be compressed by a lipoma, ganglion or even where the nerve passes through the *extensor carpi radialis* muscle, also resulting in wrist drop.

Sciatic nerve

The sciatic nerve is the largest peripheral nerve arising from the roots of L4–S3. It leaves the pelvis through the greater sciatic foramen and runs posteriorly down the thigh where, just above the knee, it divides into the tibial and common peroneal divisions. It lies close to the back of the hip joint and can be damaged if that joint suffers extensive trauma or during hip surgery. In its upper part, the sciatic nerve is covered by the *gluteus maximus* but in the inferior part of the buttock it is relatively superficial and so may be directly damaged by a buttock injection misplaced too medially. The sciatic nerve may also be damaged by direct pressure in the unconscious patient: it may also be compressed by tumours on the side of the pelvis. The peroneal nerve fibres lie more laterally in the sciatic nerve and so are more prone to compression.

A high lesion of the sciatic nerve will affect the hamstrings and all the leg muscles below the knee, the calf and anterior tibial as well as the small foot muscles. **This will produce a 'flail' foot with distal** wasting and weakness. There will be sensory loss involving the foot and posterolateral aspect of the lower leg (Figure 7.3), and sometimes also on the posterior aspect of the thigh, if the closely related posterior cutaneous nerve of the thigh is also involved. Electrically, there will be denervation of the affected muscles, with impaired conduction in the tibial and peroneal nerves and absent sural and common peroneal nerve action potentials.

Femoral nerve

The femoral nerve arises from the L2, L3 and L4 roots, passing through the *psoas* muscle and under the inguinal ligament lateral to the femoral artery, to supply the anterior thigh muscles. It may be compressed by an abscess, a haematoma (often from over-anticoagulation) in the *psoas*, or be damaged acutely by fractures of the pelvis, traction during surgery, knife wounds to the groin or from thrombotic lesions of the vasa nervorum, such as in diabetes mellitus.

A femoral nerve lesion will produce weakness of the knee extensors, the quadriceps group, with muscle wasting, a depressed or absent knee jerk, and sensory loss in the anterior thigh and medial part of the knee. The terminal branch of the femoral nerve is the saphenous nerve, which supplies the medial side of the lower leg. There may be mild weakness of the hip flexors, and patients will experience difficulty walking, particularly going up stairs, and the leg may seem to buckle. On EMG there may be denervation in the *quadriceps* and a prolonged distal motor latency when the nerve is stimulated in the groin.

Tarsal tunnel

Rarely, the posterior tibial nerve may be compressed in the tarsal tunnel in the sole of the foot. Usually this will provoke tingling, pain and sometimes 'burning' in the sole and toes which may be worse at night and aggravated by inversion of the ankle. Such symptoms may be provoked by standing or walking. In severe cases, there is weakness of *abductor hallucis* and sensory loss distally over the soles and toes. On EMG, there may be a prolonged distal motor latency to *abductor hallucis* and in younger patients the medial plantar sensory action potential will be absent. Surgical decompression is sometimes effective.

The long thoracic nerve (of Bell)

The long thoracic nerve (of Bell) supplies the *serratus anterior* muscle arising from C5, C6 and C7 roots. A lesion of this nerve leads to a winged scapula with inability to fix the scapula on the chest wall when the arm is being forcefully flexed, abducted or pushed forward. It may follow an injury, carrying a heavy weight on the shoulders (e.g. rucksack) or from an acute inflammation (see below under Brachial neuritis). Most recover with time.

BRACHIAL PLEXUS LESIONS

The brachial plexus is formed from the spinal roots of C5–T1 and extends from the spinal canal to the axilla. The roots of C5 and C6 join to form the upper trunk, from C7 the middle trunk, and from C8 and T1 the lower trunk (Figure 7.5). From there they separate into anterior and posterior divisions. The three posterior divisions join to form the posterior cord, the anterior divisions of the upper and middle trunks join to form the lateral cord, and the anterior division of the lower trunk to form the medial cord. These cords pass through the thoracic outlet, between the first rib and clavicle.

Damage to the plexus may arise in a number of ways (Table 7.1). Trauma from acute stretching or traction is common and when severe may result in actual avulsion of a nerve root from the spinal cord, most commonly caused by motorcycle accidents. The upper trunk is most often affected. Penetrating injuries may also affect the plexus, for example, knife or gunshot wounds. If the lower cord is

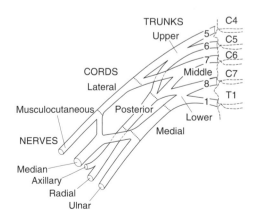

Figure 7.5 Diagram of the brachial plexus.

Table 7.1 Common causes of brachial plexus damage

Trauma	(a) Avulsion of root, stretch, traction
	(b) Penetrating injuries
Neoplastic sarcoma	Local – breast or lung infiltration carcinoma, neurofibroma
Radiotherapy	Radiation fibrosis
Inflammatory	Neuralgic amyotrophy
Diabetic plexopathy	
Mechanical	Cervical rib, fibrous band compression

involved there is often an accompanying Horner's syndrome (Figure 7.6).

The signs and symptoms reflect the motor and sensory involvement extending over more territory than that of a single nerve root or peripheral nerve (Table 7.2).

Metastatic infiltration of the plexus most often involves the lower cord, with wasting and weakness of the thenar and hypothenar muscles and also the finger and wrist flexors. The sensory loss extends from the ulnar two fingers up the medial side of the forearm. Pain as an early symptom is common. Spread from a primary breast carcinoma or from an apical lung tumour is the most common. **Radiation fibrosis** produces patchy involvement of the plexus with early sensory symptoms and weakness, progressing slowly. It can be difficult to differentiate from metastatic infiltration.

Electromyography studies will help to confirm the anatomical localization. There is often loss of sensory action potentials, prolonged F-wave latencies, small muscle action potentials and even signs of denervation. Electrical myokimia is a feature of radiation damage. Plain x-rays may show cervical

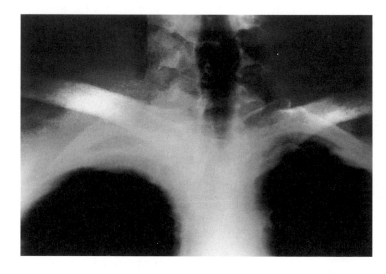

Figure 7.6 Apical chest x-ray to show shadowing at the right apex. This patient presented with wasting of the small muscles of the right hand and had a right Horner's syndrome. The shadow was caused by a lymphoma.

Table 7.2 Clinical features of disturbances of the brachial plexus

	Pain and sensory symptoms	Sensory loss	Motor loss	Reflex
Upper C5/C6	Lateral shoulder, scapula, supraclavicular fossa, arm to elbow	Deltoid and upper arm	*Deltoid, biceps brachioradialis*	BJ, SJ
Middle C7	Shoulder to hand of index, middle and ring fingers	Palmar and dorsal surfaces	*Triceps*, extensors of wrist and fingers	TJ
Lower C8/T1	Shoulder to hand	Ulnar surface of hand, forearm and arm	Long finger and wrist flexors, intrinsics	FJ
All	Neck to hand	Upper limb	Complete flaccid paralysis	

ribs, an elongated transverse process on C7 or even an apical shadow. MRI with gadolinium enhancement or computed tomography (CT) may show the presence of tumours.

Thoracic outlet compression

The lower cord of the brachial plexus passes across the posterior triangle of the neck behind the subclavian artery running between *scalenus anterior* and *medius*. If there is an extra cervical rib attached to the transverse process of C7 or a fibrous band attached to an elongated transverse process, either of these may compress the lower cord of the plexus. They may also compress the subclavian artery, producing **vascular symptoms**. These include Raynaud's phenomenon with complaints of coldness and colour changes in the fingers or more severe symptoms from arterial or venous obstruction. The radial pulse may disappear in certain arm positions on the affected side and a bruit may be audible in the supraclavicular fossa. Rarely, distal emboli may affect the fingers. **Neurological features** include aching and pain radiating down the inner forearm to the ulnar side of the hand, associated with tingling and sometimes numbness.

Sensory loss can be demonstrated on the medial side of the forearm proximal to the wrist, unlike that found in an ulnar nerve lesion. There is often wasting and weakness involving all the intrinsic muscles of the hand, the thenar and hypothenar pads and the medial forearm muscles.

Investigations

Investigations include electrophysiological studies, evoked potentials, x-rays, MR imaging and occasionally arteriography, if compression of the subclavian artery is suspected.

In severe symptomatic cases, surgical treatment may be necessary. It is important to choose a surgeon experienced in the exploration of this region.

Brachial neuritis (neuralgic amyotrophy, Parsonage–Turner syndrome)

Neuralgic amyotrophy is an acute inflammatory disturbance causing a patchy plexopathy, due to demyelination and axonal degeneration in more severe lesions. It is uncommon. The aetiology is unknown, although it may follow a viral infection, immunization or, on rare occasions, be linked with a hereditary liability to pressure palsies.

The onset is with excruciating severe pain, usually in the shoulder, at the base of the neck or in the arm. Initially, this is unremitting, keeping the patient awake and requiring strong analgesics.

The pain typically lasts for about 10 days, but sometimes as long as 3 weeks, and as it remits the patient becomes aware of weakness of the affected muscles. The most commonly affected muscles are innervated by the axillary, long thoracic and suprascapular nerves. Winging of the scapula is a frequent and characteristic finding in this condition. There is associated depression or loss of reflexes and varied sensory loss, most often in the territory of the axillary nerve. The pattern of the weakness is patchy and a whole muscle may be affected, which may help to differentiate this from an acute cervical root lesion arising from a disc prolapse. **In most patients over a period of months, often six months, there is recovery, but in others the progress is slow, up to 18 months, indicating that repair here is by axonal regeneration. About 90 per cent of patients show functional recovery after three years.**

Electrical studies will confirm denervation in affected muscles, commonly with slowing in affected motor nerves with prolonged or absent F-waves. The cerebrospinal fluid may be normal, although a mild lymphocytic pleocytosis and protein rise have been found.

Treatment is symptomatic: analgesics and rest until the acute pain has settled. Corticosteroids have been advocated, but there is no good evidence that these are effective. Physiotherapy directed towards strengthening the affected muscles is helpful.

CERVICAL ROOT PROBLEMS

The muscles of the arm are supplied by the C5, C6, C7, C8 and T1 roots. These leave the spinal canal through the intervertebral foramina and may be irritated or compressed, causing symptoms and signs referred to that root. It should be emphasized that the pain from such a lesion is referred into the myotome, which may be different from the site of the sensory symptoms (paraesthesiae, numbness), which are referred to the dermatome (see Figure 4.19). In the cervical spine, there are eight exiting nerve roots from the seven vertebrae so that the root exits above the body of the vertebra concerned; that is, the C6 root exits between C5 and C6. Below T1 the roots exit below; that is, T1 exits between T1 and T2.

Causes of cervical root damage

The most common causes of cervical root damage are:

- compression by an acute soft disc prolapse;
- compression by a hard bony spur in degenerative spondylosis;
- compression by a neuroma, lymphoma, extradural tumour or metastasis.

CERVICAL ROOT SYMPTOMS

Pain in the neck or arm is very common, affecting over 10 per cent of the population. However, only a small number of patients have pain arising from cervical root irritation. More often, pain arises from the soft tissues and joints. With cervical root disturbances the initial symptoms are usually increasing pain, often referred to the base of the neck, shoulder, scapula or upper arm. Root pain is often described as shooting, burning or like an electric shock. Later there may be weakness of affected muscles, depression or loss of appropriate reflexes, tingling and numbness.

Commonly affected roots compressed by spondylotic spurs or disc protrusions are C6 (C5/C6 disc space), C7 (C6/C7), C5 (C4/C5) and C8 (C7/T1).

In younger patients, there may be an acute soft disc prolapse. If this extends laterally, it will compress the affected root. The root is initially irritated causing referred pain, but if the compression is more severe, the nerve root may infarct, leading to loss of pain but more severe weakness with signs of denervation in the affected muscles, reflex loss and sensory impairment (Table 7.3).

A large central disc protrusion in the neck will lead to compression of the spinal cord, producing a myelopathy with spastic leg weakness, sensory changes in the feet and sometimes disturbed bowel and bladder function. These will be accompanied by long tract signs, brisk reflexes, clonus, extensor plantar responses and sensory loss in the feet – most often posterior column impairment.

Most patients with neck problems, particularly root irritation, show pronounced spasm of the nuchal muscles causing greatly limited neck movements. Lateral flexion is particularly affected, for most rotation occurs at the atlanto-axial joint and proximally. Sometimes a 'wry' neck may develop. Lateral flexion or rotation of the neck,

Table 7.3 Localizing features of cervical root disturbances

Root	Pain	Dermatome	Muscle	Reflex
C5	Neck, shoulder, lateral arm to elbow	Lateral deltoid	*Deltoid, spinati, biceps*	BJ, SJ
C6	Neck, lateral arm to thumb and index	Lateral arm, forearm,	*Biceps, brachioradialis*	BJ, SJ
C7	Neck, lateral arm to middle finger	Lateral forearm, index, middle and ring fingers	*Triceps*, finger and wrist	TJ
C8	Medial forearm and hand	Medial forearm, ring and little fingers	Finger flexors, abductor of thumb	FJ
T1	Medial arm	Medial arm	Intrinsics – all. Horner's syndrome	

BJ, biceps jerk; FJ, finger jerk; TJ, triceps jerk.

which aggravates ipsilateral pain referred down the shoulder or arm, suggests root compression on that side. Neck pain that is worsened on the side contralateral to the lateral flexion or rotation suggests a muscular origin to that pain.

In older patients, degenerative changes in the spine lead to narrowing of the intervertebral space, with bulging of the disc and hypertrophy of the surrounding ligaments causing these to thicken. The bony margins of the vertebrae become raised, producing hard osteophytic spurs, which may compress nerve roots, the spinal cord or both. The latter causes a **spondylotic radiculo–myelopathy**. Again, symptoms and signs depend on the root involved and whether there is spinal cord compression. Failure to recognize spinal cord compression may lead to irreversible damage, with even a tetraplegia and lost sphincter control.

Cervical spondylosis may be aggravated by trauma, particularly extension injury and if this is repeated. Occasionally, patients may give a highly relevant history of trauma causing acute but transient neurological symptoms, for example, paresis in an arm or leg with sensory upset, which recover only to be followed some time later by further symptoms, which may slowly progress.

Investigations

Plain x-rays are of limited value because with increasing age all will show some spondylotic changes in the cervical spine to some extent, so it is important to put all these in the clinical context of the patient's symptoms and signs before attributing all arm and neck pain to the blanket term 'cervical spondylosis' (Table 7.4).

The sagittal diameter of the cervical canal is an important factor in the possible development of a myelopathy. A diameter of 10 mm or less on a true lateral film suggests the cord may be compromised.

> Scanning with MRI is the investigation of choice when radiculopathy and or myelopathy are suspected. Sagittal and axial views will show most acute root or cord compressive lesions. It will also show any intramedullary lesion.

Again, the results of MRI must be put into clinical context as many compressive lesions may be asymptomatic and what looks 'mild' on MRI may be clinically severe.

In patients where MRI is contraindicated, CT scanning with contrast may be useful in delineating root disturbances. Open MRI scanners have largely eliminated fears of claustrophobic patients. Electrical studies may show denervation in appropriate root territories and help to exclude peripheral nerve entrapment or more widespread neuropathic disorders, such as motor neurone disease.

Treatment

Treatment is covered in detail in Chapter 15.

Table 7.4 Investigations of root or plexus lesions

Blood tests	Full blood count, ESR, fasting glucose, serum proteins and 'strip', calcium, phosphatases, CRP
X-rays	Spinal – for collapse, malalignment, pedicle erosion
	Chest – primary tumours, metastases
Imaging	MRI – excellent for cord and root lesions with gadolinium enhancement for neoplastic, infective/inflammatory processes
	CT – for bony lesions
	CT with contrast, intrathecal – for roots and cord lesions myelography (non-ionic contrast) if MRI not possible or not available
Electrodiagnostic	Denervation, neuropathy or myopathy, evoked potentials
Isotope scans	Bone (metastases), infective lesions (gallium)
CSF	Presence of infection/inflammation; demyelination (oligoclonal bands)

CRP, C-reactive protein; CSF, cerebrospinal fluid; CT, computed tomography; ESR, erythrocyte sedimentation rate; MRI, magnetic resonance imaging.

Many older patients with cervical spondylosis and a mild radiculo-myelopathy may be managed conservatively using a cervical collar and physiotherapy.

LUMBOSACRAL PLEXUS

The lumbosacral plexus is formed from the T12–S4 roots and is situated within the substance of the psoas muscles. It is divided into an upper part, L1–L4, and a lower part, L4–S4. Over 50 per cent of damage arises in the lower part, about 30 per cent in the upper part, and some 18 per cent involves the whole plexus. Causes of damage are given in Table 7.5.

Retroperitoneal haematoma (often from excessive anticoagulant treatment or a bleeding diathesis) and a diabetic plexopathy (femoral amyotrophy) are common causes of upper plexus lesions. Malignant infiltration, particularly from pelvic tumours, is a common cause of a lower plexus lesion. Radiotherapy may lead to the late development of a slowly progressive lumbosacral plexopathy, as in the brachial plexus (Table 7.5).

Again, pain, weakness and sensory loss are common symptoms in one leg, extending outside the territory of a single root or peripheral nerve. **Bilateral leg symptoms suggest a lesion within the spinal canal (cauda equina or lower spinal cord).** If the pudendal nerve is damaged, there may be some impairment of bladder or bowel function. Sympathetic involvement may cause a warm dry foot. If the lymphatics or venous drainage are obstructed, the leg will swell.

A rectal and/or pelvic examination is an essential part of the clinical assessment of a patient presenting with a lumbosacral plexopathy.

LUMBAR ROOT LESIONS

In the other mobile part of the spine, the lumbar region, nerve roots may be irritated, stretched or compressed, provoking symptoms and signs in the territory of the affected root (Table 7.6).

Sciatica describes the pain referred down the course of the sciatic nerve from the back to the buttock, and down the back of the leg to the foot. Mechanical back pain alone without radiculopathy commonly radiates down as far as the knee. This pain most commonly arises from compromise of the L5 and S1 roots.

Table 7.5 Common causes of lumbosacral plexus damage

Trauma	Fracture of the pelvis
Haematoma	Psoas – anticoagulant excess, bleeding diathesis
Diabetic plexopathy	
Infection	Herpes zoster
Neoplastic infiltration	Pelvis – uterine, ovarian carcinoma
	Colonorectal carcinoma
	Lymphoma, sarcoma
Radiation plexopathy	
Retroperitoneal fibrosis	
Mechanical compression	Traction at surgery

Note: bilateral involvement suggests cauda equina/conus lesion within the spinal canal.

Lumbar disc prolapses
In the lumbosacral region, a lateral disc prolapse may compress a nerve root or sometimes more than one. A central disc prolapse will extend into the lumbar sac compressing the cauda equina and producing symptoms and signs in both legs, and more alarming disturbances of bowel and bladder control. Such symptoms of sphincter upset are a medical emergency and patients require urgent hospital admission with a view to imaging the canal and surgical decompression before irreversible damage occurs.

Over 95 per cent of lumbar disc protrusions occur at L4/L5 and L5/S1 levels affecting the L5 and S1 roots, less often the L4 roots. In the lumbar region, roots can be involved at a higher

Table 7.6 Localizing features of lumbar and sacral root lesions

Root	Pain	Dermatome	Muscle	Reflex
L3	Front of thigh	Anterior thigh	*Quadriceps, adductors*	
L4	Front of thigh, knee and medial shin	Anteromedial shin	*Quadriceps, tib. ant. Hamstrings ext. hall. longus*	KJ
L5	Back of leg, lateral lower leg, dorsum foot to great toe	Dorsum of foot to great toe	evertors, hamstrings	Inner hamstring jerk
S1	Sole of foot, lateral side of foot back of thigh and leg	Sole	Plantar flexors, toe flexors, hamstrings	AJ
Lower sacral	Buttocks, saddle area	Saddle area, perianal	Anal muscles	Anal

AJ, ankle jerk; KJ, knee jerk.

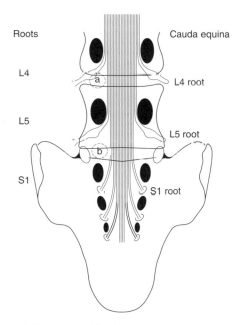

Figure 7.7 Diagram of lumbosacral roots. (a) Posterolateral disc protrusion; (b) medial disc protrusion.

level (Figure 7.7) so imaging is essential before deciding on surgery; for example, an L4/L5 disc protrusion can involve the L5 or L4 root. Many patients have a preceding history of low back pain and intermittent sciatica, which in the past has responded to rest or physiotherapy. Small disc protrusions will settle with rest but a large extruded fragment is likely to give continuing trouble (Table 7.7).

Other causes of root pain need consideration, although these are less common. **Diabetic infarction** of nerve roots, the plexus or femoral nerve, may present with acute pain in the thigh and be accompanied by wasting, impaired reflexes and sensory loss. **Neoplastic involvement** of nerve roots may arise in the spinal canal, often secondary to bony metastases with collapse of the vertebrae, most often from primary tumours of bronchus, breast, prostate, kidney, gastrointestinal tract or lymphomas. The lumbosacral plexus on the side wall of the pelvis may be involved with gynaeco-

Table 7.7 Clinical features of disturbances of the lumbosacral plexus

	Pain	Sensory loss	Weakness	Reflex
Upper	Groin, anterior thigh, lateral thigh, hip	Medial and lateral thigh, anterior thigh, medial leg	*Psoas, quadriceps, adductors*	KJ
Lower	Posterior thigh, leg and foot	Foot, lateral ankle lateral and posterior leg	Hamstrings evertors, invertors, flexors toes and ankle	AJ

AJ, ankle jerk; KJ, knee jerk.

logical or colonorectal malignancies. Such tumours cause severe pain, which is often not relieved by rest, unlike the pain from a disc. In time, the lymphatic pathways and even the iliac veins may be obstructed, leading to swelling of the leg.

Root symptoms

Root symptoms are shown in Table 7.6.

S1

S1 root lesions produce pain down the back of the buttock, thigh and leg to the heel. There will be tingling and numbness in the sole of the foot and weakness of plantar flexion (inability to stand on tiptoe), and to a lesser extent the hamstrings and glutei. The ankle jerk will be depressed or absent and there will be sensory loss on the sole and lateral border of the foot.

L5

L5 root lesions produce pain down the postero-lateral side of the leg to the ankle with sensory upset on the dorsum of the foot including the great toe. Weakness involves the dorsiflexors of the great toe (*extensor hallucis longus*, which has an exclusive L5 innervation) and, to a lesser extent, the dorsiflexors of the ankle, evertors and hamstrings. The patient may show difficulty walking on their heels. The ankle jerk is usually preserved and there is sensory impairment over the dorsum of the foot, extending onto the lateral side of the lower leg.

L4

L4 root lesions produce pain radiating down the front of the thigh, over the knee, shin and medial side of the calf. There may be tingling and numbness on the medial side of the calf, weakness of the ankle dorsiflexors (*tibialis anterior*) and the *quadriceps*. The knee jerk is usually reduced or absent.

Root tension signs are commonly associated with L4, L5 and S1 root lesions. These include the inability to raise the fully straightened leg to a right angle at the hip. In older patients, there may be local hip joint disease, which may prevent this. If nerve roots are stretched by a disc protrusion, then straight leg raising is commonly limited on the affected side with pain referred in a sciatic radiation. Such pain may be aggravated by dorsiflexion of the foot. It should be noted that in patients exaggerating their symptoms with the suspicion of a functional component, straight leg raising may be grossly restricted lying on the couch, yet if the patient is asked to sit up to demonstrate the site of their back pain, they may be able to do this with the legs flexed at the hip to 90 degrees and the knees fully extended. Spinal movements are often restricted with lumbosacral root lesions, particularly trunk flexion. There may sometimes be a scoliosis or pelvic tilt.

Upper plexus or lumbar root lesions are uncommon but produce weakness in the hip flexors, adductors and *quadriceps*. Such patients have difficulty rising from a low chair, bath or climbing stairs. If the upper lumbar roots are stretched (L2, L3) the presence of root tension signs may be detected by the femoral stretch test. Here the patient lies prone with the knee flexed to a right angle, and the thigh is then extended at the hip. A positive test will produce pain in the front of the thigh.

All patients with lumbosacral root symptoms should be specifically questioned about their bowel and bladder function, and in the male about erectile function. A rectal examination, or pelvic examination, where appropriate, should be undertaken to exclude any palpable mass. At the same time, this will enable sensation to be checked in the lower sacral dermatomes, the tone of the anal sphincter assessed and the anal reflex elicited. The last is tested by pricking or scratching the pigmented perianal skin and eliciting a local contraction of the muscle, which can be seen.

A cauda equina lesion usually affects both legs with lower motor neurone pattern weakness affecting distal muscles more than proximal ones, although this is often asymmetric. The weakness is usually accompanied by sensory changes, reflex loss and sphincter dysfunction.

Investigations

Blood should be taken for a full blood count, erythrocyte sedimentation rate, fasting blood glucose, and, where appropriate, estimation of the acid phosphatase and prostatic-specific antigen (PSA), serum proteins and electrophoresis. Plain x-rays of the spine may show degenerative changes, a narrowed disc space, or occasionally point to other pathology by the appearance of vertebral collapse, loss of a pedicle or abnormal density. However, MRI scanning will cover these aspects. A chest x-ray is appropriate in adults (Table 7.4).

If there is progressive or persistent neurological deficit, continuing pain, or diagnostic doubt, imaging should be undertaken to visualize the spinal cord and roots. **This is best achieved by MRI scanning with gadolinium enhancement if there is any suggestion of an infective/inflammatory or neoplastic process.**

Spinal CT scans, best with intrathecal contrast, may also be helpful in selected patients. The cerebrospinal fluid (CSF) obtained at the same time should be examined in the usual way but should also be sent for cytology to look for malignant cells, and for electrophoresis for the detection of oligoclonal bands. Isotope bone scans may be useful in showing bony lesions, particularly the presence of widespread spinal metastases. Electrodiagnostic studies may be useful in confirming the presence of denervation, pointing to more central conduction delays, or indicating the presence of an underlying neuropathy.

Treatment

Treatment will depend on the cause, but most acute disc lesions respond to analgesics (non-steroidal anti-inflammatory drugs) and muscle relaxants. Early mobilization with greater emphasis on exercise and return to normal activities is now being promoted, although acute pain with severe muscle spasm usually results in a period of enforced rest. Traction has its advocates but clinical trials do not support the efficacy of traction, specific exercises, bed rest or acupuncture in the relief of acute low back pain. In more chronic low back pain, exercises, multidisciplinary treatment and even behavioural therapy have been shown to help. Surgery may prove necessary where medical treatment has failed, where there is progressive or persistent neurological deficit and where a large disc is demonstrated, or there is persistent unremitting root pain. This is discussed further on p. 174.

Surgical referral

Indications for **surgical referral** include:

- cauda equina symptoms and signs (bowel and bladder disturbance) – urgent;
- progressive or severe neurological deficit;
- persistent neurological deficit after 4–6 weeks;
- persistent sciatica accompanied by root signs after 6 weeks.

SUMMARY

Common sites of peripheral nerve entrapment include the median nerve in the carpal tunnel and the ulnar nerve at the elbow.

At the more mobile parts of the spine, the neck and lumbar regions, nerve roots may be irritated or compressed. The signs and symptoms from these include:

- pain;
- loss of use;
- sensory impairment;
- reflex changes.

'Red flags'

'Red flags' indicating the need for further investigation in patients with a history of back pain include:

- age <20 and >55 years;
- a history of trauma;
- a constant progressive non-mechanical pattern of pain;
- a past history of serious illness (cancer), recreational IV drug use or steroid therapy;
- features of systemic illness, such as weight loss, malaise;
- fever;
- widespread neurological signs affecting more than one root territory;
- structural spinal deformity;
- difficulty in bladder emptying, the presence of faecal soiling, loss of anal sphincter tone, or saddle anaesthesia (requires urgent referral and investigation).

Pain and sensory symptoms may be referred into the appropriate root sclerotome or dermatome. These sites are not always identical.

A basic working knowledge of the anatomy of such nerve and root lesions allows their recognition.

REFERENCES AND FURTHER READING

Biller J (2002) *Practical Neurology*, 2nd edn. Philadelphia, PA: Lippincott-Raven.

Brazis PW, Masdeu JC, Biller J (2001) *Localisation in Clinical Neurology*, 4th edn. Boston, MA: Lippincott, Williams & Wilkins.

Mumenthaler M (1992) *Neurologic Differential Diagnosis*, 2nd edn. Stuttgart: Georg Thieme.

Nachemson AL, Jonsson E (2000) *Neck and Back Pain*. Philadelphia, PA: Lippincott, Williams and Wilkins

Seddon H (1972) *Surgical Disorders of the Peripheral Nerves*. Edinburgh: Churchill Livingstone.

Seimon LP (1995) *Low Back Pain – Clinical Diagnosis and Management*, 2nd edn. New York, NY: Demos Vermande.

Staal A, van Gijn J, Spaans F (1999) *Mononeuropathies – Examination, Diagnosis and Treatment*. London, UK: WB Saunders.

CHAPTER 8

NEUROGENETICS

Sonia Gandhi, Sarah Tabrizi and Nicholas Wood

INTRODUCTION

There has been a revolution in our understanding of the molecular genetic basis of neurological disease and there is now no area of neurology that has not been impacted by genetic discoveries. Principally, this has been as a result of the identification of genes inherited in a simple, 'Mendelian' fashion, but in the last few years, insights into the genetic bases of common sporadic neurological diseases have also been reported.

This chapter confines itself to a summary of the major findings of **Mendelian neurological disease** and, although these diseases are individually rare, cumulatively they account for a very substantial neurological burden and many cases find their way into general neurological practice.

It is therefore incumbent on the neurologist to be acquainted with this rapidly advancing area. This chapter seeks to give the general neurologist a comprehensive understanding of the broad principles of neurogenetic disease.

The recent technological advances in DNA typing have had a great practical impact. The first human genome cost approximately 3 billion dollars to sequence 3 billion base pairs, but the cost of sequencing the genome at the time of writing this chapter is less than £10000 and is decreasing. It can therefore be seen that the possibility of assaying all the genetic variants in any given patient's genome will soon be feasible. At first, such extensive genetic testing will enter the research field but it can be envisaged that a complete DNA analysis on a complex patient might be undertaken as part of a relatively routine investigation. However, it is the clinician's role to be able to interpret this wealth of data in a clinically reliable and informed way. Even now, a large number of genes can be assayed. This chapter attempts to provide a guide to the clinician through this increasingly complex area.

There has also been substantial progress in the ability to track **genetic variants underlying susceptibility to sporadic common neurological disease**. These genome-wide association studies have now been conducted in virtually all the major common neurological conditions. It remains unclear how much of the disease aetiology will be explained by these genetic variants, and the molecular role for these variants in the pathogenesis of disease remains uncertain. There is much to be done in this field before testing genetic susceptibility becomes a useful part of clinical practice. These findings are not discussed in this chapter, as they are not of clinical utility at the moment.

GENETICS FOR THE NEUROLOGIST

Deoxyribonucleic acid (DNA) provides the molecular basis for the genes that encode all proteins. DNA is made up of two helical polynucleotide chains that form a double helix. The bases of the nucleotides adenine, cytosine, guanine and thymine are arranged in a highly specific manner such that the sequence of bases encodes the sequence of amino acids in a protein. DNA consists of discrete functional units called genes, which is a segment of DNA that encodes a polypeptide chain. The DNA code is organized into three letter '**codons**' such that one codon determines one amino acid. As there are four potential bases for any position, this gives rise to 64 codons that code for the 21 amino acids.

The genome describes the DNA content of the cell, and is made up of two separate genomes: the nuclear genome and the mitochondrial genome. The nuclear genome comprises approximately 3 billion basepairs. The mitochondrial genome is much smaller with only about 16 500 basepairs and encodes a minority of the subunits of the respiratory chain.

The functional role of large amounts of the nuclear genome remains unknown, and only a fraction of it is involved in the production of functional protein.

The goal of the human genome project was to determine the sequence of the entire genome and identify all genes. It showed that there are only 23 000 human genes, which is far fewer than originally predicted. We produce far more proteins than this, with a wide range of functions.

The DNA strands are packaged into chromosomes. Humans have 23 pairs of chromosomes: 22 pairs of autosomes and one pair of sex chromosomes. Genes are arranged in a specific order on the chromosome. As one of each pair of chromosomes is inherited from each parent, then for the autosomal genes there is a one maternal copy and one paternal copy.

Most genes are encoded in blocks of basepairs termed exons, which are separated by intervening blocks of non-coding basepairs called introns.

One of the roles of introns may be to facilitate alternative splicing in which different exons of a single gene may be spliced together to create a number of different proteins from the same gene. Following translation into a protein, proteins undergo a range of other post-translational modifications such as phosphorylation or glycosylation, which are important for their functional role in the cell. Understanding the regulation of alternative splicing and post-translational modifications is a major challenge in genomics and will provide important insights into protein expression and function.

If mutation on one copy of the gene is sufficient to cause disease, then this is termed an autosomal dominant condition. The type of mutation is often due to a 'toxic gain of function' mutation whereby the mutant allele or copy results in a protein with a novel aberrant function that cannot be prevented by the presence of the normal copy.

In other situations, the mutant allele has a dominant negative effect, i.e. it exerts its influence by negatively affecting the normal allele at the DNA, RNA or protein level. In an autosomal dominant condition there is 50 per cent chance of transmitting the mutated copy to offspring.

If both copies of the gene must be mutated to cause disease, this is an autosomal recessive condition. In such cases, the gene mutation may lead to loss of function of the encoded protein.

In the carrier state (of only one mutated copy), the presence of a normal copy may compensate for the reduced function of the mutated copy. However, when both alleles are mutated, the significant loss of protein function results in disease manifestation. If two carriers of the same disease mutation have children, then the chance of offspring inheriting two mutated copies (one from each carrier parent) is 25 per cent. In cases of autosomal recessive disease, the risk of transmission to the next generation depends on the carrier state of the partner. If this is not known, then it will be predicted by the carrier frequency in the population. This is usually rare, and so there is a low recurrence risk, apart from certain circumstances such as conditions with high population carrier frequencies, or in consanguineous marriages. However, as progress is made in elucidating genetic disease, these boundaries are blurring slightly and there is increasing evidence that on occasions, being a carrier for an 'autosomal recessive' condition does increase the risk of disease, often with a phenotype different to the primary recessive condition (see below – senataxin and role in amyotrophic lateral sclerosis (ALS) and ataxia; and glucocerebrosidase (GBA) and role in Gauchers and Parkinson's disease (PD)).

If a mutation affects a gene on the X chromosome, this will result in **X-linked inheritance patterns**. Females have two X chromosomes, while males have one X and one Y chromosome. Therefore, females are relatively protected by a mutation in a gene on the X chromosome by the other normal copy. In contrast, males have only one X chromosome and therefore such a mutation will cause disease. This is termed X-linked recessive inheritance in which females are carriers, and males express. Males inevitably transmit the mutation to their daughters but never to their sons, therefore the presence of male–male transmission in a family effectively excludes this pattern of inheritance. In X-linked dominant conditions, females will manifest the condition as well as males, but the phenotype may be more severe in males.

Mitochondrial DNA is inherited from the mother, and therefore mitochondrial DNA diseases are maternally inherited. However, as the mitochondrial mutation may not be present in all mitochondria, it is difficult to predict the proportion of mitochondria with mutations that are present in offspring. It is therefore harder to predict risk recurrence estimates for such conditions. It should be remembered, however, that a significant majority of mitochondrial proteins are nuclear encoded, so an increasing number of diseases are being shown to be due to nuclear mitochondrial genes.

There are several additional factors to be considered that affect the inheritance of disease. The **penetrance** of the mutation is the proportion of mutation carriers who manifest disease. Some diseases are almost completely penetrant, e.g. Huntington's disease. However, mutations in the DYT1 (dystonia) gene exhibit reduced penetrance, such that only about 40 per cent of patients with the mutations actually manifest the disease.

Sometimes the degree of penetrance of a mutation is age-dependent. The basis for incomplete penetrance is not fully understood. Another factor is **variable expressivity**, which refers to a phenotype being expressed to different degrees in individuals with the same genetic mutation. This may occur within families. For example, duplication of part of chromosome 17 giving rise to CMT1A may cause a severe childhood neuropathy in one family member, or adult onset symptoms with pes cavus in another individual. Both penetrance and variable expressivity must be explained to patients as part of their genetic counselling.

Genetic testing and its implications

There is an ever increasing list of genes that cause neurological disease, and making sense of both the genetic complexity of a disease as well as the technical complexity of genetic testing poses a major challenge to neurogeneticists. As this chapter illustrates, the likelihood of making a definite molecular diagnosis will first depend upon an accurate determination of the clinical phenotype and a clear view of the mode of inheritance given by the family history. Once a genetic diagnosis is suspected, the second challenge is the type of genetic testing required. For example, if a mutation has already been identified in a family, or if only one type of mutation causes the disease (e.g. in Huntington's disease) then the test will be relatively straightforward and will usually involve either DNA sequencing or gel electrophoresis of a polymerase chain reaction (PCR) product from the patient's DNA.

However, if the mutation is unknown and the gene needs to be screened, the complexity of testing depends on the size of the gene. In some cases, such as the large NF1 gene, this is a difficult task. Furthermore, not all mutations are point mutations that can be detected by routine sequencing. Some mutations are gene rearrangements (exonic deletions or duplications) and these require a gene dosage assay to be performed before excluding the gene as the cause of the disease (e.g. the *parkin* gene which causes early onset Parkinson's disease).

In addition to the task of making an accurate molecular diagnosis, geneticists are faced with the challenge of giving a genetic diagnosis to an individual patient.

> Because genetic diagnoses have major implications for the family, genetic counselling is an important part of any consultation. This includes explaining the clinical features of the disease and the course, any treatment options available, the mode of inheritance and consequences to family members. Informed consent must be taken for all genetic tests.

Once the genetic mutation causing a disease is known in a family, this allows the genetic test to be offered to 'at risk' family members. Such testing is termed **predictive genetic testing** and allows a pre-manifest diagnosis to be made. Guidelines for predictive testing have been issued by the International Huntington's Disease Society, and are generally applicable for all predictive testing. These guidelines include extensive pre-test counselling to explain the disease, the risk to the individual and the implications of a positive test result, and further pre-test counselling to assess the patient's understanding of risk of disease, of the impact on employment, insurance and relationships, and assess their emotional and social support structure. Disclosure of the test result is planned, and then followed up shortly afterwards by post-test counselling.

THE DEMENTIAS

Alzheimer's disease

Mutations in the APP gene account for 10–15 per cent of early onset familial dementia. APP encodes the amyloid precursor protein, which is a transmembrane protein that is sequentially cleaved to

> Alzheimer's disease (AD) is the most common neurodegenerative disease presenting with dementia. The majority of cases are sporadic but rare autosomal dominant forms account for <5 per cent of cases. **Mutations in three genes are known to cause autosomal dominant AD with high penetrance: APP, PSEN 1 and PSEN 2.**

form Aβ fragments that can aggregate into amyloid plaques. Mutations in PSEN1 are the most common cause of early onset AD, accounting for approximately 50 per cent of cases. Mutations in PSEN 2 are rare and account for <1 per cent of early onset AD. The presenilins constitute part of the γ-secretase complex that cleaves APP. Thus the discovery of these genes and their function has strongly implicated aberrant amyloid processing to be central to the pathogenesis of AD. In addition to these genes, variation in the apolipoprotein E gene (the ApoE4 allele) is a major genetic risk factor for 'sporadic' AD. However, a significant proportion of AD patients do not possess the apoE4 allele, and similarly many people with the apoE4 allele never develop AD, and therefore predictive genetic testing for ApoE genotype is not routinely performed.

Frontotemporal lobar degeneration

> Frontotemporal lobar degeneration (FTLD) encompasses a clinically and pathologically heterogeneous group of language and behavioural disorders, associated with extrapyramidal features and amyotrophic lateral sclerosis.

Up to 40 per cent of FTLD patients report a positive family history, with approximately 10 per cent exhibiting autosomal dominant inheritance. Mutations in two genes, MAPT (microtubule-associated protein tau) and PRGN (Progranulin) account for the majority of familial autosomal dominant FTLD. MAPT encodes the tau protein which binds to microtubules and promotes their assembly and stabilization. Mutant tau protein results in aggregation and deposition of insoluble tau inclusions seen histopathologically in FTLD-TAU cases. MAPT mutations are usually missense or splice-site mutations, and are highly penetrant. However, they cause a wide clinical phenotype including behavioural variant frontotemporal degeneration (FTD), semantic dementia, progressive non fluent aphasia, corticobasal degeneration, and progressive supranuclear palsy. MAPT mutations are rarely seen in sporadic cases.

Mutations in PGRN are loss-of-function mutations leading to disease via haploinsufficiency. These cases are associated pathologically with ubiquitin positive, TDP-43 positive inclusions. PGRN mutations have a more variable penetrance than MAPT mutations, and have been detected in ~3 per cent of sporadic cases. As with MAPT mutations, PGRN mutations give rise to a variable clinical phenotype consisting of progressive aphasia, behavioural variant FTD, corticobasal degeneration (CBD), parietal syndromes or AD features.

Additional mutations have been described in CHMP2B gene (FTLD phenotype), and the VCP gene (FTLD in association with inclusion body myopathy and Paget's disease), but these are rare causes and routine testing is only performed for MAPT and PRGN.

Prion disease

The prion diseases may be sporadic, acquired or inherited. Ten to 20 per cent of cases have a positive family history displaying autosomal dominant inheritance. Clinically these present as relatively aggressive dementing illnesses, often complicated by additional movement abnormalities including ataxia and myoclonus. Mutations in the prion gene result in aggregation and deposition of the prion protein.

> **In summary**, genetic testing is recommended for PSEN 1 (and if negative, APP and PSEN2) for autosomal dominant AD, and for MAPT and PRGN for familial FTLD.

It is worth noting that there is considerable clinical heterogeneity within the dementias such that tau mutations may present with AD phenotypes, and therefore mutation screening may need to be extended to genes of other neurodegenerative disorders.

THE EPILEPSIES

The majority of epilepsy is caused by the interplay of genetic risk factors and environmental factors.

There are relatively few single gene disorders that result in inherited forms of epilepsy, and these are usually caused by mutations in ion channels or neurotransmitter genes. For example, severe myoclonic epilepsy of infancy is caused by mutations in the a1 subunit of the sodium channel gene SCN1A. Mutations in the b1 subunit of the sodium channel gene SCN1B may cause generalized epilepsy with febrile seizures-plus (GEFS+). Benign infantile neonatal epilepsy is caused by mutations in the potassium channel genes, KCNQ2 or KCNQ3. Juvenile myoclonic epilepsy has been associated with mutations in the chloride channel gene CLCN2.

Cortical development disorders that result in abnormal migration or gyration cause epilepsy and occasionally have a genetic basis. For example, one form of lissencephaly (diminished gyration) is caused by germline mutations in the double-cortin (DCX) gene and occurs mainly in females. Periventricular heterotopia is characterized by subependymal nodules of grey matter along the lateral walls of the ventricle and results in a variable degree of epilepsy. It is an X-linked dominant disorder caused by mutations in the filamin-1 (FLN1) gene. This disorder is most often lethal in males and this makes detecting a family history difficult but questioning for a history of miscarriages may be revealing.

The progressive myoclonic epilepsies are a group of phenotypically similar set of disorders but with different genetic aetiologies. Testing is more available for these than the more common primary forms of epilepsy.

The list of causes of progressive myoclonic epilepsy is long, but four of the most common causes are described here. **Unverricht–Lundborg disease** (Baltic myoclonus) is autosomal recessive and is caused by mutations in the EPM1 gene, which encodes the protein cystatin B. It is characterized by myoclonus onset in childhood associated with later onset ataxia, tremor and cognitive decline.

MERRF syndrome (myoclonic epilepsy with ragged red fibres) is caused in 90 per cent of cases by mutation 8344 in tRNA gene for lysine in the mitochondrial genome. This results in myoclonic and generalized seizures, myopathy, ataxia and dementia.

Lafora disease is an autosomal recessive disorder caused by mutations in 80 per cent of cases in EPM2A gene (encodes laforin) and less frequently in the EPM2B gene (encodes malin). It is characterized by myoclonic, generalized and partial seizures presenting in childhood, followed by dementia and ataxia. Histologically, periodic acid-Sciff (PAS) positive intracellular inclusions are found in neurones.

DRPLA (dentatorubropallido-luysian atrophy) is an autosomal dominant disorder caused by a triplet repeat expansion in the DRPLA gene. It is characterized by myoclonus, epilepsy, ataxia, choreathetosis and dementia.

Other causes of progressive myoclonus and epilepsy or ataxias include ceroid lipofuscinoses and sialidosis, but often the additional features of these conditions suggest the correct diagnosis.

MOVEMENT DISORDERS

Parkinson's disease

PD is the second most common neurodegenerative disease. The majority of cases are sporadic, although 15 per cent are inherited in a mendelian fashion. The monogenic forms are clinically and pathologically similar to the sporadic or idiopathic PD form, although they are more often associated with an earlier age of onset. The past 15 years has seen the identification of many of the autosomal dominant and autosomal recessive causes of PD.

Point mutations and gene rearrangements in the α–synuclein gene (SNCA/PARK1) cause a rare autosomal dominant form of PD. Duplications of SNCA lead to late onset autonomic dysfunction and parkinsonism, while triplications are associated with early onset PD and dementia. **Mutations in LRRK2 (leucine rich repeat kinase 2/PARK8) are a much more common cause of autosomal dominant PD**, affecting 5–15 per cent familial PD and 1–2 per cent of sporadic PD patients. The LRRK2 gene is very large and mutations have a variable penetrance. The clinical phenotype is very similar to idiopathic PD, and includes late onset disease. The most common mutation is the G2019S mutation, which has a particularly high frequency of 30–40 per cent in certain populations such as Ashkenazi Jewish people or North African Arabs. Testing for this single mutation, rather than sequencing the entire gene, is technically more feasible but does not necessarily provide a complete genetic diagnosis.

Autosomal recessive early onset PD may be caused by mutations in the parkin gene (PARK2). Approximately 80 per cent of PD patients with onset before the age of 30 have mutations in the parkin gene.

Mutations in the parkin gene may be point mutations or gene rearrangements. The next most common cause of autosomal recessive PD is mutation in the PINK1 gene (PARK6), followed by mutations in the DJ-1 gene (PARK7). All three forms of PD are characterized by early onset, a benign course and sustained response to L-dopa, but may also be associated with additional features such as dystonia and psychiatric morbidity.

Genetic testing is recommended for the LRRK2 gene in autosomal dominant cases, and parkin/PINK1/DJ-1 for early onset 'sporadic' PD or recessive cases.

It has also been recently shown that the sporadic form of PD also has genetic variants underlying it. Large genome-wide association studies have recently implicated the role of variation in α-synuclein and tau genes as significant risk factors for developing the sporadic form of PD. Although genetic susceptibility to neurodegenerative diseases does not form part of routine clinical testing, it is particularly noteworthy that the same genes are implicated both in mendelian forms of PD as well as sporadic forms, suggesting commonality in their pathogenesis.

One major genetic risk factor for developing PD is the presence of a mutation in the glucocerebrosidase (GBA) gene. Homozygous mutations in GBA cause Gaucher's disease, the most common of the lipidoses, which is particularly frequent among Ashkenazi Jewish people. However, heterozygous carriers of GBA mutations have been found to exhibit parkinsonism. The impact of heterozygous GBA mutations as a risk factor for developing 'sporadic' PD varies widely between different populations.

Several other genetic parkinsonian syndromes have been attributed PARK loci, but are not characterized by classical parkinsonism, and exhibit several atypical and more complex phenotypes. Mutations in the recessive ATP13A2/PARK9 gene have been detected in a number of families with the Kufor–Rakeb syndrome which consists of juvenile parkinsonism, early response to L-dopa, but with associated spasticity, dementia, supranuclear gaze palsy and facial myoclonus. Mutations in PLA2G6/PARK14 are a cause of adult onset dystonia and parkinsonism with a good response to L-dopa but early dyskinesias. Interestingly, mutations in PLA2G6 also cause an infantile neuraxonal dystrophy.

Dystonia

Primary dystonias are characterized by sustained involuntary muscle contraction resulting in abnormal postures and repetitive movements, in the absence of any structural or metabolic cause.

Adult onset dystonia is often focal and sporadic and requires little further investigation. However, childhood onset dystonia is more usually generalized and has a genetic basis. At least 20 monogenic forms of dystonia have been described and designated DYT loci. However, the most common genetic cause of primary dystonia is a single GAG deletion in the torsin A gene (DYT1 locus). The characteristic phenotype of DYT1 dystonia is limb onset dystonia under the age of 26, which spreads to involve the axial muscles. Due to a common founder mutation, DYT1 dystonia can be detected in 90 per cent of the Ashkenazi Jewish population with this phenotype. The GAG deletion, however, has a reduced penetrance and therefore genetic testing should be performed even in the absence of a clear family history.

In patients with dystonia that is highly L-dopa responsive, a diagnosis of dopa-responsive dystonia (DRD/DYT5) should be considered. DRD is most commonly autosomal dominant with reduced penetrance, and caused by mutations in the gene for GTP-cycohydrolase 1, the enzyme required for tetrahydrobiopterin synthesis. This biopterin is in turn the cofactor for tyrosine hydroxylase, the enzyme required for dopamine synthesis. Mutations in the gene for tyrosine hydroxylase have also been identified that give rise to an autosomal recessive form of DRD.

Dystonia-plus syndromes

In these disorders, dystonia presents with additional features. For example, familial cases of dystonia in association with myoclonic jerks affecting the trunk, neck and proximal extremities may be due to 'myoclonus-dystonia', caused by mutations in the epsilon-sarcoglycan gene (DYT11). DYT 3/Lubag dystonia is an X-linked recessive dystonia caused by mutations in the TAF1 gene. It is predominantly found in the Filipino population, presenting with adult onset dystonia followed by parkinsonism. DYT12 or rapid-onset dystonia-parkinsonism is a rare disorder characterized by dystonia manifesting over hours to weeks, and may be associated with parkinsonism that is not L-dopa responsive. It is caused by mutations in the ATP1A3 gene (the Na+/K+ ATPase α 3 gene), and is autosomal dominant with reduced penetrance.

Mixed movement disorders

Wilson's disease is a treatable autosomal recessive disorder presenting with early onset mixed movement disorder, psychiatric features and liver damage.

It is caused by impaired copper excretion resulting in copper accumulation and deposition in the brain, liver and cornea. Mutations in the ATP7B gene cause Wilson's disease and identification of a mutation is particularly useful for presymptomatic testing in at risk family members in order to guide therapy. **However, the main diagnostic test remains measurement of urinary copper excretion and serum caeruloplasmin.**

Neurodegeneration with brain iron accumulation may present with a mixed movement disorder. Pantothenate kinase associated neurodegeneration (PKAN) is due to mutations in the PANK2 gene, which encodes pantothenate kinase, which is key in regulating coenzyme A synthesis. The condition typically presents in the first decade of life with progressive and severe extrapyramidal features, corticospinal signs and cognitive decline. An atypical form is seen that presents in early adulthood with parkinsonism and slow progression. Iron accumulation in the basal ganglia results in the classic radiological feature of bilateral hypointensity in the median globus pallidus with a central area of hyperintensity (the eye of the tiger sign) on T2-weighted magnetic resonance imaging (MRI).

Neuroferritinopathy is a rare condition caused by mutations in the ferritin light chain gene (FTL1) resulting in neurodegeneration with iron accumulation. It is an autosomal dominant condition that presents in adult life with progressive dystonia or chorea.

Neuroacanthocytosis is an umbrella term for syndromes that consist of red blood cell abnormalities (acanthocytes) and neurological features. Of these, chorea-acanthocytosis is an autosomal recessive disorder that presents in early adulthood with dystonia, chorea, tics and psychiatric features. Parkinsonism may become a prominent feature later in life. Mutations have been identified in the CHAC gene encoding a protein called chorein. There is also an X-linked form associated with the presence of Kell antigen – clinically this is indistinguishable from the recessive form.

CHOREA

Huntington's disease is a neurodegenerative disease that is characterized by the classic triad of chorea, cognitive decline and personality change in the adult onset form.

The juvenile onset form may display additional features such as parkinsonism and seizures. **The mutation underlying Huntington's disease is a CAG–triplet repeat expansion in the first exon of the HTT gene**. The CAG repeat is normally polymorphic, ranging from 10 to 28 copies. In Huntington's disease (HD), the CAG repeat expands to 36-121 repeats, and becomes fully penetrant over 40 repeats. The size of the CAG repeat correlates with the age of onset of the disease such that the larger the repeat size, the earlier the age of onset. The CAG repeat length may increase from one generation to the next, particularly when transmitted in the paternal line. This results in the phenomenon of **anticipation** whereby the disease manifests with an earlier age of onset and increasing severity from one generation to the next due to the expansion of the CAG repeat.

There are a number of disorders that have a similar clinical phenotype to HD but do not harbour the CAG repeat mutation. These disorders have been termed HD phenocopies. Huntington's disease-like 2 (HDL2) is caused by CTG/CAG triplet repeats in the junctophilin 3 gene and have only been described in patients of African ancestry. The most common HD phenocopy is SCA17 (HDL4), which is caused by a CAG repeat in the TBP gene. DRPLA (dentatorubropallidoluysian atrophy) is caused by a CAG repeat in the atrophin-1 gene. Familial prion disease, neuroacanthocytosis, neuroferritinopathy and PKAN may also mimic the HD phenotype.

Tremor

Despite a high heritability for essential tremor, no genes have been identified that underlie this condition.

THE ATAXIAS

Ataxia can be inherited in an autosomal recessive or dominant fashion. The differentiation between these two modes is based on the family history and the age of onset, such that onset below the age of 20 is extremely likely to be autosomal recessive, while onset over the age of 20 is more likely to be autosomal dominant.

Friedreich's ataxia (FRDA) is the most common cause of recessive ataxia, accounting for approximately 40 per cent of cases. It is characterized by progressive limb, trunk and gait ataxia, neuropathy and pyramidal dysfunction. Additional features include cardiomyopathy, pes cavus, optic atrophy and diabetes.

A triplet repeat expansion in intron 1 of the **frataxin gene** is found in 97 per cent of cases; the remaining 3 per cent of cases harbour an expansion in association with a point mutation. Therefore, the absence of an expansion on either allele effectively excludes this diagnosis (there are no reported cases of compound heterozygous point mutations). Despite some understanding of the mitochondrial dysfunction caused by deficiency of frataxin, no therapies have emerged.

There is a very long list of other recessive ataxias and numerically the most important is senataxin, mutations in which cause ataxia with oculomotor apraxia type 2 (AOA2). This accounts for approximately 8 per cent of autosomal recessive ataxia. This is one of a series of genes implicated in DNA fragility that includes the aprataxin gene (AOA1) and the ataxia telangectasia gene (ATM). It is worth noting that not all cases display the oculomotor apraxia or the telangectasia and therefore genetic testing is worth considering for these genes in all FRDA-negative cases.

Extremely rare but clinically important is a deficiency of vitamin E causing ataxia. This may be caused by a range of malabsorption states, for example cystic fibrosis, bowel resection. Genetically this is caused by autosomal recessively inherited mutations in the gene encoding the a-tocopherol transporting protein. It is diagnosed by demonstration of very low vitamin E levels in serum and treated with vitamin E supplementation. Restitution of vitamin E levels helps stop progression and in some cases produces improvement.

> The autosomal dominant ataxias generally start in adulthood but the age range can vary from infancy to old age. In approximately 50 per cent of cases, a precise genetic diagnosis is readily achievable by assaying for mutations in SCA 1,2,3,6,7. In each of these genes, the common mutation is an expanded CAG repeat, which when translated produces a polyglutamine tract in the aberrant protein. There are now more than 25 identified dominant SCA loci, but these are very rare causes of ataxia, and genetic testing for them is not part of routine clinical practice.

Clinically, it is worth considering whether the ataxia is pure or complicated by additional neurological features. When exploring the family history, it is important to note that the clinical phenotype may vary between family members and the non-ataxic features may be predominant. **SCA6** patients exhibit a 'pure' cerebellar ataxia. **SCA7** is associated with macular degeneration as the main additional feature and blindness may present in advance of the ataxia. **SCA 1, 2 and 3** may be associated with extrapyramidal features and involvement of the peripheral nervous system. In SCA 3, parkinsonism may actually predominate and may be to some degree dopa-responsive.

Until recently, X-linked forms of ataxia were considered to be vanishingly rare. However, the recognition of a novel syndrome has emerged. The presence of a premutation expansion in the frag-ile X gene (an expansion that is just outside the normal range but not in the pathogenic range) has been shown in elderly patients to cause a tremor-ataxia syndrome. This is much more common in males than females. Imaging demonstrates symmetrical T2 signal change in the middle cerebellar peduncles.

> Paroxysms of ataxia occur in a number of families. Brief attacks of ataxia lasting seconds or minutes are most typically found in episodic ataxia type 1 (EA1) caused by mutations in the KCN1A gene. Episodic ataxia type 2 (EA2) has much longer attacks lasting hours and is further characterized by profound vertigo, nausea, vomiting and occasionally migrainous headache.

This is due to mutations in the CACNA1A gene. Interestingly, mutations in the CACNA1A gene account for a number of different disorders: episodic ataxia, familial hemiplegic migraine and SCA 6, which are termed 'allelic'. Although distinct disorders, patients with CACNA1A mutations may exhibit overlapping features. Both EA1 and EA2 are inherited in an autosomal dominant fashion and treatment with acetazolamide brings relief in some patients. Recently, it has emerged that there are other patients with episodic ataxia that do not fit into either subgroup and there remain more episodic ataxia genes to be found.

Mitochondrial DNA mutations may also present with ataxia. Mitochondrial DNA is inherited in a matrilineal fashion and a point mutation at 8993 produces a neurogenic ataxia with retinitis pigmentosa (NARP). There are other mitochondrial mutations that can produce ataxia but these are invariably complicated phenotypes with other pointers to their mitochondrial aetiology (see also Chapter 21).

HEREDITARY SPASTIC PARAPLEGIA

The age of onset is highly variable but most commonly occurs in the second to fourth decade. The mode of inheritance may be autosomal dominant, autosomal recessive or X-linked. As a broad rule, the autosomal dominant forms of HSP are relatively 'pure' whereas the autosomal recessive HSP

Hereditary spastic paraplegia (HSP) is a heterogeneous group of disorders characterized by progressive spasticity and weakness of the lower limbs. HSP may be clinically classified into 'pure' HSP in which progressive spasticity and hyperreflexia predominates with minimal weakness or other neurological features, and 'complicated' HSP in which the spastic paraparesis may be associated with optic atrophy, retinopathy, extrapyramidal features, ataxia, peripheral neuropathy, amyotrophy and epilepsy.

presents with the complicated phenotype. Many distinct forms of HSP are now recognized and 17 genes have been so far identified. Here we concentrate on the numerically most important of the HSP genes. Ultimately, the clinical features and the family history will guide genetic testing for HSP.

Of the autosomal dominant HSP, approximately 50 per cent of cases are caused by mutations in the SPAST gene (SPG4) encoding the protein spastin. Mutations may be either point mutations or deletions and therefore both sequencing analysis, as well as gene rearrangements, must be tested for. Onset before the age of 35 years is generally associated with a slower disease progression than a later age of onset.

The second most common cause of autosomal dominant HSP (~10 per cent of cases) is mutation in the SPG3A gene encoding the protein atlastin. This gives rise to an earlier childhood onset spastic paraparesis, often with a benign course. Mutations in the REEP1 gene (SPG31) underlie 8 per cent of cases of autosomal dominant HSP.

The most frequent cause of autosomal recessive HSP in Europe is SPG11 caused by mutations in the gene KIAA1840 encoding the protein spatacsin. Onset occurs before the age of 25 years and the spastic paraparesis is complicated by cognitive impairment, dysarthria, distal amyotrophy and a thin corpus callosum seen by imaging. Complicated HSP in association with a thin corpus callosum may also be caused by mutations in the gene ZFYVE26 (SPG15/Kjellin syndrome) encoding the protein spastizin. Mutations in the SPG7 gene encoding the protein paraplegin result in either a pure HSP phenotype or a complicated HSP phenotype with

optic atrophy and cerebellar atrophy. Of note, SPG7 has been reported to account for 7 per cent of adult onset 'sporadic' HSP cases in one study.

Two genes have been identified that cause X-linked HSP. Mutations in the L1-CAM gene (SPG1) encoding a cell adhesion molecule result in an infant onset HSP. Mutations in the proteolipid protein gene (PLP gene/SPG2) cause abnormal myelination. Such mutations result in a spectrum of disease that may include adult onset spastic paraparesis or the severe Pelizaeus–Merzbacher disease comprising infant onset spasticity, ataxia, movement disorder, optic atrophy and psychomotor retardation (see also Chapter 21).

DISEASES OF MOTOR NEURONS

Amyotrophic lateral sclerosis

Amyotrophic lateral sclerosis (ALS) is a neurodegenerative disease that progressively affects the upper and lower motor neurons of the bulbar, upper and lower limb territories, resulting in severe disability and death. **The majority of cases are sporadic although 10 per cent of cases are familial.** The familial cases are clinically very similar to sporadic ALS but have an earlier age of onset in the fourth decade. The first gene to be identified to cause ALS was superoxide dismutase 1 (SOD1/ALS1).

Mutations in SOD1 usually cause autosomal dominant ALS and have a variable penetrance. They account for 15–20 per cent of autosomal dominant familial ALS, and 1–2 per cent of all ALS cases.

The protein TDP-43 has been identified to be the major aggregating protein in inclusions seen in both sporadic and familial ALS (and also a group of FTLD cases). The gene encoding this protein is TARDP and dominant mutations in TARDP have been identified in a minority (1–3 per cent) of ALS cases. Mutations in the FUS gene have also been discovered to cause autosomal dominant ALS. The FUS protein and the TDP-43 protein have the common characteristics of being an RNA/DNA-binding protein that is mainly nuclear. The other ALS genes are very rare, but include the ALS2 gene encoding alsin, mutations (recessive) in which cause a juvenile primary lateral sclerosis or infantile ascending spastic paralysis phenotype. Mutations in the senataxin gene cause a dominantly inherited juvenile onset ALS (while recessive mutations in the same gene cause AOA2). Mutations in the VAPB gene, angiogenin gene and the dynactin gene have also been implicated in adult onset familial ALS.

Spinal muscular atrophy

Spinal muscular atrophy (SMA) is the second most common autosomal recessive disease of childhood (after cystic fibrosis), and is characterized by the progressive degeneration of anterior horn cells resulting in muscle atrophy and weakness.

> Four clinical types of SMA are distinguished: SMA type 1 the infantile form, also termed Werdnig–Hoffmann disease; SMA type 2 is an intermediate form presenting at six months of age; SMA type 3 is the juvenile form, also termed Kugelberg–Welander disease; SMA type 4 is the adult onset disease (onset between the third and fifth decade).

Ninety-five per cent of SMA cases (SMA type 1–3 and some of type 4) are caused by mutations in the SMN1 gene encoding the protein survival motor neurone. The mutation is frequently a homozygous deletion of exon 7. The remainder of cases are compound hereterozygotes with the exon 7 deletion on one chromosome and a point mutation, or small deletion/insertion on the other.

> Spinal and bulbar muscular atrophy (SBMA/Kennedy's disease) is an X-linked recessive disorder, affecting males aged 15–50 years.

It is characterized by progressive proximal limb and bulbar weakness, fasciculations of the facial musculature and tongue, sensory neuropathy and androgen insensitivity, leading to gynaecomastia, testicular atrophy and diabetes mellitus. A CAG triplet repeat expansion in the first exon of the androgen receptor gene causes SBMA. The repeat length in normal individuals ranges from 9 to 34 repeats, while abnormal disease causing repeat length ranges from 35 to 62 repeats (see also Chapter 17).

PERIPHERAL NEUROPATHIES

Progress in understanding the molecular genetic basis of the inherited neuropathies in which the neuropathy is the sole or major feature has been significant, and there are currently over 30 identified causative genes (see also Chapter 16).

> The classification of inherited neuropathies is complex but five groups are recognized: Charcot-Marie-Tooth disease (CMT), hereditary neuropathy with liability to pressure palsies (HNPP), hereditary sensory and autonomic neuropathy (HSAN), distal hereditary motor neuropathies (dHMN) and hereditary neuralgic amyotrophy (HNA). Clinically inherited neuropathies may be determined by the age of onset, the long gradual history, the presence of pes cavus in adults, and the family history. Electrophysiology is important in directing genetic testing.

CMT

> CMT is the most common inherited neuropathy with a prevalence of 1:2500. It is further subdivided into CMT1 and CMT2 depending on whether the neuropathy is demyelinating (median nerve conduction velocity <38 m/s) or axonal (conduction velocity >38 m/s).

The majority of CMT in Europe and the US is autosomal dominant or X-linked; autosomal recessive forms are found in areas of high consanguinity. **CMT1 (autosomal dominant demyelinating neuropathy) is the most common form of CMT.** Among these, the most frequent subtype is CMT1A which is caused by a duplication of the PMP22 gene (peripheral myelin protein gene) on chromosome 17p11.2 in 43 per cent of CMT cases, which results in the classic phenotype of difficulty walking in the first two decades with distal sensory loss and foot deformity. CMT1B is less common than CMT1A and is caused by mutations in the myelin protein zero (MPZ) gene.

X-linked CMT (CMT1X) is the second most common form of CMT, accounting for 10 per cent of CMT. It affects males more than females and is caused by mutations in the gap junction protein beta 1 gene encoding the protein connexin 32. The nerve conduction velocity is slowed as with all forms of CMT1, but the velocity tends to be in the intermediate range at 25–40 m/s rather than the severe range. Connexin 32 is expressed also in the CNS and therefore occasional features, such as deafness or extensor plantars, may be observed.

CMT2 is the autosomal dominant axonal neuropathy, for which the currently identified genes account for only 25 per cent of the disease. There are three clinical subtypes within CMT2. CMT2A is the 'classic' CMT phenotype (with axonal neuropathy) and is caused by mutations in the mitofusin 2 (MFN2) gene, which account for 20 per cent of CMT2 cases. Such mutations may also result in optic atrophy. Mutations in GJB1 and MPZ may also cause CMT2. CMT2B is associated with profound sensory involvement that leads to ulceration and amputation. Mutations in the gene RAB7 (Ras-associated protein) cause CMT2B. Finally, CMT2D is an upper limb dominant form in which patients present with wasting of the intrinsic muscles of the hand initially and later have lower limb involvement. Such cases are caused by mutations in GARS (glycyl tRNA synthetase).

The autosomal recessive forms of CMT1 and CMT2 have been grouped (confusingly) together under CMT4. In general, the autosomal recessive CMT are associated with an earlier age of onset and greater severity resulting in loss of ambulation when compared to the autosomal dominant forms. Mutations in the genes that cause autosomal dominant CMT1 (PMP22, MPZ) may also cause autosomal recessive CMT. Other genes that cause autosomal recessive CMT1 include the GDAP1 gene, which is associated with neuropathy with diaphragmatic and vocal cord involvement, and the KIAA1985 gene, which is associated with neuropathy and early scoliosis. Genes that cause autosomal recessive CMT2 include the lamin A/C gene and the GDAP1 gene.

HNPP

HNPP presents with episodic attacks of weakness or sensory loss in the distribution of a particular nerve that is liable to compression. It is an autosomal dominant condition that is caused by a deletion on chromosome 17p (the same area that is duplicated in CMT1A). Point mutations in the PMP22 gene as well as deletions may cause this condition.

HSAN

HSAN is rarer than CMT and is characterized by prominent sensory loss that may result in mutilation, and autonomic features; motor involvement may also be present. **HSAN1** presents in the second decade with lower limb sensory loss and lancinating pain. It is autosomal dominant and largely caused by mutations in the SPTLC4 gene. The phenotype shows considerable overlap with CMT2B caused by RAB7 mutations. **HSAN II** is caused by mutations in the HSN2 gene and is an early onset autosomal recessive sensory neuropathy. **HSAN III** is caused by mutations in the IKBKAP gene and presents in infancy and childhood with an autonomic and sensory neuropathy. It is an autosomal recessive condition seen in Ashkenazi Jewish people (Riley–Day syndrome). **HSAN IV and V** are autosomal recessive conditions that are characterized by congenital insensitivity to pain. HSAN IV is caused by mutations in the NTRK 1 (neurotrophic tyrosine kinase receptor type 1) gene and is associated with anhidrosis and mental retardation, as well as congenital insensitivity to pain. HSAN V is caused by mutations in either NTRK1 or NGFB genes and does not exhibit any additional features other than congenital insensitivity to pain. Mutations in the voltage gated sodium channel SCN9A have been shown to cause a phenotype similar to HSAN V.

dHMN

The dHMNs typically present with length-dependent weakness and preserved sensory action potentials on neurophysiology testing. They show considerable clinical and genetic overlap with forms of CMT and with SMA. dHMN II is an autosomal dominant form of the disease which presents as classic CMT without sensory involvement. It is caused by mutations in the HSP22 and HSP27 genes. dHMN V may be caused by mutations in GARS or BSCL2 (which also cause CMT2D). dHMN VI is also called SMARD1, which is a spinal muscular atrophy with respiratory distress and is caused by mutations in the IGHMBP2 gene. Mutations in the dynactin gene and the senataxin gene cause forms of dHMN/SMA.

HNA

HNA is characterized by attacks of brachial neuritis that are clinically indistinct from the sporadic form, except that attacks tend to be recurrent. It is an autosomal dominant condition caused by mutations in the septin 9 gene.

Currently molecular genetic testing is available for the more common CMT genes. Patients presenting with CMT1 may be tested for PMP22 duplications, followed by GJB1 mutations (if no male–male transmission observed), MPZ mutations and then PMP22 mutations. Patients presenting with CMT2 may be tested for MFN2 followed by MPZ. It is worth noting that 'sporadic' cases of CMT are caused by *de novo* mutations in the autosomal dominant genes, and are therefore considered for testing if the clinical phenotype is appropriate.

MUSCLE DISEASE

There has been rapid progress in our understanding of the genetic muscle diseases, with a large number of newly identified genetic factors. A detailed clinical assessment taking into account the age of onset, progression, distribution of disease, family history and additional features, such as myotonia, contractures or cardiac/respiratory involvement, is vital in directing the genetic diagnosis. Indeed, in cases of the dystrophinopathies, facioscapulohumeral dystrophy and myotonic dystrophy, genetic testing may be the first line of investigation. Muscle biopsy with careful immunoanalysis for protein expression patterns helps to further direct genetic testing in the limb girdle muscular dystrophies, congenital muscular dystrophies and congenital myopathies (see also Chapter 18).

Muscle dystrophies: X-linked

Duchenne muscular dystrophy (DMD) and Becker muscular dystrophy (BMD) are X-linked recessive conditions with DMD affecting 1:3500 live male births, and BMD affecting 1:20000.

In DMD, the age of onset is usually below the age of five years and the condition is characterized by progressive proximal weakness leading to loss of ambulation by the early teens and cardiac and respiratory failure in early adulthood. In BMD, the onset is later and the course of the disease less aggressive. **DMD is caused by the absence of the dystrophin protein, while BMD is caused by reduced expression of the protein.** The dystrophin gene is a large 83 exon gene. Seventy to 80 per cent of the mutations in BMD and DMD are due to multiple exon deletions. Approximately 10 per cent of cases are due to small exon duplications and the rest are due to point mutations. The effect of the mutations on the reading frame of the gene and hence the translation of the protein is important in determining the severity of the phenotype (i.e. absence of protein compared to semi-functional protein) and in prognosis. In the absence of a family history, the mutation in dystrophin may be *de novo* (or *de novo* in the maternal carrier).

X-linked Emery–Dreifuss type muscular dystrophy (EDMD) is a condition characterized by early joint contractures and a pattern of weakness and wasting affecting the proximal muscles of the upper limb and the distal muscles of the lower limb. It is caused by deletions in the Emerin gene.

An autosomal dominant form of EDMD is now recognized which is caused by mutations in the lamin A/C gene.

Muscle dystrophies: autosomal dominant

Facioscapulohumeral dystrophy (FSHD) is characterized by asymmetric weakness affecting the face and progressively descending to affect the shoulder girdle, hip girdle and anterior tibial and peroneal muscles. More than 95 per cent of cases are associated with a deletion on chromosome 4q35. Although the gene accounting for FSHD is still unknown, it is thought most likely that the shortening of the telomeric end of chromosome 4 results in a genomic dysregulation of the causative gene(s).

Myotonic dystrophy (DM1) is an autosomal dominant multisystem disorder. The neuromuscular manifestations are wasting and myotonia in the temporal, masseter, sternocleidomastoid and distal limb muscles. Other features include male baldness, cataracts, diabetes mellitus, cardiomyopathy, cognitive slowing and respiratory muscle weakness.

Muscular dystrophy (MD) is caused by a CTG triplet repeat expansion in the myotonin kinase gene (DMPK) on chromosome 19. The normal triplet repeat length varies from 5 to 37 CTGs; 38–39 is termed the subclinical premutation; >50 CTGs is associated with the clinical disease. As with other trinucleotide repeat disorders, genetic anticipation may be seen with DM1. In mutation-negative DM1 cases, consideration may be given to DM2, which is an autosomal dominant disorder resembling DM1 but with proximal myopathy. It is caused by an expansion of CCTG repeats in the zinc finger protein gene.

Bethlem myopathy is an autosomal dominant disorder with onset at any age. It is characterized by a proximal myopathy and joint contractures, which clinically overlaps with the EMDM phenotype. It is caused by mutations in one of three different genes for collagen type 6: COL6A1, COL6A2 or COL6A3.

Oculopharyngeal muscular dysytrophy (OPMD) is an uncommon late onset disorder characterized by pharyngeal muscle weakness and ophthalmoplegia. It may be autosomal dominantly or autosomal recessively inherited. The most common mutation is an expansion in a GCG repeat in the poly-A binding protein 2 (PAB2) gene.

The limb girdle muscular dystrophies (LGMD) are a group of disorders characterized by the phenotype of limb girdle weakness without facial involvement. Some subtypes may be associated with cardiomyopathy or respiratory muscle weakness.

Of the autosomal dominant LGMD, three genes have been identified. LGMD1A may be caused by mutations in the myotilin gene. LGMD1B is caused by mutations in the lamin A/C gene (which also cause AD-EDMD), and is associated with significant cardiac and respiratory involvement. LGMD1C is caused by mutations in the caveolin 3 gene.

Muscle dystrophies: autosomal recessive

The autosomal recessive forms of LGMD are in fact more common than the autosomal dominant forms, and present between two and 40 years of age. The most common form of adult onset LGMD in Northern Europe is LGMD2I, which is caused by mutations in the gene fukutin-related protein (FKRP). LGMD2I presents with axial, neck flexor and proximal girdle weakness, associated with hypertrophy of muscles such as the tongue, and calves. Respiratory muscle weakness leading to nocturnal hypoventilation is common, and a cardiomyopathy occurs in a third of cases. LGMD2B is caused by mutations in the dysferlin gene. This may present either as a proximal LGMD subtype or a distal lower limb posterior calf compartment weakness (also known as Miyoshi myopathy). LGMD2A is caused by mutations in the calpain gene. It presents with a typical LGMD phenotype but is associated with atrophy of muscles rather than hypertrophy. Cardiac involvement is rare in LGMD2A and 2B.

The congenital muscular dystrophies (CMD) are a group of autosomal recessive disorders that present in infancy with hypotonia, weakness and contractures. Four different subtypes are recognized, and nine genes that cause CMD have been identified: (1) CMD with a deficiency in laminin α2; (2) CMD with abnormal glycosylation of α-dystroglycan (caused by mutations in fukutin, FKRP, POMT1 and POMT2); (3) CMD with defects in the extracellular matrix (caused by mutations in selenoprotein N, SEPN1, or collagen type 6; and (4) CMD with reduction in integrin α7.

Distal myopathies

Most of the inherited muscle diseases have proximal presentations. However, the distal myopathies are a group of rare diseases characterized by progressive weakness that begins in the feet and hands. Several primary genetic distal myopathies are now described, but all of them are very rare. Mutations in the dysferlin gene (Miyoshi myopathy) and the GNE gene (Nonaka myopathy) cause autosomal recessive distal myopathies.

Congential myopathies

The congenital myopathies are a group of rare diseases characterized by congenital floppiness, muscle weakness and skeletal dysmorphism. The diagnosis is usually based on the morphological abnormalities found on muscle biopsy. Two forms are described here. **Central core disease (CCD)** is an autosomal dominant condition, with features of central amorphous areas within the muscle fibre. It is caused by mutations in the ryanodine receptor and is allelic to one form of malignant hyperthermia susceptibility. Patients with CCD are at risk of malignant hyperthermia. **Nemaline myopathy (NM)** is a condition characterized on biopsy by rod-shaped structures in the muscle fibres. It may be autosomal dominant or autosomal recessive and has three forms: severe congenital, typical congenital and adult onset. The genes that underlie this condition encode sarcomeric thin filament proteins: mutations in α and β tropomyosin genes cause autosomal dominant NM; mutations in nebulin, troponin-I, NEM1 and NEM2 cause autosomal recessive NM. Mutations in a actin have been reported with both autosomal dominant and recessive NM.

Channelopathies

Mutations in the ion channel genes results in alteration of the excitability of the skeletal muscle membrane, and gives rise to two groups of disorders: the periodic paralyses and the myotonias.

The periodic paralyses are autosomal dominant conditions characterized by episodic weakness. **Hyperkalaemic periodic paralysis** causes short-lived attacks precipitated by rest after exercise, stress or potassium ingestion. It is caused by mutations in the muscle sodium channel SCN4A. **Hypokalaemic periodic paralysis** causes longer attacks of weakness precipitated by carbohydrate ingestion or rest following exercise. It is caused mainly by mutations in the L-type calcium channel gene CACNA1S, or rarely mutations in the SCN4A gene.

Myotonia is a disorder in which muscle stiffness occurs as a result of failure of muscle relaxation. **Myotonia congenita may be dominant (Thomsen's disease) or recessive (Becker's disease)**. Myotonia may be detected clinically or on electromyography (EMG). Both types are caused by mutations in the muscle chloride channel gene (CLCN1). **Paramyotonia congenita** is a myotonic autosomal dominant disorder that occurs during exercise and, in contrast to myotonia congenita, worsens with activity. This disorder is caused by mutations in the muscle sodium channel SCN4A, which also causes hyperkalaemic periodic paralysis.

Metabolic myopathies

This is a heterogeneous group of myopathies characterized by a defect in muscle energy metabolism leading to skeletal muscle dysfunction. They may be caused by mitochondrial respiratory chain diseases (see later section) or by mutations causing specific enzymatic defects either in the metabolism of glucose (glycogen storage disorders) or in the metabolism of fat (lipid storage disorders). **The most common glycogen storage disorder is McArdle's disease, which is an autosomal recessive disorder that results in deficiency of myophosphorylase**. This results in muscle pain on exercise, myoglobinuria and rhabdomyolysis. The forearm ischaemic lactate test and muscle biopsy for staining of the myophosphorylase enzyme are useful tests to diagnose the metabolic defect and are usually undertaken before genetic testing.

MITOCHONDRIAL DISORDERS

Mitochondrial function is essential to the energetic balance of all cells. The respiratory chain/oxidative phosphorylation mechanism is encoded by two separate genomes: the mitochondrial genome and the nuclear genome. Mutations in mitochondrial DNA or in nuclear DNA encoding mitochondrial proteins can therefore result in mitochondrial disorders. Mitochondrial DNA mutations are either sporadic or maternally transmitted while nuclear DNA mutations are sporadic or autosomal dominant or recessive. There is a wide spectrum of phenotypes associated with mitochondrial disorders.

> Mitochondrial disorders are multisystem diseases and the presence of CNS abnormalities together with myopathy, neuropathy, optic/retinal abnormalities, deafness, cataracts, short stature and diabetes mellitus is suggestive of these conditions.

The clinical phenotype associated with a mutation is dependent on a number of factors: the inherent pathogenicity of the mutation, the tissue distribution of the mutated gene, and the vulnerability of different tissues to energy demands.

Disorders due to mtDNA mutations

> Mitochondrial DNA rearrangements are usually sporadic events in the germline, although maternal transmission of duplications and deletions has been reported in a small number of cases. Single mtDNA deletions result in three disorders: Kearns–Sayre syndrome (KSS), sporadic progressive external ophthalmoplegia (PEO) and Pearson's syndrome.

KSS is characterized by PEO, pigmentary retinopathy and has an onset at <20 years. It may be associated with a cerebellar syndrome, myopathy and endocrine dysfunction. **Sporadic PEO** is characterized by bilateral ptosis and external ophthalmoplegia and muscle weakness. **Pearson's syndrome** is characterized by the infantile onset of pancytopenia, pancreatic insufficiency and, subsequently, features of KSS.

Mitochondrial DNA point mutations are usually maternally inherited mutations. Some mutations in mtDNA may affect protein synthesis genes, i.e. tRNA and rRNA genes. In such cases, translation of all mitochondria-encoded proteins is perturbed and this leads to multiple defects in the respiratory chain. **MELAS (mitochondrial encephalomyopathy, lactic acidosis and stroke–like episodes) is caused most commonly (in 80 per cent of cases) by the A3243G mutation in the tRNA gene for leucine.** This condition presents with stroke-like episodes that may start with headache and vomiting and progress to encephalopathy, seizures and a focal neurological deficit. The stroke may be parieto-occipital and may not conform to classic vascular territories. Other features of MELAS include deafness, ataxia, dementia and myopathy. The 3243 mutation described here can also cause other phenotypes: KSS, maternally inherited PEO and Leigh syndrome.

MERRF (myoclonus epilepsy with ragged red fibres) is caused by the A8344G mutation in the lysine tRNA gene. MERRF has been described earlier. Of note, the 8344 mutation may also cause Leigh syndrome. NARP (neurogenic weakness, ataxia and retinitis pigmentosa) has been described elsewhere, and is caused by a T8993G mutation in the ATPase 6 gene. LHON (Leber's hereditary optic neuropathy) is characterized by subacute loss of vision bilaterally. Several mtDNA mutations can cause LHON, although the three most common are 11778 (ND4), 3460 (ND1) and 14484 (ND6). The age of onset is in the second to third decade and the penetrance is 40 per cent in males and only 10 per cent in females.

Disorders due to nuclear DNA mutations

Several proteins that are critical to mitochondrial function are encoded by nuclear genes rather than mitochondrial genes. Therefore, nuclear DNA mutations may cause an array of mitochondrial phenotypes. Broadly, mutations occur in genes that are involved in subunits of the respiratory chain, genes that encode proteins essential for the assembly and turnover of the respiratory chain, genes that control the maintenance and integrity of mitochondrial DNA, genes involved in mitochondrial biogenesis, genes involved in mitochondrial transport and trafficking, and coenzyme Q pathway genes. A few illustrative examples of nuclear DNA giving rise to mitochondrial disorders are given below.

Mutations in the SURF-1 gene result in **Leigh syndrome**. SURF1 is a COX assembly factor. Leigh syndrome is a subacute encephalomyopathy, which presents as an early onset neurodegenerative disorder with cerebellar and pyramidal signs, seizures, dystonia and myopathy. MRI shows symmetric lesions in the basal ganglia. It has several genetic causes, all of which result in a defect in oxidative metabolism. The mutation may be in a nuclear gene, such as SURF-1, or in the mitochondrial DNA (e.g. 8993).

Nuclear factors are essential in mitochondrial DNA replication. Such factors include POLG1, which encodes the catalytic subunit of the mtDNA specific polymerase gamma, and TWINKLE, which encodes a mtDNA helicase. Mutations in POLG1 or TWINKLE result in mtDNA breakage syndromes such as autosomal dominant PEO. Mutations in POLG1 also underlie SANDO (sensory ataxia, neuropathy, dysarthria and ophthalmoplegia).

Mitochondria are organelles that undergo fission and fusion. Mitochondrial fusion requires the action of a GTPase called OPA1. Mutations in OPA1 cause an autosomal dominant optic atrophy, which is the most common inherited optic neuropathy.

An approach to genetic diagnosis in mitochondrial disorders must begin with ascertaining the full clinical neurological and non-neurological phenotype, as well as family history. For a phenotype suggestive of mtDNA point mutations, the common mutations (3243, 8344 and 8993) may be screened for in blood samples. If this is negative, a muscle biopsy may be taken to look for the presence of ragged red fibres, perform respiratory chain enzymology, and analyse for mtDNA deletions. In the presence of multiple deletions, sequencing of nuclear genes involved in mtDNA maintenance (such as POLG1) may be considered. In appropriate cases, total sequence analysis of the mitochondrial genome may be undertaken in specialist centres.

THE PHAKOMATOSES

This group of neurocutaneous syndromes includes **neurofibromatosis (NF) 1 and 2, tuberous sclerosis (TS) and Von Hippel–Lindau (VHL) disease**, all of which share the common feature of predisposition to development of tumours. These are autosomal dominant conditions, and in the case of NF and VHL, there is a high rate of new mutations and therefore these conditions may occur in the absence of a family history. In addition, somatic mosaicism may occur in which there may be a variable distribution of the mutations in different tissues and, if the gonadal tissue is spared, the risk to offspring is minimized.

NF1

NF1 has an incidence of 1:3–4000 and manifests with café-au-lait patches (>5 lesions >1.5 cm in adult), Lisch nodules in the iris, axillary/groin pigmentation and the presence of cutaneous and/or plexiform neurofibromas. Associated features include scoliosis, renal artery stenosis, phaeochromocytomas, optic nerve tumours, rhabdomyosarcoma and peripheral nerve sheath tumours.

Surveillance for visual acuity, blood pressure, and 24 hour catecholamine tesing should be performed regularly. Mutations in the NF1 gene include both deletions, rearrangements as well as point mutations. As the NF1 gene is so large, genetic testing without knowledge of the mutation in other family members is difficult.

NF2

NF2 is less common than NF1, with an incidence of 1:30000. It is characterized by bilateral vestibular schwannomas. Patients with NF2 may also develop meningiomas, including spinal meningiomas, ependymomas and astrocytomas. The NF2 gene encodes a protein called schwannomin, and mutations may be detected in 60–80 per cent of cases. Tumours in NF2 manifest two mutated copies of the gene, one of which is inherited, and the second is an acquired somatic mutation.

VHL

VHL is an autosomal dominant condition associated with a susceptibility to benign and malignant tumours that include retina, cerebellar and spinal cord haemangiomas, renal cysts, adenomas and carcinoma, pancreatic cysts and adenomas, and phaeochromocytomas. Annual surveillance therefore requires MR imaging of the kidneys, pancreas and adrenals, 24-hour urine catecholamine testing, and a baseline MR of the neuraxis. Mutations in the tumour suppressor gene (VHL gene) cause this condition, and a mutation can be detected in >90 per cent of cases.

TS

TS has an incidence of 1:10 000. It manifests with angiofibromas around the nose, ash leaf macules and shargreen patches, and ungual fibromas. TS increases the susceptibility to a range of tumours: renal angiomyolipomas, cardiac rhabdomyomas, lung lymphangioleiomyomatosis, and retinal giant cell astrocytomas. In the CNS cortical tubers (which may lead to seizures) and subependymal hamartomas are seen. Mutations in the genes TSC1 (encoding hamartin) and TSC2 (encoding tuberin) account for most cases of TS.

CONCLUSION

This chapter provides a brief outline of the major issues and developments in the rapidly expanding field of neurogenetics. As can be appreciated, it is increasingly complex but also increasingly comprehensive, and it is certainly possible that within the next few years a precise diagnosis will be possible for the majority of neurogenetic diseases. These advances bring with them new challenges: first, the ethical issue of diagnosing (sometimes before manifesting) currently incurable disorders; second, the drive to use these discoveries to understand the molecular pathogenesis of these disorders with the aspiration of more rational design of therapies; third, it is also likely that genetic classification of disease will blur the margins of our traditional views of disease. To enable these developments to be maximized, clinicians will need to be able to appreciate the huge potential and the limitations of both the clinical framework and genetic diagnostics.

REFERENCES AND FURTHER READING

www.geneclinics.org/

www.ncbi.nlm.nih.gov/omim/

Burgunder JM, Finsterer J, Szolnoki Z *et al.* (2010) EFNS guidelines on the molecular diagnosis of channelopathies, epilepsies, migraine, stroke and dementias. *European Journal of Neurology*, **17**:641–648.

Burgunder JM, Schols L, Baets J *et al.* (2011) EFNS guidelines for the molecular diagnosis of neurogenetic disorders: motoneuron, peripheral nerve and muscle disorders. *European Journal of Neurology*, **18**:207–217.

Clarke C, Howard R, Rossor M, Shorvon SD (ed.) (2009) *Neurology: A Queen Square Textbook.* London: Wiley.

Dion PA, Daoud H, Rouleau GA (2009) Genetics of motor neuron disorders: insights into pathogenic mechanisms. *Nature Reviews Genetics*, **10**:769–782.

Finsterer J, Harbo HF, Baets J *et al.* (2009) EFNS guidelines on the molecular diagnosis of mitochondrial disorders. *European Journal of Neurology*, **16**:1255–1264.

Fogel BL, Perlman S (2007) Clinical features and molecular genetics of autosomal recessive cerebellar ataxias. *Lancet Neurology*, **6**:245–257.

Gasser T, Finsterer, Baets J *et al.* (2010) EFNS guidelines on the molecular diagnosis of ataxias and spastic paraplegias. *European Journal of Neurology*, **17**:179–188.

Klein C, Schneider SA, Lang AE (2009) Hereditary Parkinsonism: Parkinson Disease Look-Alikes – an algorithm for clinicians to 'PARK' genes and beyond. *Movement Disorders*, **24**:2042–2058.

Reilly MM, Shy ME (2009) Diagnosis and new treatments in genetic neuropathies. *Journal of Neurology, Neurosurgery and Psychiatry*, **80**:1304–1314.

Wild EJ, Tabrizi SJ (2007) Huntington's disease phenocopy syndromes. *Current Opinion in Neurology*, **20**:681–687.

Wood NW (ed.) (2011) *Neurogenetics for Clinicans.* Cambridge: Cambridge University Press.

CHAPTER 9

RAISED INTRACRANIAL PRESSURE

Laurence Watkins

BASIC PRINCIPLES

The Monro–Kellie model

The modified Monro–Kellie model of factors contributing to intracranial pressure (ICP) is based on a number of simplifying hypotheses. The skull is a fixed volume box (except in young children) so the intracranial volume is assumed to have a fixed overall value. Therefore, any change in volume of intracranial components (blood, brain parenchyma, cerebrospinal fluid (CSF)) or the addition of abnormal volume (tumour, haematoma, air) must be offset by equal change in another component, or the pressure will rise.

In an adult, the normal composition is approximately 87 per cent brain parenchyma, 9 per cent CSF, 4 per cent blood. The brain parenchyma can be further divided into an intracellular and an extracellular compartment. The typical adult intracranial volume of 1500 mL consists of about 1100 mL intracellular space, 200 mL extracellular space, 140 mL of CSF and 60 mL of blood.

The assumption that the skull is a closed, fixed box is an approximation: some displacement can occur through the foramen magnum, as well as the other cranial foramina, to a lesser extent. Each of these can be considered clinically important in some circumstances; for example, displacement of the cerebellar tonsils caudally through the foramen magnum. In some situations, therefore, it is necessary to consider the whole neuraxis, including cranial and spinal components, in order to fully understand the variables involved.

Another simplifying hypothesis is that ICP is a single value; in fact, pressure gradients exist (if only that as a result of the hydrostatic effect of gravity) and are clinically significant under some circumstances.

The craniospinal contents are approximately 80–90 per cent water. Even excluding the fluid components (blood and CSF), brain parenchyma contains 75–80 per cent water. The addition of abnormal amounts of water to any physiological compartment can thus lead to a rise in ICP; for example, brain oedema and hydrocephalus.

ICP and cerebral perfusion pressure

Given the above hypotheses, it can be seen that ICP will be dynamic: fluctuating rhythmically with the cardiac and respiratory cycles (mainly by altering the intracranial blood volume), and with gravitational effects depending on the orientation of the craniospinal axis.

> ICP most importantly is a major independent factor in determining cerebral perfusion pressure and the critical factor for tissue survival is not ICP per se, but the maintenance of adequate cerebral blood flow (CBF) to meet metabolic requirements.

Secondary brain injury (i.e. not resulting from the primary pathological process) is of enormous importance for prognosis after any brain injury and is most commonly caused by cerebral ischaemia.

However, CBF is difficult to monitor in a clinical environment. In practice, ICP is monitored (see below) and cerebral perfusion pressure (CPP) is derived (cerebral perfusion pressure = mean arterial pressure – intracranial pressure).

Even CBF is only an indirect measure of substrate delivery for energy required to match metabolic requirements and thus to maintain membrane integrity.

> 'Normal' blood flow can be insufficient to maintain cellular integrity if the blood is hypoxic or severely hypoglycaemic. Furthermore, metabolic requirements can also change; for example, they are decreased by hypothermia and increased by epileptic activity.

Homeostatic responses

With gradually increasing volume of a pathological component, ICP is first stabilized by displacement of fluid from the various compartments mentioned above: a process known as 'volume buffering'. The most immediate volume buffering response is a result of displacement of CSF through the foramen magnum into the spinal thecal sac. Intracranial blood volume can also be rapidly decreased by displacement of blood from the venous sinuses.

The above components account for the initial part of the pressure–volume curve. In this part of the curve, increasing lesion volume leads to almost no increase in ICP. Once these rapid components of volume buffering are exhausted, however, the curve becomes progressively steeper, but the exact gradient depends on the speed of addition: rapid additional volume cannot be buffered adequately, but if the addition is sufficiently slow, the extracellular space is capable of shrinking by about 50 per cent, giving considerable additional homeostatic capacity.

Once ICP begins to rise, autoregulation triggers vasodilatation, maintaining stable CBF. The autoregulation response can also compensate, to some extent, for falls in arterial pressure.

Once volume buffering and autoregulation have been exhausted, CBF begins to be compromised as ICP rises and CPP falls below 50 mmHg.

CLINICAL PRESENTATION OF RAISED ICP

Headache

The most common symptom of raised ICP is headache. The onset can be slow; for example, as a result of gradual growth of a tumour. Alternatively, the onset can be sudden, if the causation is of sudden onset (e.g. haemorrhage), or rapid (e.g. hydrocephalus from occlusion of the third ventricle by a colloid cyst) (Box 9.1).

Typically, the headaches are worsened by factors that would be expected to further increase ICP: coughing, straining, bending forwards or lying flat, though these can be reported in benign migraine type heacahe).

> The most common time to lie flat is in bed at night, so this often leads to a diurnal pattern: the headache is worst on waking, but improves after the patient has been sitting or ambulant for a while. The observation of the diurnal pattern appears to be mainly a result of the simple effect of gravity: patients often discover that they can gain some relief by sleeping with their head propped up or even in a sitting position.

However, there may also be some contribution from the normal diurnal variation of cortisol production.

Vomiting

Vomiting is also characteristic of raised ICP. Like the headache, it is typically worse in the morning after lying flat overnight. One diagnostic pitfall is

Box 9.1 Symptoms of raised intracranial pressure

> Headache
> Vomiting
> Altered conscious level
> Visual disturbances – obscurations, blurring, double vision
> Focal signs – speech, movement, sensation

that vomiting can occur in the absence of nausea, and even in the absence of headache. This presentation of 'pure' vomiting is most often caused by a brainstem lesion affecting the floor of the fourth ventricle; it may be a result of local stimulation of vomiting reflexes before the tumour has caused much increase in ICP. Vomiting with a diurnal pattern, or if sudden and 'effortless' in nature, is highly suspicious of raised ICP.

If the vomiting is accompanied by headache, the patient often notices that the headache worsens as they vomit (because this further raises ICP due to straining). Each bout of vomiting increases ICP, so the patient may reach a crescendo of vomiting, often leading to presentation at an emergency department.

Visual symptoms and signs

Visual obscuration

Raised ICP, particularly if rapid in onset, may lead to transient blackout of vision lasting seconds, referred to as visual obscuration and often precipitated by straining or bending.

Papilloedema

As ICP progressively rises, fundoscopy will often reveal loss of the normal venous pulsations in the retinal veins around the optic disc. With a further increase, axonal transport in the optic nerve becomes compromised, leading to the characteristic swelling of the disc: initially progressive loss of the cup and then the more obvious 'heaped up' appearance. Severe venous obstruction can then lead to retinal haemorrhages around the disc.

> **Presence or absence of papilloedema**
> Although papilloedema is a significant sign, it is important to realize that it is frequently not present. Fewer than half of patients with raised ICP will demonstrate papilloedema. **Thus, papilloedema is diagnostic, but lack of papilloedema should never be taken as reassurance.**

Apart from its usefulness as a sign of raised ICP, papilloedema is also significant because it represents a risk to vision. Left unresolved, papilloedema can lead to expansion of the blind spot,

loss of visual acuity and eventually to optic nerve infarction and blindness.

It should be noted that fundoscopy to check for papilloedema should not require a mydriatic to dilate the pupil (this is usually performed in the context of full retinal screening). Indeed, in many contexts where papilloedema is relevant, it will also be important to preserve normal pupil reactions as a part of the clinical assessment.

In some cases of hydrocephalus, or space-occupying lesions in the region of the optic chiasm, visual deterioration can occur even in the absence of papilloedema because of the direct effect of pressure on the chiasm. Thus, in some patients with obstructive hydrocephalus, visual deterioration can sometimes occur even without characteristic symptoms or papilloedema.

> For this reason, patients with CSF shunts should have regular visual checks as part of their ongoing surveillance; visual deterioration may sometimes be the first and only sign that their shunts are malfunctioning.

Abnormalities of eye movements

Raised ICP, particularly if a result of obstructive hydrocephalus, can lead to distortion or 'kinking' of the tectal plate region, producing a loss of up-gaze. In infants with severe hydrocephalus, this can lead to the characteristic sign of 'sunsetting', where the iris is displaced downwards and partially obscured by the lower lid, like the sun disappearing over the horizon at sunset. In the very elderly, there is sometimes a physiological loss of up-gaze and so it is a less useful sign in that age group.

Diplopia can be a symptom of raised ICP. This is sometimes caused by an abducens palsy, probably as a result of a non-specific pressure effect on the brainstem. It is thus a 'false localizing' sign, because there is usually not a lesion pressing directly on the abducens nerve, and it does not provide useful information as to the location of an intracranial lesion. On the other hand, diplopia can be caused by an oculomotor palsy from herniation of the uncus over the tentorial edge and this is a 'localizing' sign, because it occurs as a result of the direct pressure on the nerve and is usually ipsilateral with the lesion producing the mass effect.

Decreased level of consciousness

A decreased level of consciousness implies severely raised ICP. Either the homeostatic mechanisms have been exhausted and overall CBF has fallen too low to maintain brain function, or specific areas critical to maintaining arousal (reticular formation, midbrain) have been compromised by brain shift. In either case, the situation is serious and further rises in ICP can lead to deterioration into coma and death.

Pressure gradients, shifts and herniations

The intracranial space is divided by incomplete partitions formed from folds of dura. The tentorium separates the cerebral hemispheres from the cerebellum, medulla and pons; the falx separates the two cerebral hemispheres. The midbrain straddles the tentorial hiatus, with the medial part of the temporal lobe (uncus) adjacent on each side. This basic anatomy helps us to understand the three main patterns of brain shift: subfalcine, transtentorial (or uncal) and foramen magnum (or tonsillar). Each of these patterns is sometimes referred to as 'coning' (Figure 9.1).

Subfalcine herniation

A unilateral supratentorial lesion produces an asymmetrical mass effect and, as it increases, leads to progressive displacement of midline structures towards the contralateral side, forcing brain tissue to herniate underneath the edge of the falx. If there is decreased conscious level or an accompanying focal deficit, urgent treatment to reduce mass effect will be required. **Even in an otherwise well patient, if the midline displacement is more than 5 mm, the patient is at significant risk of rapid deterioration.** As the medial surface of the cerebral hemisphere herniates under the tentorial edge, bridging veins, draining blood from the hemisphere into the sagittal sinus, can become kinked leading to sudden worsening of swelling and rapid decompensation; for example, a small chronic subdural haematoma would require urgent burr-hole drainage if there was decreased conscious level, focal deficit or midline shift of >5 mm. On the other hand, in a well patient with less than 5 mm of midline shift, a small chronic subdural haematoma might be considered for conservative management.

Transtentorial/uncal herniation

Kernohan's notch describes the situation in which lateral displacement of the midbrain by a supratentorial mass leads to impingement of the opposite cerebral peduncle onto the hard tentorial edge. This produces an indentation or 'notch' in the contralateral cerebral peduncle and can produce a hemiparesis ipsilateral to the causative supratentorial mass. Thus, hemiparesis can be misleading as a localizing clinical sign. Occasionally, a posterior

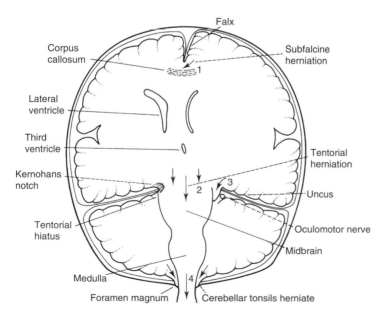

Figure 9.1 Coronal section of the brain to show the sites of possible herniation. Note: the oculomotor nerve (III) lies by the free edge of the tentorium cerebelli. (1) Subfalcine herniation; (2) transtentorial herniation; (3) uncal herniation; (4) tonsillar herniation (foramen magnum).

As supratentorial pressure increases, structures begin to herniate through the tentorial hiatus. In the case of a unilateral supratentorial mass, the first structure to herniate will be the uncus on the medial aspect of the temporal lobe. The oculomotor nerve running along the free edge of the tentorium is compressed by the herniating uncus leading to the **cardinal sign of an ipsilateral increase in pupil size. As the effect increases the pupil becomes fully dilated and unreactive.** As the uncus herniates, it also presses on midbrain structures leading to a **decrease in conscious level.** Eventually, the compressed tissue within the tentorial hiatus also compromises the contralateral oculomotor nerve, leading to bilateral fixed dilated pupils.

fossa mass can produce transtentorial herniation upwards. Thus, there is a small but definite risk of producing this complication when associated obstructive hydrocephalus is relieved by shunting fluid from the lateral ventricles in the presence of a posterior fossa mass.

Foramen magnum/tonsillar herniation

Once all the compensatory intracranial mechanisms are exhausted, the only further displacement possible is through the foramen magnum. At this stage, the cerebellar tonsils are displaced downwards and, as they become crowded into the foramen magnum, they cause compression of the medulla. Because this is usually the final stage of ICP decompensation, the patient is likely to be comatose, but, **if conscious, the patient will complain of severe occipitocervical pain and neck stiffness.** Typically, the patient will find a particular head position in which the pain is minimized (this can be flexed, extended or neutral) and will then resolutely hold their head fixed in that position.

Brainstem reflexes may become compromised, leading to cardiorespiratory irregularities. However, these signs are very late, usually occurring just prior to respiratory arrest, and so their absence should not be taken as reassurance.

It is important to note that performing lumbar puncture in the presence of brain shift either with a supratentorial or a posterior fossa mass can be rapidly fatal.

The sudden reduction of pressure within the spinal CSF can worsen the displacement, leading to further compression of vital structures. It is therefore critical to differentiate between possible meningitis and headache/neck stiffness caused by an intracranial mass. This will usually be suspected on clinical features, but if there is any doubt an urgent computed tomography (CT) scan should be performed prior to any attempt at lumbar puncture.

CAUSES OF RAISED ICP

Head injury

Head injury is a common problem. In terms of overall numbers, it is the most common cause of raised ICP.

Although it is an oversimplification, brain damage from head trauma is customarily divided into primary and secondary injury: primary injury is the damage at the moment of impact, whereas secondary injury results from ongoing causes. The most potent causes of secondary injury are hypoxia and hypertension (often sustained before the patient even reaches hospital). Intracranial causes of secondary injury predominantly act by raising ICP, decreasing CBF and thus causing brain tissue metabolic failure.

Raised ICP following trauma can be the result of haematoma (extradural, subdural or intracerebral), contusion or diffuse brain swelling. It is particularly important not to miss the diagnosis of an intracranial haematoma, because such lesions are often eminently treatable by surgery, but such treatment needs to be instituted quickly.

Hydrocephalus

Basic principles

CSF is continuously produced by the choroid plexus, mainly in the lateral ventricles but also, to a lesser extent, in the third and fourth ventricles. An even smaller amount is produced directly by the ependymal lining of the ventricles. The daily rate of production varies very little for a particular individual. It is generally around 500 mL per day in an adult and does not change, even with quite wide variations of other physiological parameters. It is very difficult to reduce CSF production, although carbonic anhydrase inhibitors, such as acetazolamide, can achieve minor reduction.

The CSF leaves the ventricular system through the foramina of Magendie and Luschka to enter the subarachnoid space. Some fluid will flow around the spinal cord, while some will enter the basal subarachnoid spaces (cisterns), but eventually all CSF circulates over the surface of the cerebral hemispheres to be reabsorbed through the arachnoid granulations into the intracranial venous sinuses.

> The production of CSF being essentially fixed, hydrocephalus (the abnormal accumulation of CSF) is caused by impairment of flow somewhere in the pathways outlined above. If blockage occurs within the ventricular system (e.g. a tumour occluding the fourth ventricle, or aqueduct stenosis), this leads to 'obstructive' or 'non-communicating' hydrocephalus. If, however, impairment of flow is a result of scarring of the arachnoid granulations or the cisternal subarachnoid spaces (e.g. following meningitis or subarachnoid haemorrhage), the resulting hydrocephalus is said to be 'communicating'.

Clinical presentation

In children, hydrocephalus can be caused by congenital malformations (e.g. aqueduct stenosis or malformations associated with dysraphism) or can be produced by perinatal intracranial haemorrhage. Raised ICP in infants produces bulging of the fontanelles and increasing head circumference. Depending on the severity, this may be less apparent and may merely cause delayed closure of the fontanelles. In an older child, hydrocephalus can present gradually with decreased educational achievement and subtle cognitive decline. In addition, any of the features of raised ICP discussed above can be present.

In adults, the presentation is more likely to be with the general features of raised ICP. In addition, middle-aged and elderly adults can present with a disorder known as **normal pressure hydrocephalus (NPH)**. This is probably a misnomer, because it is thought to be a result of intermittently raised ICP: such patients were found to have 'normal' pressure at lumbar puncture, but subsequent studies using

24-hour ICP monitoring have shown that plateau waves of raised ICP do occur.

> Patients with NPH classically present with the triad of dementia, gait apraxia and urinary incontinence (Box 9.2). It is not necessary, however, for all the features to be present. Some patients present with an akinetic-rigid Parkinsonian gait.

The diagnosis of NPH may be supported by magnetic resonance imaging (MRI), in which dilatation of the temporal horns is more likely to represent a hydrocephalic process rather than atrophy or small vessel disease, both of which are also common in the elderly. Additionally, ICP monitoring may demonstrate characteristic plateau waves, and some clinicians rely on careful and objective clinical assessments (timed walk, neuropsychometry), before and after therapeutic high volume lumbar puncture or preferably prolonged lumbar drainage. However, all of the above methods of assessment have a significant false-negative rate and so, if the clinical presentation is convincing, it is worth considering the insertion of a CSF shunt, even though improvement cannot be guaranteed and shunting can result in other significant morbidities (e.g. subdural collection). Gait apraxia alone is more likely to respond to shunting. **Neurodegeneration and small vessel vascular disease can produce identical clinical pictures to NPH.**

Treatment of hydrocephalus

> As with other causes of raised ICP, there are two aspects of treatment of hydrocephalus: treating the causative lesion and directly reducing ICP, in this case by draining CSF (usually by insertion of a CSF shunt, although acutely an external ventricular drain may be used).

Box 9.2 Symptoms and signs of normal pressure hydrocephalus

> Impaired cognitive function
> Gait disorder – short shuffling steps, unsteady, falls, 'magnetic gait', astasia-abasia
> Urinary incontinence – urgency, frequency, then incontinence with lack of concern

A catheter is inserted into the ventricle and linked via a subcutaneous tube to another body cavity, generally the peritoneal cavity, but sometimes the right atrium or, more rarely, the pleural cavity or the transverse venous sinus. The system will contain a valve to regulate the CSF flow, with various degrees of sophistication depending on the type of valve.

Some valves are now capable of being adjusted non-invasively after insertion, allowing a variety of pressure settings to be tried without requiring revision surgery. Such valves can be reset by strong magnetic fields and so, if a patient requires MRI, it is important to ascertain whether their shunt system is MR compatible and, if it is an adjustable valve, it will need to be checked and possibly reset immediately after the imaging. Thus, such patients should be dealt with at a centre familiar with hydrocephalus and shunt problems. Complications from the use of shunts include blockage, infection and the development of a subdural collection.

Obstructive hydrocephalus, particularly as a result of aqueduct stenosis, is increasingly treated by endoscopic third ventriculostomy, whereby the floor of the third ventricle is punctured to allow CSF to 'bypass' directly to the basal cisterns, avoiding the blockage in the aqueduct or fourth ventricle. Such operations are only indicated if the ventricular system is sufficiently dilated to allow safe introduction of the endoscope, and only achieve a 60–70 per cent rate of independence from subsequent CSF shunting. However, if successful, the patient then generally remains shunt-independent indefinitely, and is therefore spared the many possible complications of lifelong shunting.

It has often occurred to clinicians that hydrocephalus could also be treated by reducing the production of CSF. In practice, this is of little clinical value: acetazolamide can produce a minor reduction in CSF production; endoscopic coagulation of the choroid plexus is also sometimes used in cases where other therapeutic options have been exhausted, but it has a low rate of success. However, research is currently exploring molecular approaches aimed at selectively destroying the choroid plexus and such techniques may become available in the future.

Tumour

Glioma

Gliomas are the most common primary brain tumours (see also Chapter 14). As the name implies, they can arise from any of the glial components of the brain: astrocytoma, oligodendroglioma and ependymoma. Gliomas are classified into one of four grades (The World Health Organization system being the most widely accepted), depending on histological characteristics such as anaplasia, presence of necrosis and vascular proliferation.

- Grade 1 gliomas correspond to a specific entity known as pilocytic astrocytoma; this occurs almost exclusively in children and has a very good prognosis.
- Grade 2 gliomas are generally referred to as 'benign' and tend to be slow growing; often the history extends to many years and they may present with epilepsy rather than mass effect.
- Grade 3 and 4 gliomas are referred to as 'malignant' because they are fast growing and have a worse prognosis (Figure 9.2). In this case, however, 'malignant' does not imply metastatic potential: gliomas metastasize only very rarely outside the central nervous system.
- The most malignant grade 4 gliomas are commonly known as glioblastoma multiforme, because the cells may take on multiple forms as they dedifferentiate into more primitive tumour cells (Figure 9.3).

The earliest presentation is often with **epilepsy** and this may be associated with a relatively better prognosis because the diagnosis is being made at an early stage before the onset of mass effect. Later presentation can be with **focal effects**, such as hemiparesis or dysphasia, depending on the site of the tumour, or with the more generalized features of **raised ICP**.

If the presentation is with symptoms of mass effect, **surgery** can provide a useful palliative role, particularly if the tumour is in a non-eloquent area. However, there has been little definitive evidence that surgery improves life expectancy (this remains controversial) and so, if symptoms are not attributable to mass effect or are easily controlled by medical means, then surgery is usually limited to biopsy to establish diagnosis.

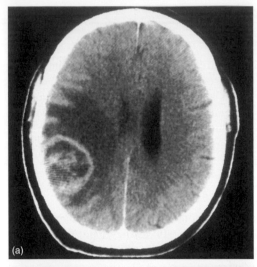

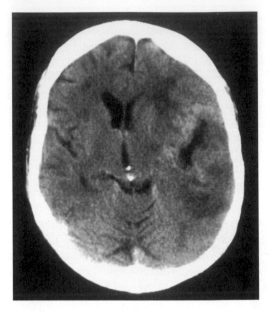

Figure 9.3 CT brain scan showing a left-sided glioblastoma multiforme with slight enhancement by contrast and considerable midline shift.

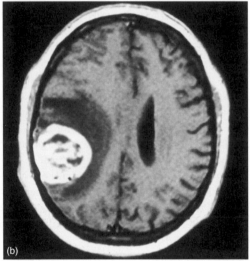

Figure 9.2 Right parietal glioma: (a) contrast-enhanced CT brain scan; (b) T1-weighted MRI brain scan with contrast enhancement.

Surgery, of whatever extent, is generally followed by **cranial radiotherapy**, which has been shown to extend survival (although overall prognosis remains poor), and sometimes by **chemotherapy**, which has also been shown to have a relatively small but positive effect. The selection of patients for radiotherapy depends on their 'performance status' by the degree of pre-existing disability; a significantly disabled patient may be more appropriate for palliative measures rather than radical radiotherapy.

Peritumoural oedema can often be dramatically relieved by **high-dose steroids**, and often the

terminal phases of the disease are marked by balancing the beneficial effect of steroids against their increasing side-effects, until eventual inevitable decompensation occurs.

Grade 2 gliomas generally present with much more subtle symptoms and signs, often with epilepsy alone. Usually a biopsy is performed to establish diagnosis. Thereafter, some clinicians recommend surgery to remove as much abnormal tissue as possible, but generally it is thought that such a radical approach has no effect on outcome. Instead, simple surveillance and symptomatic treatment (e.g. anticonvulsants to control epilepsy) is widely practised. In the case of oligodendroglioma, such tumours often respond well to chemotherapy. For astrocytomas, radiotherapy remains the best option but is usually reserved for tumours that have shown definite increasing size; irradiation at the time of diagnosis may have little biological effect if the tumour is 'quiescent', but then leaves no good therapeutic option if the tumour later increases its rate of growth.

Grade 1 (pilocytic) astrocytoma is generally removed as extensively as possible and then has a very good prognosis; life expectancy is near normal.

Meningioma

Meningioma is the most common extrinsic intra-cranial tumour, but is much less common than a glioma. Meningiomas arise from the meninges, commonly in the region of the arachnoid granulations, although they can arise from any part of the dura, or indeed can occasionally arise inside the cerebral ventricles. They are almost always histologically benign.

As with other tumours, the presenting symptoms and signs will depend on possible **focal effects** (epi-lepsy or focal neurological deficit depending on site) or worsening oedema may lead to presentation with the symptoms of **raised ICP**. Subfrontal meningioma classically presents with progressive cognitive impairment and anosmia (although the latter can be difficult to detect, particularly in a demented patient).

Very small, incidental meningiomas can often be treated conservatively with serial imaging surveillance. However, if treatment is required, surgery is generally the best option. Meningiomas are slow growing, so they tend to be resistant to radiotherapy and to cytotoxic chemotherapy.

Surgery aims to completely remove the tumour and its origin, but this can be difficult to achieve, depending on the location. A convexity meningioma (Figure 9.4) is generally the least complicated to remove and so tends to have a lower rate of recurrence, compared to skull base meningiomas (Figure 9.5). The overall recurrence rate depends on whether atypical histological features are seen, as well as the location, but most clinical series using follow-up imaging find approximately 10 per cent recurrence at ten years.

Preoperative particle embolization is often employed to reduce the blood supply to these tumours, which are often very vascular.

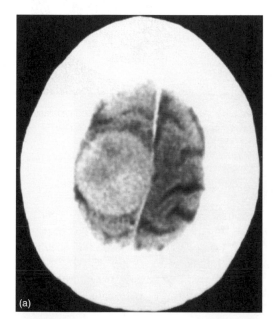

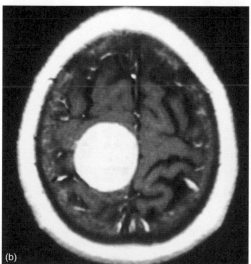

Figure 9.4 Right-sided convexity meningioma: (a) contrast-enhanced CT scan; (b) T1-weighted MRI scan with contrast.

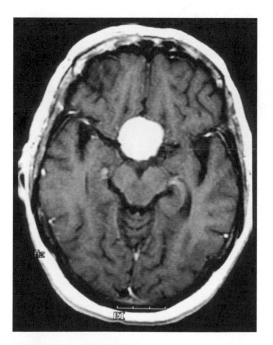

Figure 9.5 T1-weighted MRI scan, axial view, to show a suprasellar meningioma (contrast enhanced).

Despite the poor response, patients with multiple recurrent meningiomas (particularly in syndromes such as neurofibromatosis) sometimes undergo radiotherapy when repeated surgery has been unsatisfactory or is considered too high a risk. In similar circumstances, chemotherapy with hydroxyurea is sometimes tried, again with generally poor response.

Pituitary region tumours

Pituitary tumours and craniopharyngiomas are often grouped together, because they both occur in the sellar region (Figure 9.6) and clinical features are often similar: neurological, visual and endocrine.

Mass effect from a tumour in this region can produce optic nerve and/or chiasmal compression, leading to progressive visual field loss, with a bitemporal hemianopia, often asymmetric or with atypical patterns. Some patients may be unaware of such visual deterioration until central vision is affected.

With further expansion of the tumour, there may be involvement of the cavernous sinus (leading to lesions of the cranial nerves passing through the sinus) or impingement on the medial aspect of the temporal lobe, producing epilepsy. Upwards expansion can lead to obstruction of the anterior part of the third ventricle and the foramina of Monro.

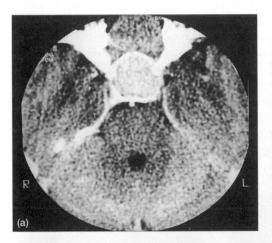

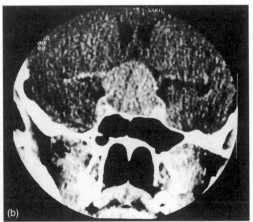

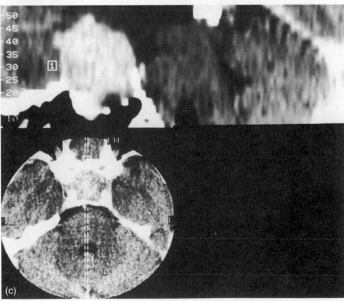

Figure 9.6 (a) Axial view of an enhanced CT brain scan to show a pituitary tumour. (b) Coronal section from the same patient to show the tumour rising well above the pituitary fossa. (c) Sagittal reconstruction from the same patient taken at the level indicated.

Endocrine manifestations are the result of production of excess hormones by the tumour itself (e.g. excess growth hormone leading to acromegaly), or non-productive tumour cells can gradually impair the production of hormones by the rest of the pituitary, leading to hypopituitarism. Any tumour with sufficient mass effect may impair the function of the pituitary stalk, producing increased prolactin (although usually not of such a high level as produced by an active prolactinoma) and may also cause diabetes insipidus.

Craniopharyngiomas possibly arise from embryonic rest cells from Rathke's pouch. These form an expanding cyst in the suprasellar region. They can produce all of the features associated with mass effect in that area: all the features mentioned above, including the endocrine effects of pituitary stalk compression, but of course they do not actually produce hormones.

Investigations

- Endocrine studies
- Visual fields
- Imaging – usually MRI (Figure 9.7).

Treatment of pituitary tumours

Relief of any optic nerve or chiasmal compression is urgent. Modern surgical treatment relies on a trans-sphenoidal approach with removal of the

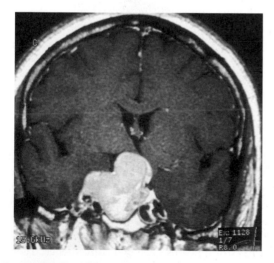

Figure 9.7 T1-weighted MRI brain scan, coronal view, to show a large pituitary tumour rising well above the sella and extending laterally on the right side (gadolinium-enhanced image).

tumour by this route. Huge tumours may require a subfrontal craniotomy. In some patients, postoperative radiotherapy may be necessary.

Bromocriptine and other prolactin inhibitors, such as octreotide, or lanreotide (analogues of somatostatin) have been used in the treatment of acromegaly and may shrink the tumour.

Following any therapy, the patient will require regular follow-up with: assessment of endocrine function (with a view to any replacement therapy); measurement of the visual acuity and charting the visual fields; and often imaging.

Metastases

Metastases are very common at post-mortem, but may present in neurological practice, because they often occur in the context of terminal widespread metastatic carcinoma, where palliation is the major concern. However, a cerebral metastasis can occasionally be the first presentation of carcinoma, even when the patient was not known to have a pre-existing primary tumour. Naturally, if the patient has a main primary tumour, the appearance of cerebral lesion is highly suspicious of metastatic disease. Also, the appearance of multiple intrinsic lesions increases the likelihood of this diagnosis (Figure 9.8). **Common primary sites include the lung and breast; other sites are the kidney, gastrointestinal tract, malignant melanomas and lymphomas.**

Metastatic deposits in the brain can occur in any location and can present either with mass effect or with epilepsy. Mass effect may manifest as focal neurological impairment, or with the general features of raised ICP.

Although it is not possible on imaging appearances to make the diagnosis, multiple well-defined lesions would certainly raise this possibility. Clinical examination to check for a possible primary site is obviously important, as well as chest x-ray, because lung carcinoma is common (Table 9.1).

If the diagnosis cannot be readily made by other means, biopsy often becomes necessary to establish diagnosis. Furthermore, surgical removal of a single intracranial metastasis can often be justified, because it produces good palliation (although no increase in life expectancy).

Further treatment will obviously depend on the underlying primary tumour, because different types of carcinoma may respond to radiotherapy and some to chemotherapy. Resection of the primary may also be indicated.

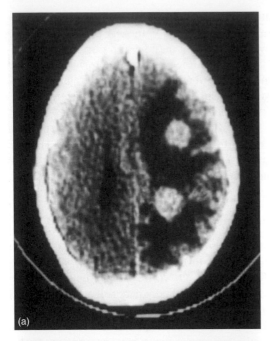

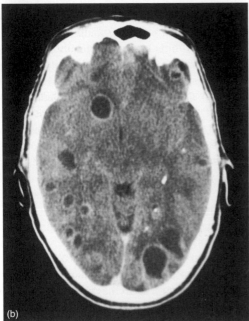

Figure 9.8 (a) Enhanced CT brain scans to show solid metastatic lesions with considerable surrounding oedema (low density). (b) Multiple cystic metastatic lesions with ring enhancement.

If the patient's general condition is good, cranial irradiation will usually be indicated, whether or not surgery has been performed. As always, decisions concerning further treatment will depend on the prognosis of the primary carcinoma, the degree of dissemination elsewhere and the general condition of the patient.

Lymphoma

Primary cerebral lymphoma can occur, or lymphoma deposits may appear in the context of known lymphoma elsewhere in the body. Typically, cerebral lymphoma appears diffusely in the white matter surrounding the ventricles. There is a marked increasing incidence among immunocompromised patients: about 5 per cent of patients with acquired immunodeficiency syndrome (AIDS) eventually develop cerebral lymphoma (see also Chapter 26).

The history is usually short and often symptoms are a subtle behavioural/personality change, although focal epilepsy and progressive hemiparesis can also occur. Later, all the features of generalized raised ICP will appear.

Biopsy generally establishes the diagnosis and treatment then usually involves radiotherapy and treatment of any underlying condition. Cerebral lymphoma often has a marked short-term response to steroids, to such an extent that steroids instituted at presentation may be so effective that the lesion is hard to locate even a few days later when biopsy is attempted. It is therefore important to repeat the scan prior to biopsy to check that the lesion has not become invisible on CT scan.

Pineal region tumours

Tumours of the pineal region are very rare. They occur most commonly in males between the ages of 15 and 25 years. The most common histological type is the germinoma, which is locally malignant and may also seed through the CSF pathways.

True pinealomas, arising from the pineal tissue itself, are very rare and when they occur may be

---

Clinical features of pineal region tumours

Tumours in the pineal region generally present by obstruction of the aqueduct, leading to hydrocephalus (Figure 9.9), or present with raised ICP. There may also be the local effects of pressure on the midbrain and tectal plate. This can present with **Parinaud's syndrome** with defects of upwards gaze and convergence. There may also be large poorly reacting pupils with light-near dissociation. Sometimes there is convergence nystagmus.

Table 9.1 Investigation of patients suspected of having a cerebral tumour

Blood tests	Full blood count, ESR
	Endocrine tests – pituitary lesions
	Special markers, e.g. chorionic gonadotrophin
Imaging	MRI scan (often with gadolinium enhancement) – particularly posterior fossa, craniocervical junction, parapituitary region. CT brain scan (enhanced) – particularly if MRI is not possible. MRA or angiography to identify vascular tumours or show blood supply
To exclude metastases or show primary:	
Blood tests	Liver function, prostatic-specific antigen
Chest x-ray	
Isotope scans	Bone, liver
PET scans	

CT, computerized tomography; ESR, erythrocyte sedimentation rate; MRI, magnetic resonance imaging; MRA, magnetic resonance angiography; PET, positron emission tomography.

either a pineocytoma or a more malignant pineoblastoma.

Other very rare tumours in this region include chorion carcinoma (of embryonic yolk sac origin) and dermoids.

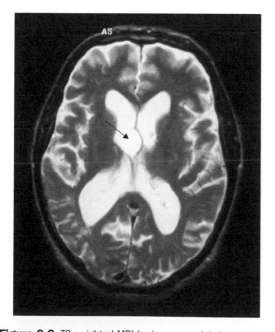

Figure 9.9 T2-weighted MRI brain scan, axial view, to show a colloid cyst slightly to the right of the midline causing an obstructive hydrocephalus.

Treatment

Treatment is primarily the treatment of hydrocephalus, by CSF shunting and sometimes a biopsy to establish the diagnosis. Sometimes the diagnosis can be indicated by blood and CSF tumour markers such as alpha-fetoprotein (in germinoma) and chorionic gonadotrophin (in chorion carcinomas). Radiotherapy is generally useful in germinomas, whereas tumours of yolk sac origin tend to be more chemosensitive. Tumours that disseminate along CSF pathways often require full craniospinal irradiation for secondary deposits.

Posterior fossa tumours

Medulloblastoma and ependymoma

Medulloblastomas are histologically malignant tumours that are the most common intrinsic brain tumour in children, although they can also occur in adults. Tumours typically arise in the vermis of the cerebellum, adjacent to the fourth ventricle. Thus, the presentation is often with obstructive hydrocephalus, as a result of impingement on the fourth ventricle. Occasionally, invasion of the floor of the fourth ventricle may cause vomiting as the primary symptom. If vomiting occurs in the absence of other symptoms, suggesting raised ICP, the diagnosis may be difficult and the patient may often have remained undiagnosed for several months, leading to dehydration and undernutrition.

Other frequently seen features are papilloedema and truncal ataxia. Medulloblastomas may also spread along CSF pathways and so, rarely, presentation can be with secondary deposits (for example in the cauda equina).

Ependymomas also occur mainly in childhood, but are much rarer than medulloblastomas. Ependymomas also commonly arise in the region of the fourth ventricle (although they can occur anywhere there is ependyma) and so it is difficult to distinguish between medulloblastomas and ependymomas on clinical or radiological grounds. Ependymomas, however, tend to be less malignant and to have a generally better prognosis. Both types of tumour are treated by relief of any associated hydrocephalus, surgery to remove as much of the mass as possible, and then radiotherapy. Early surveillance for secondary deposits elsewhere in the craniospinal axis is essential for planning treatment.

Cerebellar astrocytoma

Cerebellar astrocytoma is another tumour of childhood, although rarer than the medulloblastoma and relatively benign. It can be either cystic or solid, and more typically is located in the cerebellar hemisphere rather than the midline. A childhood cerebellar astrocytoma arising in a hemisphere may cause ipsilateral clumsiness or a habitual tilt of the head. Although relatively benign and slow growing, it may also eventually impede CSF drainage and so present with hydrocephalus and raised ICP. The basis of treatment is surgery: to relieve hydrocephalus, establish the histological diagnosis and to debulk the tumour mass. In the case of a cystic type, the solid nodular part is removed but the cystic wall is generally left in place.

Haemangioblastoma

Another tumour arising in the cerebellar hemisphere is a haemangioblastoma. It is generally cystic, with an enhancing nodule in the wall (Figure 9.10). It sometimes occurs as part of von Hippel–Lindau disease, where cerebellar haemangioblastoma may be associated with retinal angiomas and occasionally malignant renal and adrenal tumours. There may thus be a family history.

None of the above features can, however, be relied upon for diagnosis; surgery will be necessary to establish the diagnosis and remove the solid part, if possible. Once the diagnosis is established, the

patient will require ongoing surveillance for further haemangioblastomas, or the development of associated lesions. The patient and their family will also require genetic counselling.

A small, cystic lesion in the cerebellar hemisphere may be an isolated finding and relatively easy to remove at surgery. This may effectively cure the patient, if it is not part of an underlying syndrome. However, large solid lesions may be difficult to remove and extremely vascular.

Cerebellopontine angle tumours

Acoustic neuroma or schwannoma is more accurately called a vestibular neurinoma. It arises from the vestibular part of the eighth cranial nerve. True acoustic neuroma (i.e. arising from the acoustic part of the nerve) may arise in patients with hereditary type 2 neurofibromatosis, an autosomal-dominant inherited disorder. In those cases, the acoustic neuroma is often bilateral.

The common sporadic type of acoustic neuroma is typically unilateral and presents with progressive unilateral hearing impairment; often the patient will notice that they can use a telephone only on

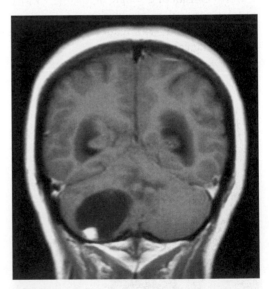

Figure 9.10 MRI bran scan, coronal view, to show a cystic area of low density in the right cerebellar hemisphere. Note the enhancing nodule inferiorly (gadolinium used). This was a haemangioblastoma.

one side. The hearing impairment will eventually progress to complete **sensorineural deafness**. Other associated symptoms may include vertigo, unsteadiness, ipsilateral facial sensory symptoms and facial weakness. As the tumour further enlarges, it may cause brainstem compression, leading to rapidly worsening ataxia and eventually CSF obstruction and presentation with hydrocephalus. By this late stage, headaches are typically severe and brainstem impingement may also have produced limb ataxia or even weakness. Nystagmus is often present as a result of associated peripheral vestibular disturbance. The ipsilateral corneal reflex may also be reduced with later facial sensory loss and facial weakness.

Unilateral sensorineural deafness will usually lead to an ear, nose and throat (ENT) referral assess-

ment. The best definitive imaging is currently gadolinium-enhanced MRI (see Figure 2.14 and Figure 9.11). Where MRI is unavailable, contrast CT scanning will show most tumours over 1 cm diameter. Smaller tumours may be indirectly demonstrated on CT scan (Figure 9.12) by observing enlargement of the internal auditory meatus (although this is only present in about 60 per cent of cases).

Rarely, other tumours can arise in the cerebellopontine angle: including meningiomas, epidermoids, trigeminal neuromas or metastases (Figures 9.13 and 9.14). Any of these tumours can present with local cranial nerve impairment, symptoms and signs of raised ICP and, later, brainstem impairment.

Large tumours with significant mass effect will require **surgery** aimed at removing the tumour if possible. The challenge is to preserve facial nerve function and any residual hearing. This is not always possible, depending on the size of the tumour. Increasingly, small tumours can be treated by **focused radiotherapy** (e.g. gamma knife). Very small tumours may not require any immediate treatment but merely ongoing surveillance. In elderly or frail patients, it may be worth considering simple debulking or intracapsular removal to produce satisfactory relief of mass effect, but with reduced risk of increasing neurological deficit.

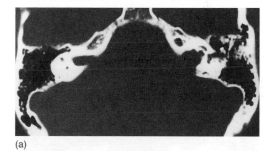

(a)

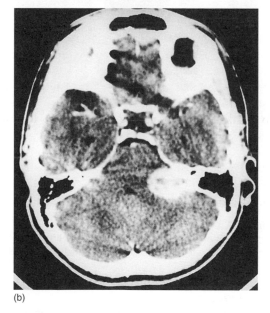

(b)

Figure 9.12 CT brain scan with adjusted window width (a), showing a very widened internal auditory meatus on the left side. (b) The enhanced view delineating the acoustic neuroma, which is displacing the fourth ventricle.

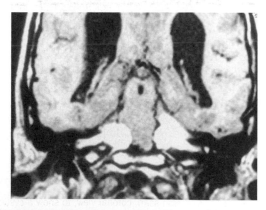

Figure 9.11 MRI brain scan, coronal view, with contrast, to show bilateral acoustic neuromas in a patient with neurofibromatosis type 2.

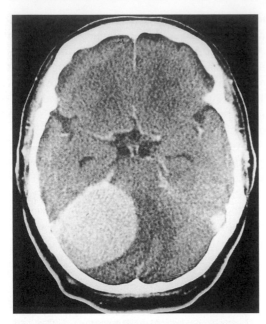

Figure 9.13 Enhanced CT brain scan to show a large posterior fossa meningioma.

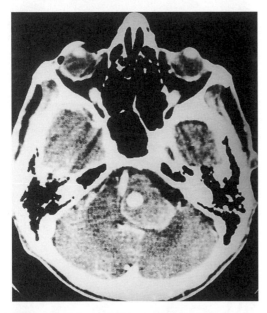

Figure 9.14 Enhanced CT brain scan showing a very large aneurysm arising from the basilar artery. This was compressing the fourth ventricle and presented as a posterior fossa mass.

Chordoma

Chordoma is a brain tumour arising from noto-chordal remnants and so can occur either in the sacrococcygeal region or in the clivus. At the skull base, such tumours can present with local impinge-ment on cranial nerves or with brainstem dysfunction. Such tumours are slow growing and so CSF obstruction and raised ICP tend to occur only very late. Scanning with CT, and sometimes plain x-ray, often show bone destruction in the skull base. The lesion will usually be defined in more detail by MRI. Subtotal removal is sometimes possible, often via the transoral route, but complete curative removal is very seldom possible.

Infection

Abscess

The two most common forms of intracranial abscess are intracerebral and subdural (empyema). Extradural abscess is rare, although it occurs particularly in association with skull osteomyelitis. Infection spreads locally, for example from a chronic ear infection or air sinus disease, or it may be blood-borne from chronic suppuration elsewhere, for example bronchiectasis or dental abscess. Subacute bacterial endocarditis may also lead to septic emboli and thus to brain abscess. Brain abscesses are more common in patients with immune compromise or in those who misuse intravenous drugs; these factors should be considered.

Any bacteria can produce abscess, because the brain is an immune privileged site, and so even low virulence organisms can establish an abscess. Sometimes even fungi or toxoplasma can be responsible, particularly in patients with AIDS.

A cerebral abscess produces an intracranial mass and so can present in any of the ways tumours present (Figures 9.15 and 9.16). In addition, cerebral abscesses often produce a florid reactive oedema and so tend to be an even more potent cause of raised ICP. The rapidity of onset may mean that papilloedema has not yet developed and so the clinical pitfall is to suspect meningitis and erroneously perform a lumbar puncture, exacerbating brain shift and causing clinical deterioration.

The symptoms and signs are generally those of raised ICP with the possible addition of focal neurological effects as a result of mass effect. In general, the patient appears very ill and there are signs of infection (pyrexia, raised inflammatory markers), although clinicians should be aware that abscesses can be well 'walled-off', and the patient may therefore appear misleadingly well.

The basis of treatment is drainage of any large

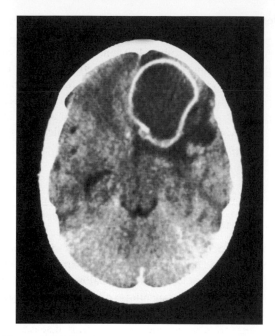

Figure 9.15 Very large ring enhancing left frontal abscess with considerable surrounding oedema (CT brain scan, axial view).

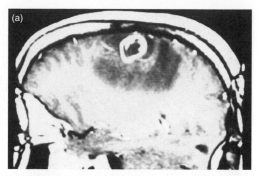

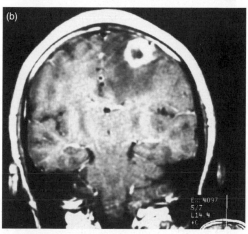

Figure 9.16 T1-weighted MRI brain scan: (a) sagittal and (b) coronal views, to show an abscess with surrounding oedema (gadolinium-enhanced scan).

abscesses (to establish the microbiological diagnosis and to decrease the bacterial load) and then prolonged antibiotic therapy with serial scanning to ensure that the abscess has fully resolved before the relevant antibiotics are discontinued. Epilepsy is a common complication.

Parasitic cysts

Parasitic cysts are most commonly caused either by hydatid disease or cysticercosis.

Hydatid disease is the result of infection by *Echinococcus granulosus* and generally occurs in rural regions where sheep are common as intermediate hosts. Treatment of the cyst is by careful removal, avoiding spillage of the contents and then appropriate chemotherapy: praziquantel or albendazole have proved most useful.

Cysticercosis is caused by larvae from the pork tapeworm *Taenia solium* and may produce multiple encysted lesions. These often occur in the muscles, and x-ray of the thighs may reveal multiple calcified lesions. The most common presentation of cerebral cysticercosis is with epilepsy, but cysts may also produce mass effect or block CSF pathways, leading to obstructive hydrocephalus. Diagnosis

can often be made on specific serological tests, or good quality MRI may reveal the diagnostic appearance of the cysts (Figure 9.17). Treatment generally includes anticonvulsants and a course of specific chemotherapy with drugs, such as albendazole or praziquantel with steroid cover (because treatment often exacerbates the tissue oedema as the cysts begin to necrose). The associated hydrocephalus may require treatment by removal of the obstructive cyst or a CSF shunting procedure.

Idiopathic intracranial hypertension

Idiopathic intracranial hypertension is of uncertain aetiology but is most frequent in young, overweight females. This led to the hypothesis that the cause is endocrine, and certainly there appears to be an association with the oral contraceptive pill and with endocrine diseases supporting this link (Box 9.3).

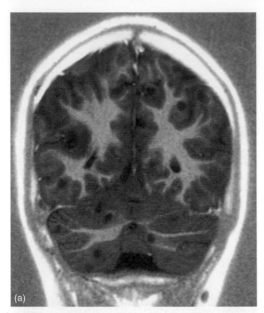

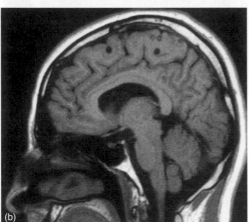

Figure 9.17 MRI brain scan: (a) coronal and (b) sagittal views, to show multiple low intensity lesions caused by cysticercosis.

Box 9.3 Causes of idiopathic intracranial hypertension

Obesity
Endocrine – amenorrhoea, Cushing's disease, hypoparathyroidism
Oral contraceptive pill
Drugs – tetracycline, minocycline, excess vitamin A, nitrofurantoin, amiodarone, lithium, retinoids, nalidixic acid, cimetidine, tamoxifen, steroid withdrawal
Severe anaemia
Always exclude venous sinus thrombosis secondary to infection, pregnancy, the oral contraceptive pill
Maximal incidence is in young overweight women, when the figure is 19:100 000 against 1:100 000 of the general population

However, the condition may not be 'benign' because if the raised ICP is allowed to continue there can be progressive visual loss and, ultimately, optic atrophy. Obscurations indicate critical optic nerve pressure relationships and may herald infarction of the optic nerve, so calls for emergency management.

The basis of treatment is therefore control of headache and careful monitoring of visual acuity and fields. Any possible causative drug should be withdrawn (oral contraceptive pill, tetracycline, nitrofurantoin, excess vitamin A supplementation) and other possible causes excluded (pregnancy, venous sinus thrombosis, intracranial mass). Overweight patients should be encouraged to lose weight.

Presentation is usually with headache, generally with the characteristics of raised ICP and often with florid papilloedema and visual obscurations. MRI may show dilatation of the optic nerve sheaths and an empty sella.

This condition rarely leads to brain shift, focal deficit, cognitive decline or decreased conscious level, hence the former label 'benign'.

Investigations should include imaging to exclude a mass lesion or venous sinus thrombosis, and CSF examination to exclude any meningitic process and to confirm the raised pressure (>250 mm).

Whereas lumbar puncture is necessary to establish the diagnosis, and may immediately relieve pressure, its effects are transient so repeated puncture is only of use to immediately reduce pressure and when the disease is self-limiting. However, if conservative measures fail or if the vision is threatened, surgical intervention must be considered. This may involve either optic nerve fenestration, which protects the optic nerve but does not improve headache, or lumboperitoneal CSF shunting.

Further treatment can be considered with aceta-zolamide (mildly effective), diuretics, or corticoster-oids (although use of the last is often limited by the side-effects and subsequent withdrawal can worsen the situation).

Venous sinus thrombosis

Obstruction of any of the intracranial venous sinuses can lead to impaired venous drainage with subsequent raised ICP and even areas of venous infarction. This can be the result of an underlying thrombotic tendency, dehydration or may be idio-pathic. It can often be diagnosed on CT imaging (producing the 'empty delta' sign on a contrast CT: the sagittal sinus in section may show contrast around its edges, but the central part of the lumen does not receive contrast, because it is obstructed by thrombus) or, more easily, on MRI. Treatment involves the correction of any underlying cause and anticoagulation.

INTRACRANIAL PRESSURE MONITORING

Standard ICP monitoring is an invasive proce-dure, usually performed by passing a monitoring catheter via a hollow bolt through the skull into either the ventricle or the brain parenchyma. There are non-invasive ways of monitoring ICP: indi-rect techniques, such as measuring the displace-ment characteristics of the tympanic membrane in response to an externally applied pressure wave, or ultrasound visualization of changes in diameter of the arachnoid sheath around the optic nerve. These non-invasive methods are, however, less well-established and more difficult to calibrate.

In common with all invasive monitoring tech-niques used in clinical medicine, use is limited by the inherent risks of insertion, as well as the risks of infection. Therefore, in practical terms, ICP moni-toring is generally used for single-event causes of raised ICP (of which head injury is by far the most frequent) that are evolving and are expected to resolve in the short term. It also tends not to be used in circumstances where clinical observation can adequately highlight any deterioration: stable, unsedated patients with a Glasgow coma score >8.

ICP monitoring is now widely established as a standard in the intensive care of severe head injury, but would not typically be used for monitoring raised ICP caused by the presence of a tumour. An exception would be, for example, where a patient is being electively ventilated overnight following surgery. In that circumstance, clinical signs in a sedated, ventilated patient tend to be very late indications of raised ICP (pupil changes, changes in pulse and blood pressure) and so short-term ICP monitoring is a useful clinical tool.

Another special circumstance is the occasional application to patients with complex shunt prob-lems, where a period of ICP monitoring can elucidate whether symptoms (typically headache) are related to changes in ICP, even if the changes are transient or related to posture.

TREATMENT OF RAISED ICP

Apart from the specifics discussed above, the gen-eral principles of treatment include the following.

Removing or directly treating the causative lesion

The most obvious examples would be removal of the haematoma in a patient with head trauma or removal of an intracranial tumour. In severe head injury, sometimes there is a decision to remove a contused area of brain to decompress the remain-ing 'healthy' brain. **More controversially, the bone flap can be removed to allow further space for brain expansion (i.e. changing the situation from a closed box to an open one).** Although sometimes this appears helpful, there is also the danger that the cortical vessels can be included at the edge of the exposed area, leading to an area of infarction and further swelling. Further trials will be necessary to ascertain whether there is any overall benefit to the patient, though in ischamic stroke producing a malignant MCA syndrome, decompression for selected patients has a very significant benefit.

Treating oedema

The treatment of oedema depends on its causa-tion. **Cytotoxic oedema (cellular swelling)** is the most common form associated with head injury and is generally thought unresponsive to steroids.

Therefore, treatment involves measures to ensure continued cerebral perfusion to support metabolic demands until the oedema subsides. **Vasogenic oedema**, on the other hand is the type most commonly associated with tumours and is often responsive to steroids. Typically, dexamethasone 4 mg q.d.s is used in the short term to relieve peri-tumoural oedema, pending definitive surgical treatment. Such high doses cannot usually be sustained in the long term without encountering unacceptable side-effects.

Manipulating physiological parameters

In the intensive care environment, ICP can be treated by sedation and neuromuscular paralysis. To some extent, ICP can also be reduced by reducing temperature and PCO_2. The scope for such manipulation is, however, very limited and usually takes the form of avoiding unhelpful elevation of the above parameters: PCO_2 is generally maintained in the region of 4.0–4.5 kPa (i.e. low physiological range) and pyrexia is treated (active hypothermia is much more controversial and may even be harmful).

Infusion with hypo-osmotic fluids is avoided, because it may exacerbate oedema. Again, active dehydration may be counterproductive because blood pressure (BP) may fall, leading to worsening of cerebral perfusion. However, it is less controversial to say that an excessively positive fluid balance should be avoided.

Mannitol, an osmotic diuretic, is sometimes used for acute treatment of life-threatening raised ICP. Its use, however, is now much more limited than previously, since it has been realized that the fluid shifts, which are helpful in the short term, inevitably lead to 'rebound' within several hours, and furthermore the associated diuresis can produce cardiovascular instability, which is even more difficult to manage. Therefore, it is now generally restricted to a single dose to 'buy time' until a definitive procedure (such as surgery to remove a haematoma) can be performed and only in life-threatening situations. Primary teams in emergency departments are not encouraged to use mannitol routinely but to reserve its use until after the case has been discussed with the appropriate neurosurgical centre and the relative risks assessed.

Draining CSF

If actual hydrocephalus exists, then CSF drainage is obviously helpful. However, in severe head injury even small amounts of remaining CSF can sometimes be drained to therapeutic advantage, if other medical means have been exhausted.

Posture

From basic principles, it should be remembered that simple elevation of the head can reduce ICP. However, the effective BP in the carotid arteries is also reduced by head elevation. Most units agree that moderate elevation (20–30 degrees) appears to be the best compromise.

Controversies in management

Considerable controversies remain in the acute treatment of raised ICP. In particular, some clinicians believe that CPP should be maintained at all costs, whereas others believe that excessive pharmacological elevation of the BP can be counterproductive, by exacerbating cerebral oedema. Certainly, it has been shown that aiming for a CPP over 70 mmHg can lead to adult respiratory distress syndrome. Current practice is therefore to aim for a CPP in the 60–70 mmHg range.

REFERENCES AND FURTHER READING

Bret P, Guyotat J, Chazal J (2002) Is normal hydrocephalus a valid concept in 2002? A reappraisal in five questions and proposal for a new designation of the syndrome as 'chronic hydrocephalus'. *Journal of Neurology, Neurosurgery and Psychiatry*, **73**:9–12.

Forsyth PA, Posner JB (1993) Headaches in patients with brain tumours: a study of 111 patients. *Neurology*, **43**:1678–1683.

McAllister LD, Ward JH, Schulman SF, DeAngelis LM (2002) *Practical Neuro-Oncology*. Boston, MA: Butterworth-Heinemann.

Pilchard JD, Czosnyka M (1993) Management of raised intracranial pressure. *Journal of Neurology, Neurosurgery and Psychiatry*, **56**:845–858.

Shakir RA, Newman PK, Posner CM (1996) *Tropical Neurology*. London: WB Saunders.

Whittle IR (1996) Management of primary malignant brain tumours. *Journal of Neurology, Neurosurgery and Psychiatry*, **60**:2–5.

Wright A, Bradford R (1995) Management of acoustic neuroma. *British Medical Journal*, **311**:1141–1145.

HEADACHE

Peter Goadsby

Headache is among the most common of neurological problems, representing between one-fifth to one-third of new presentations in outpatient clinics. This chapter will outline aspects of the key disorders, and readers are referred to larger texts for more complete accounts (Lance and Goadsby, 2005; Lipton and Bigal, 2006; Olesen *et al.*, 2005).

GENERAL PRINCIPLES

There are many types of headache, and accurate diagnosis is the key to proper management. The general concept is one of primary and secondary forms of headache, following the generic medical principle that clinical syndromes may be caused by something exogenous, secondary, or may present *de novo* as the primary disease process. Such a system is outlined in Table 10.1. The International Headache Society has developed a diagnostic system with operational definitions for most headache disorders, and this chapter will largely use those current conventions.

Broadly, primary headaches are those in which headache and its associated features are the disease in themselves - **primary headaches** and **secondary headaches** are those caused exogenously, such as headache associated with fever. Mild secondary headache, such as that seen in association with upper respiratory tract infections, is common but only rarely worrisome. The clinical dilemma remains that while life-threatening headache is relatively uncommon in western society, it nevertheless does present and requires appropriate vigilance by doctors. Primary headache, in contrast, often confers considerable disability over time and while not life-threatening certainly robs patients of quality of life. Primary headache is far more common in neurological practice than secondary headache.

SECONDARY HEADACHE

It is imperative to establish in the patient presenting with any form of head pain whether there is an important secondary headache declaring itself. Perhaps the most crucial clinical feature to elicit is the length of the history. Patients with a

Table 10.1 Common causes of headache[a]

Primary headache type	Prevalence (%)	Secondary headache type	Prevalence (%)
Migraine	16	Systemic infection	63
Tension-type	69	Head injury	4
Cluster headache	0.1	Subarachnoid haemorrhage	<1
Idiopathic stabbing	2	Vascular disorders	1
Exertional	1	Brain tumour	0.1

[a]Reproduced from Olesen *et al.* (2005) with permission from Lippincott, Williams and Wilkins.

short history require prompt attention and may require immediate investigation and management. Patients with a longer history generally require time and patience rather than alacrity. There are some important general features, including associated fever or sudden onset of pain (Box 10.1); these demand attention. Patients with a history of recent onset headache or neurological signs need a positive diagnosis that is benign or brain imaging with either computed tomography (CT) or magnetic resonance imaging (MRI). Conditions of particular concern, such as subarachnoid bleeds or arterial dissection, are dealt with elsewhere (Chapter 23). Patients with a history of recurrent headache over a period of one year or more, fulfilling International Headache Society criteria for migraine (Table 10.2) and with a normal physical examination, have positive brain imaging in only about 1/1000 images. In general, it should be noted that brain tumour is a rare cause relative to other causes of headache, and rarely a cause of an isolated long-term history of headache. A notable exception may be pituitary tumours presenting with headache, and is of particular concern in the differential diagnosis of trigeminal autonomic cephalalgias (discussed later in this chapter).

Box 10.1 Warning signs in head pain

- Sudden onset pain
- Fever
- Marked change in pain character or timing
- Neck stiffness
- Pain associated with higher centre complaints
- Pain associated with neurological disturbance, such as clumsiness or weakness
- Pain associated with local tenderness, such as of the temporal artery.

Table 10.2 Simplified diagnostic criteria for migraine adapted from the International Headache Society Classification (2004)

Repeated attacks of headache lasting 4–72 hours that have these features, normal physical examination and no other reasonable cause for the headache

At least 2 of:	At least 1 of:
Unilateral pain	Nausea/vomiting
Throbbing pain	Photophobia and
Aggravation by movement	phonophobia
Moderate or severe intensity	

The management of secondary headache is generally self-evident: treatment of the underlying condition, such as an infection or mass lesion. An exception is the condition of chronic post-traumatic headache in which pain may persist for long periods after head injury. This is an interesting generic problem that may also be seen after central nervous system infection, trauma, both blunt and surgical, intracranial bleeds and other precipitants. While the syndrome is generally self-limiting, at intervals up to 3–5 years after the event, treatment of the headache may be required if it is disabling (see below under Chronic daily headache).

PRIMARY HEADACHE SYNDROMES

Anatomy and physiology of headache

The disabling primary headaches, migraine and the TACs, have been studied extensively in recent times

The primary headaches comprise a group of disorders in which headache and associated features are seen in the absence of any exogenous cause. The common syndromes (Table 10.1) are tension-type headache, migraine and the trigeminal autonomic cephalalgias (TACs), such as cluster headache. The collection of headaches known as primary chronic daily headache form the greatest part of the neurologist's case-load. Some other less well-known, but rarer, syndromes will be mentioned because they are easily treated when recognized.

and they are now relatively well understood insofar as neurological diseases that involve the brain are concerned. In experimental animals, the detailed anatomy of the connections of the pain-producing intracranial extracerebral vessels and the dura mater has built on the classical human observations of Wolff and others. These structures, and not the brain, are responsible for generating pain from within the head.

The key structures involved in the nociceptive process are:
- the large intracranial vessels and dura mater;
- the peripheral terminals of the trigeminal nerve that innervate these structures;
- the central terminals and second order neurons of the caudal trigeminal nucleus and dorsal horns of C_1 and C_2, trigeminocervical complex.

The innervation of the large intracranial vessels and dura mater by the trigeminal nerve is known as the **trigeminovascular system**. The cranial parasympathetic autonomic innervation provides the basis for symptoms, such as lacrimation and nasal stuffiness, which are prominent in cluster headache and paroxysmal hemicrania, although they may also be seen in migraine. It is clear from human functional imaging studies that vascular changes in migraine and cluster headache are driven by these neural vasodilator systems so that these headaches should be regarded as **neurovascular**. The concept of a primary **vascular** headache should be consigned to the dustbin of history since it neither explains the pathogenesis of what are complex central nervous system disorders, nor does it necessarily predict treatment outcomes. The term **vascular** headache has no place in modern neurological practice when referring to primary headache since what is usually meant is migrainous by the adjective vascular. So it is best to refer to headache as being migrainous if indeed that is the syndrome being considered.

Migraine is an episodic syndrome of headache with sensory sensitivity, to light, sound and head movement, probably due to dysfunction of aminergic brainstem/diencephalic sensory control systems (Figure 10.1). The first of the migraine genes has been identified for familial hemiplegic migraine, in which about 50 per cent of families have mutations in the gene for the $Ca_V2.1$ (α_{1A}) subunit of the neuronal P/Q voltage-gated calcium channel. Other genes identified include those for a Na-K-ATPase and for a sodium channel mutation. These findings and the clinical features of migraine suggest it, or at least the aura features, might be part of the spectrum of diseases known as channelopathies, disorders involving dysfunction of voltage-gated channels. Functional neuroimaging has suggested that brain stem regions in migraine (Plate 3), and the posterior hypothalamic grey matter site of the human circadian pacemaker cells of the suprachiasmatic nucleus, in the TACs (Plate 4), are good candidates for specific involvement in primary headache.

MIGRAINE

Migraine is generally an episodic headache with certain associated features, such as sensitivity to light, sound or movement, and often with nausea or vomiting accompanying the headache (Table 10.2). None of the features is compulsory, and indeed given that the migraine aura, visual disturbances with flashing lights or zig-zag lines moving across the fields or other neurological symptoms is reported in only about 20 per cent of patients, a high index of suspicion is required to make a diagnosis of migraine.

A headache diary can often be helpful in making the diagnosis, although in reality usually helps more in assessing disability or recording how often patients use acute attack treatments.

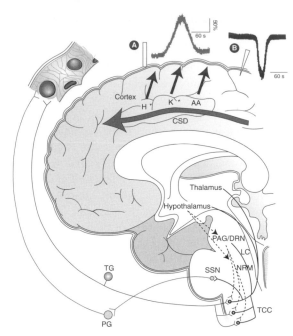

Figure 10.1 Pathophysiology of migraine. Migraine involves dysfunction of brainstem pathways that normally modulate sensory input (Goadsby et al., 2002), while aura is produced by a response almost certainly similar to the experimental changes described as cortical spreading depression (CSD). The key pathways for the pain are the trigeminovascular input from the meningeal vessels, which passes through the trigeminal ganglion (TG) and synapses on second order neurons in the trigeminocervical complex (TCC). These neurons in turn project in the quintothalamic tract, and after decussating in the brainstem, synapse on neurons in the thalamus. There is a reflex connection with neurons in the pons in the superior salivatory nucleus (SSN), which provides an efferent cranial parasympathetic outflow synapsing in the main in the pterygopalatine (PG). This trigeminal-autonomic reflex is present in normal subjects and expressed most notably in patients with trigeminal-autonomic cephalalgias, such as cluster headache and paroxysmal hemicrania; it may be active in migraine. Important modulation of the trigeminovascular nociceptive input, as suggested from brain imaging studies, comes from the hypothalamus, periadqueductal grey matter/dorsal raphe nucleus (PAG/DRN), locus coeruleus (LC) and nucleus raphe magnus (NRM). These projections are both direct and indirect with a remarkable interplay between the structures, CSD involves a passage of a way of depolarization followed by hyperpolarization that moves the cortex and has both blood flow (A) and electrophysiological (B) manifestations and is associated with changes in H+, K+ and amino acids (AA). The extent to which and mechanisms by which aura/CSD may trigger pain are hotly debated. (Image modified after original courtesy Dr Philip Holland.)

In differentiating the two main primary headache syndromes seen in clinical practice, migraine at its most simple level is headache with associated features, and tension-type headache is headache that is featureless, furthermore most disabling headache presenting to doctors is probably migrainous in biology.

The important emphasis here is the biology underlying the problem, not simply its phenotype; this is an important issue when daily headache is considered below.

If headache with associated features describes migraine attacks, then **headachy** describes the migraine sufferer over their life-time. The migraine sufferer inherits a tendency to have headache that is amplified at various times by their interaction with their environment, the much-discussed triggers. The brain of the migraineur seems more sensitive to sensory stimuli and to change; and this tendency is even more amplified in women during their menstrual cycle. The migraine sufferer does not habituate to sensory stimuli easily and so attacks can be frequently stimulated in the world in which they live and work.

Migraine sufferers may have headache when they sleep in, when they are tired, when they skip meals, with weather change, when they are under stress or when they relax. They are less tolerant to change, and part of successful management is to advise them to maintain regularity in their lives, in the knowledge of this fluctuating biology. It is this biology that marks migraine and in clinical practice must over-ride the phenotype of individual headaches.

It has been said that migraine can never occur daily, but few biological issues respect absolute rules. The syndrome of chronic migraine is now well accepted, and is part of the group of headaches known as chronic daily headache (see below). These patients have the most severe end of a spectrum of complex biology, and often require expert management. After making a diagnosis, the second step in the clinical process is to be sure that the disease burden has been captured: how much headache does the patient have and more important, what can the patient not do; what is their degree of disability? One can ask the patient directly, examine a headache diary or get a quick but accurate estimate using the Migraine Disability Assessment Scale

(MIDAS), which is well-validated and very easy to use in practice (Figure 10.2).

Management

After diagnosis, the management of migraine begins with an explanation of some aspects of the disorder to the patient. It may be useful to explain:

- migraine is an inherited tendency to headache; this is caused by the patient's genes, therefore it cannot be cured but;
- migraine can be modified and controlled by life-style adjustment and the use of medicines;
- migraine is not life threatening nor associated with serious illness, with the exception of women who smoke and are taking oestrogenic oral contraceptives, but migraine can make life a misery;
- migraine management takes time and co-operation when, for example a headache diary has to be collected, or enquiry made concerning the disability.

Non-pharmacological management

Non-pharmacological management of migraine includes helping the patient identify things that make the problem worse and encourages them to modify these. Patient associations can be very helpful with pamphlets for this form of education, and those of the Migraine Trust and Migraine Action Association are recommended. Many patients will not find any joy in this approach and should not be pilloried for this. Patients need to know the brain sensitivity that underlies migraine varies, so that the effect of triggers will vary. This fact alone may remove considerable frustration on the patient's part, will ring true to most as they will have had the experience, and is biologically plausible, since it is exactly what one would predict from a generic channelopathic theory of migraine pathogenesis.

Preventive treatments

The decision to start a patient on a preventive drug requires crucial input from the migraineur. The patient needs to have come to terms with the biology: the fact that they have an inherited, non-curable but manageable problem, and that they have

INSTRUCTIONS: Please answer the following questions about ALL your headaches you have had over the last 3 months. Write your answer in the box next to each question. Write zero if you did not do the activity in the last 3 months

1. On how many days in the last 3 months did you miss work or school because of your headaches? . . . . ☐☐ days

2. How many days in the last 3 months was your productivity at work or school reduced by half or more because of your headaches (*Do not include days you counted in* question 1 *where you missed work of school*)? . . . . ☐☐ days

3. On how many days in the last 3 months did you not do household work because of your headaches? . . . . ☐☐ days

4. How many days in the last 3 months was your productivity in household work reduced by half or more because of your headaches (*Do not include days you counted in question 3 where you did not do household work*)? . . . . ☐☐ days

5. On how many days in the last 3 months did you miss family, social, or leisure activities because of your headaches? . . . . ☐☐ days

A. On how many days in the last 3 months did you have a headache? (If a headache lasted more than one day, count each day) . . . . ☐☐ days

B. On a scale of 0–10, on average how painful were these headaches? (*where* 0 = *no pain at all, and* 10 = *pain as bad as it can be*) . . . . ☐☐

Figure 10.2 MIDAS (migraine disability assessment score) questionnaire. © Innovative Medical Research, 1997

The crucial life-style advice is to explain to the patient that migraine is a state of brain sensitivity to change. This implies that migraine sufferers need to regulate their lives: healthy diet, regular exercise, regular sleep patterns, avoiding excess caffeine and alcohol and, as far as practical, modifying or minimizing changes in stress. The balanced life with fewer highs and lows will benefit most migraine sufferers.

sufficient disability to wish to take medicine. The doctor can explain the choices available and why one might be better than another. The basis of considering preventive treatment from a medical viewpoint is a combination of acute attack frequency and attack tractability. Attacks that are unresponsive to abortive medications are easily considered for prevention, while simply treated attacks may be less obviously candidates for prevention. The other part of the equation relates to what is happening with time. If a patient diary shows a clear trend of increasing frequency of attacks, it is better to commence early with prevention than wait for the attacks to become ever more frequent.

A simple rule for frequency might be that for one or two headaches a month there is usually no need to start a preventive, for three or four it may be needed but not necessarily, and for five or more a month prevention should definitely be on the agenda for discussion.

Options available for treatment are covered in detail in Table 10.3 and vary somewhat by country, even within the European Union. The main problem with preventives is that they have fallen into migraine from other indications, so there are options, which often have troublesome side effects. It is not clear how preventives work, although it seems likely that they modify the brain sensitivity that underlies migraine. Another key clinical point is that generally each drug should be started at a low dose and gradually increased to a reasonable maximum, monitoring the side effects and clinical effect as the dose escalates.

Acute attack therapies

Acute attack treatments for migraine can be usefully divided into disease non-specific treatments, analgesics and non-steroidal anti-inflammatory drugs (NSAIDs), and disease specific treatments, ergot-related compounds and triptans (Table 10.4). It must be said at the outset that most acute attack medications seem to have a propensity to aggravate headache frequency and can induce a state of refractory daily or near-daily headache, **Medication overuse headache** (see below). Codeine-containing compound analgesics are a particularly pernicious problem when available in over-the-counter (OTC) preparations. One should advise patients with migraine who have two headache days a week or more to avoid their regular use. Probably about one-third of patients who stop taking regular analgesics will have substantial improvement in their headache with a reduction in frequency or severity. The other two-thirds will have little or no change in their headache frequency, but will still feel in some way better, especially if they have been using codeine regularly. It is crucial to emphasize to the patient that standard preventive medications will, in the main, simply not work in the presence of regular analgesic use. It is often a waste of time to start a preventive in migraine patients if they are using regular analgesics; the analgesic problem must be tackled first (see below).

A useful clinical guide here is to determine how many preventive medicines have failed in the past and if there are more than three, and there was medication overuse of acute treatments, it is highly unlikely that progress will be made until the medication overuse problem has been addressed.

Treatment strategies

Given the array of options to control an acute attack of migraine, how does one start? The simplest approach has been described as 'stepped care'. In this model all patients are treated, assuming no contraindications, with the simplest treatment, such as **aspirin 900 mg or paracetamol (acetaminophen) 1000 mg with an anti-emetic**. Aspirin has been shown to be effective in double-blind controlled

Table 10.3 Preventive treatments in migraine[a]

Drug	Dose	Selected side effects
β-Blocker		
Propranolol	40–120 mg bd	Reduced energy
		Tiredness
		Postural symptoms
		Contraindicated in asthma
Metoprolol	25–100 mg twice daily	Reduced energy
		Tiredness
		Postural symptoms
		Contraindicated in asthma
Anticonvulsants		
Valproate	400–600 mg twice daily	Drowsiness
		Weight gain
		Tremor
		Hair loss
		Foetal abnormalities
		Haematological or liver abnormalities
Topiramate	50–200 mg/day	Paraesthesiae
		Cognitive dysfunction
		Weight loss
		Care with a family history of glaucoma
		Nephrolithiasis
Gabapentin[b]	900–3600 mg daily	Dizziness
		Sedation
Flunarizine	5–15 mg daily	Drowsiness
		Weight gain
		Depression
		Parkinsonism
Antidepressants		
Amitriptyline[c]		
Dosulepin (dothiepin)	25–75 mg nocte	Drowsiness, urinary retention, arrhythmias; note: some patients are very sensitive and may only need a total dose of 10 mg, although generally 1–1.5 mg/kg body weight is required
Nortriptyline		
Venlafaxine	75–150 mg daily	Drowsiness, urinary retention, arrhythmias
Serotonin antagonists		
Pizotifen	0.5–2 mg daily	Weight gain
		Drowsiness
Methysergide	1–6 mg daily	Drowsiness
		Leg cramps
		Hair loss
		Retroperitoneal fibrosis (one month drug holiday is required every 6 months)
Single studies[d]		
Lisinopril	20 mg daily	Cough
		Dizziness

Drug	Dose	Selected side effects
Candasartan	16 mg daily	
Neutriceuticals[d]		
Riboflavin	400 mg daily	
Coenzyme Q10	100 mg three times daily or 75 mg twice daily	GI upset
Butterbur	50–75 mg twice daily	Elevation of transaminases
Feverfew	6.25 mg three times daily	Skin rash
No convincing controlled evidence		
Verapamil		
Controlled trials to demonstrate no effect		
Nimodipine		
Clonidine		
SSRIs: fluoxetine		

Commonly used preventives are listed with reasonable doses and common side effects. The local national formulary should be consulted for detailed information.
[a]Compounds not widely considered mainstream but with a positive randomized control trial against placebo.
[b]More supported by experience as the single cited study did not achieve the primary endpoint on an intention-to-treat basis.
[c]A small study although a very widely used treatment.
[d]Non-pharmaceuticals with at least one positive randomized controlled trial against placebo.

Table 10.4 Oral acute migraine treatments

Non-specific treatments	Specific treatments
Often used with anti-emetic/prokinetics, such as:	
Domperidone (10 mg)	
Metaclopramide (10 mg)	
Promethazine (25 mg)	
Aspirin (900 mg)	**Ergot derivatives**
Paracetamol (acetaminophen) (1000 mg)	Ergotamine (1–2 mg)
NSAIDS	**Triptans**
Naproxen (500–1000 mg)	Sumatriptan (50 or 100 mg)
Ibuprofen (400–800 mg)	Naratriptan (2.5 mg)
Tolfenamic acid (200 mg)	Rizatriptan (10 mg)
	Zolmitriptan (2.5 or 5 mg)
	Eletriptan (40 or 80 mg)
	Almotriptan (12.5 mg)
	Frovatriptan (2.5 mg)

clinical trials, and is best used in its most soluble formulations. The alternative strategy is known as 'stratified care', by which the physician determines, or stratifies, treatment at the start, based on likelihood of response to levels of care. An intermediate option may be described as stratified care by attack.

The latter is what many headache authorities suggest and what patients often do when they have the options. Patients use simpler options for their less severe attacks, relying on more potent options when their attacks or circumstances demand them (Table 10.5).

Table 10.5 Clinical stratification of acute specific migraine treatments

Clinical situation	Treatment options
Failed analgesics/NSAIDS	First tier
	Sumatriptan 50 or 100 mg po
	Almotriptan 12.5 mg po
	Rizatriptan 10 mg po
	Eletriptan 40 mg po
	Zolmitriptan 2.5 mg po
	Slower effect/better tolerability
	Naratriptan 2.5 mg po
	Frovatriptan 2.5 mg po
	Infrequent headache
	Ergotamine 1–2 mg po
	Dihydroergotamine nasal spray 2 mg
Early nausea or difficulties taking tablets	Zolmitriptan 5 mg nasal spray
	Sumatriptan 20 mg nasal spray
	Rizatriptan 10 mg MLT wafer
Headache recurrence	Ergotamine 2 mg (most effective pr/usually with caffeine)
	Naratriptan 2.5 mg po
	Almotriptan 12.5 mg po
	Eletriptan 40 mg
Tolerating acute treatments poorly	Naratriptan 2.5 mg
	Almotriptan 12.5 mg
Early vomiting	Zolmitriptan 5 mg nasal spray
	Sumatriptan 25 mg pr
	Sumatriptan 6 mg sc
Menstrually related headache	Prevention
	Ergotamine po nocte
	Oestrogen patches
	Treatment
	Triptans
	Dihydroergotamine nasal spray
Very rapidly developing symptoms	Zolmitriptan 5 mg nasal spray
	Sumatriptan 6 mg sc
	Dihydroergotamine 1 mg im

Non-specific acute migraine attack treatments

Since simple things, such as aspirin and paracetamol, are cheap and can be very effective, they can be employed in many patients. Dosages should be adequate and the addition of **domperidone (10 mg orally), metaclopramide (10 mg orally) or promethazine (25 mg orally)** can be very helpful. NSAIDs can be very useful when tolerated. Their success is often limited by inappropriate dosing, and adequate doses of **naproxen (500–1000 mg orally or pr, with** an anti-emetic), ibuprofen (400–800 mg orally) or tolfenamic acid (200 mg orally)** can be extremely effective.

Specific acute migraine attack treatments

When simple measures fail or more aggressive treatment is required, specific treatments are required. While ergotamine remains a useful anti-migraine compound, it can no longer be considered the treatment of choice in acute migraine. There are particular situations in which ergotamine is very useful, but its use must be strictly controlled, as overuse can produce dreadful headache in addition to a host of vascular problems. The triptans have revolutionized the life of many patients with migraine and are clearly the most powerful option available to stop a migraine attack. They can be rationally applied by considering their pharmacological, physicochemical and pharmacokinetic features, as well as the formulations that are available (Table 10.5).

TENSION-TYPE HEADACHE

As its name suggests, tension-type headache (TTH) is a term that describes the headache form most seeking understanding. Consider for a moment how hard it is to study something that is commonly considered to be well understood, and ask yourself what is the essence of TTH? TTH is diagnosed commonly, and while the phenotype is common, much of the disabling headache that goes under the name TTH is likely to be chronic migraine in terms of its biology (see below under Chronic daily headache). TTH has two clear forms, episodic TTH, where attacks occur on less than 15 days a month and chronic TTH in which attacks, on average over time, occur on 15 days or more a month. A third form of frequent episodic TTH was added in the most recent edition of the International Classification of Headache Disorders, and its place in practice is yet to be clarified. Chronic TTH is part of the broader clinical syndrome of chronic daily headache (see below), but these terms are not one and the same.

Clinical features

TTH has been defined by the International Headache Society both for its episodic and chronic forms. The definition contains problematic admixtures of nausea, photophobia or phonophobia in various limited combinations, without clear biological rationale.

A more useful clinical approach is to diagnose TTH when the headache is completely featureless: no nausea, no vomiting, no photophobia, no phonophobia, no osmophobia, no throbbing and no aggravation with movement.

Such an approach neatly divides migraine, which has one of more of these features and is the main differential diagnosis, from TTH. For research, it is best to further divide up the patients with attacks of a TTH phenotype who have migraine at other times, a family history of migraine, migrainous illnesses of childhood, or typical migraine triggers to their attacks, to try and understand what the TTH biology alone imparts to the sufferer.

For clinical simplicity, TTH is headache without other features.

Pathophysiology

The pathophysiology of TTH is poorly understood. This results from the fact that the name implies it is a product of **nervous tension**, for which there is no clear evidence, and the definitions employed have undoubtedly admitted patients with migraine to research studies. Moreover, the concept that TTH in some way involves muscle contraction is spurious since the evidence is that muscle contraction is no more likely that it is in migraine. It seems likely that TTH will be due to a primary disorder of central nervous system pain modulation alone, to contrast it with migraine, which is a much more generalized disturbance of sensory modulation. There are data suggesting a genetic contribution to TTH, but one must question these since they applied the current unclear diagnostic criteria.

Management

Adopting the clinical approach to TTH outlined above results in diagnosing a headache form that is usually less disabling, and more in the category of irritating. Its episodic form is generally amenable to simple analgesics, paracetamol, aspirin, or NSAIDs, which can be purchased over the counter. There are clear clinical studies to demonstrate that triptans in TTH alone are not helpful, although germane to the above discussion, triptans are effective in TTH where the patient also has migraine. For chronic TTH, **amitriptyline** is the only treatment with a clear evidence base; the other tricylics, selective serotonin reuptake inhibitors (SSRI) or the benzodiazepines have been shown to be ineffective in controlled trials. Similarly, there is no controlled evidence for the use of electromyography (EMG) biofeedback, relaxation therapy or acupuncture. Botulinum toxin has been shown to be ineffective, while **stress management** has been shown to be an effective approach, in controlled trials.

TRIGEMINAL-AUTONOMIC CEPHALALGIAS: I CLUSTER HEADACHE

Cluster headache is a relatively rare form of primary headache with a population frequency of 0.1 per cent. It is about as common as multiple sclerosis in the UK, and must be regarded as a disorder best managed by neurologists. It is perhaps the most painful condition of humans; in the cohort of more than 1000 patients seen by the author, not a single one has had a more painful experience, including childbirth, multiple limb fractures and renal stones. It is one of a group of conditions known now as trigeminal-autonomic cephalalgias (TACs), and needs to be differentiated from other TACs and the short-lasting headaches without cranial autonomic symptoms, such as lacrimation or conjunctival injection (Table 10.6).

The core feature of cluster headache is periodicity, be it circadian or in terms of active and inactive bouts over weeks and months (Table 10.7). The typical patients with cluster headache are male (men to women 3:1), with one or two attacks of relatively short duration unilateral pain every day in bouts totalling 8–10 weeks a year. They are

Table 10.6 Primary headache – cluster headache, other TACs and short-lasting headaches

Trigeminal autonomic cephalalgias (TACs)	Other short-lasting headaches
Cluster headache	Primary stabbing headache[b]
Paroxysmal hemicrania	Trigeminal neuralgia
SUNCT[a]/SUNA[b] syndrome	Benign cough headache
Hemicrania continua	Primary exertional headache
	Primary sex headache
	Hypnic headache

[a]Short-lasting unilateral neuralgiform headache attacks with conjunctival injection and tearing.
[b]Cranial autonomic features.

Table 10.7 Simplified diagnostic criteria for cluster headache (after ICHD-II (2004))

> Cluster headache has two key forms-
>
> **Episodic**: Occurs in periods lasting 7 days to one year separated by pain-free periods lasting one month
>
> **Chronic**: Attacks occur for more than one year without remission or with remissions lasting less than one month
>
> Diagnostic criteria for attacks:
>
> A. At least five attacks fulfilling B–D.
> B. Severe or very severe unilateral orbital, supraorbital and/or temporal pain lasting 15 to 180 minutes untreated.
> C. Headache is accompanied by at least one of the following signs that have to be present on the side of the pain:
>   1. Conjunctival injection
>   2. Lacrimation
>   3. Nasal congestion
>   4. Rhinorrhoea
>   5. Forehead and facial sweating
>   6. Miosis
>   7. Ptosis
>   8. Eyelid oedema
>   or
>   Headache is associated with a sense of restlessness or agitation.
> D. Frequency of attacks: from one every other day to eight per day.

generally completely well between bouts. Patients with cluster headache tend to move about during attacks, pacing, rocking or even rubbing their head for relief. The pain is usually retro-orbital, boring and very severe. It is associated with ipsilateral symptoms of cranial (parasympathetic) autonomic activation: a red or watering eye, the nose running or blocking, or cranial sympathetic dysfunction (Horner's syndrome). Cluster headache is likely to be a disorder involving central pace-maker regions of the posterior hypothalamus (Plate 4).

The TACs – cluster headache, paroxysmal hemicrania and short-lasting unilateral neuralgiform headache attacks with conjuntival injection and tearing (SUNCT) syndrome – present a distinct group to be differentiated from short-lasting headaches that do not have prominent cranial autonomic features, notably trigeminal neuralgia, idiopathic (primary) stabbing headache and hypnic headache. By determining the cycling pattern, length, frequency and timing of the attacks, most patients can be classified. The importance of clinical classification of this group is three-fold. First, the clinical phenotype determines the likely secondary causes that must be considered and prompt appropriate investigations. In general terms for TAC presentations, a minimum is to exclude underlying pituitary pathology. Second, the appropriate classification gives clarity to the patient about the diagnosis and allows the physician to draw on available literature to advise on natural history. Third, the correct diagnosis determines the correct therapy, which can be very different in these conditions, being highly effective if the diagnosis is correct but ineffective if it is not (Table 10.8).

Management

Cluster headache is managed using acute attack treatments and preventive agents. Acute attack treatments are usually required by all cluster headache patients at some time, while preventives can almost be life-saving for the patients with chronic cluster headache, and are often needed to shorten the active periods in patients with the episodic form of the disorder.

Preventive treatments

The options for preventive treatment in cluster headache depend on the bout length (Table 10.9). Patients with short bouts require drugs that act quickly but will not necessarily be taken for long periods, whereas those with long bouts or indeed those with chronic cluster headache require safe, effective drugs that can be taken often for long periods. Most experts would now favour **verapamil** as the first-line preventive treatment when the bout is prolonged, or in chronic cluster headache, whereas limited courses of oral **corticosteroids** or **methysergide** can be very useful strategies when the bout is relatively short.

Verapamil has been suggested as a useful option for the last decade and compares favourably with lithium. What has clearly emerged from clinical practice is the need to use higher doses than had initially been considered, and certainly higher than those used for cardiological indications. Although most patients will start on doses as low as 40–80 mg twice daily, doses up to 960 mg daily and greater are now used.

Adverse effects, such as constipation and leg swelling can be a problem, but more difficult is the issue of **cardiovascular safety**. Verapamil can cause heart block by slowing conduction in the atrioventricular node as demonstrated by prolongation of the A-H interval. Given that the PR interval on the ECG is made up of atrial conduction, A-H and His

Table 10.8 Differential diagnosis of short-lasting headaches

Feature	Cluster headache	Paroxysmal hemicrania	SUNCT	Primary stabbing headache	Trigeminal neuralgia	Hypnic Headache
Gender	M>F 3:1	F=M	M=F	F>M	F>M	M=F
Pain						
Type	Boring	Boring	Stabbing	Stabbing	Stabbing	Throbbing
Severity	Very severe	Very severe	Moderate/ severe	Severe	Very severe	Moderate
Location	Orbital/temporal	Orbital/temporal	Orbital	Any	V2/V3>V1	Generalized
Duration	15–180 min	2–30 min	5–240 s	Secs–3 min	<5 s	15–30 mins
Frequency	1–8 per day	1–40 per day	1/d–30/hr	Any	Any	1–3/night
Autonomic	+	+	+	–	–	–
Alcohol	+	–	–	–	–	–
Indomethacin	–	+	–	+	–	?

SUNCT, short-lasting neuralgiform headache attacks with conjunctival injection and tearing.

Table 10.9 Preventive management of cluster headache

Short-term prevention	Long-term prevention
Episodic cluster headache	Episodic cluster headache and prolonged chronic cluster headache
Greater occipital nerve injection	Verapamil
Prednisolone	Lithium
Methysergide	Methysergide
Daily (nocturnal) ergotamine	Melatonin
Verapamil	?Topiramate
	?Gabapentin

? = unproven but promising.

bundle conduction, it may be difficult to monitor subtle early effects as verapamil dose is increased. This question needs study in this group of patients, but for the moment it seems appropriate to do a baseline ECG and then repeat the ECG 10 days after each dose change, usually in 80 mg increments, when doses exceed 240 mg daily. It is clear that the cardiac slowing effect can occur even with a stable high dose of verapamil, so that checking the PR interval every six months while on therapy is essential.

Acute attack treatment

Cluster headache attacks often peak rapidly and thus require a treatment with quick onset. Many patients with acute cluster headache respond well to treatment with **oxygen inhalation**. This should be given as 100 per cent oxygen at 10–15 L/min for 15–20 minutes. It is important to have a high flow and high oxygen content. **Injectable sumatriptan 6 mg** has been a boon for many patients with cluster headache. It is effective, rapid in onset and with no evidence of tachyphylaxis. **Sumatriptan 20 mg or Zolmitriptan 5 mg nasal sprays** are effective in acute cluster headache, and offer useful options for patients who may not wish to self-inject daily. Sumatriptan is not effective when given pre-emptively as 100 mg orally three times daily, and there is no evidence that it is useful when used orally in the acute treatment of cluster headache.

Medically intractable chronic cluster headache

In recent years, **neuromodulation** approaches to this group of highly disabled patients have been devised. The functional imaging finding of thalamic change in patients with chronic migraine treated with occipital nerve stimulation (ONS) led to its study in cluster headache. Initial open-label experience suggests that two-thirds of otherwise medically-intractable patients will have substantial improvement with ONS. Similarly, functional imaging changes in cluster headache (Figure 10.3) led to trials of deep brain stimulation that have also seen up to three-quarters of otherwise intractable sufferers respond. Neuromodulation is an area of active research for the treatment of medically refractory cluster headache.

TRIGEMINAL-AUTONOMIC CEPHALGIAS: II PAROXYSMAL HEMICRANIA

Eight patients were reported with frequent unilateral severe but short-lasting headache without remission, coining the term **chronic paroxysmal hemicrania (CPH)**. A large personal series of 31 cases demonstrated a mean duration of attack of 17 and a daily attack frequency of 11. By analogy with cluster headache, the patients with remission have been referred to as **episodic paroxysmal hemicrania**, about 20 per cent of our series, and those with the non-remitting form **chronic paroxysmal hemicrania**. The overall syndrome can be simply called **paroxysmal hemicrania**.

The essential features of paroxysmal hemicrania are (Table 10.8):
- short-lasting attacks averaging about 20 minutes;
- very frequent attacks typically ten or more per day;
- marked cranial autonomic features ipsilateral to the pain;
- robust, quick (less than 72 hour), excellent response to indometacin.

Treatment of paroxysmal hemicrania (PH) is complicated by gastrointestinal side effects seen

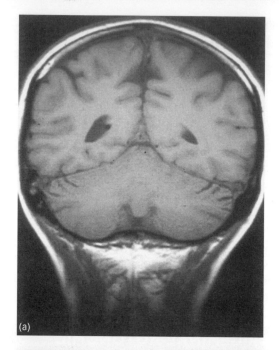

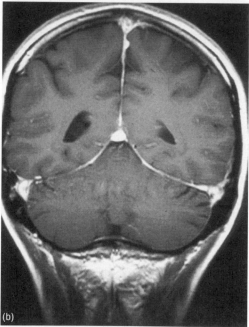

Figure 10.3 Magnetic resonance image showing MRI brain (a) and diffuse meningeal enhancement after gadolinium administration in a patient with low CSF volume (pressure) headache (b).

ache, verapamil has been used in PH, although the response is not spectacular; higher doses require exploration. We have seen **topiramate** be very helpful. PH can coexist with trigeminal neuralgia, PH-tic syndrome, just as in cluster-tic syndrome, and each component requires separate treatment. Secondary PH has been reported with lesions in the region of the sella turcica, an arteriovenous malformation, cavernous sinus meningioma and a parotid epidermoid. Secondary PH is more likely if the patient requires high doses (>200 mg/day) of indometacin. Raised cerebrospinal fluid (CSF) pressure should be suspected in apparent bilateral PH. It is worth noting that indometacin reduces CSF pressure by an unknown mechanism. It is appropriate to image patients with MRI when a diagnosis of PH is being considered, looking particularly for pituitary gland changes, and to carry out tests of pituitary function.

TRIGEMINAL-AUTONOMIC CEPHALALGIAS: III SUNCT/ SUNA

Short-lasting unilateral neuralgiform headache attacks with conjunctival injection and tearing/cranial autonomic features

In 1978, three male patients were reported whose brief attacks of pain in and around one eye were associated with sudden conjunctival injection and other autonomic features of cluster headache. The attacks lasted only 15–60 seconds and recurred 5–30 times per hour, and could be precipitated by chewing or eating certain foods, such as citrus fruits. They were not abolished by indometacin.

The paroxysms of pain in SUNCT usually last between 5 and 250 seconds, although longer duller interictal pains are recognized as have longer attacks. The conjunctival injection seen with SUNCT is often the most prominent autonomic feature and tearing may be very obvious. When both features are not present, the term **SUNA** has been proposed. SUNCT is difficult to treat, although in a large case series two-thirds of patients responded to lamotrigine and almost all patients respond acutely to intravenous lidocaine.

with **indometacin**, although thus far there is no reliably effective alternative. Piroxicam has been suggested to be helpful, although not as effective as indometacin. By analogy with cluster head-

The essential features of SUNCT/SUNA are:
- short-lasting attacks of pain typically lasting seconds;
- triggering of pain by cutaneous stimuli, such as touching, chewing or the wind;
- no refractory period to pain triggering when present;
- prominent cranial autonomic features.

Secondary SUNCT/SUNA and associations

The literature reports a number of patients with secondary SUNCT syndromes that underline the need for adequate cranial imaging in these patients. While pituitary pathology is the most commonly reported associated with SUNCT/SUNA, homolateral cerebellopontine angle arteriovenous malformations, cavernous hemangioma of the brainstem seen and structural deformity involving the posterior fossa, including osteogenesis imperfecta and craneosynostosis, have presented as SUNCT-like syndromes. Cases with both SUNCT and trigeminal neuralgia have been reported. Given that the attacks are short, this can be a challenging clinical problem. The differential diagnosis turns around the degree of cranial autonomic activation, which may be seen to some degree in trigeminal neuralgia, but is very prominent in SUNCT and the lack of a refractory period to pain triggering in SUNCT/SUNA that is typical in trigeminal neuralgia.

TRIGEMINAL-AUTONOMIC CEPHALGIAS: IV HEMICRANIA CONTINUA

Although not formally considered TACs, the accumulation of clinical and neuroimaging data in recent years suggests that **hemicrania continua (HC)** may well join the conditions considered to be TACs. Two patients were initially reported with this syndrome, a woman aged 63 years and a man of 53. They developed unilateral headache without obvious cause. One of these patients noticed redness, lacrimation and sensitivity to light in the eye on the affected side. In both patients, the headache was relieved completely by indometacin, while other NSAIDs were of little or no benefit. As with the

other TACs, HC can have remitting and unremitting forms.

The essential features of hemicrania continua are:
- strictly lateralized continuous pain;
- fluctuations of pain that can be severe and are similarly lateralized;
- pain exacerbations may be associated with cranial autonomic features in more than 90 per cent of cases;
- complete resolution of pain with indometacin.

Apart from analgesic overuse as an aggravating factor, and a report in an HIV-infected patient, the status of secondary hemicrania continua is unclear. Indometacin can be administered by injection, single-blinded with injection of saline for the placebo-controlled indometacin test, which is a safe and effective way to diagnose hemicrania continua. The alternative is a trial of oral indometacin, initially 25 mg three times daily, then 50 mg three times daily, and then 75 mg three times daily. One should allow up to 2 weeks for any dose to have a useful effect. Acute treatment with sumatriptan is of no clear benefit in hemicrania continua.

CHRONIC DAILY HEADACHE

Each of the preceding primary headache forms can occur very frequently. When a patient experiences headache on 15 days or more a month one can apply the broad diagnosis of chronic daily headache (CDH). CDH is not one thing but a collection of very different problems with different management strategies. Crucially, not all daily headache is simply tension-type headache (Table 10.10). This is a common clinical misconception in headache that confuses the clinical **phenotype** with the headache **biotype**. Population-based estimates of daily headache are remarkable, demonstrating that 4.5–4.8 per cent of Western populations have daily or near daily headache. Daily headache may again be primary or secondary, and it seems clinically useful to consider the possibilities in this way when making management decisions (Table 10.10). It should be said that population-based studies bear out clinical practice in that a large group of refractory daily headache patients overuse various over-the-counter preparations.

Table 10.10 Classification of chronic daily headache

Primary		Secondary
>4 h daily	**<4 h daily**	

Chronic migraine[a]	Chronic cluster headache[b]	Post-traumatic
		    head injury
		    iatrogenic
		    post-infectious

Chronic tension-type headache[a]	Chronic paroxysmal hemicrania	Inflammatory, such as:
		    giant cell arteritis
		    sarcoidosis
		    Behcets syndrome

Hemicrania continua[a]	SUNCT/SUNA	Chronic CNS infection
New daily persistent headache[a]	Hypnic headache	Substance abuse headache

[a]May be complicated by analgesic overuse. In the case of substance abuse headache, the headache is completely resolved after the substance abuse is controlled. Clinical experience suggests that many patients continue to have headache even after cessation of analgesic use. The residual headache probably represents the underlying headache biology.

[b]Chronic cluster headache patients may have more than 4 h per day of headache. The inclusion of the syndrome here is to emphasize that, by and large, the attacks themselves are less than 4 hours' duration.

While it is widely accepted that some of the primary headaches, tension-type headache, cluster headache and paroxysmal hemicrania, have chronic varieties, this question seems to have become unnecessarily troublesome for migraine. Considering population-based surveys, about half of the patients with daily headache have chronic migraine (**transformed migraine in the Silberstein-Lipton nomenclature**). Chronic migraine is simply the most troublesome and disabling end of the migraine spectrum, often associated with medication overuse. It seems not in question that the syndrome exists, but there continues to be argument about its prevalence. In the author's clinical experience, both in the UK and US, it is the most common problem that is sent to headache clinics.

The International Headache Society mandates 8 clear days of migraine or days treated with a triptan, out of the at least 15 days of headache to make the diagnosis. From a pragmatic viewpoint, given the advice is no different in life-style or reduction in medication overuse, a simple approach is to diagnose chronic migraine in patients with 15 days or more of headache when there are any migrainous features, throbbing, lateralization, photophobia, phonophobia or movement aggravation, to the worsenings.

Management

The management of CDH can be very rewarding. Most patients with medication overuse respond very sensibly when the problem is explained.

The keys to managing chronic daily headache are:
- exclude treatable causes (**Table 10.10**);
- obtain a clear medication use history;
- make a diagnosis of the primary headache type involved.

Management of medication overuse – outpatients

It is essential that analgesic use be reduced and eliminated. Patients can reduce their use either by, as an example, 10 per cent every week or two, depending on their circumstances, or if they wish, and there is no contraindication, by immediate cessation of use. Either approach can be facilitated by first keeping a careful diary over a month or two to be sure of the size of the problem. A small dose of an NSAID, such as naproxen 500 mg twice daily if tolerated, will take the edge off the pain as the analgesic use is reduced. It is a useful aside that NSAID overuse does not seem to be a common issue in daily headache when they are dosed once or twice daily, whereas with more frequent dosing problems may develop. When the patient has reduced their analgesic use substantially a preventive is usually introduced.

It must be emphasized that preventives generally do not work in the presence of medication overuse, so the patient must reduce the analgesics or the entire use of the preventative is a wasted effort. The most common cause of intractability to treatment is the use of a preventative when analgesics continue to be used regularly. For some patients this is very difficult and often one must be blunt that some degree of pain is inevitable in the first instance if the problem is to be controlled.

Management of medication overuse – inpatients

Some patients will require admission for detoxification. This broadly includes two groups, those who fail outpatient withdrawal or who have a significant complicating medical indication, such as brittle diabetes mellitus, where withdrawal may be problematic as an outpatient. When such patients are admitted, acute medications are withdrawn completely on the first day, unless there is some contraindication. Anti-emetics, preferring domperidone oral or suppositories, and fluids are administered as required, as well as clonidine for opiate withdrawal symptoms. For acute intolerable pain during the waking hours, intravenous aspirin (1 g intravenously) is useful and at night chlorpromazine by injection, ensuring adequate hydration. If the patient does not settle over 3–5 days, a course of intravenous **dihydroergotamine (DHE)** should be given. It is increasingly evident that DHE is indispensable in this setting; administered 8-hourly for 3 days, it can induce a significant remission that allows a preventive treatment to be established. Often $5-HT_3$ antagonists, such as ondansetron or granisetron, will be required with DHE as it is essential to ensure that the patient does not have significant nausea.

Preventive treatments

Preventive treatment is entirely dependent on the underlying clinical problem. It is essential to make a diagnosis, such as chronic migraine or chronic cluster headache, and then use the appropriate preventive, aimed at the underlying primary headache type.

New daily persistent headache

New daily persistent headache, **NDPH**, is a clinically distinct syndrome with a range of important possible causes (Table 10.11). From a nosological point of view, all that is mentioned here could be placed variously in the International Headache Society classification, however, the term serves both patients and clinicians by highlighting a group of conditions some of which are curable. NDPH can have both primary and secondary forms (Table 10.11) and neurologists will be called on to diagnose and treat these patients. It is used in this chapter more broadly than the current International Headache classification that limits the description to what is in effect primary featureless NDPH.

Clinical presentation

NDPH patients present with a history of headache on most if not all days that began from one day to the next. The onset of headache is abrupt, often moment-to-moment but at least in less than a few days where three is suggested as an upper limit. The characteristic is for the patient to recall the exact day and circumstances, so from one moment to the next a headache develops that never leaves them. This presentation should prompt certain key ques-

Table 10.11 Differential diagnosis of new daily persistent headache

Primary	Secondary
Migrainous-type	Sub-arachnoid haemorrhage
Featureless (tension-type)	Low CSF volume headache
	Raised CSF pressure headache
	Post-traumatic headache[a]
	Chronic meningitis

[a]Includes post-infective forms.

tions about the onset and behaviour of the pain. These need to be woven with the more generic questions that one asks a patient with persistent headache, to form a provisional diagnosis. The pressing issues arise from considering the differential diagnosis, particularly of the secondary headache forms. Although subarachnoid haemorrhage is listed for some logical consistency, as the headache may certainly come on from one moment to the next, it is not likely to produce diagnostic confusion in this group of patients. Suffice to say that subarachnoid haemorrhage is so important that it must always be considered, if only to be excluded, either by history or appropriate investigation.

Secondary NDPH

The secondary causes of the syndrome of NDPH are worthy of consideration, as they have a distinct clinical picture that can guide investigation.

Low CSF volume headache

The syndrome of persistent low CSF volume headache is an important diagnosis not to miss. The more immediate version of this problem is commonly encountered in neurology after lumbar puncture. In that setting, the headache settles rapidly with bed-rest. In the chronic situation, the patient typically presents with a history of headache from one day to the next. The pain is generally not present on waking, worsens during the day, and is relieved by lying down. Recumbency usually improves the headache in minutes, and it takes only minutes to an hour for the pain to return when the patient is again upright. The patient may give a history of an index event: lumbar puncture or epidural injection, or a vigorous Valsalva, such as with lifting, straining, coughing, clearing the Eustachian tubes in an aeroplane or multiple orgasms. Caffeine-containing drinks provide temporary respite. Spontaneous leaks are recognized, and the clinician should not be put off the diagnosis if the headache history is typical when there is no obvious index event.

As time passes from the index event the postural nature may be less obvious; certainly patients whose index event was several years prior to the eventual diagnosis have been reported. The term low volume rather than low pressure is used, since there is no clear evidence at which point the pressure can be called low. While low pressures, such as

0–5, are usually identified, a pressure of 16 cm CSF has been recorded with a documented leak.

The investigation of choice is MRI with gadolinium (Figure 10.3), which produces a striking pattern of diffuse pachymeningeal enhancement, although in about 10 per cent of cases a leak can be documented without enhancement. The finding of diffuse meningeal enhancement is so typical that in the clinical context immediate treatment is appropriate. It is also common to see Chiari malformations on MRI with some degree of descent of the cerebellar tonsils. This is important from the neurologist's viewpoint since surgery in such settings simply makes the headache problem worse. It seems appropriate that any patient being considered for such surgery for a headache indication should be reviewed by a neurologist first. Alternatively, the CSF pressure may be determined, or a leak sought with ^{111}In-DPTA CSF studies that can demonstrate the leak and any early emptying of tracer into the bladder, indicative of a leak.

Treatment is bed rest in the first instance. False-positive transient improvement in persistent low CSF volume headache with chiropractic and other similar therapies is recognized where the treatment necessitated the patient lying down for a prolonged period. **Intravenous caffeine** (500 mg in 500 mL saline administered over 2 hours) is often very efficacious treatment. The ECG should be checked for any arrythmia prior to administration. A reasonable practice is to carry out at least two infusions separated by 4 weeks after obtaining the suggestive clinical history and MRI with enhancement. Since intravenous caffeine is safe, and can be curative, by an unknown mechanism, it spares many patients the need for further tests. If that is unsuccessful, an abdominal binder may be helpful. If a leak can be identified, either by the radioisotope study, or by CT myelogram, or spinal T2-weighted MRI, an **autologous blood patch** is usually curative. In more intractable situations, **theophylline** is a useful alternative that offers outpatient management.

Raised CSF pressure headache

As is the case for low CSF pressure states, raised CSF pressure as a cause of headache is well recognized.

Brain imaging can often reveal the cause, such as a space-occupying lesion. The particular setting in which patients enter the spectrum of NDPH are those with idiopathic intracranial hypertension who present with headache without visual problems, particularly with normal fundi. It is recognized that intractable chronic migraine can be triggered by persistently raised intracranial pressure.

These patients typically give a history of generalized headache that is present on waking, and gets better as the day goes on. It is generally worse with recumbency. Visual obscurations are frequently reported. Fundal changes with raised intracranial pressure would make the diagnosis relatively straightforward, but it is in those without such changes that the history must drive investigation.

If raised pressure is suspected, brain imaging is mandatory, and it is best to include MR venography at the same time as MRI. The CSF pressure should be measured by lumbar puncture, taking care to do so when the patient is symptomatic, so that both the pressure and response to removal of 20 mL of CSF can be determined. **A raised pressure and improvement in headache with removal of CSF is diagnostic of the problem.** The fields should be formally documented even in the absence of overt ophthalmic involvement. Initial treatment can be with acetazolamide (250–500 mg twice daily). The patient may respond in weeks with improvement in headache. If this is not effective, topiramate has many actions that may be useful in this setting: carbonic anhydrase inhibition, weight loss and neuronal membrane stabilization, probably through actions on phosphorylation pathways. A small number of severely disabled patients who do not respond to medical treatment will come to intracranial pressure monitoring and even shunting. This is exceptional and is not undertaken without careful investigation.

Post-traumatic headache

The issue of post-traumatic headache can be vexed. The International Headache Society accepts the existence of such a syndrome. Much of the discussion degenerates because of the often-quoted medicolegal morass. The term is used here to indicate trauma in a very broad way. NDPH may be seen after a blow to the head but more commonly after an infective episode, typically viral, or in one case, malarial meningitis. A recent series identified one-third of all patients with NDPH reported the headache starting after a flu-like illness. Patients may recall a period in which they had a significant infection: fever, neck stiffness, photophobia and marked malaise. The headache starts during that period and never stops. Investigation reveals no current cause for the headache. It has been suggested that some patients with this syndrome have a persistent Epstein–Barr infection, but this syndrome is anything but clearly delineated. A complicating factor will often be that the patient had a lumbar puncture during that illness, so a persistent low CSF volume headache needs to be considered first. Post-traumatic headache is well recognized after carotid dissection, subarachnoid haemorrhage, mild head injury and following intracranial surgery for a benign mass. The common factor seems to be that a traumatic event involving the dura mater can trigger a headache process that lasts for many years after that event.

The treatment of this form of NDPH is substantially empirical. Tricyclics, notably **amitriptyline**, and anticonvulsants, **valproate and gabapentin**, have been used with good effects. The monoamine oxidase inhibitor (MAOI) phenelzine may also be useful in carefully selected patients. The headache usually runs a limited course of 3–5 years, so will eventually settle, but it can certainly be very disabling in that period.

Primary NDPH

Initial descriptions of primary NDPH recognized it to occur in both males and females. Migrainous features were common, with unilateral headache in about one-third and throbbing pain in about one-third. Nausea was reported in about half the patients, as was photophobia and phonophobia, observed again in about half. A number of these patients have a previous history of migraine but not more than one might expect given the population prevalence of migraine. It is remarkable that the initial report noted that 86 per cent of patients were headache free at 24 months.

It is general experience among those interested in headache management that primary NDPH is perhaps the most intractable and least therapeutically rewarding form of headache. In general, one can classify the dominant phenotype, migraine or tension-type headache, and treat with preventatives according to that sub-classification, as for patients with CDH. Primary NDPH with a TTH phenotype is very unresponsive to treatment.

OTHER PRIMARY HEADACHES

Primary stabbing headache

Short-lived jabs of pain, defined by the International Headache Society as primary stabbing headache, are well documented in association with most types of primary headache.

The essential clinical features are:

- pain confined to the head, although rarely is it facial;
- stabbing pain lasting from one to many seconds and occurring as a single stab or a series of stabs;
- recurring at irregular intervals (hours to days).

A series of 100 patients with sharp, jabbing pains about the head resembling a stab from an ice-pick, nail or needle has been reported. The prevalence of such pains affected only three out of 100 headache-free controls, compared to 42 of the 100 migraine patients, of whom 60 per cent had more than one attack per month. The pains affected the temple or orbit more often than the parietal and occipital areas and often occurred before or during migraine headaches. The sites of these pains generally coincide with the site of the patients habitual headache. Retroauricular and occipital region pains are also well described and these respond promptly to indometacin. Stabbing headaches have been described in conjunction with cluster headaches, and generally are experienced in the same area as the cluster pain. 'Jabs and jolts' lasting less than a minute have been described in patients with chronic paroxysmal hemicrania. These longer attacks are probably part of the spectrum of jabbing headache.

It is of interest that jabbing pains generally are not accompanied by cranial autonomic symptoms. Moreover, when seen in childhood and adolescence, the attacks are often very frequent and very disabling over months when untreated; responding rapidly to appropriate management. The response of idiopathic stabbing headache to indometacin (25–50 mg twice to three times daily) is generally excellent. As a general rule, the symptoms wax and wane and after a period of control on indometacin, it is appropriate to withdraw treatment and observe the outcome. Most patients will not want treatment when the nature of the problem is unexplained and they are reassured that the attacks are not sinister in any way.

Primary cough headache

Sharp pain in the head on coughing, sneezing, straining, laughing or stooping has long been regarded as a symptom of organic intracranial disease, commonly associated with obstruction of the CSF pathways. The presence of an Arnold–Chiari malformation or any lesion causing obstruction of CSF pathways or displacing cerebral structures must be excluded before cough headache is assumed to be benign. Cerebral aneurysm, carotid stenosis and vertebrobasilar disease may also present with cough or exertional headache as the initial symptom. The term 'Benign Valsalva's manoeuvre-related headache' covers the headaches provoked by coughing, straining or stooping but **cough headache** is more succinct and so widely used it is unlikely to be displaced.

The essential clinical features of benign cough headache are:
- bilateral headache of sudden onset, lasting minutes, precipitated by coughing;
- may be prevented by avoiding coughing;
- diagnosed only after structural lesions, such as posterior fossa tumour, have been excluded by neuroimaging.

The average age of patients with benign cough headache is 43 years older than patients with exertional headache. Indometacin is the medical treatment of choice in cough headache. Raskin followed up an observation of Sir Charles Symonds reporting that some patients with cough headache are relieved by lumbar puncture. This is a simple option when compared to prolonged use of indometacin. The mechanism of this response remains unclear.

Primary exertional headache

The relationship of this form of headache to cough headache is unclear and certainly much is shared. Indeed the relationship to migraine also requires delineation. Credit must be given to Hippocrates for first recognizing this syndrome when he wrote: 'one should be able to recognize those who have headache from gymnastic exercises, or walking, or running, or any other unseasonable labour, or from immoderate venery'.

> The clinical features of primary exertional headache are:
> - pain specifically brought on by physical exercise;
> - bilateral and throbbing in nature at onset and may develop migrainous features in those patients susceptible to migraine;
> - lasts from 5 minutes to 24 hours;
> - prevented by avoiding excessive exertion, particularly in hot weather or at high altitude.

The acute onset of headache with straining and breath-holding, as in weightlifter's headache, may be explained by acute venous distension. The development of headache after sustained exertion, particularly on a hot day, is more difficult to understand. Anginal pain may be referred to the head, probably by central connections of vagal afferents and may present as exertional headache, so-called cardiac cephalgia. The link to exercise is the main clinical clue. Phaeochromocytoma may occasionally be responsible for exertional headache. Intracranial lesions or stenosis of the carotid arteries may have to be excluded, as discussed for benign cough headache. Headache may be precipitated by any form of exercise and often has the pulsatile quality of migraine.

Management

The most obvious form of treatment is to take exercise gradually and progressively whenever possible. Indometacin at daily doses varying from 25 to 150 mg is generally very effective in benign exer-

tional headache. Indometacin 50 mg, ergotamine tartrate 1–2 mg orally, dihydroergotamine by nasal spray, or methysergide 1–2 mg orally given 30–45 minutes before exercise are useful prophylactic measures.

Primary sex headache

Sex headache may be precipitated by masturbation or coitus and usually starts as a dull bilateral ache while sexual excitement increases, suddenly becoming intense at orgasm. The term orgasmic cephalgia is not useful since not all sex headache requires orgasm. Three types of sex headache are discussed, a dull ache in the head and neck that intensifies as sexual excitement increases, a sudden severe ('explosive') headache occurring at orgasm, and a postural headache resembling that of low CSF pressure developing after coitus. The latter, in the author's clinical experience, is simply another form of low CSF pressure headache arising from vigorous sexual activity usually with multiple orgasms and is more usefully considered with NDPH as a secondary CDH (Table 10.11).

> The essential clinical features of sex headache are:
> - precipitation by sexual excitement;
> - bilateral at onset;
> - prevented or eased by ceasing sexual activity before orgasm

Headaches developing at the time of orgasm are not always benign. Subarachnoid haemorrhage was precipitated by sexual intercourse in 4.5 per cent of 66 cases in one series and 12 per cent of 50 cases in another. One young man reported developed a brainstem thrombosis and another a left hemisphere infarction. Sex headache affects men more often than women and may occur at any time during the years of sexual activity. It may develop on several occasions in succession and then not trouble the patient again, without change in sexual technique. In patients who stop sexual activity when headache is first noticed, it may subside within a period of 5 minutes to 2 hours. More frequent orgasm can aggravate established sex headache. About half the patients with sex headache have a history of exertional headaches, but there is no excess of cough headache in patients with sex headache. In about

50 per cent of patients, sex headache will settle in six months. Migraine is probably more common in patients with sex headache.

Management

Benign sex headaches are usually irregular and infrequent in recurrence, so management can often be limited to reassurance and advice about ceasing sexual activity if a milder, warning headache develops. When the condition recurs regularly or frequently, it can be prevented by the administration of **propranolol**, but the dosage required varies from 40 to 200 mg daily. An alternative is the calcium channel blocking agent **diltiazem** 60 mg three times daily. **Ergotamine** (1–2 mg) or **indometacin** (25–50 mg) taken about 30–45 minutes prior to sexual activity can also be helpful.

Hypnic headache

This syndrome was first described in patients aged 67–84 years who had moderately severe headache that typically came on a few hours after going to sleep. Hypnic headaches last from 15 to 30 minutes, are typically generalized, although may be unilateral, and can be throbbing. Patients may report falling back to sleep only to be awoken by a further attack a few hours later, with up to three repetitions of this pattern over the night. In the largest series of 19 patients reported, 16 (84 per cent) were female and the mean age at onset was 61 ± 9 years. Headaches were bilateral in two-thirds and unilateral in one-third and in 80 per cent of cases mild or moderate. Three patients reported similar headaches when falling asleep during the day. None had photophobia or phonophobia and nausea is unusual.

Management

Patients with this form of headache generally respond to a bedtime dose of **lithium carbonate** (200–600 mg) and in those that do not tolerate this, verapamil or methysergide at bedtime may be alternative strategies. Two patients who responded to flunarizine 5 mg at night have now been reported. It had been reported that one to two cups of coffee or caffeine 60 mg orally at bedtime was helpful. This is a simple approach that is effective in about one-third of patients. A patient poorly tolerant of lithium has been controlled using verapamil at night (160 mg).

Thunderclap headache

Sudden onset severe headache may occur as both a secondary headache form, and as a primary headache disorder. The differential diagnosis includes the sentinel bleed of an intracranial aneurysm, reversible cerebral vasoconstriction syndrome (RCVS), cervicocephalic arterial dissection, cerebral venous thrombosis and primary sex headache. Headaches of explosive onset may also be caused by the ingestion of sympathomimetic drugs or tyramine-containing foods in a patient who is taking monoamine oxidase inhibitors, and can also be a symptom of pheochromocytoma. Whether thunderclap headache can be the presentation of an unruptured cerebral aneurysm is unclear. A woman has been reported with three episodes of sudden-onset, very severe headache who was found to have an unruptured aneurysm of the internal carotid artery, with adjacent areas of segmental vasospasm. In the absence of a CT scan or CSF evidence of subarachnoid haemorrhage, studies indicate that such patients do very well.

In a follow-up study of 71 patients with thunderclap headache, whose CT scans and CSF findings were negative, for an average of 3.3 years. Twelve patients had further such headache, and 31 (44 per cent) later had regular episodes of migraine or tension-type headache. Factors identified as precipitating the headache were sexual intercourse in three cases, coughing in four and exertion in 12, while the remainder had no obvious cause. A history of hypertension was found in 11 and of previous headache in 22. In a study comparing the presentation of 37 patients with subarachnoid haemorrhage and 189 with a similar thunderclap headache but normal CSF examination, there was no discernable characteristics to distinguish the two conditions on clinical grounds.

Investigation of any sudden onset severe headache, be it in the context of sexual excitement or isolated thunderclap headache, should be driven by the clinical context. The first presentation should be vigorously investigated with x-ray, CT and CSF examination, and MRI/MRV/MRA. Formal cerebral angiography should be reserved for when no primary diagnosis is forthcoming, and the clinical situation is particularly suggestive of intracranial aneurysm, although with time modern techniques, including CT-angiogram, are making catheter angiography largely unnecessary.

REFERENCES AND FURTHER READING

Afridi S, Giffin NJ, Kaube H et al. (2005) A PET study in spontaneous migraine. *Archives of Neurology*, **62**:1270–1275.

Afridi S, Matharu MS, Lee L et al. (2005) A PET study exploring the laterality of brainstem activation in migraine using glyceryl trinitrate. *Brain*, **128**:932–939.

Bahra A, Matharu MS, Buchel C et al. (2001) Brainstem activation specific to migraine headache. *Lancet*, **357**:1016–1017.

Cittadini E, Matharu MS, Goadsby PJ (2008) Paroxysmal hemicrania: a prospective clinical study of thirty-one cases. *Brain*, **131**:1142–1155.

Cohen AS, Matharu MS, Goadsby PJ (2006) Short-lasting Unilateral Neuralgiform Headache Attacks with Conjunctival injection and Tearing (SUNCT) or cranial Autonomic features (SUNA). A prospective clinical study of SUNCT and SUNA. *Brain*, **129**:2746–2760.

Goadsby PJ (2002) Pathophysiology of cluster headache: a trigeminal autonomic cephalgia. *Lancet Neurology*, **1**:37–43.

Goadsby PJ (2009) Pathophysiology of migraine. *Neurologic Clinics of North America*, **27**:335–360.

Goadsby PJ, Charbit AR, Andreou AP et al. (2009) Neurobiology of migraine. *Neuroscience*, **161**:327–341.

Goadsby PJ, Lipton RB (1997) A review of paroxysmal hemicranias, SUNCT syndrome and other short-lasting headaches with autonomic features, including new cases. *Brain*, **120**:193–209.

Goadsby PJ, Lipton RB, Ferrari MD (2002). Migraine-current understanding and treatment. *New England Journal of Medicine*, **346**:257–270.

Headache Classification Committee of The International Headache Society (2004). The International Classification of Headache Disorders, 2nd edn. *Cephalalgia*, **24**(Suppl 1):1–160.

Lance JW, Goadsby PJ (2005) *Mechanism and Management of Headache*, 7th edn. New York: Elsevier.

Lipton RB, Bigal M (2006) *Migraine and other Headache Disorders*, 1st edn. New York: Marcel Dekker, Taylor and Francis Books, 2006.

Matharu MS, Bartsch T, Ward N et al. (2004) Central neuromodulation in chronic migraine patients with sub-occipital stimulators: a PET study. *Brain*, **127**:220–230.

May A, Ashburner J, Buchel C et al. (1999) Correlation between structural and functional changes in brain in an idiopathic headache syndrome. *Nature Medicine*, **5**:836–838.

May A, Bahra A, Buchel C et al. (1998) Hypothalamic activation in cluster headache attacks. *Lancet*, **352**:275–278.

Olesen J, Tfelt-Hansen P, Ramadan N et al. (2005) *The Headaches*. Philadelphia: Lippincott, Williams and Wilkins.

Tfelt-Hansen P, Saxena PR, Dahlof C et al. (2000) Ergotamine in the acute treatment of migraine – a review and European consensus. *Brain*, **123**:9–18.

CHAPTER 11

CRANIOFACIAL PAIN

John Scadding

DIFFERENTIAL DIAGNOSIS OF CRANIOFACIAL PAIN

Craniofacial pain may be caused by a wide variety of disease processes affecting the complex anatomy of the region. Diagnosis often requires a combination of specialist skills, which can include the neurologist, ENT surgeon, ophthalmologist, dental surgeon, oral medicine physician, and sometimes the psychiatrist. Patients with craniofacial pain are often referred to neurologists with a tentative diagnosis of facial neuralgia, but **it is vital that neurologists are alert to the many non-neuralgic causes of craniofacial pain (Table 11.1)**.

Meticulous history-taking is essential, because in many patients with craniofacial pain there will be no signs accompanying the symptoms and the diagnosis must be made on the history alone.

The innervation of craniofacial structures is via the sensory brances of the trigeminal, facial, glossopharyngeal and vagus nerves, and the upper cervical roots, C2 and C3. Trigeminal innervation is extensive, involving deep tissues as well as skin (Table 11.2 and Figure 3.4). Disease processes affecting the deep tissues innervated by the

trigeminal nerve can cause pain that is localized to the affected area, or pain radiating onto the face, and this can cause difficulty in diagnosis. However, conditions affecting trigeminal innervated structures usually cause facial pain that is felt within a trigeminal nerve anatomical distribution.

It is important to note that with a few exceptions, facial pain with a serious underlying structural cause is nearly always strictly unilateral. Pain that extends beyond trigeminal territory or is bilateral is much less likely to have an underlying structural basis.

A careful examination should always be performed. In addition to a detailed examination of cranial nerve function, and guided by the distribution of the patient's symptoms, some or all of the following may also require assessment:

- temporal arteries and scalp tenderness;
- temporomandibular joint movement and tenderness;
- teeth and gums – overt disease; local tenderness;
- oropharynx;
- sinuses – tenderness over frontal and maxillary sinuses, nasal obstruction;

Table 11.1 Causes of craniofacial pain excluding headache disorders

Craniofacial neuralgias	Idiopathic trigeminal neuralgia
	Symptomatic trigeminal neuralgia
	Glossopharyngeal neuralgia
	Herpes zoster neuralgia
	C2 and C3 neuralgia
	Occipital neuralgia
	Post-traumatic neuralgia
	Painful ophthalmoplegia
Cavernous sinus	Carotid aneurysm
	Meningioma
	Pituitary tumour
Meninges	Tumour – lymphoma, cancer
	Tuberculosis
	Syphilis
Trigeminal root	Tumour compression: acoustic neuroma, meningioma
	Vascular compression: arteriovenous malformation
Central nervous system	Facial anaesthesia dolorosa
	Posterior inferior cerebellar artery occlusion
	Syringomyelia, syringobulbia
	Central poststroke pain
	Brain stem tumours
	Brain stem demyelination
Musculoskeletal	Temporomandibular joint disorders
	Eagle's syndrome (elongated stylohyoid process)
	Facial dyskinesia
	Temporal bone: glomus jugulare tumours
	Metastases
	Paget's disease
Otological	Otitis externa and media
	Cholesteatoma
Sinus disease	Infection
	Sinus obstruction
Dental and oral	All causes of odontalgia
	Atypical odontalgia
	Burning mouth syndrome
Nasopharynx	Nasopharyngeal carcinoma
Salivary glands	Infection
	Duct obstruction
	Inflammation/granulomatous disease
	Tumour
Vascular	Giant cell arteritis
	Carotid and vertebral artery dissection
Referred	Ophthalmic disease
	Cervical spine disease
	Thoracic outlet syndrome
	Myocardial ischaemia
Psychogenic	Atypical facial pain

Table 11.2 Non-cutaneous trigeminal nerve sensory innervation

Ophthalmic	Cornea
	Mucosa of frontal sinus and upper nose
	Dura in anterior part of head
	Cerebral arteries and venous sinuses in anterior part of head (posterior dura and vessels supplied by upper cervical dorsal roots)
Maxillary	Lateral wall and floor of nasal cavity
	Upper jaw and teeth
	Roof of mouth
	Mucosa of maxillary sinus
Mandibular	Anterior wall of external auditory meatus
	Tympanic membrane
	Lower jaw and teeth
	Floor of mouth
	Anterior two-thirds of tongue

- external auditory meatus, tympanic membrane and pinna;
- salivary glands;
- cervical spine movement and neck muscle tenderness.

NEURALGIAS OF THE FACE AND HEAD

Trigeminal neuralgia

Definition and epidemiology

Trigeminal neuralgia is rare in younger adults; the incidence increases with age, being most common at age 75 years and above, with a prevalence of 11 per 100 000, and a female:male ratio of about 2:1.

Trigeminal neuralgia (*tic douloureux*) is pain of abrupt onset, occurring unilaterally in severe brief paroxysms, in the distribution of one or more branches of the trigeminal nerve. It tends to be over-diagnosed, as a result of failure to adhere to the strict clinical criteria for the diagnosis.

Trigeminal neuralgia occurring in younger adults should increase the suspicion of an underlying structural cause (see below).

The term **idiopathic trigeminal neuralgia** is used to denote patients with typical pain and no physical signs but, as noted below, subtle anatomical variants are probably responsible for the pain in the majority of patients.

Symptomatic trigeminal neuralgia refers to typical trigeminal neuralgia that is due to compression of the trigeminal root by a tumour or other gross lesion such as an arteriovenous malformation. However, this is rare, and most gross compressive lesions cause pain that is not paroxysmal, and is often associated with trigeminal sensory loss.

Trigeminal neuralgia is a feature of multiple sclerosis (MS). However, in MS, although the pain may be typical in the early stages, the character tends change over time, becoming less paroxysmal and responding increasingly poorly to treatment.

'**Atypical trigeminal neuralgia**' is sometimes used to describe pain that has some but not all the diagnostic features of the condition. However, a diagnosis of trigeminal neuralgia should be resisted unless the pain fulfils the diagnostic criteria, and 'atypical trigeminal neuralgia' is a term best avoided.

Cause and pathophysiology of pain

Trigeminal neuralgia and the related but much rarer glossopharyngeal neuralgia are unique among neuralgic pains in the characteristic clinical features of the pain. The pathophysiological basis remains uncertain, but recent research suggests that several properties may lead to the paroxysmal pain:

- bursting impulse discharges in mildly damaged trigeminal neurons, with prolonged afterdischarges;
- cross-talk between damaged fibres, leading to rapid recruitment of impulse activity in many fibres;

Subtle vascular compression of the trigeminal root, usually by the superior cerebellar or anterior inferior cerebellar arteries, is the most common finding in patients with trigeminal neuralgia coming to operation. However, whether or not such vascular compression is the cause in all patients remains uncertain. The success of micro-vascular decompression in relieving trigeminal neuralgia offers strong support for the vascular compression hypothesis of the causation of the condition. Histological and ultrastructural abnormalities have also been described in the Gasserian ganglion. In patients with multiple sclerosis, the pathology is plaques or atrophic areas in the trigeminal root, and central brain stem plaques are probably also responsible.

- a hyperpolarized refractory state following high frequency burst discharges, leading to termination of a paroxysm of pain.

Clinical features

The International Headache Society criteria for a diagnosis of trigeminal neuralgia are:

1 Paroxysmal attacks of pain lasting from a fraction of a second to 2 minutes, affecting one or more divisions of the trigeminal nerve and fulfilling criteria 2 and 3.
2 Pain has at least one of the following characteristics:
   a. intense, sharp, superficial or stabbing
   b. precipitated from trigger areas or by trigger factors.
3 Attacks are stereotyped in the individual patient.
4 There is no clinically evident neurological deficit.
5 The pain is not attributable to another disorder.

The clinical features are set out in Table 11.3. Trigeminal neuralgia is unilateral in 96 per cent of patients, and bilateral simultaneous neuralgia is very rare. The pain is nearly always within the second and third divisions of the trigeminal nerve.

Table 11.3 Clinical features of trigeminal neuralgia

Site	Maxillary – upper lip, nares, radiating over medial cheek to eye upper jaw teeth
	Mandibular – corner of mouth, radiating over lower jaw and cheek to ear
	Ophthalmic – eye and forehead
Nature	Paroxysmal: shooting, shock-like
Frequency	Up to several times per minute
	Often brief pain-free intervals
	Rare during sleep
Duration	A few seconds up to 2 minutes
Severity	Mild to very severe
Triggering	Innocuous trigeminal cutaneous or oral stimuli
	Movement of jaw or face
Periodicity	Bouts lasting days to months
	Tendency for periods of remission to become shorter and lost over time
Associated features	Anorexia, dehydration
	Weight loss
	Depression

The two most common sites are:
- the upper lip and nares radiating over the medial cheek towards the eye;
- the angle of the mouth radiating along the mandible towards the ear.

When the pain originates in the teeth of the upper or lower jaw, patients are likely to present initially to a dentist. Pain may also be felt along the side of the tongue and in the buccal mucosa and gingiva. Trigeminal neuralgia affecting the ophthalmic division is very uncommon; pain in this area, unless characteristic of trigeminal neuralgia, should prompt suspicion of an alternative cause.

Paroxysms of pain in trigeminal neuralgia often occur unprovoked but are characteristically triggered by normally innocuous cutaneous and oral stimuli, including touching and washing the face, shaving, wind blowing on the face, facial movement, chewing and hot or cold liquids in the mouth. The paroxysms of pain usually last for between15 and 60 seconds, but occasionally for up to 2 min-

utes. Patients dislike being examined, for fear of provocation of their pain.

Pain is sometimes described by patients as being continuous, but this may refer to very frequent paroxysms, rather than pain that is actually continuous. During a bout of neuralgia, patients may be reluctant to eat or drink, they lose weight and can become dehydrated.

In the early stages, neuralgia occurs in bouts lasting days to weeks, then may remit for months or even years. Over time, bouts tend to last longer and the periods of remission shorten or become absent. Severe pain at night is uncommon.

A background milder, non-paroxysmal dull aching or burning pain is occasionally described by some patients with longstanding trigeminal neuralgia.

Facial flushing is an occasional accompaniment to trigeminal neuralgia.

Patients with trigeminal neuralgia frequently become depressed.

Examination

In idiopathic trigeminal neuralgia, there is no sensory loss. Paroxysms of pain are likely to be provoked during facial and oral sensory examination. A reluctance to be examined and the severity and paroxysmal nature of provoked pain should leave the examiner in little doubt about the diagnosis.

The finding of trigeminal sensory loss or other abnormal signs should alert the examiner to the possibility of symptomatic trigeminal neuralgia, and prompt appropriate investigation.

Investigation

Magnetic resonance imaging (MRI) is sensitive in detecting blood vessels in contact with the trigeminal root, but this finding is not necessarily pathological, as a similar appearance is present on the contralateral, asymptomatic side in up to one-third of patients and is a frequent finding in those having MRI for other indications.

MRI is an important diagnostic investigation for the minority of patients with trigeminal neuralgia suspected of having MS. In patients with a single short-lived bout of trigeminal neuralgia, without physical signs, it is reasonable to await a further bout, which might not occur for months or years, before embarking on investigation.

Medical treatment

> **Carbamazepine** is by far the most effective drug treatment, relieving pain partially or completely in 70 per cent of patients. Treatment should start using low doses (not more than 300 mg daily), as small doses are sometimes effective and adverse effects, particularly common in older patients, are minimized.

Slow release preparations are often preferable, and measurement of blood levels can be helpful in monitoring treatment. Intolerance of even small doses limits treatment in some patients. Gradually increasing doses are required in many patients with longstanding trigeminal neuralgia, with more prolonged bouts and shorter periods of remission.

Adverse effects include an allergic rash in up to 10 per cent of patients, sedation, ataxia and, rarely, blood dyscrasias, fluid retention and hyponatraemia.

Drugs including lamotrigine, baclofen and tizanidine have been advocated on the basis of limited trials, but their efficacy remains unproven. Several other drugs have been advocated for treatment, but have not been subject to adequate trials, and thus cannot be recommended. They include phenytoin, oxcarbazepine, sodium valproate, clonazepam, topiramate and gabapentin.

Surgical treatment

> Surgical treatment should be considered in patients with frequent and prolonged bouts of pain, when medical treatment fails or only partially controls the pain, or when carbamazepine is not tolerated. Elective surgery is increasingly now offered to younger patients, for whom there is the prospect of producing long remission from pain, or permanent cure.

Alcohol injections of the peripheral branches of the affected division of the nerve or the Gasserian ganglion were frequently performed, but have now been superseded. Adverse effects include permanent facial anaesthesia, dysaesthesiae and neuroparalytic keratitis. Other ablative procedures including complete trigeminal rhizotomy and trigeminal tractotomy are no longer performed. They are often associated with severe adverse effects, particularly permanent facial anaesthesia and anaesthesia dolorosa (see Chapter 30).

Cryosurgery involves creating freezing lesions of the peripheral branches with a cryoprobe, and gives temporary pain relief for 6–12 months, and in a few patients for longer than one year.

In **controlled radiofrequency thermocoagulation**, cycles of radiofrequency induced heat are applied to the appropriate part of the trigeminal division at the level of the Gasserian ganglion, during brief periods of general anaesthesia, until partial sensory loss is detected. This results in pain relief in about 80 per cent of patients for one year, and in 50 per cent at five years. However, facial anaesthesia can be a troublesome adverse effect of the procedure. It is the preferred treatment for patients not fit enough for microvascular decompression (see below).

Transient balloon microcompression of the Gasserian ganglion is another minimally invasive treatment, though trials have been limited. Gamma knife has also been advocated as an effective treatment.

> **Microvascular decompression (Jannetta procedure)**, via a posterior fossa craniotomy, is now the surgical treatment of choice. The aim is to separate the nerve root from the vessel causing partial compression. Results are good, with 80 per cent of patients being pain free at 1–2 years, and at 8–10 years, 60 per cent remain pain free. About 12 per cent develop recurrent neuralgia that is relatively mild.

Glossopharyngeal neuralgia

Glossopharyngeal neuralgia is a paroxysmal pain felt in the distribution of the nerve, similar to trigeminal neuralgia. It is a rare condition, with an incidence of 0.8 per 100 000. The average age of onset is 50 years. It is bilateral in about 5 per cent of patients.

Clinical features

> The pain is felt in the posterior part of the tongue, tonsillar fossa, pharynx, or beneath the angle of the jaw, or in the ear. It is lancinating, lasting from seconds to 2 minutes, and is often triggered by swallowing, chewing, talking, coughing and yawning.

Patients sometimes complain of a sensation of something stuck in the throat. Glossopharyngeal neuralgia occurs in bouts, like trigeminal neuralgia, with spontaneous remissions. There is an association with sick sinus syndrome, syncope, bradycardia and occasionally asystole.

Anatomy

The somatosensory innervation of the glossopharyngeal nerve has two components: the auricular/tympanic branch, supplying the external auditory meatus and tympanic membrane, part of the pinna and the mastoid; and the pharyngeal branch, innervating the pharynx. There is a communication between pharyngeal and vagal afferents, and together, these nerves supply the soft palate, tonsil and posterior part of the tongue. The primary sensory afferents from this distribution terminate in the spinal nucleus of the trigeminal, and there are connections between this nucleus and autonomic centres in the medulla. The glossopharyngeal nerve also contains motor, somatosensory, visceral sensory and parasympathetic components, and communicates with the facial and vagus nerves and the sympathetic trunk, and this explains the autonomic features sometimes associated with glossopharyngeal neuralgia.

The glossopharyngeal nerve emerges from the anterior part of the jugular foramen, medial to the styloid process.

Cause, diagnosis and investigation

Vascular compression of the nerve is the most common cause, and this may be revealed by MRI. Other compressive causes such as tumour or an elongated styloid process are occasionally found and glossopharyngeal neuralgia occurs rarely in MS.

Diagnosis is relatively straightforward when the pain has the characteristic features and there is no neurological deficit on examination, but an ENT assessment is always advisable, to exclude other possible causes of pain in this region.

Treatment

Although there have been no randomized clinical trials of treatment in this rare condition, **carbamazepine** is often effective and should be given as for trigeminal neuralgia. Other drugs used include phenytoin, baclofen, gabapentin and lamotrigine, though these are less likely to be effective and should be considered only if carbamazepine fails.

Surgical treatment in those unresponsive to drug treatment usually involves microvascular decompression. Section of the glossopharyngeal root has also been reported to be effective, but this is associated with up to 5 per cent mortality and may be complicated by dysphagia and dysphonia.

Herpes zoster infection and postherpetic neuralgia

The ophthalmic division of the trigeminal nerve and the mid-thoracic sensory roots are by far the most common dermatomes to be affected by acute herpes zoster (shingles). The maxillary and mandibular trigeminal divisions may be involved together with the ophthalmic division, but not usually in isolation. C2 and C3 shingles is uncommon. A full account of postherpetic neuralgia is given in Chapter 30.

Clinical features and treatment

> Pre-eruptive pain in the distribution of the affected division of the trigeminal nerve or upper cervical root is frequent and may last for several days before the rash of acute herpes zoster appears. The pain is often severe and neuropathic in type (see Chapter 30). The diagnosis becomes obvious when the rash appears. Acyclovir should be given as soon as the diagnosis is suspected; this has an effect on the severity of the rash and duration acute herpetic neuralgia, but there is no convincing evidence that this treatment reduces the incidence or severity of postherpetic neuralgia.

Eye involvement in ophthalmic zoster can be severe; urgent ophthalmological advice should be obtained.

Geniculate herpes zoster: the Ramsay–Hunt syndrome

The sensory root of the geniculate ganglion, the nervus intermedius, supplies the middle and inner ear, the posterior wall of the external auditory canal, part of the pinna, the Eustachian tube and the mastoid air cells. Geniculate zoster mainly, but not exclusively, affects older people.

Acute herpes zoster affecting the geniculate ganglion causes severe pain deep in the ear, often with radiation of the pain behind the ear. Clinically, the neurological deficit is frequently more extensive than can be explained by involvement of the geniculate ganglion alone, and the infection may extend to the brainstem in some patients.

The rash affects the external auditory canal and part of the pinna, but may be subtle; a careful examination for vesicles should always be undertaken in a patient presenting with acute severe pain in the ear.

As with zoster at other sites, pre-eruptive pain may precede the appearance of a rash by several days, and this often causes diagnostic difficulty and delay, as there are many other causes of pain in the ear.

Other parts of the facial nerve are often affected. A facial palsy occurs in almost all patients, with loss of taste on the anterior two-thirds of the tongue due to involvement of the chorda tympani. Involvement of the eighth cranial nerve causes deafness and vertigo. General malaise and a low-grade fever are common associated features.

Acyclovir should be given as soon as the diagnosis is suspected, but there is limited evidence that early treatment improves the outcome. Recovery of the facial palsy is often incomplete.

C2 and occipital neuralgias

The C2 spinal nerve root passes next to the atlanto-axial joint and may be involved in inflammatory conditions affecting the joint, by tumours (neurofibromas or meningiomas), in subluxation of the atlanto-axial joint, most often seen in rheumatoid disease, and by angiomas and arterial loops. Pain from C2 root compression is felt within the distribution of the root, over the back of the head. It may be intermittent, or continuous. Depending on the degree of compression there may be demonstrable sensory impairment.

C2 neuralgia is a condition of unknown cause, which presents with intermittent, lancinating unilateral occipital pain, often associated with ipsilateral lacrymation and redness of the eye. Episodes of pain may occur several times per day, with remissions lasting for up to several months. Imaging is normal. A useful diagnostic test is a C2 root local anaesthetic block, which temporarily abolishes the pain. Longer-term relief may be achieved with root thermocoagulation.

Occipital neuralgia is due to damage or entrapment of the greater or lesser occipital nerves. It sometimes follows whiplash-type neck injuries and is also reported to be due to chronic contraction of the posterior nuchal and scalp muscles, but in many patients no cause can be found. The pain may be intermittent or persistent, either as a shooting pain starting in the occipital region and radiating towards the vertex, or as a dull, deep aching pain. It is sometimes provoked by neck movement. Often there are no signs, but there may be local tenderness over the occipital nerves, neck muscle tenderness and mild occipital sensory impairment. Local anaesthetic injections temporarily relieve the pain and corticosteroid injection can provide long-term relief.

Post-traumatic facial neuralgia

The supraorbital and infraorbital nerves may be damaged by direct trauma, with or without fractures. The inferior alveolar nerve is occasionally damaged during wisdom tooth extractions, and the lingual nerve may also be damaged as a result of dental procedures. Pain is usually continuous rather than paroxysmal, and so it is unlike trigeminal neuralgia. There is often numbness and tingling within the affected nerve territory, together with a Tinel sign at the site of nerve damage. Treatment is along the lines for other peripheral neuropathic pains (see Chapter 30).

Neck-tongue syndrome

In the rare neck-tongue syndrome, sudden turning of the head causes subluxation of the lateral atlanto-axial joint, which stretches the C2 nerve root. This leads to pain in the occipital region lasting seconds or minutes, associated with numbness or paraesthesiae on the side of the tongue, these sensory symptoms being due to compression of proprioceptive afferent fibres from the tongue, passing from the ansa hypoglossi to the C2 ventral ramus. The syndrome occurs in normal people and in patients with rheumatoid disease or congenital joint laxity.

Facial anaesthesia dolorosa

Anaesthesia dolorosa describes pain experienced in an area of decreased sensation on the face, due to either peripheral or central lesions, but is the term usually used to denote pain associated with loss of peripheral sensation. Loss of sensation in the face is particularly likely to lead to anaesthesia dolorosa, compared to other body areas. The pain is deep, diffuse, often burning, and frequently severe. In past years, trigeminal anaesthesia dolorosa was largely due to ablative procedures performed for the treatment of trigeminal neuralgia, including trigeminal rhizotomy and medullary tractotomy, operations now made obsolete by microvascular decompression, but it can occur following radiofrequency lesioning and is related to the degree of sensory impairment produced by this treatment.

PAINFUL OPHTHALMOPLEGIA

Painful ophthalmoplegia refers to all causes of ophthalmoplegia associated with pain. Pain is felt mainly in the orbital region, but may radiate widely onto the face and the head. Knowledge of the anatomy of the cavernous sinus is essential in accurate diagnosis (Chapters 2 and Chapter 3). The sinus contains the carotid artery, first division of the trigeminal nerve, third, fourth and sixth cranial nerves and the sympathetic and parasympathetic supply to the eye. Painful ophthalmoplegia can be produced by a wide range of pathologies affecting one or more of these structures, including vascular, neoplastic, granulomatous and infective processes (Table 11.4).

Anatomical and pathological subdivisions of painful ophthalmoplegia are described, including superior orbital fissure syndrome, orbital apex syndrome, cavernous sinus syndrome, parasellar syndrome and Tolosa–Hunt syndrome. However, there is frequently overlap in the characteristic clinical signs of these conditions. The inclusive term **painful ophthalmoplegia** recognizes this and encourages a systematic approach to diagnosis.

The **Tolosa–Hunt syndrome**, described in the 1960s, was thought to be exclusively the result of granulomatous infiltration of the cavernous sinus. In the International Headache Society taxonomy, it has the following diagnostic criteria:

- one or more episodes of unilateral orbital pain persisting for weeks if untreated;

Table 11.4 Causes of painful ophthalmoplegia

Neurological	Ophthalmoplegic migraine
	Diabetic third nerve palsy
Vascular	Giant cell arteritis
	Carotid, middle meningeal and posterior communicating artery aneurysms
	Carotico-cavernous fistula
	Cavernous sinus thrombosis
	Carotid artery dissection
Neoplastic	Pituitary tumours
	Retrobulbar tumours
	Skull base tumours
	Lymphoma
	Nasopharyngeal carcinoma
Infection	Tuberculosis
	Aspergillosis
	Actinomycosis
	Syphilis
Inflammatory	Sarcoidosis
	Orbital pseudotumour
	Systemic lupus erythematosus

- paresis of one or more of the third, fourth and/ or sixth cranial nerves and/or demonstration of granuloma by magnetic resonance imaging or biopsy;
- paresis coincides with the onset of pain or follows it within 2 weeks;
- pain and paresis resolve within 72 hours when treated adequately with corticosteroids;
- other causes have been excluded by appropriate investigation.

However, several variants have been described, including **Raeder's syndrome**, the combination of Horner's syndrome, pain and parasellar cranial nerve involvement; and **Gradenigo's syndrome**, a sixth cranial nerve palsy with pain due to lesions at the apex of the petrous temporal bone. In the Tolosa–Hunt syndrome itself, optic nerve involvement has been described, indicating anterior extension of the lesion responsible from the cavernous sinus, and the involvement of the maxillary division of the trigeminal nerve in some cases indicates posterior extension of pathology. Seventh cranial nerve involvement has also been described, and occasionally the eighth, ninth, tenth or twelfth cranial nerves are affected.

In addition, it is now clear that disease processes other than granulomas may cause the same clinical syndrome, and a rapid response to corticosteroid treatment is not unique to Tolosa–Hunt syndrome; it may occur in patients with painful ophthalmoplegia caused by aneurysms and tumours, including lymphoma, nasopharyngeal carcinoma, pituitary tumours and metastases, and by fungal infection in the cavernous sinus.

For all these reasons, it is appropriate to include all the previously described syndromes under the heading of painful ophthalmoplegia.

HEMIFACIAL SPASM, FACIAL PARALYSIS AND DYSKINESIA

Hemifacial spasm is sometimes painful. Patients with longstanding facial palsy sometimes complain of pain on the affected side of the face, particularly when contracture of the facial muscles develops following a lower motor neurone palsy, or when hemifacial spasm develops.

Orofacial dyskinesia (Chapter 20) affecting facial or jaw muscles can also be painful.

MUSCULOSKELETAL CRANIOFACIAL PAINS

Temporomandibular joint disorders

Transient pain in the region of the temporomandibular joint (TMJ), is often associated with limitation of jaw opening, and clicking or popping noises are commonly reported by patients.

Terminology and clinical features

Costen described TMJ pain and the term Costen's syndrome is still used today. However, three other diagnostic labels are now more commonly employed to describe the syndromes of TMJ pain:

- temporomandibular pain and dysfunction syndrome;
- oromandibular dysfunction;
- both of these are associated with dysfunction of the TMJ; and
- facial arthromyalgia, in which dysfunction may present or absent.

In neurological practice, the clinical features of these three TMJ pain syndromes can be considered together. There is aching in the muscles of mastication, exacerbated by chewing, associated with restriction of jaw movement (variably present in facial arthromyalgia) and clicking or popping sounds. Associated features include jaw clenching and gnashing of the teeth, jaw locking on opening, and other oral 'parafunction' symptoms, including biting of the tongue, lips or cheek. Women are more commonly affected than men, and the conditions may present at any age in adult life.

The pain is usually continuous, dull and aching, and is centred in the region of the TMJ, radiating to the masticatory muscles, but pain can radiate widely over the face, to the ear and occasionally onto the neck. It may be unilateral or bilateral. It is often exacerbated by jaw movement. Mental stress may be a provoking factor in some patients. Patients present with pain of several weeks', months' or even years' duration.

On examination, there is often tenderness of the TMJ and masticatory muscles, clicking of the joint on movement, subluxation, and sometimes trismus or evidence of bruxism.

Pathophysiology

Three main pathophysiological mechanisms have been proposed: psychogenic, meniscal displacement and malocclusion; these are not mutually exclusive.

The **psychogenic** theory proposes that psychological factors, including adverse life events, sleep disturbance, anxiety and stress, lead to masticatory muscle overactivity and pain, and it has been suggested that facial arthromyalgia is more common in individuals with vulnerable personality types.

The **meniscal displacement** hypothesis is based on the fact that the lateral pterygoid muscle alters the position of the meniscus within the TMJ. It is proposed that psychological stressors provoke hyperactivity of this muscle, causing the meniscus to be displaced anteromedially in the joint, with resultant loss of attachment to the lateral pole of the condyle, leading to instability in the joint and the development of pain. However, anterior displacement of the meniscus, as demonstrated by MRI, is present in a third of asymptomatic subjects, casting doubt on this hypothesis.

Costen proposed that **malocclusion** causes pain in the TMJ. However, controlled studies of devices producing occlusal equilibration have not demonstrated a clear therapeutic effect. Furthermore, there is no difference in the incidence of malocclusion in patients with facial arthromyalgia and in asymptomatic controls.

Treatment

Many treatments including physical, pharmacological and psychological measures have been advocated for the treatment of the TMJ pain disorders. There is evidence from randomized controlled trials of a therapeutic effect from antidepressants, diazepam and cognitive behavioural therapy.

LESIONS OF THE EAR, SINUSES AND ORAL CAVITY

Otalgia

Otalgia due to **otitis externa** and **otitis media** is usually well localized in the ear, but chronic otitis media can cause widely radiating pain. **Malignant** otitis media is due to chronic infection with pseudomonas aeruginosa in patients with diabetes mellitus. It presents with otalgia, followed by facial palsy and sometimes other cranial nerve palsies, developing weeks or months after the onset of the pain.

Cholesteatomas lead to destructive changes in the middle and inner ear, with secondary infection and bone erosion. They are sometimes painful.

Geniculate herpes zoster has already been discussed.

Lesions of the temporal bone may present with poorly localized pain in the region of the ear, together with conductive deafness if the middle ear is involved, as for example with **glomus jugulare tumours**. Occasionally, **metastatic deposits** in this region of the skull lead to otalgia; this occurs particularly with prostatic cancer, though any of the malignancies commonly metastasizing to bone can cause painful skull deposits. **Paget's disease** of bone involving the skull bones may cause localized pain, leading to the characteristic clinical appearance and radiological features.

Sinus disease

> **Sinusitis** is by far the most common cause of sinus pain. Bacterial **maxillary sinusitis**, unilateral or bilateral, usually follows viral upper respiratory infections, associated with nasal obstruction and discharge. There is pain in the region of the maxillary antrum, sometimes exacerbated by chewing, with tenderness over the antrum. Maxillary sinusitis is occasionally caused by a periapical dental abscess.

Frontal sinusitis causes pain and tenderness in the supraorbital region. **Sphenoid** and **ethmoid sinusitis** lead to pain felt between or behind the eyes, characteristically exacerbated by bending, and relieved by spontaneous or surgical drainage of the infected sinus.

Plain skull x-rays show opacification of the affected sinuses and sometimes a fluid level in the affected sinus. Computed tomography (CT) scans demonstrate these changes with greater sensitivity.

Fungal infection of the sinuses most commonly occurs in immunocompromised patients. In the **rhinocerebral syndrome**, seen most often in patients with diabetes mellitus, fungal infection progressively involves the sinuses, orbits and brain.

Tumours within the sinuses lead to sinus pain, and nasal polyps and severe allergic rhinitis can lead to obstruction of the sinuses causing pain in the absence of infection. A severely deviated nasal septum may obstruct sinus drainage and also cause pain due to pressure on the bony turbinates.

Dental pain

Dental pain (odontalgia) is usually well localized, but it can be diffuse and lead to diagnostic difficulty. It is appropriate for neurologists to be aware of the leading causes of odontalgia.

Dentinoenamel defects, due to caries or trauma, can occasionally lead to diffuse orofacial pain. Local dental stimulation using a wooden spatula will evoke the pain.

Pulpitis is infection of the tooth pulp due to deep caries. Pain is intermittent or continuous and may be well localized or diffuse. The typical exacerbation by chewing and hot and cold liquids in the mouth may lead to the erroneous diagnosis of trigeminal neuralgia. Without treatment, pulpitis can progress to periapical periodontitis and abscess.

Periapical periodontitis and abscess cause severe pain in the affected tooth and adjacent gingiva, which sometimes radiates widely. Examination of the affected tooth may not reveal any obvious abnormality, but the gingiva are often inflamed and a gum boil may discharge into the mouth.

Gingival pain due to local trauma or infection causes obvious gingival inflammation. **Pericoronitis** is a bacterial infection affecting the tissues surrounding an impacted or erupting tooth, and can lead to diffuse rather than localized pain.

Cracked tooth syndrome, due, as the name implies, to a crack in a tooth, causes local pain provoked by chewing; there may be an easily identifiable fracture in part of the tooth cusp.

Dry socket is a painful condition that arises following tooth extraction, usually from the lower jaw, due to localized osteitis. There is often associated submandibular lymphadenitis. After tooth extraction, clotted blood usually fills the socket, but this may not occur if excessive adrenaline has been used with the local anaesthetic. If the normal blood clot is washed out or broken down by infection, this may also result in a dry socket. Food impaction in the socket causes pain and halitosis. Treatment entails washing out and packing the socket.

Atypical odontalgia

Atypical odontalgia describes severe throbbing pain in one or more teeth, in the absence of demonstrable pathology. The pain may radiate widely, both onto the face and within the mouth. The affected tooth or teeth are often hypersensitive to stimuli, particularly heat and cold. The condition is generally considered to be of psychological origin, as in atypical facial pain (see below), with which it overlaps in its clinical features. There is sometimes obvious associated depression, but it is also considered to represent a monosymptomatic hypochondriacal disorder.

Burning mouth syndrome

Burning mouth syndrome (BMS), also called glossodynia, or burning tongue syndrome, occurs mainly in post-menopausal women over the age of 50 years.

It presents with burning pain, predominantly on the tip and lateral borders of the tongue, but also sometimes on the palate, alveolar mucosa and lips. Symptoms are often exacerbated by emotion, fatigue and hot drinks. Associated symptoms include dry mouth (xerostomia), altered or bad taste (dysgeusia) and abnormal thirst. Temporary relief is sometimes obtained by sleeping, eating, cold drinks and alcohol. Anxiety and depression are commonly associated with BMS.

The differential diagnosis includes a number of important treatable conditions causing diffuse pain in the mouth, including bacterial and fungal infection, allergies, oesophageal reflux, xerostomia as part of Sjögren's syndrome, iron, vitamin B12 and folate deficiencies and diabetes mellitus.

The pathology of BMS has remained obscure until recently. Tongue biopsies in patients with BMS, immunostained for the pan-neuronal marker protein gene product 9.5 (PGP 9.5; also known as ubiquitin C-terminal hydrolase L-1, UCHL1), have shown lower densities of unmyelinated epithelial nerve fibres compared with controls, with evidence of axonal degeneration. This indicates that BMS may be a trigeminal small fibre sensory neuropathy.

Treatment is disappointing: a recent Cochrane review revealed no evidence for effectiveness of antidepressants, iron, vitamins, zinc or antifungal drugs.

Salivary gland disease

Submandibular gland disease includes duct obstruction, inflammation, infection and occasionally tumour, all presenting with local pain, swelling and tenderness of the gland. **Parotid gland** disease can be more difficult to detect clinically as pain is often diffuse, affecting most of the side of the face, and mild to moderate gland swelling may not be clinically obvious. The development of a facial palsy suggests a mixed parotid tumour. Painful symmetrical swelling of the salivary glands occurs in mumps infection, and enlargement of one or both parotids is a feature of sarcoidosis. If facial pain is suspected to be due to parotid disease, imaging with CT or MR is indicated.

SUBOCCIPITAL AND CERVICAL DISEASE

Carotid and vertebral artery dissection

Dissection is considered fully in Chapter 23. Pain is often the first symptom of dissection and can precede the onset of symptoms and signs of cerebral ischaemia by hours or even days.

In carotid dissection, pain is usually on the same side as the dissection and is felt in the face, head or neck. Occasionally, pain is bilateral.

In vertebral artery dissection, unilateral or bilateral neck pain and headache are sometimes associated with facial pain, preceding the development of neurological deficit. However, facial pain may be a localizing symptom of brain stem ischaemia produced by the dissection.

Styloid process syndrome (Eagle's syndrome)

Eagle described the symptoms resulting from elongation of the styloid process or mineralization (calcification or ossification) of the stylohyoid ligament, now known as Eagle's syndrome. The condition is rare, but accurate diagnosis should lead to surgical treatment that is often curative.

The clinical features can be understood by reference to the complex anatomy of the styloid region: the styloid process originates from the temporal bone medial and anterior to the stylomastoid foramen. The process points anteromedially and is bordered on medial and lateral sides by the internal and external carotid arteries, respectively. Three muscles are attached to the process: stylopharyngeus (supplied by the glossopharyngeal nerve), stylohyoid (facial nerve) and styloglossus (hypoglossal nerve). The stylohyoid and stylomandibular ligaments also originate from the process. The internal jugular vein and the glossopharyngeal, vagus and hypoglossal nerves lie medial to the process.

Patients with Eagle's syndrome typically present aged 30–50 years, women slightly more often than men.

Symptoms may be intermittent or continuous and include:
- pain in the throat;
- sensation of a foreign body in the pharynx;
- dysphagia;
- otalgia;
- mandibular and facial pain;
- vertigo and syncope;
- carotidynia.

Head turning towards the side of the pain, with the neck flexed, may provoke the pain, and is a provoked symptom that should be elicited on examination in patients with pharyngeal pain of obscure origin. Less commonly, symptoms arise due to mechanical irritation of the external and internal carotid arteries (carotidynia), with a wide distribution of pain, including the eye, ear, mandible, face, soft palate and nose (distribution of the external carotid artery); and unilateral or generalized headache (internal carotid artery).

Suspicion of the diagnosis should lead to an ENT referral: symptoms can be provoked by palpation of the styloid process, which may be obviously elongated.

Plain x-rays or CT scans demonstrate an elongated styloid process and may also show mineralization of the stylohyoid complex.

The cause of elongation of the styloid process and abnormal bone mineralization in Eagle's syndrome is uncertain, but hypotheses include trauma from tonsillectomy, and recurrent trauma to the stylohyoid ligament due to neck movement.

The multiplicity and wide distribution of the often non-specific symptoms makes diagnosis of this rare condition difficult, and diagnosis is frequently delayed. The differential diagnosis includes chronic pharyngotonsillitis, otitis media, mastoiditis, pain of dental origin, pharyngeal foreign body, submandibular salivary gland disease and tumours of the pharynx or base of the tongue. A multidisciplinary approach to diagnosis is needed.

Treatment is excision of the elongated part of the styloid process, which is curative in the majority of patients.

REFERRED PAIN

Although **ophthalmic disease** causes pain that is usually centred on the eye, pain can radiate widely onto the face and head. **Cervical spine degenerative disease** frequently leads to pain in the spine radiating to the occipital region, associated with neck muscle tenderness. Pain due to **myocardial ischaemia** may be experienced in the lower jaw, anterior neck and throat, in the absence of central chest or left arm pain. **Thoracic outlet syndrome** is considered in Chapter 7. Although pain in the root of the neck, radiating down the arm, is the characteristic distribution, referred pain on the ipsilateral side of the face and head is reported by some patients.

FACIAL PAIN OF PSYCHOLOGICAL ORIGIN

Atypical facial pain

The term atypical facial pain (AFP) is used here to denote pain of psychological origin. However, AFP is sometimes used to describe atypical forms of organically determined conditions.

> The International Headache Society defines AFP as persistent facial pain that does not have the characteristics of the cranial neuralgias and is not associated with physical signs or a demonstrable organic cause. Pain may be initiated by an operative procedure or injury to the face, teeth or oral tissues.

This definition indicates an absence of organic disease, but it does not positively state that AFP is a psychologically determined condition.

There is a history of previous dental treatment or injury prior to the onset of symptoms in about 50 per cent of patients, and there is obvious associated depression and anxiety in some patients. AFP predominantly presents in middle-aged women.

Clinical features

> In AFP, pain is poorly localized, affecting non-muscular parts of the face. It is described as deep, aching or throbbing, and is often severe and debilitating. The pain tends to spread over time, and symptoms may persist for years. Pain usually starts on one side of the face, but often becomes bilateral and frequently extends beyond trigeminal territory on the head and upper neck. It may be exacerbated by fatigue and mental stress. Although provoked exacerbations occur in some patients, these do not have the characteristics of the triggered pain of trigeminal neuralgia. Symptoms indicating anxiety and depression are frequent, but depression is often denied.

There may be a history of repeated dental treatments, undertaken in attempts to relieve the symptoms. There is clinical overlap with atypical odontalgia.

Examination reveals tenderness of the face in some patients, but no other physical signs. Patients are sometimes agitated and distressed, and there may be obvious depressive features.

The differential diagnosis is potentially wide, but careful clinical assessment often permits a positive diagnosis, without the need for extensive investigation. However, by the time of presentation to a neurologist, patients with AFP have often seen a number of specialists and had a variety of investigations. Psychiatric assessment is often advisable.

Treatment

Antidepressants are often effective. Monitoring of effect is needed, with careful diagnostic review in those patients not responding to medication.

REFERENCES AND FURTHER READING

Barker FG, Jannetta PJ et al. (1996) The long-term outcome of microvascular decompression for trigeminal neuralgia. New England Journal of Medicine, 334:1077–1083.

Bogduk N (2005) Pain of cranial nerve origin other than primary neuralgias. In: Olesen J, Goadsby PJ, Ramadan NM, Tfelt-Hansen P (eds). The Headaches, 3rd edn. Philadelphia: Lippincott Williams and Wilkins. Chapter 126: 1043–1051.

Boivie J (2005) Central pain. In: SB McMahon, Koltzenburg M (eds). Wall and Melzack's Textbook of Pain, 5th edn. Amsterdam: Elsevier, Chapter 67: 1057–1074.

Costen JB (1934) A syndrome of ear and sinus symptoms dependent upon disturbed function of the temporomandibular joint. Annals of Rhinology and Laryngology, 43:1–15.

Devor M (2005) Response of nerves to injury in relation to pain. In: McMahon SB, Koltzenburg M (eds). Wall and Melzack's Textbook of Pain, 5th edn. Amsterdam: Elsevier, Chapter 58: 905–928.

Devor M, Amir R, Rappaport ZII (2002) Pathophysiology of trigeminal neuralgia: the ignition hypothesis. Clinical Journal of Pain, 18:4–13.

Eagle WW (1958) Elongated styloid process: symptoms and treatment. Archives of Otolaryngology, 67:172–176.

International Headache Society (1988). Classification and diagnostic criteria for headache disorders, cranial neuralgias and facial pain. Cephalalgia, 8(Suppl. 7):1–96.

International Headache Society (2004) The international classification of headache disorders. 2nd edn. Cephalalgia, 24(Suppl. 1):1–160.

Katusic S, Beard CM, Bergstralh E, Kurland LT (1990) Incidence and clinical features of trigeminal neuralgia, Rochester, Minnesota, 1945–1984. Annals of Neurology, 27:89–95.

Katusic S, Williams DB, Beard CM et al. (1991) Incidence and clinical features of glossopharyngeal neuralgia, Rochester, Minnesota, 1945–1984. Neuroepidemiology, 10:266–275.

Lance JW, Anthony M (1980) Neck tongue syndrome on sudden turning of the head. Journal of Neurology Neurosurgery and Psychiatry, 43:97–101.

Lopez BC, Hamlyn PJ, Zakrzewska JM (2004) Systematic review of ablative neurosurgical techniques for the treatment of trigeminal neuralgia. Neurosurgery, 54:973–982.

Nurmikko TJ, Jensen TS (2005) Trigeminal neuralgia and other facial neuralgias. In: Olesen J, Goadsby PJ, Ramadan NM, Tfelt-Hansen P (eds). The Headaches, 3rd edn. Philadelphia: Lippincott Williams and Wilkins, Chapter 127: 1053–1062.

Scadding JW (2009) Craniofacial pain. In: Donaghy M (ed.). Brain's Diseases of the Nervous System, 12th edn. Open University Press, Chapter 19: 499–514.

Scadding JW, Koltzenburg M (2005) Painful peripheral neuropathies. In: McMahon SB, Koltzenburg M (eds). Wall and Melzack's Textbook of Pain, 5th edn. Amsterdam: Elsevier, Chapter 62: 973–1000.

Wiffen P, McQuay HJ, Carroll D et al. (2000) Anticonvulsant drugs for acute and chronic pain. Cochrane Database of Systematic Reviews, (1):CD001133.

Zakrzewska JM, Harrison SD (2003) Facial pain. In: Jensen TS, Wilson PR, Rice ASC (eds). Clinical Pain Management: Chronic pain. London: Hodder Arnold, Chapter 37: 481–504.

Zakrzewska JM, Lopez BC (2004) Trigeminal neuralgia. Clinical Evidence, 11: 1755–1765.

CHAPTER 12

HEAD INJURY

Andrew McEvoy and Nick Losseff

EPIDEMIOLOGY

The estimated incidence of head injury is 430/100 000 of population. There are approximately one million patients in the UK who present to hospitals each year with head injuries. Males outnumber females by more than 2:1 and over 50 per cent of admitted patients are younger than 20 years. Of those patients with head injuries admitted to hospital, 2.5 per cent will die there. While 85 per cent of patients who sustain severe head injuries and 63 per cent of adult patients who sustain moderate head injuries remain disabled one year after their accident, patients with minor head injuries also have difficulties. Three months after sustaining mild head injuries, 79 per cent of patients have persistent headaches, 59 per cent have memory problems and 34 per cent are still unemployed. In fact, only 45 per cent of patients who have sustained a minor head injury have made a good recovery one year after admission.

While the most common cause of injury in developed countries is a road traffic accident, falls and assault are also frequent causes. Injuries at work or during sport and leisure are less common.

There are a number of associated factors – alcohol (38 per cent), drugs (7 per cent) and suicide (10 per cent). Preventive measures such as limiting alcohol consumption with driving, road improvements, speed control, better vehicle design (seats belts, airbags, windscreens), motorcycle/bicycle helmets, along with health and safety legislation in the workplace have led to a dramatic reduction in the number of serious head injuries.

Considerable progress has been made over the past 30 years in understanding the mechanisms involved in brain damage. In many series, the mortality of patients suffering a severe head injury has been reduced from 45 to 34 per cent, with a similar fall in morbidity.

The recognition of the need to deal with hypotension, hypoxia and hypercarbia, early evacuation of mass lesions and the development of modern principles of critical care have accounted for this, as well as a reduction in the number of vegetative survivors.

The major cause of death is primary brain damage, followed by multiple injuries, cerebral oedema and airway obstruction. These are the commonly recognized causes, the least common cause being intracranial haematomas.

PATHOPHYSIOLOGY OF BRAIN INJURY

The classical division of brain injury is into primary and secondary damage. This division is clinically useful.

Primary brain damage occurs at the time of the injury, produces its clinical effect immediately and has proved resistant to most treatments. **Secondary brain damage occurs some time after the primary impact and is largely preventable and treatable**. The importance of managing a head-injured patient is to recognize and document the primary brain damage and subsequently to prevent and treat secondary damage.

The pattern of brain injury following trauma is diverse. There may be focal cortical damage (e.g. after a blow to the head from a blunt instrument). Subdural and extradural haematoma may cause coning injury. Whereas a focal brain deficit is easily recognized and may dominate the clinical picture, all injuries also may produce a degree of diffuse injury to the brain. The underlying pathology of this is 'diffuse axonal injury' (DAI), resulting from acceleration/deceleration injury, and it is this that is responsible for contusional haematomas and deep white matter injury. This can be seen on t2* magnetic resonance imaging (MRI) as microhaemorrhage when it is invisible to other imaging sequences. The severity of this diffuse injury correlates with the degree of disturbance of consciousness. This should be separated from secondary injury (subdural/extradural) occurring at a later time point. The clinical effects of primary brain damage may be greatly aggravated by secondary brain damage. Diffuse axonal injury, contusions and lacerations of the brain will produce immediate clinical effects, varying from concussion with mild diffuse axonal injury, to coma and death.

The nature of progressive injury has three components:

1 Cytotoxic oedema, membrane damage and mitochondrial failure and inhibition of protein synthesis causing destruction of cells.

2 Microcirculatory disturbance leading to vasogenic oedema, loss of autoregulation and vasospasm.
3 Ischaemia, which develops in the injured brain around areas of haematoma, oedema, contusion and with local compression around mass lesions. This leads to focal ischaemia, high intracranial pressure (ICP), diminished cerebral perfusion pressure (CPP) and global ischaemia.

If global ischaemia as a result of raised ICP is associated for long periods with a low CPP (under 50 mmHg), then the mortality rate will be 90 per cent or more. The three main causes of brain ischaemia are:

1 Inadequacy of flow delivery.
2 Inadequacy of cerebral artery content of oxygen and substrate.
3 Inability of the brain to utilize oxygen, which is a cytotoxic problem.

The systemic secondary insults to be avoided/managed are listed in Box 12.1.

Pressure/volume relationship

The skull is a rigid compartment within which lies the brain, cerebrospinal fluid (CSF), blood and extracellular fluid. The volume within the cranial vault is constant and any increase in volume results in an increase in ICP. The relationship between the pressure and volume is expressed in Figure 12.1. The major intracranial volumes are brain parenchyma (1200–1600 mL), blood (100–150 mL) and CSF (100–150 mL). The latter two constitute about 20 per cent of total intracranial volume and part of each is capable of rapid extracranial displacement. An ini-

Box 12.1 Effects of hypoxia and hypotension on the outcome of brain injury (reprinted from Gentleman and Jennett, 1981, with permission from Elsevier)

Hypoxia
Hypotension
Hypercapnia
Hypocapnia
Hyperthermia
Hyperglycaemia
Hypoglycaemia
Hyponatraemia
Hypoproteinaemia

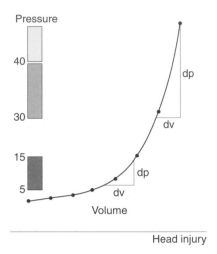

Head injury

Figure 12.1 Pressure–volume curve (see text).

tial increase in intracranial volume is compensated for by squeezing venous blood through the jugular veins or through the emissary and scalp veins. CSF is displaced through the foramen magnum into the spinal subarachnoid space. When compensatory mechanisms fail, minute changes in volume produce large changes in pressure. There is compression of brain tissue with herniation of the brain and a decrease in cerebral blood flow (CBF). The redistribution of the CSF and venous blood have little pathological consequence, but a reduction in CBF and the occurrence of brain herniation results in cerebral ischaemia and secondary cerebral damage.

Intracranial pressure

The normal range of ICP is 0–10 mmHg. Raised ICP in the head-injured patient is associated with increased mortality. Patients whose ICP remains between 0 and 20 mmHg have a mortality rate of 23 per cent while those whose pressures rise above 60 mmHg have a 100 per cent mortality. It seems likely that the level of ICP is not as important as its effect on CPP. The current consensus is to treat ICP exceeding 20 mmHg.

Continuous ICP monitoring is used to optimize CPP in comatose patients. ICP is best measured directly and continuously from the cranial cavity. There are two options in contemporary practice. First, it can be measured from a ventricular catheter. The advantage of this is that it can be used as a treatment modality allowing continuous drainage

of CSF, when the pressure exceeds physiological limits. Antibiotic and silver impregnated catheters may reduce the risk of infection. The second method is a fibreoptic transducer-tipped catheter system. Newer technologies allow the simultaneous acquisition of brain temperature, brain tissue oxygenation and cerebral microdialysis. Multimodal monitoring allows the determination of cerebral autoregulation with the goal of better MAP management. The challenge is to find a therapeutic manoeuvre that can improve cerebral autoregulation and assess the effect of such therapy on outcome.

Infection and haemorrhage associated with the placement of devices is rare, but aggressive CPP-driven protocols can result in severe cardiorespiratory complications without improving neurological outcome. There is a physiological basis for ICP-guided treatment, but there is an argument that randomized controlled trials are still to demonstrate benefit. In the absence of ICP monitoring however, late increases in the ICP in the sedated patient could only be detected by papillary dilatation or the hypertension associated with the Cushing response, making early intervention impossible. ICP monitoring not only guides medical treatment, but also triggers prompt imaging and timely evacuation of space occupying lesions, preventing surgical delays and secondary brain injury. Non-invasive methods of measuring ICP are being validated.

Cerebral perfusion pressure

This is equal to the mean blood pressure minus the mean ICP. Normally within a range of CPP of 60–160 mmHg, CBF remains constant. However, in brain injury, this autoregulatory relationship may be altered by a number of factors.

Cerebral perfusion pressure is equivalent to the transmural pressure across the cerebral vessel walls; at the arteriolar level, CPP is the stimulus for the autoregulatory response, and at the capillary level is the driving force for fluid exchange.

There are a number of observational studies with the general consensus that maintaining the CPP at 70 mmHg may be associated with a decrease in head injury morbidity and mortality. **Evidence shows that aggressive action in the head-injured patient to maintain normal blood volume or induced systemic hypertension to maintain a CPP of 70 mmHg has no deleterious effect on ICP, morbidity or mortality.**

In managing a head-injured patient, attention must be paid to both ICP and CPP. ICP control has been the primary goal in order to improve CPP and CBF. Initial steps involve simple measures such as relieving and restriction to cerebral venous drainage and head elevation, sedation and muscle relaxation, draining CSF and mild hyperventilation. Second tier management strategy involves hyperosmolar therapy to decrease cerebral oedema, moderate hyperventilation, suppression of electrical activity, induced hypothermia, and decompressive craniotomy.

Cerebral blood flow and head injury

CBF is affected by arterial PaO_2; an arterial PaO_2 of below 7 kPa produces an increase in CBF. Variations in arterial $PaCO_2$ can also cause marked changes in CBF because CO_2 is a very potent vasodilator. If the $PaCO_2$ is increased above 6 kPa, CBF increases, while it falls if the $PaCO_2$ drops below 4 kPa. The maintenance of CBF in response to various changes has been termed autoregulation and this may be impaired by ischaemia, hypoxia or brain trauma. Cerebral blood flow is the critical factor in terms of function and survival. The mean hemispheric CBF is about 55 mL/100 g per minute. A CBF of below 18 mL/100 g per minute is the threshold for global ischaemia and infarction will occur if these levels are sustained for more than 1–3 hours. While CPP would have to fall to 40 mmHg in the normal brain before CBF fell, following trauma a CPP of 50 mmHg would indicate a low CBF.

Shift and distortion

Expanding lesions in head-injured patients produce a well-established sequence of events. The ventricle on the side of the expanding lesion becomes smaller and, with distortion and compression of the third ventricle, dilatation of the opposite ventricle occurs.

If the uncus of the temporal lobe is pushed through the tentorial edge, the third cranial nerve and the posterior cerebral artery are compressed causing a third nerve palsy and a homonymous hemianopia.

A computed tomography (CT) scan shows the disappearance of the subarachnoid space in the supratentorial compartment with loss of the basal cisterns (Figure 12.2a,b); crowding of the brainstem in the tentorial hiatus occurs. Central areas of the brain are pushed in a downwards axial direction towards the foramen magnum, and coning occurs. The compression of the midbrain produces ischaemia of central areas, leading to a loss of consciousness and increasing neurological signs.

MEDICAL MANAGEMENT OF THE HEAD-INJURED PATIENT

There is a trimodal distribution of death after injury. The first peak occurs within seconds or minutes of the injury, the second peak is within several hours as a result of subdural/extradural haematomas, pneumothorax, abdominal injuries including ruptured spleen, pelvic fractures and other conditions leading to hypovolaemia and hypotension. The final peak happens several days to weeks after the injury and is caused by sepsis or multiple organ failure. The most important treatment area lies within the second peak and is termed the 'golden hour'. However, minutes count and it is now recognized that the first 20 minutes after an injury can be the most vital.

During the pre-hospital phase, the prime aim is to reduce any initial hypoxic/ischaemic damage using principles of resuscitation that have been set out in the advanced trauma life support system (ATLS – American College of Surgeons, 1993). This phase (primary survey) requires a major emphasis on airway maintenance, control of external bleeding and shock, immobilization and immediate transfer to the closest and most appropriate hospital.

The effects of hypotension and hypoxia need to be fully recognized. There is increased morbidity and mortality if the systolic blood pressure drops below 90 mmHg. The effects of hypoxia and hypotension on the outcome of head injury are shown in Table 12.1. Only in the terminal stages of medullary failure is the hypotension due to the head injury itself. More commonly, it is a marker of severe blood loss.

Resuscitation takes place with the airway secured and, if necessary, the patient intubated, paralysed and ventilated. It is critical to keep

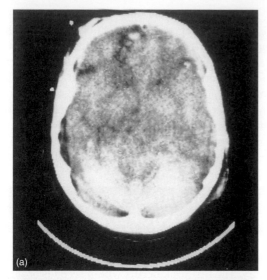

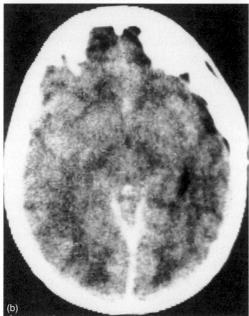

Figure 12.2 (a) and (b) CT brain scans showing raised intracranial pressure with the loss of basal cisterns.

systolic blood pressure above 90 mmHg, PaO_2 at a minimum of 9 kPa and a $PaCO_2$ maintained between 3.5 and 4.0 kPa. Venous access is achieved and volume replacement carried out if necessary. Electrocardiogram monitoring, pulse oximetry and blood pressure monitoring should be instituted. In addition, the patient's level of consciousness needs to be recorded and this is undertaken using the Glasgow Coma Scale (GCS). In the hospital emergency department, the second phase of assessment (secondary survey) is undertaken. The airway is maintained with continued control of the cervical spine. Breathing and ventilation are maintained. Circulation is maintained and haemorrhage is controlled. The patient is completely undressed and the conscious level documented. **The most important clinical assessment is the post–resuscitation GCS which is subsequently measured at regular intervals.**

Guidelines

In 2007, the National Institute for Health and Clinical Excellence (NICE) published UK guidance on the assessment, investigation and early management of head injury. This was an update of earlier recommendations where there has been a significant shift from 'admit and observe' to 'diagnose and decide'.

The guideline offers best practice for the care of all patients who present with a suspected or confirmed traumatic brain injury (TBI), with or without other major trauma, and includes separate advice for adults and children.

All patients who have sustained a head injury (HI) should be transported directly to a facility with the necessary resources to resuscitate, investigate and initially manage multiple injuries.

Table 12.1 Effects of hypoxia and hypotension on the outcome of brain injury. Reprinted from Gentleman and Jennett, 1981, with permission from Elsevier

	Patients (*n*)	Dead (%)	Good recovery (%)
Hypoxia and hypotension	5	100	0
Hypotension only	12	75	8
Hypoxia only	29	59	17
Neither factor	104	34	34

All patients presenting to an emergency department with a head injury should be assessed by a trained member of staff within 15 minutes. CT imaging of the head must be performed and analysed within 1 hour of the decision to scan.

The report also provides detailed guidance of specialized radiological imaging of the spine in head injury patients.

If the patient requires hospital admission they must be admitted under a team led by a consultant who has been trained in the management of HI during higher specialist training.

Criteria for hospital admission

- Patients with new, clinically significant abnormalities on imaging
- Patients who have not returned to GCS 15 after imaging, regardless of imaging results
- When the patient fulfils the criteria for CT scanning but this cannot be done within the appropriate period, because CT is not available or because the patient is not cooperative
- Continuing worrying signs (e.g. persistent vomiting, severe headache) of concern to the clinician
- Other sources of concern such as drug or alcohol intoxication, other injuries, shock, suspected non accidental injury, meningism and CSF leak.

For patients admitted for observation, the minimum acceptable documented neurological observations are: GCS, pupil size and reactivity, limb movements, respiratory rate, heart rate, blood pressure (BP), temperature and oxygen saturation. Observations should be performed half-hourly until GCS returns to 15. The minimum frequency of observations for patients with GCS equal to 15 is:
- half-hourly for 2 hours;
- then 1-hourly for 4 hours;
- then 2-hourly thereafter.

X-rays and imaging

In patients after major trauma, the initial plain x-rays should include a lateral cervical spine, chest and pelvis. Once all life-threatening injuries have been treated, further views of the cervical, thoracic and lumbar spine may be necessary.

Indications for CT brain scanning in adults are:
- GCS <13 on initial assessment;
- GCS <15 2 hours after the injury;
- suspected open or depressed skull fracture;
- any sign of basal skull fracture;
- post-traumatic seizure;
- focal neurological deficit;
- one or more episodes of vomiting;
- amnesia for event more than 30 minutes before impact.

Indications for CT brain scanning in children are:
- age over one year: GCS <14 on initial assessment;
- age under one year: GCS paediatric <15 on initial assessment;
- age under one year and presence of bruise, swelling or laceration (>5 cm) on head;
- dangerous mechanism of injury;
- clinical suspicion of non-accidental injury;
- loss of consciousness lasting more than 5 minutes;
- post-traumatic seizure but no history of epilepsy;
- abnormal drowsiness;
- suspected open or depressed skull fracture, or tense fontanelle;
- any sign of basal skull fracture;
- focal neurological deficit;
- three or more episodes of vomiting;
- amnesia (antegrade or retrograde) lasing more than 5 minutes.

All patients with skull fractures should be detained in hospital for observation and should undergo CT scanning prior to discharge. A patient who remains drowsy for 24 hours or more should be scanned before discharge. It is important to be aware that an early CT scan (within 6 hours) may have to be repeated to exclude a developing/enlarging haematoma in a patient failing to recover, or if there is a deteriorating level of consciousness.

Guidelines for transfer to regional neurosurgical unit

Local guidelines on the interhospital transfer of patients with HI should be drawn up between referring hospitals, the neurosurgical unit (NSU) and the local ambulance service. These should recognize the merit of transferring all patients with serious HI (GCS <8), irrespective of their need for neurosurgery. If transfer of those who do not require neurosurgery is not possible, ongoing liaison with the NSU over clinical management is essential.

There should be a designated consultant in the referring hospital with responsibility for establishing arrangements for the transfer of patients with HI to the NSU and another consultant at the NSU with responsibility for establishing arrangements for communication with referring hospitals and for receipt of patients transferred.

> Patients with HI requiring emergency transfer to a NSU should be accompanied by a doctor with appropriate training and experience in the transfer of patients with TBI. The doctor should be familiar with the pathophysiology of HI, the drugs and equipment they will use and with working in the confines of an ambulance or helicopter. They should have a dedicated and adequately trained assistant. They should be provided with appropriate clothing, medical indemnity and personal accident insurance. Patients requiring non-emergency transfer should be accompanied by appropriate clinical staff. The transfer team should be provided with a means of communication with their base hospital and the NSU during the transfer.
>
> **The patient must be resuscitated and stabilized before transfer. It is imperative that continued intensive care should continue during transfer**. A key factor in the success of a transfer is that any previous insult (hypotension, hypoxia) is predictive of further problems. Insults before and during transfer, leading to greater problems after transfer, will increase morbidity and mortality.

In the UK currently only a small proportion (3–5 per cent) of head-injured patients are transferred to a NSU, usually because of a deteriorating level of consciousness, progressive focal neurological deficits, the detection of recognized risk factors for developing intracranial haematoma or their confirmation by local CT imaging, or because of specific complications requiring neurosurgical intervention (e.g. CSF leak, depressed fracture).

Mannitol

In patients who develop a fixed dilated pupil and there is concern that this relates to a mass lesion or raised ICP, it is common practice to give a bolus of 200 mL of 20 per cent mannitol. The hyperosmolar effect of osmotic diuretics causes a transient increase in intravascular volume. However, diuresis is induced which may cause hypotension in a partially compensated multi-trauma victim. Thus, osmotic diuretics must be used judiciously to prevent the potential beneficial effects of lowering ICP being offset by hypotension and inadequate cerebral perfusion. Serum osmolarity should not be allowed to go above 320 mOsm/L to avoid systemic acidosis and renal failure.

MANAGEMENT OF SPECIFIC COMPLICATIONS OF HEAD INJURY

Skull fracture

The frequency of skull fractures increases with the severity of the TBI. A linear vault fracture significantly increases the risk of intracranial haematoma. Thus, the detection of a skull fracture generally warrants admission to hospital for observation. Clinical signs such as orbital haematoma, CSF rhinorrhoea/otorrhoea, haemotympanum or Battle's sign (bruising over the mastoid process) should be taken as presumptive evidence of a basal skull fracture.

Depressed skull fracture

Simple depressed skull fractures

Surgical elevation should be considered if the injury is cosmetically disfiguring, the depressed fragment has significant mass effect or there is an underlying haematoma. However, this approach needs to be modified if the simple depression is located over a major venous sinus. A skull fracture is considered significantly depressed if the outer table of the skull lies below the inner table of the surrounding bone.

Compound depressed or comminuted skull fractures

Surgery for patients with compound depressed or comminuted skull fractures is initially local wound closure after thorough cleaning and removal of foreign bodies. The surgical requirement is to achieve haemostasis and prevent infection. If there is no dural laceration, this may well be the definitive treatment. However, definitive surgery must be performed as soon as possible if there is a suspected dural laceration, intracranial haematoma or moderate to severe wound contamination.

Complications as a result of a depressed fracture include intracranial infection (meningitis or an intracerebral abscess) and epilepsy. Up to 30 per cent of patients with a depressed skull fracture develop epilepsy if the dura is torn or if there is an associated cortical contusion or laceration.

Haematomas

Extradural haematoma

Typically, extradural haematoma (EDH) may arise after a mild injury and more than half the patients with this complication are under the age of 20 years; it is rare after the age of 40 years (Figure 12.3). It is also rare before the age of two years when trauma tends to indent the more pliable skull and dura together so damage tends to occur to the brain and haematomas are subdural. In infants, the large head size relative to the body means that the volume of the extradural space is large in relation to the blood volume, so hypovolaemia may be the primary presenting feature with an EDH. In an adult, the blow causes the dura to become separated from the skull immediately below the point of impact and this is where the clot forms. They most commonly occur in the temporal region. Bleeding commonly arises from a torn middle meningeal artery but may also be venous. EDH is rare, with only 0.5 per cent of head-injured patients admitted to hospital developing the condition.

Acute subdural haematomas

Acute subdural haematoma (ASDH) is relatively common (Figure 12.4), occurring at any age, and tending to occur following more severe impact

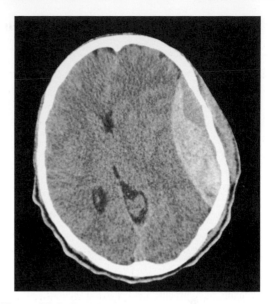

Figure 12.3 CT brain showing a large acute extradural haematoma, with marked midline shift. Courtesy of Dr Andrew MacKinnon, Consultant Neuroradiologist, St George's Hospital, London.

The single most important clinical feature is deterioration in the level of consciousness or occasionally a period of increasing restlessness. EDHs are extracerebral lesions and there may be little or no primary brain damage so that initially consciousness may recover before further deterioration in conscious level occurs, the so-called 'lucid interval'. To wait for the classic textbook description of a unilateral dilated pupil, hemiparesis, slow pulse and rise in blood pressure is to accept a high morbidity and mortality. The mortality rate is 10 per cent or less.

---

damage than occurs with EDH. Morbidity and mortality tend to be higher.

There are two common causes of traumatic ASDH. A haematoma may accumulate around a parenchymal laceration, usually frontal or temporal lobe with a severe underlying primary brain injury. Patients are more likely to present in coma in contrast to EDH and there is no 'lucid interval'. The second cause is as a result of the tearing of veins bridging the extradural space during violent head motion. In this case, primary brain damage is less severe and a lucid interval may occur followed by rapid deterioration. **Acute subdural haematoma**

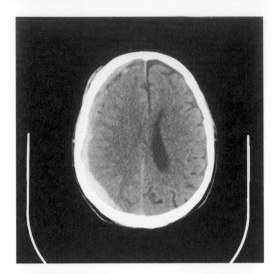

Figure 12.4 CT brain showing an acute right subdural haematoma, with effacement of the lateral ventricle and some midline shift.

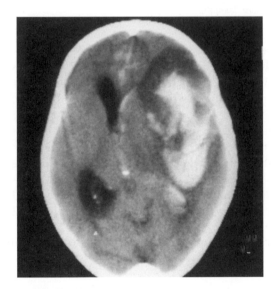

Figure 12.5 CT brain scan showing a traumatic intracerebral haematoma.

may also occur in patients receiving anticoagulation therapy, often following only minor trauma. In 15–20 per cent of cases, the haematoma may be bilateral and about 50 per cent are associated with a skull fracture. Brain scanning with CT establishes the diagnosis. Factors indicating the need for an operation include the size of the haematoma, the degree of midline shift, obliteration of the third ventricle or basal cisterns and dilatation of the con-

tralateral ventricle. ASDH often carries a poor prognosis because of delay in diagnosis and because of the severity of the underlying brain damage. The mortality rate is often over 50 per cent, with an associated high morbidity. The treatment is urgent surgical evacuation via a craniotomy.

Traumatic intracerebral haemorrhage

Traumatic intracerebral haemorrhage (ICH) may be related to cerebral contusion or result from penetrating injuries (Figure 12.5). The haematoma may remain within the parenchyma, or burst into the ventricles or extracerebral spaces. Serial CT scans show that after 24–72 hours, these haematomas are commonly surrounded by an area of oedema. Increasing mass effect will lead to a rise in ICP and a decrease in CPP and ultimately CBF. Much of the appearance on CT of the area around the haematoma is the result of ischaemia, and, although surgical removal of the mass will reduce ICP, it will do little to relieve the ischaemic neuronal damage. Surgical management will be to protect the patient from the harmful effects of raised ICP but is unlikely to improve neurological deficits. Controversy surrounds whether surgery or conservative treatment offers the best prognosis for patients with ICH. The results of the STICH (Spontaneous Supratentorial ICH) trial showed no overall benefit of conservative initial treatment over early surgery.

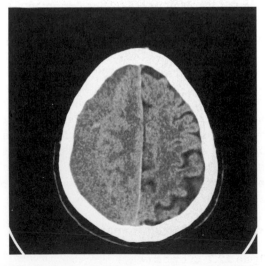

Figure 12.6 CT brain showing an isodense right subdural haematoma.

Chronic subdural haematomas

Head injury is identified in less than 50 per cent of adults who present with a chronic subdural haematoma (CSDH) and the injury is usually mild. There are a number of risk factors including cerebral atrophy, alcoholism, epilepsy, CSF shunts and coagulopathies, including patients on anticoagulant therapy, and patients with a tendency to fall.

There is a tendency for CSDH to occur in **older people** with a male preponderance. Most CSDHs are seen in the parietal region, the majority are unilateral with **20–25 per cent of cases being bilateral**. Patients usually present with minor symptoms of headache, often accompanied by a change in personality, variable drowsiness or confusion, and a hemiparesis. While it is often emphasized that major fluctuations in consciousness and neurological signs are characteristic features in CSDH, these signs only occur in about one-third of patients. A CT scan will usually show a CSDH, although isodense lesions may be difficult to identify (Figures 12.6 and 12.7), particularly if there are bilateral CSDH, in which case there may be no midline shift. A CSDH is usually drained through one or two burr holes, although in a few cases if the haematoma is clotted or multilocular, a craniotomy may be required.

Cerebrospinal fluid leaks

Traumatic CSF leaks occur in adults in about 2 per cent of closed head injuries. The risk of CSF leak is especially high in penetrating head injuries, where a frequency of 9 per cent has been reported. Traumatic CSF leaks usually appear within the first 48 hours after injury but can develop several years later.

Rhinorrhoea (via the nose) is the most common type of CSF leak. The fluid can be confirmed as CSF if the glucose level is greater than 30 mg %, identified using a dipstick. β_2-transferrin is present in CSF but is absent in tears, saliva, nasal secretion and is a useful test to employ if there is doubt. Most cases of CSF rhinorrhoea (70 per cent) stop within 1 week and the remainder usually by six months. The great risk is meningitis and the incidence is around 5–10 per cent. This increases if the leak persists for more than 7 days. In a long-term study of patients who had CSF leaks that were not repaired, 80 per cent developed meningitis over a 20-year period. Leaks of CSF should be identified and the fistula repaired if possible. The exception is CSF otorrhoea (via the ear), which usually stops spontaneously within 3 weeks. An operation is only required for persistent CSF otorrhoea.

Conscious patients are nursed head up to reduce the intracranial CSF pressure. There is no evidence supporting the use of prophylactic antibiotics.

The fistula can be localized in patients with CSF rhinorrhoea with CT, using 2 mm slices and bone windows in axial and coronal planes. Intrathecal contrast is only of value in patients with an active CSF leak. MRI scanning using T2 sequences and coronal cuts may reveal a protrusion of the subarachnoid space through an unsuspected bony defect.

Attention must be paid to the risks of passing nasal tubes (nasotracheal or nasogastric) in multitrauma patients suspected of having skull base fractures. There have been several dramatic reports of intracranial penetration of such tubes through areas of bony disruption in the anterior fossa.

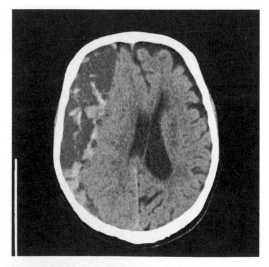

Figure 12.7 CT brain showing a right chronic subdural haematoma (SDH), together with some fresh blood (acute on chronic SDH). There is marked midline shift.

Traumatic aerocoele

Air may enter the skull after basal fractures. The air may be subarachnoid, subdural, intraventricular or intracerebral. Urgent decompression may be required if the aerocoele is responsible for a clinical deterioration, but usually a delayed dural repair is required after the patient has recovered from the acute effects of the head injury.

Craniofacial repair

Complex disruption of the craniofacial skeleton with associated cerebral and ophthalmological problems may result from severe head injury. Close cooperation between neurosurgeons, maxillofacial surgeons and ophthalmologists is required. CT scanning with bone windows in axial and coronal planes is necessary to visualize fractures of the anterior cranial fossa, orbit, skull base and facial skeleton. Three-dimensional CT scans are particularly useful in some complex cases.

Hydrocephalus

Acute obstructive hydrocephalus may develop secondary to a posterior fossa haematoma that obstructs the ventricular pathways or intraventricular haematoma. However, delayed hydrocephalus is far more common, occurring in 6 per cent of severe head-injured patients. This communicating hydrocephalus results from blood in the subarachnoid space. Ventriculoperitoneal shunting is the surgical solution.

Decompressive craniectomy

Patients with a variety of intracranial disorders (TBI, stroke, ICH, etc.) present with increased ICP leading to clinical deterioration and ultimately death. Decompressive craniectomy with durotomy has been shown to decrease ICP and is widely used in coma producing TBI. There is no evidence, however, of an association with better clinical outcome. Indeed, the recently reported Decompressive Craniectomy (DECRA) trial showed worse clinical outcomes in the surgical arm despite clinically lower ICP and fewer days on the ICU. Decompressive craniectomy shifted survivors from a favourable outcome to an unfavourable outcome (i.e. dependence on assistance to complete activities of daily living). The Randomized Evaluation of Surgery with Craniectomy for Uncontrollable Elevation of ICP (RESCUEicp) trial continues to recruit and its results are eagerly anticipated.

Hypothermia

Therapeutic hypothermia has been used to treat acute diseases of the CNS for over 60 years. Hypothermia is thought to suppress the cascade of physiological and metabolic events that result in the cytotoxic, oxidative and inflammatory injury that follows initial TBI. Surface cooling, intravascular cooling with coils and rapid intravenous infusion of cold fluids are employed. The best available evidence supports the use of mild to moderate (32–34°C) hypothermia in patients with severe TBI (GCS <=8) to decrease mortality and improve rates of good neurological recovery. Maximal benefit occurs when cooling was continued for at least 72 hours or until normalization of ICP. Avoiding temperatures below 30°C reduces the risks of serious medical complications, especially hypothermia-induced hypotension. The North American Brain Injury Study: Hypothermia IIR (NABIS:H IIR) is a randomized clinical trial enrolling 240 patients with severe brain injury between 16 and 45 years. It is due to report in 2012.

Corticosteroids

The CRASH (Corticosteroid Randomization after Significant Head Injury) trial tested whether high dose methylprednisolone sodium succinate (MPSS) administered within 8 hours of injury improved survival and outcome. Metanalysis of previously underpowered studies had suggested efficacy. CRASH planned to randomize 20 000 patients but was stopped early when mortality was greater in the MPSS-treated cohort.

NEUROLOGICAL ASPECTS OF HEAD INJURY

Considerable emphasis is given to the immediate management of head injury, mostly focused on neurosurgical aspects and specifically how to identify patients in need of decompression to prevent brain herniation. Patients with HI have often been managed (for example in the UK) through general surgical admission pathways and only to neurosurgeons if necessary. They may frequently return in an impaired state to general surgical units. Patients may then be discharged to the community or to rehabilitation facilities. There remains a void in HI treatment during and following this acute phase, and this is often not recognized by clinicians because of its predominantly cognitive presentation. Some healthcare providers have filled this void by establishing 'acute brain injury units' where further medical management is carried out using an identical principle of care to acute stroke units and filling the gap between the acute situation and early rehabilitation.

> Cognitive impairments dominate post HI, however, three-quarters of severely head injured patients have obvious physical impairment. A hemiparesis may result from a coning injury, generalized spasticity from a severe diffuse injury, quadraparesis from a brainstem injury. Loss of smell/taste is common, individual cranial nerve palsies may occur and visual impairment from ocular/oculomotor/optic nerve trauma are all possible. In some patients, a fistula may form between the carotid and the cavernous sinus (carotico-cavernous fistula) resulting in acute proptosis, chemosis of the orbit with progressive visual failure.

Vestibular damage is particularly common, and after minor head injury can accompany migrainous headache and memory difficulty. Head injury can also result in benign positional vertigo due to dislodgement of crystals into the semicircular canals. This can be detected with a Hallpike manoeuvre and is not to be missed as an Epley manoeuvre can be curative (see Chapter 3). With more fixed vestibular damage, habituation needs to take place and may be promoted by vestibular rehabilitation. In addition to vestibular failure, conductive deafness due to tympanic perforation/haemotympanum or sensineural deafness may occur.

Post-traumatic amnesia

The immediate consequence of diffuse primary injury is a confusional state (loss of orientation and awareness) and this dominates the clinical picture before fixed cognitive and behavioural consequences become apparent. This phase is termed 'post-traumatic amnesia' (PTA) and is the period following HI in which working memory fails. The length of PTA is an important measure of diffuse injury severity. Retrograde amnesia (the period before the injury) is of less use. The GCS also provides a useful initial measure of head injury severity and allows TBI to be graded as mild (admission GCS 13–15), moderate (GCS 9–12) or severe (GCS 8 or less).

The clinical picture of a patient in PTA is that of confusion, disorientation and agitation, with a disordered sleep wake cycle. PTA can be measured using specific scales or by simple bedside tests of orientation and attention. The management of PTA is to nurse the patient in a calm environment reducing external stimulation to a minimum, deal with agitation by reassurance and distraction and provide a structured day/environment. These are predominantly nursing issues. All too often the agitated, combative and highly mobile patient is dealt with using sedative drugs, although there is a role in some patients for regular carbamazepine (up to 800 mg per day) or newer antipsychotic agents (e.g. olanzapine 5–10 mg bd) if behavioural measures fail. The extreme of PTA is such profound agitation that the patient needs nursing on a mattressed floor for some weeks.

Cognitive and psychiatric impairment

Cognitive function becomes assessable when PTA has resolved. Attention, memory and executive function (the ability to plan) are preferentially affected. These need assessing by a skilled neuropsychologist and usually dominate the long-term picture after severe HI. Behavioural problems go hand in hand with these cognitive difficulties, with a spectrum from dangerous impulsive behaviour to mild personality change (e.g. irritability, aggression). It is not to be forgotten that a patient fresh out of PTA who claims to be fine may happily cross a road without looking. Depression and post-traumatic stress disorder is common and may accompany these behavioural problems.

Minor head injury and post-concussional syndrome

Post-concussional syndrome is characterized by multiple symptoms with little or no neurological signs. In the vast majority of cases, the head injury is minor. The incidence is uncertain but it is a common reason for consultation in a general neurology practice.

Headache, dizziness and tiredness are the three most common symptoms. Other troublesome symptoms include cognitive (lack of concentration, memory impairment), affective (irritability), reduced libido, sensitivity to light and noise, insomnia, anxiety and depression. The number of symptoms and their severity tend to change with time. In most patients, symptoms improve over three months but in a minority the symptom complex remains static or deteriorates (20 per cent persist at one year).

The headache may be generalized or localized and is often related to the site of injury or impact. It is most common in the younger age group and in women. It is inversely related to the severity of the injury. The headache is often migrainous in character (associated with sensory dislike). Dizziness may be described as giddiness, faintness or unsteadiness. Problems with short-term memory are also common. Poor concentration and depression frequently occur. Depression often appears worse with minor injuries, and sometimes may be linked with the premorbid state of the patient. Many of the symptoms of the post-concussional syndrome amount to a true reactive depression. When litigation or compensation is involved, symptoms are more likely to persist longer than 12 months, often accompanied by depression, stress and chronic pain.

The diagnosis is usually one of exclusion, which can usually be made confidently on the basis of the history and negative clinical findings. Special investigations such as CT or MRI scanning are of little value but do provide reassurance.

Epilepsy

There is no indication for preventative anticonvulsants following head injury. A study by Annegers on the prospective risk of seizures following brain injury shows that severity is key. Brain contusion and subdural haematoma pose particular risks. The evolving risk across the population, in this study, is summarized in Figure 12.8.

> The overall incidence of post-traumatic epilepsy in unselected head injuries, including mainly closed head injuries, is about 3–5 per cent. The incidence rises with open injuries to 8–9 per cent and in penetrating head injuries epileptic seizures may occur in 50 per cent of patients.

Post-traumatic epilepsy is usually divided into early, with seizures starting within the first week after injury, and late with seizures starting after 1 week or more. After mild head injuries (patients with no skull fractures and PTA of less than 30 minutes), the risk of late seizures is 0.1 per cent after one year and 0.6 per cent after five years – similar to the risk of developing epilepsy in the general population.

Early epilepsy occurs in 2–5 per cent of TBI patients who are admitted to hospital. Early seizures are focal in 50 per cent of cases. Early epilepsy has a higher incidence if consciousness has been lost for more than 24 hours (11–14 per cent), if a linear fracture is present (2–7 per cent), and if there is a depressed fracture (10–11 per cent). The incidence rises to 45 per cent in subdural or intracerebral haematomas.

Late epilepsy also occurs in about 5 per cent of TBI patients who are admitted. The incidence is higher in penetrating injury (53 per cent), intracerebral haematoma (39 per cent), focal brain damage seen on an early CT scan (32 per cent), following

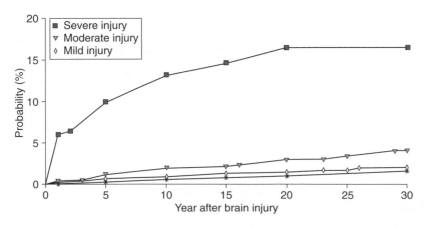

Figure 12.8 Probability of developing epilepsy, up to 30 years after mild, moderate and severe head injury. Reproduced with permission from *N Engl J Med* 1998; 338: 20-4. © 1998 Massachusetts Medical Society.

early epilepsy (25 per cent), depressed fracture/torn dura (25 per cent), extradural/subdural haemorrhage (20 per cent) and if the PTA is longer than 24 hours.

Early seizures are more common in children, particularly those under the age of five years. Children younger than 16 years are less likely to develop late epilepsy after depressed skull fractures than adults. In addition, late epilepsy may develop after a longer interval in children than in adults.

In the acute emergency situation, drugs which can be given parenterally, and which achieve therapeutic plasma levels rapidly, are most appropriate (e.g. phenytoin, phenobarbitone). In the long-term treatment of post-traumatic epilepsy, there is no evidence to suggest a differential effectiveness of the common anticonvulsants. No reliable information is available on the optimum duration of anticonvulsant treatment for post-traumatic epilepsy. Patients have a high risk for relapse if a focal brain injury has been defined. Approximately 50 per cent of patients with post-traumatic epilepsy will be in complete remission 15 years after injury.

Systemic problems

Marked weight loss from insufficient feeding and the secondary hypercatabolic state may complicate severe injury and oral feeding may be prevented by dysphagia, a tracheostomy or behavioural problems. Initial management may require PEG feeding. Malnutrition may itself then predispose to pressure sores which are avoidable with adequate nursing. Patients may later gain excessive weight and this can be correlated with endocrine dysfunction. Heterotopic ossification may occur next to large joints causing pain.

REHABILITATION

Because of the diverse impairment seen after TBI, rehabilitation can be complex. The acute stage is characterized by the management of PTA and very importantly the prevention of complications, for example contractures from spasticity, which may lock a patient into their body and take years to release. One of the most puzzling problems with the treatment of brain damage is the heterogeneous nature of recovery. Motivation, cognitive and behavioural problems in patients with brain injury seem to be a biological issue that is affected by existing cognitive and social skills.

Rehabilitation is a multidisciplinary and specialized process. There is a recognition that if it is to be successful, it needs to be started early and so minimize the development of physical and behavioural complications.

OUTCOME

There are a number of predictors of outcome after severe head injury, including the GCS after resuscitation, the pupillary responses, age, ICP and the intracranial diagnosis on CT scanning.

After a severe head injury, overall mortality at six months is 36 per cent in patients looked after in NSUs experienced in and committed to the care of head-injured patient. In non-specialist units, head injury mortality varies from 43 per cent less than expected to more than 52 per cent greater than expected. These differences are largely explained by variation in the outcome of patients with a low risk of death and not in the high risk group. There is, therefore, a compelling argument that neurosurgical assessment and supervision are as important for the less severely injured patient as for the severely injured one.

There is increasing recognition that real world outcomes after TBI require assessment beyond the Glasgow Outcome Score. An assessment of neurocognitive, social and emotional deficits can provide a better characterization of the burden of residual morbidity, while providing important therapeutic targets.

REFERENCES AND FURTHER READING

Bracken MB (2005) CRASH (Corticosteroid Randomization after Significant Head Injury Trial): landmark and storm warning. *Neurosurgery*, 57:1300–1302.

Fox JL, Vu EN, Doyle-Waters M *et al.* (2010) Prophylactic hypothermia for traumatic brain injury: a quantitative systematic review. *CJEM*, 12:355–364.

Cooper DJ, Rosenfeld JV, Murray L *et al.* (2011) Decompressive craniectomy in diffuse traumatic brain injury. *New England Journal of Medicine*, 364:1493–1502.

Gentleman D, Jennett B (1981) Hazards of inter-hospital transfer of comatose head-injured patients. *Lancet* 2:853–854.

Greenwood RJ (2002) Head injury for neurologists. *Journal of Neurology, Neurosurgery, and Psychiatry*, **73**:i8–i16.

Lavinio A, Menon DK (2011) Intracranial pressure: why we monitor it, how to monitor it, what to do with the number and what's the future? *Current Opinion in Anaesthesiology*, **24**:117–123.

McMillan TM, Greenwood RJ (2003) Head injury rehabilitation. In: Greenwood R, Barnes MP, McMillan TM, Ward CD (eds). *Handbook of Neurological Rehabilitation*. London: Psychology Press, 465–486.

Nortje J, Menon DK (2004) Traumatic brain injury: physiology, mechanisms, and outcome. *Current Opinion in Neurology*, **17**:711–718.

Yates D, Aktar R, Hill J (2007) Assessment, investigation, and early management of head injury: summary of NICE guidance. *BMJ*, **335**:719–720.

CHAPTER 13

EPILEPSY AND SLEEP DISORDERS

Matthew Walker and Ley Sander

EPILEPSY – INTRODUCTION AND CLASSIFICATION

> **Epileptic seizure**
>
> An epileptic seizure ('ictus') is a synchronous and excessive discharge of neurones in the cerebral cortex causing a clinically discernible event. The clinical manifestations of a seizure depend on where in the cortex it begins, and the speed and extent of its spread. Epileptic seizures frequently have a sudden onset and, in most instances, cease spontaneously. They are usually brief, lasting from seconds to minutes. Frequently seizures are followed by a period of drowsiness and confusion (the post-ictal period).

> Epilepsy is the propensity to have recurrent and unprovoked seizures; this propensity can result from a number of underlying aetiologies. Epilepsy is thus best considered a symptom of an underlying brain disorder.

A single seizure is not usually considered sufficient to make a diagnosis of epilepsy. Epileptic seizures occurring solely in association with precipitants or triggering factors are termed acute symptomatic or situation-related seizures. Such precipitants include fever in young children, strokes, metabolic disturbances, alcohol or drug abuse, and acute head injury. Recurrent acute symptomatic seizures are not usually considered as 'epilepsy'.

International seizure classification scheme

The International Seizure Classification Scheme divides epileptic seizures into two main groups according to the putative source of the epileptic discharge (Table 13.1).

Those originating from localized cortical areas are classified as partial (focal) seizures, and those characterized by initial synchronous discharges over both hemispheres are classified as generalized seizures.

Occasionally, seizures are 'unclassifiable', even after extensive investigation. This is especially so with tonic–clonic seizures in adults, which can be partial or generalized in nature (see below).

Partial seizures

> Partial seizures arise from a localized region of cerebral cortex. The clinical manifestations of a partial seizure depend on where in the cortex it begins, and how fast and how far it spreads.

The most common sites of origin of partial seizures are the **temporal lobes**; approximately 60 per cent of people with partial seizures have temporal

Table 13.1 Summary of International League Against Epilepsy classification of seizures (1981)

I	Partial seizures	
	A	Simple partial seizures
	B	Complex partial seizures
	C	Secondary generalized seizures
II	Generalized seizures	
	A	(1) Absence seizures ('petit mal')
		(2) Atypical absence seizures
	B	Myoclonic seizures
	C	Clonic seizures
	D	Tonic seizures
	E	Tonic–clonic seizures ('grand mal')
	F	Atonic seizures
III	Unclassified epileptic seizures	

lobe seizures. Extratemporal seizures usually originate from the **frontal lobes**; seizures originating in the **parietal** or **occipital** regions are relatively rare. The partial nature of the seizure and the location of the focus can often be identified from the symptoms and signs present either during or after the seizure. Partial seizures are subdivided into three groups: **simple partial, complex partial, and partial with secondary generalization**.

Simple partial seizures

Simple partial seizures are epileptic events in which **consciousness is fully preserved**, and in which the **discharge remains localized**.

They are usually brief (unless progression occurs) and intense. The manifestation include: focal motor signs, autonomic symptoms (e.g. flushing, sweating, vomiting), somatosensory or special sensory symptoms (e.g. flashing lights, unpleasant odours or tastes, vertigo, paraesthesiae, pain) or psychic symptoms (e.g. déjà vu, depersonalization, fear, illusions, hallucinations).

Complex partial seizures

Complex partial seizures, one of the most common types of seizure, may have similar characteristics to simple partial seizures, but by definition always involve **impairment of consciousness.**

They can start as a simple partial seizure and then progress (in this instance the simple partial seizure is often termed the 'aura'), or the patient may have alteration of consciousness from the onset.

Complex partial seizures frequently present as altered or **'automatic' behaviour**. The patient may pluck at his or her clothes, fiddle with objects and act in a confused manner. Lip smacking or chewing movements, grimacing, undressing, the carrying out of purposeless activities or of aimless wandering may all occur on their own or in different combinations. **Reactive automatisms**, determined by environmental circumstances, can also occur. During these, a patient is able to carry on with a task with very few outward signs of a seizure. The tasks are usually simple, although on occasion more complex tasks may be performed. These seizures usually last a matter of minutes, but occasionally are more prolonged. Afterwards, the patient is amnesic for the seizure, although may recollect the 'aura'. Complex partial seizures are usually followed by confusion in the post-ictal period.

Secondarily generalized seizures

Secondarily generalized attacks are partial seizures, in which the epileptic discharge spreads to both cerebral hemispheres, so that a generalized seizure, usually a tonic–clonic convulsion, ensues. The patient may experience and recollect an aura, but this is not always the case. The spread of the discharge can occur so quickly that no features of the localized onset are apparent to the patient or to an observer. On rare occasions, a secondarily generalized seizure may take the form of a tonic, atonic or unilateral tonic–clonic seizure.

Generalized seizures

Generalized seizures are characterized by the bilateral involvement of the cortex at the onset of the seizure. Patients experiencing generalized seizures lose consciousness at seizure onset, so that there is usually no warning.

Generalized tonic clonic seizures

Generalized tonic clonic convulsions, or convulsive seizures, previously termed **grand mal** attacks, are common. In this type of seizure, there is no warning, but the patient may experience a prodrome of general malaise. In some epilepsies, increasing frequency of another generalized seizure type, such as **myoclonic jerks** or **absences**, may herald a **tonic-clonic seizure**.

The initial phase (tonic phase) is marked by rigidity; often the patient will cry out as air is expelled. Apnoea occurs, and the patient often becomes cyanosed. The tongue may be bitten, usually on one side, and the patient falls. Then clonic movements, usually involving all four limbs, develop. These are followed by muscle relaxation. The frequency of these movements gradually decreases and eventually the clonic movements cease altogether, marking the end of the seizure. Incontinence can occur at the end of the clonic phase. Most convulsions last less than 2 minutes. There is then a post-ictal period characterized by drowsiness and confusion lasting a variable period (sometimes as long as 20 minutes). It is not uncommon for people to fall asleep after a convulsion and this may sometimes be misinterpreted as unconsciousness.

Although patients are unaware of what has occurred, they will often be aware that they have had a seizure because of a variety of symptoms such as lethargy, generalized muscle aching, headache, bitten tongue and incontinence.

Absence seizures

Typical **absence attacks**, previously known as **petit mal**, occur almost exclusively in **childhood** and adolescence. The child appears suddenly blank and stares: fluttering of the eyelids, swallowing and flopping of the head may occur. The attacks last only a few seconds and often pass unrecognized.

Children may have many of these attacks a day, and not infrequently they are misdiagnosed as learning difficulties at school. **Absence attacks are associated with a characteristic electroencephalography (EEG) pattern – three per second generalized spike-and-wave discharges**. They may be precipitated by **hyperventilation**, which can be a useful diagnostic manoeuvre during EEG recordings, and sleep deprivation. There are also atypical absences, which are usually associated with more severe epilepsy syndromes, such as the Lennox–Gastaut syndrome. In these, the EEG usually demonstrates less homogeneous, slower and more irregular spike/wave discharges. The onset and cessation of the seizure is not as abrupt as with typical absence seizures, and additional features such as eyelid flutter and myoclonic jerking are usually pronounced.

Myoclonic seizures

Myoclonic seizures are abrupt, very brief, involuntary movements that can involve the whole body, or just part of it such as the arms or the head. In idiopathic generalized epilepsies (see below), they occur most commonly in the morning, shortly after waking. They may sometimes cause the patient to fall, but recovery is immediate. The majority of myoclonic seizures occur in relatively **benign seizure** conditions, but sometimes they herald more severe disorders such as **the progressive myoclonic epilepsies**. These are rare, progressive conditions, which often begin in childhood. They consist of **mental deterioration** and **myoclonus** in association with other **neurological deterioration**, depending on aetiology. Not all myoclonus is the result of epilepsy: non-epileptic myoclonic jerks occur in a variety of other neurological conditions including lesions of the brainstem and spinal cord. In addition, myoclonic phenomena also occur in healthy people, particularly when they are just going off to sleep (hypnic jerk). Myoclonus is epileptic if it occurs in the context of a seizure disorder, and is cortical in origin.

Atonic and tonic seizures

Atonic and tonic seizures are very rare generalized attacks, accounting for less than 1 per cent of epileptic attacks. They are often termed '**drop attacks**' and usually occur during the course of some forms of severe epilepsy, often starting in early childhood, such as **Lennox–Gastaut syndrome** or **myoclonic astatic epilepsy**. Atonic seizures (sometimes called akinetic attacks) involve a **sudden loss of tone in the postural muscles, and the patient falls to the ground**. There are no convulsive movements. Recovery is rapid, with no perceptible post-ictal symptomatology. During tonic seizures, there is a sudden increase in the muscle tone of the body and the patient becomes rigid, usually falling backwards onto the ground. Again, recovery is generally rapid.

The International Classification of Epilepsies (ICE), epileptic syndromes and related disorders

Epilepsy syndromes are defined by the features of the seizures, the presence of characteristic structural lesions, the age of onset of the condition, the presence of a family history, and by typical changes in the EEG. It is important to categorize epilepsies according to the syndromic classification because this may have implications both for management and prognosis. The classification scheme for epileptic syndromes proposed by the International League Against Epilepsy (ILAE) is currently the most widely used (Table 13.2). This classification does have a number of limitations, in particular it does not take into account recent progress in neuroimaging and neurogenetics; this classification is thus being revised and updated. The ILAE classification divides epileptic syndromes into four groups: localization-related (partial or focal), generalized, undetermined and special syndromes. Within these groups, the syndromes are further divided into three subgroups: primary or idiopathic, secondary or symptomatic, and cryptogenic (probably symptomatic). When epileptic seizures are the only symptom of an inherited or genetic disorder, the syndrome is termed primary; when they occur as symptoms of a condition associated with structural brain lesions, the syndrome is termed secondary, and when the aetiology of the condition is unknown the term cryptogenic is used. Below, the more common epilepsy syndromes are divided by the age at which they occur.

Neonatal

Neonatal seizures (ICE 3.1)

Neonatal seizures are seizures occurring in the **first 4 weeks of life**: the syndrome is defined solely by age of onset, with no regard for the background aetiology or ictal manifestations. Causes of neonatal seizures include infection, anoxia, ischaemia, trauma, metabolic imbalance and nutritional disturbances. In around a quarter of cases, no aetiological factor is identified. In a few babies, seizures are genetically determined.

Seizures are often subtle and include clonic movements, eye deviation and blinking, usually of short duration; very rarely, more conventional seizure types may occur. These clinical features probably reflect the immaturity of the neonatal brain.

The EEG in the neonate is often difficult to interpret, but it may be possible to identify an epileptic focus. About 0.5 per cent of babies have neonatal seizures. The prognosis is related to the underlying pathology, but the **overall outcome is not good**; approximately 25 per cent die in the first year of life, and about half of those living longer either carry on having seizures into adult life or have evidence of neurological damage. Only about 25 per cent make a full recovery. Indicators of poor prognosis include prematurity, early onset of seizures (especially within the first 2 days of life), focal cerebral lesions or malformations, intracranial bleeding and the presence of a very abnormal EEG.

Infancy

West syndrome (infantile spasms) (ICE 2.2)

West syndrome is also known as **infantile spasms, salaam spasms and hypsarrhythmia**. The onset is usually around the age of six months (range 3–9 months), and the child may have identifiable brain lesions (such as tuberous sclerosis, cortical dysplasias, malformations or anoxic-ischaemic insults) prior to the onset, but in about one-third of cases no aetiology can be found. In this syndrome a **characteristic EEG pattern, termed hypsarrhythmia**, is seen. This consists of a chaotic pattern of high amplitude, irregular, slow activity intermixed with multifocal spike and sharp wave discharges.

The seizures may be flexor, extensor or mixed, the latter being most common. Flexor spasms consist of sudden flexion of the neck, arm and legs. Sudden flexion of the trunk causes so-called 'salaam' or 'jack-knife' seizures. During extensor spasms, sudden movement of the neck, trunk and legs occurs, while in mixed spasms, there is flexion of the neck, trunk and arms, and extension of the legs. Seizures often occur in clusters, particularly soon after the child has been awoken.

Table 13.2 Summary of International League Against Epilepsy classification of epilepsies, epileptic syndromes and related seizure disorders (1989)

1 Localization-related
   1.1 Idiopathic
        Benign childhood epilepsy with
            centrotemporal spikes
        Childhood epilepsy with occipital
            paroxysms
        Primary reading epilepsy
   1.2 Symptomatic
        Chronic progressive epilepsia partialis
            continua of childhood
        Syndromes characterized by seizures
            with specific modes of precipitation
        Temporal lobe epilepsies
        Frontal lobe epilepsies
        Parietal lobe epilepsies
        Occipital lobe epilepsies
   1.3 Cryptogenic
        As 1.2, but aetiology is unidentified
2 Generalized
   2.1 Idiopathic
        Benign neonatal familial convulsions
        Benign neonatal convulsions
        Benign myoclonic epilepsy in infancy
        Childhood absence epilepsy
            (pyknolepsy)
        Juvenile absence epilepsy
        Juvenile myoclonic epilepsy (impulsive
            petit mal)
        Epilepsies with grand mal seizures on
            awakening
        Other generalized idiopathic epilepsies
        Epilepsies with seizures precipitated by
            specific modes of activation (reflex
            epilepsies)
   2.2 Cryptogenic or symptomatic
        West syndrome (infantile spasms)
        Lennox-Gastaut syndrome
        Epilepsy with myoclonic-astatic seizures
        Epilepsy with myoclonic absences

   2.3 Symptomatic
        2.3.1 Non-specific aetiology
               Early myoclonic
                   encephalopathy
               Early infantile epileptic
                   encephalopathy with
                   suppression bursts
               Other symptomatic generalized
                   epilepsies
        2.3.2 Specific syndromes
               Epileptic seizures may
                   complicate many disease
                   states
3 Undetermined epilepsies
   3.1 With both generalized and focal
            features
        Neonatal seizures
        Severe myoclonic epilepsy in infancy
        Epilepsy with continuous spike-waves
            during slow wave sleep
        Acquired epileptic aphasia (Landau–
            Kleffner syndrome)
        Other undetermined epilepsies
   3.2 Without unequivocal generalized or
            focal features
4 Special syndromes
   4.1 Situation-related seizures
        Febrile convulsions
        Isolated seizures or isolated status
            epilepticus
        Seizures occurring only when there
            is an acute or toxic event as a
            result of factors such as alcohol,
            drugs, eclampsia, non-ketotic
            hyperglycaemia

The prognosis for West syndrome is poor. Overall, only about 20 per cent of children make a complete recovery, with death occurring in a further 20 per cent in childhood. Almost 65 per cent of survivors have ongoing epilepsy, and up to 50 per cent have persistent neurological handicap. The response to treatment with most anti-epileptic drugs (AEDs) is poor in West syndrome, but in some children the outcome may be improved if adrenocorticotropic hormone is given early in the condition. Vigabatrin has become the treatment of choice, particularly in children in whom the condition is associated with tuberous sclerosis.

Childhood

Lennox–Gastaut syndrome (ICE 2.2)

The **Lennox–Gastaut syndrome** is characterized by multiple seizure types including tonic and atonic seizures and complex absences. Tonic–clonic convulsions and myoclonic seizures may also occur.

It is a rare condition, accounting for perhaps 1 per cent of all new cases of epilepsy, although because of its poor outcome it may represent as many as 10 per cent of cases of severe epilepsy. Lennox–Gastaut syndrome is frequently associated with **learning difficulties** and **neuropsychiatric disturbances**. In about half of the cases, no definite aetiological factor can be identified. A past history of West syndrome is the most common identifiable cause, being present in 30–40 per cent of children. Other causes include brain damage at birth, infections, tumour and severe head trauma. The condition typically has its onset between ages three and five years, although it may start at as early an age as one year or as late as eight years of age (rarely even older). **Patients are at high risk of developing status epilepticus**, either tonic–clonic or non-convulsive. The **prognosis** of Lennox–Gastaut syndrome is **poor**, both with regard to seizure control (seizures persisting in 60–80 per cent of patients) and mental development. Cognitive and behavioural problems are very common, and it is unusual for patients ever to lead independent lives.

The EEG pattern in Lennox–Gastaut syndrome is almost invariably abnormal. The background activity is slow, and 2.0–2.5 Hz spike and wave and polyspike and wave discharges, often most marked over the anterior and posterior head regions, are characteristically seen. Such discharges may sometimes dominate the EEG for hours or days at a time. The complexes are not usually induced by hyperventilation or by photic stimulation. Rhythmic 10 Hz spikes are seen particularly during slow-wave sleep. Polypharmacy and sedation may worsen seizures. Valproate and benzodiazepines are the drugs of choice, and adjunctive treatment with lamotrigine, felbamate, rufinamide and topiramate appears to be of benefit. A ketogenic diet may also be of benefit, but compliance is usually poor.

Benign childhood epilepsy with centrotemporal spikes (ICE 1.1)

Benign partial epilepsy of childhood also known as **Rolandic epilepsy or centrotemporal epilepsy** is the most common of the idiopathic partial epilepsies. The onset of seizures is between the ages of two and 14 years, usually between five and ten years. This syndrome accounts for about 10–15 per cent of epilepsy in this age group. Children with this benign epilepsy usually have simple partial seizures, occasionally with progression to complex partial or to secondarily generalized seizures. Seizures tend to occur during the night or on awakening, and usually involve the face, lips and the tongue. Consciousness is usually preserved.

The **interictal EEG** tracing has a **characteristic appearance** in this syndrome; it consists of frequent paroxysms of slow spike and wave discharges over the centrotemporal ('Rolandic') region, with a normal background rhythm. About 30 per cent of the children have a family history of epilepsy. It has an **excellent prognosis** for complete seizure remission by puberty. Long-term treatment is usually not required, but if seizures are frequent then carbamazepine is the drug of choice. A variety of this syndrome is **benign occipital epilepsy**, in which the EEG disturbance is in the occipital lobe and the children may present with visual disturbances during the seizures.

Childhood absence epilepsy (ICE 2.1)

Childhood absence epilepsy is common, and occurs at the age of 3–13 years, more commonly in girls than boys. Typical **absences** lasting 5–15 seconds (no longer than 30 seconds) may be '**simple**' or '**complex**' and may occur many times a day. Up to 40 per cent may develop tonic–clonic seizures. The EEG shows characteristic 3 Hz spike and wave. Absence seizures are usually well controlled with valproate or ethosuximide, and they usually resolve by adult life.

Febrile convulsions (ICE 4.1)

Febrile seizures are seizures occurring in the context of a **febrile illness**, often of viral aetiology, in children **between the ages of six months and six years**. They affect as many as 3 per cent of children in the general population and there is often a **family history** of febrile convulsions or epilepsy.

The seizures usually take the form of short, generalized tonic–clonic convulsions, without other features, with body temperatures over 38°C, particularly following a rapid rise in temperature. Acute treatment, in addition to supportive treatment, consists of diazepam, either rectally or intravenously, reducing the child's temperature and treatment of the underlying condition if appropriate. **Febrile convulsions do not usually require long-term prophylactic treatment unless complications develop**. However, parents should be counselled about the risk of recurrences and measures to avoid these. Risks for recurrence include age less than 15 months, epilepsy in first-degree relatives, febrile convulsions in first-degree relatives, and first febrile seizure with partial onset. In some children, intermittent prophylaxis with a benzodiazepine is helpful. Investigation by EEG is usually not indicated. The most important differential diagnosis in this condition is with seizures that are triggered by central nervous system infections such as meningitis, encephalitis or brain abscess. If there is suspicion of a central nervous system infection, imaging, lumbar puncture (if safe) and antibiotic treatment are necessary.

In the great majority of children presenting with febrile convulsions, even if recurrent, the overall prognosis is excellent with no further seizures or other problems.

However, in a **few** children, **chronic seizures** subsequently develop, so that the risk of epilepsy occurring by the age of 25 years is about 7 per cent.

> The risk is greatest in children with prolonged convulsions (lasting more than 20–30 minutes), those with previous signs of developmental delay and those with partial seizures. The probability of epilepsy subsequently developing is also greater in children with a family history of afebrile seizures in a first-degree relative.

Adolescence

Juvenile absence epilepsy (ICE 2.1)

Juvenile absence epilepsy is similar to childhood absence epilepsy, but there is an equal sex incidence and later onset. Tonic–clonic seizures occur in 80 per cent, and are **less** likely to remit.

Epilepsies that present in both childhood and adulthood

Epilepsies occurring in both childhood and adulthood are most commonly **cryptogenic or symptomatic partial epilepsies**, and are usually divided by the cortical origin of the seizures into temporal, frontal, parietal and occipital lobe epilepsies.

Temporal lobe epilepsy

Approximately 60–70 per cent of localization-related seizures originate in the temporal lobes. Seizures commonly derive from the **hippocampus**, with **hippocampal sclerosis** (Figure 15.1) being the most common aetiology. Seizures originating from temporal neocortex are similar in nature, but it is **common** to find a **structural lesion** such as glioma,

> **Juvenile myoclonic epilepsy (ice 2.1)**
> Juvenile myoclonic epilepsy is a common disorder that is probably underdiagnosed. It begins at the age of 8–18 years, and a family history is common. Seizures consist of bilateral or unilateral myoclonic jerks, usually affecting the upper limbs. Tonic–clonic seizures may also occur and approximately 10 per cent of those affected have typical absences. Seizures often occur shortly after waking, and can be precipitated by sleep deprivation and alcohol. Investigation by EEG shows irregular spike and wave, and high frequency spikes. Approximately one-third have a response to photic stimulation. Spontaneous remission is rare, although the seizures respond well to valproate. Lamotrigine is used as an alternative but may exacerbate the myoclonic jerks. Newer AEDs, such as topiramate and levetiracetam, are also effective. Carbamazepine, vigabatrin and barbiturates may worsen the myoclonus and absences.

angioma (Figure 15.2), neuronal migrational defects (Figure 15.3), post-traumatic change, hamartoma (Figure 15.4) or dysembryoplastic neuroepithelial tumour underlying the seizure disorder.

The seizures take the form of complex partial seizures and less commonly simple partial seizures and are described in Box 13.1.

Frontal lobe epilepsy

Frontal lobe epilepsy accounts for approximately 30 per cent of partial epilepsy syndromes in adults (Figure 15.5). The clinical features of frontal lobe seizures are given in Box 13.2.

Seizures originating in the motor cortex most commonly involve the face and limbs, particularly the hands. A well-known, though rather uncommon, form of simple partial motor seizure is the 'Jacksonian seizure' (see Table 13.3). This starts as clonic jerking in one part of the body, often in a hand, which slowly spreads to contiguous muscle groups in the so-called 'Jacksonian march'. This parallels the slow progress of the epileptic discharge along the motor cortex (Figure 15.6).

Parietal and occipital lobe epilepsy

About 10 per cent of all localization-related epilepsies originate in the **parietal and occipital lobes** (Figure 15.7).

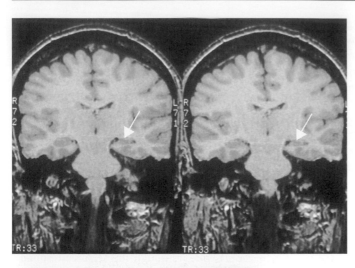

Figure 13.1 MRI brain scans, coronal views, to show hippocampal sclerosis on the left side (two contiguous cuts).

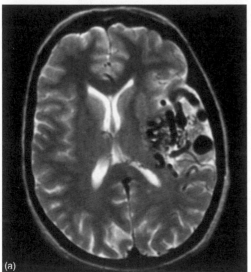

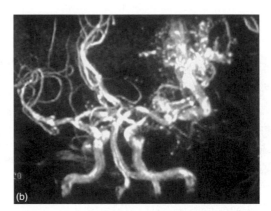

Figure 13.2 (a) MRI brain scan, T2-weighted axial view, to show large arteriovenous malformation in the left temporal lobe. (b) MRI angiogram of the same malformation.

Their clinical features are described in Table 13.4.

EPIDEMIOLOGY OF EPILEPSY

Incidence

The incidence of epilepsy in the general population has been estimated to be 80 cases per 100 000 people. No consistent national or racial differences have been found, although it is thought that the incidence may be higher in parts of the developing countries, particularly in rural areas. The **incidence**

of epilepsy has a **bimodal** distribution with a peak in the first two decades of life and a second peak in later life, over 60 years of age.

Prevalence

Most well-conducted prevalence studies of active epilepsy have found rates between **5 and 10 per 1000 people** in the population, regardless of location. Lifetime prevalence rates are much higher and it is estimated that 2–5 per cent of the population at age 70 will have had epileptic seizures at some point in their lives, men slightly more than women.

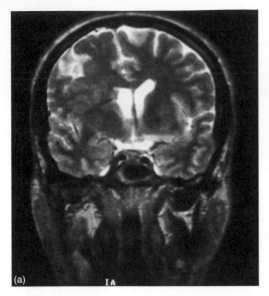

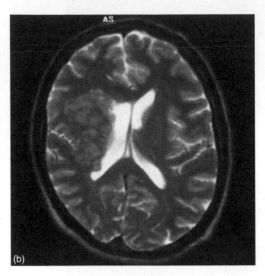

Figure 13.3 MRI brain scan, T2-weighted: (a) coronal view and (b) axial view, to show heterotopia in the right hemisphere.

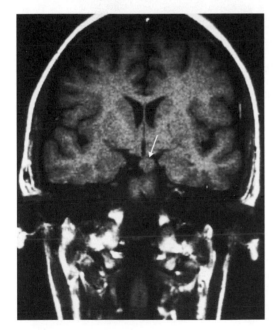

Figure 13.4 MRI brain scan, T1-weighted coronal view, to show hypothalamic hamartoma, presenting with complex partial seizures.

Box 13.1 Clinical features of temporal lobe seizures – 60–70 per cent of partial seizures

Complex or simple partial seizures
Usual duration 2–10 minutes – slow evolution over 1–2 minutes
Aura
    Epigastric – nausea, borborygmi, belching, a rising epigastric sensation
    Olfactory, gustatory hallucinations (often unpleasant)
    Autonomic symptoms – change in heart rate, blood pressure, pallor, facial flushing, pupillary dilatation, piloerection
    Affective – fear (may be intense), anger, depression, irritability, dreamy states, depersonalization
    Dysmnestic – déjà vu, déjà entendu, recall of childhood or even former lives
Motor – arrest and absence prominent
    Automatisms – oro-alimentary (lip smacking, chewing, grimacing), gestural (fidgeting, undressing, walking)
    Vocalizations common, recognizable words suggests origin in dominant temporal lobe
May be secondary generalizations
Post-ictal confusion common

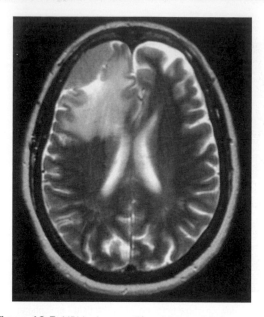

Figure 13.5 MRI brain scan, T2-weighted axial view, to show a right frontal meningioma with surrounding high signal. This patient presented with seizures suggestive of a frontal lobe origin.

Box 13.2 Partial seizures arising from the motor cortex – rare

Simple partial seizures
Duration variable – may be prolonged
Motor onset – corner of mouth, side of face, thumb, finger and hand, foot. Jacksonian march spreading proximally
Post-ictal – Todd's paresis
May have secondary generalization

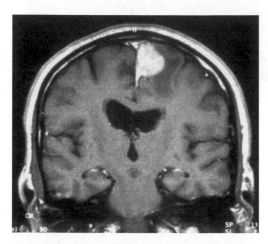

Figure 13.6 MRI brain scan, T1-weighted coronal view with enhancement, to show a meningioma. This patient presented with simple partial seizures with onset in the foot.

Table 13.3 Clinical features of frontal lobe seizures – 30 per cent of partial seizures

Complex partial	May be nocturnal
Duration very brief – c. 30 seconds	Abrupt onset
Aura	Cephalic:
	Non-specific dizziness, strange feelings in the head
	Forced thinking, ideational and emotional manifestations
Automatisms	Violent and bizarre
	Ictal posturing and tonic spasms
	Legs kick, cycle, step, dance
	Vocalization shrill loud cry, occasional speech fragments
	Version of head and eyes: version of the body causes circling
	Abduction and external rotation of the arm with flexion of the elbow in the contralateral arm with version of the eyes to the affected limb
	Autonomic symptoms may arise
	Sexual automatisms with pelvic thrusting, obscene gestures and genital manipulation
Secondary generalization common	
Post-ictal confusion brief with rapid recovery	

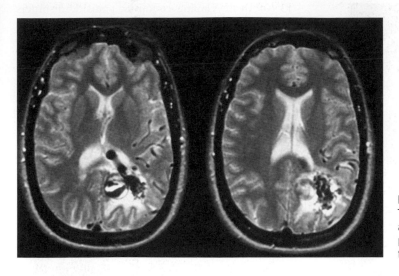

Figure 13.7 MRI brain scans, T2-weighted axial views, to show an occipital arteriovenous malformation. This patient presented with seizures with a stereotyped formed visual hallucination.

Table 13.4 Clinical features of parietal and occipital lobe seizures – 10 per cent of partial seizures

Parietal lobe	Complex and simple partial seizures
	Often non-specific sensory symptoms – commonly tingling or pain
	May include numbness, prickling, crawling or even shock-like sensations. Odd temperature sensations. May be a Jacksonian type march of sensory symptoms
	Distorted body image – floating, limb immobility or even absence of body part
	Rare apraxia, acalculia, alexia and vertiginous sensations
Occipital lobe	Complex and simple partial seizures
	Visual hallucinations – often crude sensations of light and colour, may be various patterns. Usually moving. Occasional transient amaurosis
	Eyelids may flutter, occasional eye turning or even rapid blinking

The aetiology of epilepsy

Epilepsy is a symptom of an underlying brain disorder and can present many years after the damage occurs; for example, it is not uncommon for people with a brain injury in childhood to present with epilepsy in their 20s. In approximately 40–50 per cent of cases no known cause is found, although with the advent of modern neuroimaging this number is dwindling.

The probable **aetiology depends on the age of the patient and the type of seizures**. The most common acquired causes in **young infants** are **hypoxia or birth asphyxia**, perinatal intracranial trauma, metabolic disturbances, congenital malformations of the brain, and infection. In young children and adolescents, idiopathic or primary epilepsies account for the majority of seizure disorders, although **trauma and infection** (Figure 13.8) also play a role. The range of causes of **adult–onset** epilepsy is very wide (Table 13.5). Both idiopathic epilepsy and epilepsy as a result of birth trauma can begin in early adulthood. Other important causes of seizures in adulthood are **head injury, alcohol abuse, brain tumours and cerebrovascular disease including vascular malformations** (Figures 13.9 and

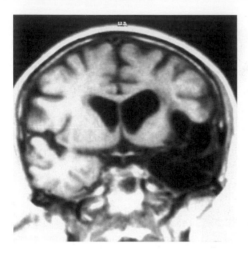

Figure 13.8 MRI brain scan, T1-weighted coronal view, to show extensive scarring in the right temporal lobe following herpes encephalitis. This patient had complex partial seizures.

13.10). In developing countries, parasitic disorders such as **cysticercosis** (see Figure 9.17) and malaria are important causal agents for epilepsy.

> **Brain tumours** are responsible for the development of epilepsy in up to **one-third of patients between the ages of 30 and 50 years. Over the age of 50 years, cerebrovascular disease** is the most common cause of epilepsy and may be present in up to half of the patients (Figure 13.11).

With modern imaging, **structural abnormalities** such as **hippocampal sclerosis** and **neuronal migrational defects** have grown in importance as causes of partial epilepsies (especially refractory partial epilepsies). Most epilepsies starting in adult

Table 13.5 Causes of epilepsy

Trauma	Perinatal insults
	Closed head injury – incidence linked to severity
	Penetrating injury – incidence about 50 per cent
Infection	Acute bacterial meningitis c. 30 per cent; post-meningitis 3–10 per cent
	Encephalitis – 10–25 per cent of herpes simplex survivors
	Brain abscess – c. 70 per cent
	Worldwide – cysticercosis, tuberculoma, malaria
	AIDS – c. 13 per cent: also with toxoplasmosis
	Prion – CJD
Tumours	Primary – particularly slow growing – oligodendroglioma, meningioma, dysembryoplastic neuroepithelial tumours
	Secondary – (20 per cent of adults presenting with epilepsy may have a cerebral tumour)
Vascular	Thrombo-embolic infarcts and cerebral haemorrhage – 5–8 per cent
	Arteriovenous malformations
	Cavernomas
	Vasculitis
	(Post-stroke most common cause of seizures in older patients)
Alcohol	Binge, withdrawal – 5–15 per cent of chronic alcoholics have seizures
Drugs	Recreational – cocaine, amphetamines, ecstasy
	Therapeutic – isoniazid, aminophylline, tricyclics, phenothiazines
Degenerative	Alzheimer's disease – 15–20 per cent have seizures
Multiple sclerosis	Some 5–10 per cent have seizures
Metabolic triggered	Hypoglycaemia, hypocalcaemia, hyponatraemia
	Hepatic and renal failure
	Porphyria
	Coeliac disease
Inherited	Down's syndrome, tuberous sclerosis, mitochondrial defects, Rett syndrome, Sturge–Weber
Idiopathic	Nearly two-thirds of adults with newly diagnosed seizures have no cause found

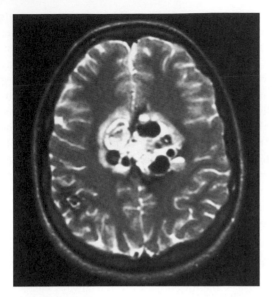

Figure 13.9 MRI brain scan, T2-weighted axial view, to show multiple cavernomas. A solitary, small right parietal cavernoma is also seen. The patient presented with right-sided motor seizures.

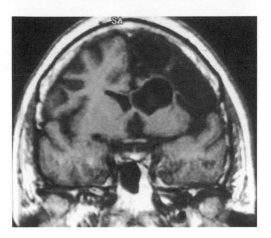

Figure 13.11 MRI brain scan, T1-weighted coronal view, to show extensive scarring from an old infarct. This had caused the development of simple partial seizures.

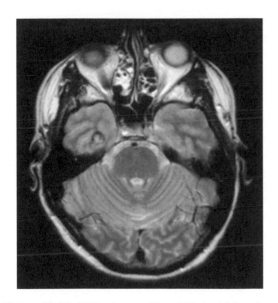

Figure 13.10 MRI brain scan, T2-weighted axial view, to show a more subtle small cavernoma in the right temporal lobe. This patient presented with complex partial seizures and occasional episodes with secondary generalization.

life are symptomatic and investigations to detect the underlying aetiology are mandatory.

Idiopathic epilepsies constitute the majority of childhood epilepsies. Many of the idiopathic epilepsies undoubtedly have a genetic basis. Thus the chance of developing idiopathic/cryptogenic epilepsy with a first-degree relative with idiopathic/cryptogenic epilepsy is three times that of the general population.

Most idiopathic epilepsies probably have polygenic inheritance and seem to show genetic heterogeneity. Single genes have, however, been identified for some rarer idiopathic epilepsies such as autosomal dominant nocturnal frontal lobe epilepsy, generalized epilepsy with febrile seizures and benign neonatal seizures.

In addition to these inherited conditions, which have seizures as their main clinical expression, there are a large number of **inherited disorders**, most of them rare, which present as neurological or systemic illness of which epileptic seizures form a part, such as tuberous sclerosis and neurofibromatosis. Other rare, inherited, degenerative brain disorders and inborn errors of metabolism such as adrenoleukodystrophy, Alpers' disease and Tay–Sachs disease, phenylketonuria, porphyria and neuronal ceroid-lipofuscinosis can also cause seizures.

DIAGNOSING EPILEPSY

Diagnosis

The diagnosis of epilepsy is mainly a clinical one based upon the history given by the patient and, importantly, by eyewitnesses. This is because epilepsy is an intermittent condition and in between seizures examination and investigations may all be normal.

Conditions that mimic seizures

In adults, **syncope, migraine, panic attacks, transient ischaemic attacks (TIAs) and non-epileptic attacks with a psychogenic** basis are the main conditions that can be confused with epilepsy (Table 13.6). **In children** there are also other conditions that can commonly be confused with epilepsy, **including breath-holding attacks and night terrors (pavor nocturnis).**

Syncope

Syncope can be differentiated from seizures by the **situation** in which the attacks occur and the prodrome and nature of the attacks. Except in those cases caused by **cardiac arrhythmias,** syncope rarely occurs in patients who are recumbent. Syncope often has a clearly identifiable precipitant.

Vasovagal attacks are almost invariably preceded by a warning in which the patient feels dizzy, hot and sometimes sick, the vision becomes blurred or goes grey, and hearing may be lost. To an observer, the patient appears pale and may sweat profusely. Consciousness is then usually lost and the patient falls to the floor; recovery is usually quick. Incontinence and injury are rare. Some jerking of the limbs can occur, especially if the person is propped up as this may prevent adequate blood flow to the brain. The jerking is occasionally prolonged, but seldom has the co-ordinated pattern of a tonic–clonic seizure; in this instance, however, confusion with an epileptic seizure is commonplace.

Furthermore, in some partial seizures, the patient may experience similar feelings to a faint prior to the seizure – an autonomic aura. Thus in a few cases the differences are not always clear-cut. After a faint, the patient usually feels nauseated and shaky, but is rarely confused.

Table 13.6 Causes of episodes that may mimic epilepsy

Circulatory	Syncope	
	Orthostatic	
	Cardiac	Changes in rate, rhythm, conduction defects
		Outflow obstruction
	TIAs	Particularly sensory attacks
		Basilar migraine
		Vertebrobasilar ischaemia
		Transient global amnesia
Neurological	Narcolepsy, cataplexy	
	Myoclonus other than epilepsy	
	Intermittent obstructive hydrocephalus	
	Vertigo (may be the aura of epileptic seizure)	
	Paroxysmal disorders, e.g. kinesigenic spasms	
	Parasomnias	
Metabolic	Hypocalcaemia,[a] hypoglycaemia, hyponatraemia	
	Renal[a] and hepatic failure	
	Porphyria	
	Phaeochromocytoma	
Drugs and alcohol		
Drop attacks	In middle-aged women ? cause	
	In elderly patients – often orthostatic or cardiac element	
	Tilt-table testing may be helpful	
Non-epileptic attacks	Psychogenic (dissociative seizures)	
	Panic attacks	
	Hyperventilation	

[a]May induce an epileptic seizure.
TIAs, transient ischaemic attacks.

Migraine

There are several reasons why **migraine** attacks may be confused with epileptic seizures. Syncope can occur during the course of migraine, particularly when vomiting occurs. **Basilar migraine** may present with loss of consciousness causing confusion with epileptic seizures. The accompanying brainstem symptoms and a family history of migraine may help in their differentiation. Migraine preceded by visual or sensory disturbances can also be mistaken for partial epilepsies, especially as seizures are commonly followed by headache in the post-ictal phase. However, the progression of visual and sensory symptoms is usually much more rapid in epilepsy than in migraine. Diagnostic difficulty occurs in a few patients, especially because migraine can be accompanied by paroxysmal **EEG** phenomena.

Hyperventilation

Overbreathing is not uncommon, especially in those under stress or in those with panic **attacks**. The immediate feeling is usually described as a sudden difficulty in catching one's breath, and a feeling of panic (although these symptoms do not always have to be present). During hyperventilation, paraesthesiae, carpopedal spasm, light-headedness and even loss of consciousness can occur.

Transient ischaemic attacks (TIAs) and transient global amnesia

TIAs may produce weakness and sensory symptoms; it is the latter that usually causes confusion with epileptic seizures. The TIAs usually last longer than epileptic seizures, and there is rarely loss of consciousness. Critical stenosis of the carotids can result in myoclonic jerks with a sudden fall in blood pressure.

Transient global amnesia occurs in middle-aged or older people. Usually this occurs as a single episode lasting several hours, in which the patient is unable to remember events. He or she remains alert and communicative throughout this period, but may repeatedly ask the same question. Recovery afterwards is complete, except for amnesia for the duration of the episode. The cause of transient global amnesia remains unclear. Migraine, epilepsy and cerebrovascular disease have been suggested, but it is thought that only a small minority of patients with such symptoms have epilepsy, and in these, the attacks are usually short-lived and recurrent.

Non-epileptic attack disorder

Other terms used to describe this condition are **pseudoseizures** and **hysterical seizures**. The preferred term is 'dissociative seizures'. In tertiary referral clinics, approximately 20 per cent of patients, newly referred for assessment, have non-epileptic attacks. **Non-epileptic attack disorder (NEAD)** (see Table 31.3) may be seen in people with genuine epilepsy.

Findings of NEAD are more common in women who may have a past or family history of psychiatric disorder, sometimes including unexplained neurological dysfunction or previous attempted suicide. The attacks tend to start in the teens or 20s, and do not respond (or respond transiently) to the introduction of anti-epileptic drugs. If the attacks have the appearance of generalized tonic-clonic seizures, measurement of serum prolactin levels 20 minutes after a seizure may help in the differentiation from genuine epileptic attacks, in which there may be an elevation of prolactin. Prolactin levels do not always rise during complex partial seizures and can rise following a faint.

Breath-holding attacks

Breath-holding usually occurs in children under the age of six years, and attacks are commonly mistaken for seizures, although if witnessed, diagnosis should be possible from the history of precipitating factors. **Cyanotic breath-holding attacks** occur when the child is frustrated or angry. A period of crying is followed by the cessation of breathing. Cyanosis follows and the child becomes limp and unresponsive; sometimes trembling or a few clonic movements occur. Unresponsiveness usually lasts for about 2 minutes and is followed by rapid recovery.

Investigations

EEG

The routine EEG is usually performed interictally, and an epileptiform abnormality is usually defined as the presence of spikes, sharp waves or spike-wave complexes (Table 13.7).

Table 13.7 Investigations used in the management of patients with a suspected seizure

Blood tests	Full blood count, ESR, creatinine, electrolytes, calcium and liver function, pregnancy test
	Fasting blood glucose. Serum prolactin level (if any doubt about veracity of attack). AED levels if compliance suspect
Urine for porphyrins	
ECG	
Chest X-ray in smokers and older patients	
EEG	Resting, sleep, prolonged, with video monitoring
Imaging	Best MRI scan with special sequences
	CT scanning if MRI not available or possible
Special tests	PET, SPECT – in selected patients
CSF examination	In patients suspected of acute meningitis, encephalitis

AED, anti-epileptic drug; CT, computerized tomography; EEG, electroencephalography; ESR, erythrocyte sedimentation rate; MRI, magnetic resonance imaging; PET, positron emission tomography; SPECT, single photon emission computerized tomography.

EEG

The EEG is an integral part of the diagnosis and classification of epilepsy, and the localization of seizures (see also Chapter 5).

Recordings can be carried out in a number of circumstances: at rest, during sleep, ambulatory monitoring, video monitoring (telemetry) and intracranial recording.

The main problem with the interictal EEG is the specificity and sensitivity. A routine EEG will detect an epileptiform abnormality (spike or sharp wave) in 50 per cent of adults with epilepsy and in less than 1 per cent of adults without epilepsy (this figure is probably higher for children). The sensitivity can be increased up to 80 per cent with repeat routine EEG and, in particular, sleep EEG. This, however, still leaves 20 per cent of patients with epilepsy in whom there are no epileptiform abnormalities in the interictal EEG, even after multiple EEGs. During a routine EEG, intermittent photic stimulation and hyperventilation may be performed in order to elicit abnormalities in specific epilepsy syndromes. These activation procedures should be avoided if the consequences of inducing a seizure will have an unacceptable impact (e.g. loss of driving licence).

The probability of recording an ictal EEG during routine EEG is small and thus **ambulatory EEG** and **video-telemetry** are used. An ictal EEG is both more specific and sensitive than the interictal EEG. Ambulatory EEG is confounded by artefact, and lack of video, which make interpretation difficult. Video-telemetry is routinely used for pre-surgical assessment in order to define accurately the point of initiation of a seizure. During pre-surgical evaluation, a patient's AEDs are often reduced in order to induce a seizure. Video-telemetry is also used in the diagnosis of epilepsy, especially in difficult patients where a NEAD is suspected or to diagnose unusual events during sleep.

However, it should be noted that not all cortical spikes are recorded by scalp EEG, and hence an absence of ictal change in the EEG does not exclude epilepsy.

This is particularly the case for simple partial seizures, seizures arising in the mesial or orbital frontal regions, and seizures in which the only manifestation is a visceral aura. Intracranial EEG is used in the assessment of patients for epilepsy surgery when the scalp EEG is not able to give adequate information for the localization of the epileptic 'focus'.

Brain imaging

> ### Imaging
>
> Magnetic resonance imaging (MRI) is the investigation of choice and ideally almost all patients with epilepsy should have an MRI scan, but the detection rate of abnormalities is substantially increased if neuroimaging is restricted to: patients with focal neurological signs; patients with seizure onset either during the neonatal period or after the age of 20 years; or patients with partial or generalized seizures that are resistant to medication.

MRI detects many more abnormalities than are apparent on computed tomography (CT) scanning. Furthermore, MRI is able to give much better views of the hippocampus and temporal lobes. This has enabled hippocampal volumes to be calculated, and has helped in the diagnosis of hippocampal sclerosis (see Figure 13.1) – a surgically resectable cause of temporal lobe epilepsy. More recently, three-dimensional reconstruction, analysis of MRI images and developments in MRI protocols and higher field strengths (3 Tesla) have increased the yield of abnormalities detected including morphological abnormalities (abnormalities of gyri and sulci).

Other imaging techniques that are increasingly being used in presurgical assessments are:

- **positron emission tomography (PET)**, which is occasionally useful for preoperative seizure localization by identifying areas of brain hypometabolism;
- **single photon emission computerized tomography (SPECT)**, which uses gamma-emitting radioisotopes in order to create three-dimensional images of cerebral blood flow. The isotopes are longer lived than in positron emission tomography, enabling ictal images to be taken. This can provide useful information for pre-operative seizure localization;
- **magnetoencephalogram (MEG)**, which measures magnetic fields rather than electrical signals;
- **EEG–fMRI**, which is a method that combines the high temporal resolution of EEG with the good spatial resolution of functional MRI to give an indication of the source of interictal EEG abnormalities.

TREATMENT STRATEGIES FOR EPILEPSY

The aim of long-term treatment is to stop all seizures, and this can be attained in the majority (approximately 70–80 per cent) of patients. The three main ways to achieve this are:

1 avoiding those factors that precipitate seizures;
2 drug treatment;
3 epilepsy surgery.

Avoidance of precipitating factors and photosensitivity

In many patients, avoiding certain factors will lessen the frequency of seizures, and in a few, will prevent them altogether. Very rarely, people can have seizures brought on by hearing particular pieces of music, by reading, by hot showers, by seeing certain patterns, and so on, and these are referred to as 'reflex epilepsies'. For most, however, there is no specific trigger.

There are, nevertheless, four factors that can induce or worsen seizures in many patients:

1 Excessive alcohol
2 Lack of sleep
3 Stress
4 Fever.

Photosensitivity to flashing lights or particular photic patterns occurs in less than 5 per cent of all people with epilepsy. The photosensitive seizures usually occur with lights that flicker at 5–30 Hz. Television and video games can induce photosensitive seizures, as can sunlight reflecting off water, passing a line of trees through which the sun is shining and stroboscopic lights.

In some patients with photosensitivity, avoidance of the triggers for their seizures is the only treatment needed, and AEDs may not be necessary. Seizures induced by watching television are reduced by viewing the television in a well-lit room, sitting at least 2.5 metres from the television set, changing channels with a remote control and covering one eye and using high frequency, 100 Hz, televisions. Seizures are rarely triggered by film in a cinema, and usually computer screens operate at a sufficiently high frequency not to provoke seizures.

When to start drug treatment

Epilepsy is the propensity to have seizures and thus, following a first seizure, the probability of having further seizures is of paramount importance in determining when to initiate treatment. **Studies have suggested that after one seizure only 30–60 per cent of people have a recurrence within two years**; if an identifiable and avoidable provoking factor (e.g. alcohol) is present, then the recurrence rates are much lower. Following two unprovoked seizures within a year, the recurrence rate is possibly as high as 80–90 per cent. In view of the impact upon a patient's life, and the side-effects of AED treatment, **many physicians do not treat unless a patient has had at least two clearly described unprovoked seizures**. In certain situations, however, patients are not necessarily treated even after two seizures. These are: a poor description of episodes (possible seizures); seizures separated by more than one year; the presence of identifiable and avoidable provoking factors; certain benign epilepsy syndromes; and patient preference.

Even after a first seizure, **treatment is effective in decreasing the risk of further seizures by approximately 50 per cent**, although early treatment does not affect long-term prognosis.

Thus in certain circumstances (unprovoked seizures), it may be prudent to start therapy after the first seizure. Indeed, treatment is often considered after one clearly described unprovoked seizure in situations in which: a seizure is associated with a neurological deficit present at birth; a seizure is associated with a clearly abnormal EEG (such as presence of 3 Hz spike and wave); and a seizure occurs in the context of a progressive neurological disorder. It is crucial to realize that the risks of recurrence following a first seizure are very different for individual patients.

There appears at present to be no place for prophylactic AED treatment to prevent the occurrence of epilepsy. Following a severe head injury, for example, phenytoin and valproate have been shown to be no better than placebo in preventing the occurrence of late epilepsy, and thus should be reserved for those who actually develop epilepsy. In the case of febrile convulsions, prophylaxis is not necessary in the majority of children.

Which drug to choose

Freedom from seizures can be achieved with monotherapy in about 80 per cent of patients developing epilepsy.

The aim must be good seizure control with minimal drug side-effects, **balancing efficacy and toxicity**. Certain AEDs are more effective in certain seizure types or certain epilepsy syndromes. First-line therapies in partial epilepsies are lamotrigine and carbamazepine, while valproate is generally the drug of choice in patients with generalized epilepsies (however, see below under Pregnancy). Overall, the established AEDs are often equally effective, and tolerability is the main determinant of 'success'. Other factors include:

- **compliance** – improved with drugs that can be taken **once or twice daily**;
- **cost**;
- **teratogenicity** – various AEDs may have different risks in pregnancy;
- **age** – this has implications for side-effects and their significance.

How treatment is started

If started at too great a dose, AEDs may result in side-effects and the abandonment of a potentially useful therapy. Therefore AEDs are introduced cautiously. The titration of an AED dose is usually symptom led, and if seizures are not controlled by an AED, it is then titrated slowly up to the maximum tolerated dose, regardless of serum concentrations. Possible dose-related side-effects are discussed with patients and carers and they are given instructions to reduce the dose if they occur.

Patients and carers should also be warned about idiosyncratic side-effects such as rash. For most AEDs, the serum concentration is linearly related to dose. The exception is phenytoin, which has saturation kinetics. Here an increase in serum concentration is not linear so a small dose increase will produce a disproportionate rise in serum concentration. Carbamazepine induces its own metabolism (autoinduction) resulting in a drop in serum concentration after 20–30 days. Occasionally, the maximum tolerated dose may be higher than that recommended under the licence. With some AEDs (notably valproate) there is little benefit in exceeding the recommended dose.

If one first-line AED fails (at the maximum tolerated dose), it is substituted by another first-line therapy. The first-line therapies are then tried in combination and finally second-line AEDs are added. The aim of AED treatment is to achieve seizure control with one drug because polytherapy leads to poor compliance, drug interactions, increased teratogenicity and increased long-term toxicity.

Pharmacokinetics and drug monitoring

Therapeutic drug monitoring

The adherence to AED 'therapeutic' serum concentrations is often misconceived, and may lead to either under-treatment or over-treatment. Of patients on phenytoin monotherapy, 20–40 per cent are well controlled with 'subtherapeutic' serum concentrations. Conversely, some patients are only controlled with phenytoin serum concentrations above the 'therapeutic' range, and yet experience no side effects. This effect is seen with other AEDs, and in some cases (notably valproate) the serum concentration bears little relationship to either efficacy or side effects.

The titration of an AED should thus be symptom led, and if seizures are not controlled by an AED, it should then be titrated up to the maximum tolerated dose, regardless of serum concentrations. Measurement of AED serum concentrations, however, is helpful under certain circumstances: if poor seizure control occurs (serum concentrations may have fallen or very high serum concentrations occasionally may cause a paradoxical decrease in seizure control); if suspected drug toxicity occurs; if there is suspected non-compliance; if concomitant drug therapy is modified (to check for drug interactions); during pregnancy and illness; and during clinical trials. Finally, in the case of phenytoin, which shows saturation kinetics, the serum concentration is a useful guide to the dosage increments that should be used.

Surgery

It has been estimated that there are approximately 750–1500 new patients per annum in the UK who could benefit from **epilepsy surgery**, and who thus require presurgical assessment. The potential and the success of surgery may increase as MRI techniques improve and the cause of seizures may be identified in more patients.

Epilepsy surgery is a major undertaking as it involves removing the part of the brain where the seizures begin and obviously carries some risks. In patients with a progressive underlying lesion (such as a tumour) or a lesion that carries other inherent risks (such as the risk of haemorrhage from an arteriovenous malformation) the need for surgery is often determined by these considerations, regardless of seizure control. In other patients, the seizure disorder is the primary determinant.

There is wide agreement that **epilepsy should have been shown to be intractable to medical treatment** before surgery is contemplated. Such a trial of therapy should include treatment separately with at least two first-line drugs appropriate to the type of epilepsy, and with adequate compliance. Although it is often reasonable to try several different drugs alone or together over a period of time, the chance of a patient becoming seizure-free diminishes if control is not achieved with initial first-line drugs, and evaluation for surgery is not usually delayed while every possible combination of medication is tried.

Patients considered for epilepsy surgery need to fulfil a number of criteria:

- it has to be felt that the seizures are one of the main causes of a patient's disability;
- similarly, it has to be considered that stopping the seizures would result in a significant improvement in quality of life (severe learning difficulties and psychiatric disease are relative contraindications);
- the patient must be able to understand the possible risks and benefits of the epilepsy surgery;
- seizure origin can be located (there should preferably be concordant data from psychometry, EEG and imaging);
- the risks of surgery do not outweigh the benefits (e.g. removal of dominant temporal lobe may result in unacceptable memory deficits even if seizures are halted).

Assessment for surgery thus involves a **multidisciplinary approach** including: neurologist, neurosurgeon, psychologist, psychiatrist, neurophysiologist and radiologist.

There are two main strategies for the surgical treatment of seizures. The first involves **resective surgery**, in which the aim of the surgery is the **removal of the epileptic focus** itself. Examples of this type of surgery are: anterior temporal lobectomy; selective amygdalo-hippocampectomy (in which only the mesial temporal structures are removed); or resection of a frontal lobe lesion. At the other extreme of resective surgery are patients in whom most or all of one hemisphere is abnormal, as in hemimegalencephaly or Rasmussen's encephalitis (an uncommon inflammatory condition causing seizures, progressive hemiparesis and intellectual deterioration), **hemispherectomy** may be necessary. The other strategy for surgical treatment is **to interrupt the pathways of seizure spread**, so isolating the epileptic focus from the rest of the brain. Examples of this type of surgery include section of the corpus callosum, and multiple subpial transection. **Callosotomy** is used to prevent secondary generalization of seizures, and its chief indication is in the treatment of intractable generalized seizures, particularly tonic seizures. **Multiple subpial transection** is a technique that relies upon the theory that seizure spread occurs tangentially through the cerebral cortex, while impulses controlling voluntary movement travel radially. In this operation, multiple cuts are made vertically in the cortex in an effort to isolate the epileptogenic area from the surrounding cortex. It may be helpful in the treatment of seizures arising in eloquent areas of the brain, such as the speech area or motor cortex.

Importantly, the social and medical results of surgery are better earlier on in the course of the epilepsy. The prognosis for epilepsy surgery depends upon the surgery and the underlying cause for the epilepsy, **but in patients in whom there is an identifiable lesion, approximately 60–70 per cent will become seizure-free following surgery.**

Temporal lobe surgery (anterior temporal lobectomy, selective amygdalo-hippocampectomy) results in approximately 70–80 per cent of patients becoming seizure-free in the first year (this drops in subsequent years), and 30 per cent are improved. The overall mortality of temporal lobectomy is less than 0.5 per cent, and the risk of permanent hemiparesis less than 1 per cent. Memory problems, depression and visual field defects are the other common morbidities. Extratemporal surgery is performed less frequently and the results are less impressive, with 40 per cent becoming seizure-free and 30 per cent improved. The morbidity is related to the site of resection. Hemispherectomy is particularly effective in controlling seizures, with approximately 80 per cent becoming seizure-free, but this operation is reserved for patients with a profound hemiplegia. Corpus callosotomy results in 70 per cent of patients having a worthwhile improvement, but only 5 per cent become seizure-free.

Other treatment modalities

Diet

It was the observation that starving patients had fewer seizures that resulted in the introduction of the ketogenic diet in the 1920s, in which most calories were given as fat. The diet comes in two main forms: (1) the classical form in which the primary fat source is long chain triglycerides and the ratio of fat to carbohydrate is maintained as 3 or 4 to one, and (2) the medium chain triglyceride (MCT) diet in which 30–60 per cent of daily calories are as MCTs. The latter diet is better tolerated because less fat is necessary to produce the same level of ketosis. These diets have been shown to be effective in children with severe refractory epilepsy (used in addition to medication). There is some evidence that they may be effective in some adults, but the diet is generally poorly tolerated.

Vagal nerve stimulation

Stimulation of the **vagal nerve** involves surgically implanting a small **stimulator** under the skin in the neck, which intermittently stimulates the nerve. Data on the vagal nerve stimulator in patients with intractable partial seizures show a significant decrease in seizure frequency, with few side-effects. The efficacy was comparable to short-term results in new AED trials, but, as described above, the impact of new AEDs on the prognosis of intractable epilepsy has been modest.

Drug treatment in special circumstances

Pregnancy

Conception

Frequent seizures may result in hormonal abnormalities that could contribute to infertility; however, AEDs possibly have a greater effect on fecundity. Some AEDs decrease libido and can induce impotence in men (e.g. phenobarbitone). There have been recent concerns of the association of polycystic ovarian syndrome and valproate, but the extent of this association is unclear; valproate should be prescribed cautiously in women who are obese or who have menstrual irregularities.

The metabolism of the contraceptive pill is increased with certain AEDs (carbamazepine, eslicarbazepine acetate, oxcarbazepine, phenobarbital, phenytoin, primidone, topiramate). Women taking these drugs should use a higher dose pill (containing 50–100 μg ethinyloestradiol is generally recommended). Breakthrough bleeding is a sign that the contraceptive dose is not adequate.

> The **fetal malformation rate** in infants born to mothers with epilepsy is: higher than that of the general population; higher in those treated with AEDs; higher in those with high plasma AED concentrations; and higher in those on polytherapy. An attempt is thus often made to reduce therapy in women who wish to fall pregnant. In addition, women should be given folate supplements (5 mg daily) prior to conception and through the first trimester.

The most common abnormality in infants born to mothers with epilepsy is cleft lip/palate, comprising approximately 30 per cent of the abnormalities. Specific syndromes have been described for different AEDs, the most well known being the fetal hydantoin syndrome, consisting of dysmorphic features and learning difficulties; other such syndromes have been described with other AEDs, in particular valproate. Also of note is the risk of spina bifida, which is most common with valproate (1–2 per cent of births), and carbamazepine (0.5–1.0 per cent of births). Women on these drugs require alpha-fetoprotein measurement and fetal ultrasound for the early detection of neural tube defects.

Recent evidence indicates that valproate has among the highest associated fetal malformation rates, and may be associated with an increase in learning difficulties and an average decrease in IQ of approximately nine points. For these reasons, use of valproate is not recommended during pregnancy unless there is no suitable alternative. Some new AEDs appear free from teratogenic effects in animals, but it is not certain that these data can be extrapolated to humans. Indeed, trials of new AEDs are not carried out on pregnant patients, and patients of child-bearing potential involved in drug trials have to be on adequate contraception. There are thus scarce data on the teratogenic potential of new AEDs, and caution is needed when new AEDs are used in women likely to fall pregnant.

The pharmacokinetics of AEDs may substantially change during pregnancy, requiring regular monitoring of seizures and serum drug concentrations. Furthermore, it is not uncommon for problems of compliance to occur during pregnancy, usually from maternal concern of the effects of AEDs on the developing fetus. It is essential to emphasize the importance of compliance, as frequent seizures may damage the fetus and seizures can complicate the puerperium. Pharmacokinetic effects that occur are: a decrease in protein binding, resulting in an increase in the 'free' plasma concentrations of drugs that are predominantly protein bound (phenytoin, valproate and diazepam); an increase in hepatic metabolism and renal clearance of drugs; an increase in volume of distribution also increases during pregnancy, and a fall in total plasma concentrations of AEDs is thus not uncommon, especially in the third trimester. In the case of phenytoin, the increase in 'free' concentrations may result in toxicity despite a fall in total concentrations, and thus monitoring of 'free' phenytoin is recommended. However, as with all treatment, the absolute indication for changing drug dosages is an increase in seizures or drug toxicity.

In the last month of pregnancy, women should be given oral vitamin K if they are taking enzyme-inducing drugs, and at birth the baby should receive vitamin K. **Breast feeding is not usually contraindicated**, except for women taking phenobarbitone or ethosuximide; other AEDs are present in insignificant amounts in breast milk. Breast feeding should only stop if the baby becomes drowsy or irritable following feeds.

Management of status epilepticus

> ### Status epilepticus
> Status epilepticus is defined as a condition in which a patient has a seizure or a series of seizures that last more than 30 minutes without regaining consciousness. Emergency treatment of convulsive seizures should, however, begin if the seizure has lasted more than 5 minutes or with repeated convulsions within an hour.

The term **status epilepticus** can apply to **all seizure types**, but it is convulsive status epilepticus (CSE) that is of most importance. The **mortality of CSE is approximately 20 per cent** and relates mostly to the underlying aetiology. Approximately half the patients with CSE have chronic epilepsy, and in these **AED withdrawal** is the most common identifiable cause. Reintroduction of a withdrawn AED often helps to terminate CSE.

> Other important causes are: cerebral trauma, cerebral tumour, cerebrovascular disease, intracranial infection, metabolic disturbances and alcoholism.

In treating CSE, there are three important considerations:

1 CSE is associated with severe physiological and metabolic compromise
2 Prolonged CSE can result in significant neuronal damage even after the clinical manifestations have halted, and there is only on-going electrographic status epilepticus
3 The longer that CSE continues, the harder it is to treat.

General measures are critical in the treatment of CSE. These are outlined in Table 13.8.

Drug treatment can be divided into stages (Table 13.8). Although opinion varies as to which are the preferred therapeutic options, the use of a protocol for the treatment of CSE is mandatory as this simple measure results in the rapid administration of adequate doses of effective drugs and thus improves prognosis.

Early status

Intravenous lorazepam. This can be repeated after 10 minutes, or intravenous diazepam. If intrave-nous access is difficult, midazolam can be given buccally (between the gum and teeth) or intramus-cularly (rectal diazepam is an alternative).

Established status

Intravenous fosphenytoin. The prodrug fosphenytoin can be used with greater speed and less risk. This is given in a dose of 20 mg/kg as PE (phenytoin equivalents – 1 mg of phenytoin being equivalent to 1.5 mg of fosphenytoin). Alternatively, phenytoin (15–20 mg/kg given at 25–50 mg/minute with EEG and blood pressure monitoring) can be used. If this has no effect, then intravenous phenobarbitone can be tried.

Refractory status

Transfer to intensive care unit. General anaesthesia is used with concomitant EEG monitoring, and continued for 12–24 hours after the last EEG/clinical seizure.

Once the patient is stable, the underlying cause needs to be identified and patients may require lumbar puncture, chest x-ray, neuroimaging and further blood tests.

To control the seizures, intravenous propofol is often used. An alternative is thiopental. Thiopental is cumulative in the body and a proportion of patients may develop hypotension. It is possible to monitor the blood level. Again a slow withdrawal of the drug is necessary.

> Seizures that do not respond to therapy should always raise the question of whether they may be non-epileptic attacks.

Non-convulsive status epilepticus

> In this condition, no convulsion is apparent. It may present with confusion, obtundation and psychiatric symptoms. Diagnosis is usually made with EEG. It usually responds well to benzodiazepines. It may be underdiagnosed in the elderly and psychiatric populations.

Furthermore 'electrical' status epilepticus (on EEG) with minimal visible signs can occur after acute hypoxic events and may be a cause of continuing coma. It is underdiagnosed and the **diagnosis should be considered in all comatose patients**. Diagnosis is by EEG.

Table 13.8 Acute management of status epilepticus

General measures

- Secure airway and resuscitate: monitor respiration, blood pressure and pulse
- Venous access
- Oxygen should be given – hypoxia is common during a convulsion
- Monitor urea, electrolytes, blood gases, pH, blood count and temperature
- Monitor neurological signs and GCS level
- ECG
- EEG (where possible)
- Intravenous glucose (25 g) and thiamine 250 mg (10 mL Pabrinex) (if poor nutrition or alcoholism suspected)
- Correct any metabolic abnormalities
- Save blood for AED levels

Medication

1 Immediate

  IV lorazepam 4 mg slowly for adults: 0.1 mg/kg for children

  or IV diazepam 10–20 mg in adults (0.25–0.5 mg/kg in children at 2–5 mg/minute as an alternative

  if difficult venous access, midazolam:

  buccally (between teeth and gum) 10 mg in adults (0.2–0.4 mg/kg)

    or IM 0.15–0.3 mg/kg

2 If seizures continue after 5–10 minutes add IV fosphenytoin (as PE 20 mg/kg) given slowly c. 150 mg/ minute (1 mg of phenytoin is equivalent to 1.5 mg of fosphenytoin) or IV phenytoin (20 mg/kg) at 50 mg/minute

  If seizures continue, try IV phenobarbitone 10 mg/kg given slowly at 100 mg/minute

  Monitor respiration and BP. **Could seizures be non-epileptic?**

  Treatment for refractory seizures – continuing after 30–40 minutes:

  - Transfer to ITU for intubation and GA
  - Continuous EEG monitoring (if possible)
  - IV propofol – loading dose 2 mg/kg – infuse 1–10 mg/kg per hour. Slow taper when all seizure activity disappeared ('burst suppression')
  - Or IV thiopental – loading dose 100–250 mg, infuse 3–5 mg/kg per hour. Cumulative drug with possible hypotension. Slow withdrawal. Can monitor blood level 40 mg/L
  - Ensure maintenance AEDs are continued

AEDs, anti-epileptic drugs; ECG, electrocardiogram; EEG, electroencephalography; GCS, glasgow coma score; ITU, intensive therapy unit; PE, phenytoin equivalents.

THE PROGNOSIS OF EPILEPSY

The prognosis for full seizure control is relatively good. **Studies have shown that about 70–80 per cent of all people developing epilepsy will eventually become seizure-free and about half will successfully withdraw their medication.** Once a substantial period of remission has been achieved, the risk of further seizures is greatly reduced. A minority of patients (20–30 per cent) will develop chronic epilepsy, and in such cases treatment is more difficult. Patients with symptomatic epilepsy, more than one seizure type, associated learning difficulties, or neurological or psychiatric disorders are more likely to develop a chronic seizure disorder. Five per cent of patients with intractable epilepsy will be unable to live in the community or will be dependent on others for their day-to-day needs. In a minority of patients with severe epilepsy, physical and intellectual deterioration may occur.

Stopping treatment

Because of the possible long-term side-effects of the drugs, it is common clinical practice to consider drug withdrawal after a patient has had a substantial period of remission (usually two years). After this period of seizure freedom, the chance of successfully coming off medication is approximately 60 per cent. Even after being seizure-free for two years, there is still a chance of relapse while continuing the same medication; this chance of relapse is about half that of withdrawing medication.

The prognosis for AED withdrawal is worse in those who:

- are 16 years or older;
- are taking more than one AED;
- have seizures after starting AEDs;
- have a history of generalized tonic–clonic seizures or of myoclonus;
- have an abnormal EEG.

The mortality of epilepsy

Epilepsy is often assumed to be a benign condition with a low mortality. Although this is usually the case, it does carry an **increased mortality**, particularly in younger patients (less than 40 years of age) and those with severe epilepsy (tonic–clonic seizures). Common causes of death in people with epilepsy include chest infections, neoplasia and deaths directly related to seizures. Deaths directly related to seizures fall into several categories: status epilepticus; seizure-related death; **sudden unexpected death**; and accidents. There is extensive literature on death in status epilepticus, which is estimated to occur in about 20 per cent of all cases of generalized tonic–clonic status. Sudden unexpected death in epilepsy is defined as a non-traumatic unwitnessed death occurring in a patient with epilepsy who had been previously relatively healthy, for which no cause is found even after a thorough post-mortem examination. Suggested explanations for the cause of death have included suffocation during a seizure, deleterious action of AEDs, autonomic seizures affecting the heart, and the release of endogenous opioids, although the pathophysiology (if indeed there is

a single mechanism) is still unknown. The annual mortality rate is one sudden death for every 1000 people with epilepsy in the community, but increase to one in 200 per year for those with refractory epilepsy and is more than 1 per cent per year for those referred to surgical programmes. Another possible cause of mortality and morbidity in people with epilepsy is as a result of accidents during seizures or as a consequence of a seizure. Mortality rates for traumatic death have been shown to be increased, indicating that accidents and trauma are a more frequent cause of death in patients with epilepsy than in the general population. There is also an increased mortality from drowning among people with epilepsy. Mortality rates also indicate that patients with epilepsy are at a higher risk of committing suicide.

SOCIAL IMPLICATIONS OF EPILEPSY

It is important to realize that there are many social implications of epilepsy; for instance, in regard to driving, schooling, employment and relationships. Unfortunately, there is still some unnecessary prejudice against those who have epilepsy, but there are also certain laws governing driving and employment for people with epilepsy.

Driving

Seizures while driving are still one of the most common preventable causes of road traffic accidents. In the UK, the rules laid down about driving are straightforward, and there is little excuse not to follow them.

Driving and epilepsy

In the UK, it is the obligation and responsibility of every person who has any condition that may impede their driving (this includes all people with epilepsy) to inform the Driver and Vehicle Licensing Authority (DVLA). Anyone who fails to inform the DVLA and continues to drive is committing a criminal offence. Furthermore, failing to inform the DVLA may invalidate the driver's insurance.

This applies to all people with seizures, and for this purpose even the smallest epileptic event (for example, an aura or a myoclonic jerk) is counted as a seizure. Once the DVLA has been informed, the patient should stop driving and can reapply for a licence only when the following criteria have been fulfilled: either that **no epileptic attacks while awake (including aura, etc.) have occurred during the past year**, or that if epileptic attacks have occurred, that these were **only during sleep and that this pattern has been present for at least three years**. Following a single epileptic seizure, or if there is loss of consciousness of no known cause, patients are barred from driving for six months (provided no abnormality on scan or EEG and assessed by an appropriate specialist) or one year.

If a patient has been seizure free, and has thus regained his driving licence, but wishes to come off medication, the advice from the DVLA is that the patient should not drive during the changes in medication and for six months after the withdrawal from medication.

The rules for heavy goods vehicle and passenger-carrying vehicle licences are much stricter, and it is not possible to hold these licences if a person has a continuing liability to epileptic seizures. This is interpreted as meaning no epileptic seizure or anti-epileptic medication for the previous ten years and no evidence of a continuing risk of seizures (e.g. three per second spike and wave on the EEG or a brain lesion). The rules for a single seizure are five years if there is no abnormality on scan or EEG and the patient has been assessed by an appropriate specialist

Employment

There are a few occupations that are barred by statutory provision for people with epilepsy and these include: aircraft pilot, ambulance driver, taxi driver, train driver, merchant seaman, working in the armed services, or fire brigade. There are also certain jobs that involve substantial risks if a seizure should occur and thus cannot be recommended (e.g. scaffolder), and common sense should apply when considering such jobs. Furthermore there are jobs in which epilepsy is not explicitly mentioned but may be considered a bar (e.g. midwifery). For insurance purposes, it is generally important that employers are aware if employees have epilepsy.

NORMAL SLEEP AND ABNORMALITIES OF SLEEP

Adults require on average 7–8 hours' sleep a night. This sleep is divided into two distinct states – rapid eye movement (REM) sleep and non-REM sleep. These two sleep states cycle over approximately 90 minutes throughout the night, with the REM periods becoming progressively longer as sleep continues and accounting for about one-quarter of sleep time. During REM sleep, dreams occur; there is hypotonia or atonia of major muscles that prevents dream enactment. REM sleep is also associated with irregular breathing and increased variability in blood pressure and heart rate. Non-REM sleep is divided into four stages (stages I–IV) defined by specific EEG criteria. Stages I/II represent light sleep, while stages III/IV represent deep, slow-wave sleep. Dreams do occur during non-REM sleep, but these tend to lack narrative structure.

Abnormalities of sleep are divided into three main categories:

1 Dysomnias or disorders of the sleep–wake cycle;
2 Parasomnias or disordered behaviour that intrudes into sleep;
3 Sleep disorders associated with medical or psychiatric conditions.

Dysomnias

Dysomnias are divided into: intrinsic sleep disorders, such as idiopathic insomnia, idiopathic hypersomnolence (a diagnosis by exclusion) or narcolepsy; extrinsic sleep disorders, in which there is an extrinsic cause for the sleep disorder such as drugs, poor sleep hygiene or high altitude; and disorders of the circadian rhythm, which can be intrinsic (e.g. delayed sleep-phase syndrome) or extrinsic (e.g. caused by shift-work).

Insomnia

Although **insomnia** can be idiopathic, in the majority of patients there is an underlying cause. This cause can be an intrinsic sleep problem, such as **periodic limb movements, restless legs or sleep**

apnoea, or an extrinsic problem, such as **high altitude, drugs** (e.g. certain AEDs, and certain anti-depressants) or **poor sleep hygiene**. This last problem is usually easy to address – no caffeine or alcohol in the evening, avoidance of exercise close to bedtime, no daytime naps, regular bedtime, and so on. Other **medical conditions**, such as chronic obstructive lung disease, asthma, cardiac failure, gastro-oesophageal reflux and nocturia can all contribute to insomnia, and certain neurological conditions can also have a significant impact (see below). Among the more common causes, however, are **depression, fibromyalgia, anxiety and old age**. The elderly tend to have more fragmented sleep patterns, with less slow wave sleep and more early morning awakenings.

The treatment of insomnia should first of all address possible underlying causes and sleep hygiene. For short-term insomnia, hypnotics can be useful, but long-term use of these drugs, especially benzodiazepines, can result in tolerance, dependence and poor sleep. Certain cases of insomnia benefit from a behavioural approach, in which the patient is retrained in normal sleep behaviour; such an approach should be considered in all with chronic insomnia.

Narcolepsy

> ### Narcolepsy
> Narcolepsy is a specific, well-defined disorder with a prevalence of approximately one in 2000; it is a lifelong condition usually presenting in the late teens or early 20s. Narcolepsy is a disorder of REM sleep and the main symptom is excessive daytime sleepiness. This is manifest as uncontrollable urges to sleep, not only at times of relaxation (e.g. when reading a book, watching television), but also at inappropriate times (e.g. when eating a meal or while talking). The sleep is usually refreshing. The other typical symptoms are cataplexy, sleep paralysis, hypnagogic/hypnapompic hallucinations, fragmented/poor nocturnal sleep and microsleeps (very brief sleep episodes).

Some of these represent REM sleep phenomena such as hypotonia/atonia, and dreams occurring at inappropriate times. **Cataplexy** is a sudden decrease in voluntary muscle tone (especially jaw,

neck and limbs) that occurs with sudden emotion like laughter, elation, surprise or anger. This can manifest as jaw dropping, head nods or a feeling of weakness or, in more extreme cases, as falls with 'paralysis' lasting sometimes for several minutes. Consciousness is preserved. Cataplexy is a specific symptom of narcolepsy, although narcolepsy can occur without cataplexy. **Sleep paralysis and hypnagogic hallucinations** are not specific and can occur in other sleep disorders and with sleep deprivation (especially in the young). Both these phenomena occur shortly after going to sleep or on waking. Sleep paralysis is a feeling of being awake, but unable to move. This can last for several minutes and is often very frightening, so can be associated with a feeling of panic. Hypnagogic/hypnapompic hallucinations are visual or auditory hallucinations occurring while dozing/falling asleep or on waking; often the hallucinations are frightening, especially if associated with sleep paralysis.

Narcolepsy in humans is rarely familial. However, the lifetime risk for developing narcolepsy is increased to 1 per cent in first-degree relatives of narcoleptic patients.

> Approximately 90 per cent of all narcoleptic patients with definite cataplexy have the human leukocyte antigen (HLA) allele, HLA DQB1* 0602, compared with approximately 25 per cent of the general population. The sensitivity of this test is decreased to 40 per cent if cataplexy is not present. The strong association with HLA type has raised the possibility that narcolepsy is an autoimmune disorder. There is a functional defect in hypocretin secretion (hypocretins are expressed in neurones in the hypothalamus) in most patients with narcolepsy with cataplexy.

Because narcolepsy is a lifelong condition with possibly addictive treatment, the diagnosis ideally should be confirmed with a **multiple sleep latency test (MSLT)**. During this test, five episodes of sleep are permitted during a day; rapid onset of sleep and **REM** sleep within 15 minutes are suggestive of narcolepsy. A low level of cerebrospinal fluid hypocretin has also been suggested as a diagnostic test for narcolepsy.

The excessive sleepiness of narcolepsy can be treated with modafinil, methylphenidate or dexamphetamine and regulated daytime naps. The cataplexy, sleep paralysis and hypnagogic/hypnapompic hallucinations respond to antidepressants (fluoxetine or clomipramine are the most frequently prescribed). More recently, a new approach has become available in which sodium oxybate is given at night; this increases slow wave sleep, and decreases both daytime somnolence and cataplectic attacks.

Sleep apnoea

Sleep apnoea can be divided into the relatively common **obstructive sleep apnoea** and the rarer **central sleep apnoea**. Obstructive sleep apnoea is more common in men than women and is associated with obesity, micrognathia and large neck size. The prevalence may be as high as 4 per cent in men and 2 per cent in women.

> The symptoms suggestive of obstructive sleep apnoea are loud snoring, observed nocturnal apnoeic spells, waking at night fighting for breath or with a feeling of choking, morning headache, daytime somnolence, personality change and decreased libido. Although the daytime somnolence can be as severe as narcolepsy, the naps are not usually refreshing and are longer.

Obstructive sleep apnoea and central sleep apnoea can be associated with **neurological disease** (see below), but central sleep apnoea can also occur as an idiopathic syndrome. The correct diagnosis requires **polysomnography** with measures of oxygen saturations and nasal airflow or chest movements. To be pathological, a sleep apnoea or hypopnoea (a 50 per cent reduction in airflow) has to last 10 seconds and there needs to be more than five apnoeas/hypopnoeas per hour (the precise number to make a diagnosis varies between sleep laboratories).

Uncontrolled sleep apnoea can lead to hypertension, cardiac failure, pulmonary hypertension and stroke. In addition, sleep apnoea has been reported to worsen other sleep conditions, such as narcolepsy, and to worsen seizure control.

Treatment of sleep apnoea should include avoidance of alcohol and sedatives and weight reduction. Pharmacological treatment is not particularly effective. Dental appliances to pull the bottom jaw forward can be effective in mild cases. The mainstay of treatment for moderate/severe obstructive sleep apnoea is **continuous positive airway pressure** administered by a nasal mask. In cases with neuromuscular weakness (see below), intermittent positive pressure ventilation is often necessary. Surgical treatments, including tonsillectomy, adenoidectomy and procedures to widen the airway, are effective in selective cases.

Restless legs syndrome/periodic limb movements in sleep

Restless legs syndrome (RLS) and periodic limb movements in sleep (PLMS) can occur in association or separately. Most people with RLS also have PLMS, but the converse is not true and most people with PLMS do not have RLS.

> RLS is characterized by an unpleasant sensation in the legs, often described as tingling, cramping or crawling, and an associated overwhelming urge to move the legs. These sensations are worse in the evening, and movement provides temporary relief. About 5 per cent of the population is affected by RLS. Periodic limb movements in sleep are a brief, repetitive jerking of usually the legs or arms that occurs every 30–90 seconds. These occur in non-REM sleep and can cause frequent arousals.

Approximately 50 per cent of people over 65 years are affected by PLMS. These conditions can also be associated with daytime jerks. The two conditions of RLS and PLMS are included as dysomnias as they present as insomnia and daytime tiredness and disrupt the sleep–wake cycle. Both RLS and PLMS can be familial, but can be secondary to peripheral neuropathy (especially diabetic, uraemic and alcoholic neuropathies), iron deficiency, pregnancy and, rarely, spinal cord lesions.

Symptoms may be relieved by benzodiazepines, gabapentin and opioids, and L-DOPA; dopamine agonists are, however, the mainstay of treatment.

Parasomnias

There are a number of common parasomnias that will not be discussed, including bruxism and enuresis. Other parasomnias can be divided into those that occur at sleep–wake transition and those that occur during sleep. The latter can be further divided into non-REM and REM parasomnias.

Sleep–wake transition disorders

The most common of the sleep–wake transition disorders are **hypnic jerks** or **myclonic jerks** that occur on going to sleep or on waking. They are entirely benign in nature and require no treatment. They can occur in association with other sleep disorders. Rhythmic movement disorder is a collection of conditions occurring in infancy and childhood, characterized by repetitive movements occurring immediately prior to sleep onset that can continue into light sleep. One of the most dramatic is head banging or jactatio capitis nocturna. Persistence of these rhythmic movements beyond ten years of age is often associated with learning difficulties, autism or emotional disturbance, but can occur in other groups.

Non-REM parasomnias

Non-**REM** parasomnias usually occur in slow-wave (stage III/IV) sleep. These conditions are often termed arousal disorders and indeed can be induced by forced arousal from slow wave sleep. There are three main non-**REM** parasomnias – **sleep walking, night terrors and confusional arousal**. These disorders often have a familial basis, but can be induced by sleep deprivation, alcohol and some drugs. They can also be triggered by other sleep disorders, such as sleep apnoea, medical and psychiatric illness. Patients are invariably confused during the event, and are amnesic for the event. These conditions are most common in children, but do occur in adults.

Sleep walking may occur in up to 25 per cent of children, with the peak incidence occurring from the age of 11–12 years. The condition is characterized by wanderings, often with associated complex behaviours such as carrying objects and eating. Although speech does occur, communication is usually impossible. The episode usually lasts a matter of minutes. Aggressive and injurious behaviour is uncommon, and should it occur then polysomnography may be indicated to exclude a REM sleep parasomnia (see below) and to confirm the diagnosis. **Night terrors** are less common and are characterized by screaming and prominent sympathetic nervous system activity – tachycardia, mydriasis and excessive sweating. Both these conditions are usually benign and rarely need treatment. If dangerous behaviour occurs, then treatment may be indicated. If very frequent then polysomnography may be required to exclude precipitating conditions (such as obstructive sleep apnoea) and nocturnal seizures. Benzodiazepines, especially clonazepam, are usually very effective. Otherwise antidepressants, especially selective serotonin reuptake inhibitors, can help.

REM parasomnias

Nightmares are REM phenomena that can occur following sleep deprivation, with certain drugs (e.g. L-DOPA) and in association with psychological and neurological disease. Sleep paralysis (see above under Narcolepsy) is also an REM parasomnia, and may be familial.

Of more concern are **REM sleep behaviour disorders**. These consist of dream enactment. They are often violent and tend to occur later in sleep when there is more REM sleep. These are rare and tend to occur in the elderly. In over one-third of cases, REM sleep behaviour disorders are symptomatic of an underlying neurological disease such as dementia, multisystem atrophy, Parkinson's disease, brainstem tumours, multiple sclerosis, subarachnoid haemorrhage and cerebrovascular disease. In view of this, a history of possible REM sleep behaviour disorder needs to be investigated by polysomnography and, if confirmed, then possible aetiologies need to be investigated. REM sleep behaviour disorders usually respond very well to clonazepam.

Sleep disorders and neurological disease

Neurological diseases can disturb sleep indirectly through nocturnal spasms (e.g. in multiple sclerosis), nocturia or pain (e.g. painful neuropathies). Neurological disease can, however, disturb sleep in more specific ways. Insomnia can occur following strokes, but more specifically occurs in fatal familial insomnia (an autosomal-dominant prion disease) and in Alzheimer's disease when there can be reversal of the day–night cycle. Narcolepsy can be symptomatic, especially with lesions affecting the third ventricle or hypothalamus. Hypersomnolence can occur following head injury, with strokes, especially those affecting the diencephalon, and in multiple sclerosis. Encephalitis can also cause hypersomnolence and can occur in epidemics such as encephalitis lethargica and also sleeping sickness (trypanosomiasis).

Neuromuscular disease, especially myopathies, myotonic dystrophy, myasthenia gravis, motor neurone disease, poliomyelitis and some neuropathies, can lead to sleep apnoea. Myotonic dystrophy is also associated with primary hypersomnolence. Strokes can cause sleep apnoea, and also are more frequent in those with sleep apnoea. Multisystem atrophy and some other neurodegenerative diseases are associated with central sleep apnoea. In addition, brainstem strokes can result in Ondine's curse, in which automatic respiratory control is lost, resulting in severe nocturnal apnoea. The two syndromes of RLS and PLMS can be associated with neuropathies, spinal cord lesions and Parkinson's disease.

Perhaps one of the disorders that is most indicative of an underlying neurological cause is **REM sleep behaviour disorder**, which is most commonly associated with extrapyramidal syndromes such as Parkinson's disease, multisystem atrophy and cortical Lewy body disease, but is also associated with other neurodegenerative conditions, strokes and brainstem tumours. Dopaminergic agents used to treat parkinsonism are also associated with REM sleep disorders, especially nightmares.

Epilepsy has a complex association with sleep. Certain seizures are more common during sleep, such as frontal lobe seizures, which occur during non-REM sleep. Rarely, nocturnal seizures may be the only manifestation of an epileptic disorder and these can be confused with a parasomnia – this has been especially true for autosomal-dominant nocturnal frontal lobe epilepsy, the seizures of which were thought originally to represent a nocturnal paroxysmal dystonia. Activation of EEG in epilepsy commonly occurs during sleep, so that sleep recordings are much more likely to demonstrate epileptiform abnormalities. Rarely, non-convulsive status epilepticus can occur during slow wave sleep; the clinical manifestation of this is usually intellectual regression and autism. Lack of sleep can precipitate seizures, especially in the idiopathic generalized epilepsies, and sleep apnoea has been reported to worsen seizure control. Sleep disturbances also commonly occur in people with epilepsy in whom there is a higher incidence of sleep apnoea, fragmented sleep and insomnia as well as daytime somnolence (often drug related).

Specific clinical approach to patients with sleep disorders

As in most neurological conditions, **the history of patients with sleep disorders is paramount**. In the history of the presenting complaint, it is often important to have a witnessed account and to determine at what stage of the night the sleep disturbance is occurring or under what circumstances daytime somnolence occurs. Sleepiness at times of relaxation may be as a result of sleep deficit, but sleepiness at inappropriate times is much more likely to be indicative of a condition such as narcolepsy. A history of a typical night is often helpful, as are sleep diaries and an exploration of sleep hygiene. Family history can be informative, as many sleep disorders such as insomnia, restless leg syndrome and parasomnias run in families. Alcohol and drug history are critical as many drugs can influence sleep and can contribute to or trigger sleep disorders. Specific scales have been developed to assess somnolence, and the **Epworth sleepiness scale** (Table 13.9) is one of the most common and most frequently used.

The mainstay of sleep investigation is **polysomnography**. Full polysomnography measures EEG to sleep stage, respiration either by chest movements or nasal airflow, electrocardiography and oxygen saturations. For suspected cases of sleep apnoea, an overnight measure of oxygen saturations is a cheap and effective screening process that can be carried out at home. Polysomnography is indicated for the investigation of all patients with suspected narcolepsy, sleep apnoea and REM sleep disorders. It can be used to monitor treatment in these conditions, and this is especially useful for obstructive sleep apnoea treatment with continuous positive airway pressure in order to optimize the machine settings. In addition, **multiple sleep latency tests** are used for the diagnosis of hypersomnolence. The patient is permitted to sleep for up to 15 minutes on five occasions through a day. Short latency to sleep indicates hypersomnolence; REM sleep occurring in two or more of the sleep episodes is indicative of narcolepsy. Other investigations are determined by the clinical picture.

As well as the treatment suggested above. Social aspects should be discussed, as sleep disorders can have a considerable psychosocial impact. Depression, anxiety and loss of libido can result directly from sleep disorders. In addition, driving

Table 13.9 Epworth Sleepiness Scale (ESS)

How likely are you to doze off or fall asleep during the following situations, in contrast to just feeling tired? For each of the situations listed below, give yourself a score of 0 to 3 where 0 = would never doze; 1 = slight chance; 2 = moderate chance; 3 = high chance. Work out your total score by adding up your individual scores for situations 1 to 8.	
Situation	**Chance of dozing**
Sitting and reading	
Watching television	
Sitting inactive in a public place, e.g. theatre, meeting	
As a passenger in a car for an hour without a break	
Lying down to rest in the afternoon	
Sitting and talking to someone	
Sitting quietly after lunch (when you have had no alcohol)	
In a car while stopped in traffic	
An ESS score of greater than 10/24 or more is considered abnormally sleepy	

should be discussed and patients with daytime somnolence should not drive unless their condition is being adequately treated. This is especially important for those with narcolepsy and sleep apnoea in whom naps at inappropriate times can occur.

REFERENCES AND FURTHER READING

NICE (October 2004) *The Epilepsies: Clinical Practice Guidelines.* Available from: www.NICE.org.uk/nicemedia/live/12108/55689/55689.pdf.

Sander JW, Hart YM (2007) *Epilepsy: Questions and Answers.* Basingstoke: Merit.

Schneerson J (2005) *Sleep Medicine: A Guide to Sleep and its Disorders.* Oxford: Blackwell.

Wallace H, Shorvon S, Tallis R. (1998). Age-specific incidence and prevalence rates of treated epilepsy in an unselected population of 2,052,922 and age-specific fertility rates of women with epilepsy. *Lancet,* 352:1970–1973.

Walker MC (2005) Status epilepticus: an evidence based guide. *BMJ,* 331:673–677.

CHAPTER 14

NEURO-ONCOLOGY

Jeremy Rees and Naomi Fersht

INTRODUCTION

Neuro-oncology is the study of tumours of the nervous system and of the neurological complications of cancer. Because of the rising incidence of brain tumours and the improvements in treatment for systemic cancers, this subspecialty is becoming increasingly important and relevant to physicians in a variety of different fields.

The effects of brain tumours on patients, their families and carers are enormous. Not only is survival with a malignant primary brain tumour poor, with only 15 per cent of patients still alive five years from diagnosis, but the neurological effects (cognitive and functional) are devastating.

EPIDEMIOLOGY

Incidence

Central nervous system (CNS) tumours may be primary, arising from the intracranial structures and the spine, or metastases from malignancy outside the CNS.

Brain tumours occur at any age, and are the most common solid malignancy in children (20 per cent). This peak drops through teenage and young adult years, before slowly rising again from the mid-twenties to reach a second major peak in the eighth decade. There is a clear distinction in both tumour type and site with age. Most adult brain tumours are supratentorial, 70 per cent in childhood are infratentorial. Brain metastases in adults are seen four times more frequently than primary brain tumours and are ten times more common than gliomas.

The most frequent tumours in children are low-grade glioma, ependymoma and medulloblastoma, in adolescents germ cell tumours (GCTs) and astrocytomas, while in adults, meningiomas, pituitary tumours and astrocytomas are the most common primary tumours. Meningiomas are far more frequent in women, pituitary tumours equal in women and men, and astrocytomas are more common in men.

Around 300 children and 8500 adults each year in the UK are found to have primary brain tumours (non-invasive and malignant). This accounts for 3

per cent of all new cancers presenting that year. However, they are responsible for more years of life lost per cancer than any other adult tumour.

Survival

Treatment outcome and survival is dependent on tumour type and grade; tumour location and size; patient age and performance status at diagnosis. **Patients with benign tumours, such as pituitary tumours and meningiomas, are usually cured**. Around a third of adults diagnosed as having a malignant brain tumour will live at least one year, but only 15 per cent will survive more than five years with only a small percentage cured. Germinomas are rare in adults, but with appropriate treatment have almost 100 per cent survival. Children fare much better than adults, with an overall 65 per cent five-year survival (5YS), and a 90 per cent cure rate in low-grade gliomas.

> Histological grade is an extremely important prognostic factor, with the 5YS falling from over 85 per cent in a WHO Grade I (Gd1) astrocytoma, through 50 and 20 per cent for Gd2 and Gd3 respectively, to an average life expectancy of less than a year in the Gd4 Glioblastoma multiforme (GBM).

Risk factors

The cause of most primary brain tumours is unknown. Risk increases with age. Radiation exposure, either therapeutic or following nuclear contamination, is the only proven environmental factor.

Meningiomas and gliomas are more common after
- previous cranial radiotherapy in adults for pituitary tumours, and in childhood for craniopharyngiomas;
- treatment for acute lymphoblastic leukaemia, and for benign conditions such as tinea capitis and haemangioma.

Radiation-induced tumours may take up to 40 years to develop, and are usually found in the lower dose areas at the edge of the treatment field.

Family history and genetic factors are rare but important. Hereditary syndromes with increased incidence of CNS tumours include the following:

- tuberous sclerosis and subependymal giant cell astrocytoma;
- Von Hippel Lindau and haemangiomablastoma;
- neurofibromatosis types 1 and 2 and optic nerve glioma, meningioma and vestibular schwannoma;
- Li-Fraumeni syndrome (inherited germline mutation in p53) and astrocytoma and medulloblastoma;
- Gorlin's (naevoid basal cell carcinoma) and Turcot's syndromes and medulloblastoma.

PATHOLOGY

The 2007 WHO classification of CNS tumours (Table 14.1) is the standard definition worldwide. Primary CNS tumours are heterogeneous and are defined very differently to tumours arising outside the neuraxis. The TNM staging system is not applicable to CNS tumours and tumour grade reflects local growth and behaviour, rather than the ability to metastasize. Haematogenous spread is extremely uncommon, although some tumours may metastasize within the craniospinal axis. The pathology of individual tumours is discussed below.

CLINICAL FEATURES

> The presentation of brain tumours is dependent on site and rate of growth. Rapidly growing malignant tumours usually present with features of raised intracranial pressure (ICP) and/or localizing neurological deficits. In contrast, low-grade tumours are more likely to present as seizure disorders due to their slower, more infiltrative behaviour.

In a retrospective study of over 300 patients with a radiological space-occupying lesion, headaches and seizures were the most frequent symptoms at diagnosis. Headaches may be due to raised ICP, or stretching or distortion of the meninges, and have few specific features with the evolution of associated neurological symptoms often prompting the diagnosis.

Raised ICP can be due to mass effect (direct tumour infiltration and vasogenic oedema), haem-

Table 14.1 Classification of primary brain tumours – summary of WHO 2007 classification

	Grade
Tumours of neuroepithelial tissue	
Astrocytic tumours	
Pilocytic astrocytoma	I
Diffuse astrocytoma	II
Anaplastic astrocytoma	III
Glioblastoma	IV
Oligodendroglial tumours	
Oligodendroglioma	II
Anaplastic oligodendroglioma	III
Mixed gliomas	
Oligoastrocytoma	II
Anaplastic oligoastrocytoma	III
Ependymal tumours	
Ependymoma	II
Anaplastic ependymoma	III
Choroid plexus tumours	
Choroid plexus papilloma/carcinoma	
Neuronal and mixed neuronal-glial tumours	
Pineal parenchymal tumours	
Embryonal tumours	
Tumours of meninges	
Meningiomas	
Primary CNS lymphomas	
Germ cell tumours	
Tumours of the sellar region	
Tumours of cranial and peripheral nerves	
Metastatic tumours	

optic atrophy. Tumours in the pineal region may cause Parinaud's syndrome (paralysis of upward gaze, convergence retraction nystagmus, light-near dissociation), tumours in the thalamus and basal ganglia produce pain, sensory loss and memory disturbance. Base of skull tumours (primary and metastatic) may cause cranial nerve palsies.

Para- and suprasellar tumours (such as pituitary tumours and craniopharyngiomas) may present with endocrine dysfunction as well as bitemporal hemianopia secondary to compression of the optic chiasm. Craniopharyngiomas and low-grade gliomas (LGG) in children can lead to delayed or precocious puberty. Non-functioning tumours may cause pituitary failure, while the clinical effects of pituitary hormone oversecretion may be observed in the functional pituitary adenomas (such as acromegaly and Cushing syndrome).

Infratentorial tumours in the posterior fossa present with ataxia and nystagmus, those in the brainstem result in multiple cranial nerve palsies, hemiparesis and spasticity. Children with medulloblastoma usually present with features of raised ICP from compression of the IV ventricle rather than cerebellar signs.

Both primary intramedullary spinal tumours and spinal metastases can present with pain (local back and root pain), motor and sensory disturbance, sphincter disturbance and reflex changes.

Cognitive and behavioural changes occur only in a small number of patients, but are well recognized. They range from psychiatric disturbances (personality change, psychosis and depression) through behaviour disorders (for example abulia with frontal lobe tumours), to specific focal cognitive deficits (for example aphasia, alexia, acalculia or apraxia).

orrhage into the tumour, or obstruction of the cerebrospinal fluid (CSF) pathways. The classical features are headache (waking with pain during the night, headache worst in the morning, and improving with an upright posture during the day), and nausea and vomiting (also usually worse in the morning). A sixth cranial nerve palsy may be a false localizing sign due to the vulnerability of the nerve in its long intracranial course.

Focal neurological signs may help to localize the tumour prior to imaging. Supratentorial tumours may present with hemiparesis, spasticity and seizures (focal, generalized), optic pathway tumours with visual field and acuity deficits and

IMAGING OF BRAIN TUMOURS

Imaging is an essential component in many aspects of brain tumour management – at diagnosis, guiding the surgical approach, assessing the response to treatment and in surveillance. Modern radiotherapy planning techniques rely on both computed tomography (CT) and magnetic resonance imaging (MRI) images, and surgeons are increasingly using intraoperative imaging, both ultrasound scanning and MRI, to define extent of resection.

MRI is the most sensitive technique currently available and the gold standard in neuro-oncology imaging. It is better than CT in terms of soft tissue and tumour delineation, whereas CT provides more information about calcification, bony structures and abnormalities.

MR imaging for brain tumours includes differently weighted sequences before and after the injection of intravenous contrast, gadolinium: T1-weighted (T1); T2-weighted; and fluid attenuated inversion recovery (FLAIR) sequences. The majority of brain tumours are hypodendense on CT, hypointense on T1-weighted MRI images, and hyperintense on T2 and FLAIR MRI sequences.

Contrast enhancement on both CT and MRI is generally seen with high-grade tumours, metastases and with highly vascular tumours, such as meningiomas. However, up to 15 per cent of low-grade gliomas, particularly pilocytic astrocytomas, may also enhance.

Modern imaging techniques such as functional and physiological MRI and positron emission tomography (PET) are becoming more widely available, and provide complementary biological information about blood flow and cellular ultrastructure that may help choice of treatments and assessment of response.

Functional magnetic resonance imaging (fMRI) is used in brain tumours to assess the risk of neurosurgical treatment for tumours in eloquent cortices controlling language, motor and memory functions. Localizing the motor strip and coregistering the results to a structural scan prior to surgery can help guide the extent of resection aided by direct cortical stimulation during an awake craniotomy. In some cases, using fMRI to confirm the expected location of the motor strip may remove the need for awake neurosurgery.

MRI lacks specificity in two key areas: the prediction of tumour grade and the distinction between recurrence and radiation necrosis (becoming increasingly important with the increasing use of high-dose, small field radiation treatments using gamma and cyberknife). Physiological imaging techniques (MRI perfusion and diffusion-weighted imaging) and metabolic imaging (^{18}F-fluorodeoxyglucose positron-emission tomography (FDG-PET) scanning) can potentially differentiate neoplastic from non-neoplastic brain tissue based on physiological rather than structural features.

Magnetic resonance spectroscopy (MRS) identifies metabolites involved in physiological or pathological processes and can be used to provide semi-diagnostic data for brain tumours: choline and myo-inositol peaks are seen with gliomas; free lipids in necrotic tumour (metastases and GBM); and alanine in meningiomas. However, it is not sufficiently sensitive to be used in isolation for histological grading.

Dynamic susceptibility-weighted contrast-enhanced MRI measures relative cerebral blood flow (rCBV), which has been shown to have a good correlation with WHO tumour grade (high rCBV is seen in areas of high capillary density thought to reflect tumour aggressiveness) and may help distinguish tumour recurrence (high rCBV) from radiation necrosis (low rCBV). It is also used to assess the risk of malignant transformation in adult low-grade gliomas.

The apparent diffusion coefficient (ADC) describes water diffusion: the more cellular the tumour, the greater the barrier to diffusion, the lower the ADC measurement. This can be used to demonstrate tumours with tightly packed cells and very little extracellular matrix, for example primary CNS lymphomas and primitive neuroectodermal tumours (PNET).

Diffusion tensor imaging (DTI) can provide information about white matter connections among brain regions and the influence of the tumour on white matter integrity. White matter neuronal axons have an internal fibrous structure. Water diffuses more rapidly along white matter pathways than across pathways and this property, known as fractional anisotrophy, can be used to select and follow neural tracts through the brain – a process called tractography. This in turn can help determine whether a tumour is displacing or destroying a white matter tract and the anatomical relationship between the tumour boundary and the fibre pathways.

^{18}F FDG accumulates in areas of high glucose metabolism, and is trapped within metabolically active tumour cells. However, it is difficult to distinguish tumour from normal grey matter struc-

tures due to the high glucose utilization. FDG-PET scanning is used in the differential diagnosis of radiation necrosis versus tumour progression and in grading tumours which are too dangerous to biopsy. PET scanning based on amino-acid metabolism, for example ^{11}C-methionine PET is more sensitive for distinguishing low-grade gliomas from other non-neoplastic lesions.

MANAGEMENT

The multidisciplinary team
Multidisciplinary teamworking is central to the current management of patients with brain tumours. Its core members are neurosurgeons, clinical oncologists, neurologists, neuropathologists, neuroradiologists, clinical nurse specialists, physiotherapists, occupational therapists and neuropsychologists, and the involvement of palliative care services.

The team discusses diagnosis and management options, both at presentation, postoperatively and at progression or recurrence. It ensures that appropriate care and rehabilitation is in place, and that good communication occurs between patient and carers, and between different specialties within the hospital and between secondary care and primary care. Patients with neurological tumours have a wide range of issues that necessitate the input of the multidisciplinary team aside from the management of their malignancy, including intellectual and personality change, disabling motor and visual deficits, seizures and adverse effects of steroid use including weight gain and muscle wasting.

Surgery

Surgery lies at the core of management for brain tumours. It provides tissue for histological diagnosis, allows rapid relief from the symptoms due to mass effect, may improve focal neurological defects, and allow cure in certain cases. For many CNS tumours, the extent of surgical resection is an important prognostic factor that needs to be balanced against neurological deficit.

At presentation, or at any stage in their disease, some patients will require urgent surgical CSF diversion by insertion of external ventricular drains or a ventriculoperitoneal shunt. In certain cases, third ventriculostomy is an alternative to shunt insertion and spares the patient from potential complications of shunt blockage and infection.

New techniques and technologies are available which improve surgical outcomes and reduce neuro-disability. Biopsies (and definitive surgery) are usually performed by open methods (craniotomy) but tumours that are difficult to access may undergo an image-guided biopsy. Ventricular tumours can be biopsied endoscopically.

Biopsy and definitive surgery may involve frameless neuro-navigation, which utilizes MRI scanning with fiducial markers placed on the patient's scalp, to identify preoperatively structures and accurate localization of the tumour and to enable the surgeon to register in real time the incision with the location of the underlying tumour. However, the main drawback is the lack of real-time information once the dura has been opened and the tumour has been partly resected, as there is considerable shift of brain tissue. Intraoperative scanning techniques, both ultrasound scanning (USS) and MRI, are now helping to overcome this. USS informs on tumour depth, cystic components and extent of resection. Intraoperative MRI can update the surgeon on the extent of residual tumour that can still be resected, reducing the need for second procedures.

Other neurosurgical techniques include transphenoidal surgery and neuro-endoscopy for access to sellar tumours. Awake craniotomy with cortical pathway mapping and neurophysiological monitoring is used in low-grade glioma surgery to maximize tumour resection while minimizing neurological deficits. During the operation, a dedicated team carries out cortical stimulation, and assesses language and motor and sensory tasks.

Radiotherapy

Radiotherapy for brain and spinal tumours is often given as short palliative courses, between two and six treatment fractions, aimed at symptom relief, steroid weaning and prevention of further neurological decline. Treatment courses are usually 6 weeks long when given with curative or radical (prolongation of survival) intent.

Radiotherapy is now planned based on CT and MRI images with the aim of sparing normal brain tissue and more accurately localizing tumour boundaries. The patient is immobilized, as for treatment, in a plastic shell and CT slices are obtained. MRI data are then fused with the CT data and used to define the 'volumes' to be treated to high dose. The beam arrangement is chosen to encompass the treatment volume with maximal sparing of surrounding brain. Shielding is designed to conform the fields more closely to the actual tumour volume, and protect critical structures (such as the optic apparatus) from doses exceeding their known radiation tolerance.

The next technical step up from this is to combine conformal planning with stereotactic techniques for immobilization and tumour localization, allowing further reduction in treatment volume due to increased accuracy. Stereotactic shells (unlike the frames used in radiosurgery discussed below) enable the dose to be given in a conventionally fractionated regime. **Stereotactic radiotherapy is useful for treating small benign tumours, such as pituitary adenomas, rather than gliomas – where the aim is to encompass a large target volume that includes likely microscopic tumour invasion.**

Intensity modulated radiotherapy (IMRT) is a further refinement of conformal radiotherapy in which the radiation beam intensity can be modified across the treatment volume. This allows greater conformity to tumour anatomy, and for treatment of concave volumes with sparing of critical structures (such as the spinal cord or optic pathways and retina) lying within these tumour concavities.

Radiosurgery uses stereotactic positioning to define a highly conformal high dose volume that is treated with one or several large dose fractions of radiotherapy. These large single doses are safe and possible due to a steep dose gradient sparing normal brain tissue. The gamma knife uses a cobalt source of gamma rays to deliver a single high-dose treatment to small (<3 cm) lesions in the brain, such as brain metastases, meningiomas and acoustic neuromas. The Cyberknife utilizes a relocatable immobilization system that can be used to treat intra- and extracranial sites, and allows the high-dose treatments to be fractionated over 1–5 days. This means larger tumour volumes can be treated with the gamma knife, and those closer to critical structures.

Proton therapy

This is a form of particle therapy that allows high intensity highly localized deposition of energy at a fixed depth, enabling treatment of tumours to a high dose despite close proximity of critical surrounding structures. Protons are preferable in the management of radioresistant clival chordomas and base of skull chondrosarcomas close to the brainstem. **Protons have benefits over IMRT in children, as there is no associated low–dose radiation 'bath' considered to carry a higher risk of second tumour development.** There is currently no proton facility in the UK that can treat these tumours, but there are clear national referral pathways to send these patients to Europe and the USA.

Radionuclide therapy

This involves using radiation as a drug. A radionuclide is an atom with an unstable nucleus, which undergoes radioactive decay emitting gamma rays and/or subatomic particles. Radionuclides are a source of radiation that can be targeted to specific tumours when given orally or intravenously (for example radioidine concentrates only in thyroid and thyroid cancer cells) or instilled into cavities to give high-dose, localized treatment (such as in the management of cystic craniopharygiomas).

Chemotherapy

Although surgery and radiotherapy are central to management, chemotherapy also has a role to play in several CNS malignancies.

> Chemotherapy can be curative or palliative. Neoadjuvant chemotherapy is given before definitive treatment with surgery and/or radiotherapy. Concomittant chemotherapy is given during radiotherapy, while adjuvant chemotherapy is given after definitive treatment.

Chemotherapy is now standard treatment of GBM in good performance status patients under the age of 70 (both concomitant with radiation, and then adjuvantly). It is considered at relapse for all high-grade gliomas (Gd3 and Gd4), and also for previously irradiated low-grade gliomas, or those that are too extensive to be encompassed within a radiation field. All children with PNET and medulloblastoma routinely receive chemotherapy during and after radiotherapy, but there is currently no role for chemotherapy in adult PNET outside the context of a clinical trial. Chemotherapy is a key part of the management of primary CNS lymphoma and intracranial GCTs.

PRIMARY CNS TUMOURS

Glioma

Two-thirds of new neuro-oncology referrals are gliomas, and half of those are GBM.

Low-grade glioma

LGG (WHO grade I and 2) account for 20 per cent of gliomas and are seen in both children and adults with a median age at diagnosis around 35 years. They are a diverse group of tumours and are named according to the presumed cell of origin – 85 per cent are astrocytomas, 10 per cent are oligodendrogliomas and the rest are of mixed lineage (oligoastrocytomas). LGG are slow growing and diffusely infiltrating, and usually present with seizures. Median survival is 5–10 years.

The astrocyctic LGGs are pilocytic astrocytoma (Gd1) and diffuse astrocytoma (Gd2). Pilocytic astrocyomas are mostly seen in children and young adults, either infratentorially or along the optic pathways and thalamic regions. There is a 90 per cent cure rate with surgery and/or radiotherapy. In contrast, the grade 2 gliomas (Figure 14.1) are usually supratentorial within the temporal and frontal lobes and are less histologically stable than the Gd1 tumours, with the majority transforming to higher grades over time. LGG differ markedly in their response to treatment, with oligodendroglial tumours having a better prognosis than astrocytic tumours.

Radiologically, LGG are hypo- or isointense compared to normal brain tissue on T1 MRI images. They are best seen on T2 and FLAIR images, where there are hyperintense. Pilocytic astrocytomas usually show contrast enhancement within a mural nodule. About 20–30 per cent of Gd2 gliomas enhance, more commonly with oligodendrogliomas, and contrast enhancement at presentation is a poor prognostic sign, and it is an indication of malignant transformation if it develops during surveillance.

In the infratentorial childhood LGG, maximal resective surgery (with minimal morbidity) is the mainstay of treatment and results in a 90 per cent ten-year survival. The choice between focal radiotherapy and chemotherapy, where indicated, depends upon the age of the patient and consequent risk of radiation-induced cognitive deficits. Chemotherapy is preferred up to the age of eight (previously the cut off was three years).

The childhood visual pathway tumours, especially in NF-1, may follow a very indolent course. Surveillance is preferred, with surgery and radiotherapy or chemotherapy reserved for pro-

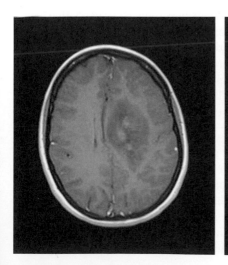
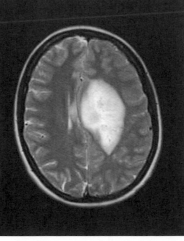

Figure 14.1 Left frontal oligodendroglioma. A 34-year-old man presenting with a generalized tonic-clonic seizure and frontal adversive seizures. Axial T1W post-gadolinium and axial T2W MRI of left frontal subcortical tumour showing typical radiological features of low-grade glioma – well circumscribed homogeneous lesion, absence of oedema and central necrosis. There is patchy low-level contrast enhancement which is often seen in grade II oligodendrogliomas.

gression with symptomatic visual impairment. Children with NF-1 have a higher risk of long-term effects of radiation, especially vasculopathy and second tumours, so radiation is avoided where possible.

In adults, the optimal management of cerebral LGG is uncertain. The typical patient is a young adult presenting with seizures without neurological deficit or raised intracranial pressure.

Surgery is considered if the tumour is well demarcated and away from eloquent brain structures, for example primary motor or speech area. Thus only about 30 per cent of adult LGG are resectable in their entirety and as partial resection has not been shown to be of prognostic benefit, many patients are treated medically with anti-epileptic drugs and monitored closely with imaging surveillance, usually at six-month intervals.

Treatment at progression may include biopsy and radiotherapy/chemotherapy or partial resection, particularly when there is mass effect.

The role of radiotherapy early in the course of LGG is still not clear. Some argue that radiotherapy will be more effective while a tumour is small, others feel that early intervention is not warranted given the long natural history. Recent data suggest that radiotherapy immediatcly after diagnosis or initial surgery can significantly prolong the time to progression, but does not affect overall survival.

Patients considered to have a higher risk of recurrence or progression are usually treated with radiotherapy early on. Adverse prognostic factors include two or more of the following: age over 40, tumour diameter greater than 6 cm, astrocytic histology, neurological deficit before surgery and tumour crossing the midline or causing midline shift. There is a lower threshold for early treatment of tumours in eloquent areas (where progression would lead to significant disability). Radiotherapy may improve neurological deficits, and also epilepsy control in 50 per cent of patients.

The role of chemotherapy in LGG has not yet been established, and is usually reserved for large tumours requiring extensive radiation fields. However, both low- and high-grade oligodendro-gliomas are more chemo- and radiosensitive than astrocytomas, attributed to a specific chromosomal loss of both 1p and 19q found in about 70 per cent. This genetic change is associated with a longer time to progression following radiotherapy and an almost 100 per cent response rate to subsequent chemotherapy.

High-grade glioma

High-grade glioma (HGG) (Gd3 and Gd4) may arise *de novo* (primary), or by transformation of a LGG (secondary). These are considered different entities, and can be distinguished genetically by the presence of IDH1 mutations (present in most secondary HGG but very rarely in primary HGG). Primary HGG are found in older patients (peak incidence 60–70 years), secondary HGGs are seen in younger patients, often with a known LGG.

Age, performance status and neurological impairment are strong determinants of survival in this group, and must be considered when deciding on treatment recommendations. The addition of radiotherapy to surgical management is standard management for HGG, regardless of whether an extensive debulking or a diagnostic biopsy has been performed. Surgery alone is never curative, but craniotomy and debulking will relieve pressure symptoms, reduce steroid dependence, and is an independent prognostic factor for survival. However, all benefits are modest and measured in months.

Radical radiotherapy should be restricted to younger patients (less than 70 years) with excellent performance status. In the elderly and poorer prognostic groups, shorter course, high-dose palliative radiotherapy regimes are preferred as they impinge less on the patients remaining quality of life and are equivalent dose-wise to the longer conventional courses.

The Gd3 anaplastic astrocytomas (Figure 14.2) have a better prognosis than GBM: good performance status patients have a median survival of 3–5 years, but this falls to 18 months in the elderly with poor performance status. The Gd3 oligodendrogliomas are more chemo- and radiosensitive than other anaplastic gliomas, with a longer time

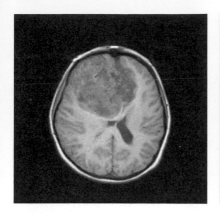

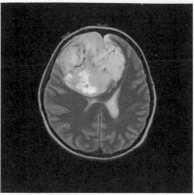

Figure 14.2 Bifrontal anaplastic oligodendroglioma. A 28-year-old woman presenting with symptoms of raised intracranial pressure during the second trimester of pregnancy. Axial T1W post-Gd and axial T2W MRI shows minor contrast enhancement and a heterogeneous tumour through which vessels are running. There is effacement of sulci and frontal horns. Histology revealed anaplastic oligodendroglioma (WHO grade III).

to progression following radiotherapy and an almost 100 per cent response rate to subsequent chemotherapy. However, large clinical studies have not demonstrated a survival benefit of neoadjuvant or adjuvant chemotherapy over first chemotherapy given at relapse. This is probably due to their radio-sensitivity, and current practice is to assess chromosome loss as a prognostic rather than predictive factor. All anaplastic gliomas are, therefore, treated with adjuvant radiotherapy following surgery, with chemotherapy reserved for disease progression.

> However, the gold standard management of GBM (Figure 14.3) in good performance status patients under 70 years, is surgery followed by adjuvant radical radiotherapy with temozolomide chemotherapy (given concurrently with the radiotherapy and adjuvantly for 6–8 months). Recent randomized controlled trial data showed an increase in two-year survival from 10 to 26 per cent with chemoradiation and an increase in median survival from 11 to 14 months and an increase in four-year survival from less than 2 to 13 per cent.

GBMs with high levels of the O^6-methylguanine-DNA methyltransferase (MGMT) DNA repair enzyme are less likely to benefit from the addition of temozolomide and this is assessed using methylation of the MGMT promoter sequence (hypermethylation of the promoter sequence turns off the gene and reduces levels of MGMT production). **It is highly likely that molecular and chromosomal analysis of HGG will become a standard part of diagnosis and will influence treatment decisions.**

When good performance status patients relapse, the treatment options include further surgery, chemotherapy or reirradiation (if sufficient time has elapsed for the benefits of further radiotherapy to outweigh the risks of late effects of high-dose treatment). Chemotherapy response rates (in the absence of chromosomal loss of 1p 19q) are low, at around 20–30 per cent in terms of symptomatic benefit, radiological improvement and increased time to progression. The appropriateness of continuing treatment with potentially serious adverse effects must always be considered.

There are ongoing phase 1, 2 and 3 trials of new agents in HGG, including tyrosine kinsase inhibitors, epidermal growth factor receptor antagonists and anti-angiogenic drugs, but their role in improving survival is as yet unproven.

Brainstem glioma

Brainstem gliomas are mainly seen in children aged 5–10 years and in young adults. Most are high-grade astrocytomas arising in the pons, extending into the medulla and midbrain, presenting with a short history of ataxia, long tract signs and cranial nerve palsies. This typical history with the characteristic MRI features of a diffuse, poorly T1-enhancing lesion, is considered diagnostic of the high-grade diffuse intrinsic pontine glioma, and obviates the need for a brainstem biopsy, with its high morbidity and failure rate.

Diffuse intrinsic pontine gliomas have a median survival of nine months, with only 5 per cent long-term survivors (usually low-grade variants). As they are inoperable, radical radiotherapy is the standard treatment, usually starting urgently due to rapidly progressive brainstem deficits.

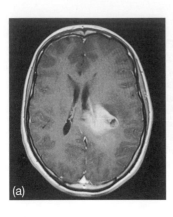
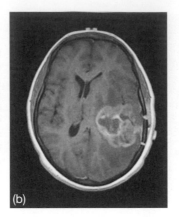
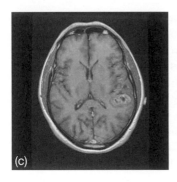
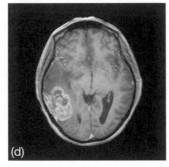

Figure 14.3 Glioblastoma multiforme (GBM). Four patients showing characteristic appearances of a high-grade intrinsic tumour with irregular rim enhancement and central necrosis. (a) Deep left frontal with ependymal enhancement. (b) Left frontal with surrounding oedema and mass effect. (c) Left post frontal presenting with seizures and dysphasia. (d) Right parieto-occipital presenting with headache and dyspraxia. All tumours were biopsied and showed vascular proliferation and necrosis consistent with GBM.

When there is a longer history, and radiology suggests a low-grade, more discrete lesion, efforts should be made to obtain histology if possible, to confirm the improved prognosis.

Gliomatosis cerebri

Gliomatosis cerebri is an unusual manifestation of glioma characterized by extensive involvement of at least three lobes of the brain by glial cell neoplastic proliferation (Figure 14.4). It is most common in middle age, often with delayed presentation due to variable features and lack of localizing neurological signs. It may be low or high grade, and a biopsy is required for diagnosis. It is usually too extensive for surgical treatment, and is managed by large radiation fields and temozolomide chemotherapy.

Ependymoma

Ependymomas (Figure 14.5) are found anywhere along the ventricular system and occur at any age. There are three grades – Gd1 (myxopapillary and subependymal), Gd2 (ependymoma) and Gd3 (anaplastic ependymoma). The difference in prognosis between Gd2 and Gd3 is not as pronounced as that

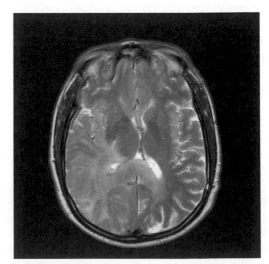

Figure 14.4 Gliomatosis cerebri. A 67-year-old man presenting with cognitive decline and seizures. Axial T2W MRI showing diffusely infiltrating high signal change in both cerebral hemispheres compressing the right posterior horn. Biopsy showed gliomatosis cerebri.

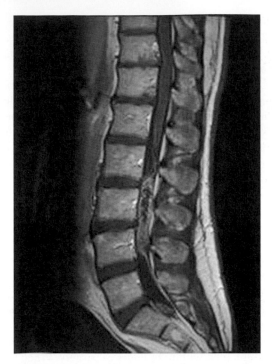

Figure 14.5 Intramedullary spinal cord tumour. Sagittal MRI showing a well-demarcated tumour in the lumbar region. Histology showed a WHO grade II ependymoma.

between Gd2 and Gd3 astrocytomas. They are more common in children, with two-thirds in the posterior fossa, presenting with focal neurology and obstructive hydrocephalus. Spinal ependymomas are more common than intracranial ependymomas in adults, usually in the cervical spine or the conus medullaris. Adult ependymomas have better survival rates than other gliomas (over 50 per cent are curable), with survival related to age, performance status, extent of resection and grade.

Craniospinal dissemination can occur, so imaging of the entire craniospinal axis is required at diagnosis and on follow up. Ependymoma is primarily managed surgically, with the extent of resection determining prognosis, and the natural history being a prolonged one characterized by local recurrence, usually after incomplete resection.

Adjuvant radiotherapy is indicated after subtotal resection of Gd2 tumours (and should always be discussed after complete resection) and in all Gd3 tumours. Historically, craniospinal radiotherapy was used for posterior fossa lesions, but has been replaced by focal radiotherapy after studies demonstrated only a 3 per cent relapse rate outside the primary site. Ependymomas are not chemosensitive,

with vincristine-based regimes being used with only modest benefit for inoperable relapses following radiotherapy.

Spinal tumours

Primary spinal tumours may be intramedullary (ependymomas and astrocytomas) or more frequently extramedullary. Extramedullary tumours are either intradural (schwannomas, meningiomas) or extradural (e.g. metastases).

Spinal ependymomas present in middle age and have a better prognosis than when intracranial, but there is the risk of significant neurological morbidity with complete surgical resection. The diagnosis is often made after months or years of slowly progressing symptoms. MRI demonstrates a well-defined, brightly enhancing lesion. Recurrence rates are around 5–10 per cent in low grade, fully resected tumours. As with intracranial ependymomas, adjuvant radiotherapy should be considered after incompletely resected Gd1, and for all Gd2 and Gd3 tumours. Localized radiotherapy is used except when lumbosacral. Tumours at this site may spread with a 'sugar coating' of ependymoma along the nerve roots below the primary site, thought to be secondary to gravity. Standard practice is therefore to encompass the whole thecal sac within the radiation field.

Spinal astrocytomas are usually the fibrillary, low-grade subtypes, presenting in a similar manner to ependymomas. Prognosis is less good than for ependymoma. The median survival of spinal high-grade gliomas is about 20 months. Surgery is the mainstay of treatment but needs to be carefully considered in high-grade lesions or in patients with significant neurological deficit. Radiotherapy is indicated as for the low- and high-grade intracranial astrocytomas.

Meningiomas

There are two main predictors of increased rate of recurrence: atypical and malignant histology, and residual disease following surgery. Adjuvant radiotherapy has been shown to reduce local recurrence, but without a survival advantage. There is also the issue of the long-term side-effects of radiation,

Meningiomas (Figure 14.6) account for about 20 per cent of all intracranial tumours, peak in the sixth decade and are more common in women. Many are asymptomatic when they are discovered as an incidental finding. They are slow growing and only rarely invade brain. They can involve bone and cause hyperostosis (best demonstrated on the CT bone windows). They often have a dural tail visible on MRI. Common intracranial sites are parasagittal, olfactory groove, tuberculum sellae and the sphenoid wing. Most are benign, but up to 5 per cent will be histologically atypical (WHO grade II) and 2–3 per cent anaplastic (malignant, WHO grade III). Treatment is surgical, with recurrence rates less than 10 per cent in the benign lesions.

especially pertinent when treating younger patients with a long life expectancy. Radiotherapy is usually given after the first relapse, unless the neurological cost of local progression is high, or as primary treatment in inoperable cases (with local control rates over 90 per cent in Gd1 tumours).

Primitive neuroectodermal tumours

PNETs are generally childhood tumours, responsible for only 1 per cent of CNS tumours in adults (mainly younger adults). Most PNETs are medulloblastomas (the most common childhood CNS tumour at 20 per cent) arising in the cerebellum. PNETs arising in the cerebral hemispheres are called supratentorial primitive neuroectodermal tumours (sPNET), and in the

pineal area called pineoblastoma. The sPNET have a significantly worse outcome than medulloblastoma, possibly due to complete surgical resection being more difficult and to biological differences.

PNETs are all histologically similar with small round cells with larger hyperchromatic nuclei clustered into rosettes. There are distinct subtypes of medulloblastoma, all highly malignant WHO grade IV tumours with a propensity for spread via the CSF. A third will have radiological evidence of leptomeningeal disease at presentation. About 5 per cent disseminate outside the CNS (most commonly to bone), a phenomenon not seen with other primary CNS tumours.

Staging requires preoperative MRI of the brain and whole spine. In children, they appear as well-defined, enhancing midline tumours whereas in adults they are poorly defined masses in the cerebellar hemispheres. Residual postoperative disease, an important prognostic factor, is best demonstrated by comparing the preoperative MRI with one obtained within 24 hours of surgery. When the residual exceeds 1.5 cm^2 (maximum cross-sectional area), further 'second look' surgery should be considered. Unless there is evidence of meningeal/metastatic disease on the preoperative imaging, a lumbar puncture for CSF cytology is necessary. This must be performed at least 15 days following surgery to avoid false positives due to contamination.

Poor prognostic factors are metastatic disease, postoperative residual greater than 1.5 cm^2, anaplastic or large cell pathology, age (children under 36 months and adults). These divide patients into two treatment groups: standard risk, medulloblastoma, no metastases, residual less than 1.5 cm^2,

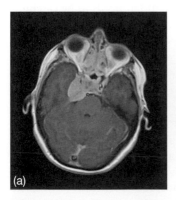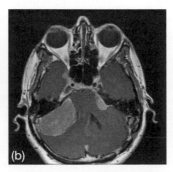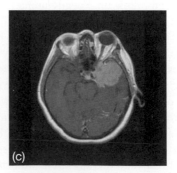

Figure 14.6 Meningioma. MRI showing skull base meningiomas in three patients. (a) Right cavernous sinus. (b) Bilateral posterior fossa. (c) Left lateral sphenoid and middle cranial fossa with intra-orbital extension causing visual loss in left eye.

children; and high risk, sPNET (including pineoblastoma), M1-4, anaplastic/large cell, residual greater than 1.5 cm², adults.

Surgical resection of a medulloblastoma may result in cerebellar mutism syndrome. This occurs in up to 8 per cent of all posterior fossa craniotomies but most commonly after resection of a medulloblastoma extending into the brainstem, thought to be caused by damage to the dentate nuclei.

Following maximal resection, craniospinal axis radiation (CSA) must be given and has been the standard management for decades. This is complex and the technical quality of radiotherapy is closely related to outcome in PNET. It should therefore only be delivered in designated paediatric and young adult radiotherapy centres. An 85 per cent 5YS is now seen in standard risk patients given 35 Gy to the whole CSA, followed by a boost to 55 Gy to the primary tumour.

There is now an increasing focus on quality of survival, in addition to cure. CSA radiotherapy leads to significant endocrine, growth and cognitive deficits in children. Multimodality treatment has been introduced for standard risk children, which enables the dose of CSA radiotherapy to be safely reduced, with the addition of a 'Packer' chemotherapy regimen (weekly vincristine during radiotherapy, followed by eight cycles of CCNU, cisplatin and vincristine). However, chemotherapy brings its own adverse effects including peripheral neuropathy, hearing loss, renal failure and myelosupression.

In the high risk group of children, the priority is still to improve survival. The 5YS rates are still 30–50 per cent despite the addition of chemotherapy to CSART. The optimal chemotherapy regimen has yet to be defined, with new high-dose regimens promising improved survival.

However, there are few clinical data to help define treatment strategies in adults and young people, and this patient group does not have the same issues with the harmful late effects of CSA radiotherapy. Chemotherapy should not be used routinely outside the context of a clinical trial.

Primary CNS lymphoma

Most patients are over 60 years with a male predominance. Immunosupressed patients, mostly HIV positive, are at far greater risk (up to 1000 times) than the general population. It is usually

Primary central nervous system lymphoma (PCNSL) is a rare form of non-Hodgkin's lymphoma (NHL), accounting for only 5 per cent of all primary brain tumours (Figure 14.7). It arises in, and is confined to, the brain, spinal cord and leptomeninges, with 20 per cent of patients having intra-ocular involvement at diagnosis. Over the last three decades survival has improved, mainly because of the introduction of methotrexate-based combination chemotherapy. Long-term treatment-related neurological toxicity remains a major problem.

an aggressive high-grade malignant lymphoma, mainly B-cell, and patients typically present with focal neurological symptoms developing over a few weeks. Behavioural changes and seizures are also common.

Characteristic brain imaging features are of solidly enhancing mass lesions; typically in the periventricular regions, deep grey matter structures and corpus callosum. Lesions are more frequently frontal and multifocal.

Corticosteroid treatment usually results in marked initial reduction in mass effect and contrast enhancement, and can confound radiological diagnosis and localization of targets for stereotactic biopsy. Wherever possible, corticosteroid therapy should be avoided prior to biopsy.

A neuropsychological baseline evaluation should be carried out before treatment and repeated during and after treatment. Cognitive dysfunction is present in 83 per cent of patients at the time of diagnosis, but improvement is seen in up to 60 per cent of patients who achieve clinical remission after primary chemotherapy. However, radiotherapy and chemotherapeutic agents are neurotoxic and the neurocognitive risk is increased when these treatment modalities are combined. The aim is to achieve the right balance between long-term disease control and neurotoxicity. This is a particular issue with older patients.

Treatment options include steroid therapy, whole brain radiotherapy (WBRT) and chemotherapy. Surgery has no role apart from diagnostic biopsy.

WBRT has limited long-term efficacy and causes delayed neurotoxicity (at around 1–2 years). Neurotoxicity presents as dementia, ataxia and urinary incontinence. WBRT is not recommended as

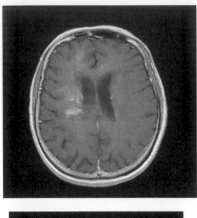
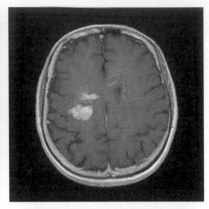
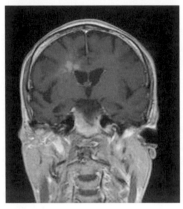
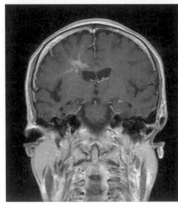

Figure 14.7 Primary CNS lymphoma. A 56-year-old woman presenting with visuospatial disorientation and headache. Contrast enhanced MRI (axial and coronal slices) show a homogeneously enhancing periventricular lesion; biopsy revealed a high-grade B cell lymphoma. There was no evidence of systemic lymphoma.

first-line treatment except as palliation in patients unfit to receive chemotherapy. All good performance status patients should be offered high-dose methotrexate chemotherapy regimes. For patients who achieve a complete response, consolidation WBRT can increase 5YS to 65 per cent. However, in patients over 60 years, neurocognitive adverse effects are more likely to outweigh potential benefits

Relapsed or refractory disease should be treated with salvage radiotherapy. Dexamethasone should be considered for short-term palliation.

Pineal tumours (including GCTs)

GCTs (Figure 14.8) are derived from pluripotential primordial germ cells, most commonly seen as gonadal (ovary/testis), mediastinal and intracranial tumours. They arise in the midline structures of the brain: pineal, third ventricle, suprasellar region and basal ganglia. Two-thirds are germinomas, one-third are NGGCTs made up of secreting GCTs (embryonal, yolk sac tumours and choriocarcino-

Pineal tumours, of a variety of different histological types, make up 1–2 per cent of all CNS tumours. There are around 50 cases per year in the UK. The majority are germinomas (45 per cent), then astrocytomas (17 per cent), non-germinomatous germ cell tumours (NGGCTs) (16 per cent) and pineal parenchymal tumours (pineocytoma and pineoblastoma) (15 per cent). Meningiomas, pineal cysts and metastases are also seen.

ma), teratomas (mature and immature) and mixed GCTs.

Intracranial germinomas are histologically identical to testicular seminoma, do not usually have raised CSF and/or serum tumour markers and are extremely radiosensitive. The secreting GCTs are characterized by significant secretion of alpha-fetoprotein (AFP) or human choriogonadotropin (β-HCG) detectable in the CSF and blood.

Since they are more frequent in children (up to

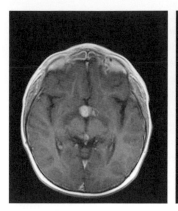
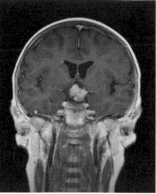
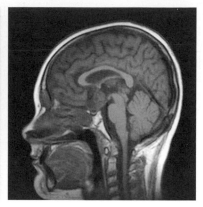

Figure 14.8 Germ cell tumour. An eight-year-old boy presenting with diabetes insipidus. Tumour markers revealed elevated beta-human chorionic gonadotrophin. Axial, coronal and sagittal MRI shows a contrast-enhancing midline suprasellar tumour typical of a germ cell tumour.

8 per cent of childhood CNS tumours), many of the principles of adult management have been adapted from current childhood guidelines.

Diagnosis, immediate management and staging requires craniospinal MRI, relief of hydrocephalus, CSF sampling for tumour markers and cytology. High levels of AFP/β-HCG are pathognomic of secreting NGGCTs, replace the need for biopsy and can be used to monitor response to chemotherapy or remission status on surveillance. Biopsy and endocrine assessment are indicated for all other cases.

Treatment and prognosis are diagnosis-dependent. Germinomas have a 90 per cent cure rate with craniospinal radiotherapy alone. NGGCTs have a worse prognosis and require multi-modality therapy with platinum-based chemotherapy, resection of any residual tumour and then focal radiotherapy. Teratomas require surgery only. Pineocytomas are treated with maximum tumour resection and adjuvant radiotherapy. Pineoblastomas are managed as all other supratentorial PNETs. Astrocytic tumours are managed as astrocytomas elsewhere.

Pituitary tumours

Pituitary adenomas (Figure 14.9) arise from the anterior pituitary and account for 10 per cent of intracranial tumours. Most are benign, but atypical tumours occur. Pituitary carcinoma is exceedingly rare, diagnosed by the presence of craniospinal or systemic metastases rather than local invasion, with a poor prognosis. It is thought to arise from a benign adenoma rather than *de novo*, and there is no obvious link between previous radiotherapy and

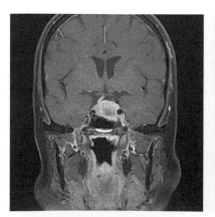
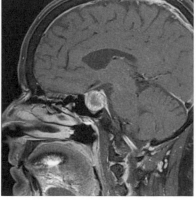

Figure 14.9 Pituitary adenoma. A 70-year-old man presenting with bitemporal hemianopia. Coronal and sagittal MRI show a large peripherally enhancing pituitary macroadenoma invading the left cavernous sinus. Histology revealed a silent corticotroph.

malignant transformation. Rarely, metastases and lymphoma are found in the pituitary fossa.

Pituitary adenomas are classified according to:

1 Size: microadenomas (more common) or macroadenomas depending on whether the tumour is less than or greater than 10 mm in diameter.

2 Histology: acidophilic, basophilic or chromophobic derivation and hormonal staining.

3 Hormonal function: functional (hormone-secreting) or non-functional (30 per cent).

Prolactinomas are the most common secreting adenomas (70 per cent), 15 per cent secrete GH causing acromegaly and 5 per cent secrete adrenocorticotropic hormone (ACTH) causing primary Cushing syndrome. Thyroid-stimulating hormone (TSH) or gonadotroph hypersecretion is rare.

> They present with hormonal effects, either over- or underproduction, or mass effect on the pituitary stalk with visual defects, typically a bitemporal hemianopia due to optic chiasm compression. Rarely, there may be cranial nerve palsies from cavernous sinus involvement (III, IV, V1 and V1,2) causing ptosis and double vision, or visual loss due to direct compression of the optic nerve. Temporal lobe epilepsy occasionally occurs due to direct extension. Hypothalamic disturbances including diabetes insipidus (DI) and (rarely) pituitary apoplexy also occur. They are sometimes seen as incidental findings on MRI.

> Pituitary apoplexy occurs when there is acute infarction or haemorrhage into the pituitary, and causes abrupt onset of headache, diplopia, visual loss and impaired consciousness, followed by panhypopituarism. It is more common in pregnancy and following trauma and diabetic ketoacidosis. Management requires steroids and occasionally decompressive surgery.

Initial investigation includes MRI of the pituitary region, full endocrine assessment (many patients will require life-long hormonal replacement, which may start at presentation, or years later) and careful charting of the visual fields. The majority will undergo surgery. However, medical therapy alone with dopamine agonists may be sufficient in prolactinomas, and, in tumours found as incidental findings which are non-functioning and not causing mass effect, no therapy may be necessary.

The role of surgery is to obtain the histological diagnosis, to achieve decompression of the optic chiasm and to produce an early reduction in hormone levels if required. Surgery is usually via the trans-sphenoidal route (which is well tolerated and allows visualization of the gland and tumour). More extensive tumours may require a frontal craniotomy.

Radiotherapy is given following surgery to reduce the risk of recurrence, and contributes to control rates of around 95 per cent at ten years. The broad indications for radiotherapy are for non-functioning tumours with incomplete removal (especially around the cavernous sinus), a large mass at diagnosis (the large silent corticotroph especially prone to early recurrence), recurrence after surgery alone, and failure of surgery to produce a hormonal 'cure' in functional tumours.

Radiotherapy carries an increased risk of hypopituitarism and the need for full hormonal replacement. This tends to develop many years after radiotherapy, but this will depend on the 'reserve' left by the tumour and the extent of surgical excision. The risk of recurrence (which may well be managed by further surgery) needs to be balanced against the risk of pituitary hypofunction. In young patients, radiotherapy can be delayed to maintain reproductive capabilities. Similarly, it can be avoided in older patients with normal pituitary function as they may die from other causes before recurrent tumour develops. The risk to visual function from conventionally fractionated radiotherapy is very low.

Surgery will cure 60–80 per cent of acromegalics. Radiotherapy is necessary in the surgical failures but produces a slow fall in GH levels, which may continue over many years. About 80 per cent are cured at ten years, particularly those with lower GH levels at presentation. Symptomatic patients will require medical therapy with somatostatin analogues in the meantime.

Surgery will cure 80 per cent of Cushing's, and again radiotherapy is indicated for the surgical failures. The fall in ACTH occurs over many months with radiotherapy. Excess ACTH can be acutely life-threatening and patients with significant hyper-secretion after surgery should be considered for adrenalectomy.

Up to 90 per cent of prolactinomas will respond to cabergoline, which produces a fall in prolactin and a reduction in tumour mass. The clinical picture, with a markedly raised prolactin and subsequent response to cabergoline, is diagnostic, and biopsy is not indicated for small tumours confined to the pituitary fossa. However, macroadenomas threatening vision require surgery and radiotherapy. It is important to be aware that any pituitary tumour may cause a moderate rise in prolactin due to pituitary stalk compression.

Craniopharyngiomas

Craniopharyngiomas are slow growing, benign tumours but can cause significant morbidity, especially in younger patients with hypothalamic involvement. They account for 2 per cent of all adult CNS tumours, but 8 per cent of those in childhood (median age of eight years at presentation).

They originate from the remnants of Rathke's pouch and most are suprasellar, though they may occur within the sella or adjacent to it. Over half are entirely cystic (containing cholesterol-laden fluid), 15 per cent are solid, and the rest are mixed.

Adults usually present with headaches and visual field defects (typically a bitemporal hemianopia due to chiasmal compression), while children present with diabetes insipidus, endocrinopathies, behavioural disturbances and visual failure. Involvement of the hypothalamus can lead to hyperphagia and obesity. Compression of the third ventricle causes hydrocephalus and raised ICP.

Preoperative opthalmological and endocrine work-up is essential. Imaging is usually diagnostic: calcification is seen on CT; MRI will distinguish the solid and cystic components.

Surgery is the mainstay of treatment, usually via a transphenoidal route. Progression-free survival is greatly improved with complete rather than subtotal resection (60–90 versus 30–50 per cent), but may cause increased neuroendocrine, neurocognitive and visual deficits. Adjuvant radiotherapy will improve performance-free survival after a subtotal resection. The tumour capsule may be difficult to resect as it is usually adherent to the adjacent brain tissue. **Cyst rupture may cause a chemical meningitis.**

Currently, adjuvant radiotherapy is recommended in all adults. In children, radiotherapy is only given routinely to older children after subtotal resection in an attempt to balance the neurocognitive and neuroendocrine morbidity of radiotherapy.

Chordomas and chondrosarcomas

Chordomas are thought to arise from the remnants of the primitive notochord, and may arise anywhere within the axial skeleton. However, the base of skull, clivus and the sacrococcygeal regions are the most frequent sites. Childhood chordomas are more aggressive than in adults, and may metastasize to bone, lung and skin. The overall 5YS is around 65 per cent.

They present with symptoms related to local invasion. A chordoma arising in the clivus will produce lower cranial nerve palsies, dysphagia, dysarthria and motor weakness. A chordoma arising in the sacrum will involve the sacral nerve roots, causing pain and sphincter disturbance.

Surgery via 'open door maxillotomy' is the mainstay of treatment, but the location and invasive nature often prevents complete resection necessitating adjuvant radiotherapy. Chordomas are radioresistant, requiring doses up to 70 Gy, which is not possible, even with IMRT, due to the proximity of critical structures (the brainstem for clival lesions, the bowel for sacrococcygeal lesions). There is now an established role for proton therapy for base of skull chordoma.

Base of skull chondrosarcomas present clinically like chordomas but, despite their name, behave in a more benign fashion. Treatment is also radical surgery followed by adjuvant radiotherapy, again preferably with protons due to radioresistance.

Nerve sheath tumours

Benign tumours of Schwann cells are called schwannomas, and may involve any cranial nerve, spinal root or peripheral nerve. Most commonly, they occur on the vestibulocochlear, trigeminal and facial cranial nerves. Bilateral acoustic neuromas are seen in neurofibromatosis type 2.

Vestibulocochlear schwannomas (Figure 14.10) present with progessive unilateral hearing loss, tinnitus and vertigo. Facial sensory loss and facial weakness, due to compression of the trigeminal and facial nerves, develop when the tumour extends beyond the internal auditory meatus. Eventually, with neglected tumours, brainstem compression and obstructive hydrocephalus develop.

Treatment is required for progressive tumours, either surgery or radiotherapy. Complete excision of small tumours, with microsurgical dissection techniques, is curative with low morbidity **although there is now a greater trend to treating these tumours with stereotactic radiosurgery**. However, only surgery can relieve brain stem compression. Large acoustic neuromas lead to severe or complete sensorineural deafness, and this is inevitable following surgical excision. Salvage surgery is used for recurrence following radiotherapy.

Radiotherapy for these tumours is either conventionally fractionated (as stereotactic radiotherapy or IMRT) for larger lesions or single fraction gamma knife **or linear accelerator based** radiosurgery for smaller lesions. Control rates for all types of radiotherapy are consistently above 90 per cent, with hearing preservation at 75 per cent with radiosurgery and 85 per cent with fractionated regimes.

Malignant peripheral nerve sheath tumour (MPNST) originates from peripheral nerve sheaths, with up to 20 per cent associated with neurofibromatosis type 1. The most common sites are the trunk and extremities, but, extremely rarely, they may be seen in association with a cranial nerve (VIII, V and VIIth) and the spinal column. Despite surgery and radiotherapy, the overall survival is only around 66 per cent.

NEUROLOGICAL COMPLICATIONS OF CANCER

Direct infiltration

Certain cancers may directly affect the nervous system by direct spread, for example breast cancer invading the brachial plexus, or lung cancer infiltrating the C8/T1 cervical roots with deficit including a Horner's syndrome (Pancoast tumour). This is usually a painful subacute presentation with clear imaging evidence of tumour on MRI, best seen after contrast is given. NHL can rarely present with direct infiltration into the peripheral nervous system (neurolymphomatosis) either as a mono- or polyneuropathy, cranial neuropathy or painful radiculopathy.

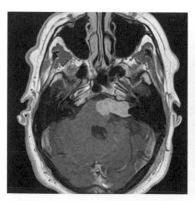
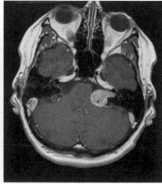
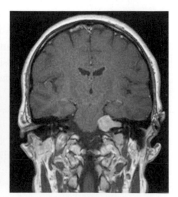

Figure 14.10 Vestibular schwannoma. A 60-year-old man with progressive left-sided sensorineural hearing loss. Contrast enhanced axial and coronal MRI shows a large, enhancing cerebello-pontine angle tumour extending into the internal auditory meatus, typical of a vestibular schwannoma.

Neurological complications of cancer (NCC) are the second most common reason for admission to oncology beds (after elective chemotherapy), are potentially disabling and usually treatable when correctly diagnosed. NCC are due either to direct, metastatic or paraneoplastic involvement of the nervous system, or to adverse effects of cancer treatment. Knowledge of the wide range of neurotoxic effects of cancer treatments, particularly the newer chemotherapuetic and biological agents, is essential. While chemotherapy usually produces toxicity during administration, radiation treatment may lead to neurotoxicity many years after the original treatment when the cancer has been cured and so present to a neurologist without the benefit of detailed oncological information. It is therefore essential to adopt a systematic approach to the patient with cancer and a neurological problem – the history should document the type and stage of the cancer, treatments received and the evolution of neurological symptoms in relation to those treatments.

Brain metastases are the most common adult intracranial malignancy and a significant cause of morbidity and death. They occur up to four times more frequently than primary brain tumours and are seen in 30 per cent of patients with systemic malignancy. They usually present alongside known metastatic disease, but may also be the first site of relapse or the presenting site of an occult cancer.

Lung cancers most frequently metastasize to the brain (45–50 per cent) followed by breast cancer (10–30 per cent). Other common primaries are colorectal cancer (10 per cent), melanoma (5–20 per cent) and renal cancer (5–10 per cent). Up to 5 per cent are due to an unknown primary. The cerebral hemispheres are the usual site of metastases (80 per cent), with only 15 per cent of lesions in the cerebellum and 5 per cent in the brainstem.

Brain metastases

Historically, brain metastases were regarded as an end-of-life event in the context of untreatable widespread disease. Treatment was palliative, with quality of life being the main issue. Patients with brain metastases were excluded from the majority of studies.

However, the incidence of brain metastases has doubled over the last two decades, due to higher overall cancer incidence in the ageing population, improved systemic cancer treatments with longer survival from primary diagnosis, and increased detection with more sophisticated imaging techniques. This new patient group is younger and fitter, with a low burden of extracranial disease, suitable for aggressive management of their brain metastases.

Patients may present with changes in cognitive status, headaches, focal neurology (such as weakness, visual change, ataxia), seizures, and nausea and vomiting. MRI scanning usually demonstrates contrast-enhancing lesions with significant associ-

ated oedema. **CT scanning can fail to identify up to 30 per cent of small metastases.**

Initial management is with corticosteroids, and anticonvulsants in those presenting with seizures.

Brain metastases from rare chemosensitive diseases, such as GCTs, may be cured with aggressive local and systemic treatment. However, in the overwhelming majority of cases, the treatment of brain metastases is palliative, and great emphasis must be put upon balancing treatment options with quality of life. Clinicians need to be able to identify which patients are most likely to benefit from treatment, so as to avoid unnecessary treatment-related morbidity in those with a short life expectancy.

Standard treatment for good performance status patients, without active systemic disease, presenting with multiple brain metastases is WBRT. Treatment is likely to be of limited benefit in other patients, but one advantage to giving radiotherapy is that it decreases the requirement for steroid treatment.

However, with the emergence of the younger, fitter patient group with limited or no extracranial disease, treatment of brain metastases is moving from WBRT to more aggressive focal management involving surgical resection or radiosurgery for solitary or oligometastases (<4).

Surgical intervention ranges from biopsy necessary for diagnosis through debulking for symptom relief, particularly in posterior fossa lesions causing obstructive symptoms, to surgical excision of solitary metastases (or up to three resectable lesions) in the setting of controlled systemic disease. Complete resection aids neurological recovery and helps control neurological deterioration.

All patients presenting with a solitary brain metastasis on MRI should be considered for either surgical excision or radiosurgery. Radiosurgery may be appropriate in patients with up to three inoperable lesions, but is limited by a 3–4 cm maximum target size due to the high single doses administered. The overall 12-month local progression-free survival is in the region of 60–80 per cent.

> Radiation-induced neurocognitive adverse effects must be considered when managing these patients, leading to greater use of surgery or radiosurgery approaches alone. A recent randomized study has shown that following surgery or radiosurgery with WBRT reduces the frequency of intracranial relapses but has no effect on prolonging either functional independence or overall survival, at the expense of radiation-induced neurocognitive decline. For this reason, many patients are not given WBRT and are monitored with three-monthly imaging to detect early asymptomatic recurrence.

Recurrent brain metastases should be managed in the same way as at initial presentation. Management should always take performance and extracranial disease status into account. Solitary metastases may be considered for aggressive local treatment with surgery or radiosurgery, and multiple lesions for WBRT. Occasionally, despite the lack of supporting evidence, patients with good performance status and late relapse are retreated with WBRT.

There is no established role for systemic treatments, but they should always be considered in chemosensitive tumours. It is probably most useful in chemonaive patients with concurrent extracranial disease, although most patients will already have received appropriate treatment. Responses to hormone therapy have been reported for breast cancer brain metastases. Penetration of chemotherapeutic agents may be restricted by the blood–brain barrier, though there is evidence for its disruption by the presence of metastases.

Spinal metastases and metastatic spinal cord compression

> Metastatic spinal cord compression (MSCC) is a neurological emergency. Untreated, irreversible neurological damage ensues with resulting paraplegia or tetraplegia.

The true incidence of MSCC is unknown due to the lack of a recognized coding system, but there are probably 4000 cases each year in the UK. It is found at post-mortem in 5–10 per cent of advanced cancer cases. However, the incidence is expected to rise as cancer patients live longer. The median age is 65 years.

> MSCC is the compression of the dural sac and its contents (spinal cord or cauda equina) by an extradural mass that threatens or causes neurological disability. There are three mechanisms of compression: haematogenous spread to the vertebral column causing collapse and compression (85 per cent), direct tumour extension and the direct deposition of tumour cells. The main risk factors for developing MSCC are the underlying primary (breast, prostate or lung primary), the presence of widespread malignancy, known spinal bony metastatic disease and the duration of malignant disease.

The cause of damage to the spinal cord from compression is complex and multifactorial. Direct compression causes oedema, venous congestion and demyelination. Gradual compression of recent onset is often reversible. In contrast, meaningful recovery is unlikely with prolonged compression resulting in vascular injury and spinal cord infarction.

> Unlike brain metastases, spinal cord metastases usually cause compression of the cord from the epidural space (they are usually due to haematogenous dissemination to the vertebral bodies). As a result, most patients have identifiable abnormalities of the affected vertebral body or bodies on plain x-ray at the site of compression prior to the development of neurological symptoms.

Up to two-thirds of MSCC occurs in the thoracic spine, with 17 per cent of patients presenting with multiple levels of compression.

Pain is the most frequent presenting symptom followed by limb weakness, sensory loss and sphincter disturbance. Rarely, cord compression presents as gait ataxia without pain, particularly posterior compression of the dorsal columns. Sensory symptoms include paraesthesiae and a sensory level, and autonomic dysfunction, including impotence and bladder and bowel disturbance, which is unusual in the absence of other major deficits. Cervical cord compression may present with a rotating paresis, i.e. starting in one arm and then affecting the ipsilateral leg, then contralateral leg and then the other arm.

About 95 per cent of patients have back pain, either localized spinal or neurogenic radicular pain at diagnosis. Weakness of the limbs is seen in 85 per cent, with only 18 per cent able to walk unaided.

The median survival is three months, in comparison to the three years now seen with bony metastases (all diagnoses). The one-year survival is 50 per cent (treated) versus 13 per cent (untreated). Survival is significantly linked to the ability to walk at diagnosis. Other independent predictors of improved survival are primary tumour histology (haematological malignancies and prostate cancer) and surgical treatment.

Spinal instability may result from metastases. This presents with acute severe back pain on the background of previous pain, which is markedly worse on movement, escalation of previous stable back pain or the development of rapid neurological deficit. These patients must not have decompressive posterior laminectomies if there is anterior cord compression because of the risk of development of complete paraplegia following surgery. Patients should be nursed flat and log-rolled until spinal stability has been established by specific radiological findings and clinical features.

For the purposes of radiographic assessment of spinal stability, the vertebrae are divided into front (anterior), middle and rear (posterior) columns. If any two of the three columns are disrupted, the spine is considered unstable.

Dislocations and fracture-dislocations are by definition unstable.

As soon as the diagnosis is suspected, the patient should be treated with high-dose dexamethasone (100 mg IV followed by 8 mg bd). MR imaging of the entire spine (to exclude or demonstrate multiple levels of compression) should be performed as an emergency and, ideally, definitive treatment undertaken within 24 hours of confirmation of MSCC.

Radiotherapy is the treatment of choice for the vast majority of patients with MSCC, with the aims of preventing neurological progression and promoting neurological recovery. There are situations in which primary chemotherapy may be appropriate, such as in NHL or GCTs. Management of all patients should be discussed with a spinal surgeon: some may have gross spinal instability that requires surgery; those with a localized block and no metastatic disease elsewhere benefit from initial surgical decompression followed by radiotherapy.

Decompressive laminectomy, the removal of the posterior elements of the spinal column, was previously the operation for MSCC. However, as 85 per cent of spinal metastases are located in the vertebral body, the risk of destabilizing the spine by removing the only intact parts of the vertebra was considered far too great to justify surgery, except in carefully selected cases. This led to a period of 'therapeutic nihilism' among neurosurgeons but in the 1980s a new operation was developed – tumour removal and circumferential spinal decompression, with intraoperative spinal reconstruction where necessary to achieve immediate stability. A multicentre randomized trial showed that significantly more patients treated with this type of surgery plus radiotherapy (versus radiotherapy alone) were able to walk after treatment, maintain the ability to walk for longer, and regain the ability to walk, together with a reduced need for steroids and opioid analgesia.

Leptomeningeal metastases

Leptomeningeal metastases (LM) are rare in comparison to brain and spinal cord metastases but are increasing in incidence as the survival from solid tumours continues to increase. The most common associated cancers are breast, small cell lung cancer (SCLC), lymphoma and melanoma.

They present with a multitude of symptoms and signs reflecting the potential for all regions of the CNS to be involved and the multifocal distribution of tumour cells (Box 14.1). The diagnosis should be suspected if there is clinical involvement of more than one anatomical area or cranial nerve/ root lesions in the absence of any obvious mass on standard imaging.

Cytological examination of the CSF is the most valuable diagnostic test but only 50 per cent of patients with LM will have malignant cells in the first CSF examination. A minimum of 10 mL should be collected and immediately taken to the laboratory to minimize the time for autolysis of malignant cells to occur. At least three samples should be taken, if necessary, to increase sensitivity but examination remains negative in up to 50 per cent of patients with LM demonstrated at autopsy. Other characteristic abnormalities, in the absence of malignant cells, include a raised opening pressure, raised CSF white cell count and protein concentration, and reduced glucose concentration.

Imaging with gadolinium-enhanced MR is indicated to exclude intraparenchymal mass lesions. This shows nodular or linear 'tramline' meningeal enhancement in the basal cisterns, around the brainstem or along the spinal cord. However, the false-negative rate of imaging is still about 30 per cent when compared to CSF cytology.

Box 14.1 Leptomeningeal metastases – spectrum of clinical presentations

Headache, nausea and vomiting
Confusion
Seizures
Cranial nerve palsies
Meningism
Myelopathy
Cauda equina syndrome
Radicular pain, sensory loss and weakness
Gait ataxia

Treatment is dependent on the clinical presentation and status of the patient. As a general rule, focal radiotherapy is used in patients with bulky nodular disease, whole brain radiotherapy for diffuse brain disease and intrathecal chemotherapy reserved for high performance patients to treat the entire subarachnoid space.

NON-METASTATIC COMPLICATIONS OF CANCER

Toxic/metabolic encephalopathy

Toxic/metabolic encephalopathy is a frequent occurrence in cancer patients, particularly in the terminal phases of the disease. It presents, when fully developed, as delirium (acute confusional state). There are numerous causes, mostly reversible (Box 14.2). The earliest manifestations are subtle deficits of concentration and attention which progress through inappropriate behaviour and cognitive disturbance into a full-blown state of delirium, characterized by either a state of lethargy and apathy (quiet delirium) or by hyperactivity, hallucinations and restlessness, similar to that seen in

Box 14.2 Causes of delirium in cancer patients

Tumour
    Brain metastases
    Leptomeningeal metastases
Toxic/metabolic encephalopathy
    Organ failure (renal, hepatic)
    Hypoxia
    Infection
    Electrolyte disturbance
    Hypoglycaemia
Drug induced
    Chemotherapy toxicity
    Opioids
    Sedatives/anxiolytics
    Anticholinergics
Paraneoplastic neurological syndromes
    Limbic encephalitis
    Encephalomyelitis
Other
    Drug/alcohol withdrawal
    Endocrinopathy

the delirium tremens of alcohol withdrawal. These symptoms may be initially mistaken for a primary psychiatric problem, particularly as neurological signs are often absent and rarely focal (except in hypoglycaemia which may cause hemiplegia).

Neurological examination usually reveals deficits in orientation, attention, concentration as well as language, short-term memory and visuospatial orientation. Tremor, myoclonus and asterixis are also sometimes seen. Investigation consists of excluding a primary oncological cause, such as brain or leptomeningeal metastases, and then identifying a treatable condition. A careful drug history is mandatory – patients with advanced disease are frequently taking several drugs including opiates and other psychotropic medication, which may trigger an encephalopathy in the presence of another cause such as infection or metabolic disturbance.

Vascular disorders

Cerebrovascular complications are relatively common in cancer patients and are either due to a direct effect of tumour or its treatment on blood vessels or due to a coagulopathy indirectly caused by the neoplasm. **Cerebral haemorrhage** may be the presenting symptom of a primary intracranial tumour or, more commonly, metastases, particularly melanoma, GCTs or colonic carcinomas. The most common primary brain tumours associated with intratumoural haemorrhage are oligodendrogliomas, glioblastomas and GCTs, but bleeding has also been reported in meningiomas, medulloblastomas, choroids plexus papillomas and ependymomas.

Intracerebral haemorrhage may also occur due to thrombocytopenia caused by either tumour invasion of bone marrow, replacement of normal bone marrow by leukaemia or due to the effects of chemotherapy or radiotherapy.

A hypercoagulable state leading to cerebral thrombosis is sometimes seen in patients with widespread metastatic disease due to the multiple procoagulant effects of cancer on platelet function and coagulation factors. Haemostatic abnormalities occur in more than 90 per cent of cancer patients, most commonly presenting as **deep vein thrombosis, or disseminated intravascular coagulation (DIC)** characterized by a depletion of platelets and clotting factors. In general, venous thromboembolism is more frequent with solid tumours, while DIC is more common in widespread metastatic can-

cer and haematological malignancies and causes both venous and arterial occlusions. Occasionally, drug therapy causes abnormal coagulation, for example cerebral vein thrombosis associated with L-asparaginase in acute leukaemia.

Rarer causes of cerebral infarction include **tumour emboli** (usually intracardiac tumours, e.g. atrial myxoma), **non-bacterial thrombotic endocarditis (NBTE)** and **cerebral vasculitis.** All of these can present with a diffuse brain syndrome caused by multiple small infarcts. **Venous cerebral sinus occlusion** may also result from compression or invasion by metastatic tumour, particularly breast cancer and lymphoma. Other causes of hypercoagulability include **hyperfibrinogenaemia** (seen in up to 50 per cent of cancer patients) and **antiphospholipid syndrome** (up to 17 per cent of cancer patients).

NBTE is the most common cause of ischaemic stroke in the cancer population, particularly patients with mucinous adenocarcinomas from a variety of organs, including the lung, pancreas, stomach and ovary. This condition is poorly understood and results in a predisposition for platelets and fibrin plugs to deposit on cardiac valves (usually aortic and mitral valves) giving rise to sterile vegetations, which may break off and cause arterial emboli.

One-third of patients have a purely neurological presentation as either a focal or diffuse encephalopathy including transient ischaemic attacks and rarely spinal cord infarction. Coagulation testing is usually normal, although a few will have evidence of DIC. In some cases NBTE may precede the diagnosis of malignancy and may be the first presentation of an occult tumour. Treatment is directed to the underlying cause and the benefits of anticoagulation have to be carefully weighed against the risks of haemorrhage.

Infections

Infections of the nervous system are one of the least common NCC and are almost always seen in patients suffering from haematological malignancies. Nevertheless, they are important to remember because these patients rarely have the florid symptoms and signs seen in immunocompetent patients.

The most common presentation of CNS infection in a cancer patient is altered mental state while headache and fever may be mild and neck stiffness absent, so there should be a low threshold for imaging and CSF examination in patients presenting with drowsiness and irritability.

In addition, the causative organisms are different and in up to 40 per cent of patients there may be multiple pathogens infecting the CNS simultaneously. *Cryptococcus neoformans* and *Listeria monocytogenes* are the major causes of meningitis in cancer patients while enteric Gram-negative bacilli, *Toxoplasma gondii*, *Aspergillus fumigatus* and *Nocardia asteroids*, are the major causes of brain abscesses. Gram-negative rods, for example *Pseudomonas aerogenes* and *Escherichia coli*, are common causes of meningitis in neutropenic patients. The paranasal sinuses should always be considered as a possible source of CNS infection, especially in neutropenic patients. It is essential to make an accurate microbiological diagnosis in order to institute vigorous and appropriate antibiotic therapy. Even so, the treatment of CNS infections in this patient group is less successful than in immunocompetent patients with a mortality of up to 85 per cent in neutropenic patients with CNS infection. Survival largely depends on bone marrow recovery and even when antibiotic treatment cures the infection, relapse and superinfection are common.

PARANEOPLASTIC NEUROLOGICAL DISORDERS

Paraneoplastic neurological disorders (PND, Box 14.3) are rare neurological complications of cancer, occurring in less than 1 per cent of patients with cancer, but are important because they frequently present before the cancer becomes symptomatic and because they cause severe neurological disability. They encompass several rapidly progressive central and peripheral nervous system disorders that result from indirect immune-mediated effects of systemic cancer.

Box 14.3 Classification of paraneoplastic neurological syndromes by anatomical site

Brain
    Encephalomyelitis
        Limbic encephalitis
        Brainstem encephalitis
    Cerebellar degeneration
    Opsoclonus-myoclonus
Spinal cord
    Sensory neuronopathy (dorsal root ganglionitis)
    Necrotizing myelopathy
Peripheral nerve
    Sensori(motor) neuropathy
Neuromuscular junction
    Lambert–Eaton myasthenic syndrome
    Myasthenia gravis
Muscle
    Polymyositis/dermatomyositis
Retina
    Cancer-associated retinopathy

By definition, these disorders do not arise out of direct or metastatic invasion of the nervous system, rather they are triggered by expression of antigens by tumours which are common to the tumour and to the nervous system (onconeural antigens).

There is now strong evidence that most of these syndromes arise out of a cell-mediated immune response directed against one or more targets in the nervous system, caused by presentation of apoptotic tumour cell antigens by dendritic cells and activation of systemic T-cell based response in lymph nodes. These immune responses are often associated with specific antineuronal antibodies in CSF and serum.

The underlying pathology in most CNS PND is a combination of inflammatory CD4+ and CD8+ T cell infiltrate, microglial activation and neuronal death. Patients dying of PND often have extensive inflammatory disease and neuronal loss, which accounts for the relative lack of response seen after treatment with immunosuppressive treatment, including plasma exchange, steroids and cyclophosphamide, or immunomodulation with, for example, intravenous human immunoglobulin (IVIg).

PND may be either focal affecting one system (for example cerebellar degeneration) or diffuse (for example encephalomyelitis). The classification of PND is based on the anatomical structures affected (Box 14.3).

Following a workshop of European experts, formal diagnostic criteria for PND have been drawn up that determine whether a neurological syndrome is a definite or possible PND on the basis of the following:

Syndrome

Classical or non-classical syndrome – 'classical' because their presence strongly suggests an underlying cancer and 'non-classical' because they are frequently not associated with cancer, for example myasthenia gravis is only associated with thymoma in 10 per cent of cases.

Anti-neuronal antibodies

This workshop determined that patients with well-characterized anti-neuronal antibodies (anti-Hu, anti-Yo, anti-CV2/CRMP5, anti-Ri, anti-amphiphysin and anti-Ma2) have a definite PND irrespective of whether a cancer is found. Only patients with proven cancer and non well-characterized antibodies can be said to have a definite PND.

Cancer

In a patient with a non-classsical syndrome and negative anti-neuronal antibodies, a possible PND can still be diagnosed if the neurological condition improves after treatment of the underlying tumour.

Recently, the spectrum of paraneoplasia has been broadened to include ovarian teratoma (a benign tumour in young women) presenting with prodromal flu-like symptoms, psychiatric disturbance progressing to coma, movement disorders, autonomic instability and respiratory failure. These are treatable disorders associated with antibodies directed against N-methyl-D-aspartate (NMDA) receptors in the hippocampi and improve with removal of the teratoma and plasma exchange.

Clinical features

PND affecting the CNS usually present as a **subacute encephalomyelitis or cerebellar syndrome**,

in which neurological investigations, for example MRI scanning and CSF examination, are normal or non-specifically abnormal. Examples of MRI abnormalities including high-signal within the hippocampi in limbic encephalitis and cerebellar atrophy in established paraneoplastic cerebellar degeneration (PCD). Almost all patients with PND have abnormal CSF (pleocytosis, raised protein or oligoclonal bands). Pleocytosis occurs early in the evolution of the illness and becomes less common after three months. In 10 per cent of patients, CSF oligoclonal bands are the only abnormality found and can be helpful when attempting to distinguish an immune process from a neurodegeneration, for example encephalomyelitis from Creutzfeldt–Jakob disease (CJD).

Paraneoplastic encephalomyelitis

Paraneoplastic encephalomyelitis (PEM) presents as a multifocal CNS disorder involving the limbic system (severe amnesia, confusion, seizures, personality changes), brainstem/cerebellum (vertigo, ataxia, eye movement abnormalities, jaw spasms), spinal cord (myelopathy), dorsal root ganglia (loss of joint position and vibration sense and sensory ataxia) and autonomic system (orthostatic hypotension, gastric paresis and intestinal pseudo-obstruction).

The clinical presentation is determined by which of these anatomical sites is preferentially affected, but pathological studies may show inflammatory infiltrates in asymptomatic regions.

This syndrome is most frequently associated with SCLC and the presence of anti-Hu antibodies. Other associated antibodies include anti-CRMP5/CV2 and anti-amphiphysin antibodies.

PEM responds poorly to treatment with the exception of limbic encephalitis. In one large series of anti-Hu PEM, only treatment of the underlying tumour with or without associated immunotherapy led to neurological improvement or stabilization.

Paraneoplastic cerebellar degeneration

In contrast to PEM, PCD is usually a unifocal pancerebellar syndrome manifesting as severe gait ataxia, nystagmus, dysarthria and impaired limb coordination, often preceded by vestibular symptoms, for example nausea, vomiting, vertigo and blurred vision.

PCD is associated with breast and gynaecological malignancies (anti-Yo antibodies), Hodgkin's disease (anti-Tr antibodies) or SCLC (anti-Hu antibodies). Imaging is usually normal or subtly abnormal at the onset of the condition, including transient enhancement of the cerebellar cortex, but in most cases cerebellar atrophy develops within the first six months, corresponding to severe Purkinje cell loss and thinning of the molecular and granule cell layers. PCD rarely responds to treatment and in cases of metastatic ovarian cancer, may deteriorate after chemotherapy.

Paraneoplastic opsoclonus/ myoclonus

Paraneoplastic opsoclonus (POM) presents with prominent truncal ataxia and opsoclonus/myoclonus. Opsoclonus or 'dancing eyes' refers to an eye movement disorder characterized by multidirectional involuntary large amplitude saccades with no intersaccadic interval. This is a rare disorder most frequently associated with breast cancer and anti-Ri antibodies.

Lambert–Eaton myasthenic syndrome

Lambert–Eaton myasthenic syndrome (LEMS, see Chapter 18) is paraneoplastic in about 60 per cent of cases when it is almost always associated with SCLC. The non-paraneoplastic cases are clinically indistinguishable. As about 3 per cent of patients with SCLC have LEMS, this is the most common PND. It presents non-specifically with leg weakness, which may become more obviously fatiguable over time and spread to involve oculobulbar and upper limb muscles. There are also autonomic features (dry mouth, impotence and constipation) and these should be specifically enquired about. The diagnosis is made by identifying characteristic neurophysiological abnormalities on repetitive nerve stimulation (small CMAPs which decrease in amplitude at low frequency stimulation but increase at high frequency stimulation) and by the detection of antibodies directed against voltage-gated calcium channels (VGCC).

Diagnosis and treatment of PND

PND are associated with several different serum anti-neuronal antibodies directed against intracellular neuronal antigens or membrane components (Table 14.2). Antibodies in CNS syndromes are so specific for PND that their detection should prompt a detailed search for an underlying malignancy. Not uncommonly, the tumours are too small to be detected by conventional imaging, for example CT scanning and ultrasound. For this reason, metabolic imaging, such as whole body FDG-PET scanning, may be helpful as this can identify tumours down to a resolution of 6–8 mm anywhere within the body.

The majority of PND affecting the CNS respond poorly to immunomodulatory treatments such as plasma exchange, suggesting that anti-neuronal antibodies are diagnostic markers rather than pathogenic effectors of the immune attack. The results are particularly disappointing in PCD in which only 5 per cent of patients improve after anti-tumour therapy, while the majority show further progression of cerebellar symptoms. Occasionally, stabilization and improvement occur when the underlying tumour is treated, particularly with PEM. In contrast, LEMS responds well to removal of anti-VGCC antibodies by plasma exchange or intravenous immune globulin and may go into remission when the underlying tumour is removed.

NEUROTOXICITY OF CHEMOTHERAPY AND RADIOTHERAPY

Iatrogenic neurotoxicity is common and may severely affect patients' quality of life long after they have been 'cured' of their underlying cancer. Both chemotherapy and radiotherapy can cause neurotoxicity, and with the increasing use of multimodality therapy, for example chemoradiation, the neurotoxic effects may be synergistic.

Table 14.2 Anti-neuronal antibodies in paraneoplastic neurological disorders

Site	Syndromes	Tumour	Antineuronal antibody
Brain	Limbic encephalitis	SCLC[a]	Anti-Hu
Testis	Anti-Ma2		
Brainstem encephalitis	SCLC	Anti-Hu	
		Testis	Anti-Ma2
	Cerebellar degeneration	SCLC	anti-Hu
	Breast, ovary	Anti-Yo	
	Hodgkin's	Anti-Tr	
	Opsoclonus-myoclonus	SCLC	
Breast	Anti-Ri		
DRG[b]	Sensory neuronopathy	SCLC	Anti-Hu
NMJ[d]	LEMS	SCLC	Anti-VGCC[c]
	Myasthenia gravis	Thymoma	Anti-AchR[e]
Muscle	Polymyositis/dermatomyositis	Many	

[a]Small cell lung cancer
[b]Dorsal root ganglia.
[c]Anti-voltage-gated calcium channel antibodies.
[d]Neuromuscular junction.
[e]Anti-acetylcholine receptor antibodies.

Neurological complications of chemotherapy

Certain cytotoxic drugs cause neurological toxicity which can be dose-limiting.

The most frequent neurological adverse effect of older chemotherapeutic agents is **peripheral neuropathy**. This is particularly seen with vincristine, taxols, cisplatin and oxaliplatin. The neuropathy is almost always sensory axonal, involving small and large fibres and occasionally autonomic nerves. Patients with predisposing factors, such as diabetes, alcohol, hereditary neuropathy, are particularly vulnerable. Neuropathic symptoms usually settle over time but in rare cases, particularly after cisplatin and oxaliplatin, may deteriorate after completion of chemotherapy, a phenomenon known as 'coasting'. Oxaliplatin is associated with a reversible unpleasant sensory disturbance, often triggered by cold (cold dysaesthesiae) such that patients sometimes have to wear gloves when taking food out of the fridge or driving on a cold day. Laryngospasm may be provoked by breathing cold air. These symptoms subside with dosage reduction. Oxaliplatin also causes a persistent painful sensory neuropathy.

CNS disorders are rarer manifestations of chemotherapy toxicity and are usually reversible after discontinuation of the agent. Examples include ifosfamide and encephalopathy, 5 fluorouracil and cerebellar syndrome, methotrexate and encephalopathy or aseptic meningitis (when given intrathecally), cisplatin and ototoxicity and rarely a posterior reversible encephalopathy syndrome. These usually occur during or immediately after treatment.

Methotrexate is particularly neurotoxic – it can cause an acute encephalopathy developing up to 14 days after intrathecal administration, particularly in children with acute lymphoblastic leukaemia (ALL). The clinical features are characteristic, consisting of alternating hemiparesis, dysphasia, emotional lability and drowsiness. The standard T2W MRI may be normal but the diagnosis is usually made on diffusion-weighted MRI, showing symmetrical areas of restricted diffusion usually within subcortical white matter.

Neurological complications of radiotherapy

In contrast to chemotherapy where neurotoxicity is closely temporally related to the administration of the drug, radiotherapy may lead to neurological toxicity many weeks, months or even years after treatment, through long-term effects on vascular endothelium and oligodendrocytes. **A number of factors determine the likelihood of radiation toxicity including the total dose delivered, the dose per fraction and the total volume of nervous tissue irradiated.** For the brain, a dose of 60 Gy delivered with 1.8–2 Gy fractions represents the upper limit of the safe dose. Patient factors include the length of survival after completion of radiotherapy, the presence of other systemic diseases that predispose to atherosclerosis (e.g. diabetes, hypertension) and concomitant administration of chemotherapy.

Radiation neurotoxicity is usually classified into acute, early delayed and late delayed according to the timing of clinical symptoms in relation to when radiation was given. **Acute radiation toxicity** is unusual and presents as an encephalopathy of varying severity, ranging from mild drowsiness and lethargy to life-threatening brain herniation. Predisposing factors include the presence of large metastases, posterior fossa tumours and high radiation dosages per fraction.

Early delayed radiation toxicity is more common – so called because it starts soon after the end of the radiotherapy course and lasts up to three months. In severe cases, patients experience the somnolence syndrome (particularly children) characterized by severe drowsiness, hypersomnia and irritability. More commonly, the symptoms are milder and may be associated with worsening of pre-existing focal deficits. Early delayed toxicity usually responds to steroids and recovers fully.

In contrast, **late delayed radiation toxicity** is untreatable and irreversible and may begin many years after radiotherapy. It thus tends to affect patients with benign tumours or low-grade gliomas, in whom the prognosis is considerably better than that of patients with brain metastases and high-grade gliomas. Symptoms of late delayed radiation toxicity include progressive memory loss leading to dementia, urinary incontinence and gait apraxia, i.e. similar to the symptoms of normal pressure hydrocephalus. To date, no treatment exists to arrest the course or to improve function.

An example of cumulative toxicity caused by the synergistic reaction between radiotherapy and chemotherapy is that which occurs with methotrexate in the treatment of CNS lymphoma, where a rapidly progressive dementia may develop, particularly when methotrexate is administered after the brain has been irradiated. It is thought that the latter causes damage to the blood–brain barrier, promoting the development of the condition.

Radiotherapy is also neurotoxic to the pituitary gland, the lens of the eye (cataract) and cranial nerves (particularly the vestibulocochlear) and peripheral nerves. It may cause optic neuropathy when used for the treatment of pituitary tumours and therefore great efforts are taken to ensure that the optic nerves are decompressed prior to radiotherapy and that they do not receive a dose above their known tolerance using highly focussed radiation delivery techniques, such as fractionated stereotactic radiotherapy (FSR).

Brachial plexopathy following radiation administered to the chest wall and axilla as adjuvant treatment of breast cancer is becoming much less common but is important to recognize and to distinguish from local recurrence of the underlying disease. Radiation-induced plexopathy is usually painless, in contrast to direct tumour infiltration of the plexus, and associated with myokymic discharges on EMG studies.

Radiation damage to the vasculature may result in large arterial stenoses which may present many years after treatment of suprasellar tumours, particularly in childhood. Patients may present with transient ischaemic attacks (TIAs) and strokes or less commonly with moyamoya disease (a progressive occlusive cerebral arteriopathy affecting the distal internal carotid arteries near the circle of Willis, particularly common in children with neurofibromatosis and optic pathway gliomas).

The spinal cord is less commonly affected by delayed radiation toxicity when compared to the brain, but progressive cervical myelopathy after treatment of head and neck cancer and Hodgkin's lymphoma is recognized. More commonly, patients may experience a transient myelopathy presenting with Lhermitte's sign, which usually resolves spontaneously.

Radiation to the brain can also predispose to the development of secondary tumours including gliomas, meningiomas and cavernomas. These present at an interval of 5–50 years after treatment, and are usually located in areas of the radiation field that have received a lower dosage.

Neurological complications of bone marrow transplantation

Bone marrow transplantation (BMT) is now established as a standard treatment for haematological malignancies and some solid tumours. BMT is either allogeneic (from an HLA-matched sibling or unrelated donor), or autologous (from the patient)

Patients receiving BMT are at risk of encephalopathy, CNS infections and cerebrovascular disease, particularly haemorrhagic complications including subarachnoid and subdural haemorrhage. Diffuse encephalopathy may be an adverse effect of drugs used in conditioning regimes, for example cytarabine, high-dose busulphan, methotrexate and ifosfamide. More commonly it is seen after transplantation and may be an early manifestation of multiple organ dysfunction.

---

and may consist of peripheral blood stem cells (PBSCT) rather than bone marrow. Autologous BMT or PBSCT is generally associated with a lower frequency of complications than allogeneic transplants, particularly graft versus host disease (GvHD). This is important to neurologists as treatments used to prevent or reduce GvHD are common causes of neurological adverse effects.

CNS infections in BMT patients are usually caused by opportunistic pathogens as a result of impaired cell-mediated immunity. Examples include cerebral abscesses caused by nocardia, aspergillus and toxoplasma, encephalitis affecting medial temporal lobes caused by herpes simplex and human herpes virus type 6 and progressive multifocal leucoencephalopathy caused by John Cunningham virus.

REFERENCES AND FURTHER READING

Rees J, Wen PY (eds) (2010) *Neuro-oncology Series: Blue Books of Neurology*, Saunders. Philadelphia, PA: Elsevier.

Schiff D, Wen PY (eds) (2003) *Cancer Neurology in Clinical Practice*. Totowa, NJ; Humana Press.

CHAPTER 15

SPINAL DISEASE

James Allibone and Vivian Elwell

INTRODUCTION

This chapter aims to give an overview of the presentation, diagnosis and management of diseases of the spine, and in particular those disease processes that affect the enclosed spinal cord and nerve roots. Traumatic spinal injury is not considered here.

Anatomical considerations

The spine is a two-part structure. First, the vertebral column, which must support the upright stance of the body and protect the neural contents, while remaining flexible to allow for bending and twisting. Second, the neural contents, the spinal cord and nerve roots. The pathological processes that affect the spine are legion and may be focal, multifocal or diffuse. Some pathologies affect the vertebral column alone, with no consequence for the neural contents: these conditions will not be addressed in this chapter. Some pathologies affect the spinal cord or nerve roots directly, while others cause problems by means of external compression of these neural structures. The spinal cord extends from the foramen magnum to approximately L1.

The spinal cord is vulnerable to injury for a number of reasons. First, within the spinal cord, there is precious little neurological tissue that can be considered functionally redundant. Thus, even small insults to the cord, whether of intrinsic or extrinsic origin, may result in major functional consequences. Second, the arterial supply of the cord, in particular of the thoracic spine, is vulnerable. Third, the ability of the cord to repair itself after injury is negligible.

SYMPTOMS AND SIGNS OF SPINAL DISEASE

Spinal disease presents with pain and/or loss of neurological function. Pain may be felt in the spine itself, at the site of the pathology or, in those cases with neurological involvement, in the dermatome/sclerotome of the affected nerve roots – so-called 'referred pain'.

While modern imaging technology, particularly magnetic resonance imaging (MRI), has dramatically improved our ability to accurately diagnose spinal disease, skilful history taking and clinical examination remain crucial for appropriate decision-making in the management of spinal conditions. The history and clinical examination should allow the physician to establish whether the disease process is unifocal, multifocal or diffuse in terms of its neurological involvement. If the clinical picture can be explained by a single lesion, neurological examination should then be able to localize this lesion with reasonable accuracy. The evolution of the neurological history and associated features will provide crucial clues about the pathology, for example, pyrexia and night sweats suggesting infection or the ascending picture of neurological loss after a viral illness, suggesting inflammatory myelitis or Guillain–Barré syndrome (GBS).

> **Myelopathy**, the term used to describe any pathological process of the spinal cord, may result from either an intrinsic spinal cord lesion or from external compression of the cord within the cervical or thoracic regions. The cardinal neurological features of myelopathy include hypertonia, pyramidal (upper neurone) distribution of weakness, hyperreflexia and extensor plantar responses, combined with loss of sensation in one or more modalities, loss of sphincter control and sometimes autonomic dysfunction.

A number of partial spinal cord syndromes are described, depending on the site of the lesion within the spinal cord (Table 15.1).

Table 15.1 Partial spinal cord syndromes

Syndrome	Description
Anterior cord syndrome	Motor loss with a dissociated sensory level below the lesion. There is loss of pain and temperature with preservation of the posterior columns (proprioception and vibration sense)
Brown Sequard syndrome	Ipsilateral loss of motor function and posterior column sensation with contralateral spinothalamic loss (pain and temperature) below the lesion
Central cord syndrome	Ipsilateral loss of motor function and posterior column sensation with contralateral spinothalamic loss below the lesion

Radiculopathy is the term used to describe a pathological process of an exiting nerve root. Single or multiple roots may be affected, most commonly by a compressive lesion. Radiculopathy is characterized by reduced tone, muscle wasting within the affected myotome, weakness, sometimes fasciculation, loss of the deep tendon reflexes (lower motor neurone pattern weakness) and loss of sensation within the affected dermatome. A compressive radiculopathy is often also associated with severe pain in the distribution of the affected nerve root.

> **Radiculopathy** may affect a cluster of lumbar and sacral roots alone to produce a cauda equina syndrome characterized by paraparesis, saddle and lower limb anaesthesia. A combination of these signs together with upper motor neurone signs in the legs indicates a lesion at the level of the conus medullaris, the termination of the spinal cord.

INVESTIGATION

The principle tool for imaging the spine is the MR scan, which has superceded all other imaging techniques as the first-line investigation for spinal symptoms. **Plain x-rays** can give additional useful information about the bony structure of the spine, and are particularly useful for assessing spinal alignment and for the postoperative assessment of patients with implanted metalwork. **Computed tomography (CT) scans** are primarily used to delineate the fine details of the bony components of the spine, but are less useful for the neural structures unless combined with myelography. **CT myelography** still has an occasional role, for the assessment of persisting symptoms following surgery and in those patients for whom MRI is contraindicated, such as patients with a cardiac pacemaker. Blood tests, neurophysiological studies (electromyography and nerve conduction studies, sensory evoked potentials) and cerebrospinal fluid (CSF) examination will be required in selected cases.

Both CT and MRI angiography can be used for non-invasive assessment of the vascular supply of a lesion, but there remains a place for digital subtraction spinal angiography (DSA), via a catheter inserted into the femoral artery. DSA is used for the investigation of arteriovenous malformations, dural fistulas and tumours. Embolization using balloons, coils, microparticles or glue can be carried out at the same time as the diagnostic angiogram. Embolization may be the definitive treatment for an arteriovenous malformation (AVM) or a haemangioma and can be invaluable, when used preoperatively, for reducing intraoperative bleeding from very vascular tumours, such as a renal metastasis.

Congenital anomalies of the spine and spinal cord

The nervous system develops from the ectodermal neural plate, which appears during the third week of gestation and whose formation is induced by the underlying notochord and adjacent mesoderm. The process of infolding of the neural plate to form the neural tube is termed primary neurulation. It commences at the fourth somite and progresses cranially and caudally with closure of the cranial and caudal neuropores at 25 and 27 days, respectively. Failure of this infolding leads to neural tube defects, known as spinal dysraphism or spina bifida.

- *Spina bifida occulta* (congenital absence of a spinous process and variable amounts of lamina with no visible exposure of meninges or neural tissue). This presents with a cutaneous dimple or tuft of hair. Typically asymptomatic, it may occur in up to 10 per cent of the population.
- *Spina bifida aperta* (protrusion of the meninges with or without the neural tissues through the defective neural arch).
- *Meningocoele* (meningeal protrusion, but no abnormality of neural tissue).
- *Myelomeningocoele* (neural tissues also protrude and typically there is a marked neurological deficit).
- *Myeloschisis* (open spinal cord due to the failure of the neural folds to fuse).

In the embryo, the spinal cord occupies the entire length of the canal, but differential growth causes ascent of the conus during fetal development. At birth, the conus lies at the level of L2. After a further two months, it lies at its final position, at the level of L1. Disturbance of this process may lead to tethering of the spinal cord leading to a low-lying conus and, in a minority of cases, neurological disturbance, which typically presents with symptoms during the adolescent growth spurt (Figure 15.1).

A number of other congenital anomalies of the spine and spinal cord are also seen including arachnoid cysts, neurenteric cysts, Klippel–Feil syndrome and split cord malformations (Figure 15.2).

SPINAL NEOPLASIA

Traditionally, spinal tumours are classified by their site of origin, whether extradural or intradural and, if intradural, whether intra- or extramedullary.

Extradural tumours

The great majority of extradural spinal tumours are metastases (particularly prostate, lung and breast)

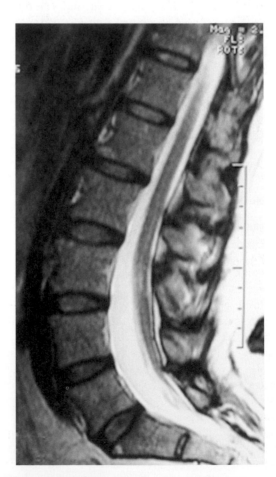

Figure 15.1 Sagittal T2-weighted MRI showing cord tethering. The conus lies at the level of L5. The normal position is at approximately L1.

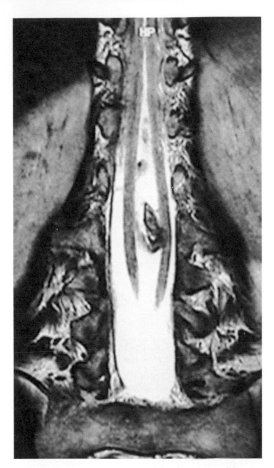

Figure 15.2 Coronal and axial T2-weighted MRI showing a split-cord malformation or diastematomyelia. In this example, the split cord is separated by a bony bar.

Box 15.1 Spinal cord tumours

Extradural spinal tumours (arising in the vertebral body or epidural tissue)
Metastatic spinal tumours
    Lung
    Breast
    Prostate
    Kidney
    Lymphoma
Primary vertebral tumours
    Osteoid osteoma/Osteoblastoma
    Aneurysmal bone cyst
    Osteochondroma
    Giant cell tumour
    Osteosarcoma
    Chondrosarcoma
    Chordoma
Haemopoietic malignancy
    Plasmacytoma/myeloma
    Lymphoma
Intradural extramedullary spinal tumours
    Meningioma
    Neurofibroma
    Myxopapillary ependymoma
    Ependymoma
Intradural intramedullary spinal tumours
Glial tumours
    Astrocytoma
    Ependymoma
Others
    Dermoid
    Epidermoid
    Cavernoma
    Teratoma
    Hemangioblastoma
    Intramedullary metastasis

or tumours of lymphoid origin (Box 15.1). In most cases, the tumour takes root in the region of the pedicle/vertebral body junction and then spreads through the vertebral body and into the posterior elements. Initially asymptomatic, they become painful as the tumour distorts the periosteum. Neurological compromise follows if the tumour erodes into the vertebral canal, compressing the spinal cord or exiting nerve roots. As the vertebral body is weakened, collapse and instability may occur, typically manifesting with severe pain on movement and neurological loss as a result of spinal cord compression. Initially, by means of clinical and radiological assessment, one should attempt to identify the site of the primary tumour and the site and extent of any other skeletal or visceral metastases. Diagnosis and the initial management decisions should be conducted through a multidisciplinary team approach. In one-third of patients presenting with a spinal metastasis, there will be no known primary lesion; on occasion, investigations do not reveal one either. In cases of diagnostic doubt, a CT-guided biopsy may be appropriate.

The decision to perform surgery for a spinal metastasis will depend on the diagnosis, the patient's performance status, the extent of the spinal disease, the number and sites of visceral metastases, the overall prognosis and a careful risk to benefit analysis for the individual patient.

In selected cases, surgery can have a locally curative role and can prolong survival. In most cases, however, the role of surgery is palliation with one or more of the following goals: relief of neurological compression, relief of pain and maintenance of spinal alignment and stability (Figure 15.3). Radiotherapy may be used as a primary treatment or as an adjunct to surgery, either delivered traditionally or by a number of focused stereotactic methods, such as the Cyberknife. For some tumours, chemotherapy will also be appropriate.

> **Primary vertebral tumours, both benign and malignant, are rare** and if suspected radiologically, the patient should be referred promptly to one of the specialist bone tumour units, prior to any further investigation. The diagnosis and management (both surgical and oncological) of primary malignant tumours of the spine is demanding and highly specialized. Inappropriate early management may prejudice the patient's chance of survival.

Intradural tumours

These may be extramedullary or intramedullary. **The most common extramedullary tumours are meningiomas and nerve sheath tumours (schwannomas or neurofibromas).** By contrast to extradural tumours, intradural extramedullary tumours are nearly always benign, encapsulated tumours. They exert their effect by slowly progressive compression of the spinal cord or nerve roots, resulting in distal loss of neurological function. One characteristic feature is nocturnal back pain. **Meningiomas** arise from arachnoid cells near the attachment of the dentate ligament. They occur mainly in the thoracic and cervical spine with a female preponderance. Nerve sheath tumours arise from the sensory nerve roots and occur throughout the spine (Figure 15.4). They may lie purely intraspinally or may extend through the intervertebral foramen to produce a 'dumb-bell' appearance. Typically, they are solitary, but can be multiple and in some cases are a manifestation of neurofibromatosis (Figure 15.5). They occur equally in both sexes and typically affect a younger group of patients than meningiomas. In the lumbar spine, a nerve sheath tumour may be difficult to distinguish from a myxopapillary ependymoma, a variant of ependymoma, which

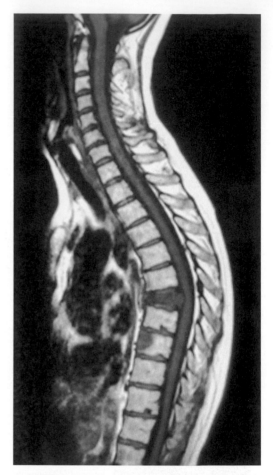

Figure 15.3 Sagittal T1-weighted MRI showing disseminated carcinoma of the breast. There are multiple foci of tumour within the spine. At T7, there is vertebral body collapse, kyphosis and cord compression. The postoperative lateral x-ray shows decompression and stabilization by means of a posterior construct using hooks, rods and screws.

arises from the filum terminale, typically just below the conus. The treatment of all of these tumours is surgical removal, which is usually curative.

Most intradural intramedullary tumours are of glial origin and of low histological grade. They typically present with very slowly progressive neurological loss; the diagnosis often being delayed by months or years. **Ependymomas** (Figure 15.6) are the most common, closely followed by astrocytomas. Intramedullary ependymomas are typically well demarcated, expand the cord over several levels and occur most commonly in the cervical region. The goal of treatment is to attempt curative surgical removal. **Astrocytomas** are typi-

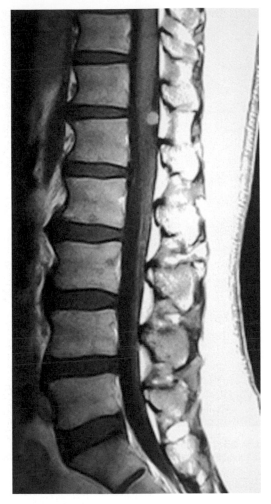

Figure 15.4 Capital T1-weighted MRI demonstrates a solitary schwannoma lying at the tip of the conus at T12/L1.

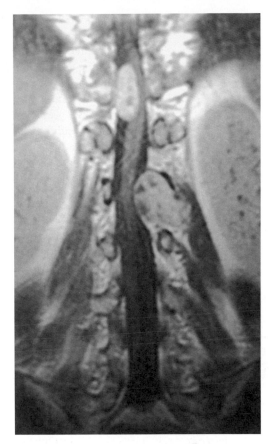

Figure 15.5 Multiple neurofibromata associated with neurofibromatosis. A coronal T1-weighted MRI demonstrates an intradural tumour compressing the cord from the right side. Two levels below, a slightly larger tumour is seen extending out through the intervertebral foramen on the left.

cally less defined than ependymomas and are also slow growing. Surgery for an astrocytoma usually has poorer outcome than for an ependymoma, as establishing a clear surgical plane between tumour and normal tissue is usually not possible. A number of rarer intramedullary tumours are also seen, of which the most common is a **haemangioblastoma**. This is a benign tumour derived from malformed elements of primitive vessels within the spinal cord. Haemangioblastomas are common in the cervical region and may have a large cystic component. Again, the definitive treatment is surgical resection. The role of radiotherapy remains unclear for any of these tumours.

SPINAL INFECTION

Acute pyogenic infection

The typical presentation is with fever and localized pain. Referred pain and neurological deficit will follow if neurological compression occurs. The diagnosis is established with imaging (usually MRI) and microbiological cultures of blood and likely sites of primary infection. The mainstay of treatment is appropriate antibiotics, based on the advice of a microbiologist and, if needed, surgical debridement. In the presence of neurological dete-

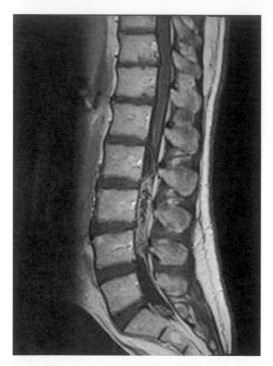

Figure 15.6 Sagittal T1-weighted MRI showing an ependymoma in the lumbar region.

rioration, surgical decompression may be required as a matter of urgency. Surgical spinal stabilization may be required.

Pyogenic bacterial infection may be iatrogenically and directly introduced to the spine during invasive procedures, such as surgery or needling (e.g. CT-guided biopsy, nerve root injections and epidural injections) or indirectly by haematogenous spread from an infected intravenous cannula. The site of infection may be a disc (discitis) (Figure 15.7), a facet joint (septic arthritis), the epidural space (epidural abscess) or less commonly a vertebral body (osteomyelitis). The intradural space is much less commonly infected (meningitis) as the dura usually acts as a very resistant barrier to spread of infection. Pyogenic infection may also reach the spine by haematogenous spread from any systemic infected focus. *Staphylococcus aureus* is the most common organism, but haematogenous spread of coliform organisms from the urinary tract is not uncommonly seen, especially in the elderly.

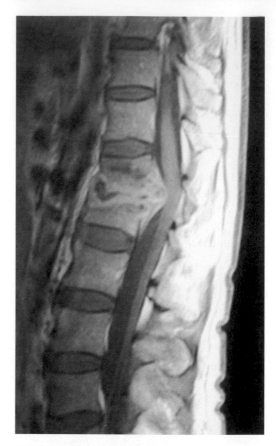

Figure 15.7 Sagittal T1-weighted MRI demonstrating a lower thoracic MRSA discitis. The disc has been virtually destroyed with expansion of the infected material into the canal resulting in compression of the thoracic spinal cord. A postoperative lateral x-ray. The patient collapsed in kyphosis, requiring surgery. An anterior debridement of the infected disc was performed followed by an anterior column reconstruction using cylindrical cages and posterior pedicle screw/rod stabilization.

Tuberculous infection (Pott's disease)

The incidence of spinal TB is increasing in the UK. The typical presentation is with local pain, systemic disturbance and sometimes neurological deficit.

The diagnosis is based on MRI appearances and blood tests (ELISA and PCR). A *Brucella* complement fixation test should also be considered in patients from endemic areas, as *Brucella* can clinically mimic tuberculosis. In some cases, a CT-guided biopsy will be required. Most commonly, the infection starts in a disc space and spreads behind the anterior and posterior longitudinal ligaments, to form an epidural or paravertebral abscess (Figure 15.8). Neurological compromise occurs as a result of epidural abscess formation or following vertebral body collapse. Treatment is with antituberculous drugs, based on expert microbiological advice, given typically for 9–12 months, and immobilization. This will usually take the form of a period of bed-rest followed by external bracing with an orthosis. Surgery may be required for neurological decompression, debridement of infection or stabilization of the spine.

> Both pyogenic infection and TB can lead to major destruction of the spine and in some cases the radiological appearances can mimic a malignant process. Typically, however, infection is centred on the disc space while tumours, at least initially, leave the disc spaces intact.

HIV

There is an increased risk of pyogenic spinal infection in immunocompromised HIV-positive patients. *Staphylococcus aureus* remains the most common organism, followed by *Mycobacterium tuberculosis*. In addition, there is also a risk of hitherto rare fungal, viral and atypical bacterial infections from organisms that are usually nonpathogenic. A low threshold should be maintained for investigation for patients with HIV presenting with back pain. Patients with HIV infection are also at risk of developing spinal cord disease as a result of demyelination or vacuolar myelopathy.

Tabes dorsalis

Tabes dorsalis is a progressive demyelination of the posterior columns, as a result of untreated syphilis. Clinical features, which may not appear for decades after the initial infection, include weakness, paraesthesia, dysaesthesia, formication (a sensation like that produced by small insects crawling over skin) and episodes of intense pain. 'Tabetic ocular crises' are characterized by intense ocular pain, lacrimation and photophobia. Patients may demonstrate a

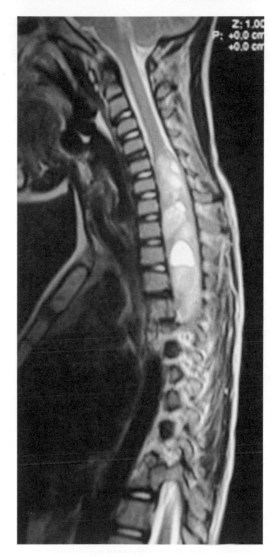

Figure 15.8 Sagittal and axial T2-weighted images showing TB. At T5, there is partial collapse of the vertebral body with expansion of the posterior vertebral body wall into the spinal canal. There is destruction of the right pedicle and posterior elements. A focal collection of pus lies within the canal, compressing the spinal cord. At T8/9, a further collection can be seen, demonstrating the often multifocal nature of the disease. (An incidental congenital fusion at C5 and C6 is seen.)

high steppage 'tabetic gait' or have Charcot joints. Dementia, deafness and visual impairment may also be seen, as well as light-near dissociation (Argyll Robertson pupil). The treatment includes antibiotics (e.g. penicillin), but existing neural damage cannot be reversed (see also Chapter 25).

INFLAMMATORY AND DEMYELINATING CONDITIONS

Subacute combined degeneration of the spinal cord

Subacute combined degeneration is a progressive degeneration of the spinal cord due to vitamin B12 deficiency. 'Combined' refers to the fact that demyelination affects the lateral columns in addition to the posterior columns. It presents with progressive leg weakness and paraesthesia in the extremities, over weeks or months. Examination reveals spastic weakness in the legs, with loss of vibration and joint position sense, sometimes profound. There may also be cognitive impairment, optic atrophy, and there are often signs of a peripheral sensory neuropathy. A combination of extensor plantar responses and absent ankle jerks is characteristic.

Vitamin B12 deficiency usually develops as a result of lack of intrinsic factor (pernicious anaemia (PA)), and less commonly as a result of inadequate intake or malabsorption. Nitrous oxide anaesthesia may precipitate deficiency in depleted patients. Treatment with vitamin B12 injections prevents progression and may lead to neurological recovery. Treatment is more successful if started early, and in the case of PA must be continued for life.

Transverse myelitis and multiple sclerosis

Transverse myelitis is a term encompassing at least two distinct conditions. In partial transverse myelitis, the whole axial section of the cord is not affected, the deficit may be mild, and the usual aetiology is multiple sclerosis (MS) or a clinically isolated syndrome (see below). However, a complete (whole axial section) transverse myelitis may also occur as an inflammatory, demyelinating condition of either unknown aetiology (usually secondary to a presumed but unidentified viral infection) or in some cases clearly secondary to herpes zoster infection. Symptoms may develop over hours or a few days, with variable loss of distal motor, sensory and sphincter function. In complete transverse myelitis, there may be loss of all neurological function below the affected spinal level. The diagnosis is based on the clinical picture, MR scan appearances and CSF examination. Treatment consists of corticosteroids followed by rehabilitation. The prognosis for complete myelitis may be poor.

MS is an inflammatory condition of immune but ultimately unknown aetiology, characterized by patchy demyelination in the central nervous system. MS can mimic a number of other neurological diseases and should be considered in the list of differential diagnosis of patients with symptoms of spinal cord pathology, especially if the disease appears multifocal. The clinical diagnostic criteria, the MR scan appearance of plaques in the brain and spinal cord and the identification of oligoclonal bands in the CSF are described further in Chapter 22. In addition to MS, myelitis may occur in sarcoidosis, antiphospholipid syndrome, lupus, Sjögren's syndrome and neuromyelitis optica.

Guillain–Barré syndrome

GBS is an acute inflammatory demyelinating polyneuropathy (AIDP), typically triggered by antecedent bacteria of viral infection (see Chapter 16). It is very variable in its presentation, often not conforming to the classical 'ascending weakness' starting in the lower limbs. Sensory disturbance is often mild and affects the extremities. Cranial involvement is common and there is usually areflexia. There may be a genuine suspicion of spinal pathology, as acute or subacute spinal lesions can present with flaccid weakness ('spinal shock'), the typical signs of spastic weakness developing only after an interval. Bladder function is usually normal in GBS (though may be disturbed in patients with associated autonomic involvement – see Chapter 16), and this is often a helpful distinguishing feature.

Fever is unusual and should raise the possibility of another cause. The diagnosis is essentially clinical, supported by CSF examination, MR imaging (if a cord lesion is suspected) and most importantly neurophysiological studies. Treatment consists of high-dose intravenous immunoglobulin. Plasma exchange and ventilatory support may be required. Approximately 80 per cent of patients make a complete recovery within a few months to a year, but 10 per cent are left with long-standing disability and the mortality remains at 2–3 per cent.

Acute spinal cord haemorrhage is usually due to an AVM or cavernoma. These lesions may also lead to spinal damage due to progressive or episodic ischaemia.

Vascular lesions

The blood supply of the cord is predominantly from the anterior spinal artery fed by segmental vessels throughout the length of the spine. **Anterior spinal artery occlusion** is caused by thrombus or embolism leading to sudden loss of the anterior cord function – an anterior spinal infarct. Occlusion due to atherosclerotic disease occurs most frequently in middle-aged and elderly people, and is often associated with evidence of other cardiovascular disease. It often occurs at mid-thoracic level where the spinal vascular borderzone lies and is characterized by acute flaccid paraparesis with dissociated sensory loss. Examination reveals a striking preferential loss of spinothalamic modalities, often with intact dorsal column function. In the acute stage, the weakness is usually flaccid due to spinal shock, and this gives way to spasticity, developing over days or weeks.

AVMs are congenital abnormalities comprising an arterial feeding vessel and dilated, tortuous veins, which contain high pressure arterialized blood. They may remain asymptomatic or present with sudden, sometimes catastrophic, loss of neurological function (often associated with severe pain) below the level of the lesion as a result of haemorrhage or infarction. They may also present with subtly progressive or step-wise development of neurological symptoms, due to spinal cord ischaemia, as a result of vascular steal and venous hypertension.

Dural arteriovenous fistulas (AVF) are rare, probably acquired lesions, most commonly seen in elderly men. These lesions often affect the lower part of the spinal cord and involve the conus medullaris. The typical presentation is a **conus syndrome**, with gradually progressive loss of lower limb function, with combined upper and lower motor neurone signs and mixed cord and root sensory loss, with saddle anaesthesia and loss of bladder and bowel sphincter control.

The diagnosis of AVMs and AVFs is established with MRI and spinal angiography. The treatment is endovascular embolization or surgical occlusion. Either treatment modality carries considerable risk and treatment planning and requires a multi-disciplinary collaboration between interventional radiologist, neurologist and neurosurgeon.

Cavernomas (cavernous haemangiomas) are capillary malformations which may occur within the spinal cord. Typically, they comprise multiple small blood-filled cavernous structures lined by endothelium. In 20 per cent of cases, they are familial and if so may be multiple. The whole spine and brain should be imaged to exclude this possibility. Sudden catastrophic haemorrhage can occur, but more typically there are small repeated bleeds with subtle and gradual loss of cord function distal to the lesion. They are angiographically occult with no demonstrable pathologic circulation. The diagnosis is made from MRI alone. The treatment, if appropriate, is surgery.

Spontaneous haemorrhage may also occur in the spine, due to a bleeding diathesis, or iatrogenically, in patients who are anticoagulated. The most common site of bleeding is in the extradural space. A spontaneous extradural (or epidural) haemorrhage typically presents with severe pain and neurological loss distal to the lesion. The treatment is surgical decompression, following correction of the underlying clotting disorder.

SYRINGOMYELIA

This is a condition in which cystic cavitation (syrinx) develops in the spinal cord. In most cases, syringomyelia is associated with brainstem herniation, in which the cerebellar tonsils become impacted in the foramen magnum – the **Chiari malformation**. Four types of Chiari malformation have been described, depending on the degree of hindbrain abnormality. Types 3 and 4 are not compatible with life. The type 2 abnormality (also termed the Arnold–Chiari malformation) is associated with a myelomeningocoele. The more minor degree of tonsillar descent that is commonly associated with a syrinx is termed the Chiari 1 malformation (Figure 15.9).

Symptoms usually develop slowly over several months or years. The classical picture is one of predominant upper limb neurological loss; wasting of the muscles of the hand and a cape-like dissociated sensory loss in the limbs and the upper trunk (a

The pathophysiology of syrinx formation remains poorly understood but, in principle, the herniated tonsils occlude the foramen magnum, leading to a pressure differential between the CSF surrounding the brain and the CSF surrounding the spinal cord. The pressure differential drives the accumulation of fluid within the cord leading to the formation of a syrinx, which may subsequently expand and extend downwards in the cord or upwards into the brainstem. It is the neurones lying in the centre of the cord that are damaged first. At the level of the syrinx, the anterior horn cells are lost, producing lower motor neurone signs in the upper limbs. The syrinx also interrupts the central decussating fibres of the spinothalamic tracts, producing dissociated loss of thermal and pain sensation. The posterior columns are spared, at least initially.

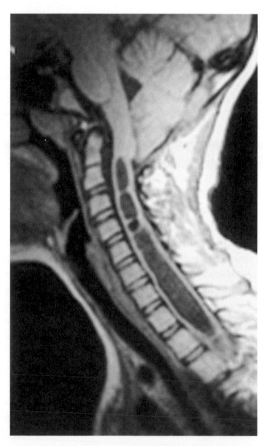

Figure 15.9 Sagittal T1-weighted MRI demonstrating a Chiari 1 malformation and a large syrinx.

'suspended' sensory loss). The signs are sometimes unilateral, particularly at the time of presentation, and there is usually asymmetry when the signs are bilateral. In advanced cases, all cord function may be lost and the severe impairment of pain sensation may lead to the development of neuropathic joints (Charcot joints) in the hand, elbow or shoulder joints.

The treatment of a syrinx associated with a Chiari malformation is foramen magnum decompression.

This aims to equalize the pressure differential across the cranio-cervical junction and remove the driving force for fluid accumulation in the syrinx. If the syrinx does not collapse over the subsequent few months, a shunt may be placed to drain the syrinx to either the subarachnoid space or pleural cavity.

Syrinx formation may also follow spinal cord injury, in which case the cavity occurs at the site of injury. A traumatic syrinx may expand and extend, causing a severe rostral extension of the level of neurological loss. Deterioration of neurological function following spinal injury, at an interval ranging from a few months up to many years following the original trauma, should always the possibility of the development of a post-traumatic syrinx, prompting reimaging with MRI.

DEGENERATIVE DISEASE

Spondylosis is the term used for the ubiquitous, age-related degenerative changes that occur throughout the spine. The most important predisposing factor for the development of these degenerative changes is genetic. It is the most mobile parts of the spine, the subaxial cervical spine and the lumbar spine, that are principally affected. While for the most part degenerative changes are asymptomatic, episodes of low back and neck pain are very common and virtually all of the adult population, at some point in their lives, will experience them. For a few individuals, these degenerative changes, either as a result of pain or neurological disturbance, will result in significant disability.

The process of degeneration starts with dehydration and subsequently disintegration of the nucleus pulposus, leading to loss of disc height. Tears may subsequently develop in the annulus fibrosus. The loss of disc height causes increased loading of the facet joints and, especially in those with a pre-existing constitutionally narrow spinal canal, the degenerative changes that ensue (disc bulge, facet joint hypertrophy and ligamentum flavum hypertrophy) summate to cause **spinal canal stenosis**. In the cervical and thoracic spines, central canal stenosis will result in compression of the spinal cord, in the lumbar spine, compression of the cauda equina. Localized areas of narrowing may result in compression of an individual nerve root, causing a painful radiculopathy. The pain, which is termed **brachalgia** in the upper limbs and **sciatica** in the lower limbs, often develops acutely or subacutely, is typically severe, lancinating or burning in nature and is referred into the dermatome/sclerotome of the affected root. The distribution of any neurological deficit (motor, sensory and tendon reflex loss) will be determined by the root or roots affected. Disc degeneration may also manifest acutely with herniation of the nucleus pulposus through a defect in the annulus fibrosis (colloquially termed a 'slipped disc').

Conservative treatment options for degenerative spinal disease include: analgesia, anti-inflammatories, exercise and physiotherapy.

> Most back pain occurs through postural and other mechanical factors that lead to agonizing muscle spasm, and this is best dealt with physically, i.e. physiotherapy.

For acute painful episodes, a brief period of bed-rest may be helpful, but early mobilization should be the aim. Injections, which may have both a diagnostic and a therapeutic role, can be used, targeted at the facet joints, dorsal root ganglia or the epidural space. Surgery may be required for patients with pain, neurological deficit that does not improve with conservative management and for those with spinal cord compression.

Cervical spine

In the cervical spine, central canal stenosis may lead to symptomatic compression of the spinal cord, termed **cervical spondylotic myelopathy**

(CSM). Movement is an important component of the pathogenesis of the spinal cord injury seen in CSM. Movements of the neck cause dynamic narrowing of the spinal canal, at the extremes of flexion and extension. At the same time during flexion, there is relative movement between the spinal cord and the vertebral canal, such that the spinal cord is dragged upwards through the narrowed area of the canal. In this way, the repetitive movements of normal daily life cause repeated microtrauma to the cord.

Rapid or acute neurological deterioration may be seen, but the more typical pattern is one of progressive step-wise neurological deterioration, interspersed with relatively stable periods. In the lower limbs, the initial symptom is unsteadiness, progressing to difficulty walking. Characteristically, the lower limbs may jerk at night. Upper limb involvement will depend on the level of cord compression, and it is common for cervical cord compression to lead to symptoms and major neurological deficit being confined to the legs, with only mild and sometimes subtle signs in the arms. It is important to recognize this when requesting imaging studies, ensuring that the cervical spine is adequately investigated.

In the syndrome of 'numb clumsy hands', there is initial numbness later accompanied by increasingly severe, intrusive burning pain in the hands, associated with dysaesthesia or allodynia.

CSM will usually require surgical decompression to arrest the neurological loss. Neurological improvement is seen in around 60 per cent following decompressive surgery, the prognosis being better for the lower limbs than for 'numb clumsy hands', which are particularly resistant to recovery. As neurological recovery is often incomplete, surgery should be performed early, preferably prior to the development of significant neurological loss. The surgical approach depends on the precise details of the compression, the number of spinal levels involved and the overall spinal alignment. In most instances, for single or two-level disease, an anterior cervical decompression and fusion is performed, with removal of the causative discs and occasionally the intervening vertebral body. For longer segments of compression, either an anterior or posterior approach may be used.

Compression of an individual exiting nerve root in the neck may cause brachalgia. The causative lesion in the cervical spine is usually a combination of disc and bony osteophyte, the so-called osteophytic disc bar or hard disc, although acute soft disc prolapses also occur, typically in a younger age group. The peak age for presentation with spondylotic radiculopathy is the sixth decade, ten years earlier than for CSM. The C5/6 level is the most commonly affected, followed by C4/5 and C6/7. Brachalgia can be extremely severe and resistant to analgesia. Targeted nerve root injections can be extremely useful in the early stages. Approximately 60 per cent will settle over three months. Surgical decompression of the affected root by anterior discectomy or posterior foramenotomy is reserved for persisting pain or neurological deficit.

Thoracic spine

The thoracic spine is relatively immobile due to the bracing effect of the thoracic cage; as a result, symptomatic degenerative disease is uncommon and canal stenosis, as found in the cervical region, is very rare. On occasion, the spinal cord is compressed by a thoracic disc, presenting with localized back pain, signs of myelopathy and a sensory level. Typically, such a disc is calcified or ossified and often represents a significant surgical challenge. In most cases, a thoracic disc is best removed transthoracically to minimize the chance of further, iatrogenic injury to the cord.

Lumbar spine

In the lumbar spine, canal stenosis leads to compression of the cauda equina and may cause limitation of walking as a result of progressively worsening calf pain, weakness and sensory disturbance; a pattern of symptoms termed **neurogenic claudication**. Typically, the symptoms are slowly progressive. A characteristic feature is that the symptoms are eased by bending forward, as bending enlarges the diameter of the lumbar canal. Patients can therefore cycle with relative ease and find walking much easier with a shopping trolley, allowing a flexed posture of the spine.

The main differential diagnosis is vascular claudication due to iliac or femoral artery occlusion. Decompressive surgery by means of laminectomy or more focused microsurgical decompression is the only successful treatment. Laterally placed degenerative changes, such as lateral recess stenosis, foraminal stenosis, or a degenerative facet joint

cyst, may cause compression of an individual nerve root resulting in sciatica and radiculopathy.

A prolapsed lumbar disc may present acutely with sciatica. There may be little in the way of back pain once the sciatica starts, but a prodromal period of back pain is common. **The levels most frequently affected are L4/5 and L5/S1.** A relatively minor physical event may precipitate the attack. The pain is usual severe with the distribution reflecting the affected root. For example, L5 pain radiates posterolaterally down the thigh and calf and across the dorsum of the foot to the great toe. The prolapse is usually posterolateral, trapping the traversing nerve root under the facet joint in the lateral recess. At L4/5, for example, the traversing L5 nerve root is compressed. Less commonly, a disc prolapse occurs laterally, compressing the exiting nerve root in or lateral to the foramen. At L4/5, it is the exiting L4 nerve root that is compressed (Figure 15.10). The management of sciatica will be one or more of: conservative measures, targeted nerve root injections or surgery, depending on circumstances, duration of symptoms, the presence of neurological deficit and patient choice.

A large acute disc prolapse may have serious consequences. In the cervical or thoracic spine, a large, centrally placed disc prolapse will compress the spinal cord, leading to myelopathy and will require urgent surgical attention. In the lumbar spine, a large, centrally placed disc prolapse may compress all the lumbar nerve roots causing a **cauda equina syndrome** (Figure 15.11). In most cases, cauda equina syndrome from disc prolapse evolves over a few hours or days. Accurate clinical diagnosis and urgent investigation and treatment are crucially important. Sudden bilateral sciatica, perineal or perianal sensory loss and bladder dysfunction are all highly suggestive symptoms, which should lead to careful examination. Decompression is a surgical emergency to restore neurological function, particularly bladder and bowel control. Unfortunately, once sphincter control is lost for even a few hours, even prompt surgical intervention may not rescue this aspect of cauda equina function.

As a result of spinal degeneration, deformity may occur, which complicates the management. In the lumbar spine, this may take the form of a degenerative spondylolisthesis (anterior slip) or scoliosis. A degenerative spondylolisthesis is most commonly seen at the L4/5 level. The presentation is with back pain, or a painful radiculopathy, as a

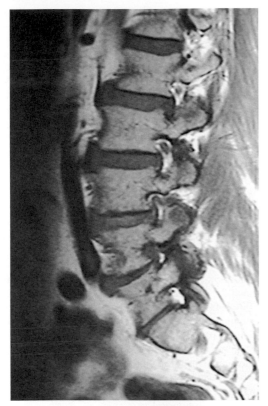

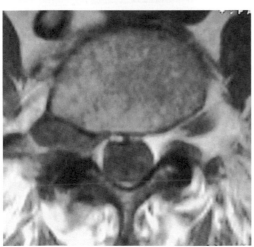

Figure 15.10 Sagittal and axial T1-weighted MRI showing a foraminal L4/5 disc herniation compressing the right L4 nerve root.

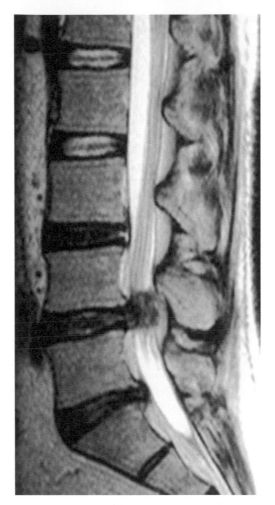

Figure 15.11 Sagittal T2-weighted MRI demonstrates a huge central disc prolapse at L4/5, severely compressing the cauda equina and causing a cauda equina syndrome with loss of sphincter control.

result of compression of the L5 nerve root in the lateral or with neurogenic claudication. In a few cases, the L4 nerve roots are also compressed in the exiting foramina. Once neurological symptoms and signs develop, surgery will usually be required. Although the choice of operation remains controversial, in some cases a simple microsurgical decompression or laminectomy is appropriate, but, in the majority, the best result will be achieved by decompression and fusion of the affected level. However, surgery for degenerative scoliosis is complex and carries a high morbidity. Where possible, treatment should rely on conservative measures.

Rheumatoid arthritis

The incidence of spinal rheumatoid disease is decreasing, probably due to better disease control and the reduced use of steroids. The C1/2 level is predominantly involved, in contrast to spondylosis, which typically affects the subaxial spine. Myelopathy occurs as a result of **basilar invagination, atlanto-axial subluxation** and less commonly sub-axial disease. Myelopathy will usually require surgery, but the management of these patients is particularly challenging.

Surgery of the spine – recent advances

The spine lies centrally within the trunk and may be accessed circumferentially from all directions, most commonly posteriorly for the lumbar spine and anteriorly in the cervical spine. A thorough knowledge of the underlying pathology and the anatomy of the various approaches will guide the direction of access in an individual case. There is a progressive shift in spinal surgery, which started in the 1960s with the popularization of the operating microscope and which was followed in the 1970s with the introduction of microdiscectomy, towards minimally invasive surgery. In contrast to this, rapid advances in the technology available to reconstruct or stabilize the spine and parallel advances in anaesthesia have resulted in surgeons being able to perform very complex spinal procedures, such as the resection of very large tumours and the correction of very significant spinal deformities which previously would have been viewed as unsafe or impossible.

REFERENCES AND FURTHER READING

Devo RA, Weinstein DO (2001) Low back pain. *New England Journal of Medicine*, 344:363–370.

Findlay GF (1984) Adverse effects of the management of malignant spinal cord compression. *Journal of Neurology, Neurosurgery and Psychiatry*, 47:761–768.

Junge A, Dvorak J, Ahrens ST (1995) Predictors of bad and good outcomes of lumbar disc surgery: a prospective clinical study with recommendations for screening to avoid bad outcomes. *Spine*, 20:460–468.

Lees F, Aldren-Turner JW (1963) Natural history and prognosis of cervical spondylosis. *British Medical Journal*, 2:1607–1610.

Menezes AH, Sonntag VKH (1996) *Principles of Spinal Surgery*. New York: McGraw-Hill.

Mixter W, Barr J (1934) Rupture of the intervertebral disc with involvement of the spinal canal. *New England Journal of Medicine*, 211:210–214.

Nussbaum ES, Rigamonti D, Standiford H *et al.* (1992) Spinal epidural abscess: a report of 40 cases and review. *Journal of Neurosurgery*, 38:225–231.

Peul W, van Houwelingen HC, van den Hout WB *et al.* (2007) Surgery versus prolonged conservative treatment for sciatica. *New England Journal of Medicine*, 356:2245–2256.

Rosenblum B, Oldfield EH, Doppman JL, Di Chiro G (1987) Spinal arteriovenous malformations: a comparison of dural arteriovenous fistulas and intradural arteriovenous malformation in 81 patients. *Journal of Neurosurgery*, 67:795–802.

Souweidane MM, Benjamin V (1994) Spinal cord meningiomas. *Neurosurgery Clinics of North America*, 5:283–291.

Symon L, Kuyama H, Kendall B (1984) Dural arteriovenous malformations of the spine. *Journal of Neurosurgery*, 60:238–247.

Weinstein JN, Tosteson TD, Lurie JD *et al.* (2006) Surgical vs nonoperative treatment for lumbar disk herniation: the Spine Patient Outcomes Research Trial (SPORT): a randomized trial. *JAMA*, 296:2441–50.

Williams B (1978) A critical appraisal of posterior fossa surgery for communicating syringomyelia. *Brain*, 101:223–250.

Young S, O'Laoire S (1987) Cervical disc prolapse in the elderly: an easily overlooked, reversible cause of spinal cord compression. *British Journal of Neurosurgery*, 1:93–98.

CHAPTER 16

PERIPHERAL NEUROPATHIES

Gareth Llewelyn and Robert Powell

INTRODUCTION

Due to the varied manifestations of neuropathy (Box 16.1), clinical assessment can be difficult, and planning appropriate investigations challenging. The first step is an accurate history of the tempo, pattern and severity of the neuropathy, followed by a careful examination and a selective approach to investigations, leading to a diagnosis and a treatment plan. It is unfortunately still the case that even after extensive testing, the cause of about 30-40 per cent of neuropathies remains uncertain, leading to the unsatisfactory diagnostic labels of cryptogenic or idiopathic neuropathy.

Focal, multifocal and symmetric neuropathies

The first step in diagnosis is to identify the pattern of a neuropathy as focal, multifocal or symmetric. While the history and examination often make this obvious, nerve conduction studies (NCS) can add valuable information in many instances.

Focal involvement of a single nerve is termed a **mononeuropathy**, and usually results from local compression or direct injury. Common examples include ulnar neuropathy at the elbow, median neuropathy (carpal tunnel syndrome) at the wrist and common peroneal neuropathy at the knee. Isolated cranial nerve palsies are termed 'cranial mononeuropathies'.

A diagnosis of **multifocal neuropathy** (also termed 'multiple mononeuropathy' or 'mononeuritis multiplex') is established when there is involvement of separate nerves, occurring either simultaneously or sequentially. The nature and distribution of the symptoms and signs will reflect the nerves affected, and depending on the underlying cause, evolution of the deficit may be over days or as long as years. With progression, the clinical pattern may become more symmetric in its appearance and can become difficult to distinguish from a polyneuropathy. It is therefore important to establish in any patient with a clinically symmetric neuropathy whether the evolution of symptoms indicates a patchy evolution (multifocal) or symmetric progression (polyneuropathy).

The term **polyneuropathy** generally refers to a neuropathy that has evolved in a symmetric

Box 16.1 Clinical pattern and causes of neuropathies

- Sensory polyneuropathy
  - Diabetes, uraemia, hypothyroidism
  - Amyloidosis
  - Paraneoplastic, paraproteinaemic
  - Thallium, isoniazid, vincristine, cisplatin, metronidazole
  - Sjögren's syndrome
  - Leprosy
  - HIV, Lyme disease
  - Hereditary sensory and autonomic neuropathies
  - Fabry's disease
  - Vitamin B_{12} deficiency
- Sensorimotor polyneuropathy
  - Charcot–Marie–Tooth disease
  - Alcohol
  - Guillain–Barré syndrome (GBS); chronic inflammatory demyelinating polyneuropathy (CIDP)
  - Vasculitis
  - Paraneoplastic, paraproteinaemic
  - Diabetes, uraemia, hypothyroidism, acromegaly
  - Sarcoidosis
- Motor neuropathy
  - GBS/CIDP
  - Porphyria, diphtheria, lead
  - Hereditary motor neuropathies (HMN)
- Focal and multifocal neuropathies
  - Entrapment/compression syndromes
  - Polyarteritis nodosa
  - Connective tissue disorders
  - Non-systemic (tissue-specific) vasculitis
  - Wegner's granulomatosis
  - Infiltration of nerve by lymphoma or carcinoma
  - Neurofibromatosis
  - Tuberculoid leprosy, herpes zoster, human immunodeficiency virus, Lyme disease
  - Sarcoidosis
  - Hereditary neuropathy with liability to pressure palsies
  - Multifocal motor neuropathy with conduction block

fashion. Polyneuropathies are 'length-related' conditions, starting distally in the toes and feet with sensory symptoms, developing into the typical 'stocking and glove' pattern of numbness. Motor symptoms and signs reflect a similar length-related progression, initially with distal weakness and wasting, the legs almost always being more affected than the arms. The rate of progression, prominence of sensory or motor features, with or without pain, depends on the cause. The challenge for the clinician is to use these clinical features to help narrow the list of possible causes.

CLINICAL FEATURES

There are negative and positive symptoms related to neuropathies (Table 16.1). Numbness is the most common sensory symptom, with associated loss of all sensory modalities. Sometimes the sensory loss is confined to pain and temperature sensations with preservation of light touch, vibration and joint position sense; this pattern would indicate a predominant loss of small fibres – a small fibre neuropathy (for example, due to diabetes or amyloidosis). The loss of pain and temperature sensations predisposes the patient to the risk of painless injuries, including the development of **neuropathic ulcers and neuropathic (Charcot) joints**. Such neuropathies are also likely to be associated with autonomic symptoms and signs including postural hypotension, impotence, constipation, loss of bladder control, abnormal sweating and occasionally blurring of vision. It is therefore important to check

Table 16.1 Symptoms of peripheral neuropathy

Sensory symptoms	
Negative	Numbness
Positive	Paraesthesiae (tingling, pins and needles)
	Pain (burning, shooting, stabbing, 'like walking on pebbles', 'like walking on hot sand', may be induced by non-painful stimuli, allodynia, hyperalgesia)
Motor symptoms	
Negative	Weakness and wasting
Positive	Fasciculations
	Myokymia
	Cramps
	Restless legs
	Tremor

Table 16.2 Clinical signs associated with a peripheral neuropathy

	Clinical sign
Skeletal abnormalities	Pes cavus
	Clawing of toes
	Scoliosis/kyphoscoliosis
Change in skin, nails and hair	Foot ulcers
	Loss of hair to mid-calf region
	Thin dry skin
	Hypopigmentation of the skin
Motor	Normal tone with distal wasting and weakness
Reflexes	Absent or depressed
Sensory	'Stocking and glove' loss of sensation

for postural hypotension and pupillary reactions in every patient with a neuropathy.

The other cardinal sign of neuropathy is absent or depressed reflexes (Table 16.2). When a neuropathy develops during the early growth period, skeletal deformities may be seen (clawed toes, pes cavus and kyphoscoliosis). Sometimes a clue to the cause of a neuropathy may come from thickening of peripheral nerves. Nerves that can be examined for evidence of thickening include the radial nerve at the wrist, ulnar nerve at the elbow, common peroneal nerve at the knee and the superficial peroneal nerve on the dorsum of the foot.

Conditions that may cause nerve thickening include:
- Leprosy
- Charcot–Marie–Tooth disease type I and II
- Acromegaly
- Amyloidosis
- Neurofibromatosis
- Refsum's disease

APPROACH TO INVESTIGATION AND MANAGEMENT

No battery of laboratory tests is going to make up for a haphazard history and examination. The pattern of the neuropathy (Box 16.1), established by history and examination, provides important clues as to aetiology. This allows appropriate investigations to be undertaken (Table 16.3) to confirm the cause. Most blood tests and urinalysis are straightforward. Certain investigations, for example anti-neuronal antibodies, should only be requested when there is strong suspicion of a paraneoplastic neuropathy. DNA analysis in suspected inherited neuropathy will require the patient's consent and in some circumstances genetic counselling, before the sample is taken.

Nerve conduction studies (NCS) and electromyography (EMG) are an extension of the clinical examination and are crucial in distinguishing between an axonal and a demyelinating process (see Chapter 5). In the latter, the conduction velocities are reduced (less than 35 m/s and often in the range 20–30 m/s). The causes of chronic demyelinating neuropathies are shown in Box 16.2.

Sensory threshold tests (thermal and vibration) can be helpful when the standard nerve conduction tests are normal, but the clinical picture suggests a small fibre neuropathy. Thermal threshold tests should only be performed in a laboratory used to

---

Box 16.2 Chronic demyelinating neuropathies

- Immune mediated
  - CIDP and MMN
- Paraproteinaemic
  - Benign paraprotein (IgM, G or A)
  - Myeloma (IgM,G or A)
  - Waldenström's macroglobulinaemia (IgM)
  - POEMS syndrome (IgG or A)
- Hereditary
  - CMT disease (type 1, Dejerine-Sottas,/CMT3, X-linked CMT)
  - HNPP
  - Refsum's disease
  - Metachromatic leukodystrophy
  - Globoid cell leukodystrophy
- Toxic
  - Amiodarone, perhexiline, suramin
  - Diphtheria

CIDP, chronic inflammatory demyelinating polyneuropathy; CMT, Charcot-Marie-Tooth disease; Ig, immunoglobulin (M, G, A); HNPP, hereditary neuropathy with liability to pressure palsies; MMN, multifocal motor neuropathy; POEMS, polyneuropathy, organomegaly, endocrinopathy, monoclonal protein and skin changes.

Table 16.3 Investigation of a neuropathy

Blood	**FBC, ESR/CRP, U&E, LFT**
	Glucose (+GTT if borderline)
	Serum protein electrophoresis
	Autoantibodies, T4/TSH
	Vitamin B$_{12}$, folate
	Genetic testing – e.g. PMP22, Po for CMT type 1
Urine	**Glucose, protein**, Bence–Jones protein, porphyrins
Cerebrospinal fluid	Rarely indicated. May be helpful in acute neuropathy (GBS)
Nerve conduction studies	Slowing of motor and sensory conduction velocities (moderate in axonal neuropathy; severe in demyelinating neuropathy)
Sensory threshold test	Only in suspected small fibre neuropathy when nerve conduction studies may be normal
Autonomic function tests	Lying and standing BP is useful. More detailed testing requires specialist input
Imaging	Skeletal survey for myeloma
	Chest x-ray for suspected carcinoma or sarcoidosis
	MRI of plexus or nerves requires specialist input
Nerve biopsy	Rarely indicated. May be useful in a mononeuritis multiplex or when the cause of a progressive neuropathy has not been revealed by other investigations. It is useful to confirm the presence of vasculitis or other inflammatory infiltration. Only sensory nerves are biopsied (sural, superficial peroneal or superficial radial nerves)

Initial screen is in bold type.

BP, blood pressure; CSF, cerebrospinal fluid; CMT, Charcot-Marie-Tooth disease; CRP, C-reactive protein; ESR, erythrocyte sedimentation rate; FBC, full blood count; GBS, Guillain-Barré syndrome; GTT, glucose tolerance test; MRI, magnetic resonance imaging; TSH, thyroid stimulating hormone.

interpreting these measurements as they are prone to wide variability. Cerebrospinal fluid (CSF) analysis is helpful, but only in specific situations – when there is no clear answer from blood tests and NCS and the neuropathy is progressing rapidly.

Nerve biopsy should only be considered in certain situations, for example, if there is suspicion of a vasculitis in a patient with a mononeuritis multiplex, with non-contributory blood test results. In this example, confirmatory evidence from a biopsy will guide treatment. Careful planning is needed in selection of which nerve to biopsy (the most common is the sural nerve at the ankle), the choice of nerve being guided by evidence of clinical involvement, supported by neurophysiological investigation. Examination of biopsies by light and electron microscopy should be undertaken by a pathologist with special experience of the interpretation of peripheral nerve pathology.

Treatment of specific neuropathies is discussed below, but some aspects of management are common to many patients with neuropathies. These include:

- Foot care
- Physiotherapy advice regarding use of walking aids or ankle-foot orthoses
- Occupational therapy for advice on seating, hand rails, utensils.

Neuropathic pain presents a particular therapeutic challenge. This topic is considered in detail in Chapter 30.

DIABETIC NEUROPATHIES

Due to life-style issues (sedentary existence and over-eating, resulting in obesity), the number of people affected by diabetes mellitus (mainly type 2) across the world is projected to increase exponentially over the next 20 years from 220 million to 500 million in 2030. Peripheral neuropathy occurring as a complication of both type 1 and type 2 diabetes will present an increasing problem. Occasionally, the neuropathy appears before diabetes becomes evident, but in such cases, the diagnosis is suggested by evidence of impaired glucose metabolism (prediabetes).

The most common form is **distal sensorimotor polyneuropathy**. There is evidence of a neuropathy in about 10 per cent of patients at the time of diagnosis of their diabetes, increasing to 50 per cent after more than five years of diabetes, but the frequency of neuropathy depends on whether patients are assessed clinically, or by the use of more sensitive NCS. **Multifocal neuropathies** are also common in diabetes and often coexist with the distal symmetric neuropathy.

A number of aetiological factors have been proposed for the range of diabetic neuropathies (see below), including oxidative stress, ischaemia, inflammation and microvasculitis (Box 16.3). The only treatment with demonstrated benefit is strict diabetic control with maintenance of normal blood glucose levels.

Diabetic neuropathies

- Usually progressive:
  - distal symmetric sensory and sensorimotor neuropathies
  - autonomic neuropathy
- Potentially reversible:
  - acute painful neuropathy
  - cranial neuropathy (VIth, IIIrd and IVth nerve palsies)
  - thoraco-abdominal neuropathy
  - lumbosacral radiculoplexus neuropathy (diabetic amyotrophy).

Box 16.3 Possible mechanisms in the pathogenesis of diabetic neuropathy

---

- Metabolic hypothesis
  - Polyol accumulation, myo-inositol depletion, reduced Na1K1-ATPase
  - Advanced glycosylation end-product formation
  - Altered neurotrophic factors
  - Oxidative stress
  - Altered fatty acid metabolism
- Vascular hypothesis
- Altered protein synthesis and axonal transport
- Immunological mechanisms

Distal sensory and sensorimotor polyneuropathy

For most patients with **distal sensory or sensorimotor polyneuropathy**, the symptoms are mild, and consist of numbness and minor tingling. Pain is a troublesome and sometimes debilitating symptom in 10 per cent of cases, and is described as aching, burning, stabbing or shooting.

Tactile hypersensitivity (allodynia, see Chapter 30) is often present in these patients, and despite the severity of the symptoms the neurological deficit on examination may be relatively minor.

Examination reveals distal weakness and loss of ankle reflexes. The sensory loss affects all modalities and begins at the toes and evolves into a 'sock' distribution. It follows a length-related pattern, so that when the sensory extends up to knee or mid-thigh level, sensory loss will begin to develop in the fingers. Uncommonly, the neuropathy becomes so severe that sensory loss develops on the anterior chest and abdominal wall. Sensory symptoms and signs dominate in this form of neuropathy, and if there is evidence of more severe distal weakness with wasting, or additional proximal weakness, then the coexistence of another neuropathy, such as chronic inflammatory demyelinating polyneuropathy (CIDP), vasculitis or paraproteinaemic neuropathy, should be considered.

With a typical clinical picture, there is a need for only a few simple blood tests (see Table 16.3). NCS add little unless the neuropathy evolves in an unexpected way. Nerve biopsy is rarely indicated and should not be done without a specialist opinion.

The **painful small fibre neuropathy** is a clinical variant in which pain in the feet is the main symptom. Examination may be normal, but careful testing of pain and temperature sensations often reveals subtle impairments. Likewise, standard NCS, which reflect function of large nerve fibres, may also be normal. Thermal thresholds are likely to be abnormal. Skin biopsies show loss of small epidermal nerve fibres, but this remains largely a research investigation at present, and is not available in routine practice.

Diabetic autonomic neuropathy is also length-related, causing loss of sweating in the feet as an early feature. Autonomic involvement is associated with an increased mortality rate. Treatment of autonomic symptoms is outlined in Table 16.4.

These slowly progressive neuropathies show an

Table 16.4 Diabetic autonomic neuropathy

Cardinal symptoms	Treatment
Impotence	Counselling. Sildenafil. Penile papaverine injection. Mechanical prosthesis
Postural hypotension (<30 mmHg drop)	Fludrocortisone ± indometacin
Abnormal sweating	
Gastroparesis	Metoclopramide, domperidone, erythromycin
Diarrhoea	Tetracycline with loperamide/codeine
Decreased awareness of hypoglycaemia	

association with diabetic retinopathy and nephropathy, and are more likely to occur with longer duration of diabetes, in men, taller subjects, and in those who are overweight. In addition to blood glucose, elevated triglyceride level is a consistent risk factor.

Acute painful neuropathy

Acute painful neuropathy appears to be a distinct entity, with the onset of severe pain distally in the legs associated with progressive weight loss. The burning pains and contact hyperaesthesiae are often particularly troublesome at night, causing insomnia and depression. With continued good diabetic control and adequate pain relief, improvement does occur, but often takes several months. Regaining body weight is an early indicator of improvement. This syndrome can be triggered following the institution of tight glucose control with either insulin or oral hypoglycaemic drugs. The specific pathogenesis of this type of neuropathy is not known.

Cranial neuropathies

There is an increased incidence of **IIIrd and VIth cranial nerve palsies** in diabetic patients. In a IIIrd cranial, there is aching pain around the affected eye in half of those affected, **usually with sparing of the pupil,** in contrast to the majority of patients

with compressive IIIrd nerve palsies, in which the pupil is involved. The diabetic IIIrd nerve palsy is thought to be caused by ischaemia of the central core of the IIIrd nerve. The prognosis is excellent, most recovering within three to four months.

Thoracoabdominal neuropathy

An acute onset of pain in a localized area over the anterior chest or abdominal wall, associated with sensory loss, may appear to be odd unless one is aware of **thoracoabdominal neuropathy**. The pattern of sensory loss, sometimes accompanied by allodynia and hyperpathia (see Chapter 30) produced is consistent with a lesion of the spinal nerve or its branches. The pain resolves within a few days and the numbness recovers over 4–6 weeks. On the abdominal wall, muscle weakness may present as a hernia. The pathogenesis is not known.

Lumbosacral radiculoplexus neuropathy

Often termed **diabetic amyotrophy, lumbosacral radiculoplexus neuropathy** occurs in older people with type 2 diabetes, affecting men more often than women. There is lumbar or proximal leg pain from the outset – which may be acute or subacute – followed a week or so later by an asymmetric onset of lower limb weakness and wasting which is most striking proximally, but which may be global. The knee jerk is depressed or absent on the affected side, and often both ankle jerks are absent because of the coexistence of a distal symmetric sensorimotor neuropathy. There is often marked weight loss. Leg weakness becomes the dominant feature as the pain resolves, and there may be progression over weeks and months.

Recovery occurs slowly over many months or years, but a number of patients have moderate or severe residual neurological deficit. Recent studies have demonstrated either microvasculitis or non-vasculitic epineurial and endoneurial inflammatory infiltration in about one-third of cases. Whether lumbosacral radiculoplexus neuropathy would respond to immunotherapy is not known. Treatment is based on achieving good glucose control, paying close attention to pain relief and physiotherapy.

GUILLAIN–BARRÉ SYNDROME AND OTHER IMMUNE-MEDIATED NEUROPATHIES

Guillain–Barré syndrome

Guillain–Barré syndrome (GBS), also called acute inflammatory demyelinating polyradiculoneuropathy (AIDP), is the most common subacute neuropathy, with an incidence of 1.5–2.0:100 000 population per year. About 4 per cent of cases will have a second episode.

Clinically, it usually reaches its peak within 4 weeks of the onset of symptoms. When there is ongoing progression for between 4 and 8 weeks, this is termed subacute IDP/GBS to distinguish it from chronic inflammatory demyelinating polyradiculoneuropathy, in which, by definition, there is neurological progression beyond 8 weeks from the onset of the illness. Although tingling, shooting pains and numbness in the feet and hands are the first symptoms, the predominant feature is weakness, which initially appears in the legs, often producing a symmetric distal pattern that progresses to involve the arms (so-called 'ascending paralysis'). Only in 10 per cent of cases does weakness start in the arms. The clinical variants of GBS are outlined in Figure 16.1 and Box 16.4. Facial weakness is often asymmetric and is present in just over 50 per cent of cases. Ophthalmoparesis occurs in 15 per cent of patients with typical GBS.

Features suggesting a diagnosis other than GBS
- Sensory level: spinal cord syndrome
- Severe bladder or bowel dysfunction: spinal cord syndrome
- Marked asymmetry: vasculitis
- CSF >50 WBC/mm$_3$: HIV, Lyme disease, polio
- Very slow nerve conduction velocities (<32 m/s): CIDP.

In patients with cranial nerve involvement, bulbar weakness or neck and proximal arm weakness, there is a high risk of developing intercostal muscle and diaphragmatic weakness leading to potentially fatal respiratory failure.

The reflexes are depressed or absent from an early stage, but may be normal in the first 2 days of the illness.

Autonomic function is abnormal in two-thirds of patients.

Sinus tachycardia is common, but rarely needs treating. Bradycardias, heart block, paroxysmal atrial tachycardia and periods of sinus arrest and asystole are life threatening and require urgent cardiological assessment and treatment. Labile blood pressure may also need treatment. Urinary retention occurs in 10–15 per cent of cases, but urinary incontinence is rare. Constipation is far more common than diarrhoea.

During the course of the illness, almost 75 per cent of patients will complain of deep muscle pains, mainly in the lower back and legs, which can be severe.

A slow but steady recovery over weeks and up to six months is seen in 80 per cent of GBS cases. A more aggressive course is seen in 10–15 per cent of patients, who have a prolonged stay on the intensive therapy unit and a recovery period extending up to two years (usually acute motor and sensory axonal neuropathy variant). Even with optimal management, about 5 per cent of patients with GBS die from complications of the illness.

Poor prognostic factors in GBS are:
- Older age
- Rapid onset (<7 days)
- Requiring ventilatory support
- Previous diarrhoeal illness (*Campylobacter jejuni*)
- Small distal compound muscle action potentials
- No treatment given (intravenous immunoglobulin (IVIg) or plasma exchange)

Confirmation of the clinical diagnosis comes from NCS and examination of the CSF. Both may be normal early on in the illness, but later the

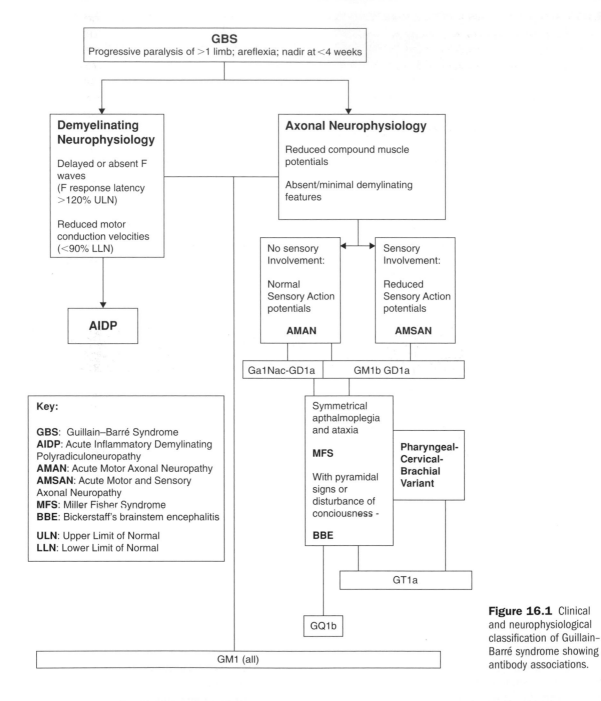

Figure 16.1 Clinical and neurophysiological classification of Guillain–Barré syndrome showing antibody associations.

CSF shows a raised protein, usually with a normal white cell count. A mild lymphocytosis (10–30 cells/mm3) is seen in some patients with GBS, but a higher cell count raises the possibility of an underlying infective cause, such as HIV infection.

NCS show slowing of velocities with patchy conduction block in the common AIDP variant. Important blood tests are listed in Table 16.5.

Management and treatment

It is vital that the patient has adequate monitoring of respiratory and cardiac function (Box 16.5). If this cannot be undertaken on the general medical ward, the patient must be transferred either to a high dependency unit or to a regional neurology unit.

Box 16.4 Guillain–Barré syndrome (GBS) and variants

- Acute inflammatory demyelinating polyradiculoneuropathy (AIDP)
  - 60 per cent will have antecedent illness
  - Progression is over days up to 4 weeks
  - Recovery usually starts at 4 weeks
  - 20 per cent will have significant neurological disability
  - Mortality rate is about 5 per cent
- Acute motor and sensory axonal neuropathy (AMSAN)
  - Diarrhoeal illness is common trigger (*Campylobacter jejuni*)
  - Acute onset of weakness, rapid progression
  - Often there are early respiratory difficulties
  - Longer recovery and more severe residual disability than AIDP
  - Mortality rate is 10–15 per cent
- Acute motor axonal neuropathy (AMAN)
  - Diarrhoeal illness (*Campylobacter jejuni*) is usual trigger
  - Rare in Western world
  - Most commonly affects children in northern China and is seasonal
  - Recovery and mortality rates are similar to AIDP
- Miller–Fisher syndrome (MFS)
  - Accounts for 5 per cent of all GBS cases
  - Begins with diplopia, followed 3–4 days later by gait ataxia
  - Evolves to complete ophthalmoplegia with areflexia
  - Sometimes mild limb weakness is present
  - >80 per cent have IgG antibodies to ganglioside GQ1b
  - Monophasic course with excellent recovery
  - Intravenous immunoglobulin or plasma exchange is appropriate for those who cannot walk
- Bickerstaff's brainstem encephalitis
- Acute panautonomic neuropathy
- Pure sensory neuropathy

Table 16.5 Blood tests that may be abnormal in Guillain–Barré syndrome (GBS)

Full blood count	White blood count may be raised
	Lymphoma and CLL linked with GBS
Electrolytes	Sodium may be low due to SIADH
T4/TSH	Hypothyroidism linked to GBS
ANA	Collagen vascular disease linked with GBS
Porphyrin screen	AIP may mimic GBS
HIV test (when indicated)	Increased white cells in the cerebrospinal fluid (>50/mm^3)
Anti-GQ1b	For MFS variant
Infection screen	*Campylobacter* serology (and stool culture), CMV, EBV, hepatitis A and C, Mycoplasma

AIP, acute intermittent porphyria; ANA, anti-nuclear antibody; CLL, chronic lymphatic leukaemia; CMV, cytomegalovirus; EBV, Epstein–Barr virus; HIV, human immunodeficiency virus; SIADH, syndrome of inappropriate antidiuretic hormone; TSH, thyroid stimulating hormone.

Monitoring of respiratory function in GBS is essential. Peak expiratory flow rate (PEFR) measurements are not just unhelpful, they are misleading and dangerous. PEFR is appropriate in airways obstruction, but in GBS (and other neuromuscular causes of ventilatory failure) the problem is not obstruction, but an underlying pathology that leads to muscular weakness. This should be monitored by serial measurement of vital capacity. PEFR may remain relatively normal when the vital capacity is critically low.

Intravenous immunoglobulin is the first-line immunomodulating treatment, and although there are no strict guidelines as to when to start treatment, it is reasonable to consider IVIg (0.4 g/kg body weight per day for 5 days) if the patient has difficulty with walking. It is recommended that the patient or next of kin be fully informed of the 10–20 per cent risk of relapse after IVIg, and of the small but theoretically possible risks of transmission of hepatitis A, B and C viruses and HIV and of transmission of prion proteins; a consent form should be completed before treatment is started.

Box 16.5 Management of Guillain–Barré syndrome

- Early
  - 4–12 hourly recording of VC and oxygen saturation
  - Continuous electrocardiogram
  - Low molecular weight heparin and compression stockings
  - Daily clinical assessment of facial, neck and limb strength
  - Regular chest physiotherapy, turning and mouth care
  - Nasogastric tube if there are swallowing problems
  - Intravenous immunoglobulin (0.4 g/kg body weight per day for 5 days) or
  - Plasma exchange – five exchanges of 50 mL/kg over 5–10 days
  - Pain control – opiate analgesia may be required
- Late
  - Ventilatory assistance if VC is falling rapidly or is below 24 mL/kg
  - Tracheostomy – if ventilation is needed for more than 10 days
  - Cardiac pacemaker – for bradyarrhythmias or episodes of asystole
  - PEG – if recovery of bulbar function is delayed
  - Mobilization; prevention of contractures and bed sores
  - Nutritional advice
  - Monitor pain control

PEG, percutaneous endoscopic gastrostomy; VC, vital capacity.

Supportive care remains the most important component of treatment and the patient needs to be monitored carefully until the illness has stabilized for at least 3 weeks.

If the patient relapses after IVIg, a second treatment (further IVIg or plasma exchange) should be given. However, if there has been no improvement after 2 weeks, with a steady deterioration, there are currently no trial data supporting any specific additional intervention.

With early diagnosis and treatment and appropriate measures to prevent thromboembolism, aspiration and pressure sores, most patients with GBS recover satisfactorily. The GBS support group provides information and important contact with patients.

Pathogenesis of GBS

Antibodies generated by the immune response to infection and directed against neural epitopes (the molecular mimicry hypothesis) may be the basis of axonal GBS and Miller–Fisher syndrome (MFS). Strains of *Campylobacter jejuni* which trigger GBS are more likely to possess lipo-oligosaccharide epitopes similar to gangliosides GM1, GD1a or GQ1b. These antigens induce neuropathy-causing ganglioside antibodies in animal models. The titre of anti-GQ1b antibody correlates with disease severity in MFS, and the GQ1b ganglioside is concentrated in nerves supplying extra-ocular muscles.

The pathophysiology of the more common AIDP is less well understood. T cells appear to play an important part in inducing macrophage attack against Schwann cells or myelin. The correlation between NCS and clinical and immunological markers is only approximate.

Chronic inflammatory demyelinating polyradiculoneuropathy

CIDP is considered to be uncommon – between 1 and 8/100 000 population depending on how the diagnosis is established, but it is probably under-diagnosed. To consider CIDP, a chronic form of GBS is probably too simplistic, and it is important to distinguish between the two conditions as there are important differences in their treatment and outcome. The main clinical feature is that AIDP worsens over 4 weeks and CIDP worsens over any length of time beyond 8 weeks.

The typical pattern is that of a symmetrically progressive sensorimotor neuropathy that often gives rise to proximal and distal weakness with loss of reflexes.

CIDP is predominantly a symmetric polyradiculoneuropathy with symptoms of weakness, sensory loss and paraesthesiae. Both proximal and distal muscles may be affected early on in the illness, and although the weakness can be severe, muscle wasting is not a major feature, because the pathology

Table 16.6 Clinical and neurophysiological features of CIDP subtypes and their response to immunotherapy

		Chronic inflammatory demyelinating polyradiculoneuropathy (CIDP)	Distal acquired demyelinating symmetric neuropathy (DADS)	Multifocal acquired demyelinating sensory and motor neuropathy (MADSAM)	Multifocal motor neuropathy (with conduction block) (MMN)
Pattern	Weakness	S; p > d	S; d	A; d > p	A; d > p
	Numbness	++	+/–	++	++
	Reflexes	+	++	+	–
		+/–	+/–	Patchy +/–	Patchy +/–
	MCS	Conduction block ++	Conduction block +/–	Conduction block ++	Conduction block ++
	SCS	Symmetric	Symmetric	Asymmetric	Normal
Response to treatment					
	IVIg	Good	Poor	Variable	Good
	Plasma exchange	Good	Poor	Good	None
	Steroids	Good	Poor	Good	None

A, asymmetric; S, symmetric; d, distal; p, proximal.
MCS, motor conduction studies; SCS, sensory conduction studies.

Several clinical subtypes are now recognized (see Table 16.6). These include:

- CIDP – symmetric with proximal and distal weakness
- DADS (distal acquired demyelinating symmetric neuropathy) – symmetric distal weakness and numbness
- MADSAM (multifocal acquired demyelinating sensory and motor neuropathy) – asymmetric weakness and sensory loss
- MMN (multifocal motor neuropathy) – asymmetric weakness with normal sensation.

is demyelination with areas of conduction block, rather than marked loss of axons. Neck weakness is common, but facial weakness is rare (<15 per cent) and is usually mild. Respiratory muscle weakness does not occur. There is hyporeflexia or areflexia and sensory loss in a stocking-and-glove distribution with an emphasis on loss of large fibres, leading to a sensory ataxia. Autonomic features can occur, but are uncommon.

The clinical course may be slowly progressive, stepwise progressive (66 per cent), or relapsing (33 per cent). The CSF protein is elevated with normal cells. NCS show demyelination, which is patchy, with regions of conduction block. Although there is no other specific diagnostic for CIDP, the clinical features, detailed neurophysiology and CSF examination, are usually enough to make a diagnosis without any need for a nerve biopsy, which is only of value in those cases where either the neurophysiology is not typical or where the clinical picture suggests that vasculitis is a possibility.

Treatment of CIDP

The variability of response to treatment in CIDP and its subtypes is shown in Table 16.6.

CIDP usually responds to IVIg, plasma exchange and oral corticosteroids. In practice, the choice of treatment is between IVIg and corticosteroids. As a general rule, those with more severe disability are given IVIg (0.5 g/kg body weight per day for 5 days) and if there is a good response, a repeat course of IVIg can be given if there is a relapse.

Oral prednisolone is given at a dose of 1–1.5 mg/kg body weight per day for 4 weeks, then gradually reducing the dose by 10 mg every 4 weeks to 30 mg/day and then reducing by 5 mg every 4 weeks until the lowest effective dose is reached.

This is often combined with bisphosphonate treatment, calcium supplements and a preventative treatment for gastritis. The use of alternate day steroid dosing for long-term treatment reduces adverse effects.

For patients who relapse early after IVIg or steroids or whose initial response has been modest, the next option is to consider long-term treatment (12–24 months) with an alternative oral immunosuppressant. Unfortunately, there is currently no evidence to support any of the standard options available (azathioprine, methotrexate, ciclosporin and cyclophosphamide) and the potential benefits and adverse effects need to be clearly discussed with the patient before embarking on treatment. The role of newer agents, such as the monoclonal antibodies rituximab and alemtuzumab is under investigation.

Multifocal motor neuropathy with conduction block

> MMN is an uncommon disorder, but is important as it may resemble the lower motor neurone variant of motor neurone disease. Unlike motor neurone disease, MMN is potentially treatable, with good response.

MMN is characterized by **progressive and asymmetric weakness without sensory involvement.** Unilateral grip weakness, wrist drop or foot drop are common presenting features. Cranial nerve and respiratory involvement are rare. Cramps and fasciculations are common and the reflexes are asymmetrically depressed.

The electrophysiological hallmark is the presence of persistent **multifocal conduction block** – where the transmission of electrical impulse is blocked due to an area of loss of myelin somewhere along the nerve (see Chapter 5). Evidence of more widespread peripheral nerve demyelination is also often found. Unlike CIDP, the CSF protein is usually normal. Elevated anti-GM1 ganglioside antibody titres are of no diagnostic or prognostic value.

Treatment with IVIg is effective in most patients, but the duration of benefit is variable (2–12 weeks), and patients require regular maintenance doses. The

periods between treatments may get shorter as the disease continues. There is no clear evidence to support the use of oral immunosuppressants, such as cyclophosphamide. Corticosteroid treatment should be avoided as this may worsen the condition.

NEUROPATHIES WITH MONOCLONAL GAMMOPATHIES

> Serum protein electrophoresis should be performed on every adult patient with a neuropathy, but immunofixation is required to detect low concentrations of paraprotein (<0.2 g/L). A monoclonal paraprotein is associated with 10 per cent of otherwise cryptogenic neuropathies. The level of paraprotein can vary, but does not correlate with the severity of the clinical picture.

Detection of a paraprotein (IgM, IgG or IgA) raises the possibility of underlying myeloma, lymphoma, macroglobulinaemia or systemic amyloidosis, but if the appropriate investigations are negative, then the diagnostic term used is **benign monoclonal gammopathy of unknown significance (MGUS).**

Screening tests for a monoclonal gammopathy
- Full blood count, erythrocyte sedimentation rate (ESR), creatinine, calcium
- Paraprotein concentration (<3 g/dL indicates a benign paraprotein)
- Urinalysis for Bence–Jones protein
- Skeletal survey
- Bone marrow examination – request a haematology opinion, as this is often not required providing the other tests are normal.

Monoclonal gammopathy of unknown significance

The chance finding of a monoclonal paraprotein increases with age (present in 1 per cent of those aged over 50 years and 3 per cent of those over 70 years) and the vast majority have no evidence of a neuropathy. The most common paraprotein type is IgG, accounting for up to 61 per cent of cases. However, in those with MGUS the prevalence of a neuropathy is variable (1–36 per cent), and highest in those with an IgM paraprotein.

Clinical features of MGUS neuropathy

- Symmetric distal sensorimotor neuropathy; 20 per cent have a pure sensory neuropathy
- Paraesthesiae is a prominent early symptom
- Prominent ataxia (especially IgM-MGUS)
- Postural tremor in 49–90 per cent of cases (especially IgM-MGUS)
- Slowly progressive over many years with evolving motor weakness
- Males more frequently affected than females
- Peak incidence 50–70 years old
- Antibody to myelin-associated glycoprotein (MAG) – in 50 per cent of IgM-MGUS cases.

NCS show a demyelinating neuropathy in 40 per cent of cases.

MAG accounts for 1 per cent of peripheral nerve myelin. Although strongly associated with IgM paraproteinaemia, and often separated into an 'anti-MAG syndrome' as immunotherapy results in a reduction in anti-MAG antibodies, the clinical response to treatment is small which raises questions about the proposed pathogenesis. IVIg does not appear to help and the role of newer immunosuppressants, such as rituximab, remains unclear. There is no effective immunotherapy for IgM MGUS.

For IgG- and IgA-MGUS neuropathies, the response to immunotherapy (prednisolone with or without cyclophosphamide, IVIg or plasma exchange) is more encouraging, but supporting evidence from controlled trials is inadequate. Any potential benefit of immunotherapy should be weighed against adverse effects.

All MGUS neuropathies tend to be chronic and very slowly progressive. For this reason, the decision to start immunotherapy can be difficult.

Occasionally, patients with MGUS can have a clinical pattern similar to CIDP. Whether this is a distinct entity from CIDP is not known. The treatment should be as for CIDP, although the feeling is that these neuropathies (CIDP-MGUS) have a more protracted clinical course and are less responsive to therapies than standard CIDP.

VASCULITIC NEUROPATHIES

The vasculitides are a heterogeneous group of disorders that may affect different, sometimes multiple, organ systems. Peripheral nerve involvement may be seen as part of a systemic vasculitis or as an isolated finding (Box 16.6).

Clinical features

Vasculitic neuropathies typically present with multiple mononeuropathies. The progression of mononeuropathies may be rapid and therefore the presentation may be confused with that of a polyneuropathy unless a careful history is taken of the initial deficits. The most commonly affected nerves are the common peroneal, posterior tibial, ulnar, median and radial in descending order of frequency. Around 25 per cent of patients present with a symmetric sensorimotor polyneuropathy. Other features suggestive of a vasculitic aetiology include subacute onset, asymmetric distribution, dysaesthetic pain, lower limb involvement and the presence of constitutional or systemic symptoms.

Box 16.6 Classification of vasculitic neuropathies

Systemic

- Primary
  - Polyarteritis nodosa
  - Wegener granulomatosis
  - Churg–Strauss syndrome
  - Microscopic polyangiitis
- Secondary
  - Connective tissue disorders
    - o Rheumatoid arthriits
    - o Systemic lupus erythematosis
    - o Sjogren syndrome
  - Drugs
  - Viral infections – Hepatitis C, HIV, CMV
  - Malignancy

Non-systemic

- Isolated peripheral nerve vasculitis

Primary systemic vasculitides

Polyarteritis nodosa

This affects the medium and small muscular arteries, and patients are usually found to be ANCA (anti-neutrophil cytoplasmic antibody) negative. A characteristically painful and asymmetric neuropathy occurs in up to 75 per cent of patients, associated with hepatitis B antibodies in 30–50 per cent of cases.

Churg–Strauss syndrome

Churg–Strauss syndrome usually causes asthma, pulmonary infiltrates, fever and eosinophilia. Neuropathy is common, occurring in 65–80 per cent of patients. ANCA is positive in around 50 per cent of patients.

Microscopic polyangiitis

Patients with microsopic polyangiitis usually present with systemic, renal or cutaneous manifestations. ANCA is positive in 60 per cent of patients and a peripheral neuropathy is seen in over 50 per cent.

Wegener's granulomatosis

Wegener's granulomatosis typically affects the upper and lower airways, with peripheral nerve involvement in up to 40 per cent of patients, including cranial neuropathies.

Secondary systemic vasculitides

Rheumatoid disease

Multiple mononeuropathies associated with a necrotising vasculitis can occur as a late manifestation of severe seropositive rheumatoid disease (RD), although its incidence is declining with the advent of modern disease-modifying drugs. In addition, many patients with RD develop a mild, symmetrical, distal sensory or sensorimotor polyneuropathy that is not caused by vasculitis. Carpal tunnel syndrome and other entrapment neuropathies are also common.

Systemic lupus erythematosus

Involvement of the peripheral nervous system is less common than that of the central nervous system in systemic lupus erythematosus (SLE), with a neuropathy occurring in about 10 per cent of patients. This is usually a distal symmetric sensorimotor neuropathy, but more rarely can present as multiple mononeuropathies, an acute/subacute inflammatory demyelinating polyneuropathy (GBS or CIDP-like), or a trigeminal sensory neuropathy. As with rheumatoid disease, it may be vasculitic and needs nerve biopsy confirmation.

Sjögren's syndrome

Peripheral nervous system complications, which may precede the onset of other symptoms, are seen in 10–50 per cent of patients with primary Sjögren's syndrome, and are more variable than those encountered in other connective tissue diseases. The most common type is a distal axonal sensorimotor neuropathy, with autonomic features. Vasculitic changes may be seen on nerve biopsy, but the response to corticosteroid treatment is variable, and in general treatment is only considered if this usually slowly changing neuropathy progresses more rapidly than expected. A sensory neuronopathy is a much rarer complication, resulting from lymphocytic infiltration of dorsal root ganglia. Patients present with paraesthesiae affecting the limbs, trunk and face, with loss mainly of large fibre function and areflexia, progressing to a severe sensory ataxia. The differential diagnosis lies between a paraneoplastic and idiopathic sensory neuronopathy. As the clinical features are very similar, the diagnosis depends on the relevant antibody tests (anti-Hu or extractable nuclear antigens (ENA)) being positive or negative, a positive Schirmer test and biopsy evidence of inflammation in a salivary gland to confirm the diagnosis of Sjögren's syndrome. There is no convincing evidence supporting the role of immunosuppression. Case reports document benefit with IVIg, but it is well recognized that this neuropathy can show recovery without treatment. As with SLE, trigeminal neuropathy or CIDP may occur.

Hepatitis C and mixed cryoglobulinaemia

Raised concentrations of serum cryoglobulins may be secondary to chronic infection, autoimmune disease or haematological disease. Type 2 cryoglobulinaemia has a strong association with hepatitis C virus infection, and neuropathy is reported in 30–70 per cent of cases of cryoglobulinaemic vasculitis, either as a symmetric sensorimotor polyneuropathy or multiple mononeuropathies.

Investigation of suspected vasculitic neuropathy

In isolated peripheral nerve vasculitis, the ESR and CRP may be slightly raised, but other serological markers are usually normal (Box 16.7). In systemic vasculitis, serological tests may help identify the underlying syndrome. CSF analysis is rarely helpful, other than in excluding other causes, such as infections and malignant infiltration. Because of the need for long-term treatment with potentially toxic medication, **the diagnosis of vasculitis usually needs histological confirmation**. The patchy nature of the neuropathy means that it can easily be missed on a sural nerve biopsy. Recent studies have suggested a modest increase in diagnostic yield from a combined nerve and muscle biopsy, compared to nerve alone. A kidney biopsy is likely to yield the diagnosis in cases where there is renal involvement.

Treatment

Management should be coordinated with physicians treating other manifestations of the vasculitis (often the rheumatologist or nephrologist). Careful documentation of the response to treatment using reliable, objective, clinical and laboratory measurements is essential. In general, **corticosteroids remain the first-line treatment for systemic vascu-** litis, either alone or combined with other immunosuppressants, together with prophylactic treatment for osteoporosis. There are few controlled trials looking at dosing regimens and titration should be based on the patient's disease severity and response to treatment (Table 16.7).

In most patients, a second immunosuppressive drug is required. **Cyclophosphamide** seems to be the most effective drug in systemic vasculitis, although may not be required in isolated peripheral

---

Most patients need between three and 12 months of cyclophosphamide before they can be switched to an alternative maintenance immunosuppressant (methotrexate, azathioprine or mycophenolate), which is then continued for at least a year before the dose is tapered.

Despite small open label trials and case reports suggesting that IVIg may be effective in the acute stages of vasculitic neuropathy, its use is not yet approved for this indication. In vasculitis associated with hepatitis C, there is evidence for the use of interferon-alpha, ribavirin and rituximab, with plasma exchange in patients with systemic vasculitis secondary to cryoglobulinaemia. In hepatitis B-associated polyarteritis nodosa (PAN), a short course of corticosteroid is usually followed by six months of antiviral treatment.

Box 16.7 Investigations in suspected vasculitic neuropathies

- Blood tests
  - FBC, ESR, CRP
  - Renal and liver function
  - Glucose
  - ANA, dsDNA, ENA, ANCA, RF
  - C3, C4
  - Cryoglobulins
  - Hepatitis B, C and HIV
  - ACE
  - Lyme serology
- Urinalysis and chest x-ray
- Nerve conduction tests
  - Patchy, asymmetric distribution
  - Motor and sensory axonal loss
  - Clinically asymptomatic lesions

Tissue biopsy – nerve ± muscle biopsy, or a kidney biopsy if there is renal involvement.

Table 16.7 Immunosuppressive treatment for vasculitic neuropathy

Mild/moderate neuropathy	Oral prednisolone 1.5 mg/kg per day for 14 days (or until clear clinical response), switching to alternate day regimen thereafter for 4–6 weeks
	Dose to be slowly reduced, e.g. by 5–10 mg/month
Severe neuropathy	i.v. methyl prednisolone 1 g/day for 5 days with oral cyclophosphamide 2.0–2.5 mg/kg per day
	i.v. pulsed cyclophosphamide is of equal efficacy to oral treatment
	Also start on oral prednisolone 1.5 mg/kg per day

nerve vasculitis. It may cause haemorrhagic cystitis and transitional cell carcinoma of the bladder, and patients need to be advised of the importance of good hydration. Urinalysis should be performed every three to six months and, if haematuria is present, the drug should be discontinued and the patient referred for urological investigation. Intravenous pulsed cyclophosphamide is as effective as continuous oral treatment (dose typically 2 mg/kg per day) and is believed to be associated with fewer adverse effects, including bladder toxicity.

NEUROPATHIES ASSOCIATED WITH INFECTION

HIV neuropathy

Peripheral nerve disorders related to HIV infection develop due to a number of factors, including HIV infection itself, immune suppression and dysregulation, comorbid illnesses and infections, and side effects of medications.

A number of different peripheral nerve syndromes are recognized and given the high prevalence of a distal symmetric polyneuropathy, these may coexist in the same patient. This is discussed in more detail in Chapter 26.

Peripheral nerve syndromes in HIV
- Distal symmetric polyneuropathy
- Mononeuropathies
- Mononeuritis multiplex
- Inflammatory demyelinating polyneuropathy (acute or chronic)
- Autonomic neuropathy
- Radiculopathies

Lyme disease

Infection of the peripheral nervous system with *Borrelia burgdorferi* presents as a **cranial neuropathy** (mainly VIIth cranial neuropathy) or **radiculopathy** with CSF pleocytosis (and antibodies against *B. burgdorferi* can be detected in the CSF) – (**Banwarth syndrome**) or as an **asymmetric peripheral neuropathy** with acrodermatitis chronica atrophicans and normal CSF examination.

Serological testing is complicated by the fact that a small percentage of healthy individuals have positive results with enzyme-linked immunosorbent assay (ELISA), and any other infection or inflammatory condition. A confirmatory Western blot test is therefore recommended. A negative result of testing does not exclude the condition.

Early treatment with antibiotics **(amoxicillin, doxycyclin/tetracyclin, cephalopsporin (second and third generation)) for 10–21 days** is indicated and, in those with neurological manifestations, should be administered intravenously.

Diphtheria

In the Western world, neuropathy related to diphtheria is very rare because of the success of immunization programmes, and artificial ventilaton and use of antitoxin has reduced mortality rates.

Following a throat infection, paralysis of pharyngeal and laryngeal muscles develops, and some weeks later a generalized sensorimotor neuropathy appears with prominent paraesthesiae and sensory loss often leading to a sensory ataxia. Weakness may be severe and autonomic features are common. In patients who have already been immunized, a more prolonged neuropathy may be encountered with less prominent bulbar problems.

The nerve conduction velocities may be very slow (15–20 m/s) confirming a demyelinating process. Diphtheria antitoxin should be given as early as possible (within 48 hours of onset), and the treatment thereafter is supportive.

Leprosy

Peripheral nerve damage in all forms of leprosy is caused by direct invasion by the bacillus *Mycobacterium leprae* and the immune reaction that follows. Although there are clinical and pathological differences between the various forms, the **main common feature is sensory loss**. Early on, the sensory impairment does not conform to a peripheral nerve distribution as the damage is in the intracutaneous nerves. Pinprick and temperature loss predominate, with loss of sweating. Neuropathy related to leprosy is a readily treatable condition, and must be considered in the differential diagnosis of any neuropathy – but particularly **mononeuropathy** or **multiple mononeuropathy** – in anyone who has come from or travelled in an endemic area. If infection is suspected, the patient should be referred to a tropical disease unit where the diagnosis can be confirmed by skin or nerve biopsy. Treatment is with dapsone, rifampicin and clofazimine. A hypersensitivity reaction to treatment is a potentially serious complication.

Tuberculoid leprosy causes a localized neuropathy. There may be one or two patches of cutaneous sensory loss at the site of entry of the bacillus and if it multiplies and invades a nearby nerve trunk, then a mononeuropathy will develop. The median, ulnar, peroneal and facial nerves are most frequently affected.

In the **lepromatous** (or low resistance) form, there is a more widespread loss of sensation, beginning distally in the limbs in an asymmetric manner eventually coalescing to produce a more symmetric pattern. The bacilli proliferate in cool areas, and so the ears are often the first area to be affected by numbness. Haematogenous spread of bacilli in this low-resistance type contributes to the eventual symmetric distribution of the neuropathy, which in the later stages has a prominent motor component. The **peripheral nerves become thickened**, but reflexes are retained, often until the neuropathy is advanced. **Borderline leprosy** shows a variable spectrum of clinical features between the tuberculoid and lepromatous types.

Because of the loss of pain sensation, foot ulcers are common, and other destructive changes occur, including Charcot (neuropathic) joints.

PARANEOPLASTIC NEUROPATHIES

These arise as a result of the remote effect of cancer, and represent an autoimmune phenomenon.

Detailed screening for underlying malignancy should only be undertaken if the neuropathy has features consistent with one of the syndromes outlined below (Box 16.8). The most frequent are **sensorimotor** and **pure sensory neuropathies**. The latter is the best defined paraneoplastic neuropathy, resulting in a severe sensory ataxia with relatively normal muscle strength. It is also called a **sensory neuronopathy**.

Box 16.8 Paraneoplastic neuropathies

- Demyelinating sensorimotor
  - Acute (GBS-like) neuropathy associated with Hodgkin's disease
  - Chronic form (CIDP-like), associated with non-Hodgkin's lymphoma and osteosclerotic myeloma
- Axonal sensorimotor – less well defined, associated with CV2 antibodies (typically linked to a cerebellar ataxic syndrome)
- Microvasculitic
  - A hypersensitivity reaction related to some haematological malignancies
  - Immune-complex mediated with cryoglobulin production – related to chronic lymphocytic leukaemia, lymphoma, Waldenström's macroglobulinaemia
  - Also related to cancers of the prostate, stomach, uterus, lung and kidney
- Sensory
  - May precede finding of malignancy (small cell lung tumour) by up to two years Subacute in onset with pain a marked sensory ataxia
  - Associated with antineuronal antibodies (anti-Hu, anti-amphiphysin)
  - Females more frequently affected than males

The most common underlying tumour is a small cell lung carcinoma, and anti-Hu (ANNA-1) antibodies may be present, but are more likely to be positive in the more complex syndrome of **paraneoplastic encephalomyelitis/sensory neuronopathy ('anti–Hu syndrome')**. Some of these patients also develop an autonomic neuropathy.

Treatment with IVIg has no benefit. Removal of the primary tumour does not ameliorate the neuropathy.

Direct infiltration of nerve, root or plexus is well recognized, but uncommon and chemotherapy agents used to treat cancer can also produce a neuropathy.

CRITICAL ILLNESS POLYNEUROPATHY

An **acute primarily axonal sensorimotor polyneuropathy, critical illness polyneuropathy (CIP)** occurs in critically ill patients, most of whom have a combination of adult respiratory distress syndrome, organ failure and infection. CIP leads to severe limb weakness and difficulty in weaning from artificial ventilation. The pathogenesis of CIP is unknown.

In some patients with critical illness, the problem of weakness is muscular– a **critical illness myopathy (CIM)**.

The clinical signs of CIP and CIM are similar – flaccid weakness of the limbs, and because the two conditions often coexist, it is difficult to distinguish clinically between them. Deep tendon reflexes are usually absent in CIP, but may be normal or reduced in pure CIM. In CIP, distal loss of all sensory modalities may also occur. Weakness affects the legs more often than the arms; facial weakness and ophthalmoplegia may occur, although these are uncommon features. Involvement of the phrenic nerves and diaphragm is the main cause of ventilator weaning problems.

In any patient remaining ventilator dependent, EMG and NCS are vital in establishing the diagnosis, and important in excluding myasthenia gravis and Guillain–Barré syndrome. Clinical and neurophysiological assessment can be difficult in patients who are sedated and ventilated.

Other than the main risk factors of sepsis, systemic inflammatory response syndrome and multiple organ failure, independent risk factors for CIP include female sex, severity of illness, duration of organ dysfunction, renal failure and hyperglycaemia. The last factor has led to the use of intensive insulin treatment for CIP. This has been shown to improve neurophysiological abnormalities, but its effect on strength and outcome is less clear. There is no role for corticosteroid or IVIg treatment.

There are important consequences of CIP/CIM, including impaired rehabilitation, prolonged mechanical ventilation and increasing duration of stay on the intensive care unit, together with an overall increase in mortality. Improvement occurs within weeks in mild cases and within months in severe cases. In the most severe cases, recovery may be incomplete or even not occur at all.

TOXIC NEUROPATHIES

Peripheral nerve damage caused by drugs (see Box 16.9) should always be considered when assessing a patient with a neuropathy. In general, toxic neuropathies result in painful paraesthesiae with distal sensory loss, but variable degree of distal lower limb weakness.

The neuropathy caused by **alcohol** is in part a result of its toxic effect, but is also caused by an associated thiamine deficiency. There is distal sensory loss, particularly involving small fibre function in the early stages, with painful, burning or aching feet. There is often marked allodynia, with superficial and deep tenderness in the feet and calves. Distal leg weakness is uncommon in the early stages, but may develop in chronic alcoholic neuropathy. Very occasionally, the neuropathy can be acute in onset. Nerve conduction studies show an axonal process and the CSF is usually normal. Treatment is cessation of all alcohol consumption,

Box 16.9 Drugs which cause peripheral neuropathy

- Adriamycin
- Amiodarone
- Bortezomib
- Chloroquine (with myopathy)
- Dapsone
- Disulfiram
- Ethambutol
- Gold
- Isoniazid
- Metronidazole
- Misonidazole
- Nitrofurantoin
- Nitrous oxide (with a myelopathy)
- Nucleoside analogue reverse transcriptase inhibitors: zalcitabine, didanosine and stavudine
- Phenytoin
- Platinum: cisplatin and carboplatin
- Podophyllin
- Pyridoxine
- Suramin
- Taxanes: paclitaxel and docetaxel
- Thalidomide
- Vincristine

generous vitamin supplementation (often parenterally initially) including thiamine, and ensuring adequate nutrition.

Neuropathy as a result of **metal toxicity (thallium, mercury, arsenic and lead)** is very uncommon and unless there is a specific risk that exposure has occurred a 'routine metal screen' should not be requested.

PORPHYRIC NEUROPATHY

The hepatic porphyrias are genetically transmitted as autosomal dominant disorders with variable expression that produce a particularly **severe acute axonal motor polyradiculopathy or neuronopathy** that is clinically similar to GBS, including CSF changes. Features that suggest a porphyric neuropathy include asymmetry of the weakness and predominance of proximal rather than distal weakness. In addition, when there is sensory involvement, this may also have a rather unusual proximal distribution ('bathing trunk' and 'breast plate'). Like GBS, porphyric neuropathy can involve respiratory, facial, ocular and bulbar muscles, and autonomic involvement. Porphyric neuropathy is commonly associated with abdominal pain, psychiatric disturbance and sometimes epileptic seizures.

The underlying pathophysiology has not been established, but it may be related to direct neurotoxicity of elevated levels of δ-aminolevulinic acid. The severity of the neuropathy and the availability of potential treatments, including avoidance of provocative factors, make identification important, and so a porphyria screen should always be undertaken in cases of GBS.

Management is initially focused on withdrawing or avoiding any drugs that might exacerbate the porphyria. Adequate hydration and continuous i.v. glucose infusion are important. If the weakness progresses, it is worth considering i.v. haematin (2–5 mg/kg per day for 10–14 days depending on the clinical response), which suppresses the haem biosynthetic pathway. The rate of recovery is variable.

INHERITED NEUROPATHIES

Inherited neuropathies comprise a clinically and genetically heterogeneous group of conditions. The field is a complex one and is constantly evolving as new genes are discovered. As a result, the classification systems used can prove daunting for both trainees and experienced neurologists (Box 16.9, and Tables 16.8 and 16.9).

Charcot–Marie–Tooth disease

Charcot–Marie–Tooth disease (CMT) is the most common inherited neuromuscular disorder with a prevalence of one in 2500. The classification of CMT is partly genetic, partly clinical and partly based on electrophysiological findings. The CMT terminology is now favoured in the classification system over the previously used hereditary motor and sensory neuropathy (HMSN). The main division, based on motor (usually median) conduction velocities (MCV), is between demyelinating (MVC <38 m/s) and axonal (MCV >38 m/s) neuropathies; however, some variants have intermediate MCVs (25–38 m/s). Most cases can be classified as either CMT1 (autosomal dominant and demyelinating) or CMT2 (mostly dominant and axonal), with a smaller number of cases of CMT4 (recessive and demyelinating). Each of these can be further subdivided depending on the underlying genetic defect (Table 16.8). To complicate matters, considerable clinical variation can be seen within families with the same genetic defect.

Diagnostic approach

It is important to adopt a logical approach that involves a thorough clinical assessment to define the phenotype, including a detailed family history. Neurophysiology is used to divide cases into demyelinating or axonal forms, which then guides the approach to genetic testing. The algorithms shown in Figures 16.2 and 16.3 suggest the diagnostic approach, but referral to a specialist unit should be considered if one of the more common genetic diagnoses cannot be made.

CMT1

CMT1 is characterized by autosomal dominant inheritance and MCVs in the demyelinating range.

Table 16.8 Charcot–Marie–Tooth neuropathies

Type	Locus	Gene	Inheritance
CMT 1 (demyelinating)			
CMT1A	17p11	PMP22 dupication	Dominant
CMT1B	1q22	MPZ point mutation	Dominant
CMT1D	10q21	EGR2 point mutation	Dominant
CMT1F	8p21	NEFL point mutation	Dominant
CMT3 (Dejerine–Sottas disease)	17p11	PMP22 point mutation	Dominant or recessive
		MPZ point mutation	
CMT 2 (axonal)			
CMT2A	1p36	MFN 2 mutation	Dominant
CMT2E	8p21	NEFL point mutation	Dominant
CMT2I/2J	1q22	MPZ point mutation	Dominant
CMT2K	8q21	GDAP1 point mutation	Recessive
CMT4			
CMT4A	8q21	GDAP1	Recessive
X-linked dominant CMT			
CMTX	Xq13	GJB1 (Connexin 32)	Point mutation

EGR, early growth response, GDAP, ganglioside-induced differentiation-associated protein; GJB, gap junction; MFN, mitofusin; MPZ, myelin protein zero; PMP, peripheral myelin protein.

Table 16.9 Hereditary sensory and autonomic neuropathies

Type	Inheritance	Gene	Clinical features
HSAN I	Autosomal dominant	SPTLC1	Painful sensory loss
			Ulceration, arthropathy and amputation
			Motor involvement
			Autonomic features not prominent
HSAN II	Autosomal recessive	NK	Early onset
			Painless sensory symptoms
			Later autonomic features
HSAN III (Riley–Day syndrome)	Autosomal recessive (Ashkenasi Jews)	IKAP gene	Prominent autonomic symptoms
			Sensory and motor involvement
HSAN IV	Autosomal recessive	TRKA gene	Congenital insensitivity to pain
			Anhidrosis
			Recurrent fevers
			Self-mutilating behaviour
			Mental retardation
HSAN V	Autosomal recessive	TRKA gene	Clinically similar to HSAN IV

IKAP, IKB kinase complex-associated protein; NK, not known; SPTLC, serine palmitoyltransferase, long chain base subunit; TRKA, neurotrophic tyrosine kinase receptor type 1.

Symptoms may appear in infancy, with subsequent delayed motor milestones and participation in sports in school. Because of this early onset, skeletal abnormalities, such as pes cavus and clawed toes, are prominent and may be the first obvious clinical feature. There is distal wasting

Demyelinating neuropathy with clinical features of CMT (AD or sporadic)

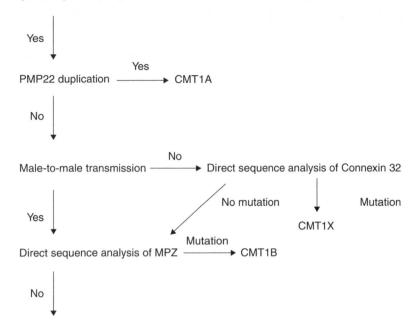

Figure 16.2 Diagnostic algorithm for CMT1. Consider referral to a specialist clinic for direct sequence analysis of PMP22, ERG2 and NFFl (see **Table 16.8** for details).

Axonal neuropathy with clinical features of CMT (AD or sporadic)

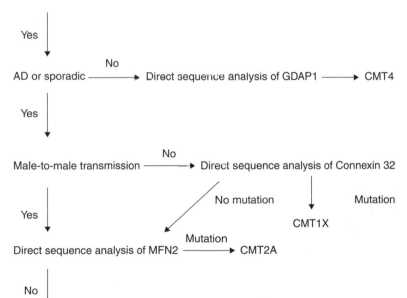

Figure 16.3 Diagnostic algorithm for CMT2. Consider referral to a specialist clinic for direct sequence analysis of MPZ and NEFL (see **Table 16.8** for details).

and weakness in the legs and also in a majority of cases involving the hands, with more severe cases having clawing of the fingers. Tendon reflexes are depressed or absent and distal sensory loss affects all modalities. About one-third of patients will have a positional upper limb tremor. Palpable thicken-ing of peripheral nerves occurs in 50 per cent of patients. Sensory symptoms are not a major feature, although patients may complain of musculoskeletal pain. The presence of prominent positive sensory symptoms should prompt consideration of alterna-tive causes of neuropathy.

> **Most common CMT1 subtypes**
> - CMT1A. Accounts for 70 per cent of CMT1 cases; caused by a duplication of the gene for peripheral myelin protein 22 (PMP 22) on chromosome 17. Molecular testing is readily available.
> - CMT1B is caused by mutations in the human myelin protein zero (MPZ) gene.

A more severe demyelinating form, Dejerine–Sottas disease (previously known as CMT3, but now recognized as a severe variant of CMT1) is characterized by early childhood onset, and can be due to point mutations in PMP22 and MPZ.

CMT2

> CMT2 is clinically similar to CMT1 but less common. Inheritance is mostly autosomal dominant and nerve conduction velocities (NCVs) are in the axonal range.

Fewer genes have been identified than for CMT1. A mutation in the gene for mitofusin 2 (MFN2) accounts for 20 per cent of cases and is characterized by the presence of brisk tendon reflexes in some patients.

X-linked CMT

> X-linked CMT (CMTX) is the second most common form of CMT and accounts for around 10 per cent of cases. It is caused by a mutation in the gap junction *B1* gene for the protein connexin 32, located on the X chromosome.

It is clinically similar to CMT1, but there is no male-to-male transmission. The neuropathy is more severe and demyelinating, in males than in females, in whom it is usually axonal.

Autosomal recessive CMT

Autosomal recessive CMT is rare and may be axonal (CMT2) or demyelinating (CMT4). In both, the most common cause is mutation in the gene for ganglioside-induced differentiation-associated protein (GDAP1).

Hereditary neuropathy with liability to pressure palsies

> Hereditary neuropathy with liability to pressure palsies (HNPP) is an autosomal dominant condition caused by deletion of the same *PMP22* gene involved in CMT1A.

Patients typically experience recurrent pressure palsies after minor compression or trauma. The nerves most frequently involved are the ulnar nerve at the elbow, the common peroneal nerve at the head of the fibula, and carpal tunnel syndrome. There may also be an associated mild sensorimotor polyneuropathy with pes cavus and recurrent painless brachial plexopathy. Neurophysiology shows a patchy demyelinating neuropathy.

Hereditary sensory and autonomic neuropathies

The hereditary sensory and autonomic neuropathies (HSAN) are much less common than CMT. Five different types are recognized as outlined in Table 16.9.

Familial amyloid neuropathies

> Dominantly inherited amyloid neuropathies are rare and mostly caused by mutations of the transthyretin (*TTR*) gene on chromosome 18, with other cases due to mutations in the apolipoprotein A1 on chromosome 11, and gelsolin on chromosome 9.

The clinical picture can be extremely variable, with onset between the age of 30 and 60 years. A predominantly small fibre neuropathy or painful sensorimotor neuropathy with autonomic involvement develops. There may be palpable nerve thickening. There is an increased incidence of carpal tunnel syndrome. There is often vitreous opacification, nephropathy and cardiomyopathy, and the latter is the most common cause of death. As most *TTR* is produced in the liver, liver transplantation has been clearly shown to halt the progression and even improve the neuropathy. This, however, is not curative as cardiac function continues to deteriorate.

The cornerstone for diagnosis of amyloid neuropathy, familial or acquired, is finding amyloid deposition in tissue biopsy (rectum, kidney, skin or sural nerve). Antibody kits can identify *TTR*. Because of patchy deposition, a negative biopsy does not exclude the diagnosis. The advent of DNA testing has not made establishing the diagnosis that much easier, as most routine laboratories will only offer screening of the most common mutations.

Distal hereditary motor neuropathies

The distal hereditary motor neuropathies (HMNs) usually present with progressive weakness and wasting of the extensor muscles of the toes and feet without sensory symptoms, followed later on by upper limb involvement. The distal HMNs are clinically and genetically heterogeneous and are subdivided according to the mode of inheritance, age at onset and clinical features. Additional features, such as vocal cord and diaphragmatic involvement, and pyramidal signs may also be present. Clinically, it can be difficult to distinguish distal HMN from CMT, and neurophysiological testing is essential. Inheritance can be either autosomal dominant or recessive and a number of different genetic mutations have been identified.

REFERENCES AND FURTHER READING

Albers JW, Fink JK (2004) Porphyric neuropathy. *Muscle and Nerve*, 30:410–422.

Burns TM, Schaublin GA, Dyck PJ (2007) Vasculitic neuropathies. *Neurology Clinics*, 25: 89–113.

Dyck Peter J, Thomas PK (2005) *Peripheral Neuropathy*, 4th edn. London: Elsevier Saunders.

European Federation of Neurological Societies; Peripheral Nerve Society, Hadden RD, Nobile-Orazio E, Sommer C *et al.* (2006) European Federation of Neurological Societies/Peripheral Nerve Society Guideline on Management of Paraproteinaemic Demyelinating Neuropathies: report of a joint task force of the European Federation of Neurological Societies and the Peripheral Nerve Society. *European Journal of Neurology*, 13:809–818.

Freeman R (2009) Not all neuropathy in diabetes is of diabetic etiology: differential diagnosis of diabetic neuropathy. *Current Diabetes Reports*, 9:423–431.

Howard RS, Tan SV, Z'Graggen WJ (2008) Weakness on the intensive care unit. *Practical Neurology*, 8:280–295.

Hughes R (2008) The bare essentials: peripheral nerve diseases. *Practical Neurology*, 8:396–405.

Lawson V, Gharibshahi S (2010) Alphabet soup: making sense of genetic testing in CMT. *Seminars in Neurology*, 30:373–386.

Pareyson D, Marchesi M (2009) Diagnosis, natural history and management of Charcot–Marie–Tooth disease. *Lancet Neurology*, 8:654–667.

Rudnicki SA, Dalmau J (2005) Paraneoplastic syndromes of the peripheral nerves. *Current Opinion in Neurology*, 18:589–603.

Schaublin GA, Michet CJ, Dyck PJB, Burns TM (2005) An update on the classification and treatment of vasculitic neuropathy. *Lancet Neurology*, 4:853–865.

Tesfaye S, Boulton AJ, Dyck *et al.* (2010) Diabetic neuropathies: update on definitions, diagnostic criteria, estimation of severity, and treatments. *Diabetes Care* 33:2285–2293.

Vallat JM, Sommer C, Magy L (2010) Chronic inflammatory demyelinating polyradiculoneuropathy: diagnostic and therapeutic challenges for a treatable condition. *Lancet Neurology*, 9:402–412.

Winer JB (2008) Guillain–Barré syndrome. *British Medical Journal*, 337:a671.

CHAPTER 17

MOTOR NEURONE DISEASE AND SPINAL MUSCULAR ATROPHY

Katherine Sidle

INTRODUCTION

The motor neurone diseases encompass a number of conditions that affect the motor neurones. These include **amyotrophic lateral sclerosis (ALS), progressive bulbar palsy (PBP), primary muscular atrophy (PMA) and primary lateral sclerosis (PLS)**, in addition to **spinal muscular atrophy (SMA)** and **Kennedy's disease**.

ALS, also (rather confusingly) often referred to as motor neurone disease (MND) is the most common variant and is a progressive neurodegenerative disease often causing death within a few years of onset. It is one of the most common adult onset neurodegenerative conditions. Once thought to be a disease affecting exclusively the motor neurons, it is now increasingly recognized that its pathological effects extend beyond motor neurons, to involve other systems including sensory, cerebellar and extrapyramidal pathways, together with centres involved in cognitive function. There is also evidence of involvement of non-neuronal cell populations. This has given rise to the concept of MND being a multisystem disease with a 'relative' rather than 'absolute' predilection for motor neurons.

The reader should be aware when reviewing the wider literature that terminology in this field may be a little confusing. The terms 'motor neurone disease' and 'amyotrophic lateral sclerosis', are often used interchangeably, and in the United States, the condition is also called 'Lou Gehrig disease', the latter being named after the famous 1930s American baseball player who later developed MND. However, the term motor neurone disease may also be used in the literature as an umbrella term to refer to a group of diseases affecting the motor neurons, of which ALS is the most common subtype. In this chapter, we will use the terms motor neurone disease and ALS synonymously.

EPIDEMIOLOGY

MND/ALS is a heterogeneous disorder, both clinically and genetically. **The incidence is 1.5–2 per 100 000 per year** with a slight male predominance with a male:female ratio of 1.7:1, higher in younger onset cases. The mean duration of illness is three years, although approximately 10 per cent of patients have a slower course of disease with survival extending beyond ten years. Because of the relatively short duration of illness, the **prevalence is low at 3–8 per 100 000**. This means that at any one time, there are approximately 5000 people suffering from MND/ALS in the UK. This rate is uniform throughout the world with the exception of a few clusters notably on the island of Guam in the Western Pacific and also in the Kii peninsula in Japan, for reasons that have not been satisfactorily explained. The mean age of onset is 60 years, with a wide range of 20–90 years. Rare juvenile forms are also recognized. The life-time risk of developing MND/ALS is one in 2000. Approximately 5–10 per cent of ALS cases are familial, inherited mostly as an autosomal dominant mode of inheritance and this is discussed in more detail later in this chapter. A summary of epidemiological features of ALS is seen in Table 17.1.

PBP has a worse prognosis with a median survival of 2–2.5 years and this is likely to reflect the increased risk of aspiration. Conversely, patients with PLS may commonly survive beyond 20 years and can have a normal life span.

Despite many studies attempting to ascertain environmental risk factors in the development of MND, none to date has shown convincing, reproducible results and this may, in part, reflect the inherent difficulties in undertaking such studies in a rare, heterogeneous group. However, there appears to be a very weak association with athletic activity, although it remains unclear whether this may be due to musculoskeletal injury precipitating disease or whether, for example, there may be a genetic profile that confers athletic advantage in youth but renders the individual more susceptible to MND in later life.

CLINICAL PHENOTYPES

ALS/MND

> The World Federation of Neurology diagnostic criteria for ALS/MND require the presence of both upper and lower motor neurone degeneration, with evidence of progression and in the absence of other possible disease processes.

Involvement of the upper motor neurones, which arise in the precentral gyrus of the cerebral cortex and project on to the lower motor neurones in the spinal cord, results in upper motor neurone (UMN) clinical features of spasticity, brisk tendon reflexes and extensor plantars. If there is bulbar involvement, UMN signs may also include a spastic dysarthria, dysphagia, hypersalivation, laryngospasm and emotional lability. The latter is also called 'pseudobulbar affect' where patients find themselves laughing or crying uncontrollably. Degeneration of the lower motor neurones, which arise in the anterior horn of the spinal cord or brainstem motor nuclei, results in lower motor neurone (LMN) features including muscle cramps, fasciculations, wasting and weakness.

Cognitive involvement has long been recognized in MND, although previously thought to occur only rarely. However, there is increasing evidence that cognitive involvement is far more common than had previously been appreciated and systematic studies have demonstrated cognitive impairment may be present in more than half of cases of MND, with 10 per cent of cases fulfilling the diagnostic criteria for frontotemporal dementia (FTD). This has lead to the concept that MND and FTD may represent two ends of a continuum with frequent MND/FTD overlap.

Despite the relentless progression of this disease, some groups of motor neurones appear to be relatively spared, although the reason for this remains unknown. Those spared include the motor nerves arising from the oculomotor nuclei responsible

Table 17.1. Summary of epidemiology in motor neurone disease

Epidemiology of ALS	
Incidence	1.5–2 per 100 000 per year
Prevalence	3–8 per 100 000 = 5000 (UK)
Familial cases	5–10% of cases
Mean duration of illness	3 years
Mean age of onset	60 years (range, 20–90 years)
Life-time risk of developing MND/ALS	1 in 2000
Male:female	1.7:1

ALS, amyotrophic lateral sclerosis; MND, motor neurone disease.

Typically, onset is with muscle cramps, which may become less severe as the disease progresses, and fasciculations, with focal, asymmetrical and distal weakness and wasting. It is very unusual for patients to present with isolated cramps and fasciculations without evidence of accompanying weakness. Disease progression is typically segmental, i.e. starting in, for example, the right arm, then right leg, followed by left arm then left leg. Approximately 60–85 per cent of patients present with limb onset weakness with the remainder presenting with bulbar involvement, although 90 per cent of patients will eventually develop bulbar symptoms. These may be particularly problematic for patients, impairing their ability to communicate and also swallowing, causing both poor nutritional intake and increased risk of aspiration, as well as troublesome drooling and sialorrhoea. Management of these symptoms is discussed below. Rarely, patients may present with isolated respiratory failure although, as the disease progresses, respiratory muscle weakness is common and, indeed, respiratory failure is the most common cause of death.

for eye movements, and those arising from Olaf's nucleus in the sacral spinal cord and responsible for bladder and bowel control. Although sensory nerves are not typically involved, up to 25 per cent of patients describe mild sensory symptoms.

Flail arm variant

Approximately 10 per cent of patients with MND present with a symmetrical flaccid weakness of the arms with prominent proximal involvement and with sparing elsewhere in the body, giving rise to the name 'flail arm' or 'man in a barrel' syndrome. It is more common in men with a 9:1 male to female predominance. UMN signs often develop later in the disease course, giving rise to the view that it is simply a variant of more classical MND/ALS, although the prognosis tends to be more favourable with a median survival of 57 months.

Progressive muscular atrophy

In the initial stages, progressive muscular atrophy (PMA) presents with only lower motor neurone

features, but as the disease progresses UMN signs frequently develop. It is likely that in at least some patients, the UMN features are simply masked by the severity of the lower motor neurone involvement. This variant appears to have a favourable prognosis and represents approximately 10 per cent of all MND cases.

Progressive bulbar palsy

Approximately 25 per cent of MND patients present with a bulbar onset, with symptoms limited to the tongue, and muscles innervated by the lower cranial nerves ('bulb' is an old name for the brain stem). Most of these later develop more widespread involvement, although they may remain 'bulbar predominant' and the term progressive bulbar palsy (PBP) therefore remains a clinically useful descriptive term, with these cases representing a further variant of ALS/MND. However, there does appear to be a small proportion of patients in whom the symptoms remain limited to the bulbar region. Those affected tend to be female and are older, with a worse prognosis, with a median survival of two years. This is likely to be due, in part, to the increased risk of aspiration and poorer nutritional intake.

Primary lateral sclerosis

In primary lateral sclerosis (PLS), 1–5 per cent of patients present with pure UMN signs. Typically, these start in the lower limbs and progress to involve the arms and the bulbar muscles. According to the currently accepted diagnostic criteria, signs are required to remain exclusively UMN for a minimum period of three years before the diagnosis can be made. Unlike the other regional variants, PLS appears to have a distinct prognostic phenotype with slow progression and near normal life span.

DIAGNOSIS OF MOTOR NEURONE DISEASE

History

Typically, there is a history of progressive symptoms, **most commonly, distal, asymmetrical muscle wasting and weakness** with a segmental progression, the pattern of involvement varying as described above. Enquiry should be made about muscle

The diagnosis of MND/ALS remains essentially a clinical one and there is no single specific diagnostic test. Diagnosis may be particularly difficult in the early stages when the characteristic combination of UMN and LMN features may be absent and up to 30 per cent of patients who may be initially thought to have MND will be found to have other conditions. Even within a specialist neurology clinic, this figure may be as high as 10 per cent. Often, repeated follow up is required in order to allow the disease to declare itself. As a result, there may be considerable delay from onset of symptoms to diagnosis, with an average delay of 14 months.

cramps and fasciculations (although patients are frequently unaware of the latter), and the absence of diplopia, prominent sensory signs and bladder/bowel involvement, the presence of which will suggest alternative diagnoses.

Twenty per cent of patients present with bulbar symptoms, the majority of patients developing bulbar involvement later in their clinical course. Specific enquiry should therefore be made regarding difficulties with swallowing and speech. A history of orthopnoea and morning headaches suggests incipient respiratory failure secondary to respiratory muscle weakness and hypoventilation. A detailed family history should be obtained, bearing in mind that 5–10 per cent of cases are familial, and a suggestion of this in the history may necessitate consideration for genetic counselling.

Cognitive difficulties have not previously been considered to be a common component of MND, and are therefore frequently not specifically sought in the history, perpetuating this view and leading to a probable underestimate of cognitive involvement. Enquiry should therefore be made, although not necessarily at the first meeting.

Examination

Careful inspection is needed to look for fasciculations and wasting, which may lie outside the region of symptomatic involvement, indicating a more widespread disease process. More than 70 per cent of patients present with distal, asymmetric wasting and weakness of the upper limbs. Examination should include a detailed assessment of the cranial nerves, with particular attention to the tongue and bulbar muscles. Lying and sitting vital capacity (FVC) should be measured, looking for evidence of possible respiratory muscle involvement.

The presence of a combination of mixed upper and lower motor neurone features, in particular, the presence of LMN features caudal to UMN ones, in the absence of sensory abnormalities, is highly suggestive of MND. As presentation may be so variable, attempts have been made to produce a set of useful diagnostic criteria. The '**El Escorial**' criteria (Box 17.1) were developed primarily as a research tool in order to try and standardize patients entering into research trials. These criteria stratify patients into 'definite', 'probable' and 'possible' MND/ALS based on clinical demonstration of both LMN and UMN in four possible anatomical regions (brainstem, cervical, thoracic, lumbar sacral) in addition to supportive electromyogram (EMG) findings. While these criteria are useful to bear in mind when examining a patient, and may be helpful in developing a sense of diagnostic certainty, it should be noted that these criteria do not cater for the other motor neurone diseases, such as PMA, PLS or bulbar onset. In addition, they have a low sensitivity in the early stages of disease; a stage when diagnosis is often most important so that patients receive optimal management.

Box 17.1 Revised El Escorial criteria for the diagnosis of ALS (Data from Brooks *et al.*, 2000)

- Definite ALS
  - Progressive with both UMN and LMN features in three out of four regions (brainstem, cervical, thoracic, lumbosacral)
- Probable ALS
  - Progressive with both UMN and LMN features in two regions
- Clinically probable, laboratory-supported ALS
  - UMN signs in at least one region plus LMN signs or LMN EMG features in two or more regions
- Clinically possible ALS
  - UMN and LMN signs in only one region, or
  - UMN signs in two or more regions, or
  - UMN and LMN signs in two regions with LMN signs found rostral to UMN signs

ALS, amyotrophic lateral sclerosis; LMN, lower motor neurone; UMN, upper motor neurone.

Investigations

While MND/ALS is essentially a clinical diagnosis, investigations are important to both support the clinical picture and to exclude conditions that may mimic the motor neurone diseases (Table 17.2). Almost invariably patients will undergo brain and cord imaging to exclude skull base lesions and cervical myeloradiculopathies which may give rise to mixed UMN and LMN features and therefore may mimic MND. Imaging is mandatory in patients presenting with only UMN features. The choice of further investigations will depend on the clinical features and useful investigations are summarized in Table 17.2.

Neurophysiological assessment

While there is no single diagnostic test available, all patients suspected of having MND will undergo

Table 17.2 Differential diagnosis of motor neurone disease

	Differential Diagnosis	Clinical features	Investigations
Central lesions	Multiple sclerosis	History of relapse and remitting symptoms	MRI brain and cord, CSF, evoked potentials
	Skull base lesions	Bulbar symptoms (often asymmetrical)	MRI brain
Spinal cord lesions	Cervical spondylotic radiculomyelopathy	Lower limb spasticity and LMN features in upper limbs ± pain and stable symptoms	MRI cord and EMG
	Syringomyelia	Dissociated sensory loss	MRI cord
	Conus lesions	Sensory and bladder involvement	MRI cord
	Vitamin B12 deficiency	Dorsal column involvement	Low vitamin B12
	HIV/HTLV1/VDRL/Lyme infection	History of risk factors ± pain, sensory symptoms	Serological testing
	HSP	Spastic paraparesis with normal MRI imaging	HSP genetic testing
	Post-irradiation lumbosacral radiculopathy	Relevant history	MRI cord and EMG
Neuropathy/ neuronopathy	Multifocal motor neuropathy with conduction block/CIDP	Pure LMN, focal onset, IVIg responsive	Conduction block on NCS, anti GM1 antibody
	Spinal muscular atrophy	Pure LMN	*SMN1* gene deletion
	Kennedy's disease	Males, slow, bulbar and limb, gynaecomastia, perioral fasciculations	Androgen receptor gene, CAG expansion
	Heavy metal poisoning	History of exposure	Urine and blood screen
	Hexosaminidase A deficiency	Young onset	White cell enzymes
Neuromuscular junction	Myasthenia gravis	Fatiguable weakness	EMG, Ach receptor abs
	Lambert–Eaton syndrome		
Myopathy	Inclusion body myositis	Volar, quadriceps weakness	EMG, muscle biopsy
Other	Benign fasciculations	No weakness or progression	No denervation on EMG
	Cramp fasciculations		EMG, VGKC abs

CSF, cerebrospinal fluid; EMG, electromyogram; HSP, hereditary spastic paraparesis; LMN, lower motor neurone; MRI, magnetic resonance imaging.

EMG/nerve conduction study (NCS) to aid diagnosis (see Chapter 5). These are particularly important tests in patients presenting with only UMN features in order to assess for the presence of possible subclinical LMN involvement. In addition, neurophysiological assessment is essential in patients presenting with pure LMN features in order to exclude mimics of MND, such as multi focal motor neuropathy with conduction block, which may be amenable to effective treatment.

Typically, **nerve conduction** will be normal in the early clinical course of the disease. However, as the disease progresses, a mild reduction in the compound muscle action potential (CMAP) may be seen due to loss of motor axons. The reduction in CMAPs is less than perhaps expected, due to collateral sprouting of neighbouring surviving motor axons which reinnervate the nearby denervated muscle fibres, and increase the size of the surviving motor units. There may be a mild slowing of motor conduction velocities (MCVs), although these should remain a minimum of 70 per cent of the lower limit of normal. Distal motor latencies (DMLs) and F-waves may be mildly prolonged (no more than 30 per cent of the upper limit of normal) and mild sensory abnormalities should not necessarily exclude a diagnosis of MND although if severe, should raise the possibility of conditions such as B12 deficiency or Kennedy's disease. In patients with a predominantly LMN presentation, a careful search for conduction block or temporal dispersion should be sought away from the common sites of nerve compression, to exclude multifocal motor neuropathy (see Chapter 16).

EMG demonstrates fasciculations with evidence of acute denervation, indicated by fibrillation potentials and positive sharp waves. Demonstration of these findings in clinically unaffected muscles may allow a more definite diagnosis of MND using the El-Escorial criteria (Box 17.1). In addition, evidence of chronic reinnervation should be sought in the form of very large amplitude motor unit potentials with markedly decreased recruitment. A minimum of two of the four El-Escorial body regions should be examined (more if those tested are uninformative) with at least two muscles, innervated by different root and peripheral nerves in the cervical and lumbosacral regions. Only one muscle need be tested in the bulbar region. Abnormalities found in this region are highly specific for MND and are particularly useful if there is concomitant cervical spondylotic myelopathy. EMG of the thoracic paraspinal muscles should be routinely performed. Lumbar paraspinals are not helpful and may be abnormal in lumbosacral polyradiculopathy.

Central motor conduction times (CMCTs) may be useful for detecting clinically silent UMN involvement which may be masked clinically, by profound LMN weakness.

DIFFERENTIAL DIAGNOSES AND MND MIMICS

Establishing a diagnosis of MND early in the course of the disease can be difficult, so regular clinical review and a thorough approach to investigation is required to reduce the risk of misdiagnosis. Despite this, initial diagnosis may be incorrect in up to 30 per cent of patients initially diagnosed as having MND. A list of the major differential diagnoses is listed in Table 17.2.

PATHOGENESIS

Much of our understanding of the pathogenesis of motor neurone disease is derived from studies focusing on familial ALS. Although these cases represent only 5–10 per cent of total cases of ALS, interest intensified following demonstration of linkage to chromosome 21, followed by identification of mutations arising in the copper/zinc superoxide dismutase (*SOD1*) gene. Since then, more than 120 mutations have been found in the *SOD1* gene.

These are the most common mutations found in familial ALS representing approximately 20 per cent of all familial cases, i.e. 2 per cent of ALS cases in total. However, the mechanisms by which mutations in the *SOD1* gene lead to the development of degenerative changes leading to clinical MND are complex. Several candidate cellular mechanisms have been identified, but pathogenesis remains only partly understood. *SOD1* is a ubiquitously expressed, mostly cytosolic protein that works as a free radical scavenger, converting free radical oxygen species to hydrogen peroxide. While there is some relationship between some of the mutations and clinical severity, this does not correlate with the mutation's effect on enzyme activity. In addition, knock-out animal models of *SOD1* (i.e. mice that have had the *SOD1* gene removed and therefore have no *SOD1* activity) do not recapitulate disease phenotype, while models overexpressing wild-type (i.e. normal) *SOD1* do.

These findings indicate that loss of *SOD1* enzyme activity alone is not responsible for disease development. However, mutations that cause more severe disease are more likely to cause abnormal *SOD1* protein aggregation and this is also seen in *SOD1* transgenic mouse models. This suggests that *SOD1* acts through a 'toxic gain of function' rather than a loss of its normal physiological role. There are likely to be several mechanisms by which *SOD1* protein aggregates are toxic. The aggregates appear to sequester other proteins required for normal cell function, such as molecular chaperones, anti-apoptotic proteins and glutamate transporters. They also appear to interfere with mitochondrial activity by a number of mechanisms and in addition, they interfere with normal axon transport. *SOD1* may exert a toxic gain of function by aberrant enzyme activity by the mutant *SOD1* protein, causing oxidative stress by reversal of its normal function and therefore producing, rather than eliminating, damaging free radical species.

While many of these mechanisms have been demonstrated in sporadic cases of ALS, they are not consistent and *SOD1* protein deposition is rarely found. Furthermore, attempts to modulate disease in humans through drugs acting on these mechanisms have been disappointing.

However, one of the pathological hallmarks for both familial and sporadic ALS is the presence of insoluble ubiquitin-positive neuronal cytoplasmic inclusions (NCIs) within the motor neurons. Recently, these inclusions have been found to contain a ubiquitously expressed nuclear protein, TDP-43. This protein also appears to form the major component of the ubiquitin-positive inclusions seen in frontotemporal lobar degeneration, with ubiquitin-positive inclusions (FTLD-U). This feature, common to both conditions, mirrors the recognition of clinical overlap of ALS and FLTD-U. At least 30 mutations have now been identified within the *TDP-43* gene (TAR DNA binding protein, *TARDBP*) on chromosome 1 within familial ALS and FTD cases. Transgenic mice expressing mutant *TDP-43* have recapitulated clinical and pathological features of ALS, and it currently appears that *TDP-43* is the major proteinopathy underlying both ALS and FTLD-U.

TDP-43 appears to play several roles in RNA processing and more recently, a further gene has been identified in familial ALS involved in RNA processing, named FUS (fused in sarcolemma), suggesting a role for RNA processing in the pathogenesis of ALS. The survival motor neuron (SMN) protein appears to have a similar role and loss of function of SMN activity leads to autosomal recessive spinal muscular atrophy.

MANAGEMENT

Breaking bad news

With the availability of the internet, many patients may already suspect the diagnosis prior to specialist review and it is therefore vital to explore the patient's understanding and, indeed, misunderstanding, surrounding the diagnosis. For this reason, it is important that patients are seen in a timely fashion; the recommendation from the Motor Neurone Disease Association (MNDA) is that all patients are seen within 4 weeks of referral. It may be appropriate to discuss a potential diagnosis even prior to organizing investigations if the patient has concerns. Conversely, it is important to gauge how much information the patient really wants to receive; offering a prognosis based on statistics is rarely helpful for an individual. Regardless of their suspicions, receiving a diagnosis of MND is inevitably a devastating event and its handling invariably shapes the subsequent patient–doctor relationship.

As MND is a clinical diagnosis, it may not be possible to offer a definitive diagnosis on initial consultation, so that an honest approach is generally appreciated. However, it should be remembered that the El Escorial criteria are predominantly a research tool, to facilitate recruitment of homogeneous populations for clinical trials. Many patients with a bulbar or lower motor neuron presentation never fulfil these criteria, although the treating physician will have little doubt about the diagnosis. Giving a patient a diagnosis of 'probable' or 'possible' MND is therefore generally unhelpful.

Multidisciplinary team management

Once a diagnosis has been given, it is important that patients are managed within a multi-disciplinary team setting as their needs may rapidly change, requiring a well-coordinated approach. Health professionals likely to be involved include neurologists, specialist nurses, physiotherapists, occupational therapists, speech and language therapists, dieticians, respiratory physicians, gastroenterologists, palliative care and, of course, the primary care physician. In the UK, the MNDA provides a network of regional care advisors who can provide support for patients and their families. Many specialist MND clinics will have a nurse specialist care coordinator who, in the author's experience, plays one of the most vital roles in managing patients' care.

Genetic counselling

Between 5 and 10 per cent of ALS cases are familial and, of these, 20 per cent are due to *SOD1* mutations. All patients with a familial history should be given the opportunity for formal genetic counselling. However, the picture is complicated by the fact that many of the known mutations demonstrate variable penetrance. This is particularly important when considering predictive testing in family members of those with a known SOD1 mutation, as a positive test may not necessarily indicate that the individual will develop ALS. For this reason, *SOD1* testing is not recommended in sporadic cases. As 80 per cent of familial cases will be due to mutations in genes other than *SOD1*, counselling should emphasize that a negative test for *SOD1* does not exclude the possibility of familial ALS.

Pharmacotherapy

Riluzole, a glutamate receptor antagonist, is the only drug licensed in the UK for the treatment of ALS. A number of trials have been undertaken to assess its effectiveness. The 2009 Cochrane systematic review concluded that riluzole at 100 mg daily prolongs survival by approximately three months,

when assessed at 18 months' duration of illness. However, there are few data on its effects across the entire duration of illness as studies have not proceeded beyond the 18-month median. The UK National Institute for Health and Clinical Excellence (NICE) concluded that the beneficial effects are modest and the cost per quality adjusted life year (QALY) expensive at around £43 500, although adverse effects are minor and reversible. The UK NICE guidelines recommend the use of riluzole, but restrict its use to those with probable or definite ALS. However, increasingly, both genetic and pathological studies demonstrate that both bulbar onset and pure lower motor neuron variants almost certainly share a common pathogenesis with ALS. So it would seem reasonable to extend this prescribing practice to those patients. Other pharmacological agents used in the symptomatic management of patients with MND are outlined in Table 17.3.

Bulbar symptoms and nutrition

Bulbar symptoms may be particularly distressing for patients, resulting in a range of difficulties including dysarthria, poor saliva control causing either constant drooling or pooling of secretions at the back of the mouth, dysphagia, laryngospasm and choking episodes. Despite patients' fears, choking is not, in fact, a cause of death in this patient group. Sialorrhoea can be managed by anticholinergic agents such as 1 per cent atropine eye drops used sublingually, Hyoscine patches, glycopyrrolate or low-dose amitriptyline, and also beta-blockers. Tenacious secretions are treated with carbocysteine, and pineapple juice may also be of value. Parotid botulinum toxin or even irradiation may be used to manage sialorrhoea unresponsive to pharmacological management.

The majority of patients will develop communication difficulties and in those with a bulbar onset, anarthria may occur relatively soon after disease onset. A number of communication strategies and aids are available including vocal output communication aids (VOCAs), which generate a synthetic voice output from typed words. However, as limb impairment ensues, these aids may become impractical. Advanced planning is particularly important in the subgroup of patients in whom early anarthria is anticipated.

Patients should be managed closely with both

Table 17.3 Symptom management in motor neurone disease

Symptoms	Drugs	Other treatments
Cramps	Carbamazepine	Physiotherapy
	Phenytoin	Physical exercise
	Quinine	Massage
Spasticity	Baclofen	Physiotherapy
	Tizanidine	Hydrotherapy
	Dantrolene	
	Botulinum toxin type A	
Laryngospasm	Lorazepam	
Pain	Simple analgesics	
	Non-steroidal anti-inflammatory drugs	
	Opioids	
Emotional lability	Tricyclic antidepressant	
	Selective serotonin-reuptake inhibitors	
Sialorrhoea	Anticholinergics	Parotid botulinum toxin
	β-blockers	Home suction/cough assist

dieticians and speech and language therapists as weight loss is inversely correlated with survival. Indicators for consideration for percutaneous endoscopic gastrostomy (PEG) include weight loss of more than 10 per cent of baseline weight, evidence of aspiration and patient preference. Evidence suggests that PEG prolongs survival by approximately eight months. Complication rates of PEG insertion are primarily related to impaired respiratory function, with an FVC <50 per cent of predicted associated with a higher mortality rate. Patients with an FVC of <50 per cent of predicted should be considered for radiologically inserted gastrostomy (RIG) in preference, as this has a lower complication rate in this patient group.

Respiratory symptoms

The use of **non-invasive ventilation (NIV)** often improves quality of life and prolongs survival in patients with MND and it is therefore important to assess for symptoms and signs of respiratory insufficiency regularly. This is most commonly performed within the clinic setting using vital capacity (VC, lying and sitting) and serial measurements may provide useful in predicting the onset of respiratory insufficiency. However, VC may prove inaccurate (and therefore misleading) in

Patients invariably develop respiratory insufficiency as the disease progresses. It is a strong predictor of quality of life and survival and it is the most common cause of death in patients with motor neurone disease. Rarely, this will be the patient's presenting complaint. Respiratory difficulties may arise from a combination of respiratory muscle and diaphragm weakness, impaired bulbar function, obstructive sleep apnoea and central involvement. Interestingly, patients may not necessarily describe breathlessness, but report a range of symptoms including poor sleep, nocturia, day-time somnolence and fatigue, and morning headache. Impaired sleep quality may be one of the earliest indicators of respiratory insufficiency.

patients with bulbar onset disease, or facial weakness leading to leakage of air when performing the test. This may also be a problem in patients with cognitive impairment (although this, itself, may be a manifestation of respiratory impairment and can improve following NIV). Sniff nasal pressures (SNP) may provide a more accurate assessment in those with bulbar dysfunction, although they are still not widely used. Patients with a VC of <50 per cent (or <80 per cent if they report symptoms) or a SNP of <40 cm H$_2$0 should certainly undergo overnight oximetry, which can be carried out at home. In the author's experience, all patients reporting symptoms, regardless of respiratory function, should undergo overnight oximetry, as a normal study is reassuring for both patient and physician. In July 2010, UK NICE developed guidelines for the use of NIV in patients with MND, although the lack of high quality evidence on the indications for the use of NIV in patients with MND is emphasized. It should be borne in mind, when commencing a patient on NIV, that patients with bulbar palsy due to MND may be poorly tolerant and are at increased risk of aspiration.

Tracheostomy may be considered in patients requiring prolonged ventilatory support, although this is generally not recommended, due to the concern of prolonging survival to the point of severe disability, when the patient becomes unable to express his or her wishes by any means.

Cognition

As discussed above, cognitive impairment may occur in up to half of all patients presenting with ALS, typically a mild frontal lobe impairment. It is important to address cognitive issues and this may require discrete enquiry with the carers, who will often be relieved simply by its acknowledgement. Emotional lability is a frequent problem, particularly in patients with a pseudobulbar clinical picture. Symptoms may be helped by a selective serotonin reuptake inhibitor (SSRI) antidepressant.

Palliation

Involvement of palliative care services should be encouraged, and is increasingly being offered in the earlier stages of the disease course, prior to the patient entering the terminal phase. Palliative care services can provide a range of help to both patients and carers, including symptomatic management, for example for sialorrhea and pain. Explaining the benefits of an early referral to patients is usually well received. Importantly, palliative care includes opportunities for respite, psychological support, advanced care planning and, following death, bereavement support for family and carers.

SPINAL MUSCULAR ATROPHY AND KENNEDY'S DISEASE

The spinal muscular atrophy (SMA) disorders represent a group of inherited conditions characterized by progressive degeneration of anterior horn cells and brain stem nuclei. The incidence is 1/6000–8000 live births and SMA represents the second most common autosomal recessive disease of childhood after cystic fibrosis (see also Chapter 8). SMA is classified into four types based on the age of onset and clinical course. Patients with all forms of SMA have diffuse symmetric proximal muscle weakness that is greater in the lower than upper limbs, and absent or markedly decreased deep tendon reflexes. All SMA types are associated with progressive respiratory insufficiency. Cardiac muscle is not affected.

Type 1 (infantile spinal muscular atrophy or Werdnig–Hoffmann disease)

This is the most common and severe type of SMA. Mothers of affected individuals may describe reduced fetal movements in late pregnancy. Infants fail to develop a normal sitting posture and may suckle poorly and have a weak cry due to bulbar and respiratory muscle involvement. The majority of infants die before one to two years of age from respiratory failure.

Type 2 (intermediate form)

Onset of muscle weakness develops later, typically between six and 12 months. Affected individuals will achieve a sitting position, although they do not normally manage to walk. However, motor development is variable. Death is usually in early adulthood from respiratory failure.

Type 3 (juvenile, Kugelberg–Welander disease)

SMA 3 is the least severe, and typically presents with signs of weakness at or after one year of age and is slowly progressive. The outcome depends primarily upon the severity of muscle weakness at presentation rather than the age of onset, although earlier onset tends to correlate with greater weakness. In addition to weakness, symptoms may include cramps and fasciculations and some develop a fine tremor. Weakness is more evident in proximal muscles, affecting the legs more than the upper limbs. Patients with type 3 SMA may have a normal life expectancy.

Type 4 (adult onset)

Adult onset SMA usually presents in the second or third decade of life, although onset up to the sixth decade is reported. Weakness is proximal with distal sparing and respiratory muscle involvement is rare. Thirty per cent of cases demonstrate an autosomal dominant mode of inheritance.

Diagnosis of SMA

The different forms of SMA are caused by biallelic deletions or mutations in the survival motor neuron 1 (*SMN1*) gene on chromosome 5q13. The SMN protein, like TDP-43 and FUS in MND, appears to play a role in mRNA processing in motor neurons. However, SMA is largely an autosomal recessive condition and levels of SMN protein expression are correlated with a severity of disease, with lower levels causing a more severe phenotype. However, the related *SMN2* gene which lies close to the *SMN1* gene appears to have a modifying effect on disease severity. This gene is largely deleted in most SMA type 1 chromosomes, the most severe phenotype. However, the presence of three or more copies of *SMN2* is associated with a milder phenotype.

Genetic testing involves screening for the most common deletions. However, point mutations also occur and therefore sequencing of the *SMN1* gene should be pursued if the diagnosis is typical of SMA and only a single deletion is identified. Occasionally, genetic testing is unhelpful, in which case diagnosis rests on EMG testing and muscle biopsy.

Kennedy's disease

Symptoms present as a slowly progressive lower motor neuron syndrome with predominant bulbar and facial muscle involvement in addition to both axial and limb weakness. Characteristic features include prominent perioral fasciculations and mus-

Occurring at a frequency of 1/50 000, Kennedy's disease, also known as spinal bulbar muscular atrophy (SBMA), has a frequency similar to that of ALS and shares a number of clinical features. Onset is typically in the third decade, although may be later. It is due to a CAG trinucleotide expansion in the androgen receptor gene and is X-linked recessive. Symptoms are therefore only manifest in males, with females acting as asymptomatic carriers.

cle cramps. Patients often have gynaecomastia, testicular atrophy and infertility. There is a recognized association with diabetes mellitus. Unlike typical ALS, patients may have sensory symptoms, there are no UMN features and disease progression is slower, with respiratory muscle involvement being less common. Nerve conduction studies show evidence of both motor and sensory neuropathy (even in the absence of sensory symptoms) with evidence of diffuse, chronic denervation on EMG. The diagnosis is confirmed by genotyping.

SUMMARY

The motor neurone diseases are a group of heterogeneous conditions. Attempts to produce effective therapeutic interventions have, to date, been disappointing. Recently, the discovery that TDP-43 is central to the majority of sporadic cases has given new hope to achieving an effective treatment within the next decade. For the time being, however, management relies on a vigorous multidisciplinary approach to symptom control.

REFERENCES AND FURTHER READING

Bach JR (2002) Amyotrophic lateral sclerosis: prolongation of life by non invasive respiratory AIDS. *Chest*, 122:92–98.

Bensimon G, Lacomblez L, Meininger V (1994) A controlled trial of riluzole in amyotrophic lateral sclerosis. *New England Journal of Medicine*, 330:585–591.

Brooks BR, Miller RG, Swash M (2000) El Escorial revisited: revised criteria for the diagnosis of Amyotrophic Lateral Sclerosis. *Amyotrophic Lateral Sclerosis and Other Motor Neurone Disorders*, 1:293–299.

Cheyne G (1733) *The English Malady; or, a Treatise on Nervous Diseases of All Kinds.* London: Strahan.

Gordon PH, Cheng B, Katz IB *et al.* (2009) Clinical features that distinguish PLS, upper motor neuron-dominant ALS, and typical ALS. *Neurology*, **72**:1948–1952.

Kahana E, Alter M, Feldman S (1976) Amyotrophic lateral sclerosis: a population study. *Journal of Neurology*, **212**:205–213.

Kwong LK, Neumann M, Sampathu DM *et al.* (2007) TDP-43 proteinopathy: the neuropathology underlying major forms of sporadic and familial frontotemporal lobar degeneration and motor neuron disease. *Acta Neuropathologica*, **114**:63–70.

Lijima M, Arasaki K, Iwamoto H *et al.* (1991) Maximum and minimal motor nerve conduction velocities in patients with motor neuron diseases: correlation with age of onset and duration of illness. *Muscle and Nerve*, **14**:1110–1105.

Logroscino G, Beghi E, Zoccolella S *et al.* (2005) Incidence of ALS in southern Italy: a population based study. *Journal of Neurology, Neurosurgery and Psychiatry*, **76**: 1094–1098.

Lomen-Hoerth C, Murphy J, Langmore S *et al.* (2003) Are amyotrophic lateral sclerosis patients cognitively normal? *Neurology*, **60**:1094–1097.

Lunn M (2009) Nerve and muscle disease. In: Clark C, Howard R (eds). *Neurology, A Queen Square Handbook.* Oxford: Wiley-Blackwell, 337–410.

Mazzini L, Corrà T, Zaccala M *et al.* (1995) Percutaneous endoscopic gastrostomy and enteral nutrition in amyotrophic lateral sclerosis. *Journal of Neurology*, **242**:695–698.

Miller RG, Mitchell JD, Lyon M, Moore DH (2007) Riluzole for amyotrophic lateral sclerosis (ALS)/motor neuron disease (MND). *Cochrane Database of Systematic Reviews*, (1):CD001447.

National Institute for Health and Clinical Excellence. Motor neurone disease; the use of non-invasive ventilation in the management of motor neurone disease. July 2010. Available from: www.nice.org.uk/guidance/CG105.

Rothstein JL (2009) Current hypotheses for the underlying biology of amyotrophic lateral sclerosis. *Annals of Neurology*, **65**(Suppl. 1):S3–S9.

Traynor BJ, Codd MB, Corr B *et al.* (2000) Amyotrophic lateral sclerosis mimic syndromes: a population-based study. *Archives of Neurology*, **57**:109–113.

Vance C, Rogelj B, Hortobágyi T *et al.* (2009) Mutations in FUS, an RNA processing protein, cause familial amyotrophic lateral sclerosis type 6. *Science*, **323**:1208–1211.

CHAPTER 18

DISEASES OF MUSCLE AND THE NEUROMUSCULAR JUNCTION

Chris Turner and Anthony Schapira

INTRODUCTION

Neuromuscular disorders have been at the vanguard of the translation of the clinical neurosciences from a purely clinically descriptive to an evidence-based and molecularly driven discipline. The **hereditary muscular dystrophies** and **channelopathies** have provided fertile ground for modern molecular genetics to define aetiology, and for cell biology to investigate the molecular pathogenesis in a tissue that can be readily biopsied and cultured. Neuromuscular disorders have therefore become one of the most exciting and rapidly advancing areas of clinical neurology and have provided an insight into the understanding of other neurological diseases. Molecular genetic analysis has allowed genetic counselling and firm diagnosis to be made. Specific treatments are being developed and muscular dystrophies are leading the way in genetic treatments for neurological disease. The next 20 years will see the development of gene therapies and will revolutionize our management and understanding of many neuromuscular disorders.

- Muscular dystrophies
  - Dystrophinopathies (Duchenne/Becker) (X-linked)
  - Facioscapulohumeral (autosomal dominant (AD))
  - Limb girdle (AD and autosomal recessive (AR))
  - Emery–Dreifuss (X-linked, AR and AD)
  - Oculopharyngeal (AD)
- Metabolic muscle disorders
  - Glycogen storage diseases (**Table 18.1**)
    - Acid maltase deficiency
    - Myophosphorylase deficiency
  - Defects of fatty acid metabolism
    - Carnitine palmitoyl transferase deficiency
    - Acyl co-enzyme A dehydrogenase deficiency

Table 18.1 Glycogen storage diseases

Type	Enzyme deficiency
II	Acid maltase
III	Debrancher
IV	Brancher
V	Myophosphorylase
VIa	Phosphorylase b kinase
VII	Phosphofructokinase
IX	Phosphoglycerokinase
X	Phosphoglyceromutase
XI	Lactate dehydrogenase

- Mitochondrial myopathies
  - Chronic progressive external ophthalmoplegia (CPEO)
  - Kearns–Sayre syndrome
  - Myopathy, encephalopathy, lactic acidosis and stroke-like episodes (MELAS)
  - Myoclonic epilepsy with ragged red fibres (MERRF)
- Dystrophic myotonias
  - Myotonic dystrophies (AD)
  - Schwartz–Jampel syndrome (AR)
- Channelopathies
  - Periodic paralysis (AD)
  - Non-dystrophic myotonias (AD and AR)
  - Paramyotonia congenita (AD)
- Congenital myopathies
  - Central core disease
  - Nemaline myopathy
  - Centronuclear myopathy
- Inflammatory muscle disorders
  - Polymyositis
  - Dermatomyositis
  - Inclusion body myositis.
- Neuromuscular junction disorders
  - Myasthenia gravis
  - Lambert–Eaton syndrome

CLINICAL EXAMINATION

Muscle dysfunction manifests within a limited spectrum of clinical presentations. Muscle disease typically presents with muscle wasting and weakness and is often proximal. Muscle disease can also cause pain or 'myalgia', pseudohypertrophy/hypertrophy, rhabdomyolysis and abnormal muscle contraction.

Clinical history and examination remain fundamental in establishing the diagnosis in muscle diseases. The onset and course of the weakness may be important but the pattern of wasting and weakness of muscles is often more important in establishing the aetiology of the muscle disorder.

Symptoms of muscle disease

- Proximal weakness: working above head, lifting objects, standing up, getting out of the bath, climbing stairs
- Distal weakness: difficulty with hand dexterity, e.g. writing, buttons, eating and catching of toes
- Face: characteristic myopathic facies, drooling of food out of the mouth, collection of food in the mouth
- Eyes: ptosis and diplopia (rare)
- Bulbar: dysarthria, dysphagia
- Neck and spine: 'dropped' head, scoliosis
- Chest: breathless, especially on lying flat
- Heart: exercise intolerance, palpitations, blackouts

Weakness of the shoulder girdle may result in difficulty for patients in raising their arms above their head. These patients may complain of problems with washing or drying their hair, storing items in overhead cupboards and hanging out the washing. Weakness of the pelvic girdle is often manifested by difficulty rising from a chair, climbing stairs and getting in or out of a bath. In comparison, distal weakness results in problems such as difficulty opening bottles and jars and turning taps and in the feet, weakness frequently results in foot drop and catching of the toes especially on curbs. Weakness of the cranial musculature may produce symptoms such as diplopia, dysphagia, dysarthria and occasionally of neck weakness. Facial weakness may be suggested by a history of difficulty whistling, using a straw, blowing up balloons or blowing out candles.

Muscle cramps or pain may suggest a metabolic myopathy. It is always important to ask for a history of pigmenturia or 'coca cola' urine which would indicate myoglobinuria secondary to rhabdomyolysis.

Deciding that a patient has a muscle disorder as a cause of their weakness in comparison to an

The onset of muscle weakness is important to establish, in particular the length of history and whether the patient's weakness can be traced back to early childhood. A history of motor development, if available from a parent, is often useful as difficulty feeding and delayed sitting or walking would indicate congenital muscle disease. Difficulty playing sports and keeping up with peers are often important clues to early muscle problems.

upper motor neuron, lower motor neuron or neuromuscular junction disorder can sometimes be difficult. Upper motor neuron disorders, such as stroke and multiple sclerosis (MS), are often associated with stiffness due to spasticity, weakness of limbs, and not part of a limb as in muscle disease, and sensory symptoms. Lower motor neuron disorders, such as motor neurone disease or the Guillain–Barré syndrome, may be associated with prominent cramps and fasciculations. Neuromuscular junction disorders often present with fatigable weakness. A careful clinical history will delineate these disorders from primary myopathies.

The **family history** is an important part of making a diagnosis in muscle disease and it is often useful to draw out a family tree. Expression of the same genetic defect may vary within a single family. This is typically seen in myotonic dystrophy where the disease may be worse with subsequent generations especially when inherited from the mother ('genetic anticipation', see Chapter 8). Grandparents may only have a history of cataracts at a young age, whereas the mother may have stiffness in the muscles due to myotonia and mild handgrip weakness, while the child has the severest form of myotonic dystrophy or congenital myotonic dystrophy which can be fatal. Carriers of X-linked diseases may be picked up through affected relatives of the maternal carrier. Mitochondrial myopathies may be suggested by strictly maternal inheritance.

A **drug history** is also important. Statins are uncommonly associated with an acute severe myopathy, but commonly cause myalgia. The prolonged administration of steroids leads to a proximal myopathy. Pencillamine causes a myasthenic-like syndrome.

A **systemic review** is important as many diseases can present with muscle weakness or fatigue.

Endocrine disorders, such as thyrotoxicosis, myxoedema, Cushing's or Addison's disease, for instance, may present with fatigue or proximal weakness. A history of fevers, weight loss, skin rash and arthritis may suggest a connective tissue disorder in association with a myopathy.

A neurological history is helpful in deciding that a patient's symptoms are likely to be due to a muscle disease, but **a full examination** is essential to confirm this and the identification of the type of muscle disorder. Simple observation of the patient will identify the frontal balding and myopathic facies of a patient with myotonic dystrophy; the bilateral ptosis of myasthenia or CPEO; the heliotrope discoloration around the eyes of dermatomyositis, and head drop in myasthenia gravis, inflammatory muscle disease (this mat also occur in motor neurone disease). Winging of the scapulae suggests periscapular weakness which is usually caused by a dystrophic process. Alternatively, there may be pseudohypertrophy, such as in the calves of patients with Becker's muscular dystrophy. There may be signs of multisystem disease, such as hypothyroidism or Cushing's disease.

Examination of the cranial nerves may show some specific abnormalities. Visual acuity is not impaired in muscular disorders except with the development of cataracts in myotonic dystrophy. Retinal examination may demonstrate retinitis pigmentosa of the 'salt and pepper type' as seen in some mitochondrial disorders or the microangiopathy of facioscapulohumeral dystrophy. Ptosis may be unilateral or bilateral and symmetrical or asymmetrical. Ptosis is indicative of weakness of *levator palpebrae superioris* and is a common finding in myopathic disorders or diseases of the neuromuscular junction. The latter may be signified by fatigue and can be demonstrated by asking the patient to look at a fixed point above their head while gradual descent of the eyelids is observed. Alternatively, the patient is asked to look at the examiner's finger, which is held in a position to allow the patient to look down. The finger is then brought abruptly upwards to above the patient's head. The eyelids in myasthenia gravis may twitch in such circumstances as elevation is initially normal before fatigue sets in and the eyelids begin to droop (Cogan's lid twitch). Examination of eye movements is important and the examiner must ask the patient whether diplopia is experienced at any time. **Ophthalmoplegia** may occur in ocular myasthenia, mitochondrial disorders, or the ocular dystrophies, such as oculopharyngeal muscular dystrophy.

There may be wasting and weakness of temporalis, sternomastoid or trapezius. Facial weakness is demonstrated by attempting to open the eyes against resistance and opening the mouth against pursed lips. The patient may also be asked to blow out their cheeks or to whistle; these actions are often difficult with marked facial weakness. Bulbar weakness may be suggested by a nasal quality to the voice and coughing or nasal regurgitation when drinking a glass of water offered by the examiner. Neck weakness is an important sign in myopathies and is usually demonstrated by overcoming the patient's forced neck flexion. Examination of the tongue may show wasting and fasciculations, which are more commonly a result of lower motor neuron disorders, such as motor neuron disease. Enlargement of the tongue may be seen in amyloidosis or acid maltase deficiency. Tongue myotonia may be demonstrated in myotonic dystrophy. This is achieved by striking a tongue depressor laid edge on across the protruding tongue with a patella hammer.

Muscle wasting, fasciculations, myokymia and contractures may be seen on inspection of the muscles. Fasciculations are uncommon in muscle disease and are usually the result of denervation of the muscle. Myokymia, which is a persistent worm-like motion of muscle fibres underneath the skin, is also usually caused by denervation. It may be a physiological symptom of fatigue especially when it occurs around the eye. The myokymia in Whipple's disease tends to occur in the face. Neuromyotonia can cause stiffness in the muscles and be associated with myokymia. Contractures are an indication of long-standing muscle weakness and can be seen in several dystrophies. The pattern of muscle wasting and weakness is important. It is usually symmetrical and proximal in the limb girdle dystrophies. Proximal muscle wasting is common in inflammatory myopathies and sometimes the muscles have normal bulk but can take on a 'woody' feel caused by oedema. In facioscapulohumeral dystrophy (FSHD), muscle wasting and weakness is often strikingly asymmetrical and may affect the face, proximal upper limbs and distal lower limbs. Inclusion body myositis may lead to focal wasting especially in the flexor compartment of the forearms and thighs in an asymmetric pattern.

On examination, muscle tone is either normal or reduced in muscle disease. The results of testing muscle strength can be documented according to the Medical Research Council grading system (see Chapter 3). It is important to look for fatigue through repetitive movement. This is usually seen in neuromuscular junction disorders, such as myasthenia gravis or the congenital myasthenias, but can also occur in myopathies. Alternatively, increasing strength through repetition would suggest a rarer disorder of the neuromuscular junction, the Lambert–Eaton myasthenic syndrome.

It is crucial to ask the patient to walk, as this may demonstrate the typical waddling gait of pelvic girdle weakness or the dropped foot of FSHD or myotonic dystrophy type 1. Truncal weakness may be tested by asking the patient to sit up from lying flat on the couch, and pelvic girdle weakness may be tested by asking the patient to stand from a crouch. Muscle weakness in children is often best observed while they are at play and seeing them stand up from lying on the floor. This may reveal the typical Gower's manoeuvre seen in pelvic girdle weakness whereby the child climbs up his extended legs. This is most commonly seen in Duchenne's muscular dystrophy.

The tendon reflexes are often depressed in muscle disease in proportion to the muscle wasting and weakness. Isometric contraction will increase tendon reflexes in the Lambert–Eaton myasthenic syndrome.

Plantar responses should be flexor in pure myopathic disorders unless there is associated central nervous system (CNS) involvement. Sensory examination should also be normal unless there is associated neurogenic disease.

INVESTIGATION

The following outlines the range of investigation of patients with suspected muscle disease and is summarized in Box 18.1.

Blood tests

A full blood count is typically normal in myopathic disorders, although there may be a mild leukocytosis in inflammatory muscle disease or eosinophilia in, for instance, trichinosis. The erythrocyte sedimentation rate (ESR) is usually elevated

Box 18.1 Investigation of patients with suspected muscle disease

- Blood
  - Full blood count, urea, electrolytes, calcium, creatine kinase, liver function tests
  - Endocrine - thyroid, Cushing's, diabetes mellitus
  - Antibodies - connective tissue disorders
  - DNA testing - Duchenne, myotonic dystrophy
- ECG
  - Cardiac involvement
- EMG
  - Muscle sampling
  - Nerve conduction studies
- Biopsy
  - Needle sample
  - Open biopsy
- Ischaemic forearm lactate test

in the inflammatory myopathies. Electrolytes are typically normal unless there is some other underlying endocrine disorder, such as Cushing's disease or Addison's disease. Diabetes mellitus may be seen in myotonic dystrophy or the mitochondrial myopathies as part of more widespread systemic involvement. Calcium levels are typically normal. Thyroid function studies should be undertaken to exclude myxoedema or thyrotoxicosis. Liver function tests may reveal a mild elevation of aspartate aminotransferase (AST) or alanine aminotransferase (ALT) from muscle rather than liver. **The most useful blood test is** creatine kinase **(CK)**. This muscle enzyme leaks into the blood when there is muscle breakdown or a defect of the plasma membrane. Levels of CK are usually in the high hundreds or thousands in the muscular dystrophies. CK may reach very high levels when there is severe muscle breakdown in rhabdomyolysis. Elevation of CK is common in the inflammatory myopathies and usually in the high hundreds, although levels may occasionally be normal. CK levels are normal in neuromuscular junction defects and in several of the congenital myopathies. A mild increase to approximately twice the normal upper limit may be seen in individuals of West Indian extraction. High CK levels may be seen in otherwise apparently normal women who are carriers of mutations in the dystrophin gene.

The **ischaemic forearm lactate** test may be used to detect disorders of glycogenolysis or glycolysis. This involves the contraction of a muscle undergoing anaerobic metabolism. It is usually tested by inflating a sphygmomanometer to above arterial pressure and collecting blood samples in the forearm following contractions of the hand. In the normal individual, energy requirements will come from the breakdown of glycogen and glucose to pyruvate, which subsequently accumulates as lactic acid. In a patient with an enzyme defect of either of these pathways, there will be a failure to accumulate lactic acid following exercise. This is interpreted as a positive test. A defect of aerobic metabolism as occurs in patients with mitochondrial myopathies will result in an elevation of lactic acid. This will be exacerbated by exercising the patient. Typically, lactic acid levels will rise to several times the upper limit of normal, while pyruvate levels will usually remain low. This results in a substantial increase in the lactate:pyruvate ratio.

Nerve conduction studies (NCS) and electromyography (EMG) are important investigations in making the diagnosis of muscle disease or disorders of the neuromuscular junction (see Chapter 5). Nerve conduction studies are usually used to exclude diseases of the peripheral nerves, although peripheral nerve abnormalities may be seen in a proportion of patients with mitochondrial disorders and incidentally in patients with myopathy, such as those with myotonic dystrophy. Measurement of the compound muscle action potential (CMAP) may reveal a reduction in amplitude in muscle disease, including dystrophies and inflammatory myopathies. Repetitive nerve stimulation at 3 Hz may demonstrate a decrement in the CMAP in myasthenia gravis or an increment in the CMAP in the Lambert–Eaton myasthenic syndrome. Single fibre EMG studies may demonstrate neuromuscular junction blockade with 'jitter' and block in myasthenia gravis.

A coaxial needle is used for EMG, which examines muscles for insertional activities, spontaneous activity and in measuring motor unit action potentials. A short burst of electrical activity following insertion of the needle is normal. This activity may be reduced when muscles are replaced by fat or connective tissue and increased when muscle membranes are unstable, such as with the inflammatory myopathies. A myotonic syndrome may produce typical 'dive bomber' sounds when the needle is moved.

Spontaneous activity may appear as fibrillation potentials or positive sharp waves and these are a result of depolarization of single muscle fibres and are seen typically in the primary myopathies and in inflammatory muscle disease. They are probably caused by functional denervation resulting from fibre necrosis or atrophy.

Motor unit action potentials become polyphasic and of short duration and low amplitude where there is loss of muscle by necrosis. Denervation and hypertrophy of muscle fibres may result in polyphasic motor unit action potentials, but with prolonged duration and high amplitude components. Sometimes these findings may occur simultaneously.

Muscle biopsy remains the gold standard for the diagnosis of muscle disease. Two techniques are available to obtain muscle for examination. The first involves open biopsy under local anaesthesia and the second is taken by a needle biopsy. Each method has its advocates and in practice, both are widely used. The selection of muscle for biopsy is important. The muscle should be affected but not too severely as muscle fibres may be replaced by fat and connective tissue and therefore not provide a diagnosis. Biceps, triceps and vastus lateralis are the muscles most frequently biopsied. In each case, it is essential that the biopsy is subjected to a full range of histochemical stains. Immunohistochemistry involving antibodies to proteins within the muscle fibres, such as dystrophin and sarcoglycans, are now becoming an important part of the diagnosis of muscle disease. The most frequent patterns of abnormality on muscle biopsy are those that involve dystrophic processes, inflammatory processes, enzyme deficiencies or structural changes indicative of mitochondrial disorders or the congenital myopathies. Occasionally non-specific changes are seen, such as type II muscle fibre atrophy which may result from immobility. Alternatively, the muscle biopsy may demonstrate fibre type grouping or atrophy indicative of a neurogenic disorder. Electron microscopy can also be used in the diagnosis

of muscle diseases. This may show the typical vacuolar contents in inclusion body myositis, the paracrystalline inclusions of mitochondrial disorders or the rods and filaments of nemaline myopathy (a congenital myopathy).

Magnetic resonance imaging (MRI) and magnetic resonance spectroscopy (MRS) are increasingly being used to investigate muscle disease. MRS can be used to identify defects of energy metabolism. MRI can be used to demonstrate the pattern of muscle involvement which may be helpful in the differentiation of dystrophies. MRI may also be helpful in guiding which muscle to biopsy and possibly whether there is an ongoing inflammatory process.

Genetic testing has provided the greatest developments in refining diagnoses, especially in the dystrophies, mitochondrial cytopathies and channelopathies. The testing of white blood cell DNA may even occur before a muscle biopsy is performed especially if the phenotype is characteristic, e.g. FSHD, channelopathies, myotonic dystrophies. The limb girdle dystrophies, Duchenne and Becker muscular dystrophy, some congenital myopathies, disorders of the neuromuscular junction and the mitochondrial encephalomyopathies are increasingly diagnosed by genetic testing.

DUCHENNE AND BECKER MUSCULAR DYSTROPHY

Duchenne and Becker muscular dystrophies are X-linked genetic disorders and are associated with mutations in the dystrophin gene at the Xp21 locus and are therefore called the 'dystrophinopathies'. They are usually associated with a reduction or loss of expression of dystrophin at the sarcolemma. **Duchenne muscular dystrophy (DMD) is the most common of the dystrophies** with an incidence of approximately 1:3500 live male births and a prevalence of approximately 6:100 000 total male population. Becker muscular dystrophy (BMD) is less common at approximately 1:18 000 live male births and a prevalence of 2:100 000 total male population. DMD is usually associated with a complete loss of dystrophin and a severe phenotype, whereas BMD is associated with a partial reduction in dystrophin and a milder phenotype.

Dystrophinopathies are X-linked recessive traits. Males carrying the abnormal dystrophin gene are always affected, while heterozygous females are carriers but usually unaffected. Carrier females will pass on the condition to 50 per cent of their sons and 50 per cent of their daughters will be carriers. Female carriers can be affected clinically with mild proximal weakness or calf pseudohypertrophy. These patients are known as 'manifesting carriers' and are the result of asymmetrical Lyonization of the maternal X chromosome towards the affected allele. Other female carriers may only have elevated CK levels and mild EMG changes.

Approximately 30 per cent of patients with DMD have no family history and therefore appear as sporadic cases. The mutation may have arisen in the mother's gametes or in the affected embryo. However, new techniques to identify carrier status suggest that a significant proportion of apparently sporadic cases are in fact the offspring of previously unrecognized carriers.

Clinical and molecular features of dystrophin deficiency

The weakness of DMD usually presents at an early age with **delayed motor milestones**. The child is often unable to walk until the age of two or three years. There is **bilateral symmetrical proximal limb weakness, usually more profound in the pelvic girdle**. The child may exhibit Gower's sign (described above under Symptoms of muscle disease). The gait is waddling and the child has difficulty rising from sitting, crouching or lying. Most patients have pseudohypertrophy of the calves as a result of accumulation of fat and connective tissue (Figure 18.1). Progression of the disease leads to marked wasting of the limb girdles with accompanying progressive weakness. Paraspinal weakness may result in kyphoscoliosis, particularly once the patient is confined to a wheelchair. This, together with weakness of the intercostal and other respiratory muscles, may result in muscular respiratory failure, although because of relative preservation of diaphragmatic function, this becomes severe only relatively late in the course of the disease.

The CK is usually very high and is often in the thousands. The EMG is abnormal and the muscle biopsy shows a dystrophic pattern with a wide variation in fibre size, central nuclei muscle, fibre necrosis and increased endomysial connective tis-

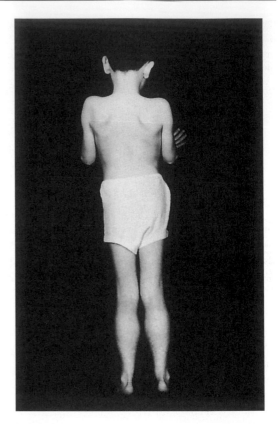

Figure 18.1 Prominent calves, wasted thighs and thinning of scapulohumeral muscles in Duchenne dystrophy.

sue and fat (Figure 18.2). **Immunostaining with dystrophin antibodies** often shows absence of expression of the protein at the sarcolemmal membrane.

Cardiac involvement is common in DMD and may result in arrhythmias, impaired contractility and, occasionally, progressive cardiac failure. Abnormalities on ECG are also common and include conduction defects, tall R waves and deep Q waves. One intriguing aspect of DMD is that approximately one-third of patients have associated mental retardation. This particularly seems to affect verbal abilities. Brain MRI may show mild generalized cerebral atrophy.

Diagnosis

The specific diagnosis of DMD or BMD rests upon demonstrating complete or partial dystrophin deficiency in the muscle biopsy using immunocytochemical techniques. Molecular genetic diagnosis can be made by demonstrat-

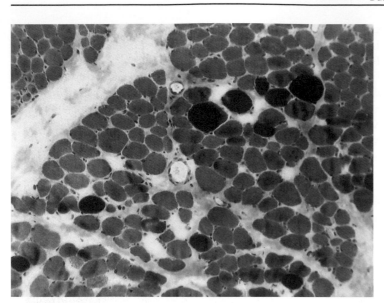

Figure 18.2 Duchenne muscular dystrophy (H&E frozen section ×120) shows large 'waxy' strongly eosinophilic (black) fibres together with great variation in fibre size. The large areas without muscle fibres are fat replacement and fibrosis as a result of progressive fibre loss.

The onset and rate of progression of BMD are usually slower than in DMD. Patients may present in early adolescence, although there is often a history of delayed motor milestones and difficulty keeping up with their peers at school, although some patients may not present until adulthood. The pattern of muscle weakness is similar to that of DMD (Figure 18.3) and muscle hypertrophy is often a prominent feature, particularly affecting the calves. Spinal contractures are uncommon in BMD. Most patients are able to continue walking into adulthood. Whereas patients with DMD often die before the age of 25 years, those with BMD may survive much longer. The heart may be involved in BMD patients although usually this is less severe than in DMD. Abnormalities of ECG are seen in about half the cases of BMD. Intellect is not affected in BMD. Pathological features are similar to those seen in DMD, but are usually much less severe.

are found in skeletal and cardiac muscle, brain, retina and peripheral nerves. This may explain why mental retardation may accompany the myopathy in some patients. Two-thirds of patients have an out-of-frame deletion, which results in a small truncated, unstable protein with poor function. The remaining DMD patients have point mutations or duplications, which also result in an unstable protein. Becker muscle dystrophy usually results from in-frame deletions that lead to a truncated protein which is present in reduced quantity and function.

There is no specific treatment to cure DMD or BMD, although recent advances in gene transfer may change this in the future. Some clinicians advocate the use of steroids in young boys with DMD and clinical trials will aim to determine optimal dosing ing a mutation in the dystrophin gene although, especially in BMD, this can sometimes be difficult to demonstrate. Genetic diagnosis may be used in prenatal and preimplantation diagnosis.

The *Xp21.1* gene is the largest known gene and contains 2.4 million base pairs. At least seven protein isoforms are encoded by this gene and these

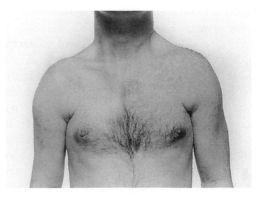

Figure 18.3 Asymmetric wasting of pectoral muscles in a man aged 40 years with Becker dystrophy.

and duration of treatment. Management is directed towards supportive care and maintaining function including treatment with an ACE inhibitor, treatment of arrhythmias, and non-invasive respiratory support. Moderate physical exercise is often helpful, avoidance of contractures is important and prevention of scoliosis crucial when the patient is no longer able to walk. This often requires a thoracic support, breathing exercises and postural drainage.

FACIOSCAPULOHUMERAL DYSTROPHY

FSHD is probably a molecularly heterogeneous group of disorders with a similar clinical phenotype. Transmission is usually autosomal dominant, although both autosomal recessive and X-linked cases have been described. One locus at chromosome 4q35 has been identified and accounts for the majority of cases, but the responsible gene and its protein product remain unknown.

Onset is usually insidious and often occurs in late childhood or adolescence, although diagnosis in later adulthood is not uncommon. Weakness usually begins in the face and progresses to the periscapular region with winging of the scapulae and wasting in the arm. Difficulty with eye closure may be the symptom that precipitates medical attention, although some patients experience minimal face weakness. Weakness may subsequently develop in the lower limbs with foot drop in approximately half of patients. Pelvic girdle weakness occurs later. Weakness in FSHD is often strikingly asymmetrical initially and then becomes more symmetrical with disease progression.

Creatine kinase is usually elevated in the high hundreds or above 1000 and EMG is myopathic. Muscle biopsy can show typical myopathic features with increased variation in fibre diameter, occasional necrosis and regeneration, and an increase in connective tissue and fat. Rimmed vacuoles and endomysial inflammatory cells are not uncommon findings. However, in some cases, the biopsy shows only mild changes, which may include scattered atrophic angulated fibres suggestive of a neurogenic component.

FSHD tends to be slowly progressive, with only modest shortening of lifespan. This is in part due to the relative absence of cardiac and respiratory involvement. Early onset typically leads to more severe subsequent involvement. Studies with the β-agonist, albuterol, have demonstrated a significant increase in lean body mass and muscle strength and this may be a useful drug in the management of FSHD.

LIMB GIRDLE MUSCLE DYSTROPHIES

The limb girdle muscular dystrophies (LGMD) are a clinically and genetically heterogeneous group of disorders that manifest predominantly as gradually progressive weakness affecting shoulder and pelvic girdles.

LGMD vary in severity from very mild to severe. The mild forms usually become apparent in the second or third decade with slow onset and progression of proximal upper and lower limb involvement. Muscles of the face and hands are rarely affected. Mobility is often maintained into late adulthood. The CK is moderately elevated and EMG is often characteristic of a myopathy. Muscle pathology shows histological changes typical of a

Significant advances have been made in the identification of the underlying molecular genetic bases of the LGMDs. Recent classification has divided the LGMDs into autosomal dominant (type 1) and autosomal recessive (type 2). Mutations in the genes *calpain-3* (2A), *dysferlin* (2B), the sarcoglycans (2C-F) and FKRP (2I) are some of the more common genes causing autosomal recessive LGMD. These mutations usually manifest in childhood or early adolescence, although occasional late-onset cases have been described. The mutations cause deficiency of the respective proteins and this can be demonstrated immunohistochemically on muscle biopsy and the mutation confirmed with genetic testing. Mutations in the genes *myotilin* (1A), *lamin A/C* (1B) and *caveolin-3* (1C) are some of the more common genes causing autosomal dominant LGMD.

dystrophy with variation in fibre size, occasional necrosis, fibre splitting and replacement with fat, central nuclei and increased endomysial connective tissue. The severe forms of LGMD may be indistinguishable from DMD in male patients. Onset is in early childhood with early loss of ambulation. The pelvic girdle is usually most affected and intellectual function is retained.

Dilated cardiomyopathy and neuromuscular respiratory failure may develop in some patients with LGMD, usually after the onset of limb girdle weakness. Other muscle groups may also be affected such as periscapular involvement in LGMD caused by mutations in FKRP or *calpain-3*.

EMERY–DREIFUSS MUSCULAR DYSTROPHY

There are six types of Emery–Dreifuss muscular dystrophy (EDMD). The classic form, or Emery–Dreifuss muscular dystrophy type 1 is linked to Xq28, the *STA* gene, whose product is called emerin. This is a 34-kDa protein, which is ubiquitously expressed at the nuclear membrane, but the precise function of which remains unclear. Antibodies are available to emerin and a mutation in the emerin gene usually leads to loss of immunoreactivity. The diagnosis of Emery–Dreifuss muscular dystrophy may be made by observing the absence of immunostaining for emerin protein in peripheral whole blood cells or muscle biopsy.

> There is insidious onset of wasting and weakness involving mainly the scapulohumeral muscles in the upper limbs and the peroneal muscles in the lower limbs. A typical feature is the development of contractures with flexion at the elbows, equinovarus deformities at the ankles and limitation of neck flexion. Symptoms usually begin in early childhood with a waddling gait.

Cardiac involvement is invariable with conduction defects and low amplitude P waves on ECG. Cardiac involvement may become symptomatic, with syncope or progressive cardiac failure. The CK is modestly elevated, the EMG is myopathic and the muscle biopsy shows typical changes of a dystrophy. There is no evidence of involvement

of higher mental function. Management should include supervision by a cardiologist and treatment for dysrhythmias. Avoidance of contractures may be helped by physiotherapy.

Other patients with a similar Emery–Dreifuss phenotype have dominant/recessive mutations in other genes, such as lamin A/C, SYNE1 and SYNE2.

OCULOPHARYNGEAL MUSCULAR DYSTROPHY

> Oculopharyngeal muscular dystrophy (OPMD) is an autosomal dominant inherited disorder with complete penetrance and only a few sporadic cases have been described. **It is characterized by onset in the fifth or sixth decades with ptosis and dysphagia.** There is slow progression and involvement of other muscles, such as the limb girdle, occurs in the later stages.

Oculopharyngeal muscular dystrophy has been linked to chromosome 14q11 and an abnormally expanded triplet GCG repeat expansion identified in the polyA binding protein 2 gene (*PABP2*). Normal individuals have six repeats in comparison to patients who have eight to 13.

Although ptosis is more commonly the first symptom of OPMD, dysphagia has been reported early in some patients. The ptosis often requires the patient to compensate by overactivity of the frontalis muscle and extension of the neck to enable them to see. External ocular movements are normal in the early stages of the disease, but an ophthalmoplegia may develop later. Dysphagia can become severe enough to cause malnutrition and require parenteral feeding, such as via a gastrostomy. Dysphonia may also occur as a result of laryngeal weakness. Later in the disease, weakness and wasting may occur in the limb girdle muscles.

Levels of CK may be normal or only modestly elevated and EMG is usually myopathic. Barium swallow may reveal weak prolonged and repetitive pharyngeal contractions with delayed sphincter relaxation. The ECG may be abnormal in a proportion of cases and usually shows a conduction defect.

Muscle biopsy shows a characteristic picture of generalized dystrophic change in addition to the presence of rimmed vacuoles within muscle fibres.

These contain membranous structures and debris from the breakdown of muscle. Electron microscopy also shows the presence of intranuclear tubular filaments. There is no specific treatment for OPMD. Supportive and palliative treatments are important and may include eye props, pharyngeal myotomy and gastrostomy.

THE GLYCOGEN STORAGE DISEASES

The glycogen storage diseases are listed in Table 18.1. They are a heterogeneous group of disorders of glycogen metabolism. **They generally present as liver or muscle disease,** reflecting the different functions of glycogen in these tissues. In the liver, glycogen is mainly utilized to keep blood glucose constant, while in the muscle it provides a substrate for energy production during high intensity acute exercise. This chapter will deal with those disorders that predominantly affect muscle.

Acid maltase deficiency

Acid maltase deficiency may present at any time from infancy to late adulthood. In the **infantile form (Pompé's disease)** glycogen accumulates, particularly in the heart, skeletal muscle, liver and brain. The baby presents with hypotonia, respiratory failure and hypoglycaemia. Early death is usual.

Childhood-onset acid maltase deficiency presents with delayed motor milestones and proximal weakness. Occasionally, the respiratory muscles can be selectively affected and calf enlargement can sometimes occur. This picture can simulate muscular dystrophy. Progression is slow but inexorable and death usually results from respiratory failure in the second decade.

> **Adult acid maltase deficiency** can present in the third decade or later as a slowly **progressive proximal limb girdle myopathy** with symptoms of **respiratory failure**. Prognosis is usually good for several years, with many patients maintaining ambulation. Cardiac involvement is uncommon.

Acid maltase deficiency causes an elevation of CK and AST. Myopathic changes are demonstrated

on EMG. Muscle biopsy shows a vacuolar myopathy. The vacuoles contain glycogen and are strongly reactive for acid phosphatase, indicating that they are secondary lysosomes. Acid maltase can be assayed in muscle fibroblasts or lymphocytes and prenatal diagnosis can be undertaken on amniotic fluid cells. Electron microscopy can also show lysosomes filled with glycogen. Gene deletions or missense mutations in the acid maltase gene have been identified. A family history, if present, usually suggests an autosomal recessive inheritance. Some investigators have suggested that a high protein diet may result in increased strength and exercise tolerance in patients with acid maltase deficiency. Intravenous recombinant α-glucosidase therapy is increasingly used especially in the severe early onset cases and may improve limb weakness and respiratory function.

Myophosphorylase deficiency

Myophosphorylase deficiency (McArdle's disease) is a predominantly autosomal recessive disorder and in approximately half of those affected there is no positive family history. The myophosphorylase gene has been localized to chromosome 11q13 and mutations in this gene have been identified in patients.

> Onset may be variable, with a fatal infantile form with progressive weakness and respiratory failure leading to death within a few months, a milder childhood-onset form with delayed motor development and proximal weakness, and an adult-onset form with muscle cramps, exercise intolerance, proximal muscle wasting and weakness and myoglobinuria. Muscle pain and stiffness are induced by exercise of short duration and high intensity. Following a brief period of rest, the pain may resolve and lead to a 'second wind' phenomenon in which the patient has a marked improvement in exercise capacity.

Elevated CK levels over 1000 are seen in most patients at rest. Electromyography is myopathic and ECG occasionally shows abnormalities. The forearm ischaemic lactate test demonstrates a failure in the rise in lactic acid following exercise. Muscle biopsy shows periodic acid-Schiff-positive glycogen deposits in subsarcolemmal 'blebs'. The histochemical reaction for phosphorylase is absent. Regenerating muscle fibres may express phosphorylase which may represent expression of a fetal isoform. No effective therapy is available for patients with McArdle's disease. A high protein diet has been suggested to be beneficial, although this has been useful in only a few patients.

DEFECTS OF FATTY ACID METABOLISM

Defects of fatty acid metabolism may present with muscle pain and weakness. Infants usually have generalized profound hypotonia and fail to thrive, while adults complain of proximal muscle weakness. Symptoms are provoked by prolonged exercise, fasting or cold, as these are occasions when lipids become an important source of ATP. An acute energy crisis in muscle in these patients may lead to rhabdomyolysis with myoglobinuria. Abnormalities of liver and heart may coexist. Central nervous system disease has been seen in some patients with long-chain fatty acid deficiencies.

Typically, the symptoms are episodic, although a chronic progressive history can occur. A history of hypoglycaemia, encephalopathy or cardiorespiratory arrest should alert the physician to the possibility of a fatty acid defect. Hypoglycaemia and elevated ammonia levels, together with a high CK, are strongly suggestive of a fatty acid metabolic defect. Additional important investigations include urinalysis for organic acids and measurement of plasma and tissue carnitines which may be low in total form, but high in esterified (acetylated) form.

Carnitine palmitoyl transferase (CPT) deficiency was the first of the β-oxidation defects to be described in fatty acid metabolism. The most common form of CPT deficiency presents in adolescence or early adulthood with recurrent episodes of muscle pain, rhabdomyolysis and myoglobulinuria. These episodes may typically be induced by prolonged exercise or by fasting and occasionally by infection. The enzyme defect is located in CPT II and results in a severe deficiency of lipid in muscle. The inheritance pattern is autosomal recessive. Most patients are clinically normal between attacks, although recurrent episodes may lead to persisting weakness.

Acyl coenzyme A (CoA) dehydrogenase defi-ciency may be classified into long-chain, medium-chain or short-chain varieties. Generally, these disorders present in early childhood with recurrent hypoglycaemia, vomiting and coma induced by fasting. A later onset form may be seen and is characterized by muscle pain and myoglobinuria.

Primary carnitine deficiency may be associated with a myopathy and is caused by defective carnitine uptake. It may be diagnosed in skin fibroblasts or blood leukocytes. Patients respond to carnitine supplementation. Secondary carnitine deficiency occurs in some patients with respiratory chain defects, acyl CoA dehydrogenase deficiencies and methylmalonyl CoA mutase deficiency. Sodium valproate may also deplete carnitine stores. Carnitine-deficient myopathy usually presents in childhood or adolescence with proximal limb weakness, although facial and bulbar weakness may also occur. Muscle biopsy may show increased accumulation of lipid, especially in type 1 fibres.

Diagnosis of patients with defects of fatty acid metabolism is important, as treatment is available for some of these disorders. Beta-oxidation defects may be diagnosed by random mass spectrometric analysis of blood or urine, carnitine estimation in blood and muscle, studies of cultured cells or molecular genetic analysis, e.g. CPT II deficiency where one mutation accounts for about 50 per cent of cases. Avoidance of prolonged fasting and a diet high in carbohydrate and low in fat are important. Additional carbohydrates must be given if there is any coexisting illness and in coma intravenous glucose must be administered in high quantities. Carnitine supplementation is helpful for those with carnitine deficiency and riboflavin has been beneficial in patients with multiple acyl CoA dehydrogenase deficiencies.

MITOCHONDRIAL MYOPATHIES

The mitochondrial myopathies are often one feature of a multisystem disease, the mitochondrial cytopathies which can potentially affect the central and peripheral nervous systems, muscle and most other organs. These disorders have in common a defect of oxidative phosphorylation resulting from a deficiency of one or more of the respiratory chain enzyme activities. Although there is considerable overlap between patients, the mitochondrial cytopathies may be grouped into a number of phenotypes with often several different genotypes. Mutations in mitochondrial (mt) and genomic DNA are increasingly being associated with the mitochondrial cytopathies.

Chronic progressive external ophthalmoplegia (CPEO). Patients usually present in childhood or early adult life with slowly progressive bilateral, often asymmetric, ptosis with ophthalmoplegia. Patients occasionally complain of diplopia as the ophthalmoplegia is usually slowly progressive. The CPEO may be a sporadic isolated finding when it is associated with a single mtDNA deletion or associated with maternal (mitochondrial) inheritance when it is caused by a single mtDNA point mutation.

Kearns–Sayre syndrome. This is defined as CPEO and 'salt and pepper' retinitis pigmentosa with onset before the age of 20 in association with elevated cerebrospinal spinal fluid (CSF) protein, cardiac conduction defect, hearing loss, proximal myopathy and/or ataxia. These patients usually have a single large mtDNA deletion.

MELAS. These patients present in early childhood with shortness of stature and any one of the features contained within the acronym. The myopathy is usually proximal and associated with muscle thinning. CNS features include epilepsy, dementia and deafness. Lactic acidosis may be provoked by exercise or intercurrent illness and induce nausea, vomiting and coma. The stroke-like episodes may cause hemianopia or hemiparesis and, interestingly, do not appear to conform to standard cerebrovascular territories. Diabetes, hearing loss and cardiomyopathy are frequent findings in these patients. MELAS is usually caused by the common point mutation (A3243G) in the transfer ribonucleic acid (tRNA) gene for leucine in mtDNA.

MERRF. These patients may present in adolescence or early adulthood with proximal muscle weakness, ataxia, deafness and seizures and the disease is often caused by a mtDNA point mutation (A8344G) in the gene that encodes the tRNA for lysine.

Patients may also present with a pure myopathy or with multisystem disease, which may include liver failure, Fanconi syndrome, pancreatic insuf-

ficiency and sideroblastic anaemia. This wide spectrum of presentation reflects the ubiquity of mitochondria and their pivotal role in cellular metabolism.

Mutations of mitochondrial DNA have been identified in most of the phenotypes. However, a specific mutation may be associated with different phenotypes and the same phenotype may be caused by different mutations. Thus, our understanding of the pathogenesis of these disorders is far from complete. More recently, mutations in nuclear genes which are involved in mitochondrial function, such as DNA polymerase gamma or POLG, have been described in association with mitochondrial cytopathies.

Investigation of these patients may demonstrate multisystem abnormalities; for example, diabetes, sideroblastic anaemia, basal ganglia calcification on computed tomography (CT) scan or EEG abnormalities. The CK is often normal or only mildly elevated and the EMG may be normal or mildly myopathic. **Muscle biopsy is often characteristic** and histochemical stains show dense aggregates of mitochondria located throughout the fibres or in subsarcolemmal regions on transverse section. The Gomori trichrome stain, which produces a red colour with mitochondria, has given rise to the term **'ragged red fibres' because of the characteristic subsarcolemmal red accumulations of mitochondria**. Staining for succinate dehydrogenase (an integral part of the respiratory chain) is more sensitive in identifying abnormal fibres which are intensely stained. A proportion of patients, particularly those with CPEO, have a significant number of cytochrome oxidase (another integral part of the respiratory chain) negative fibres. Electron microscopy may show intramitochondrial paracrystalline inclusions in a proportion of patients.

Molecular genetic diagnosis of these patients is best undertaken on muscle biopsies as not all the mitochondrial DNA mutations appear in blood. Genetic counselling is difficult as, although the mtDNA **point mutations are transmitted in a maternal fashion**, it is difficult, if not impossible, to predict clinical involvement because of the variation in the number of copies of mtDNA affected in an individual. Treatment is unsatisfactory but includes ubiquinone, riboflavin and carnitine, as well as the avoidance of drugs which can inhibit mitochondrial function, such as sodium valproate.

THE MYOTONIAS AND PERIODIC PARALYSES

Myotonic dystrophy

Myotonic dystrophy type 1 (DM1) is the most common adult muscle disease with a prevalence of approximately 1:7000 in the UK. **It is an autosomal dominant disorder caused by an expanded trinucleotide (CTG) repeat sequence in the 3′ untranslated region of the gene myotonin protein kinase (DMPK) on chromosome 19q13.** Normal individuals have between five and 37 repeats, whereas myotonic dystrophy (MD) patients typically have greater than 50. There is a general relationship between repeat length and disease severity, but this does not allow accurate prognostic information on an individual basis. The repeat lengths show instability such that the size may vary from one tissue to another. Myotonic dystrophy also shows anticipation, subsequent generations being more severely affected, probably as a result of intergenerational expansion of the CTG repeat, especially when the abnormal gene is inherited from the mother.

It is uncommon to find a case of DM1 without a family history, although some patients can develop the disease from an unaffected parent who has an expansion between 38 and 49 CTGs or 'premutation allele' and this expands to greater than 50 in their offspring.

Myotonia is usually worse in the cold, especially in the hands. Myotonia can be elicited either following voluntary contraction or through percussion myotonia. Percussion myotonia may be demonstrated by tapping the thenar eminence with a tendon hammer. This results in the thumb being drawn across the palm followed by a slow relaxation. Tongue myotonia may also be demonstrated using a tongue depressor and tendon hammer (Figure 18.4). Muscle wasting and weakness causes myopathic facies, weakness of neck flexion and distal weakness in the limbs. Bilateral ptosis is common and is occasionally associated with ophthalmoplegia. The jaw often hangs open and there may be laryngeal weakness of the bulbar muscles

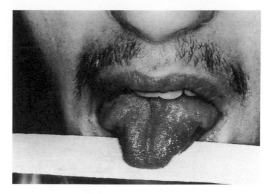

Figure 18.4 Percussion myotonia of tongue in myotonic dystrophy.

causing dysarthria, dysphagia and an increased risk of aspiration pneumonia. The respiratory muscles can often be affected and increase the risk of pneumonia especially when swallowing is impaired.

Abnormalities on ECG are found in the majority of symptomatic patients and usually consist of a prolonged QRS duration and PR interval. These are caused by specific degeneration of the conduction system with relative sparing of the heart muscle. These abnormalities are usually asymptomatic, but paroxysmal tachyarrhythmias and bradyarrhythmias may lead to sudden death, and so the early involvement of a cardiologist in management is vital.

Myotonic dystrophy is a multisystem disease, examination often showing frontal balding, bilateral ptosis, myopathic facies (Figure 18.5) and wasting of the small hand muscles. Cataracts, insulin resistance and testicular atrophy are all common features. Smooth muscle may also be involved and result in impaired gastrointestinal motility, which usually presents with irritable bowel-like symptoms. Many patients with DM1 appear apathetic and lethargic. Excessive daytime sleepiness is very common. Several studies have documented mild cognitive impairment. MRI brain scans may show cerebral atrophy and white matter lesions. Positron emission tomography has shown reduced cerebral glucose utilization.

The definitive investigation in patients with a typical phenotype is genetic testing. Relatives of affected patients should be offered genetic counselling. Appropriate investigation is needed for associated diabetes mellitus, cataracts, cardiac dysrhythmias and neuromuscular respiratory weakness. The CK is usually normal; EMG shows typical

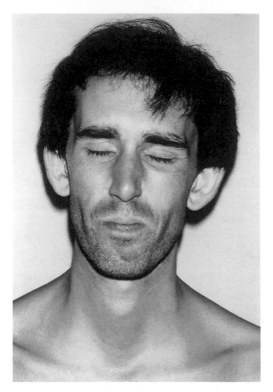

Figure 18.5 Dystrophia myotonica: facial appearance and inability to close eyes tightly.

myotonic discharges in association with positive sharp waves and complex repetitive discharges. A myopathic pattern may develop with time. Muscle biopsy should not be routinely performed and often does not demonstrate any specific features, but can show a range of abnormalities including increased central nuclei, muscle atrophy and ringed fibres.

Management includes treatment of the associated disorders. Regular testing for glucose, cataracts and cardiac involvement are important. Patients may need insertion of a pacemaker or an implantable cardioverter defibrillator. An overnight sleep study can detect abnormalities of nocturnal ventilation which can reflect the severity of neuromuscular respiratory involvement or coexisting sleep apnoea which should be treated with non-invasive ventilation. Daytime sleepiness is treated with the psychostimulant, modafinil. Foot drop is often successfully managed with ankle-foot orthoses. Myotonia is rarely severe enough to warrant pharmacological treatment.

General anaesthesia should be undertaken with care in patients with DM1 and unnecessary operations should be avoided. Patients have a high risk

of postoperative aspiration pneumonia and cardiac dysrhythmias.

Congenital MD is an early onset form with bilateral facial weakness, feeding difficulties, delayed motor and cognitive milestones, mental development and severe hypotonia. Surviving children are often severely affected. It is not uncommon for such infants to be born to mildly affected mothers, in whom the diagnosis has not yet been made. Approximately 25 per cent of affected infants die before the age of 18 months and only 50 per cent survive to the third decade.

Non-dystrophic myotonias and paramyotonias

Congenital myotonias or 'myotonia congenita' fall into two main types – the autosomal dominant (Thomsen) and autosomal recessive (Becker). Patients usually experience generalized myotonia with onset in childhood or adolescence. Clinical features outside skeletal muscle are rare.

In **Thomsen's disease**, the myotonia is provoked by voluntary muscle contraction and is most severe after a period of rest, stress, fatigue, cold or hunger. **The patient interprets the myotonia as stiffness.** Repeated attempts at movement will initially cause the myotonia to worsen, but then to improve after a few contractions – this is the 'warm-up phenomenon'. The legs are more frequently affected than the arms, but hands and the cranial musculature may be significantly affected causing mild swallowing difficulties. Muscle hypertrophy is common. The CK is normal or slightly elevated. EMG demonstrates myotonia. Muscle biopsy may show type II atrophy, hypertrophied fibres and increased numbers of central nuclei.

Becker's disease is similar in its clinical features to the Thomsen type, although onset may be a little later and the myotonia is usually more severe. Transient weakness on muscle contraction is more obvious. The EMG, CK and muscle biopsy are similar.

Defects in the skeletal muscle chloride channel protein (CLCN1) have been identified in patients with myotonia congenita. Several different mutations in the gene can cause either the dominant or recessive forms. Treatment of myotonia congenita consists of antiarrhythmic agents, such as mexiletine and procainamide, often significantly improve myotonia, but side effects can limit the use of these drugs. Other drugs that are used include phenytoin, carbamazepine, quinine and acetazolamide. Mexiletine tends to produce the best reduction in myotonia with the fewest side effects, although it can prolong the QTc interval and therefore regular ECG monitoring is mandatory. General measures, such as avoidance of cold and an understanding of the 'warming up' phenomenon, may be of practical benefit. Drugs that exacerbate myotonia, such as fenoterol, a β2-agonist, and certain β-blockers and diuretics, should be avoided if possible. Myotonia is exacerbated by all depolarizing muscle relaxants and anaesthetics, and these can impair intubation or ventilation.

Paramyotonia congenita is an autosomal dominant disorder caused by mutations in the muscle sodium channel SCN4A and occasionally CLCN1. Patients with this disorder develop **myotonia during exercise and this increases with continuing exercise**. The myotonia is exacerbated by **cold**. The distribution of myotonia particularly affects the face and hands. This may produce pseudo lid lag. Patients usually present in early life with attacks of weakness. Exposure to cold may produce immobility of the face and stiffness in the hands. This may subsequently lead to weakness, which persists for several hours after warming. Although generalized myotonia can be reported in some circumstances, for example, swimming in cold water, respiratory involvement has not been reported. Serum CK is often elevated and the EMG typically shows myotonic discharges. Cooling reduces the amplitude of the evoked compound muscle action potential. Muscle biopsy can show non-specific myopathic changes and a few vacuolated fibres can be seen. Treatment with mexiletine has been used with success. During recovery from anaesthesia, there may be prolonged weakness and depolarizing muscle relaxants can lead to muscle stiffness.

The **Schwartz–Jampel syndrome** is a rare disorder which usually presents within the first three years of life, with muscle stiffness, particularly affecting the face and thighs. Children, who are often of small stature, have multiple skeletal deformities including platyspondylosis, muscle contractures, facial features, including blepharophimosis, pursed lips, small mouth and micrognathia, myopia and cataracts, and myokymia of the chin. Other dysmorphic features include low set ears, a crouched stance and a waddling gait. The disorder may be associated with mild mental retardation.

Persistent spontaneous activity is shown on EMG with continuous muscle discharges, myotonia and complex repetitive discharges. Levels of CK are normal or only mildly elevated. Muscle biopsy does not identify any specific changes. The syndrome is usually caused by mutations in the gene *perlecan* and is autosomal recessive. Perlecan is a major component of basement membranes and interstitial matrix in cartilage.

Periodic paralysis

Hypokalaemic periodic paralysis

Hypokalaemic periodic paralysis is an autosomal dominant disorder, although 30 per cent of cases are sporadic. Prevalence is approximately 1:100 000. Point mutations have been identified in the genes for the skeletal muscle calcium channel (CACNA1S), but also in the skeletal muscle sodium channel (SCN4A) and potassium channel (KCNE3).

Onset is usually in adolescence or early childhood, although rare adult-onset cases have been described. The patients complain of **attacks of weakness** which most often occur late at night or on waking. Large carbohydrate-rich or sodium-rich meals and rest after exertion are common precipitating factors. Cold and alcohol ingestion may occasionally induce an attack. Symptoms begin with stiffness and heaviness of the limbs, followed by weakness, usually in the legs. Severity is variable and may involve only mild loss of power, but can lead to profound generalized weakness. Attacks usually last hours, but can last several days with an extremely variable frequency of up to one per day to only a few attacks in a lifetime.

The frequency and severity of attacks usually diminish with advancing years. Respiratory and bulbar muscles are only occasionally involved. Myotonia usually does not occur except occasionally to affect the eyelids and muscle hypertrophy is very rare. Some patients over 40 begin to develop fixed weakness which progresses slowly over years. Cardiac involvement is very uncommon. Secondary forms of hypokalaemic periodic paralysis occur and are usually the result of chronic potassium depletion, such as severe diarrhoea, or thyrotoxicosis. The latter is most frequently seen in Japanese or Chinese people and is rare outside East Asia. The paralytic episodes may occasionally occur before the diagnosis of thyrotoxicosis.

The diagnosis of hypokalaemic periodic paralysis used to depend on the documentation of hypokalaemia during an attack. Hypokalaemia may be provoked with a glucose load with or without insulin, followed by careful monitoring of the serum potassium and ECG. Muscle strength is examined clinically for up to 6 hours. This type of provocation test can carry risks and should not be performed unless absolutely necessary and always with a physician in attendance. Monitoring by EMG may be useful in demonstrating a sustained fall in compound muscle action potential amplitude following isometric exercise. This methodology has recently been formalized into the McManis protocol EMG (see Chapter 5) which can provide electrophysiological evidence of a disorder of muscle membrane ion channels (channelopathy). Electrical myotonia is not seen in hypokalaemic periodic paralysis. Muscle biopsy may reveal the characteristic central vacuoles, sometimes filled with material staining on periodic acid-Schiff reaction (glycogen). Additional non-specific myopathic changes may also be seen on the biopsy.

In current practice, **diagnosis is made from a combination of a typical clinical phenotype, McManis protocol EMG and genetic testing.** The potassium levels can be normal during an attack and it is often practically difficult to coordinate taking a blood sample during an attack. There are patients with a clinical picture typical of a channelopathy, but in whom these tests are normal or inconclusive. These are probably patients with as yet undetected novel mutations.

The **treatment** of an acute attack of hypokalaemic periodic paralysis requires oral potassium replacement (0.23 mEq/kg body weight) given every 30 minutes until muscle strength improves. Serum potassium levels must be carefully monitored. Intravenous replacement can be used if the oral route is impractical. Intravenous potassium should be given with 5 per cent mannitol, as combination with glucose or normal saline will cause a drop in plasma potassium. Prophylactic treatment of acute attacks may involve the use of potassium supplements at bedtime or thiazide diuretics. Acetazolamide is the treatment of choice for prophylaxis and reduces attack frequency and severity, although, in about 10 per cent of patients, its use may actually exacerbate attacks, especially when associated with thyrotoxicosis. Dilchlorphenamide is an alternative carbonic anhydrase inhibitor that has greater efficacy and/or fewer side effects in some patients. An uncommon complication of carbonic anhydrase inhibitors is renal stone formation and a yearly ultrasound of the kidneys is recommended in all patients.

Hyperkalaemic periodic paralysis

Hyperkalaemic periodic paralysis is much less common than the hypokalaemic form and is associated with an elevation of serum potassium during an attack. The disorder is transmitted as autosomal dominant and sporadic cases have been described. Mutations in the gene encoding the alpha subunit of the skeletal muscle sodium channel (SCN4A) on chromosome 17q35 have been identified in patients with hypokalaemic periodic paralysis.

Attacks of generalized weakness usually begin in childhood. The attacks most commonly start in the morning and last less than an hour. Serum potassium becomes elevated, usually to greater than 5 mmol/L. Recovery is often improved by exercise, although some mild weakness may continue for several days. Between attacks, the patient and serum potassium are normal. The frequency of attacks is very variable and they are generally not as severe as those with hypokalaemic periodic paralysis. They may be triggered by muscular exercise with subsequent rest, alcohol, fasting, pregnancy and potassium loading. Myotonia may be seen in some but not all patients. Some mutations in SCN4A are associated with the development of fixed weakness.

As with hpokalaemic periodic paralysis, the diagnosis is established with a combination of a typical clinical phenotype, McManis protocol EMG and genetic testing.

Neuromyotonia

Neuromyotonia (Isaac's syndrome) is the result of hyperexcitability of peripheral nerves leading to spontaneous and continuous muscle activity. This may be triggered by muscle contraction and results **in muscle stiffness, cramps, myokymia and delayed muscle relaxation.**

Symptoms may begin at any age but occur most often in late childhood or early adulthood. Muscle stiffness is usually the first symptom and appears in distal limb muscles, slowly spreading over months or years to involve the axial and cranial muscles. Movement becomes slow. Myokymia can be seen in overactive muscles. Muscle relaxation after contraction is slow and percussion myotonia is absent. Increased sweating and muscle weakness with hyporeflexia is seen in some patients. Examination demonstrates mild weakness, which can be proximal, distal or both. Hallucinations, insomnia, seizures and intellectual impairment have been reported in some patients in conjunction with neuromyotonia, a polyneuropathy and sometimes an underlying thymoma (Morvan's syndrome).

Electromyography is diagnostic and reveals bursts of motor unit potentials firing at high rates. These discharges are often provoked by voluntary activity. The abnormal activity continues during sleep and is abolished by neuromuscular blockade. Nerve conduction studies themselves show no evidence of a peripheral neuropathy. Neither muscle nor nerve biopsies show any specific features. Increased CSF protein and oligoclonal bands have been described in some patients.

Neuromyotonia has occasionally been seen as a paraneoplastic disorder in association with tumours of the lung and thymus and Hodgkin's lymphoma. Antibodies to voltage-gated potassium channels are found in a high proportion of patients. Plasma exchange has resulted in clinical improvement in some patients.

MALIGNANT HYPERTHERMIA

Malignant hyperthermia (MH) is usually an autosomal dominantly inherited disorder and is most commonly caused by mutations in the ryanodine receptor gene on chromosome 19q (RYR1). Mutations in sodium ion channel gene, SCN4A, and two calcium channel genes have been described, as well as other cases where the gene has not been found.

> Malignant hyperthermia is characterized by a hypercatabolic reaction to **triggering factors**. These include **inhalation anaesthetics, such as halothane and depolarizing muscle relaxants, such as succinylcholine.** Physical exercise, trauma, heat, alcohol excess and infections have also been recorded as triggering MH. Approximately 50 per cent of patients with an MH reaction will have undergone previous anaesthesia without side effect.

MH is rare and is said to occur in about 1:15 000 anaesthetics in children and 1:50 000–200 000 anaesthetics in adults. Males are affected more than females and reactions occur most frequently between the ages of three and 30 years.

Muscle rigidity may begin shortly after infusion of the triggering agent. This makes intubation difficult as the rigidity of the masseter muscles is often intense, rendering it impossible to open the jaw. Cardiac dysrhythmias, labile systolic blood pressure, hyperventilation, fever and mottling cyanosis are all common features. A rise in pCO_2 or core temperature are probably the earliest signs of MH. An increasing pCO_2 and oxygen consumption, rising CK, calcium, magnesium, glucose and urea, as well as a lactic acidosis are common. Subsequent damage to the skeletal muscle membranes results in myoglobinuria. These changes are usually maximal 1–4 days after the start of the reaction. Late complications include renal failure, clotting disorders, cerebral and pulmonary oedema.

Muscle biopsies from individuals suspected of having MH can be investigated with the caffeine halothane contracture test. For the most part, muscle biopsies appear normal on light microscopy, although there is an association of MH with central core disease, a congenital myopathy. Treatment of MH is with dantrolene and this can also be used in the prevention of acute MH reactions. Treatment of acute MH also involves lowering of body temperature, correction of blood gases and appropriate management of other associated organ failure.

THE CONGENITAL MYOPATHIES

The congenital myopathies are disorders of skeletal muscle present at birth or early infancy which do not show dystrophic features, i.e. muscle cell death. They are associated with delayed motor milestones and disorders of other organs.

Central core disease

Central core disease is an autosomal dominant disorder associated with mutations in the ryanodine receptor gene (*RYR1*). It often presents with hypotonia and muscle weakness at birth followed by developmental motor delay. However, some patients have mild symptoms and are subsequently diagnosed on muscle biopsy with a raised CK only. The pattern of muscle weakness may be proximal or generalized and is not usually associated with significant wasting. There may be associated kyphoscoliosis or pes cavus. Cardiac and respiratory involvement can occur. The EMG shows a myopathic pattern. Muscle biopsy shows myopathic features, but the most prominent abnormality is the presence of central cores in muscle fibres, which probably comprise eccentric myofibrils. The cores are most easily seen in histochemical stains of oxidative enzymes, where the cores appear as regions of negative staining. There is often associated type I fibre predominance. Some patients also have malignant hyperthermia.

Minicore/multicore disease

Minicore/multicore disease is an autosomal recessive, sporadic and possibly dominant disorder characterized clinically by a slowly progressive or non-progressive childhood-onset myopathy. Weakness may involve axial muscles, the extraocular muscles and muscles of respiration. Kyphoscoliosis is common. The disease is associated with mutations in several genes including *RYR1*, *SEPN1* and *Titin*, although all causative genes are not known. There is characteristic muscle pathology of multiple small cores in individual muscle fibres.

Nemaline myopathy

There are three forms of nemaline myopathy:

Severe neonatal nemaline myopathy presents with cyanosis at birth, marked hypotonia, joint contractures and foot deformities. Feeding is poor. Swallowing difficulties may result in pneumonia. Respiratory involvement is often severe and may be associated with a dilated cardiomyopathy. Most affected infants die in the first weeks or months of life.

Mild non-progressive or slowly progressive nemaline myopathy presents with hypotonia and feeding difficulties in early life, but is less severe than the neonatal form. There is generalized muscle thinning but without focal wasting. Proximal weakness produces a waddling gait and there is often weakness of neck and trunk muscles. Facial muscles are often significantly affected, producing myopathic facies. Ocular muscles are rarely affected. Involvement of the bulbar muscles may produce

dysphonia and dysphagia. Mental development is usually normal. Many patients retain a reasonable degree of motor activity, but kyphoscoliosis may develop later in childhood. Approximately 20 per cent of children die in the first six years of life.

Both severe neonatal and mild nemaline myopathy are most commonly associated with mutations in the α-actin or nebulin genes.

Adult onset nemaline myopathy presents with weakness in adulthood, although an accurate history will often reveal some deficits in childhood. Cardiomyopathy is often associated with the proximal greater than distal limb weakness, posterior neck weakness and dysphagia which often develops from the fourth decade onwards. There are no known genetic associations and the disease is sporadic.

Serum CK is usually normal in the nemaline myopathies and EMG may be normal or mildly myopathic. Skeletal muscle biopsy reveals changes that are common to all the three main types of nemaline myopathies. In addition to general myopathic features, rods may be seen to be distributed at random throughout muscle fibres but particularly show clustering under the sarcolemma and around nuclei. Type I fibre type predominance is common. Electron microscopy reveals an accumulation of the rods, with localized enlargement and streaming of the Z lines. The rods themselves appear to originate from the Z discs.

Centronuclear myopathies

Centronuclear myopathy may be an X-linked, recessive or dominant disease. Early onset disease is the most common presentation with hypotonia, weakness and respiratory distress at birth. Dysmorphic features, including a thin face and high arched palate, may be present. There is often ptosis and facial asymmetry. Motor milestones are delayed and children are rarely able to run. Muscles are generally thin and there is diffuse weakness with easy fatigability. Muscle weakness usually progresses and most patients are wheelchair-bound by adolescence. Early onset cases tend to be caused by X-linked mutations in the *MTM1* gene or recessive mutations in the *BIN1* gene.

Dominant mutations in the *MYF6* and *DNM2* genes cause later onset disease with a milder phenotype. Slow progression of muscle weakness is usual and patients are often wheelchair-bound by the sixth decade.

Serum CK is usually normal and the EMG is myopathic. The main abnormality on muscle biopsy is the central position of nuclei in the majority of muscle fibres. Longitudinal sections may show long chains of nuclei in the centre of fibres. A small perinuclear halo, with absent histochemical enzyme activity, is often seen. There is usually a preponderance of type I fibres.

THE INFLAMMATORY MYOPATHIES

The idiopathic inflammatory myopathies include polymyositis, dermatomyositis and inclusion body myositis. Inflammation of muscle may also occur in response to certain bacterial, viral or parasitic infections. Inflammatory changes may be seen on the muscle biopsy in some muscular dystrophies, especially FSHD. Inflammatory changes can also be seen in muscle in response to certain drugs or graft-versus-host disease.

Polymyositis and dermatomyositis

Polymyositis and dermatomyositis may occur at any age, although most cases of dermatomyositis in childhood present between the ages of five and 15 years, while most adult cases of polymyositis present between the ages of 50 and 70 years. Females are more often affected than males and the annual incidence is between 0.5 and 1:100 000.

Childhood-onset dermatomyositis is associated with a slow progressive onset of a photosensitive, purple or heliotropic skin rash over extensor surfaces of the limbs, anterior chest and neck and periorbital regions. A scaly purple/red rash may also be seen over extensor joints (Gottron's papules). Proximal upper and lower limb muscle weakness typically occurs simultaneously with the rash. Changes in the finger nails include cuticular overgrowth and nail bed telangiectasia. Digital ulcerations may also be seen. Progression of symptoms is variable, but may advance to involve all muscles, including those of swallowing and respiration. Flexion contractures and calcification in subcutaneous tissues and muscle may develop in up to half of affected children. Arthralgias, myalgias and arthritis are also common.

In **adult patients with dermatomyositis and polymyositis,** weakness progresses insidiously and mainly involves the proximal upper and lower limb muscles. Dysphagia and neck flexion weakness may follow and involve muscles of respiration in severe cases. Skin lesions are similar to those seen in childhood in dermatomyositis. Cardiac involvement is relatively uncommon but can lead to cardiac dysrhythmias and congestive cardiac failure in severe cases. Pulmonary complications most commonly cause a restrictive defect as a result of respiratory muscle involvement causing type 2 respiratory failure.

Patients with polymyositis may also develop interstitial fibrosing lung disease, most frequently in the lung bases, causing type 1 respiratory failure. Symptoms include fever, cough and dyspnoea, and lung infiltrates are visible on chest x-ray. It is often associated with anti-Jo-1 antibodies in serum.

Polymyositis and dermatomyositis may be associated with malignancy. Reports of the incidence of underlying carcinoma vary between 6 and 45 per cent for dermatomyositis and 0 and 28 per cent for polymyositis. This association has no gender preference, but is more frequent in patients over the age of 40 years. In one study, an underlying carcinoma was found in 40 per cent of patients over the age of 40 years with dermatomyositis, although another study found only 8.5 per cent of similar patients to have an underlying carcinoma. Identification of the malignancy may precede or follow the diagnosis of polymyositis or dermatomyositis, although onset of each disorder is usually within 12 months of the other.

Investigations often demonstrate an elevated serum CK and ESR, although these may be normal in a proportion of cases. Approximately half of the patients have a significantly important positive ANA (anti-nuclear antibody) test. EMG usually shows decreased motor unit potentials together with reduced amplitude. There is increased insertional activity with fibrillation potentials and positive sharp waves (see Chapter 5).

Muscle biopsy is essential for the diagnosis of dermatomyositis or polymyositis. There is often an intense inflammatory infiltrate with lymphocytes, plasma cells and macrophages. These cells may be endomysial or invading muscle fibres especially in polymyositis (Figure 18.6). Necrotic muscle fibres are

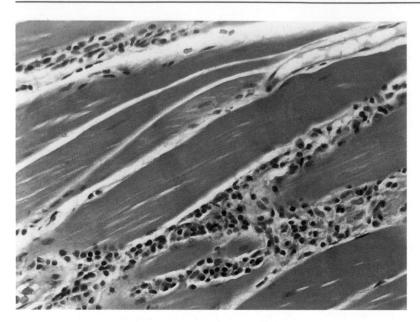

Figure 18.6 Polymyositis (paraffin section, H&E ×300): portion of three necrotic fibres with many large nuclei and macrophages and slightly more numerous round dark nuclei of lymphocytes. The intervening fibres are microscopically normal.

seen together with some evidence of regenerating fibres. Other non-specific changes include variation in fibre diameters and some increase in connective tissue. In dermatomyositis, perivascular collections of inflammatory cells may be seen and capillaries often have complement deposition; endothelial hyperplasia and small infarcts are often detected in childhood dermatomyositis. Perifascicular atrophy may also be a feature of dermatomyositis.

The mainstay of **treatment is immunosuppression**, starting with pulsed methyl prednisolone if the disease is severe and then prednisolone at 0.75–1 mg/kg per day. This is often followed by a steroid-sparing agent, such as azathioprine, methotrexate and mycophenalate, as the clinical and laboratory features of the disease are beginning to improve. Intravenous immunoglobulin may be used in patients with dermatomyositis especially when the disease is severe and affects respiratory and swallowing muscles.

The prognosis in childhood dermatomyositis is variable. In one study, approximately 15 per cent of children died in spite of adequate therapy, 50 per cent recovered incompletely and the remainder returned virtually to normal. The prognosis is more favourable in adults without an underlying malignancy. Eighty per cent of patients survive five years.

Inclusion body myositis

Inclusion body myositis (IBM) exists in two forms, a relatively common sporadic form and rare familial forms. Sporadic IBM occurs in those over 50 years in 80 per cent of cases. There is a 3:1 male:female preponderance. IBM is the most common late onset muscular degenerative disease and it is probably under-recognized.

Patients present with muscle weakness of insidious onset and progression. The weakness typically affects the quadriceps causing knee extension weakness and difficulty climbing stairs. Ankle dorsiflexors are also commonly affected causing foot drop. A common clinical feature is forearm wasting with finger flexor weakness which causes difficulty in grasping objects. Facial muscles are involved in a minority of patients and bulbar weakness becomes more common as the disease progresses. Extraocular muscle involvement is rare. Respiratory and abdominal muscles may be affected in about 10 per cent of patients. Cardiac involvement is rare. Wasting is often seen and is proportionate to the weakness. Tendon reflexes may be retained until late in the disease.

There is an association of IBM with diabetes mellitus, but there is no association with underlying malignancy.

The ESR and CK are usually normal or only mildly elevated, EMG shows motor unit potentials of short duration and a high proportion of polyphasic units. There are frequent fibrillation potentials and positive sharp waves (see Chapter 5). Muscle biopsy shows a variable degree of inflammatory infiltration and muscle fibre necrosis. The characteristic finding is rimmed vacuoles within muscle fibres. Immunohistochemistry shows that these contain a variety of proteins including ubiquitin, β-amyloid, desmin and prion protein. Mitochondrial changes can also be seen with ragged red fibres and occasional excess of cytochrome oxidase negative fibres. Inflammatory infiltration is predominantly with endomysial CD8-positive T cells. MHC class 1 is often significantly elevated on the sarcolemmal membrane. An additional feature on light microscopy is of several small, often angulated, fibres suggesting a neurogenic component. Electron microscopy shows abnormal accumulations of filaments within the nucleus and the cytoplasm.

Inclusion body myopathy with dementia and Paget's disease of the bone has been described in association with Valosin-containing protein (VCP). The onset is often earlier than sporadic IBM and tends to affect distal and respiratory muscles more often. Other hereditary forms of IBM have been described caused by mutations in muscle proteins, such as desmin.

There is no specific treatment for IBM. Many patients are treated with steroids or intravenous immunoglobulin, but response is usually poor. Nevertheless, those with evidence of a significant inflammatory infiltrate on biopsy and in the early stages of the disease should be offered a trial of immunosuppression.

DEFECTS OF THE NEUROMUSCULAR JUNCTION

Myasthenia gravis

Myasthenia gravis (MG) is an autoimmune disorder caused by the production of antibodies against the nicotinic acetylcholine receptor at the post-synaptic membrane of the neuromuscular junction. The aetiology underlying the generation of these antibodies is unknown, but there is a clear association with other autoimmune disorders, particularly thyroid disease, and with abnormalities of the thymus gland, including thymic hyperplasia or thymoma. MG tends to affect young women in their 20s and older men in their 70s.

> **The characteristic clinical feature of MG is fatiguable weakness following contraction of voluntary muscles.** Patients often present with episodic diplopia and ptosis. There may be facial weakness (Figure 18.7), slurring of **speech, dysphagia and dyspnoea** as a result of respiratory muscle involvement. **Limb weakness is usually proximal and neck flexion weakness** is common. There is often a clear diurnal variation in that patients may start the morning feeling normal, but gradually fatigue through the day.
>
> Examination may reveal ptosis and ophthalmoplegia, which are the presenting features in 50 per cent of patients and eventually develop in 90 per cent. Fatiguability of *levator palpebrae superioris* may be demonstrated by Cogan's lid twitch (see above under Symptoms of muscle disease) and by asking the patient to sustain upward gaze. Fatiguability of the proximal muscles should be tested before and following repeated contractions, such as shoulder abduction. Wasting of muscles is unusual, although it can develop in advanced cases. Tendon reflexes are normal or brisk. Sensation is normal.

Myasthenic symptoms

- Ocular
  - ptosis
  - diplopia
  - weak eye closure
- Bulbar
- Neck
- Respiratory
- Proximal muscle weakness

The investigation of MG (Box 18.2) involves the demonstration of **acetylcholine receptor (AchR) antibodies**, although these are absent in 15 per cent of patients. Patients who have only ophthalmoplegia (ocular MG) have a lower incidence of antibodies (50 per cent). About 85 per cent of patients with more generalized myasthenia have acetylcholine receptor antibodies (seropositive). More recently, 50 per cent of patients who are seronegative have

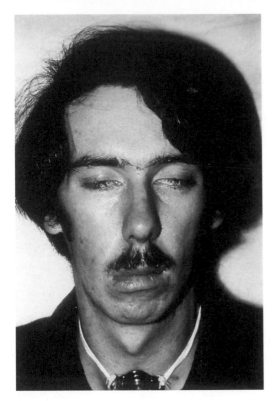

Figure 18.7 Bilateral ptosis and facial weakness in myasthenia gravis.

Box 18.2 Investigation of myasthenia gravis

- Blood
  - Full blood count, ESR
  - Creatine kinase
  - TSH, T4
  - Acetylcholine receptor antibodies (+ve in 85% generalized myasthenia)
- Muscle-specific kinase antibodies (found in c.50% of sero-negative myasthenics)
  - Striated muscle antibodies (+ve with thymoma)
  - Voltage-gated calcium channel antibodies
  - (Lambert–Eaton)
- Imaging
  - Chest x-ray, CT scan chest (thymoma)
- Electrodiagnosis
  - Before and after exercise
  - Repetitive stimulation (proximal muscle)
  - Single fibre EMG – 'jitter'
- Pharmacological
  - Edrophonium test

ESR, erythrocyte sedimentation rate; TSH, thyroid stimulating hormone; CT, computerized tomography; EMG, electromyography.

been found to have antibodies to muscle-specific kinase (anti-MUSK) antibodies. Other organ-specific autoimmune disorders may occur with MG especially affecting the thyroid. **Electrophysiological studies** show a decrement in the CMAP on repetitive stimulation and the presence of jitter and block on single fibre studies (see Chapter 5).

The **edrophonium (Tensilon) test** is an important diagnostic investigation and should always be undertaken in a double-blind fashion in hospital, with appropriate resuscitation facilities immediately available, because edrophonium can cause bradyarrhythmias. Useful clinical measures to judge the effectiveness of edrophonium include improvement in ptosis, diplopia and proximal limb fatigability. The patient is given a covering dose of atropine and then a test dose of 2 mg of edrophonium intravenously. If this produces no effect, then the remaining dose, up to 10 mg, is given. A positive effect is usually seen within a few seconds and lasts for a few minutes.

CT **or** MRI **scan of the thorax** is undertaken to help exclude a **thymoma, which especially in the elderly, may have undergone malignant transformation.** Thymoma is associated with **anti-striated muscle antibodies**.

Anti-acetylcholine esterase drugs, pyridostigmine and neostigmine, are symptomatic treatments for myasthenia gravis, but do not treat the underlying disease process. Pyridostigmine acts within 60 minutes and lasts for 3–6 hours. Typical dosages may be 30–90 mg every 6 hours, but doses in excess of this should be used with caution, as the drug may lead to an exacerbation of weakness (cholinergic crisis). The edrophonium test is useful to distinguish myasthenic weakness from a cholinergic crisis due to treatment. Again, ventilatory support must be immediately available.

Plasmapheresis or IVIg are used in acute severe exacerbations of myasthenia gravis.

Immunosuppressive therapy with alternate-day corticosteroids will induce improvement over several weeks and are given in combination with daily steroid-sparing immunosuppressants, such as azathioprine, mycophenalate cyclophosphamide or cyclosporin. Steroids should be started at a low dose and gradually increased as there may be an initial deterioration with steroids. Complete remission in response to steroids and other immunosuppressant therapy has been reported in 40–70 per cent of patients. Certain drugs (Table 18.2) may aggravate myasthenia gravis.

Thymectomy may induce remission in approximately 50 per cent of selected patients within seven to ten years. Young women with high titres of AchR antibodies and thymic hyperplasia respond more rapidly than men, but at ten years there is no difference between male and female groups. Thymectomy is usually undertaken through a mediastinal approach as a transcervical approach may not remove all thymic tissue, and it is important that all thymic tissues is removed. The presence of a thymoma is an absolute indication for thymectomy as malignant transformation may occur. The removal of a thymoma does not improve the MG.

Lambert–Eaton myasthenic syndrome

Lambert–Eaton myasthenic syndrome (LEMS) is an autoimmune disorder caused by antibodies against the presynaptic voltage-sensitive calcium channel of the motor nerve terminal. The male:female ratio is approximately 5:1 and 75 per cent of males and 25 per cent of females have an underlying malignancy, although this is uncommon under the age of 40 years. The majority of malignancies are small cell carcinomas of the lung.

Patients present with weakness and fatigability, particularly of the lower limb muscles. Seventy per cent of patients have mild ocular symptoms, such as ptosis or diplopia, but patients never present with ocular weakness. There may be autonomic nervous system abnormalities including decreased salivation, lacrimation, sweating, postural hypotension and impotence. There may be weakness at rest, particularly in the lower limbs, but isometric muscle contraction improves strength, although power may subsequently fatigue. Tendon reflexes are usually absent, but are briefly restored following sustained contraction for a few seconds, a useful diagnostic sign (post-tetanic potentiation).

AchR antibodies are not present and an edrophonium test usually produces no improvement in the weakness. EMG shows increased jitter and block with single fibre studies. Repetitive stimulation at 10 Hz or higher produces a gradual increase in the compound muscle action potential (see Chapter 5).

Treatment of LEMS includes appropriate management of any underlying malignancy. Specific treatment is with 3,4-diaminopyridine, which improves strength by prolonging the duration of the presynaptic action potential and increases calcium entry into the nerve terminal. Plasmapheresis and IVIg can sometimes be helpful.

Table 18.2 Drugs that aggravate myasthenia gravis

Type of medication	Drug name
Neuromuscular block	Succinylcholine, vercuronium, D-tubocurarine
Cardiac drugs	Procainamide, quinidine, quinine
Calcium channel	Verapamil, diltiazem blockers
Beta blockers	Atenolol, metoprolol, propranolol, timolol eye drops
Aminoglycoside	Gentamicin, streptomycin – antibiotics rarely, ampicillin, tetracycline, ciprofloxacin
Miscellaneous	Chloroquine, ketoprofen, lithium, phenytoin
D-penicillamine	May induce or aggravate

FURTHER READING

Hart PE, De Vivo DC, Schapira AHV (2002) Clinical features of the mitochondrial encephalomyopathies. In: Schapira AHV, DiMauro S (eds). *Mitochondrial Disorders in Neurology*, 2nd edn. London: Butterworth Heinemann, 35–68.

Karpati G, Hilton Jones D, Bushby K, Griggs RC (eds) (2010) *Disorders of Voluntary Muscle*, 8th edn. Cambridge: Cambridge University Press.

Katirji B, Kaminski H, Preston D et al. (eds) (2002) *Neuromuscular Disorders in Clinical Practice*. London: Butterworth Heinemann.

Rahman S, Schapira AHV (1999) Mitochondrial myopathies clinical features, molecular genetics, investigation and management. In: Schapira AHV, Griggs RC (eds). *Muscle diseases*. London: Butterworth Heinemann, 177–223.

Schapira AHV (2002) The 'new' mitochondrial disorders. *Journal of Neurology, Neurosurgery and Psychiatry*, 72:144–149.

DEMENTIA

Catherine Mummery

INTRODUCTION

Dementia is common and places a tremendous burden on patients, their carers and society. This burden will only increase as our society ages. There are approximately 700 000 people with dementia in the UK today, a number forecast to double within a generation. Forty-two per cent of the UK population are affected by dementia by knowing a friend or family member with the condition. In spite of this, until recently, dementia attracted remarkably little scientific resource.

In recent years, there has been a major shift in recognition of the problem. Public awareness has been greatly enhanced by government initiatives, such as the National Dementia Strategy. Considerable advances have been made in our understanding of the epidemiology, pathogenesis and diagnosis of different forms of dementia. New biomarkers are being developed, better able to predict pathology, which are changing the way we classify dementia. Furthermore, emergent agents, such as immunomodulation therapies, will be able to alter the course of diseases, such as Alzheimer's disease (AD) in the foreseeable future.

Definition of dementia as yet lags behind. According to the International Classification of Diseases, 10th edn (ICD10), dementia 'is a syndrome due to disease of the brain, usually of a chronic or progressive nature, in which there is impairment of higher cortical functions, includ-ing memory, thinking, orientation, comprehension, calculation, learning capacity, language and judgement. The cognitive impairments are commonly accompanied, and occasionally preceded, by deterioration in emotional control, social behaviour or motivation.'

Within this 'catch-all' definition, myriad presentations occur. The dominant symptoms depend on the brain regions most affected by the disease.

- Dementia describes a clinical syndrome of progressive cognitive impairment.
- It has numerous causes (**Table 19.1**), and clinical diagnosis should always prompt careful investigation.
- Topography determines phenotype.

Fortunately, for diagnostic purposes, certain pathologies have predilection for certain brain areas (e.g. Alzheimer's and the entorhinal cortex), frequently allowing prediction of the likely disease process responsible for a particular syndrome.

Epidemiology and classification

The risk of developing dementia increases dramatically with age (Table 19.2).

Early attempts to classify dementia distinguished between presenile and senile dementia. However, the same pathological processes can afflict the elderly and the relatively young: these

Table 19.1 Causes of dementia

	Sporadic		Genetic
Degenerative	Alzheimer's disease		Familial AD: PSEN-1/PSEN-2/APP
	Frontotemporal lobar degeneration – FTD/SD/PNFA		FTDP-17
	Parkinsonian 'plus' syndromes – DLB/PDD		HD/DRPLA/SCAs
		MSA/CBD/PSP	Neuroacanthocytosis
		Neurofilamentopathy	PKAN – Hallervorden Spatz
Vascular	Strategic infarct	CADASIL	
	Multiple cortical infarcts	Fabry's	
	Small vessel disease	Cerebral amyloid angiopathy	
Inflammatory	MS/neurosarcoidosis/Behçet's disease		
	Vasculitis, e.g. PAN; SLE; primary CNS vasculitis		
Infective/ transmissible	HIV/AIDS–dementia complex		
	CJD – variant; sporadic; iatrogenic	Familial prion GSS/FFI	
	Neurosyphilis; TB; fungal		
	PML; SSPE		
	Whipple's disease; Lyme disease		
Neoplastic/ paraneoplastic	Tumour (primary or metastatic)		
	Limbic encephalitis – classical/ VGKCA/ANMDA		
Metabolic/ nutritional	Hypothyroidism; B12 deficiency; uraemia, hepatic	Wilson's disease; CTX	
Epilepsy			
Toxins	Alcohol; heavy metal poisoning; organic solvents		
	Drugs, e.g. lithium; CO poisoning		
Head injury	Dementia pugilistica		
	Chronic subdural haematoma		
Other cause	Normal pressure hydrocephalus		
	Obstructive sleep apnoea		
Lysosomal and other storage disorders	Metachromatic leukodystrophy		
	Neimann Pick – type C		
	Kuf's/Batten's/Krabbe's disease		
	Mitochondrial		

CJD, Creuzfeldt–Jakob disease; CNS, central nervous system; CO, carbon dioxide; CTX, chemotherapy; DLB, dementia with Lewy bodies; DRPLA, dentatorubro-pallidoluysian atrophy; FFI, fatal familial insomnia; FTD, frontotemporal dementia; GSS, Gerstmann–Straussler–Scheinker; HD, Huntington's disease; PAN, polyarteritis nodosa; PDD, Parkinson's disease with dementia; PNFA, progressive non-fluent aphasia; SCA, spinocerebellar ataxia; SD, semantic dementia; SLE, systemic lupus erythematosus, TB, tuberculosis.

Table 19.2 Prevalence of dementia in UK

Age (years)	Prevalence	Prevalence
40–65	0.1%	(1 in 1000)
65–70	2.0%	(1 in 50)
70–80	5.0%	(1 in 25)
80 plus	20.0%	(1 in 5)

terms are no longer favoured. The description **young onset dementia** is used to depict those under 65 years of age presenting with dementia. This group have a different disease profile and must be thought of separately.

There are many causes of dementia; the most common are degenerative. However, many are treatable and even reversible, particularly in younger patients, e.g. Wilson's disease, porphyria and cerebral vasculitis. In the under-40 age group, inherited errors of metabolism, mitochondrial and other genetic disorders are over-represented.

CLINICAL ASSESSMENT

Dementia may present in a variety of ways: as a complaint of impaired performance or behaviour, in association with neurological or psychiatric symptoms, or as a part of a widespread disease process (Table 19.3). The onset and progression process can be either insidious, or alternatively a rapidly progressive deterioration can occur, with development of neurological and cognitive abnormalities in parallel.

Key questions in defining the problem include:
- Organic or psychiatric?
- Delirium, dementia, both or neither?
- Earliest symptoms?
- Length of history?
- Tempo? Fluctuation/gradual progression/stepwise?
- Impact on social and occupational functioning?

Dementia must be distinguished from acute confusional states and psychiatric disorders. The term 'acute confusional state' refers to a neurobehavioral disorder characterized by an acute change in mental status, fluctuation and deficits in attention. Acute confusional states (delirium) account for 10–25 per cent of all hospital admis-

Table 19.3 Dementia and other causes of cognitive impairment

	Dementia	Acute confusional State	Learning difficulties	Depression
Conscious state	Alert	Impaired	Alert	Alert
Onset	Acquired; insidious	Acquired; abrupt	Developmental	Acquired; variable
Progression	Yes	Fluctuation; circadian disruption	No	Fluctuation; improvement with treatment
Orientation	Initially preserved	Early prominent disorientation	Preserved	Variable
Hallucinations	Late	Prominent	Absent	Auditory possible
Behaviour	Depends on topography	Marked restlessness	May show static behavioural disturbance	Withdrawn
Other characteristic features	Depends on pathology	Identifiable systemic or CNS disorder	History of developmental disorder	Withdrawn; other features of depression; psychomotor retardation

CNS, central nervous system.

sions over 65 years old. It is important to realize that the cognitively impaired brain has a much lower threshold for developing delirium, hence dementia is a major risk factor for delirium.

History

Obtaining a reliable history is the key to diagnosis. It is essential to obtain a collateral history, as patients often lack insight. Independent discussion with a carer or relative assists understanding of the extent of problems and prevents fear of embarrassment or contradiction.

Earliest symptoms correlate with the area of the brain first affected; subsequent symptoms parallel the march of the disease through the brain. The pattern of spread is dictated to some extent by pathology and gives an indication as to aetiology. For example, **in Alzheimer's disease, recent memory impairment is the most common initial complaint**, and probably reflects early degeneration of hippocampal regions. In **frontotemporal dementia (FTD), changes in personality** are initially reported, mirroring early involvement of frontal structures.

The mode of onset and progression are important in diagnosis. A gradual onset with steady evolution implies degeneration or a structural cause, while abrupt onset and stepwise progression can suggest a cerebrovascular origin. Rapidly progressive dementia with psychiatric features might suggest spongiform encephalopathy or a vasculitic cause. Specific precipitants, such as significant life events, should be sought especially with a fluctuating or static history of cognitive deficit. Additional neurological features are common in many causes and should be specifically asked for, such as fasciculations in a patient with a progressive behavioural disorder, indicative of frontotemporal dementia, associated with motor neurone disease (FTD-MND). Table 19.4 highlights 'red flags' in rapidly progressive dementias.

In the past, the occurrence of relevant previous events, such as head injury, should be sought, as well as vascular risk factors and malignancy. A detailed history of drugs, alcohol consumption and lifestyle risk factors should be obtained. Enquiry into the family history should include psychiatric and neurological disorders, even if unspecified; the possibility of family history being 'masked' by young deaths should be considered.

Examination

Examination should attempt to answer the following questions:
- What is the pattern of cognitive impairment?
- Are there any abnormalities of the nervous system apart from dementia?
- Are there any relevant findings on general examination?

Careful general examination must be performed. Neurological examination may reveal pointers to the aetiology. For example, anosmia with frontal lobe features may point to an inferior frontal meningioma. Visual field abnormalities can imply occipital lobe dysfunction. Eye movements may be abnormal when there is basal ganglia or cerebellar involvement. A pseudobulbar palsy can occur with brainstem involvement due to vascular disorders or, rarely, Wilson's disease. Dysarthria may indicate brainstem involvement if explosive, cerebellar if slurring and can suggest a specific disorder, e.g. in progressive supranuclear palsy (PSP) speech becomes distinctively slow, hoarse and effortful.

In the limbs, the presence of a peripheral neuropathy may indicate alcoholism, or disorders such as metachromatic leukodystrophy. Fasciculation with wasting may occur in FTD-MND (see also Chapter 17), while asymmetric long tract signs may suggest cerebrovascular disease. Early chorea in Huntington's disease may be subtle, but the characteristic jerks and facial grimaces may become more noticeable when the patient is distracted.

Gait disturbance may be revealing. The festinant, shuffling gait of the parkinsonian patient contrasts with the ramrod axial rigidity in patients with progressive supranuclear palsy. Gait apraxia (seen in vascular disease and 'normal pressure hydrocephalus') may result in an inability to put one foot in front of the other, yet when lying on the bed, walking movements may be mimed satisfactorily.

Cognitive evaluation

Observation provides a wealth of information. Restlessness and stereotypical movements while sitting in the waiting room may suggest a frontal disorder. Head-turning – constantly looking to the carer for answers to questions – may be seen in Alzheimer's disease. Bedside testing can be used to

Table 19.4 Causes of rapidly progressive dementia

	Cause		
Reversible	Non-convulsive status epilepticus	Episodic, fluctuation, topographical amnesia	
	Cerebral vasculitis	Rapid, headache, seizures	
	Paraneoplastic limbic encephalitis	Rapid, complex neurology, behavioural change, smoker	
	VGKCAB/ANMDA encephalitides	Rapid, severe, seizures, psychiatric, hyponatraemia	
	Cerebrovascular e.g. SLE, APL	Brisk facial reflexes, flexor plantars, risk factors	
	Drug toxicities (especially lithium)	Rapid, neurological features, altered csness, tremor	
	Tuberculous and fungal meningitides	Systemic features, immunosuppression	
	Parenchymal Whipple's disease	GI symptoms	
	Chronic subdural haematoma	Rapid, HX falls, fluctuation	
	?Hashimoto's encephalopathy	Stroke-like episodes, migraine	
Irreversible	Rapidly progressive neurodegenerative variants:	DLB/AD	Accelerated decline; neurological signs, e.g. myoclonus
	Sporadic CJD	Rapid, myoclonus, global impairment	
	Variant CJD		Psychiatric, dysaesthesiae, ataxia, (rapid, young)

AD, Alzheimer's disease; ANMDA, anti-NMDA encephalitis; CJD, Creuzfeldt–Jakob disease; DLB, dementia with Lewy bodies; GI, gastrointestinal; SLE, systemic lupus erythematosus; VGKCAB, voltage-gated calcium channel antibody.

test the preserved and affected cognitive domains, although this does not obviate the need for detailed neuropsychological testing, which delineates the precise pattern of deficit, thus providing pointers towards certain types of disease.

The Mini-Mental State Examination (MMSE) (see Chapter 3) is performed as a screen of cognitive impairment in most clinics. It is valuable as a measure of change in illnesses such as Alzheimer's disease, but is insensitive and user-dependent. For example, a patient with FTD may score normally for many years despite having significant cognitive disturbances. Additional bedside tests with the rest of the assessment give a profile of the affected brain areas and hence the likely pathology. Table 19.5 gives examples of syndromes suggesting location of the disease process.

It can also be useful to distinguish between **cortical and subcortical presentations**. The terms do not imply that pathological changes are limited to cortical or subcortical structures, but provide a guide to the dominant brain regions involved.

Cortical dementias typically cause selective changes in memory function or other focal cognitive domains in the early stages, depending on the main site of pathology. The subject's processing speed may be normal, the level of motivation unchanged, and many aspects of executive function intact. There are seldom focal neurological signs or evidence of extrapyramidal dysfunction. The term **subcortical dementia** indicates a syndrome in which slowness of mental processes, decreased initiative, and mood changes dominate over impairment of intellectual functions. Disorders producing this syndrome tend to cause subcortical damage with extrapyramidal or pyramidal signs. A typical subcortical pattern is found in diseases such as Parkinson's disease with dementia.

Table 19.5 Patterns indicating location of pathology

History	Examination	Location
Change in behaviour, personality or mood	Executive dysfunction Apathy/disinhibition	Frontal/subcortical
Difficulty in word-finding, expression or comprehension	Fluent/nonfluent aphasia	Dominant – ? FTLD
Ever become lost? Facial recognition poor?	Topographical confusion Episodic amnesia	Mesial temporal – AD
History of visual misperceptions or hallucinations	Visuoperceptual deficit Attentional deficits Extrapyramidal	Posterior – ? PDD/DLB
Misidentification, e.g. Capgras syndrome?	Reading Writing	Posterior hemisphere
Are there motor or autonomic features?	Extrapyramidal	Subcortical
Are there extra-neurological physical symptoms?	Bradyphrenia, e.g. Livedo reticularis	Systemic disorder

AD, Alzheimer's disease; DLB, dementia with Lewy bodies; FTLD; frontotemporal lobar degeneration; PDD, Parkinson's disease with dementia

Memory testing can help determine whether the dementia is cortical or subcortical. In cortical disorders, memory shows a 'storage deficit' – once the memory is gone, it cannot be recalled (the 'file' has been lost; no amount of searching will find it); in subcortical pathology, memory may be impaired but can often be recalled eventually (the 'filing system' is disorganized – the search takes longer and is unreliable, but may eventually be successful) – an 'access deficit' (Table 19.6).

INVESTIGATION

Clinical assessment (Box 19.1) is diagnostically more useful than an unconsidered battery of tests. The aim of investigation is to identify the pathological process as accurately as possible. Paramount is the identification of any treatable cause of dementia.

Table 19.6 Dementia: cortical versus subcortical

	Cortical	Subcortical
Speed of cognition	Normal	Slow
Attention	Relatively intact	Impaired
Memory	Prominent deficit	Variable
	Lost file	Lost filing system
Executive	Less prominent	Often prominent
Behaviour/affect	Often normal	Often abnormal
Language	Aphasic features	Word retrieval difficulties
For example	Alzheimer's disease	Huntington's disease

Box 19.1 Investigations in dementia

- Essential investigations to delineate problem and exclude treatable conditions:
  - Blood tests: FBC, ESR, CRP, B12/folate, TSH, treponemal serology, renal and liver function, calcium
  - Chest x-ray
  - Imaging – MRI
  - Psychometry
- Investigations dependent on age and clinical features:
  - Blood tests – autoantibody studies including antineuronal Abs, VGKCAbs, thyroid microsomal abs, anti-NMDA abs, HIV serology, serum copper and caeruloplasmin
  - Urine – urinary copper
  - EEG
  - CSF examination to exclude treatable causes: cells, protein, oligoclonal bands
    - for dementia specific proteins: tau, abeta 1-42, 14-3-3 and S100
    - for virology, e.g. JC, HIV, HHV; cytology
  - Functional imaging – SPECT (DaT); FDG PET
- Investigations occasionally indicated:
  - Blood tests: white cell enzymes, e.g. metachromatic leukodystrophy
  - Neurogenetics: HD, familial prion, familial AD
  - Biopsy of peripheral tissues, e.g. muscle, peripheral nerve; small bowel biopsy in Whipple's disease; tonsillar biospy in nvCJD
  - Brain biopsy (highly selected group) younger patients in whom all other tests have been negative, or when a histological diagnosis may determine a specific therapy

Blood tests

In all patients, a screen of bloods should be performed. Routine haematology and biochemistry often detect comorbidity, but of particular importance in dementia is the presence of anaemia, and evidence of inflammatory or vasculitic disorder, B12 deficiency and thyroid dysfunction. Neurosyphilis, although uncommon, is so protean in its manifestations that serology should be sent. Tests for more complex inflammatory, endocrine or metabolic causes of dementia should be undertaken where clinically indicated. HIV testing should be considered at any age if there are appropriate clinical indicators. Autoantibodies, antineuronal antibodies and those implicated in limbic encephalitis should be performed in rapid onset dementia or evidence of systemic disease. In early adulthood, white cell enzymes and very long chain fatty acid assays may be relevant.

Neurogenetics

Genotyping is labour-intensive and expensive so should be selectively performed and based on a full, accurate family history.

Lumbar puncture

Guidelines recommend cerebrospinal fluid (CSF) examination in the under 65s. It is obligatory if a treatable cause is possible. A lymphocytosis may point to an infective, inflammatory or vasculitic disorder; the presence of oligoclonal bands may suggest an immune process, e.g. limbic encephalitis. CSF determination of tau and abeta 42 can help predict a diagnosis of AD. S100 and protein 14.3.3 are measured when Creutzfeldt–Jakob disease (CJD) is considered; although not specific, they can provide supportive evidence.

Electroencephalography

In most dementias, electroencephalography (EEG) findings are non-specific. However, in some situations the EEG may be revealing, e.g. subclinical epilepsy and CJD, in which periodic sharp wave complexes are typical in later stages. Loss of normal rhythms with diffuse slowing usually indicates a diffuse or metabolic disorder. Loss of alpha rhythm supports a diagnosis of Alzheimer's disease; a normal EEG in the face of significant behavioural and language change is consistent with frontal temporal lobar degeneration.

Imaging

Magnetic resonance imaging

Brain imaging is obligatory in a patient with dementia. The primary goal is to exclude structural lesions (Figure 19.1); additionally, magnetic resonance imaging (MRI) allows assessment of signal change and patterns of atrophy consistent with particular forms of dementia. Signal change can suggest underlying inflammatory disorders or

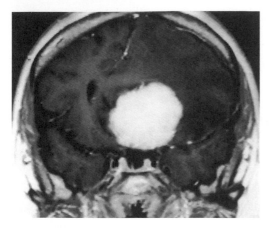

Figure 19.1 Gadolinium-enhanced coronal view magnetic resonance brain scan: large subfrontal meningioma presenting with dementia and apathy.

prion disease. For example, increased signal in the thalami on T2-weighted MRI scans is characteristic of variant CJD (Figure 19.2). Some patterns of atrophy are predictive of pathology, for example, early atrophy of hippocampal regions is characteristic of Alzheimer's disease; knife-edge atrophy in the temporal lobes suggests frontotemporal lobar degeneration (FTLD) (Figure 19.3). In cerebrovascular disease, imaging can delineate multiple infarcts or significant small vessel disease (Figure 19.4). Serial scanning can demonstrate progressive loss in

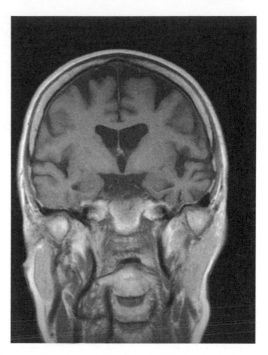

Figure 19.3 Coronal T1-weighted MRI, showing knife-edge atrophy in semantic dementia.

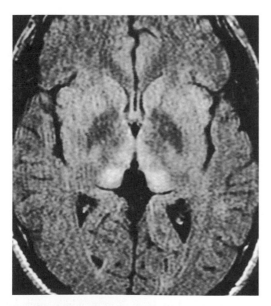

Figure 19.2 Axial FLAIR image showing symmetrical signal abnormality in the pulvinar nuclei and dorsomedial thalami in variant CJD.

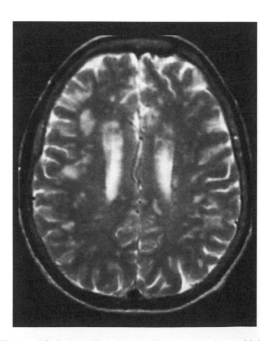

Figure 19.4 Axial T2-weighted MR scan, showing multiple small patches of high signal in the periventricular white matter consistent with small vessel disease.

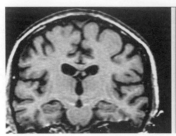
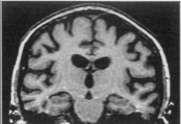
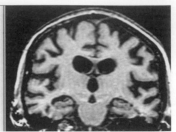

Figure 19.5 Serial T1-weighted coronal MR scans showing progressive shrinkage of the hippocampus bilaterally in Alzheimer's disease.

focal areas strengthening a clinical suspicion of a particular disease, e.g. AD (Figure 19.5).

Positron emission tomography

The measurement of cerebral metabolism using FDG positron emission tomography (PET) can reveal focal metabolic changes before structural changes are evident on MRI and may help determine the disease process or point towards an organic disorder rather than psychological cause.

Ligand scans, e.g. PET imaging with PIB (Pittsburgh B compound), may delineate amyloid deposition (Figure 19.6). The ability to measure amyloid in patients with memory problems has huge potential in the early diagnosis of AD, but as yet this remains a research tool.

Tissue biopsy

In selected cases, tissue biopsy is required to confirm diagnosis. For example, skin biopsy may detect

pathological accumulations in storage diseases; muscle biopsy may detect mitochondrial disorder. Tonsillar biopsy can confirm variant CJD.

Brain biopsy may be occasionally necessary in young onset dementia with a possible treatable process. A full thickness biopsy is taken from the nondominant frontal lobe. A specific diagnosis is made in about 50 per cent of cases, and 10 per cent are potentially treatable.

TYPES OF DEMENTIA

Degenerative

Alzheimer's disease

AD is the most common of the primary degenerative dementias: AD pathology, in part or in whole, underlies at least 50 per cent of all cases of dementia.

Pathology
The pathological hallmarks comprise extracellular amyloid plaques and intracellular neurofibrillary tangles. Plaques are composed of beta-amyloid, a peptide formed by cleavage of a precursor polypeptide called amyloid precursor protein (APP). In established disease, amyloid plaques are widely distributed throughout the cortex. Amyloid can also be deposited in cerebral blood vessels leading to amyloid angiopathy. The proportion of parenchymal and vascular amyloid varies between patients. Neurofibrillary tangles result from the breakdown of microtubule. Tau is a protein which normally promotes and stabilizes microtubule assembly. In AD, tau becomes hyperphosphorylated and aggre-

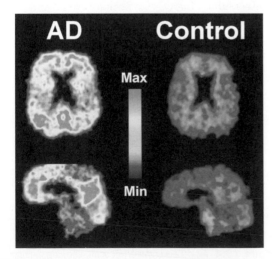

Figure 19.6 PiB scan showing amyloid deposition in a patient with Alzheimer's disease.

gates into an insoluble tangle within the neurone. The tangles first appear in the entorhinal cortex, then spread to other limbic structures; eventually they become widely distributed in the cortex, sparing primary motor and sensory cortex.

Clinical

Symptoms start insidiously and progress gradually. The most common complaint is of 'problems with memory'. Patients become repetitive in their questioning. They forget to relay messages or items are misplaced around the house. These symptoms reflect deficits in episodic memory.

It is important to remember that an isolated memory deficit is not sufficient for a clinical diagnosis of AD. Diagnostic criteria require deficits in multiple cognitive domains, severe enough to impair activities of daily living. By this stage, disease has been established for some time. Therefore, the concept of **amnestic mild cognitive impairment (MCI)** has been introduced to indicate early stages of selective episodic memory deficit and no difficulty performing activities of daily living. Between 10 and 15 per cent of patients with MCI develop AD per annum. However, progression to AD is not inevitable: MCI includes a heterogeneous group of problems including depression, anxiety or static deficits from some other insult.

Other early features in AD include a **loss of confidence and of interest in activities**. Commonly initial problems are put down to depression or anxiety. It is helpful to ask relatives whether they believe the individual's personality to be the same underlying these problems. In contrast to FTLD, patients with AD usually retain their premorbid personality and social facade.

As pathology progresses, so do cognitive deficits. **Loss of concentration** is often an early feature. Other deficits include **difficulty with topographical sense** – patients may fail to recognize a previously familiar environment. Facial recognition may be impaired. Typically, deficits are cortical, symmetrical and generalized. Patients develop **language problems** including naming deficits, and **visuo-perceptual deficits**. Later, using implements such as remote controls becomes difficult. Visuospatial difficulties may cause errors in driving. These can lead to accidents, compounded by the tendency to

get lost and errors in judgement. Often, the patient self-regulates their driving to short distances. **Praxis disturbances** increase and cause problems with dressing and other activities of daily living. There may be difficulties in **executive function**, such as planning, decision making and sequencing. In later stages, **agitation** is common and patients can exhibit **aggression associated with frustration**. **Delusions** are common, often paranoid in ideation.

Neurological examination is usually normal in the early stages. **Myoclonus** can be present later in the disease. This often forewarns of **seizures** later on. Ultimately, patients cannot self-care but can still wander with **disturbance of sleep–wake cycle** common. Swallowing difficulties can develop and precipitate pneumonia. Survival is typically 5–15 years from onset of symptoms.

Atypical presentations of AD
- **Posterior cortical atrophy.** Initial distribution of pathology lies in the posterior visual and parietal cortex. Patients have relatively spared episodic memory, in contrast to typical AD. They complain of visual symptoms, such as blurring, or inconsistency of images (typewriter keys 'vanishing and reappearing'); early problems with reading and writing are noted. They develop marked visuospatial problems, causing difficulty with locating items and themselves in space – visual disorientation.
- **Language dominant presentation – fluent or nonfluent aphasia.** Patients develop agrammatical, often nonfluent speech with mixed phonological and semantic deficits. In contrast to FTLD, they also show episodic impairment. Communication is rapidly impaired leading to significant distress as insight is retained.
- **Frontal AD.** Behavioural problems are seen early and dominate the presentation; however, episodic memory deficits are also present.

Familial Alzheimer's disease

Between 5 and 10 per cent of patients with AD have a family history suggestive of an autosomal dominant mode of inheritance. Clinically, presentation at a younger age, myoclonic jerks, seizures and depression are more common than in non-familial AD.

Mutations in three genes are known to cause autosomal dominant AD. However, together these mutations only account for 1 per cent of all cases of AD. Mutations of the *APP* gene were first to be discovered, and produce symptom onset between 45 and 60 years of age. Mutations in the *presenilin-1* gene on chromosome 14 account for about 50 per cent of all autosomal dominant familial AD. They often have the youngest age at onset, usually between 35 and 50 years. Mutations in *presenilin-2* on chromosome 1 are relatively rare; cases have a young but variable age at onset.

Risk factors in development of AD

A family history of AD in a first-degree relative confers a two-fold increase in the lifetime risk of developing AD. This is mainly due to the risk-modifying effect of the apolipoprotein E gene (*ApoE*). *ApoE* exists in three allelic variants: E2, E3 and E4. The most common allele is E3; E4 is less common; E2 is relatively rare. Inheriting a single E4 allele increases the risk of AD two- to three-fold and is associated with earlier age of onset. E4 homozygosity is associated with a four- to eight-fold increase in risk and age at onset five to ten years earlier. However, possession of the E4 allele is not sufficient to cause AD: 20–30 per cent of the population have one or more E4 alleles and only 60 per cent of AD cases have one or more E4 alleles.

Vascular risk factors are associated with an increased risk of AD, as well as of vascular dementia. Previous head trauma may increase the risk of AD.

Investigations

There are currently no definitive laboratory tests, but a number have positive predictive value for AD. **Neuropsychometry** establishes the cognitive profile, showing deficits in a broad range of cognitive functions, with dominant problems in episodic memory and including symmetrical posterior and anterior dysfunction. **MRI (coronal T1-weighted)** can identify a pattern of disproportionate medial temporal lobe atrophy (Figure 19.3) and may show generalized, symmetrical cortical atrophy. **FDG–PET** may demonstrate symmetrical temporoparietal hypometabolism. However, these investigations can be normal in the early stages of AD. PIB scans are promising but still a research tool. **EEG** typically shows generalized slowing and loss of alpha rhythm, though may be normal.

In AD, the CSF is usually acellular with normal protein. Determination of **CSF tau and abeta 42** is increasingly used in young cases with possible AD, as decreased amyloid b 1–42 and increased tau levels has good sensitivity and specificity for AD.

Treatment

Cholinesterase inhibitors

Symptomatic treatment with **cholinesterase inhibitors (AChEIs)** is the primary mode of pharmacological management. In AD, there is reduced activity of the enzyme choline acetyltransferase, with reduction in cortical levels of acetylcholine. AChEIs inhibit breakdown of ACh and enhance levels. **Three drugs are licensed for treatment of AD: donepezil, rivastigmine and galantamine.** They are all similarly efficacious and have similar side effects, commonly gastrointestinal and sleep disturbance. However, they are usually well tolerated.

Clinical trials have shown statistically significant, modest, symptomatic benefits of AChEIs on measures of cognitive function over six months. This translates to a delay in symptomatic cognitive decline and temporary stabilization of clinical and functional state. These effects have been reported to last up to five years. Clinical experience suggests that up to 20 per cent of patients have dramatic improvements which are concealed in averaged responses across the patient group.

Current NICE (National Institute of Health and Clinical Excellence) guidelines recommend prescription to moderate AD (defined as MMSE 10–20 out of 30), but are likely to be extended to those with mild AD (MMSE 21–27) in the near future. Treatment should be stopped when no longer demonstrating benefit – this decision is made with the patient and carer based on MMSE deterioration or global impression. The drug is tailed off and if a rapid deterioration is noted, it can be reintroduced.

Memantine

Memantine has an entirely different mode of action. It is a voltage-dependent N-methyl-D-aspartate receptor (NMDA) receptor antagonist and blocks the effect of elevated levels of glutamate. It is licensed for use in moderate to severe AD and is currently used in the UK when AChEIs are thought to have lost efficacy or cannot be used. Elsewhere, it is much more widely used in conjunction with AchEIs.

One promising strategy is a-beta immunotherapy, currently undergoing stage III clinical trials. In mice, this has been shown to clear amyloid plaques in the brain and be neuroprotective if given early.

Vascular cognitive impairment

> **Cerebrovascular disease** is a major cause of cognitive impairment in its own right and in association with AD ('mixed dementia'). It is the second most frequent cause of dementia; in spite of this, there is little agreement on how 'vascular dementia' should be defined. **Vascular cognitive impairment (VCI)** may be a more appropriate term as it reflects the range of presentations including static syndromes, mild cognitive impairment due to vascular disease and progressive dementia.

Pathology

There are no absolute criteria for a diagnosis of VCI. A spectrum of pathological changes occurs. Large vessels may show atheromatous change, although small vessel disease is usually prominent. Ischaemia is the most common pathology. There may be lacunar and larger infarcts, typically in watershed regions. Microscopically, leukoariosis is seen – atrophy and cavitation of white matter due to nerve fibre degeneration, gliosis and demyelination plus microinfarcts. Haemorrhage can cause VCI if multiple. Recurrent lobar haemorrhage may suggest cerebral amyloid angiopathy (CAA). Genetic factors influence the development of CAA; it is associated with ApoE e4 and e2.

Clinical

Presentation is diverse, dependent on location and type of vascular change. Historically, emphasis was placed on stepwise deterioration with recurrent cortical strokes – 'multi-infarct dementia'. However, VCI comprises a number of other presentations. A frontosubcortical pattern is common, leading to executive and attentional impairments, behavioural change and cognitive slowing with relative sparing of memory. This reflects the relative vulnerability of these structures to vascular damage.

Strategic infarcts cause focal cognitive deficits, dependent on location. For example, an infarct affecting the medial frontal lobe may have disproportionate effects on executive function. Single subcortical infarcts can damage corticosubcortical connections leading to multiple cognitive impairments. For example, focal infarction in the anteromedial thalamus can produce profound memory loss and marked apathy.

More commonly, VCI results from diffuse small vessel disease causing widespread white matter change. This used to be called 'Binswanger disease'. Patients present with gradual cognitive decline and no history of vascular episodes, and it may mimic AD. Clues include bradyphrenia and prominent frontal deficits with subcortical pattern of memory impairment. Neurological examination may reveal focal signs, such as hemiparesis, brisk facial and limb reflexes, vascular parkinsonism (gait apraxia) or pseudobulbar palsy.

A history of vascular risk factors should be obtained. Evidence suggesting antiphospholipid antibody syndrome or sickle cell disease should be sought in younger patients. Genetic vasculopathies should be excluded. For example, CADASIL (cerebral autosomal dominant arteriopathy with subcortical infarcts and leucoencephalopathy, see Chapter 23) may present with psychiatric disturbance, acute encephalopathy or adult onset migraine.

Investigations

Thrombophilia and other haematological/metabolic screens may be indicated. MRI findings are important in diagnosis. Other causes of white matter change must be excluded, e.g. multiple sclerosis, progressive multifocal leukoencephalopathy, HIV, lymphoma, post-radiotherapy changes, leukodystrophies, etc. The pattern of change can indicate likely diagnosis: for example, in CADASIL, MRI shows white matter involvement in the temporal pole with microhaemorrhages. However, there is no agreement on the extent of vascular lesion load required to cause cognitive impairment. Vascular changes are common on MRI and determining their clinical significance can be difficult.

Assessment of extracranial vessels is indicated if imaging suggests large vessel involvement. Intracranial magnetic resonance angiography (MRA) may show beading or irregularity of vessels in vasculitis, but this and formal angiography are neither sensitive or specific with regard to a diagnosis of vasculitis. EEG often shows non-specific slowing bitemporally, but preseved alpha rhythm. CSF is indicated in younger patients to exclude inflammation or infection. Brain biopsy may be indicated if cerebral vasculitis is a possibility and its positivity is predicted by the presence of headache or an abnormal CSF. Diagnosis of CADASIL is confirmed by screening the *Notch3* gene.

Management

Primary and secondary prevention of vascular damage is the main thrust of management; control of hypertension and other vascular risk factors is core. The benefit of statins is not clear. Current NICE guidelines do not recommend prescribing CHEIs in VCI.

Frontotemporal lobar degeneration

> **Frontotemporal lobar degeneration** is a term used to describe the clinical features of a group of neurodegenerative disorders affecting the frontal and/or temporal lobes. The group accounts for 20 per cent of young-onset dementia and 5–10 per cent of dementia overall. Nosology in this group is confusing. Pick first clinically described cases that would fit within FTLD, with aphasia and frontotemporal atrophy. The term 'Pick's disease' was therefore initially used to describe the clinical syndrome, but when neuropathological Pick bodies were described (by Alzheimer) the term became synonymous with the pathology of characteristic neuronal inclusions found in a subgroup of patients with FTLD. However, multiple pathologies can cause the clinical syndromes of FTLD. Therefore, it is best to avoid the term Pick's disease when referring to the clinical disorder.

Three syndromes are recognized, each with a distinct clinical profile and distribution of atrophy. Onset usually occurs between 50 and 65 years; survival is between six and 12 years. A large proportion of FTLD patients (35–50 per cent) have a family history of dementia.

Pathology

Cortical atrophy is usually confined to the frontal and/or anterior temporal lobes (Figure 19.7). In some frontal cases, atrophy may be mild; the most common focus of frontal atrophy is the orbitome-

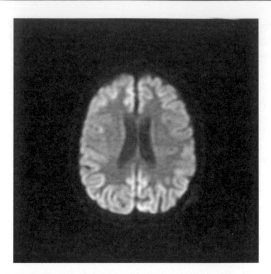

Figure 19.7 Axial diffusion weighted image MR showing 'ribboning' in sporadic Creutzfeldt–Jakob disease.

dial region. Temporal lobe involvement is focused on the anteromedial regions especially the fusiform gyrus, inferior and lateral regions. It can be striking: so called 'knife-edge atrophy'.

There are three broad groups of associated histopathology:

1 Tau positive inclusions (Pick bodies) are found in 20 per cent of cases. A larger proportion has distended neurons but no inclusions. This is most common in FTD and progressive non-fluent aphasia (PNFA).
2 Inclusions negative for tau, positive for ubiquitin (first described in motor neurone disease): now known to be common with no neuromuscular involvement. Disproportionately common in semantic dementia (SD) cases.
3 Neuronal loss and gliosis unaccompanied by any specific histological features. Accounts for a small and diminishing number of cases as diagnostic tools improve.

Familial FTLD

There have been major advances in the understanding of genetics and neuropathology of FTLD. In tau-positive FTLD, microtubule associated protein tau (MAPT) mutations cause FTD and parkinsonism linked to chromosome 17 (FTDP-17). These mutations have also been linked to syndromes resembling PSP, corticobasal degeneration and Pick's disease. A large proportion of familial cases with tau-negative ubiquitin-positive inclusions (FTLD-U) have been associated with mutations in the pro-granulin gene. Recent work has identified tau DNA-binding protein 43 (TDP-43) as a key protein in the ubiquitin inclusions of FTLD-U and in motor neurone disease (MND), constituting a common pathological substrate linking the two disorders.

Clinical features

The three syndromes have distinct presentations, but progressively merge with time. In the later stages, patients develop features of Kluver–Bucy syndrome, comprising hyperorality including excessive smoking, drinking or eating. Severely affected patients may try to eat non-food items.

FTD is the most common presentation, accounting for over half of all cases. Patients typically present with personality change and breakdown in behaviour, manifesting as apathy or disinhibition, sociopathy and euphoria. Invariably, there is loss of insight and self-care early on. Later changes include altered food preference and hyper-religiosity. Within this group, a distinction has been made between patients exhibiting disinhibition, distractibility and overactivity, and those presenting with apathy, inertia and withdrawal. These two presentations seem to reflect distribution of pathology with damage to dorsolateral and orbital regions of the frontal cortex, respectively. As disease progresses, behavioural disruption increases. In disinhibited patients, behaviour may become antisocial; forensic involvement is frequent. Angry outbursts and aggression become common. Emotional lability may be seen with rapid changes from inappropriate jocularity to passivity or anger. In apathetic patients, there is increasing inertia, child-like behaviour and emotional detachment. Patients may develop utilization behaviour (inability to inhibit interaction with an item within reach), repetitive behaviours such as checking or stereotypical gestures. These changes are distressing for the family, greatly increasing caregiver burden; unfortunately they do not often respond to treatment.

Neuropsychometry may reveal executive impairment as the sole finding. Patients are commonly impaired on verbal fluency and perseverate across items and tasks; they are unable to plan or problem-solve and are concrete in responses. Memory may be impaired, but improves with cueing.

Primary progressive aphasia

The two remaining FTLD syndromes are language dominant disorders, although the prototypical presentations of the two are distinct; together they are known as primary progressive aphasia. While most cases are due to FTLD, this presentation can also be associated with AD or corticobasal degeneration (CBD) pathology.

Semantic dementia

The onset of SD is insidious with a prodrome of five years or more. Patients typically complain of difficulty remembering words or names. Spontaneous speech is fluent and grammatically correct but 'empty' of content, with word finding difficulties, circumlocution, impaired naming and reduced category fluency. Disintegration of general knowledge becomes apparent – patients cannot understand single words ('what's a holiday?'). In contrast, other aspects of language are relatively preserved including phonology, prosody and grammar. When reading, patients regularize words, for example, 'sew' is read as 'soo'. Later changes include echolalia (automatic repetition of words/phrases) and bruxism. Other cognitive domains are relatively preserved although verbal memory is often impaired due to loss of understanding of the meaning of words. Later on, behaviours such as rigidity and obsessive-compulsive behaviour may be seen.

The disease is asymmetrical. Left temporal atrophy (more common) dominates when the patient presents with semantic loss; right temporal atrophy when there is initial behavioural or social change.

Progressive non-fluent aphasia

PNFA presents with a non-fluent insidious language disorder, often remaining circumscribed for many years. This can lead to significant delay in presentation. Speech becomes increasingly effortful with increasing phonological disruption and decrease in quantity. This is associated with preserved ability to understand words, but not sentences. Sentence production is telegraphed and disjointed. Writing is similarly affected leading to severe difficulty in communication. This along with retained insight leads to extreme distress in many cases. Patients become virtually mute while other functions are relatively preserved.

There may be associated buccofacial apraxia, exacerbating speech disturbance and causing swallowing disturbance. Behavioural features do not appear until late in the course of the disease, but can include rigidity and loss of empathy.

Examination

Neurological examination is usually normal in FLTD. A subgroup of cases develop additional signs of weakness and wasting in bulbar and/or limb muscles in a pattern identical to that in amyotrophic lateral sclerosis (ALS). These cases have ubiquitin positive pathology and are termed FTD-MND (frontotemporal dementia associated with MND). The dementia may precede or follow the evolution of MND (see Chapter 17).

Primitive reflexes such as snout, suck and grasp may become prominent in mid to late stages. Urinary and faecal incontinence occur in the final stages. Basal ganglia involvement can cause parkinsonism in some and dysfunction of the frontal eye fields can cause abnormal eye movements (frontal impersistence of gaze).

Investigation

There are no diagnostic investigations, although often imaging strongly supports the diagnosis.

MRI can be normal in FTD. In semantic dementia, it usually reveals knife-edge atrophy in the anterior temporal lobes, left more commonly than right, particularly involving the fusiform gyrus (Figure 19.3). In PNFA, MRI brain reveals atrophy in left inferior frontal and anterior insular cortex.

Functional imaging (FDG-PET) may reveal regional hypometabolism and can be useful in making a diagnosis in FTD when structural imaging is normal. EEG has traditionally been thought of as remaining normal in contrast to AD. However, over half of FTLD cases show abnormalities on EEG. These may be non-specific slowing or findings, such as FIRDA. The CSF is usually normal.

Dementia with Lewy bodies and Parkinson's disease dementia

Dementia with Lewy bodies (DLB) and Parkinson's disease dementia (PDD) together make up the third most common cause of dementia in later life. The two disorders form a continuum, pathologically and clinically. Dementia occurs in about 40 per cent of patients with idiopathic Parkinson's disease (IPD) at some point during the course of the disease. Risk factors for development of PDD are increasing age, disease duration, motor disability, early visual hallucinations, decreased levodopa response and drug-induced confusion.

Pathology

The pathological hallmark is the formation of Lewy bodies: eosinophilic intraneuronal inclusions containing the protein alpha-synuclein, aggregated with abnormally phosphorylated neurofilaments and ubiquitin. These are most commonly found in pigmented neurones of the substantia nigra in idiopathic Parkinson's disease. No pathological features reliably separate DLB, PDD and IPD – the phenotype depends on the pattern of spread of the pathology. Additionally, in DLB, AD pathology often coexists at post-mortem, which has led to the concept of 'Lewy body variant of AD', intermediate between AD and DLB.

Clinical

The distinction between DLB and PDD is made temporally: DLB is diagnosed when dementia occurs before or with parkinsonism, and PDD when dementia develops in established IPD. DLB is typically a sporadic disease of later life with survival similar to AD, but young onset, rapidly progressive and familial cases have been described.

Core features are progressive cognitive decline with fluctuations, visual hallucinations and parkinsonism. Cognitive problems are primarily executive, attentional and visuospatial, with apraxia and spatial disorientation. The fluctuations in attention are marked and often recurrent within a 24-hour period – they can manifest as drowsiness, poor response or altered behaviour. Clinically, it may mimic delirium. Visual hallucinations are often circumscribed and do not upset the patient; directed questioning is necessary as they may not spontaneously offer them as a symptom. The hallucinations are generally of animals or people, vivid, stereotyped and silent. They may form a tableau and they often emerge from background features or in low light and disappear if the patient turns away and looks back. In contrast, drug-induced visual hallucinations in IPD are often frightening and accompanied by paranoid delusions. Memory is often patchily affected, showing improvement with cueing and variability in performance, in a subcortical pattern.

Although a core feature in diagnostic criteria, parkinsonism is not recorded in a significant number of autopsy-proven cases, suggesting that a lack of extrapyramidal features does not exclude the diagnosis.

Other characteristic features include **marked neuroleptic drug sensitivity leading to profound**

rigidity and akinesia, REM sleep behaviour disorder, recurrent syncope and falls, significant autonomic dysfunction, early prominent delusions, including misidentification disorders, e.g. Capgras phenomenon, apathy and depression.

In PDD and DLB, parkinsonism may mimic uncomplicated IPD, although postural instability, axial involvement, absence of tremor and limited response to levodopa are more common.

Investigations

No specific diagnostic biomarkers have been identified. Brain MRI may show generalized atrophy or be normal. Dopaminergic ligand single photon emission computed tomography (SPECT) scanning (DaT) may show reduced strial dopamine transporters uptake and can differentiate between AD and DLB (although cannot differentiate between IPD, PDD and DLB); FDG-PET may show global reduction in cortical perfusion, often with posterior emphasis.

Treatment

No specific treatments are available. AChEIs modestly improve attention, alertness and hallucinations in a proportion of patients, and can be more effective than in AD. Extrapyramidal symptoms can occasionally worsen and therefore should be monitored carefully. **Neuroleptics must be avoided as they can cause severe, often life threatening, rigidity and akinesia.** New generation agents, e.g. olanzapine, are given cautiously if required for behavioural problems. Management of parkinsonism follows similar lines to that in IPD, although dopamine agonists are best avoided due to the risk of exacerbation of behavioural symptoms. Levodopa may have less benefit than in IPD and can lead to exacerbation of cognitive problems. In practical terms, the balance between motor and cognitive problems is often difficult to achieve and requires careful monitoring.

Dementia with other movement disorders

Cognitive decline in other movement disorders commonly manifests as a subcortical dementia due to involvement of frontosubcortical circuits. The severity and pattern of cognitive deficits may assist diagnosis, although this rests on non-cognitive aspects.

In the early stages of **Huntington's disease**, patients show attentional deficits and behavioural

or executive dysfunction; often presenting to psychiatric services. Visuospatial deficits are frequent. The cognitive decline correlates with caudate atrophy and frontal hypometabolism, consistent with disruption of frontosubcortical circuits.

Progressive supranuclear palsy is accompanied by profound bradyphrenia and executive deficits including perseveration of response, utilization behaviour or environmental dependency.

Severe cognitive decline is an exclusion criterion for **multiple system atrophy (MSA)**, but patients often show mild executive deficits and cognitive slowing.

In contrast to other 'Parkinson-plus' syndromes, CBD is associated with early cortical deficits such as limb and buccofacial apraxia, parietal signs and impaired speech production. The 'alien-limb' phenomenon is characteristic. The profile may overlap with disorders in the FTLD spectrum.

In the **spinocerebellar ataxias** (see Chapter 8 and Chapter 21), cognitive deficits vary with the underlying genetic abnormality. They include executive, memory, affective disorders and personality change.

Transmissible diseases and infections

Prion disease

Prion diseases are neurodegenerative diseases that affect humans and animals, including sheep (scrapie) and, notoriously, cattle (bovine spongiform encephalopathy (BSE)). **Spongiform encephalopathy** was first recognized as a cause of dementia by Creutzfeldt in 1920 and Jakob in 1921. Human prion diseases have been classified as sporadic, familial and iatrogenic. The disorder is rare, with an incidence of one per million.

Pathogenesis

Prions are transmissible agents with unique properties. An abnormal isoform of a host-encoded glycoprotein, prion protein (PrP), accumulates in the brain. This protein is widely expressed throughout the body, but in the disease form it is altered and becomes resistant to protease digestion. This then acts as a template to promote conversion of normal isoform to abnormal, causing misfolding of host proteins and aggregation.

Transmission was first demonstrated in 1966 with inoculation of brain from a patient with kuru into chimpanzees. Kuru was a form of spongiform encephalopathy that occurred in the Fore people of Papua New Guinea, and is thought to have been transmitted by **ritual cannibalism**. Clinically, it was characterized by emotional lability, behavioural changes and progressive ataxia, with dementia as a late feature. Cultural changes have led to its disappearance.

Sporadic CJD

This accounts for the majority of prion disease. Onset is between 45 and 75 years, with a peak onset around 60 years. Patients develop a non-specific prodrome with behavioural change or depression, insomnia, weight loss, general malaise and ill-defined pain sensations. The core clinical syndrome is a rapidly progressive multifocal dementia, usually with startle myoclonus. Often, there are additional neurological features with extrapyramidal and pyramidal signs, and cerebellar ataxia. Ten per cent present initially with cortical blindness (Heidenhain's variant). The disease progresses rapidly to akinetic mutism and death, often within two to three months and usually within six months. However, 10 per cent have a much more prolonged course with disease duration of over two years.

Pathology
The characteristic changes comprise spongiform degeneration with neuronal loss in the cerebral cortex together with positive immunohistochemistry for PrP. Most cases are homozygous with respect to the 129 polymorphism of PrP and MM is the most common genotype in classical subacute CJD.

Investigations
Routine bloods are normal. CSF examination is normal apart from an elevated 14-3-3 protein concentration. However, this is non-specific and the protein can be elevated in rapidly progressive AD, which may be difficult to distinguish from CJD. MRI is useful in diagnosis, showing high signal in the striatum or cortex (ribbon sign) on FLAIR or DWI (Figure 19.7). In around 70 per cent of cases, EEG shows characteristic pseudoperiodic sharp wave activity (Figure 5.26). Serial EEG increases sensitivity. Brain biopsy may be considered in selected cases to exclude treatable alternatives.

Acquired prion diseases: iatrogenic CJD

Evidence for transmissibility derives from patients who developed iatrogenic CJD following **neurosurgical procedures**, such as dural grafts, or **corneal grafts**, and in people who received **cadaveric pituitary hormones** for childhood endocrine disturbances, or blood transfusion. Patients develop a progressive cerebellar syndrome and behavioural disturbance or a classic CJD-like syndrome. This can occur in any age group. Intracerebral inoculation typically manifests as classic CJD, with a short incubation period (two to four years). Peripheral inoculation typically causes a progressive cerebellar syndrome after a longer incubation period (15 years or more).

Secondary iatrogenic CJD: Since 2004, four transfusion-related cases of vCJD prion infection have been recognized among patients identified as having received blood from a donor who developed vCJD.

Investigations
EEG, CSF and MRI are less helpful in this group. Brain biopsy may be considered to exclude treatable diagnosis; confirmation of diagnosis is by PrP immunocytochemistry of brain tissue.

Acquired prion diseases: variant CJD

In the mid-1990s, recognition that a novel human prion disease, variant Creutzfeldt–Jacob disease (vCJD), was caused by the same prion strain as BSE raised major public health concerns. The number of cases to date has been modest, but uncertainty with respect to incubation period and widespread population exposure suggest the need for caution.

The most prominent early feature is depression with anxiety and social withdrawal. Delusions are common. Patients may show emotional lability, aggression, insomnia and auditory and visual hallucinations. A common early feature is limb dysaesthesiae. In most cases, neurological features are not apparent until months into the clinical course. In most, a progressive cerebellar syndrome develops with gait and limb ataxia. Cognitive impairment occurs with progression to mutism. Myoclonus and chorea are often present. Age at onset ranges from 12 to 74 years; the clinical course is relatively prolonged.

Investigations

The EEG is abnormal, most frequently showing generalized slow wave activity. MRI, especially FLAIR, will show bilateral increased signal in the posterior thalamus (pulvinar sign) in the majority of cases (Figure 19.2). Tonsillar biopsy is a sensitive and specific diagnostic procedure for vCJD and obviates the need for brain biopsy. CSF 14-3-3 may be elevated or normal; PRNP (PrP) analysis is essential; to date all cases of vCJD have been PRNP 129 MM genotype.

Inherited prion disease

These are adult onset autosomal dominant conditions associated with PRNP coding mutations. **Gerstmann–Sträussler syndrome** is associated with a slowly progressive ataxia, pyramidal features and late dementia (as in kuru). Onset is usually in the third or fourth decade. **Fatal familial insomnia** is characterized by untreatable insomnia with progressive autonomic and motor dysfunction. Age at onset varies from 20 to 70 years. Duration varies from less than a year to over 20 years.

Treatment

There is no treatment that will alter the course of these disorders.

HIV/AIDS dementia complex

Patients with HIV infection are at risk of opportunistic infections and neoplasms, which can both cause cognitive impairment. In addition, patients may develop encephalopathy associated with cognitive decline, known as 'AIDS–dementia complex'. This term encompasses cognitive deficits, behavioural changes and motor involvement. Affected individuals may manifest deficits in each of these three aspects, with varying severity.

Clinical features

Patients typically develop a 'subcortical dementia' with poor concentration, forgetfulness and psychomotor slowing. Sometimes, they present to psychiatrists with behavioural symptoms. A third group develop extrapyramidal features, such as tremor or ataxia. As the disease progresses, speech is affected and motor abnormalities become marked. In one-fifth of patients, it is rapidly progressive.

Investigations

Increased CSF protein and a mild pleocytosis may be seen, often with oligoclonal bands. White matter changes and cortical atrophy are prominent on MRI.

Pathology

HIV enters the CNS by infecting macrophages and monocytes which then cross the blood–brain barrier, carrying the virus with them. Immunohistochemistry reveals dense concentrations of virus in basal ganglia, subcortical regions and frontal cortex, correlating with areas of pathological change. Infected cells lead to accumulation of neurotoxins, which create an inflammatory environment and then damage surrounding astrocytes and neurons.

Other infections

In most infections, cognitive decline is acute and consistent with delirium. However, occasionally decline is insidious. Clues include an aggressive course, evidence of active systemic disease and young age. Risk factors include ethnic origin, occupation, travel or sexual habits, clinical infection or contacts, immunosuppression.

A static cognitive deficit may be seen following recovery from **herpes simplex encephalitis**. In **subacute sclerosing panencephalitis**, a chronic reaction to the measles virus in brain parenchyma causes behavioural change, leading to generalized cognitive and neurological decline, with prominent myoclonus and death within months. **Lyme disease** (*Borrelia burgdorferi*) can cause cognitive and behavioural disturbance; fatigue and mild memory deficits are common post-acute illness.

Progressive multifocal leukoencephalopathy (PML) is caused by viral infection with a papovavirus (JC virus) which, in the presence of immunocompromise, causes widespread demyelination resulting in focal neurological and cognitive abnormalities. It is most commonly seen in AIDS, but may complicate lymphoma, sarcoidosis or long-term immunosuppression. Antiviral treatment is unhelpful and death is usually within one to two years.

Neurosyphilis is now a rare cause of dementia. Patients may develop dementia 15–20 years after initial infection. In the preparalytic phase, insidious memory failure is the only feature and can cause diagnostic confusion. Later patients show apathy, seizures, tremor, hypertonia and dysarthria. Cortical features develop, e.g. dyspraxia. Blood and CSF serology are positive. MRI brain may show increased signal on T2-weighted images and atrophy. Treatment with penicillin may improve the course.

Dementia may arise from **chronic meningitis due to tuberculosis or cryptococcosis** with secondary damage to the brain often associated with impaired immunity. Inflammation and thickening of meninges can cause cerebral infarction or hydrocephalus.

Whipple's disease is a rare multisystem disorder that is seen in middle-aged men, usually with gastrointestinal malabsorption. Jejunal biopsy can show abnormal macrophages and the presence of *Tropheryma whippleii*. Polymerase chain reaction (PCR) may show bacilli in CSF. Rarely, neurological disease occurs, without systemic features. There are usually associated ocular palsies and ataxia or hypothalamic syndrome. Antibiotic treatment can reverse the dementia.

Immune-mediated dementia

Limbic encephalitis

There is increasing recognition of this group of disorders. A number of patients with autoimmune limbic encephalitis may improve if correctly diagnosed and treated, making awareness of this group vital. Patients usually present with rapidly progressive amnesic deficit, psychiatric syndromes and seizures.

There are two broad categories:

1   directed against intracellular, classic paraneoplastic antigens, e.g. Hu, Ma2, tend to associate with cancer (lung, testis, etc.) and have a limited response to treatment
2   directed against cell membrane antigens – e.g. voltage-gated potassium channels (VGKCA), NMDA. Less frequently associated with cancer (thymoma, teratoma); respond better to immunotherapy.

Investigations
CSF shows inflammatory changes. On MRI, there is non-enhancing increased signal on FLAIR sequence in the mesial temporal lobes (Figure 19.8), and EEG reveals diffuse slowing with epileptiform discharges.

Paraneoplastic 'classic' limbic encephalitis (PLE)

In approximately 60 per cent of patients with paraneoplastic limbic encephalititis (PLE), neurological presentation occurs before a diagnosis of cancer is made. The mechanism is likely to be related to cell-mediated immunity developing against cancer cells. Patients develop subacute memory impairment over several months, associated with temporal lobe seizures and psychiatric symptoms. The most common associated tumour is small cell bronchial carcinoma (50 per cent; anti-Hu Ab positive); testicular (>20 per cent; anti-Ma2 positive); breast (>13 per cent; VGCC Ab-positive). Lymphoma and thymoma have also been associated.

CSF reveals pleocytosis and raised protein in 80 per cent of patients. In 40 per cent, serum antineuronal antibodies are negative. Whole body FDG-PET is sensitive in detecting occult underlying tumours.

PLE may improve following removal of the primary tumour or with immunosuppression, but there is often considerable residual deficit.

Anti-NMDA encephalitis

This is potentially lethal, but usually reversible if promptly recognized and treated. It should be suspected in young women with prominent psychiatric symptoms accompanied by seizures, autonomic instability, hypoventilation and dyskinesias. Less frequently, it presents as classical limbic encephalitis.

NMDAR antibodies are present in serum and CSF. The CSF usually shows inflammatory abnormalities. The most common tumour association is ovarian teratoma.

Up to 75 per cent of patients recover with treatment, in spite of the severity of the illness, often requiring extensive intensive care support. Optimal management is removal of tumour, but in a proportion of cases, no tumour is found. Immunomodulation with IVIg, plasma exchange, or steroids may result in improvement or stabilization.

VGKC Ab limbic encephalitis

This may be indistinguishable from 'classical' paraneoplastic limbic encephalitis, but in some patients the condition is associated with REM sleep behaviour disorder or seizures. Hyponatraemia is often seen and is a clue to aetiology.

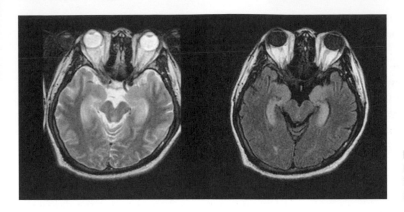

Figure 19.8 Axial T2-weighted (left) and FLAIR MRI (right) showing non-enhancing increased signal in both mesial temporal lobes, in a patient with limbic encephalitis.

There can be a dramatic response to steroid treatment, plasma exchange or IVIg, suggesting a direct role for the antibody.

Hashimoto encephalopathy (steroid-responsive encephalopathy with autoimmune thyroiditis)

This condition is more frequent in women (4:1). Presentation is variable with seizures, psychosis and stroke-like episodes. Occasionally, there may be tremor, myoclonus or sleep disturbance. Investigation typically shows elevated CSF protein and abnormal EEG with slowing and epileptiform discharges. MRI is usually normal. The neurological presentation is associated with the presence of thyroid autoimmunity often without clinical or biochemical evidence of thyroid dysfunction. Discussion is ongoing as to whether association with antibodies is an epiphenomenon, or whether the antibody is pathogenic. Treatment with corticosteroids can be effective, although it may need to be prolonged.

Other **inflammatory/granulomatous diseases** associated with cognitive decline include multiple sclerosis, vascular disorders, such as Behçet's disease and systemic lupus erythematosus, and granulomatous disorders such as sarcoidosis (see Chapter 27).

Metabolic, nutritional and toxic causes of dementia

Toxins

Alcohol causes approximately 10 per cent of young-onset cases of dementia. It is unclear how much of the cognitive decline is due to ethanol versus associated factors such as malnutrition (e.g.

thiamine deficiency, hepatic encephalopathy), head trauma, or is multifactorial. It is likely that chronic heavy alcohol intake alone can produce dementia including frontal deficits, with generalized cerebral atrophy. It is thought that abstinence may lead to some improvement, although the time course and extent are unknown.

Heavy metal poisoning, although rare, causes intellectual deterioration. 'Mad as a hatter' describes the mental disturbance, ataxia and restlessness found in workers who dressed hats with **mercury**. Chronic exposure to **lead** is still occasionally implicated as a cause of dementia.

Therapeutic agents have been implicated. Immunosuppressant drugs allow development of opportunistic central nervous system infections. Some **antiepileptic drugs**, especially phenytoin and barbiturate, in long-term high dosage can cause irreversible intellectual impairment. Topiramate can cause speech disturbance; valproate can lead to hyperammonaemic encephalopathy. Cytotoxic drugs, in particular methotrexate, especially when given in combination with cranial irradiation, can cause a decline in cognitive function several years post-therapy.

Endocrinopathies and metabolic causes of dementia

Chronic disturbance of electrolyte balance, particularly **hyponatraemia**, may disturb brain activity through the development of cerebral oedema. Metabolic abnormalities, e.g. renal or liver failure, may cause neuropsychiatric disturbance, often with **movement disorders** including myoclonus and asterixis.

Five per cent of patients with **hypothyroidism** have non-specific slowing of cognition and apathy (myxoedema madness). The features indicate a sub-cortical disturbance. Treatment must be prompt to reverse the impairment.

Chronic recurrent hypoglycaemia may cause gradual intellectual decline. Usually the patient also develops ataxia and involuntary movements.

Hypercalcaemia may result in reversible neuropsychiatric disturbance, while **hypocalcaemia** is rarely associated with subcortical dementia with extrapyramidal features. Behavioural abnormalities and even psychosis may occur with Cushing's syndrome. In Addison's disease, personality may change and apathy develop.

Deficiency diseases

Thiamine deficiency causes a profound amnesia with intact long-term and procedural memory (**Korsakoff's psychosis**). This is most commonly seen in alcoholism but also with hyperemesis gravidarum. **B12 deficiency** commonly causes spinal cord and peripheral nerve changes (subacute combined degeneration). Additionally, there are often cognitive changes, ranging from apathy to gradual intellectual decline. Early B12 replacement can reverse the disorder. **Pellagra** (niacin deficiency) leads to extrapyramidal rigidity, primitive reflexes and cognitive dysfunction.

Inborn errors of metabolism

Patients with certain inborn errors of metabolism may present with a **dementia–plus syndrome**, usually with a subcortical pattern of dementia or even psychosis.

In trying to determine the cause, several factors are important:

- Is the cognitive impairment progressive?
  - Often congenital brain damage or static early life insult
- Is there a family history? Any consanguinity?
  - Many of these disorders have an autosomal recessive inheritance
- Look for other neurological and systemic clues
  - Neurological: pyramidal, extrapyramidal, cerebellar, peripheral
  - Additional: deafness, retinopathy, seizures
  - Systemic: hepatomegaly
  - Pathognomonic: Kayser–Fleicher rings in Wilson's disease

- Confirm associated laboratory findings
  - Specialized processing of tissue samples often required.

Wilson's disease may present in adulthood with tremor, dysarthria and dystonia. Impaired cognition is occasionally an early feature; behavioural and cognitive changes are common in established disease.

Metachromatic leukodystrophy can present with cognitive impairment early. Extensor plantars and absent tendon reflexes suggest the diagnosis. There is reduced activity of arylsulphatase A in white blood cells. Rarely, **adrenoleukodystrophy** causes dementia in adult life. **Kuf's disease** (neuronal ceroid-lipofuscinosis) presents with behavioural and personality changes leading to dementia with extrapyramidal features.

Lysosomal storage disorders, e.g. Niemann-Pick disease, cerebrotendinous xanthomatosis, may present in early adulthood with cognitive impairment. The other neurological features provide clues to diagnosis. The **mitochondrial encephalopathies** are commonly associated with cognitive impairment in childhood, but in the context of widespread neurological dysfunction.

Other causes of cognitive impairment

Neoplasms and other space occupying lesions

Between 5 and 10 per cent of patients with dementia have intracranial neoplasms (Figure 19.1). The site of the lesion determines the presentation. Slowly growing tumours are more likely to cause diagnostic difficulty. Tumours arising in the frontal lobe, corpus callosum or midline thalamus can cause prominent cognitive impairment. Cognitive impairment may result from compression or infiltration, oedema or impairment of CSF circulation causing hydrocephalus, metabolic disturbances, paraneoplastic syndromes and meningeal infiltration. Cerebral lymphoma, especially intravascular lymphoma, is notoriously good at mimicking other disorders, is extremely aggressive and requires brain biopsy for diagnosis.

Subdural haematomas have varied presentations. They can mimic other causes of dementia and are most commonly seen in the elderly. Suspicion should be aroused by fluctuations in cognitive and neurological findings (see Chapter 12).

Head injury

Typically, a closed-head injury causes contusions to the frontal and temporal poles, which may lead to widespread cognitive deficits. The length of retrograde amnesia and degree of anterograde amnesia indicate extent. The resulting organic cognitive disturbance may not always be easy to separate from secondary psychological response to the injury.

Repetitive head trauma is linked with 'dementia pugilistica', a syndrome associated with boxing and repeated 'minor' head injuries. Patients develop progressive cognitive decline, behavioural change, parkinsonism, ataxia and dysarthria. Pathologically, many features are shared with AD. The level of risk is influenced by the severity and number of traumatic insults to the head.

Epilepsy and dementia

Several mechanisms may cause cognitive impairment in epilepsy. In addition, cognitive function may be impaired by some antiepileptic drugs.

Seizures themselves may cause cognitive deficits. **Transient epileptic amnesia** is recognized as a cause of cognitive impairment, producing discrete episodes of amnesia for events. It primarily affects middle-aged people. Episodes are brief and recurrent, often on waking. EEG may show temporal lobe spikes; MRI may show evidence of hippocampal damage. The episodes respond to antiepileptic drugs, but there may be residual interictal deficits.

Some disorders lead to both cognitive dysfunction and seizures. These include alcohol intoxication and withdrawal, intracranial infections, head trauma, stroke, space-occupying lesions, cerebral vasculitis, limbic encephalitis and degenerative disorders. It is important to distinguish cognitive effects of seizures from those of the underlying disease.

Certain rare epilepsy syndromes are associated with primary disease processes also causing cognitive decline: for example, epilepsia partialis continua in Rasmussen encephalitis, progressive myoclonic epilepsy associated with inborn errors of metabolism.

Normal pressure hydrocephalus

Normal pressure hydrocephalus (NPH) is usually listed as a reversible cause of dementia. The char-

acteristic presentation is a triad of gait apraxia, urinary incontinence and cognitive decline. The mechanism is uncertain, although it is suggested that impaired CSF resorption at the arachnoid granulations is responsible. MRI shows ventricular enlargement disproportionate to the degree of gyral atrophy, with no evidence of obstruction to CSF flow (Figure 19.9). Clinical improvement following removal of 20 mL of CSF, and monitoring of CSF

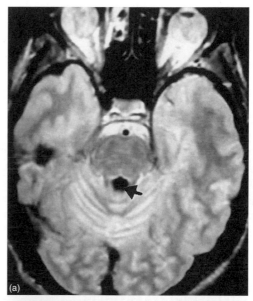

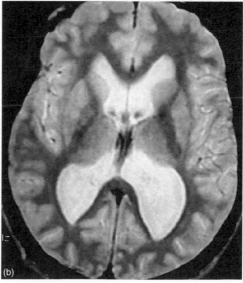

Figure 19.9 (a, b) Normal pressure hydrocephalus. T2-weighted axial MR scans, showing ventricular enlargement and flow void (arrowed in (a)), which has similar low signal to that seen in the basilar artery. The flow void lies in the bottom of the aqueduct.

pressure changes are used as criteria for shunting. However, the relationship between NPH and cognitive decline remains unclear. Many patients also have changes of small vessel disease and/or AD at post-mortem. It has been shown that patients with AD may improve transiently following ventricular drainage. Patients with long-standing symptoms, established dementia or radiological evidence of cerebral atrophy or cerebrovascular disease generally fail to improve following CSF shunting. The benefit–risk balance therefore needs careful discussion with the patient and family prior to operation.

Sleep apnoea

Patients with sleep apnoea may present with memory complaints and show objective deficits. This is not uncommon – one series found up to 8 per cent of young-onset patients had sleep apnoea. Typical symptoms such as snoring, morning headache and daytime somnolence should be enquired about. Nocturnal 'seizures' may be a clue. The mechanism of cognitive dysfunction may be intermittent hypoxaemia or sleep deprivation; diagnosis and treatment may reverse the problem.

MANAGEMENT: GENERAL CONSIDERATIONS

Comorbidity of dementia

Behavioural management

Behavioural changes have an enormous impact on the carer. These include loss of insight, personality change and impaired social behaviour, and can cause relationship difficulties, legal issues and loss of social contacts. Treatment requires a **multidisciplinary approach**, combining behavioural modification with pharmacological intervention. Areas to be considered include sleep cycle, agitation and incontinence.

Safety

A home safety evaluation determines necessary modifications to optimize patient independence. Patients may be unaware of certain risks due to lack of insight. Wandering is a frequent problem which

Demented patients are prone to develop **acute confusional states (ACS)**; up to 20 per cent of acute admissions in the elderly involve ACS. These may be precipitated by intercurrent infection, dehydration, poor nutrition, medication and trauma. The cause should be elicited carefully. If sedation is required, the smallest effective dose should be used. Benzodiazepines may be helpful; neuroleptics should be avoided if possible, using newer agents instead, such as olanzapine.

Depression is a treatable cause of dementia and often coexists with other causes. Over 50 per cent of patients with dementia experience depressive symptoms at some stage. Appropriate and active treatment makes a significant difference to quality of life, using drugs such as selective serotonic reuptake inhibitors (SSRIs) in preference to older tricyclics with anticholinergic effects.

Seizures occur more frequently in patients with dementia than in controls. In AD, 10–20 per cent have at least one seizure, usually later in the course of the disease. When treating, side effects of antiepileptic drugs should be taken into account.

can be helped by increasing daytime stimulation, but may require locating devices.

Fitness to drive is a source of huge anxiety to patients with dementia. Patients with AD tend to self-regulate; however patients with frontal impairment can lack insight and continue driving when no longer safe. The relationship between dementia and driving ability is complex. The patient is required to inform the Driver and Vehicle Licensing Agency (DVLA) of their diagnosis; if ability to drive is in doubt, assessment at a mobility centre may be appropriate.

The majority of patients are cared for in the community, with family shouldering the considerable burden of care. Assistance and adaptation of environment via social services is variable and even under optimum conditions demands substantial family commitment. As the dementia progresses, the carer has to curtail their outside work and independence. Nevertheless, multidisciplinary input can make the difference between coping at home and institutional care. Finally, the patient will require long-term residential care.

REFERENCES AND FURTHER READING

Dubois B, Feldman H, Jacova C *et al.* (2007) Research criteria for the diagnosis of Alzheimer's disease: Revising the NINCDS-ADRDA criteria – a position paper. *Lancet Neurology*, **6**:734–746.

Galton CJ, Patterson K, Xuereb JH *et al.* (2000) Atypical and typical presentations of Alzheimer's disease: a clinical, neuropsychological, neuroimaging and pathological study of 13 cases. *Brain*, **123**:484–498.

Harvey RJ, Skelton-Robinson M, Rossor MN (2003) The prevalence and causes of dementia in people under the age of 65 years. *Journal of Neurology, Neurosurgery and Psychiatry*, **74**:1206–1209.

Moorhouse P, Rockwood K (2008) Vascular cognitive impairment: current concepts and clinical developments. *Lancet Neurology*, **7**:246–255.

Rossor MN, Fox NC, Mummery CJ *et al.* (2010) The diagnosis of young onset dementia *Lancet Neurology*, **9**:793–806.

Smith SJ (2005) EEG in neurological conditions other than epilepsy: when does it help, what does it add? *Journal of Neurology, Neurosurgery and Psychiatry*, **76**(Suppl. 2):ii8–ii12.

Vincent A, Buckley C, Schott JM *et al.* (2004) Potassium channel antibody-associated encephalopathy: a potentially immunotherapy-responsive form of limbic encephalitis. *Brain*, **127**:701–12.

Warren JD, Schott JM, Fox NC *et al.* (2005) Brain biopsy in dementia. *Brain*, **128**:2016–25.

MOVEMENT DISORDERS

Niall Quinn

INTRODUCTION

Movement disorders comprise two main categories:

1 Akinetic-rigid syndromes and
2 Dyskinesias.

AKINETIC-RIGID SYNDROMES

These are characterized by akinesia and rigidity, the most common degenerative cause being Parkinson's disease (PD). Other causes are given in Table 20.1.

Parkinson's disease

PD is a slowly progressive, degenerative disease involving the basal ganglia, as well as many other brain areas. In the motor system, it causes an akinetic-rigid syndrome, usually with rest tremor, accompanied later in the disease by a flexed posture, shuffling gait, impaired balance, freezing of gait and falls.

In addition, it causes a variety of non-motor symptoms.

Epidemiology

Parkinson's disease is a common illness – one in 40 people will develop it in their lifetime. The preva-lence rate in the UK is about 170 per 100 000 of the overall population, but much higher in older subjects. There are about 100 000 patients with PD in the UK. Most series show a slight male prepon-derance and the illness occurs in all races. While there are no striking differences in overall inci-dence among most populations of the world, this may be somewhat lower in sub-Saharan Africa and China. The relative frequency of causative genes varies between populations. Average age at disease onset is about 60 years. Survival is only modestly reduced.

Pathology

The characteristic main pathological finding in PD is loss of pigmented neurones in the brain-stem, particularly those in the substantia nigra, with the presence in some of the surviving neurones of intracytoplasmic eosinophilic inclu-sions, known as Lewy bodies.

The substantia nigra pars compacta projects to the striatum (the caudate nucleus and putamen) via the nigrostriatal pathway, which utilizes dopamine as its neurotransmitter. Parkinson's disease is asso-ciated with a considerable loss of striatal dopamine content, 80 per cent or more, proportional to the loss of substantia nigra neurones. **Striatal dopamine deficiency is thus a central biochemical conse-**

Table 20.1 Causes of an akinetic-rigid syndrome

Idiopathic sporadic Parkinson's disease[a]		
Parkinson's disease dementia (PDD) or dementia with Lewy bodies (DLB)[a]		
Genetically determined Parkinson's diseases	Dominant	α-synuclein mutations, duplications or triplications[a]
		LRKK2 mutations[a]
	Recessive	Parkin, PINK1 or DJ1 mutations or associated with glucocerebrosidase (GCB) mutations[a]
Reversible drug-induced due to dopamine receptor blockade or dopamine depletion		
Vascular parkinsonism		
Toxic as a result of MPTP/carbon monoxide/methanol/manganese		
Post-encephalitic as a result of encephalitis lethargica, streptococcal infections or Japanese B encephalitis		
Post-traumatic from repeated head trauma ('punch-drunk syndrome')		
Hydrocephalus or tumour		
Psychogenic (rare)		
Other neurodegenerative diseases:	Classically sporadic	Multiple system atrophy (MSA)
		Progressive supranuclear palsy (PSP)
		Corticobasal degeneration (CBD)
Other genetic	Dominant	Huntington's disease
		Spinocerebellar ataxias 2 and 3
		FDTP 17
	Recessive	Wilson's disease
		NBIA1 (formerly Hallervorden–Spatz disease)
		Kufor–Rakeb disease
	X-linked	Lubag (in Philippinos)
		FXTAS
	Uncertain	Parkinsonism – dementia – ALS complex ofGuam
		PSP-like atypical parkinsonism of Guadeloupe

[a]Classically with Lewy body pathology.

ALS, amyotrophic lateral sclerosis; FTDP 17, frontotemporal dementia with parkinsonism linked to chromosome 17; FXTAS, fragile X tremor ataxia syndrome; MPTP, 1-methyl-4-phenyl-1,2,3,6-tetrahydropyridine; NBIA1, neurodegeneration with brain iron accumulation type 1 (PKAN, PANK 2).

quence of PD. This discovery led to the introduction of treatment with levodopa, the amino acid precursor for dopamine synthesis in the brain. However, the nigrostriatal dopamine deficit, while important in causing akinesia and rigidity, is only one of a number of brain regions and neurotransmitters that are affected in PD. Other dopaminergic neuronal systems also degenerate, including mesocortical, mesolimbic and tubero-infundibular pathways.

Degeneration of the locus ceruleus leads to the loss of noradrenergic pathways to the cerebral cortex and other brain regions. There is also degeneration of cells in the raphe complex, which leads to deficiency of serotonin neurotransmission, and

of cells in the substantia innominata, or nucleus basalis of Meynert, which project acetylcholine-containing pathways to the cerebral cortex. Other structures affected include cerebral cortex, olfactory pathways, dorsal motor nucleus of vagus, sympathetic ganglia, and Meissner's and Auerbach's plexuses. At autopsy, some 'control' individuals have been shown to have Lewy bodies and neuronal loss in the substantia nigra. Such cases have been called incidental Lewy body disease (ILBD).

More recently, Braak has proposed six pathological stages of Lewy body spread in the brain. In stage 1, Lewy bodies are present in the dorsal vagal nucleus in the medulla and in anterior olfactory structures. In stage 2, they have spread to raphe nuclei and locus ceruleus. It is only by stage 3 that nigral neurones are involved. This was previously the definition of ILBD, but if one includes Braak stage 1 and 2 brains, then the incidence of ILBD becomes considerably higher. Stage 4 sees involvement of temporal mesocortex and allocortex, and stages 5 and 6 progressive spread into cerebral neocortex. This proposal would provide a pathological substrate for gastrointestinal symptoms, such as constipation, and for olfactory impairment and REM sleep disorder, which are all non-motor symptoms, commonly preceding the first motor deficits that only arise at stage 3.

Aetiology

The cause of most cases of PD is not known.

About one in seven (14 per cent) PD subjects have another first- or second-degree relative affected by PD. Some instances may be due to chance co-occurrence of a common disease, but in others **genetic factors** may be important. Initial clinical studies of twin pairs, one of whom had PD, showed a very low concordance rate. However, subsequent 18F-fluorodopa positron emission tomography (PET) studies revealed abnormalities in clinically normal co-twins which, if considered as evidence of subclinical disease, considerably increased concordance. A subsequent large study of American Second World War veteran twin pairs showed significant heritability where one twin had developed PD before the age of 50.

In 1994, the first monogenic cause of 'PD' was identified in the Contursi American–Italian–Greek kindred, members of which presented clearly autosomal dominant inheritance of clinically and pathologically (with Lewy bodies) fairly typical PD, apart from young age at onset (average 43 years) and shorter survival (average nine years). In this family, the condition is the result of a mutation in the α-synuclein gene on chromosome 4, and another German family with a different mutation in the same gene also has familial PD. However, the Lewy bodies of all other PD patients, familial or sporadic, all stain heavily with anti-α-synuclein antibodies, yet no pathological mutations have been found in their α-synuclein gene.

Interestingly, individuals in some other families have been identified with parkinsonism due to duplications and triplications of a normal α-synu-clein gene, demonstrating that not only mutant α-synuclein but also a 50 or 100 per cent excess of normal α-synuclein can cause Lewy body parkinsonism. These cases have more frequent dementia and earlier onset than most PD patients, particularly in the triplication cases.

> A second gene, *LRKK2*, mutations in which are responsible for many more cases of Lewy body parkinsonism, was identified in 2004.

The frequency of *LRKK2* mutations varies greatly between different populations, but is particularly high in North African Arabian and Ashkenazi Jewish people. The mutations are dominant, but with incomplete penetrance: individuals with the most common G2019S mutation have a 28 per cent risk of PD at age 59 years, 51 per cent at age 69, and 74 per cent at age 79. Clinically and pathologically, these cases resemble classical PD.

> There are also a number of autosomal recessive gene mutations causing parkinsonism. The 'parkin' mutation on chromosome 6 was first discovered in 1998 in Japanese families with young-onset Parkinson's disease (YOPD), frequently consanguineous and containing affected siblings.

Since then, it has been found all over the world, often in sporadic cases, without consanguinity. Subsequently, two more recessive loci for YOPD have been identified – PINK 1 and DJ1.

Recently, heterozygous mutations in the glucocerebrosidase gene that in homozygous form causes Gaucher's disease, again particularly in Ashkenazi Jewish people, have been shown to confer increased risk of PD, and in some homozygotes may cause atypical PD. Importantly, parkin, PINK1 and DJ1 brains typically do not contain Lewy bodies.

> Thus, what was previously considered as one disease, PD, is in fact a number of diseases, some strongly genetic, others perhaps not, some with, and some without Lewy bodies.

In sporadic patients, might some **environmental agent** be responsible? In the early 1980s, a small outbreak of an illness clinically indistinguishable from PD, but again without Lewy bodies, occurred among drug addicts in California. The cause was a contaminant, MPTP (1-methyl-4-phenyl-1,2,3,6-tetrahydropyridine) produced during the synthesis of a designer drug. MPTP is in fact a protoxin, converted in the brain by monoamine-oxidase B in glia into the toxic form MPP+ (1-methyl-4-phenylpyridinium), which is then taken up into dopaminergic neurones by their dopamine reuptake mechanism, where it is trapped by binding to neuromelanin. MPP+ poisons mitochondria to cause death of pigmented dopaminergic neurones in the brain.

This, albeit imperfect, model of PD shows that environmental toxins can cause selective nigral cell death, and has also provided an, again imperfect, animal model of PD in MPTP-treated primates which develop a parkinsonian syndrome that responds to levodopa and to other antiparkinsonian drugs. To date, no toxin has been definitely identified in the causation of PD. MPTP is one of a number of toxic species, and there have been suggestions that the incidence of PD may be higher in populations exposed to cumulative poisoning with pesticides or contaminated well water. On the other hand, smoking is strongly negatively correlated with subsequent development of PD. The single most important risk factor for PD, and for those with PD to develop dementia, is advancing age.

The above discoveries have pointed towards a number of intracellular mechanisms that might mediate neuronal injury and death in PD: increased accumulation or decreased clearance of misfolded proteins, free radicals, mitochondrial damage and apoptosis. Each of these can potentially be targeted in order to develop neuroprotective therapies.

Main clinical features

There is no laboratory test for PD itself, so the diagnosis depends on clinical signs of akinesia, plus rigidity, tremor or postural abnormalities. The illness usually commences on one side of the body, typically in an arm, less frequently in a leg – and remains asymmetric, even when the opposite side becomes affected.

Akinesia is usually the most important disabling motor feature of PD for the patient, at least in early disease stages. Akinesia is a symptom complex including bradykinesia (slowness of movement, but with additional fatiguing and decrement of repetitive alternating movements), hypokinesia (reduced amplitude of movement), difficulty initiating movement and in doing more than one movement simultaneously, and a general poverty of spontaneous and automatic or associated movements.

Akinesia accounts for many characteristic features of PD – the masked expressionless face, reduced blinking, absence of arm-swing when walking, small cramped handwriting, soft monotonous speech, and difficulties with walking.

Rigidity of muscles is detected clinically by resistance to passive manipulation of the limbs and neck. The examiner encounters uniform resistance throughout the range of passive movement, fairly equal in agonists and antagonists (hence the terms 'plasticity' or 'lead-pipe rigidity'). When tremor is also present, rigidity is broken up ('cog-wheel' rigidity).

Tremor is an initial complaint in about two-thirds of subjects with PD, and occurs eventually in many of the remaining one-third. The characteristic tremor is present at rest at a frequency of 3–6 Hz; it is most common in the arms, where it can produce the typical 'pill-rolling' movement between index and thumb. The jaw and legs may shake as well. The tremor is intensified by mental or emotional stress but disappears during deep sleep. It also lessens or disappears during voluntary movement, for example when raising the arms in front of the body, only to reappear in the new position after a delay ('re-emergent tremor'). Some patients also, or instead, exhibit a postural tremor of the hands, at a faster frequency of 6–8 Hz.

Postural abnormalities are typical of PD. Rigidity contributes to the characteristic flexed posture. Many patients, especially later in the illness, also exhibit postural instability, with a tendency to fall.

The gait of PD is characteristic. Arm-swing is impaired, and joints slightly flexed. The feet may shuffle, and there may be a tendency to fall forward, with the result that the steps become increasingly fast in order to catch up (festination). Later in the disease, the patient has difficulty initiating gait (start hesitation), and may 'freeze' during walking and become rooted to the spot, particularly when passing through doorways, in a narrow passage, or when attempting to turn.

Non-motor symptoms

Patients with PD frequently exhibit additional non-motor symptoms, which can be their most distressing problem. Many are a result of the illness itself, but the side effects of drug therapy, intercurrent illness and changes related to ageing must also be taken into account.

Mental disturbances are common. Although the intellect and senses are usually fairly well preserved in the initial stages, most patients develop some degree of intellectual deterioration as the disease progresses. A certain slowness of thought and of memory retrieval (bradyphrenia), is common. The cumulative incidence of dementia is ultimately about 80 per cent. In such cases, the brain always contains increasing numbers of Lewy bodies in the cortex, and often additionally plaques, or sometimes plaques and tangles. When dementia supervenes after more than one year of PD, it is known as **PD dementia** (**PDD**). When the interval is less than a year, or when dementia precedes, or occurs without spontaneous, parkinsonism, it is called **dementia with Lewy bodies** (**DLB**). Clinically, patients with **PDD and DLB** can look very similar, particularly in respect to the frequent presence of hallucinations (usually visual) and fluctuating attention, alertness and cognition. The extent to which they are separate conditions or simply represent a continuum is not known. Acute toxic confusional states are often precipitated by intercurrent infections or by drug therapy, particularly in those subjects who already show evidence of cognitive decline.

Depression affects one-third of patients. It is more often minor than major, and can be either reactive, or the result of the disease causing depletion of brain monoamines. It is an important determinant of quality of life in subjects with PD, and is eminently treatable, so should not be overlooked. Apathy and fatigue are also common symptoms, but so far poorly understood.

Sensory complaints are common in PD, although bedside sensory examination is normal. Discomfort in the limbs, often amounting to pain, is frequent.

Sometimes this is associated at night with an unpleasant restlessness of the legs, although not quite the same as **idiopathic restless legs syndrome** (**RLS**) or an urge to move (**akathisia**). Curious feelings in the skin described as itching, creeping or burning can also occur.

Gastrointestinal disturbances include constipation and weight loss, which usually stabilizes at a lower weight, and (rarely) megacolon or sigmoid volvulus. Drooling of saliva is frequent in severe, advanced cases, as is dysphagia.

Urinary difficulties may be caused by PD itself, which causes detrusor hyperreflexia with frequency, urgency and sometimes urge incontinence. Prostate enlargement may complicate the picture.

Postural hypotension, worsened or unmasked by dopaminergic treatment, can be troublesome in some patients.

Assessment of the significance of many of these complaints may be difficult; for example, constipation may be the result of a combination of immobility, reduced food intake, dysphagia, anticholinergic medication, and Lewy body pathology in the gut, or may indicate the incidental development of a large bowel neoplasm. As a general principle, it is wise to investigate such complaints on their own merits before accepting them as a result of the disease or of therapy, although frequently no other pathology is discovered.

Diagnosis

Diagnosis of Parkinson's disease

The diagnosis is clinical. Typical PD is not difficult to recognize. The expressionless face, flexed posture, classical pill-rolling rest tremor, poverty and slowness of movement, small handwriting, and typical gait can be easily recognized even by the layman. However, the diagnosis is often missed in the early stages of the disease, especially if tremor is absent. The onset is typically unilateral or asymmetrical, the patient complaining of minor clumsiness of an arm, or dragging of a leg. This combination can suggest a hemiparesis; however, the tendon jerks are not usually increased, and true Babinski responses are absent.

Sensations of pain or numbness in the limbs, especially on the first affected side, may be a presenting complaint. They can arise from a frozen shoulder or lead to suspicion of other musculoskeletal disorders, such as lumbosacral degenerative disease. If generalized, such complaints may suggest rheumatism or polymyalgia rheumatica.

Fatigue is a common problem, and may be generalized or, initially, limited to one limb, or even to a single task. The picture of a general loss of vitality, aches and pains, and slowing down may simply be dismissed in the elderly as the result of 'growing old'.

Parkinson's disease can mimic depression. The patient is aware of slowing down and that life has become weary and difficult, and the loss of facial expression may be attributed to a depressive illness. Alternatively, depression can mimic PD. Often the two conditions coexist.

Investigations

Conventional brain magnetic resonance imaging (MRI) is normal in uncomplicated PD. Cardiac ^{123}I meta-iodobenzylguanidine (MIBG) scan is usually abnormal.

Dopamine transporter (DaT) single photon emission computed tomography (SPECT) scanning can reveal loss of dopamine transporter binding in putaminal, more than caudate, nigrostriatal tract nerve terminals, worse contralateral to the first affected limbs, coexisting with less severe abnormality of the other striatum even at Hoehn and Yahr stage I (unilateral clinical signs). This does not distinguish between PD, multiple system atrophy (MSA) and progressive supranuclear palsy (PSP). However, if there is clinical uncertainty between tremor-dominant PD and essential tremor, or between PD worsened by neuroleptic drugs and purely drug-induced parkinsonism, a normal scan excludes PD.

Treatment

Drug treatment may not be required in patients with mild disease. A range of drugs is available to relieve the symptoms of PD, but none is perfect.

Levodopa does not slow down the underlying pathology of the illness. Nor is there any evidence that it hastens death of nigral neurones in man. However, sooner or later most patients on levodopa develop the **long-term levodopa syndrome** (see below under Levodopa).

Accordingly, for the newly diagnosed patient with mild disability, levodopa therapy can often be held in reserve and other treatments, such as anticholinergics or amantadine (in young patients), monoamineoxidase B inhibitors (MAOBIs) or dopamine agonists, employed.

Anticholinergics

The original drugs used to treat PD before levodopa was available were the **anticholinergics**, e.g. trihexyphenidyl (benzhexol), orphenadrine, benzatropine and procyclidine. These give modest benefit, mainly for tremor, in about two-thirds of patients. Sudden withdrawal of chronic anticholinergic treatment can precipitate acute severe rebound worsening of all parkinsonian features. Unfortunately, anticholinergics cause a high incidence of unwanted side effects, including those of peripheral cholinergic blockade (dry mouth, blurred vision, constipation and urinary retention), as well as those caused by their central actions (memory impairment, difficulty concentrating, and acute toxic confusional states). For these reasons, anticholinergics are best avoided in older patients.

Amantadine is an antiviral agent which was found by chance to be of benefit in PD. It has some dopamine reuptake blocking and anticholinergic activity, and an amphetamine-like effect in releasing stored dopamine. It gives modest benefit in the early stage of the illness, but its effect often wanes with the passage of time. Side effects include ankle oedema and skin changes, in particular livedo reticularis on the legs; in high doses, it can cause a toxic confusional state and, rarely, seizures. Amantadine has also been shown to reduce levodopa-induced dyskinesias in many patients, probably through an additional N-methyl-D-aspartate receptor antagonist action, and today this is its main indication. It can also reduce freezing and falls in a minority of patients.

Levodopa

Levodopa is the most effective antiparkinsonian drug, and still the 'gold standard'. It crosses the blood–brain barrier and is converted in the brain into dopamine. The efficacy of levodopa replacement therapy is enhanced, and the incidence and severity of peripheral dopaminergic side effects, such as nausea and vomiting reduced, by

combination with a peripheral inhibitor of dopa decarboxylase. This prevents the metabolism of levodopa to dopamine outside the brain, but itself does not enter the brain so that cerebral dopamine can be replenished.

Two such extracerebral decarboxylase inhibitors are available: carbidopa, which is combined with levodopa in Sinemet (or co-careldopa), and benserazide, which is combined with levodopa in Madopar (or co-beneldopa).

There is little to choose between them, and they are both available in a variety of dosages and formulations.

With rare exceptions, levodopa helps all patients with PD. Indeed, failure to benefit from a sufficient dosage (up to 1–1.5 g/day of levodopa content, if necessary and if tolerated) and duration (ideally for two months or longer) of levodopa treatment should cast doubt upon the diagnosis. Sinemet or

However, about 10 per cent of patients per year of levodopa treatment develop features of the **long–term levodopa syndrome**. Typically, the relief from each dose of levodopa lasts for shorter and shorter periods, resulting in motor (and non-motor) fluctuations throughout the day in relation to the timing of levodopa intake ('wearing-off' or 'end-of-dose deterioration'). Over time, the amplitude and suddenness of these fluctuations increases and they become more frequent, prolonged and erratic (the 'on–off' phenomenon). In parallel, patients begin to develop levodopa-induced dyskinesias. These usually occur at the peak time of action of each dose of the drug (peak dose dyskinesias), when they are usually choreiform or mobile dystonic in nature. In some, usually younger onset, patients they may occur as the drug begins to work, or as its effect begins to wear off (beginning and/or end of dose, or biphasic dyskinesias), when they are often dystonic, stereotyped or ballistic in nature. Lower levels of dopaminergic stimulation are associated with early morning or off-period dystonia, which is relatively fixed and often painful.

Madopar is usually started in a three times a day regime, initially resulting in smooth control of symptoms, without unwanted levodopa-induced abnormal involuntary movements (dyskinesias) – the so-called 'levodopa honeymoon'.

These various dyskinesias may in themselves cause disability, such as difficulty with speaking, using the hands or walking. The relationship between individual and total daily dosages of levodopa and dyskinesias is not always clear. In general, however, peak-dose dyskinesias should improve as a result of reducing the dosage, although this may increase 'off' time. Conversely, off-period dystonia usually improves when trough levels are enhanced, but this may be at the expense of worsening peak-dose dyskinesias.

Non-motor fluctuations include wearing-off or off-period anxiety, panic, low mood, sweating, voiding dysfunction and pain.

Levodopa may also cause psychiatric side effects, such as vivid dreams and nightmares, illusions or hallucinations (usually visual), impulse control disorders including 'punding', and delusions (including morbid jealousy).

Levodopa can also cause, or worsen, postural hypotension, largely through central mechanisms.

There are no absolute contraindications to levodopa therapy, but the drug should not be given together with, or within 15 days of stopping, monoamine oxidase A inhibitors, or to those with a recent history of myocardial infarction.

Levodopa treatment for PD should be titrated in each patient individually, using the smallest dose that suffices to give adequate benefit, rather than attempting to eradicate all signs of parkinsonism. As fluctuations appear, the frequency of dosage may have to be increased, at the same time reducing the size of the individual doses, although the latter introduces the risk of 'dose failure'.

In patients with severe motor fluctuations or dyskinesias not adequately controlled despite the use or offer of apomorphine or deep brain stimulation (see below under Surgery for PD), daytime continuous intrajejunal administration of a levodopa-carbidopa gel, called Duodopa, can be helpful. However, it is invasive and extremely expensive, and system malfunctions are frequent.

Monoamineoxidase B inhibitors

Two selective monoamine oxidase B inhibitors (MAOBIs), selegiline and rasagiline, are licensed for PD. They are so-called 'suicide inhibitors' which inactivate MAOB by irreversible binding so that recovery of full enzyme activity only occurs when sufficient new enzyme has been manufactured, 6 weeks or more after stopping the drug. Both have a mild symptomatic effect and can prolong the duration of action of levodopa doses in some patients. Selegiline (usual dose 10 mg in the morning) is partly metabolized to methamphetamine, so can cause insomnia. Another, buccally absorbed, formulation of selegiline called Zelapar (usual dose 1.25 mg in the morning) avoids hepatic first-pass metabolism, so is devoid of this effect. A putative neuroprotective effect on nigral neurones (selegiline and rasagiline block MPTP toxicity in non-human primates) is unproven in humans. Delayed-start studies of rasagiline (usual dose 1 mg in the morning) suggested a possible disease-modifying effect, but this was absent at 2 mg in the morning, so is controversial.

Catechol-O-methyl transferase inhibitors (COMTIs)

The catechol-O-methyl transferase inhibitors (COMTIs) **entacapone** (peripherally acting) and **tolcapone** (centrally and peripherally acting) extend the elimination half-life, and hence the duration of action, of individual doses of levodopa. Tolcapone appears more effective clinically, but is a second-line COMTI because of a risk of potentially fatal liver failure or rhabdomyolysis, requiring frequent monitoring of liver enzymes. A combined preparation of levodopa-carbidopa with entacapone (Stalevo) is available. It was hoped that *de novo* treatment with this might delay or reduce motor fluctuations or dyskinesias relative to levodopa-carbidopa alone, but this has not occurred in a large double-blind trial.

Dopamine agonists

Another strategy in both previously untreated and fluctuating patients is the use of directly acting dopamine agonist(DA) drugs.

There are currently **five oral dopamine agonists licensed for PD in the UK. Bromocriptine, pergolide** and **cabergoline** are ergoline, and **ropinirole** and **pramipexole** non-ergoline, drugs.

Ropinirole and pramipexole are also available as prolonged-release formulations. Another non-ergoline agonist, **rotigotine**, is available as a transdermal patch.

Although none of these agonists is as effective as levodopa, their use as initial therapy is only rarely associated with fluctuations or dyskinesias. However, sooner or later an agonist alone will not give adequate benefit, at which time a levodopa preparation can be added. Such 'combination therapy' results, at least in the first few years, in an incidence of fluctuations and dyskinesias that seems intermediate between that on agonist and on levodopa monotherapy. However, over time, there is often a 'catch up' so that after a given period there is no difference in their frequency, regardless of whether treatment was originally initiated with levodopa or with a dopamine agonist. If the patient has been started on a levodopa preparation and has already developed these problems, an agonist treatment can be added. The longer duration of action of agonists helps to augment trough levels of dopaminergic stimulation, and their addition often allows the levodopa dose to be reduced, often with an associated reduction in dyskinesias.

If, despite the adjunctive use of other agonists, MAOBIs or COMTIs, the patient is still disabled by off periods, subcutaneous **apomorphine** can be added, usually tailing off an oral agonist at the same time. 'Rescue' injections of apomorphine usually reliably reverse off periods within 10–15 minutes, but their effect only lasts 40–60 minutes, by which time it is hoped the patient's levodopa dose will have taken effect. If more than six injections per day are required, it is preferable to switch to continuous daytime (approximately 12 hours) administration via a pump.

Dopamine agonists share the side-effect profile of levodopa preparations. However, they have a greater propensity to cause initial nausea and vomiting (which can be minimized by pretreatment or cotreatment with domperidone, a peripherally acting dopamine receptor blocker that does not cross the blood–brain barrier), and neuropsychiatric side effects, especially in elderly or cognitively impaired patients. All agonists can cause leg oedema.

Ergoline derivatives have long been recognized to rarely cause vasospasm, erythromelalgia, pleuropulmonary or retroperitoneal fibrosis. However, since 2004, there has been increasing concern about their capacity to cause cardiac valve fibrosis (often right-sided), so they are now second-line agonists, and rarely if ever given. This adverse effect is thought to be mediated through 5HT2B receptor agonism. All dopaminergic medications, including levodopa, can also cause drowsiness, so that patients should be instructed not to drive if they are experiencing sleepiness. Apomorphine causes fewer neuropsychiatric side effects than oral agonists, but may cause painful inflamed swellings at injection sites, which sometimes preclude further injections.

A particular area of increasing concern is the capacity of dopamine agonists, both ergoline and non-ergoline, to induce impulse control disorders to a much greater extent than levodopa. These include compulsive gambling, shopping, eating, singing and internet use, hypersexuality and paraphilias, which can have catastrophic financial and social consequences. Sometimes these occur singly, sometimes more than one at a time, and in total they affect up to 13 per cent of individuals on agonists.

Management of hallucinations, psychosis and confusion

> The management of patients with PD, or more frequently those with PDD or DLB, who develop hallucinations, psychosis or an acute confusional state is often difficult.

Alongside excluding an infection or metabolic disturbance, antiparkinsonian drugs should be gradually withdrawn in the following order: anticholinergics, then agonists, then MAOBIs, and then COMTIs, so that the patient may be left taking a levodopa preparation alone. If necessary, the dose of levodopa can then be reduced. Depending on the success of this withdrawal, or the severity or urgency of the problem, medication may need to be added to control the mental state. Conventional neuroleptics should be avoided, and atypical neuroleptics used instead. Risperidone and olanzapine may aggravate parkinsonism and are no longer used. Quetiapine does not usually worsen parkinsonism, but is not a particularly effective drug. **The best treatment is low doses of clozapine** (12.5–50 mg/day), but this needs to be carefully monitored with blood counts. Another option, especially in cognitively impaired subjects, is to use a cholinesterase inhibitor, such as rivastigmine.

Other treatments

While drugs are the mainstay of treatment in most patients with PD, many patients also gain benefit from an exercise programme, or from physiotherapy and speech therapy. Careful attention to aids to assist toileting, eating and mobility is important. Depression may require treatment with a tricyclic antidepressant drug (so far the best controlled trial favours nortryptiline), or a selective serotonin reuptake inhibitor.

Surgery for PD

The last two decades have seen a renaissance in functional stereotactic neurosurgery for PD. Previously, for many years, the only available operation was unilateral thalamotomy, which helped tremor and often rigidity, but not akinesia. From 1992, **pallidotomy** was introduced, which greatly reduced drug-induced dyskinesias, and modestly improved parkinsonian features.

> Currently, the preferred operation is bilateral deep brain stimulation **(DBS) of the subthalamic nucleus**, which seems to have a greater effect on the underlying parkinsonism and enables antiparkinsonian drug dosages to be substantially reduced, so that dyskinesias are also improved.

However, it has more adverse effects, mainly neuropsychiatric, than does bilateral pallidalDBS.

Drug-induced parkinsonism

> The neuroleptic drugs used to control psychotic illness, in particular schizophrenia, all block dopamine receptors in the brain. These include the phenothiazines (e.g. chlorpromazine), butyrophenones (e.g. haloperidol), thioxanthenes (e.g. flupentixol) and substituted benzamides (e.g. sulpiride).

About two-thirds of those taking neuroleptics show some signs of drug-induced parkinsonism. This usually remits in weeks, or sometimes months, after the offending neuroleptic drug is withdrawn or its dosage reduced. If it is necessary to continue the neuroleptic drug to control the psychotic illness, then the addition of an anticholinergic may be beneficial.

The dopamine receptor blockers metoclopramide, prochlorperazine, flunarizine and cinnarizine, commonly used to treat vertigo, migraine and gastrointestinal disturbances, can also cause drug-induced parkinsonism, as can the dopamine-depleting drug tetrabenazine.

If apparently drug-induced parkinsonism fails to resolve by three months after discontinuing the offending drug, one should suspect worsening of pre-existing nigrostriatal dopamine deficiency, in which case a DaT SPECT should be abnormal.

Post-encephalitic parkinsonism

The **encephalitis lethargica** (EL) pandemic spread throughout the world from about 1915 to 1925, but had virtually disappeared by the 1930s. Occasionally, clinically indistinguishable sporadic cases still occur today, after streptococcal throat infection, with the presence of anti-basal ganglia antibodies. Among survivors of acute EL, many developed post-encephalitic parkinsonism (PEP) within ten years of the infection. In addition to an akinetic-rigid syndrome, many of these patients also exhibited behavioural disturbances, other dyskinesias (especially dystonias), and oculogyric crises, comprising spasms of eye deviation, usually upwards or laterally, often accompanied by compulsive thoughts, lasting for minutes to hours.

Japanese B encephalitis can cause transient and sometimes persisting parkinsonism.

Progressive supranuclear palsy (Steele–Richardson–Olszewski disease)

This dissociation of voluntary from automatic eye movements confirms that the pathway from nucleus to muscle is intact, so that the problem must lie above the nucleus ('supranuclear'). Voluntary saccades are also slow in PSP, and there may be problems with opening the eyes (sometimes true blepharospasm, but more commonly levator inhibition or apraxia of eyelid opening). Diagnosis is clinical. MRI may show atrophy of the midbrain ('hummingbird sign') and superior cerebellar peduncles. The pathological changes in the brain comprise neuronal loss and gliosis, with straight

Progressive supranuclear palsy

Progressive supranuclear palsy (PSP) is a rare (prevalence six per 100 000), typically sporadic, progressive disease of middle and late life (mean onset age 63 years, rarely age <45 years, never age <40 years). Average survival from onset to death in most series is about seven years. The disease is clinically characterized by akinesia, predominantly axial rigidity, postural instability with falls, often backwards, speech and swallowing difficulties, 'frontal' symptoms and a supranuclear (upper motor neurone) palsy (paresis) of vertical, followed by horizontal, voluntary eye movements. Although PSP patients have difficulty with voluntarily moving their eyes, a full range of eye movements can be produced by the 'doll's head' manoeuvre of passive neck movement, which evokes preserved brainstem reflex eye movements.

neurofibrillary tangles, in brainstem, basal ganglia and, to a variable degree, cerebral cortex.

Recently, PSP has been divided into three forms: classical (Richardson's syndrome, mean survival six years, 54 per cent of cases), PSP-P (more resembling PD, mean survival nine years, 32 per cent of cases), and the rarer progressive akinesia with gait freezing (PAGF).

Unfortunately, PSP only responds rarely and transiently to dopaminergic drugs, but about one-fifth of patients derive useful benefit from amantadine. Posterior neck muscle spasms, pain and hyperextension, and blepharospasm, more than levator inhibition, may all be lessened by botulinum toxin injection.

Multiple system atrophy

The clinical presentation of MSA depends on the relative degree of pathological involvement of the striatonigral and olivopontocerebellar systems.

MSA-P (previously called striatonigral degeneration) presents as a progressive akinetic-rigid syndrome usually, but not always, poorly responsive or unresponsive to levodopa. Like PD, it is often asymmetric, and tremor occurs in two-thirds of cases, but is usually an irregular, postural and action tremor – classical pill-rolling occurs in <10 per cent. **MSA-C (the sporadic olivopontocerebellar atrophy (OPCA) type** presents with predominant

---

Multiple system atrophy

Multiple system atrophy (MSA) is a sporadic, adult-onset neurodegenerative disease (mean onset at age 57 years, never <30 years, prevalence four per 100 000). Average survival from first symptom to death is about seven years. Clinically, MSA can cause any combination of parkinsonian, cerebellar, autonomic and pyramidal features. Pathologically, it is characterized by cell loss and gliosis in a selection of: substantianigra, striatum, olives, pons, cerebellum, and the intermediolateral columns and Onuf's nucleus in the spinal cord (which supplies nerves to the striated external and urethral sphincters). Lewy bodies are absent, but argyrophilic, intracytoplasmic oligodendroglial inclusions, which stain positively with anti-α-synuclein antibodies, are always present.

---

cerebellar ataxia, often with the subsequent development of an akinetic-rigid syndrome. Autonomic failure accompanies both forms of MSA, and when it is the dominant feature the term **Shy–Drager syndrome** has sometimes been used. Thus, patients experience impotence and sphincter disturbances, and often symptomatic postural hypotension or loss of sweating. Many MSA patients present with autonomic failure, but develop additional neurological features within the first five years. After five years, autonomic failure that remains isolated, without additional neurology ('pure autonomic failure' – PAF), is typically associated with Lewy body pathology, and Lewy body PD can also be associated with autonomic failure, usually later in the disease course, but sometimes early on. The cardiovascular autonomic defect in PD is both preganglionic and post-ganglionic in origin, whereas that in MSA is pre-ganglionic. Urinary frequency and urgency occur in both conditions, but incontinence in MSA is largely as a result of neuronal loss in Onuf's nucleus which innervates the striated external anal and urethral sphincter muscles. Other features particularly seen in MSA are stridor, inspiratory sighs, cold violaceous extremities, myoclonus, strained speech and disproportionate antecollis. Diagnosis is clinical.

In recent years, the **fragile X tremor ataxia syndrome (FXTAS)** has been identified (see also Chapter 21). This affects (usually male) individuals who carry an intermediate length premutation in the

X-linked *FMR1* gene. The clinical picture involves cerebellar ataxia, usually with prominent tremor, but can also include peripheral neuropathy, parkinsonism and autonomic symptoms. Penetrance increases age-dependently, and in female carriers the premutation can present only as premature menopause. As in MSA, the MRI may show middle cerebellar peduncle (MCP) hyperintensity. However, because of its prominent tremor and more benign course, it is rarely misdiagnosed as MSA.

Investigations in MSA

Formal autonomic function tests may reveal several aspects of autonomic failure (AF), but the clinical documentation of otherwise unexplained postural hypotension (drop in blood pressure (BP) after 3 minutes standing of 20 mmHg systolic or 10 mmHg diastolic) alone indicates cardiovascular autonomic dysfunction. External anal or urethral sphincter electromyography is typically abnormal in MSA, but can also be abnormal in PSP and PD. However, a normal result would argue against MSA. MRI may show, supratentorially; hypointensity, or a lateral slit-like hyperintensity or putaminal atrophy (mostly in MSA-P) or, infratentorially; a 'hot cross bun' appearance of the pons or pontine atrophy, hyperintensity of middle cerebellar peduncles, or cerebellar atrophy. Cardiac MIBG scanning is typically abnormal in postganglionic (usually Lewy body pathology) and normal in preganglionic (MSA) cardiac autonomic involvement.

Corticobasal degeneration

Corticobasal degeneration (CBD) is a very rare sporadic cause of adult-onset parkinsonism, which can present as a movement disorder classically comprising combinations of unilateral upper limb fixed dystonia, akinesia, rigidity, myoclonus, apraxia, cortical sensory loss, and alien limb phenomenon, later developing dementia and a supranuclear gaze problem (difficulty and delay in initiating voluntary saccades, but normal saccadic velocity).

However, some cases begin instead in the legs, or symmetrically, and many initially present instead with primary progressive aphasia or dementia. Diagnosis is clinical. Brain MRI may reveal asymmetrical frontal and parietal atrophy.

Pathological changes (neuronal loss and characteristic ballooned achromatic neurones) involve the frontal and parietal cortices and basal ganglia. There is no effective treatment, and average survival from first symptom is five to seven years.

'Vascular parkinsonism'

Cerebrovascular disease, in the form of basal ganglia lacunes or Binswanger's subcortical white matter ischaemic changes, better visualized on MRI than on CT scanning, may produce a picture of **'lower body parkinsonism'**, without tremor. Such patients classically have an upright posture and good facial and arm mobility, but may exhibit cognitive impairment, a small-stepped 'marche à petits pas', and an unsteady, wide-based gait, with elements of freezing and start hesitation, but on close inspection do not really resemble PD. Vascular changes commonly coexist with PD, and may result in a 'top half' that is mildly affected by PD and which responds well to levodopa, associated with disproportionate problems in balance and gait. Some pathologically proven cases of 'vascular parkinsonism' without Lewy pathology have nevertheless been reported to have shown useful benefit with levodopa in life, so a therapeutic trial is reasonable.

THE DYSKINESIAS

The first step in analysing patients with abnormal involuntary movements is to decide which category of dyskinesia they exhibit. Most dyskinesias can be described using five terms: tremor, dystonia, and three types of jerk – chorea, myoclonus and tics.

Tremor is easily recognized as a rhythmic alternating sinusoidal movement. It is useful to distinguish between rest tremor (typical of PD), postural tremor (most often seen in essential tremor), and intention tremor (seen in patients with lesions of the cerebellar outflow pathways). The main causes of tremor are listed in Table 20.2.

Dystonia (athetosis) consists of sustained muscle spasms, which occur repetitively as dystonic movements, and often distort the body into characteristic postures. The neck may be affected (spasmodic

Table 20.2 Causes of tremor

	Cause
Rest tremor	Parkinson's disease > drug-induced >> other causes of akinetic-rigid syndrome
Postural tremor	Physiological tremor
	Exaggerated physiological tremor
	Thyrotoxicosis
	Anxiety states
	Alcohol withdrawal, caffeine
	Drugs (sympathomimetics, tricyclics, lithium, sodium valproate)
	Heavy metals (e.g. mercury – the 'hatter's shakes')
	Benign essential (familial) tremor
	Dystonia (primary or secondary)
	Structural brain disease (e.g. cerebellar lesions)
	FXTAS
Intention tremor	Brainstem or cerebellar outflow pathway disease
	Multiple sclerosis
	Spinocerebellar degenerations
	Vascular disease
	FXTAS
	Tumour
Holmes tremor (formerly called midbrain/rubral tremor) – a combination of rest, postural and intention tremor	
Orthostatic tremor	
Palatal tremor (also called palatal myoclonus)	
Psychogenic	

torticollis (ST)); the trunk may be forced into excessive lordosis or scoliosis; the arm is commonly hyperpronated, with the wrist flexed and the fingers extended, and the leg commonly extended with the foot plantar flexed and inturned, the great toes spontaneously dorsiflexing (the 'striatal' toe), and the other toes clenching or fanning. Dystonia can also affect the face, jaw and larynx. Initially, these dystonic muscle spasms may occur only on certain actions, so that patients may walk on their toes or develop the characteristic arm posture only on writing (action dystonia). In progressive dystonia, however, the abnormal muscle spasms and postures become apparent at rest and cause increasing movements and, usually mobile, deformity. Such dystonic spasms and postures are sometimes called 'athetosis', a term best restricted to distal mobile dystonia. Subjects often use a 'gesteantagoniste', e.g. touching the chin in ST, to help control their movements, and some with leg dystonia may find it easier to walk backwards or climb up stairs than to walk forward. Dystonia may be confined to one part of the body, as in isolated ST (focal dystonia), or affect adjacent segments of the body, e.g. the neck and one or both arms (segmental dystonia), the limbs on one side (hemidystonia, which may suggest the possibility of a contralateral structural lesion), or the whole body (generalized dystonia). The main causes of dystonia are listed in Table 20.3.

Chorea consists of a continuous flow of irregular, jerky movements that flit unpredictably from one body part to another. The main causes of chorea are listed in Table 20.4.

Myoclonus describes brief, shock-like muscle jerks, similar to the effect of stimulating the muscle's nerve with a single electric shock, or a train of shocks. The timing of the jerks may be irregular or rhythmic, and they may occur repetitively in the same muscle. Myoclonus may be confined to one part of the body (focal myoclonus), or affect many different parts at different times (multifocal myoclonus), or consist of jerks affecting all body parts (generalized myoclonus). The main causes of myoclonus are listed in Table 20.5.

Tics often resemble myoclonus because they usually consist of brief muscle contractions, but differ in that they are repetitive and stereotyped, can be mimicked by the observer, and can usually be controlled through an effort of will by the patient, often at the expense of mounting inner tension. Tics most often involve the face (e.g. blinking, nose wrinkling, sniffing), or the upper arms and neck (e.g. shrugging of the shoulders or inclination of the head). Sometimes the movements are more prolonged (e.g. neck craning), when they may be called 'dystonic tics'. The main causes of tics are listed in Table 20.6.

While most patients' abnormal movements may be categorized into one of the five major types, it must be admitted that many exhibit a 'mixed movement disorder' comprising a combination of dyskinesias. In these circumstances, it is usually best to concentrate on the most obvious abnormal movement. Having categorized the predominant dyskinesia in an individual patient, the next step is to consider the differential diagnosis of that particular form of abnormal movement, as shown in Tables 20.2, 20.3, 20.4, 20.5 and 20.6. Descriptions will now be given of several diseases in each category.

TREMOR

Benign essential tremor

Benign essential tremor

Essential tremor (ET) is considerably more common than PD. Prevalence estimates vary enormously. An autosomal dominant family history is obtained in about half of patients, and several different genetic loci are probably involved.

Pathogenesis

No consistent pathological or biochemical abnormality has been identified in the few cases that have come to autopsy, but most have some cerebellar torpedoes (possibly alcohol-related), and a few have some (probably incidental) Lewy bodies in brainstem pigmented nuclei.

Everyone has a physiological tremor of the outstretched hands at about 8–12 Hz, which can be exaggerated by adrenergic overactivity as in anxiety, thyrotoxicosis, or when taking sympathomimetic drugs. In a subject with a mild-to-moderate postural tremor, and in the absence of a family history, it can be difficult or impossible to decide whether they have enhanced physiological tremor or true ET.

Essential tremor is not usually overtly associated with any other evidence of damage to the nervous system, but possible associations with, for example, unsteady gait or cognitive impairment have been proposed. Some of these cases might be examples of FXTAS.

Clinical features

There are no signs of parkinsonism, although cog-wheeling (without rigidity) may be present. A moderate dose of alcohol often suppresses the tremor and is sometimes a helpful feature in the history.

Generally, the illness is only slowly progressive in most patients, causing predominantly a social disability, but individuals dependent upon fine manual skills may be significantly disabled.

Table 20.3 Causes of dystonia

Cause
Primary dystonia
Generalized and segmental dystonia
DYT1 (autosomal dominant – 40% of cases)
DYT 6 (dominant)
Others, either genetic or sporadic
Focal adult-onset dystonia (usually sporadic, genetic component remains undetermined in most cases)
Blepharospasm
Cranial dystonia/Meige's syndrome/Breughel's syndrome
Oromandibular dystonia (OMD)
Spasmodic torticollis (ST)
Spasmodic dysphonia/laryngeal dystonia
Axial dystonia
Writer's (and other occupational) cramps
Dystonia plus syndromes
Dopa-responsive dystonia (DRD, DYT 5, dominant)
Myoclonus dystonia (dominant – most cases DYT11)
Symptomatic dystonia
Athetoid cerebral palsy
Post-anoxic
Post-encephalitic
Drug-induced   Neuroleptics (acute dystonic reactions and tardive dystonia)
Levodopa
Manganese poisoning/other toxins
Hemidystonia (usually as a result of structural lesion in contralateral basal ganglia)
Stroke/tumour/arteriovenous malformation/trauma/encephalitis
Post-thalamotomy
Psychogenic
Heredodegenerative dystonias
Various lipid storage diseases and leukodystrophies
Acidosis (organic acidurias)
Ataxia telangiectasia (recessive)
Mitochondrial encephalopathies/Leigh's disease (mitochondrial)
Wilson's disease (recessive)
Huntington's disease (especially juvenile) (dominant)
Neurodegeneration with brain iron accumulation type 1 (NBIA 1-recessive)
Neuroacanthocytosis (recessive)
PD/PSP/MSA/CBD
Autosomal dominant spinocerebellar ataxias (especially 2 and 3-dominant)
Paroxysmal dyskinesias (sporadic or dominant)
Paroxysmal kinesigenicchoreo-athetosis (PKC/PKD
Paroxysmal dystonic choreo-athetosis (PDC, PNKD)
Paroxysmal exercise-induced dystonia (PED)
Tonic spasms in multiple sclerosis

Table 20.4 Causes of chorea

	Cause	
Heredo-degenerative		
	Huntington's disease (dominant)	
	Dentatorubropallidoluysian atrophy (DRPLA-dominant)	
	Neuroferritinopathy (dominant)	
	Benign hereditary chorea (dominant)	
	HDL-2: junctophilin-3 gene (dominant)	
	HDL-4: SCA 17 (dominant)	
	Inherited prion disease (dominant)	
	Ataxia-telangiectasia (recessive)	
	Wilson's disease (recessive)	
	Friedreich's ataxia (recessive)	
	Neuroacanthocytosis (recessive)	
	McLeod syndrome (X-linked)	
	Mitochondrial disease (mitochondrial)	
Sporadic, symptomatic		
	Drug-induced	Levodopa, anticholinergics, dopamine agonists
		Neuroleptics
		Phenytoin, carbamazepine
		Tricyclics
	Other	Thyrotoxicosis
		Systemic lupus erythematosus and the antiphospholipid syndrome
		Polycythaemia rubravera
		Hyperglycaemia
		Hypernatraemia
		Hypoparathyroidism
		Subdural haematoma
		New variant Creutzfeldt–Jakob disease
		Sydenham's chorea: variants include chorea gravidarum, 'pill' chorea, post-streptococcal chorea with anti-basal ganglia antibodies
		Cerebrovascular disease/tumour/trauma, including surgery (usually as hemichorea/hemiballism)

HDL, Huntington disease-like.

Established essential tremor always involves both hands, usually fairly symmetrically, producing a postural tremor, which can also interfere with action. Despite subsequent spread in many cases to other body parts, the part where it begins, and which remains most severely affected, is the arms. There is usually no tremor at rest, but a rhythmic vertical oscillation develops when the patient holds the arms outstretched. On movement, as in finger–nose testing, the tremor may worsen terminally, but does not progressively worsen throughout the movement. Tremor of the head (titubation) or legs may also be present, but is less severe than that in the hands.

Table 20.5 Causes of myoclonus

Generalized myoclonus		
Progressive myoclonic epilepsy[a]	Mitochondrial disease	
	Lafora body disease	
	GM2 gangliosidosis (Tay–Sachs disease)	
	Ceroidlipofuscinosis (Batten's/Kuf's disease)	
	Sialidosis (cherry red spot myoclonus syndrome)	
Progressive myoclonic ataxia[b]	Mitochondrial disease	
	Unverricht–Lundborg disease	
	Spinocerebellar degenerations	
	Coeliac disease	
Other myoclonic epilepsies[b]	First year of life:	Infantile spasms
		Opsoclonus–myoclonus syndrome
	2–6 years:	Lennox–Gastaut syndrome
	Older children and adolescents (and adults)	Photosensitive epileptic myoclonus
		Myoclonic absences
		Juvenile myoclonic epilepsy
Other causes:	Subacutesclerosingpanencephalitis (SSPE)	
	Creutzfeldt–Jakob disease	
	Alzheimer's disease	
	Corticobasal degeneration	
	Multiple system atrophy	
	Metabolic myoclonus	Uraemia/hyponatraemia/hypocalcaemia
		CO_2 narcosis
		Drug-induced (e.g. bismuth; alcohol and drug withdrawal)
Static myoclonic encephalopathies	Post-anoxic action myoclonus (Lance–Adams syndrome)	
	Post-traumatic myoclonus	
Myoclonus-dystonia (often due to epsilon-sarcoglycan mutation)		
Focal or segmental myoclonus		
Cortical reflex myoclonus		
Epilepsiapartialis continua		
Spinal and propriospinal myoclonus	Tumour	
	Infarct	
	Trauma	
Hemifacial spasm		
Palatal myoclonus/tremor		
Psychogenic		

[a]Epilepsy and mental impairment main problem, with additional myoclonus and cerebellar features.
[b]Myoclonus and cerebellar features main problem, perhaps with mild mental impairment and epilepsy.

Table 20.6 Causes of tics

	Cause
Simple tics	Transient tic of childhood
	Chronic simple tic
Complex multiple tics	Chronic multiple tics
	Gilles de la Tourette syndrome
Symptomatic tics	Encephalitis lethargica
	Drug-induced tics (e.g. cocaine)
	Neuroacanthocytosis

Treatment

About one-half of patients show some useful response to a **beta-adrenergic receptor antagonist**, such as propranolol. **Primidone**, **topimarate** or **gabapentin** help some patients. Antiparkinsonian drugs have no effect. **Unilateral or bilateral thalamic DBS** can be very effective.

Other tremors

In some cases **resembling ET**, the tremor is found to be **secondary to peripheral neuropathy** (particularly dysgammaglobulinaemic neuropathy, Chapter 16), or a **(spino) cerebellar degeneration**; and a similar postural tremor may also be seen in some patients with PD, either as well as, or instead of, a classic rest tremor. Many patients with dystonic tremor or tremor associated with dystonia are misdiagnosed as having ET. Dystonic arm tremor is often unilateral or asymmetric, position- or task-specific, and pronation–supination in type, and may be associated with dystonia in the arms, or tremor or dystonia elsewhere, most commonly neck tremor or torticollis.

A particular, rare, but functionally disabling tremor is **orthostatic tremor (OT)**. This manifests on standing, and is relieved by sitting or walking. The tremor, which is rapid at about 16 Hz, may not be visible, but can be palpated or auscultated, and is easily documented on surface EMG recordings. Treatment is difficult. Occasionally clonazepam helps, and there are recent reports that bilateral thalamic DBS may help.

DYSTONIA

Dystonia may affect the whole body (generalized dystonia, Oppenheim's dystonia or dystonia musculorum deformans), in which case onset is typically in childhood. Alternatively, it may affect only one part of the body (focal dystonia), typically with onset in adult life. Cases of segmental dystonia, involving two or more contiguous body parts, are intermediate between the generalized and focal types.

In **primary or idiopathic dystonia**, dystonia is often the only manifestation, but dystonic tremor, and rapid dystonic movements that look myoclonic, can also be present. Many patients with primary generalized or segmental dystonia give a positive family history, most commonly suggesting inheritance as an autosomal dominant trait.

Dystonia plus syndromes include dopa-responsive dystonia (DYT 5) and myoclonus dystonia (DYT-11, described above).

Secondary or symptomatic dystonia is the result of some identifiable brain disease, in which case there are likely to be other signs and symptoms of damage to the nervous system. Various heredo-degenerative diseases can include dystonia as one feature. Examples of both categories are given in Table 20.3.

Generalized or segmental primary dystonia

DYT 1 dystonia

The most commonly identified type of generalized or segmental primary dystonia is the result of a deletion in the DYT1 gene on chromosome 9.

Inheritance is dominant, with 30–40 per cent penetrance, so that a family history, although often evident, is not always present. DYT1-associated dystonia accounts for most cases of Ashkenazi Jewish patients with primary dystonia (which is common in this population as a result of a founder effect), and most cases of young-onset generalized dystonia in non-Jewish populations. This illness, with onset in childhood, usually commences with dystonic spasms of the legs on walking, or sometimes of the arms, trunk or neck. Typically the affected child begins to walk on the toes or, less commonly, develops a writer's cramp or torticollis. The illness is usually progressive when it commences in childhood. The spasms spread to involve most body parts, but usually spare the facial and bulbar muscles. The condition stops spreading as adulthood is reached. Conversely, if gene carriers have not developed symptoms by 26 years of age, they are very unlikely ever to be affected. The intellect is preserved and there are no signs of pyramidal or sensory deficit.

DYT 6 dystonia

The next most common cause of primary segmental or generalized dystonia is DYT6, due to dominant mutations in the THAP1 gene on chromosome 8, with 60 per cent penetrance.

Mean onset age is 16 years, typically with cranial, cervical or laryngeal dystonia, becoming segmental and sometimes generalized, i.e. the inverse pattern to DYT1 dystonia.

Primary generalized torsion dystonia can be distressing and difficult to treat. About 5 per cent of patients respond dramatically to a levodopa preparation (dopa-responsive dystonia, see below under Dopa-responsive dystonia). If the affected individual does not respond to levodopa, the most successful treatment is high-dose anticholinergic therapy, usually in the form of trihexyphenidyl. The aim is to start with a low dose and gradually increase to the maximum the patient can tolerate, dictated by side effects, over many months. About 50 per cent of patients with primary generalized torsion dystonia may show a useful response to such treatment. If neither levodopa nor an anticholinergic helps, other drugs are unlikely to either, but occasional patients seem to benefit from oral baclofen, carbamazepine or clonazepam. Intrathecal baclofen has been helpful in a few seriously affected subjects, typically those with additional spasticity as a manifestation of cerebral palsy, but system complications, often life-threatening, are common. Over the last decade, treatment for patients with primary generalized dystonia has been transformed by the demonstration that bilateral pallidal DBS can dramatically alleviate their dystonia.

Focal primary dystonia

The genetics of late-onset primary dystonia are less clear. DYT1 mutations are rarely found in those with adult-onset focal dystonias, but linkage to other areas of the genome has been identified in some familial cases. Most adult-onset focal dystonias occur sporadically, but genetic factors seem very likely to play a role in most of them.

Spasmodic torticollis

ST is the most common of the focal dystonias, affects women more than men, and usually occurs in the middle-aged or elderly. The onset is insidious, often with initial pain, and sometimes precipitated by local injury. The head turns to one side (torticollis), or occasionally extends (retrocollis) or flexes (antecollis). The spasms may be repetitive to cause tremulous torticollis, or sustained to hold the posture fixed.

The condition is chronic, and not to be confused with acute wry neck, which is common and transient. Although remission occurs in about one in eight cases, usually this is only temporary. Patients are usually normal apart from their torticollis, although some may exhibit a postural hand tremor similar to that of essential tremor, and in some the dystonia may become segmental.

Drug treatment is usually unrewarding. The treatment of choice is injection of **botulinum toxin type A** into the affected neck muscles, which gives most patients satisfactory relief, but requires repeating approximately every three months. Some patients, however, do not respond to injections, or lose their response to the toxin because they develop neutralizing antibodies. Such individuals may be helped by surgery (posterior primary ramicectomy or pallidal DBS) or treatment with different types of botulinum toxin (e.g. type B botulinum toxin).

Dystonic writer's cramp

A specific complaint of inability to write could be the result of any of a variety of causes, including local joint disease, carpal tunnel syndrome, a spastic or ataxic hand, PD or ET. However, in some patients none of these causes is found.

The typical presentation of writer's cramp is the development of a dystonic posture of the arm when gripping the pen, which is driven into the paper with force (simple writer's cramp). Other manual acts, such as typing or playing a musical instrument, may also be affected (dystonic writer's cramp, occupational or musician's cramp).

Isolated dystonic writer's cramp usually appears in middle or late life and does not usually progress to involve other parts of the body. Some individuals learn to write with the opposite arm, but the problem may spread to that side in up to one-third of cases. Drug treatment is disappointing. **Botulinum toxin injections**, under EMG control, can help many patients.

Blepharospasm and oromandibular dystonia

Blepharospasm refers to recurrent spasms of eye closure. The periocular muscles forcibly contract for seconds or minutes, often repetitively, and can render the patient functionally blind. Such eye spasms are commonly precipitated by reading or watching television, or by bright lights. Oromandibular dystonia (OMD) refers to similar recurrent spasms of muscles of the mouth, tongue and jaw. Blepharospasm and OMD commonly coexist, when the condition is called cranial dystonia, or Meige's or Breughel's syndrome. Some patients with cranial dystonia may also exhibit torticollis or writer's cramp (segmental dystonia).

The treatment of choice for blepharospasm is repeated injections of botulinum toxin. However, only a minority of patients with OMD are consistently helped by this treatment. Unfortunately, oral medications are not helpful.

Laryngeal dystonia (spasmodic dysphonia)

In laryngeal dystonia, dystonic spasms affect the muscles controlling the vocal cords. Usually, the adductors are involved, causing a strangled, forced voice with stops and pitch breaks. Much less commonly, the abductors are affected, causing a whispering dysphonia. Spasmodic dysphonia may be isolated, or may be part of a more widespread segmental dystonia. EMG-guided injection of botulinum toxin into laryngeal muscles is the treatment of choice.

Dopa-responsive dystonia

Dopa-responsive dystonia (DRD) (DYT5) typically presents in childhood or adolescence with dystonia of the legs and gait. Many affected individuals describe variation in the severity of their dystonia in the course of the day (diurnal fluctuation). Typically, the patient is normal or much improved in the morning, but develops increasing dystonia as the day wears on, improved after sleep. Many individuals also have unexplained falls, signs of mild parkinsonism and brisk reflexes. Adults carrying the abnormal gene may present with parkinsonism in later life.

Despite its rarity (estimated prevalence one in 2 million), it is crucial not to miss a case of dopa-responsive dystonia, because in this condition small doses of levodopa can permanently restore affected individuals to normal, without the development of the fluctuations and dyskinesias seen with chronic treatment of PD.

The condition is inherited as an autosomal dominant trait, with 40 per cent penetrance, associated with mutations of a gene on chromosome 14 that codes for the enzyme GTP cyclohydrolase I. This enzyme catalyses the first step of conversion of GTP to tetrahydrobiopterin (BH4), which is an essential co-factor for the enzyme tyrosine hydroxylase (TH), which converts tyrosine to levodopa. As a result, dopamine cannot be synthesized, although the nigrostriatal pathway is structurally intact. Levodopa treatment bypasses this metabolic block and restores brain dopamine content. Many different mutations in the gene have been identified. **A trial of a levodopa preparation is mandatory in any young person with dystonia of unknown cause.** A rarer form of DRD, usually with infantile onset, is caused by homozygous recessive mutations in the TH gene.

Wilson's disease

Wilson's disease (WD) is a rare, recessively inherited disease producing a progressive extrapyramidal syndrome with behavioural changes and liver and kidney dysfunction resulting from retention of copper in the body. It is uncommon for the neurological manifestations of WD to start after the age of 40 years.

Diagnosis

Many different mutations have been found in a gene on chromosome 13 coding for a copper-transporting ATPase, so that genetic testing is not usually practicable for diagnosis, except in populations where a particular mutation is very frequent, or in relatives when the responsible mutation(s) in the propositus are already known. For most patients, diagnosis rests on the demonstration of reduced serum caeruloplasmin or copper, increased 24-hour urinary copper excretion, and the demonstration, by slit-lamp examination, of the characteristic **Kayser–Fleischer ring** in the cornea. In cases of doubt, liver biopsy copper content should be assayed. Brain scanning with MRI may show cortical atrophy or signal change in basal ganglia, mainly putamen.

The primary abnormality in WD is a failure to excrete copper normally in bile. As a result, copper accumulates in the body, initially in the liver. Progressive liver damage occurs, and gradually the liver cannot contain the excess copper, which spills over into the circulation. Copper then accumulates in many other organs throughout the body, in particular in the brain, and especially in the basal ganglia. It is crucial not to miss a diagnosis of WD because it is treatable, and without treatment, it is ultimately fatal.

Treatment

The treatment for WD is to promote the excretion of copper from, or to reduce its absorption into the body. The most appropriate treatment is a subject of some controversy. **Penicillamine**, which chelates with copper to form a complex that is excreted in the urine, is still usually considered the drug of choice. Penicillamine treatment can effectively remove excess copper stores from the body and reverse or halt both liver and brain damage. The response to treatment may take weeks or months to appear, and some cases initially worsen before improving, but the majority of patients can be maintained healthy by such therapy, which has to be taken for life. Alternative treatments are zinc salts, trientene, tetrathiomolybdate and liver transplantation.

Fixed dystonia

Dystonia is usually mobile. Fixed dystonia often comes on acutely, mainly in young women, usually after minor peripheral trauma, and may be associated with pain, sometimes (20 per cent of cases) fulfilling criteria for complex regional pain syndrome type 1 without or, less commonly type 2 with peripheral nerve or root injury (see Chapter 30). In the largest case series, 42 per cent fulfilled criteria for documented or clinically established psychogenicdystonia, or somatization disorder, or both (24 per cent). In some of these cases, early multidisciplinary intervention and botulinum toxin injection can help, but in most patients with fixed dytonia no treatment is effective.

Paroxysmal dyskinesias

Several uncommon conditions (usually inherited as autosomal dominant traits) may cause attacks of dyskinesia (dystonic, choreic or ballistic) lasting seconds to hours, with full recovery between episodes. Some are due to channelopathies and may be associated with migraine or seizures.

Episodes of **paroxysmal kinesigenic choreoathetosis (PKC) or dyskinesia (PKD)** are brief (lasting up to 5 minutes, but usually 30–60 seconds), occur frequently during the day, and are precipitated by sudden movement. They can be prevented by low dosages of anticonvulsant drugs, typically **carbamazepine**.

Attacks of **paroxysmal dystonic choreoathetosis (PDC) or non-kinesigenic dyskinesia (PNKD)**, due to mutations in the *MR1* gene on chromosome 2, last longer (minutes to hours), are less frequent, and are not precipitated by movement, but can be brought on by fatigue, alcohol and caffeine. They are sometimes helped by clonazepam or levodopa.

In patients with **paroxysmal exercise–induced dyskinesia (PED)**, some of whom also have epilepsy, attacks are provoked by prolonged exercise, and the condition is due to mutations in a gene encoding the glucose transporter, *GLUT1*. A ketogenic diet can greatly reduce attack frequency.

Tonic spasms in multiple sclerosis comprise brief (seconds to minutes) spontaneous dystonic spasms of one extremity.

Paroxysmal nocturnal dystonia is now recognized to be nocturnal frontal lobe epilepsy.

CHOREA

Sydenham's chorea

Sydenham's chorea (St Vitus' dance) is now a rare disease. However, chorea and other movement disorders, sometimes associated with psychiatric disturbance, but without rheumatic fever, continue to be seen in some children after group A beta-haemolytic streptococcal infection, and may be associated with anti-basal-ganglia antibodies.

Huntington's disease (HD) is a rare, dominantly inherited, relentlessly progressive illness, usually starting in middle life, characterized by a movement disorder, usually including chorea, and behavioural and cognitive changes. It occurs worldwide and in all ethnic groups, with a prevalence in the UK of between five and ten per 100 000. **The mutation, caused by a trinucleotide CAG repeat expansion on the short arm of chromosome 4**, is fully penetrant, so that the children of an affected parent have a 50 per cent risk of developing the disease. About 6 per cent of cases start before the age of 21 years (juvenile HD) with an akinetic-rigid syndrome (the Westphal variant) caused by long trinucleotide repeats inherited, in 90 per cent of cases, from an affected father. The large number of cell divisions in spermatogenesis in the father allows substantial intergenerational increases in the length of the abnormal polyglutaminetrinucleotide repeat, making the disease appear at a younger age. This phenomenon, also seen in other trinucleotide repeat diseases, is called 'anticipation'. About 30 per cent of cases start after the age of 50 years (late-onset HD). 'Senile chorea' is simply chorea in an older person – once other causes are excluded, the majority of such cases turn out to have HD.

Huntington's disease

Pathogenesis

The brain is generally atrophic with conspicuous damage to the cerebral cortex and the striatum (caudate nucleus and putamen), which shows extensive loss of medium-sized spiny neurones.

Clinical features

The onset is insidious, usually between the ages of 30 and 50 years. The initial symptoms frequently are those of a change in personality and behaviour, butchorea may be the first sign. The family may begin to notice a blunting of drive and depth of feeling, irritability and truculence, or a tendency to uncontrolled aggressive or sexual behaviour. As the disease progresses, frontal lobe deficits become more pronounced and the chorea more severe and grotesque. Akinesia, rigidity and dystonia may appear and begin to dominate the picture. Finally, the patient becomes bedridden and emaciated. Death occurs on average about 17 years after onset.

Diagnosis is not difficult if the presentation is characteristic and a positive family history is available. However, often the family history is not known, or is hidden, or chorea may be absent or a relatively minor part of the patient's motor disorder. Moreover, late HD looks very different from early disease. A simple DNA test will confirm the diagnosis.

Treatment

Currently, there is no cure or disease-modifying treatment for the disease. The chorea may be reduced by dopamine receptor blocking or dopamine-depleting drugs, but these commonly cause disabling side effects, and the reduction in chorea may be only cosmetic, while the rest of the clinical state is aggravated. The mental complications of the illness often pose particular problems for the family, and eventually chronic nursing care may be required.

Genetic counselling should be made available to other family members. **Presymptomatic (predictive) and prenatal testing** are available in specialized centres.

Hemiballism

Hemiballism refers to wild flinging or throwing movements of one arm and leg. Occasionally only one (monoballism) or all four limbs (biballism) are involved. The movements are like those of chorea, but predominantly involve the large proximal muscles of the shoulder and pelvic girdle. Hemiballism is rare. It is usually seen in elderly, hypertensive or diabetic patients as a result of a **stroke affecting the contralateral subthalamic nucleus** or its connections, in which case the onset is abrupt. More recently, toxoplasma abscess secondary to HIV infection has emerged as a cause of hemiballism in younger subjects. The intensity of the movements varies from mild to severe enough to cause injury. If a result of a stroke, hemiballism often gradually remits spontaneously over a period of three to six months. In the interim, treatment with a neuroleptic or tetrabenazine may be required to damp down the movements.

MYOCLONUS

Generalized myoclonus

Generalized or multifocal myoclonus occurs in a wide variety of primary diseases of the nervous system, or as a manifestation of metabolic or toxic encephalopathy. In many of these conditions, myoclonus arises from spontaneous or reflex-triggered discharges in the cerebral cortex. Such cortical myoclonus is closely related to epilepsy. Epileptic myoclonus can be a feature of primary generalized epilepsy, or may be symptomatic of progressive brain disease as in the progressive myoclonic epilepsies (see Chapter 13).

Myoclonus may dominate the clinical picture in a number of cerebral diseases. In these conditions, myoclonus may occur spontaneously, on movement (action myoclonus), or in response to visual, auditory or somatosensory stimuli (reflex myoclonus). Severe myoclonus may be the major residual deficit after cerebral anoxia (post-anoxic action myoclonus or Lance-Adams syndrome), usually related to respiratory rather than cardiac arrest. Myoclonus may be the characteristic feature of a number of degenerative dementing illnesses, such as Alzheimer's disease, and is characteristic of Creutzfeldt–Jakob disease. When myoclonus, with occasional seizures, occurs in conjunction with a cerebellar syndrome, this combination is called 'progressive myoclonic ataxia' (one of the three Ramsay-Hunt syndromes) and caused by, for example, Unverricht–Lundborg disease, mitochondrial disease or coeliac disease. Myoclonus may also follow a variety of viral illnesses (post-infectious myoclonus). In all these conditions there are likely to be other signs of damage to the central nervous system.

Myoclonus-dystonia (DYT 11) is considered earlier(see above under Dystonia).

Focal myoclonus

There are several conditions in which myoclonic jerking is restricted to one part of the body. Such **focal myoclonus** may be a result of discharges occurring anywhere from the cerebral cortex (**epilepsia partialis continua**), the brainstem (e.g. **palatal myoclonus** or tremor), the spinal cord (**spinal myoclonus**), or even peripheral nerves and roots (**hemifacial spasm**).

Such focal myoclonus is often repetitive and rhythmic; for example, in the rare palatal tremor/myoclonus there are rhythmic contractions of the soft palate at about 2 Hz, often persisting throughout the day and night. Sometimes this rhythmic myoclonus spreads to involve the pharynx and larynx, the intercostal muscles and diaphragm, and even the external ocular muscles. Often, this condition is idiopathic, but in secondary cases the most common identifiable cause is an infarct involving the brainstem, in particular in the region bounded by the olive, dentate nucleus and red nucleus (Mollaret's triangle), and rarer cases are due to adult-onset Alexander's disease.

Much more common is **hemifacial spasm**, in which intermittent rapid twitchy movements start at the lateral border of orbicularis oculi and spread to synchronously involve orbicularis oris on the same side. In addition, the affected side of the face may be drawn up by more prolonged spasms, and often there is mild facial weakness on the same side. The cause is usually irritation of the facial nerve entry zone by a pulsatile aberrant blood vessel. Most patients are helped by botulinum toxin injections. A more invasive, but usually permanently effective, alternative is **facial nerve decompression via a posterior craniotomy**.

Drug treatment of myoclonus

Myoclonus often responds best to a combination of drugs. Clonazepam, sodium valproate, primidone, piracetam and levetiracetamare used in varying combinations.

TICS

Tics and Gilles de la Tourette syndrome

Many children exhibit simple tics transiently during development. Typically, these consist of eye blinks, grimaces, a sniff or a hand gesture. Often these transient tics of childhood disappear, but sometimes they persist into adult life as chronic simple tics.

In a proportion of patients, these chronic tics are accompanied by vocalizations, when the condition is known as **Gilles de la Tourette syndrome (GTS)**, which affects 1 per cent of the population. This illness begins before the age of 18 years with the tics affecting particularly the upper part of the body, especially the face, neck and shoulders. Their severity and distribution tend to wax and wane over time, and one tic may be replaced by another. Sooner or later, patients begin to make involuntary noises, such as grunting, squealing, yelping, throat-clearing, sniffing, coughing or barking. In about 15 per cent of cases, these noises become transformed into swear words (**coprolalia**). Often the patient recognizes an uncomfortable or even painful sensation (sensory tic) which is relieved by making the movement (itch and scratch analogy). Many Tourette patients also exhibit features of obsessive-compulsive disorder (OCD), and many affected children also display attention-deficit hyperactivity disorder (ADHD).

The illness tends to be lifelong, although its severity usually decreases in adulthood. It is strongly influenced by genetic factors which are yet to be identified.

The tics and vocalizations may cause considerable distress to the child or adolescent. Anti-dopamine drugs, such as haloperidol, pimozide, sulpiride or tetrabenazine, may control the involuntary movements and noises, although finding the appropriate dose requires careful and gradual titration in each patient. Many patients find the side effects (extrapyramidal, drowsiness, depression) from these medications unacceptable, and instead prefer to live with their tics, once they realize they are an intrinsic part of their 'motor personality'. OCD-like symptoms may be helped by selective serotonin reuptake inhibitors or clomipramine, and ADHD by methylphenidate. Some subjects with severe GTS have been helped by DBS, usually in thalamus.

NEUROLEPTIC-INDUCED MOVEMENT DISORDERS

Dopamine receptor blocking drugs used to treat psychiatric illness (neuroleptics) or as antiemetics or vestibular sedatives can cause a wide range of movement disorders.

Drug-induced parkinsonism

Drug-induced parkinsonism has been considered earlier (see above under Drug-induced parkinsonism).

Acute dystonic reactions

Some 2–5 per cent of those given neuroleptic drugs may develop acute dystonia within 24–48 hours. Typically, this consists of spasms of the jaw, mouth, tongue or neck sometimes with oculogyria, and sometimes also affecting the limbs. Such acute dystonic reactions are often accompanied by considerable distress. They can be terminated by the intravenous administration of an anticholinergic drug (e.g.procyclidine 5–10 mg).

Akathisia

Akathisia refers to a sense of motor restlessness and the inability to sit still. Sufferers are driven to stand up and walk about to gain relief. When sitting, they often exhibit stereotyped restless movements of the legs and hands. Akathisia is linked to drug-induced parkinsonism and even occurs in PD itself. It is difficult to treat, but may sometimes be attenuated by a benzodiazepine or propranolol.

Tardive dyskinesias

Tardive dyskinesias are abnormal involuntary movements that appear after months or years of neuroleptic treatment. The most common form is a choreiform orofacial dyskinesia consisting of repetitive movements of the mouth and tongue, which occurs particularly in the elderly. About 60 per cent of such cases will eventually gradually remit if the offending neuroleptic drug can be withdrawn. In younger patients, the abnormal movements of tardive dyskinesia may be dystonic (tardive dystonia).

Unfortunately, only about 15 per cent of patients with tardive dystonia remit after withdrawal of neuroleptic drugs. However, if neuroleptic therapy is required to prevent relapse of schizophrenia, withdrawal may be impractical. The best strategy to avoid the development of tardive dyskinesias is to give neuroleptics only when clinically justified, and to use the newer generation of atypical neuroleptics, which appear less likely to provoke the movements, and which may allow remission of established movements while continuing to prevent psychiatric relapse. Tardive orofacial dyskinesias may respond to treatment with **tetrabenazine**, but will be worsened by anticholinergics. In contrast, tardive dystonias may benefit from treatment with an anticholinergic drug.

Neuroleptic malignant syndrome

Dopamine receptor blocking agents of any class may occasionally provoke a life-threatening syndrome of extreme rigidity, fever (usually high), autonomic disturbances, and a fluctuating level of consciousness associated with a high serum creatine kinase concentration and often a leukocytosis. The offending drug must be withdrawn and intensive medical care given, including administration of a dopamine agonist or levodopa, together with dantrolene.

Tetrabenazine depletes presynaptic amine stores, and can also cause any of the above with the exception of tardive dyskinesia/dystonia.

OTHER MOVEMENT DISORDERS

Restless legs syndrome

RLS is common, affecting 3–10 per cent of the population to some degree. It can be familial (usually with younger onset) or sporadic. The latter is sometimes associated with iron deficiency, anaemia, pregnancy, peripheral neuropathy or uraemia. Serum ferritin is often low. It is commonly associated with periodic leg movements of sleep (PLMS).

The essential features of RLS include:
- An urge to move the legs, usually accompanied by uncomfortable or unpleasant sensations in the legs.
- These symptoms begin or worsen during periods of rest or inactivity, such as lying or sitting.
- Symptoms are partially or totally relieved by movement, at least for as long as the activity continues.
- Symptoms are worse, or only occur, in the evening or at night.

Supportive criteria are:
- Positive response to dopaminergic treatment
- Periodic limb movements during wakefulness or sleep
- Positive family history suggestive of autosomal dominant inheritance.

If drug treatment is needed, low doses of a dopamine agonist (e.g. **pramipexole**, **ropinirole** or the **rotigotine patch**) are currently favoured over levodopa because chronic levodopa treatment can lead to 'augmentation' – i.e. spillover of symptoms to the daytime, an increase in severity of symptoms, and involvement of other body parts. Second-line drugs that sometimes help are opiates, gabapentin, carbamazepine and clonazepam. If there is iron deficiency or low ferritin, iron supplementation is indicated.

Stiff person syndrome, stiff limb syndrome and encephalomyelitis with rigidity

The rare classic stiff person syndrome involves continuous paraspinal muscle activity that can be confirmed by surface EMG, and causes a sustained lumbar hyperlordosis. It is associated with the presence of autoantibodies, particularly anti-GAD, and sometimes with diabetes (but many patients with diabetes have anti-GAD antibodies without stiff person syndrome).

Patients remain ambulant, and are usually helped by high doses of diazepam and baclofen. Plasmapheresis or intravenous immunoglobulins (IVIg) are sometimes used in more severe cases.

Stiff limb syndrome is even rarer, and not usually associated with anti-GAD. It usually does not respond to any treatment and if it involves the leg most subjects become wheelchair-bound.

Encephalomyelitis with rigidity, or spinal interneuronitis, is a severe rapidly progressive inflammatory and often fatal form of stiff person associated with an inflammatory cerebrospinal fluid (CSF) picture and sometimes additional myoclonus and denervation, which can be associated with anti-amphiphysinor glycine receptor antibodies and with neoplasia.

Painful legs and moving toes

This rare condition is characterized by slow undulating flexion–extension movements of the toes, accompanied by pain in the legs, usually unilateral. There may be evidence of peripheral nerve or root lesion involving the affected leg. No treatment is effective.

Psychogenic movement disorders

Psychogenic movement disorders (PMD) can present as any movement disorder, although dystonia and tremor are the most common manifestations and psychogenic parkinsonism and chorea are rare. PMD represent 4–25 per cent of all new cases seen in specialist movement disorder clinics.

The diagnosis of a PMD is primarily clinical. Positive features suggesting the diagnosis include:

- marked fluctuations during examination
- distractibility
- increase with attention or suggestion
- incongruence with patterns of recognized movement disorders
- the presence of other non-organic signs or a psychiatric disorder
- discrepancy between objective signs and disability
- abrupt onset with rapid progression to maximum severity
- inconsistency over time
- history of previous somatizations
- sustained and substantial response to placebo or psychotherapy

While none of these features is pathognomonic, they allow a classification based on degree of diagnostic certainty into documented, clinically established, probable and possible.

Specific PMDs may have additional features that support the diagnosis. In psychogenic tremor, these include distractibility and entrainability of tremor to the frequency of contralateral hand movements. In psychogenic myoclonus, the presence of a *Bereitschaftspotential* (premovement potential) preceding myoclonic movements, of prolonged or variable duration EMG bursts, and of long latency and variable recruitment in stimulus-sensitive myoclonus, all support the diagnosis.

However, in some cases investigations may exclude a psychogenic cause. Thus, in myoclonus, consistent duration of myoclonic bursts less than 70 ms, latency to stimulus-sensitive myoclonus of less than 70 ms, or the presence of giant somatosensory evoked potentials (SEPs) or cortical correlates of myoclonic jerks on back-averaged EEG exclude a psychogenic aetiology. Similarly, an abnormal DaT SPECT scan excludes a diagnosis of psychogenic parkinsonism.

The prognosis of long-standing PMD is generally poor, although patients presenting soon after onset appear to have a better prognosis. Management is difficult but should include thorough initial investigation followed by discussion of the diagnosis in a clear but non-confrontational manner emphasizing the unconscious origin of PMD. Where appropriate, exploration of psychiatric disorders or psychological factors underlying the disorder, appropriate referral for diagnosis and treatment, initiation of pharmacological and physical therapy, and continued follow up by a multidisciplinary team (including the neurologist) should be considered.

FURTHER READING

25th Anniversary Issue, containing 23 'Milestones'reviews of all different movement disorders. *Movement Disorders* (2011) 26:947–1182.

Abdo WF, van de Warrenburg BP, Burn DJ, Quinn NP, Bloem BR. The clinical approach to movement disorders. *Nature Reviews in Neurology* (2010) 6:29–37.

Ala A, Walker AP, AshkanK *et al.* (2007) Wilson's disease. *Lancet*, 369:397–408.

Braak H, Bohl JR, Muller CM *et al* (2006) Stanley Fahn Lecture 2005: The staging procedure for the inclusion body pathology associated with sporadic Parkinson's disease. *Movement Disorders*, 21:2042–2051.

Caviness JN. (2004) Myoclonus: current concepts and recent advances. *Lancet Neurology*, 10:598–607.

Chaudhuri KR, Schapira AH. (2009) Non-motor symptoms of Parkinson's disease: dopaminergic pathophysiology and treatment. *Lancet Neurology*, 8:464–74.

Deuschl G, Bain PG, Brin M. (1998) Consensus statement of the Movement Disorder Society on tremor. *Movement Disorders*, 13:2–23.

Goetz CG, Koller WC, Poewe W *et al.* (2002) Management of Parkinson's disease: An evidence-based review. *Movement Disorders*, 17(Suppl. 4):S1–S166.

Gupta A, Lang AE. (2009) Psychogenic movement disorders. *Current Opinion in Neurology*, 22:430–436.

Horstink M, Tolosa E, Bonucelli U *et al.* (2006) Review of the therapeutic management of Parkinson's disease. Report of a joint task force of the European Federation of Neurological Societies (EFNS) and the Movement Disorder Society-European Section (MDS-ES). Part I: early (uncomplicated) and Part II: late (complicated) Parkinson's disease. *European Journal of Neurology*, 13:1170–1185 and 1186–1202

Jankovic J. (2009) Treatment of hyperkinetic movement disorders. *Lancet Neurology*, 8:844–856.

Lees AJ, Hardy J, Revesz T. (2009) Parkinson's disease. *Lancet*, 373:2055–2066.

McKeith IG, Dickson DW, Lowe J *et al.* (2005) Diagnosis and management of dementia with Lewy bodies. Third report of the DLB consortium. *Neurology*, 65:1863–1872.

Muller U. (2009) The monogenic primary dystonias. *Brain*, 132:2005–2025.

Quinn NP, Schneider SA, Schwingenschuh P, Bhatia KP (2011) Tremor – some controversial aspects. *Movement Disorders* 26:18–23

Stefanova N, Bucke P, Duerr P, Wenning GK. (2009) Multiple system atrophy: an update. *Lancet Neurology*, 12:1172–8

Trenkwalder C, Paulus W. (2010) Restless legs syndrome: pathophysiology, clinical presentation and treatment. *Nature Reviews in Neurology*, 6:337–46

Wild EJ, Tabrizi SJ (2007) The differential diagnosis of chorea. *Practical Neurology*, 7:360–73

Williams DR, Lees AJ (2009) Progressive supranuclear palsy: clinicopathological concepts and diagnostic challenges. *Lancet Neurology*, 8:270–279.

Zijlmans JC, Daniel, SE, Hughes AJ *et al.* (2004) Clinicopathological investigation of vascular parkinsonism, including clinical criteria for diagnosis. *Movement Disorders*, 19:630–640.

CHAPTER 21

THE CEREBELLAR ATAXIAS AND HEREDITARY SPASTIC PARAPLEGIAS

Nicholas Fletcher

CEREBELLAR DISORDERS

Cerebellar disorders are classified in terms of aetiology, clinical features, pathological appearances, inheritance and, increasingly, molecular genetic abnormalities. None of these approaches is entirely satisfactory for the clinician, but it is helpful to consider the cerebellar disorders with respect to age of onset and any detectable underlying cause or genetic component.

A simple classification is shown in Table 21.1. This is a guide to the conditions to be expected at different ages, but should not be interpreted rigidly, for example, paraneoplastic and drug- or toxin-induced ataxias are more common in adult life, but obviously can occur occasionally in childhood and adolescence. **A key point is that the most common cause of progressive cerebellar ataxia is a degenerative condition and that many of these conditions are hereditary.** The age of onset is particularly important in the case of the various hereditary ataxias. **Although there is some overlap, the majority of degenerative ataxias appearing before the age of 25 years are autosomal recessive, while most cases of autosomal-dominant ccrebellar ataxia develop after this age.** Genetic ataxia is much more likely in younger onset cases.

Occasionally, cervical spondylotic myelopathy, frontal lobe gait apraxia ('marche à petit pas') as a result of hydrocephalus or cerebrovascular disease, vitamin B12 deficiency, Wilson's disease and progressive supranuclear palsy (PSP) can present with a wide-based, unsteady gait, giving a false impression of a progressive cerebellar disorder. Progressive supranuclear palsy can be particularly confusing in the early stages, when there may be falling, slow eye movements and dysarthria.

There is some localizing value of cerebellar signs within the cerebellar structures. Lesions of the midline (vermis) tend to produce ataxia of gait with variable eye signs, head and body (axial) tremor; lesions of the cerebellar hemispheres are more likely to cause limb ataxia, dysdiadochokinesis and dysmetria.

CONGENITAL ATAXIAS

Developmental malformations of the cerebellum give rise to the syndrome of congenital ataxia. Pathologically, many cases show features of pontoneocerebellar or granule cell hypoplasia. In early infancy, an ataxic disorder may not be obvious but eventually nystagmus, cerebellar tremor and ataxia of the trunk and limbs become apparent. Some patients have only a mild cerebellar ataxia with or without a minor degree of learning disability. This may hardly progress or even improve with age. Other patients are severely ataxic with disabling spasticity and mental retardation. In the past, such patients were often diagnosed as cases of 'ataxic cerebral palsy' but **about 50 per cent have an autosomal recessive condition so that the recurrence risk in subsequent siblings is approximately one in eight**. In some families, there is an autosomal dominant or X-linked pattern of inheritance and many cases are idiopathic.

Autosomal recessive congenital ataxias include:
- **Gillespie syndrome** (congenital ataxia, aniridia, mental retardation)
- **Marinesco Sjögren syndrome** (mental retardation, cataracts)
- **Joubert syndrome** (retinopathy, respiratory abnormalities)
- **Disequilibrium syndrome** (gross truncal ataxia and motor delay, autism and mental retardation)
- **Paine syndrome** (congenital ataxia, seizures, developmental delay, myoclonus, optic atrophy)
- **COACH syndrome** (cerebellar hypoplasia, oligophrenia, ataxia, coloboma and hepatic fibrosis) is lethal in childhood.
- Congenital ataxias with various degrees of learning disability.
- Pontoneocerebellar hypoplasia (PCH). There are two types: PCH1 with distal wasting and PCII2 with dystonia.
- Granule cell layer hypoplasia (ataxia, strabismus, dysmorphism and short stature with learning disability).

X-linked forms include additional features such as ophthalmoplegia, learning disability, myoclonus and retinopathy.

EARLY ONSET HEREDITARY ATAXIAS

Friedreich's ataxia

Friedreich's ataxia (FA) is the most common early onset hereditary ataxia with a frequency in the UK of approximately 1–2 per 100 000. Inheritance is autosomal recessive and the gene locus is on chromosome 9q13. The mutation is a GAA trinucleotide repeat expansion in exon 1 of a gene encoding a 210 amino acid protein (frataxin). Frataxin appears to be involved in mitochondrial iron regulation. A normal repeat of 7–29 expands to a repeat length of between 29 and 1700 in Friedreich's ataxia patients. Affected individuals have two expanded alleles, but a few are compound heterozygotes with one expanded gene and a corresponding allele containing a point mutation. The FA carrier frequency in the population is about one in 110.

Pathology

The principal neuropathological changes are in the spinal cord (Figure 21.1), affecting the cervical dorsal columns and lumbar pyramidal tracts with additional involvement of the spinocerebellar tracts. Brainstem and cerebellar changes are minor. The peripheral nerves show a loss of large myelinated axons.

Clinical features

The onset is typically before the age of 15 years with the majority of cases starting by the age of 20 years. The presenting feature is almost always progressive ataxia; occasional patients present with scoliosis or cardiac disease. Cerebellar dysarthria, pyramidal weakness and areflexia of the legs, extensor plantar responses and impaired vibration and joint position sense usually develop within the first few years and Romberg's test is positive.

A cardiomyopathy occurs in about 75 per cent of cases, but is often mild. Many patients develop scoliosis (seen in 80 per cent) and pes cavus as the

Table 21.1 Classification of cerebellar disorders

Age of onset	Conditions	Inheritance
Congenital	Congenital ataxias ('ataxic cerebral palsy') with or without additional features	Autosomal recessive (50%) Autosomal dominant X-linked Non-genetic
Early onset (usually less than 25 years)	Friedreich's ataxia	Autosomal recessive
	Other early onset hereditary ataxias	Autosomal recessive X-linked
	Metabolic ataxias	Autosomal recessive X-linked
	Vitamin E deficiency	Autosomal recessive
	DNA repair defects	Autosomal recessive
	Episodic ataxia	Autosomal dominant
Late onset (usually after 25 years)	Late onset hereditary cerebellar ataxias	Autosomal dominant
	Fragile X tremor ataxia syndrome	X-linked
	Idiopathic sporadic cerebellar degenerations	Non-genetic
	Paraneoplastic	Non-genetic
	Drugs, toxins and physical agents	Non-genetic
	Tumours	Non-genetic
	Infections	Non-genetic
	Hypothyroidism	Non-genetic
	Vitamin deficiency (B1, B12)	Non-genetic
	Prion diseases	Non-genetic Autosomal dominant
	Autoimmune	Non-genetic
	Gluten ataxia	Non-genetic
Variable	Ramsay Hunt syndrome (Progressive myoclonic ataxia)	Non-genetic Autosomal recessive Mitochondrial
	Dentatorubropallidoluysian atrophy	Autosomal dominant

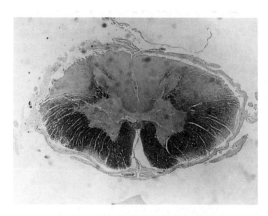

Figure 21.1 Transverse section of the spinal cord in Friedreich's ataxia (myelin stain) showing selective involvement of the dorsal columns (courtesy of Dr J Broome.)

condition progresses and distal wasting is seen in about half of cases. Diabetes (10 per cent), deafness, nystagmus and optic atrophy are less common features (Table 21.2) and cognitive function is not impaired. The progression of the disease is usually relentless, with patients losing the ability to walk after a mean of 15 years and nearly always by 45 years of age. Death often occurs in the fourth decade, but some patients survive much longer.

Clinical variants have long been recognized but their relationship to Friedreich's ataxia was questionable prior to the very recent demonstration of the Friedreich's ataxia mutation in such cases. The most important variants are:

1 **Late onset Friedreich's ataxia** may develop after the age of 25 years, often in the fourth decade and occasionally as late as 51 years of

Table 21.2 Clinical features of Friedreich's ataxia

Clinical feature	Frequency (%)
Ataxia	100
Lower limb areflexia	99
Dysarthria	96
Extensor plantar responses	89
Pyramidal weakness	88
Impaired vibration sense	84
Impaired proprioception	78
Scoliosis	80
Pes cavus	55
Distal wasting	49
Optic atrophy	30
Nystagmus	20
Diabetes	10
Deafness	8
Investigation results	
Abnormal ECG	75
Absent sensory action potentials	92

ECG, electrocardiogram.
Figures in the table based on Harding (1981).

age. There is slower progression, less skeletal deformity and lower GAA repeat numbers in the mutation.

2 **Friedreich's ataxia with retained reflexes (FARR).** The retention of lower limb reflexes was once regarded as incompatible with a diagnosis of Friedreich's ataxia, but some of these patients have a cardiomyopathy and a Friedreich's ataxia trinucleotide expansion. It is likely that early onset ataxia with retained reflexes is heterogeneous however, and that not all such patients have Friedreich's ataxia.

3 An **Acadian variant** has been described, particularly in Italy, among French Canadians and among the Acadian population of Louisiana. Onset is between the ages of 21 and 30 years, but cases with onset as late as 36 years of age have been described. Progression is slower, with less frequent scoliosis and pes cavus and survival is prolonged.

4 Occasional **atypical cases** have presented with chorea or scoliosis. Pure paraparesis or tetraparesis can also occur.

Investigations

The electrocardiogram is invaluable as FA is by far the most likely form of early onset ataxia to be associated with cardiac disease. Widespread T-wave inversion and left ventricular hypertrophy are the most common abnormalities. Cardiac arrhythmias and echocardiographic abnormalities are less common.

Most patients have reduced or absent peripheral nerve sensory action potentials as a result of degeneration of dorsal root ganglion neurones. Motor nerve conduction velocities are normal, in contrast to hereditary motor and sensory neuropathy type I, which can also present in childhood with ataxia and areflexia, but in which motor conduction velocities are slowed. Visual-evoked potentials are of reduced amplitude in many patients and somatosensory and brainstem auditory evoked potentials are frequently abnormal, but are not commonly used in clinical diagnosis of FA.

Magnetic resonance imaging (MRI) reveals atrophy of the cervical cord, but the appearance of the cerebellum is normal (Figure 21.2). Severe cerebellar atrophy, especially at clinical presentation, makes FA unlikely.

Vitamin E levels are normal, but should always be checked, as the spinocerebellar ataxia associated with vitamin E deficiency is indistinguishable on clinical grounds and is potentially treatable.

Diagnostic confirmation by DNA testing is now the usual method of confirming the clinical diagnosis. It is especially critical to pursue investigations into other causes of early onset ataxia if the FA gene DNA test is negative.

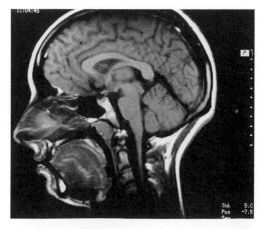

Figure 21.2 Magnetic resonance imaging scan showing cervical cord atrophy in a patient with Friedreich's ataxia.

Management

No treatment has been shown to improve the neurological deficit. Trials with L-carnitine, vitamin E, coenzyme Q10 and idebanone have not yielded significant clinical results. Annual cardiac monitoring is required; patients and families should be warned to report symptoms, such as palpitation, dyspnoea or chest pain. Cardiac symptoms are treated symptomatically and may improve with correction of scoliosis. Diabetes usually requires insulin therapy. Prevention of postural deformities by appropriate seating and physiotherapy is essential and orthopaedic correction of lower limb deformity or scoliosis is helpful in selected cases. Some patients will require hearing aids or low visual aids. The management of hypostatic oedema can be particularly difficult, but elevation is often more effective than diuretics. Depression is a common and easily overlooked treatable cause of additional morbidity.

Genetic counselling is vital, but many parents have completed their families by the time a child is affected; the risk to siblings is one in four. Affected patients survive into adult life and have children. Pregnancy does not exacerbate the disorder but the practical difficulties of caring for children are obvious. The recurrence risk in children is very low, approximately one in 220, based on the risk of a partner being a heterozygote gene carrier of one in 110. DNA testing of patients requires specialized expertise and should follow nationally agreed guidelines.

Early onset ataxia with retained reflexes and the autosomal recessive spastic ataxia of Charlevoix–Saguenay (ARSACS)

Early onset ataxia with retained reflexes is distinguished from Friedreich's ataxia by normal or increased upper limb and knee reflexes (the ankle jerks may be absent); the plantar responses are extensor. The onset is before the age of 20 years, but progression is slower than in Friedreich's ataxia. Severe skeletal deformity, optic atrophy and diabetes do not occur. Cerebellar atrophy may be revealed by brain MRI – in contrast to FA. Cardiomyopathy can occur.

Inheritance is autosomal recessive. In some families, the Friedreich's ataxia mutation has been detected and it is now clear that this condition is sometimes (but not always) a manifestation of Friedreich's ataxia.

The recessive spastic ataxia of Charlevoix-Saguenay is seen mainly in Canada. The gene encoding the protein sacsin is on chromosome 13q11 and several mutations have been associated with ARSACS.

Patients with early onset ataxia with brisk lower limb reflexes may have an X-linked ataxia and it is very important to consider adrenoleucodystrophy (see below under X-linked ataxia) in such cases, as the genetic implications for family members (including potential asymptomatic carrier females) are considerable.

Ataxia with oculomotor apraxia

Ataxia with oculomotor apraxia (AOA) is accompanied by oculomotor apraxia with abnormal restricted eye movements and head thrusting to shift gaze.

- In AOA type 1, there is a peripheral neuropathy, chorea, hypercholesterolaemia and low serum albumin; it is caused by various mutations of the aprataxin gene on chromosome 9p13.
- In AOA type 2, there is less prominent oculomotor apraxia, but more consistent peripheral neuropathy and dyskinesia (chorea or dystonia); serum alpha fetoprotein and creatine kinase levels are increased. AOA2 is caused by mutations of the senataxin SETX gene on chromosome 9q34 and accounts for 8 per cent of early onset ataxia, second only to FA.

X-linked ataxia

X-linked ataxia causes cerebellar ataxia with lower limb spasticity and hyper-reflexia. Skeletal and cardiac abnormalities are absent and progression is variable. In contrast to early onset ataxia with retained reflexes, motor conduction velocities are reduced. X-linked ataxia should be considered during genetic counselling of affected males. Ataxia of Charlevoix–Saguenay, adrenoleucodystrophy and Pelizaeus Merzbacher disease (see below under Pure hereditary spastic paraplegias (Strümpell–Lorrain disease)) must be considered.

Other early onset hereditary ataxias

A detailed discussion of other rare early onset hereditary ataxias is outside the scope of this chapter, but the clinical features seen in addition to ataxia include optic atrophy and spasticity (**Behr syndrome**, **Costeff syndrome**), hypogonadism (**Holmes' ataxia**), deafness, extrapyramidal features and retinopathy. Some patients with autosomal dominant hereditary optic atrophy due to mutations of the OPA1 or OPA3 genes can develop ataxia and other neurological signs. The syndrome of cerebellar ataxia with myoclonus (**Ramsay Hunt syndrome**) is discussed below under The Ramsay Hunt syndrome (progressive myoclonic ataxia).

EARLY ONSET METABOLIC ATAXIAS

The intermittent metabolic ataxias of childhood are rare. Affected children have a fluctuating cerebellar ataxia which tends to appear for a few weeks and then remit. Seizures, episodes of coma and cognitive impairment are often associated. Attacks may arise spontaneously or in association with infections or dietary changes. Patients with X-linked **ornithine transcarbamylase deficiency** may be only mildly affected in between attacks of severe encephalopathy and cerebral oedema. A photosensitive rash is characteristic of **Hartnup disease**. The most likely metabolic derangements are:

- **Hyperammonaemias** (several autosomal recessive forms and X-linked ornithine transcarbamylase deficiency)
- **Aminoacidurias** (Hartnup disease, maple syrup urine disease and isovaleric acidaemia)
- **Derangements of pyruvate or lactate metabolism** (various autosomal recessive or X-linked inborn errors including pyruvate dehydrogenase deficiency and pyruvate carboxylase deficiency).

Vitamin E deficiency is discussed in Chapter 7, and will be mentioned only briefly here. **Autosomal recessive ataxia with vitamin E deficiency (AVED) causes a spinocerebellar degeneration indistinguishable from Friedreich's ataxia.** Cardiomyopathy can occur, but retinopathy is extremely rare. The cause of AVED is mutations of the alpha tocopherol transfer protein (aTPP) gene on chromosome 8q13. The genetic defect causes a selective intestinal malabsorbtion of vitamin E.

Vitamin E deficiency is also associated with abetalipoproteinaemia (autosomal recessive, caused by mutations of the microsomal triglyceride transfer protein gene) and hypobetalipoproteinaemia (autosomal dominant, resulting from mutations of the apolipoprotein β-100 gene). In addition to the lipoprotein abnormalities, such patients have small stature, fat malabsorbtion with deficiencies of other fat-soluble vitamins (A, D and K). The neurological disorder is similar to Friedreich's ataxia and AVED, but a retinopathy is also seen, probably as a result of vitamin A deficiency. A similar neurological disorder may occur with intestinal malabsorbtion resulting from biliary or intestinal disease. **Vitamin E deficiency is treatable** with oral or intramuscular vitamin E supplements to prevent further neurological deterioration.

Mitochondrial diseases are characterized by defective mitochondrial respiration as a result of a complex and extensive range of mitochondrial or nuclear gene mutations. Neurological manifestations are very prominent and occur alone or in association with fatigable muscle weakness due to coexistent myopathy. Ataxia is a salient feature, often with shortness of stature, deafness, neuropathy, dementia, retinopathy, optic atrophy, ophthalmoplegia or myoclonus. Mitochondrial disease must be considered in the differential diagnosis of the Ramsay Hunt syndrome (see below under The Ramsay Hunt syndrome (progressive myoclonic ataxia)). Features suggestive of mitochondrial diseases are shown in Box 21.1.

The diagnosis may be confirmed by DNA testing or muscle biopsy, which often shows 'ragged red fibres'. Blood and especially cerebrospinal fluid (CSF) lactate levels may be elevated. Many cases are single but some affected families show maternal or occasionally autosomal dominant inheritance. Recurrence risks to siblings or children are generally low. No treatment is available.

Hexosaminidase A deficiency (GM2 gangliosidosis) is an autosomal recessive disorder, which usually causes a fatal cerebromacular degeneration of infancy (Tay–Sachs disease). However, rare patients have a later onset ataxia associated with eye movement abnormalities, facial grimacing, anterior horn cell disease or neuropathy. The diagnosis is established by measurements of hexosaminidase A.

Box 21.1 Clinical features of mitochondrial disorders

- Fatigable proximal myopathy (especially in combination with central nervous system disease)
- Ptosis, progressive ophthalmoplegia or pigmentary retinopathy, optic atrophy
- Short stature
- Deafness (sensorineural)
- Myoclonus, seizures
- Diabetes mellitus, hypoparathyroidism
- Cardiomyopathy, cardiac conduction defects
- Lipomas
- Unexplained stroke before 40 years of age
- Migraine
- Lactic acidosis
- Raised cerebrospinal fluid protein/lactate
- Muscle biopsy (ragged red fibres, COX negative fibres)

Cholestanolosis (cerebrotendinous xanthomatosis) presents as a childhood-onset cerebellar ataxia with spasticity (which may be the prime feature), epilepsy, cognitive impairment, cataracts, neuropathy and xanthomas on tendons. Magnetic resonance scanning of the brain shows lesions of the dentate nuclei, brainstem and basal ganglia. The level of CSF protein is elevated and cholestanol levels are also increased as a result of an abnormality of bile salt synthesis; early treatment with chenodeoxycholic acid is partly effective. The condition is caused by mutations of the sterol 27-hydroxylase (*CYP27A1*) gene. Limited treatment is possible with chenodeoxycholic acid and pravastatin.

Niemann–Pick disease type C (juvenile dystonic lipidosis) is characterized by ataxia, dystonia, loss of vertical eye movement (the key clinical clue) and cognitive impairment (dementia or psychosis); cataplexy can be prominent, along with dysarthria and dysphagia. Hepatosplenomegaly is not characteristic in contrast to types A and B due to sphingomyelinase deficiency. A multiple sclerosis-like presentation (on the MRI scan) with dementia has been described. Abnormal 'sea-blue histiocytes' may be seen in bone marrow biopsies, but filipin staining of cultured skin fibroblasts is more reliable. Various mutations of the *NPC1* gene on chromosome 18q have been associated with this condition.

Leukodystrophies usually present in infancy or childhood, but later onset variants may occur.

Cerebellar ataxia is accompanied by other neurological features, such as cognitive impairment, spasticity and visual loss, but is sometimes the main presenting feature. The diagnosis is suggested by an associated peripheral neuropathy, characteristic appearances in the white matter on brain MRI and the results of white cell enzyme or DNA studies.

Partial hypoxanthine guanine phosphoribosyl transferase (HGPRT) deficiency arises from point mutations of the *HGPRT* gene on chromosome Xq26. Hyperuricaemia is associated with gouty arthritis and renal stones, but about 20 per cent of affected boys have a spinocerebellar ataxia. Allopurinol is effective treatment for arthritis and nephrolithiasis, but does not help the neurological features.

DNA REPAIR DEFECTS

Ataxia telangiectasia

Ataxia telangiectasia (AT) is an autosomal recessive disorder, with an incidence of one in 100 000 births.

A progressive ataxia develops as the child starts to walk, but sometimes later. Subsequently, dysarthria and a marked eye movement disorder (oculomotor apraxia as in AOA1/AOA2 (see above under Ataxia with oculomotor apraxia)) appear along with other signs, including chorea, dystonia, myoclonus, areflexia and eventually some cognitive impairment. Telangiectasia of the conjunctivae appear at four to six years of age and may develop on the face, ears, neck and limbs. Occasionally, they are absent. Frequent infections are common as a result of impaired immunity, and malignancies, often lymphoma or leukaemia, develop in 10 per cent of patients. Survival is 20–25 years.

Characteristic laboratory findings are an elevation of alpha-fetoprotein and deficiency of IgA or other immunoglobulins. The AT gene (*ATM*) is on chromosome 11q23 and a variety of mutations have been detected in AT patients. Recurrence risk to siblings is one in four.

Xeroderma pigmentosum and Cockayne syndrome

Xeroderma pigmentosum and Cockayne syndrome are very rare autosomal recessive neurocutaneous disorders, which are caused by various mutations in the same family of DNA repair genes.

- Xeroderma pigmentosum causes a severe photosensitive rash, skin carcinomas and malignant melanoma. Neurological features appear in some patients and include ataxia, areflexia, dementia, spasticity and movement disorders; some patients have only a peripheral neuropathy.
- Cockayne syndrome produces a characteristic dwarfism with microcephaly, ataxia, spasticity, retinopathy, deafness and neuropathy. There may be a photosensitive rash and neuroimaging shows basal ganglia calcification.

EPISODIC ATAXIA

There are several forms of autosomal dominant ataxia in which ataxia occurs in intermittent attacks.

1 In **episodic ataxia with myokymia (EAM/FA type 1)**, the attacks start in early childhood and last seconds to minutes with myokymia (rippling of muscles, especially facial) evident between attacks. Persistent ataxia does not develop. Mutation analysis of the voltage gated potassium channel gene, *KCNA1*, on chromosome 12p has identified different mis-sense point mutations. The attacks may respond to acetazolamide or carbamazepine.

2 In **episodic ataxia with nystagmus (EAN/EA type 2)**, the attacks develop in later childhood or adolescence, last hours or days and may be accompanied by headache, nausea and vertigo; they are relieved by acetazolamide. There is no myokymia. In between the episodes, there may be nystagmus and mild gait ataxia; some patients do not experience any acute attacks. Cerebellar atrophy is seen on brain MRI. Similar neurological signs are seen in some patients with autosomal dominant familial hemiplegic migraine. Familial hemiplegic migraine and periodic ataxia without myokymia are allelic disorders on chromosome 19p13 caused by point mutations of the alpha 1A calcium channel gene (*CACNL1A4*). Trinucleotide CAG expansions within the same gene cause a mild autosomal dominant adult-onset cerebellar ataxia (SCA6, see below under Autosomal dominant cerebellar ataxia type III). Other point mutations of CACNL1A4 cause

familial hemiplegic migraine which has similar symptoms to EA2.

3 **Episodic ataxia type 3 is rare**; there is episodic acetazolamide-responsive ataxia, vertigo and tinnitus; myokymia can occur. There is linkage to a gene on chromosome 1q42.

4 **Episodic ataxia type 4 (periodic vestibulocerebellar ataxia)** can also be associated with a mild persistent ataxia; it is not linked to episodic ataxia type 1, 2 or 3. There are attacks of ataxia, oscillopsia, diplopia and vertigo. A persisting ataxia may develop.

5 **Episodic ataxia type 5** has been seen in one family. It was caused by a mutation of the alpha 4 subunit of the calcium channel gene *CACNB4* on chromosome 2q22-23. The same mutation rarely causes epilepsy.

LATE ONSET HEREDITARY CEREBELLAR ATAXIAS

The autosomal dominant cerebellar ataxias (ADCA) are clinically, pathologically and genetically heterogeneous and their classification is controversial. Pathologically, there is degeneration of the cerebellum, brainstem and other regions, including the optic nerves, basal ganglia, cerebral cortex, spinal cord and peripheral nerves. It is not possible to classify or define these conditions in terms of neuropathological features because these are so inconsistent, even within the same genetic type of ADCA.

Advances in molecular genetics have led to a new genetic reclassification and DNA diagnosis is now possible for some forms of ADCA. At present, there are 19 known genes underlying the autosomal dominant ataxias. There are 25 spinocerebellar ataxia (SCA) genes (an unfortunate terminology as it ignores the many earlier onset recessive genes which also cause 'spinocerebellar ataxia'), the gene for dentatorubropallidoluysian atrophy (DRPLA, see below under The Ramsay Hunt syndrome (progressive myoclonic ataxia), the fragile X gene and the five episodic ataxia genes. These are summarized in Table 21.3.

Harding proposed a clinical classification (ADCA types I–IV) in 1984 which has required revision,

Table 21.3 Autosomal dominant ataxia genes

Gene	Locus	Mutation type	Gene product	Comments or notable features
SCA1	6p23	CAG expansion	Ataxin 1	
SCA2	12q24	CAG expansion	Ataxin 2	
SCA3	14q24.3-q31	CAG expansion	Ataxin 3	
SCA4	16q22.1		unknown	Rare families with sensory neuropathy
	16q22.1		PLEKHG4 (puratrophin1)	Rare Japanese families with pure ataxia
SCA5	11cen		Ataxin 5	3 families (USA, France and Germany)
SCA6	19p13	CAG expansion	α-1A calcium channel	Allelic to EA2
SCA7	3p21.1-p12	CAG expansion	Ataxin 7	retinopathy
SCA8	13q21	CTG expansion	Ataxin 8	Unreliable DNA diagnosis
SCA10	22q13	ATTCT expansion	Ataxin 10	Rare; Mexican families; seizures
SCA11	15q14-21		Ataxin 11	1 UK family
SCA12	5q31-q33	CAG expansion	PPP2R2B (protein kinase regulator)	Several families; prominent tremor
SCA13	19q13.3-4	Point mutations	KCNC3 (potassium channel)	2 families (France, Philippines)
SCA14	19q13.4-qter	Point mutation	Protein Kinase Cγ (PKCγ)	Several families (1.4% of ADCA in France)
SCA15	3p24.2-pter			3 families (Australia, Japan)
SCA16	8q22.1-q24.1			1 family (Japan)
SCA17	6q27	CAG / CAA expansion	TATA binding protein	Several families, can resemble HD (HDL4)
SCA18	7q22-q32			1 family
SCA19	1p21-q21			2 families (Holland, China) probably alleleic with SCA22; myoclonus and tremor in some cases
SCA21	7p21-p15			1 family (France)
SCA22	1p21-q23			1 family (China) probably allelic with SCA19
SCA23	20p			1 family (Holland)
SCA25	2p15-p21			1 family (France);
SCA26	19p13.3			1 family (Norwegian); locus adjacent to SCA6
SCA27	13q34	Point mutation	FGF14 (fibroblast growth factor 14)	1 family (Holland)
SCA28	18p11.22-q11.2			1 family (Italy)
DRPLA	12p13.31	CAG expansion	Atrophin 1	
EA1	12p13	Point mutations	KCNA1 potassium channel	
EA2	19p13	Point mutations	α-1A calcium channel (CACNA1A)	Allelic with SCA6
EA3	1q42			1 family
EA4	unknown			2 families
EA5	2q22-q23	Point mutation	b4 subunit calcium channel (CACNB4)	1 family

EA, episodic ataxia; DRPLA, dentatorubropallidoluysian atrophy; SCA, spinocerebellar ataxia.

[a]SCA6 and EA-2 are allelic, resulting from different mutations of the alpha 1A calcium channel (CACNL1A4) gene.

Note: SCA9 is currently not utilized.

but is still useful in the clinic. Type IV is probably obsolete, but the ADCA types I–III are recognizable. It must be emphasized that there is a very poor correlation between the phenotype of a dominant ataxia and the genotype underlying it. The main phenotypes (ADCA types I, II and III along with Biemond's ataxia (ADCA with severe sensory peripheral neuropathy) and the episodic ataxias are summarized in Table 21.4 with the genes associated with each clinical type.

Autosomal dominant cerebellar ataxia type I

The age of onset for ADCA type I is nearly always after the age of 20 years, usually in the fourth decade, but can be as late as 65–70 years of age. Progressive ataxia with cerebellar dysarthria are the salient features.

Supranuclear eye movement disorders, eyelid retraction, nystagmus and optic atrophy are common, along with parkinsonism, chorea and dystonia. Some patients have fasciculation of the face and tongue, and occasionally the limbs. The tendon reflexes can be brisk, normal or absent, and often decline over time in the same patient. Sensory loss and pyramidal leg weakness may be seen and mild dementia occurs in about 40 per cent of cases. Retinopathy is not seen in ADCA type I and any optic atrophy is associated with mild visual loss.

No treatment is available for ADCA, which is progressive. Patients require physiotherapy, occupational therapy and speech therapy in some cases. Genetic counselling of patients and their families is important. In those with marked parkinsonian features, levodopa may be partly effective.

Cerebellar and brainstem atrophy is apparent on MRI or computed tomography (CT) scans, abnormal visual, brainstem auditory or somatosensory evoked potentials are common and there may be abnormal nerve conduction studies if a peripheral neuropathy is present.

Inheritance is autosomal dominant and the risk to children is 50 per cent. Several genes causing ADCA type I have been identified (Table 21.4), **but the clinical features are not a reliable guide to the molecular diagnosis.**

Table 21.4 Clinical and genetic classification of autosomal dominant cerebellar ataxias

Clinical type	Associated genotypes
ADCA type I	SCA1; SCA2; SCA3; SCA8; SCA12; SCA13;[b] SCA14;[b] SCA17; SCA18; SCA19; SCA21; SCA23; SCA25; SCA27; other unlinked loci
ADCA type II	SCA7; other unlinked loci
ADCA type III	SCA3; SCA5; SCA6; SCA10;[a] SCA11; SCA15; SCA16; SCA22; SCA26; SCA28; other unlinked loci
Ataxia with sensory neuropathy (Biemond's ataxia)	SCA4
DRPLA	DRPLA gene (atrophin 1)
Episodic ataxia type 1 (with myokymia)	KCNA1
Episodic ataxia type 2	SCA6/CACNL1A4
Episodic ataxia type 3 (vertigo and tinnitus)	
Episodic ataxia type 4 (vestibulocerebellar)	
Episodic ataxia type 5	CACNB4

[a]SCA10 is associated with epilepsy.
[b]SCA13 develops in early infancy and is more correctly a hereditary congenital ataxia.
[c]SCA14 can cause earlier onset ataxia with myoclonus.

Other ADCA type I genes are very rare, sometimes occurring in only single families and are not discussed further here. Some ADCA I families have no detectable SCA or other ataxia genes. The proportion is uncertain with different frequencies of the various SCA mutations in different case series.

Autosomal dominant cerebellar ataxia type II

In ADCA type II, there is progressive ataxia with visual failure as a result of a retinopathy.

- *SCA1* is reported in 15–35 per cent of ADCA I families. Larger repeat numbers are associated with earlier age of onset and increased severity. The gene product, ataxin 1, is an 8-kDa protein of unknown function. Clinically, the eye movements are affected late and reflexes are commonly brisk. A bulbar palsy often appears, along with cognitive decline. Optic atrophy, facial fasciculation and parkinsonism are less common.
- *SCA2* was first described in Cuba, but subsequently elsewhere. The clinical features are similar to SCA1 but slow eye movements and hyporeflexia are more common. This mutation has been reported in 20–40 per cent of ADCA I cases.
- *SCA3* accounts for 15–40 per cent of ADCA I cases and has also been described as Machado–Joseph disease and Azorean disease of the nervous system. Prominent dystonia or parkinsonism, facial and tongue fasciculation, a staring expression (as a result of eyelid retraction) and distal wasting are common, but are also seen in SCA1. Some patients have a parkinsonian syndrome with peripheral neuropathy but no ataxia, while others have only a spastic paraparesis.
- *SCA8* is a rare cause of ADCA type I. This mutation has also been reported as a normal polymorphism and its status as an ADCA (*SCA*) gene is controversial and it is not recommended as a diagnostic test.
- *SCA12* has been associated with an ADCA type I phenotype with prominent tremor (similar to essential tremor), parkinsonism, psychiatric features and cognitive decline.
- *SCA13* produces an ADCA I phenotype, but in some cases onset is in infancy. This gene may more correctly be placed among the congenital ataxias. Only two families have been described.
- *SCA14* is rare and can cause ataxia, myoclonus and cognitive impairment.
- *SCA17* can cause a Huntington's like picture with ataxia, chorea and mental changes.

The age of onset is highly variable, ranging from infancy to the seventh decade. Sometimes, parents develop symptoms after their affected children. There are also abnormalities of eye move-

ment and pyramidal signs in the limbs, sometimes with peripheral neuropathy. Some affected children have a severe lethal cerebromacular degeneration. In this condition, the SCA7 mutation (Table 21.4) is usually the cause. ADCA II is the exception to the generally useful rule concerning age of onset and dominant and recessive transmission (Table 21.1); all ages are affected. The visual loss may be inconspicuous or can develop much later and electroretinography may be needed in doubtful cases. Some ADCA II families do not have the SCA7 gene. It is possible to confuse ADCA II/SCA7 with multiple sclerosis given the clinical features.

Autosomal dominant cerebellar ataxia type III

In ADCA type III, there is a pure cerebellar ataxia with nystagmus and pyramidal signs in some cases. Onset is late, usually after the age of 50 years and progression is slow. Similar families have been found to have a gene locus on the centromeric region of chromosome 11 (SCA5). Some patients with SCA3 have this phenotype and the SCA6 mutation is typically associated with a mild, pure cerebellar ADCA III phenotype. Note that point mutations of the same gene (CACNL1A4) can cause familial hemiplegic migraine or episodic ataxia type 2 (see above under Episodic ataxia). Other SCA genes (listed in Table 21.4) associated with this type of ataxia are extremely rare.

Ataxia with sensory neuropathy (Biemond's ataxia)

This is a rare autosomal dominant ataxia with severe sensory neuropathy. The sensory loss is rapid and involves face and limbs. The gene on chromosome 16 (*SCA4*) has not been defined.

Fragile X tremor ataxia syndrome

The classical Fragile X tremor ataxia syndrome (FXTAS) causing learning disability in boys is associated with a CGG expansion of the normal 7–55 repeats to over 200 repeats within the *FMR-1* gene on chromosome Xq27. In about 40 per cent of males who carry a previously asymptomatic premutation of 55–200 CGG repeats, a later onset neurological disorder can develop over the age of 50 years; the features are ataxia, a postural or action tremor, cognitive impairment or parkinsonism. There may be no obvious family history of males with fragile X mental retardation. Brain magnetic resonance scanning may show lesions of the middle cerebellar peduncles. Female premutation carriers can also be affected by FXTAS (in 5–10 per cent) or premature ovarian failure.

SPORADIC DEGENERATIVE CEREBELLAR ATAXIA

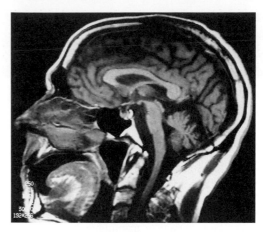

Figure 21.3 Magnetic resonance scan showing severe cerebellar and brainstem atrophy in a patient with idiopathic late onset ataxia (courtesy of Dr TP Enevoldson).

More than four out of five cases of adult-onset degenerative cerebellar ataxia are non-genetic and of unknown cause.

Pathologically, these patients have **olivopontocerebellar atrophy** or **cortical cerebellar atrophy**. However, the term 'olivopontocerebellar atrophy' should be reserved for the cerebellar presentation of multiple system atrophy (see below). Age-of-onset tends to be a little later than in ADCA. Optic atrophy and retinopathy are absent and ophthalmo-plegia is uncommon.

It is essential in late onset ataxia, where there is no family history, to exclude a posterior fossa structural lesion (such as a tumour or Chiari malformation), hydrocephalus, vitamin B12 deficiency (and vitamin E where there is any doubt), thyroid function tests and, where indicated (see below), a systemic malignancy. In most patients, these tests are all normal and a sporadic cerebellar degeneration is left as a diagnosis of exclusion. Within this group, five phenotypes are recognized:

1 **Dejerine–Thomas type**: The onset is typically between 35 and 55 years of age. There is cerebellar ataxia, and varying combinations of dementia, parkinsonism, supranuclear eye movement abnormalities and areflexia. Optic atrophy or retinopathy are rare (**Figure 21.3**).

2 **Multiple system atrophy (MSA)** may take the form of **a late onset degenerative cerebellar ataxia as well as atypical parkinsonism or primary autonomic failure. A cerebellar syndrome is associated with parkinsonism, pyramidal signs and sometimes autonomic features such as postural hypotension, bladder dysfunction and impotence.** The parkinsonism rarely responds well to levodopa. Nystagmus may occur but not severe gaze palsies, optic atrophy or retinopathy; dementia is not a feature of MSA. There is cerebellar and brainstem atrophy on MRI, which may also show an abnormal signal in the putamen. Denervation of the external urethral sphincter detected by electromyography is characteristic. Pathologically, there is degeneration of the cerebellum, brainstem (including substantia nigra), basal ganglia and sometimes the intermediolateral columns of the spinal cord with characteristic glial and neuronal cytoplasmic inclusions in these areas. Severe and early autonomic failure or bladder dysfunction is suggestive of MSA. Perhaps a quarter of those with the Dejerine–Thomas type of sporadic ataxia actually have MSA.

3 **Marie-Foix–Alajouanine type**. These patients develop ataxia later, often after 55 years of age. There is unsteadiness of gait but less limb ataxia, corresponding to a degeneration of the cerebellar vermis.

4 **Dyssynergia cerebellaris progressiva**. The onset of ataxia is between 40 and 60 years of age and is followed by increasingly severe tremor of the limbs (intention tremor with resting and postural elements).

5 A rare type with **bilateral vestibulopathy and peripheral neuropathy**.

THE RAMSAY HUNT SYNDROME (PROGRESSIVE MYOCLONIC ATAXIA)

Progressive myoclonic ataxia (Ramsay Hunt syndrome)

Progressive myoclonic ataxia (Ramsay Hunt syndrome) is a syndrome of progressive cerebellar ataxia, myoclonus and sometimes seizures. None of the disorders leading to the syndrome is treatable but myoclonus may respond to valproate, clonazepam or primidone.

Causes of progressive myoclonic ataxia include:

1 **Unverricht–Lundborg disease** (Baltic or Mediterranean myoclonus) is an autosomal recessive early onset spinocerebellar degeneration (see above under Early onset metabolic ataxias). The onset is in childhood with seizures and myoclonus, while ataxia and mild cognitive impairment appear later. The condition is caused by mutations of the cystatin B (*EPM1A*) gene on chromosome 21q22.3. There is another gene – *EPM1B* – on chromosome 12. *EPM1A* may account for a high proportion of unexplained myoclonus cases.

2 **Lafora body disease** is also an autosomal recessive disorder with onset in adolescence and severe epilepsy and dementia with milder myoclonus. A milder later onset form exists. Characteristic periodic acid Schiff-positive inclusions are seen in skin, muscle, brain and liver. Various mutations of the *EPM2A* gene on chromosome 6q24 have been identified; the function of the gene product, laforin, is unknown. Other genes can also cause Lafora body disease (malin (*NHLRC1*) and another gene referred to as *EPM2B*).

3 **Neuronal ceroid lipofuscinosis** can occur at various ages, with combinations of epilepsy, myoclonus, visual failure and ataxia. Characteristic inclusions are seen in neurones (detectable in rectal or skin biopsies). Inheritance can be autosomal recessive or dominant. An axillary skin biopsy can detect ceroid lipofuscinosis or Lafora bodies.

4 **Sialidosis** is inherited as an autosomal recessive disorder, caused by α-N-acetylneuraminidase (sialidase) deficiency. The onset is in adolescence or early adult life with epilepsy, myoclonus, visual failure (with cherry red maculae) and ataxia. Various mutations of the sialidase *NEU1* gene on chromosome 6p21 have been detected. Diagnosis is by measurement of urinary sialyloligosaccharides or neuraminidase levels.

5 **Mitochondrial disease** takes many forms including the MERRF syndrome (myoclonic epilepsy with ragged red fibres). The ragged red fibres are a muscle biopsy feature caused by an accumulation of abnormal mitochondria. In addition to myoclonic ataxia, there is often smallness of stature, deafness, dementia and sometimes subcutaneous lipomas. The majority of MERRF cases are caused by a point mutation of the mitochondrial lysine transfer RNA gene (at position 8344). A few cases have been associated with other mutations of mitochondrial DNA (at positions 8356 and 3243) and, in some, the molecular basis has not been determined.

6 **Dentatorubropallidoluysian atrophy** is described below. A Ramsay Hunt phenotype may occur.

7 **Coeliac disease** may be associated with a cerebellar ataxia with myoclonus or other neurological complications including cerebral calcification, seizures, peripheral neuropathy or a Friedreich's ataxia-like illness. Diagnosis is by antibodies (to gliadin or endomysial) or small bowel biopsy. The neurological disorder does not respond to a gluten-free diet.

8 **Whipple's disease** is associated with several neurological complications, including focal brain lesions, ataxia (with myoclonus), supranuclear eye movement abnormalities and dementia. Myoclonus may affect the eyes and face (oculomasticatory myorhythmia). Biopsy of the small bowel or detection of the organism *Tropheryma whippelii* directly or by polymerase chain reaction (PCR) analysis of DNA in bowel or CSF may allow the diagnosis. Treatment is with antibiotics.

9 **Creutzfeldt–Jakob disease** classically presents with rapidly progressive cerebellar ataxia and myoclonus, as well as dementia and sometimes cortical visual disturbances. A familial

(autosomal dominant) form, Gerstmann-Straussler-Scheinker (GSS) disease, causes a prominent ataxic presentation followed by more typical dementia and myoclonus.

DENTATORUBROPALLIDOLUYSIAN ATROPHY

The inheritance of dentatorubropallidoluysian atrophy (DRPLA) is autosomal dominant and the gene is located on chromosome 12p12-ter (ter, telomere); the mutation is a CAG trinucleotide repeat expansion. Larger repeat numbers are associated with earlier age of onset and greater severity. Onset for DRPLA is extremely variable in terms of age and clinical features, even within the same family. Childhood onset is often associated with rapidly progressive myoclonic epilepsy and dementia. Adult onset is characterized by chorea, ataxia and dementia, occasionally with dystonia. The condition may closely resemble Huntington's disease. Affected families commonly contain individuals with each phenotype. Brain MRI shows cerebral and cerebellar atrophy and abnormal lesions in the cerebral white matter and basal ganglia. DNA testing for DRPLA is useful in the investigation of families with features of Huntington's disease, but in whom the Huntington's disease mutation cannot be detected.

MISCELLANEOUS CEREBELLAR SYNDROMES

In addition to the hereditary and degenerative ataxias, the cerebellum may be affected by a wide range of pathologies (Table 21.1). Some of these, such as vascular disease, are covered in other chapters.

Paraneoplastic cerebellar degeneration

CT or MRI brain scans are normal initially, but cerebellar atrophy can appear later. The CSF usually contains a mild lymphocytic pleocytosis with elevated protein level and positive oligoclonal bands. Serum markers, such as cancer antigen 125 and carcinoembryonic antigen, may be positive. In about 50–75 per cent of cases, antineuronal

Paraneoplastic cerebellar degeneration is a rare disorder most commonly seen in association with small cell lung cancer, ovarian or uterine cancer or lymphoma and may precede the appearance of the tumour.

Severe ataxia develops rapidly, over weeks or months, along with dysarthria, vertigo, oscillopsia and nystagmus. The condition then stabilizes, but the patients are severely disabled. It is the severe subacute onset and rapid deterioration that is characteristic of paraneoplastic ataxia. Other paraneoplastic disorders, such as Lambert–Eaton syndrome, opsoclonus, peripheral neuropathy or limbic encephalitis often coexist with the cerebellar syndrome.

antibodies are detected. These react with cerebellar Purkinje cells (anti-Yo or anti-PCA1) or occasionally a wider range of neurones (anti-Hu or others such as anti-Ri, GAD, VGCC, CRMP5, Ma1, Ma2, ANNA-3 or amphiphysin). Passive transfer of anti-Yo antibodies has failed to produce cerebellar degeneration in animal studies and the role of these antibodies is unclear. Some patients have anti-VGCC (voltage gated calcium channel) or anti-Ri antibodies.

Treatment is usually unsuccessful, but improvement after treatment of the underlying tumour, plasma exchange, immunoglobulin therapy, steroids or cytotoxic drugs has been reported occasionally. Symptomatic improvement may be seen with clonazepam.

Drugs

1 **Anticonvulsants**, particularly phenytoin, carbamazepine and phenobarbitone, lead to reversible ataxia, nystagmus and dysarthria if serum levels are elevated. Permanent cerebellar damage can follow phenytoin intoxication.
2 **Lithium** toxicity can produce cerebellar ataxia, even with normal serum levels. Occasionally, a combination of ataxia with myoclonus can occur with a clinical picture very similar to Creutzfeldt–Jakob disease.
3 **Cytotoxic drugs and immunosuppressants**, such as 5-flurouracil, vincristine, cytosine arabinoside and ciclosporin, are associated with a reversible cerebellar syndrome.

4   Other causes include benzodiazepines, piperazine and amiodarone.

Toxins and physical agents

1   **Alcohol abuse** is associated with a characteristic cerebellar syndrome with similarities to that seen in Wernicke's encephalopathy. The relative roles of thiamine deficiency and direct toxicity are unclear (see below under Thiamine deficiency).
2   **Organic solvents** are highly lipid soluble and so are potent neurotoxins. Prominent cerebellar features may occur, but a diffuse encephalopathy is more common.
3   **Organic mercury** causes a cerebellar syndrome with optic neuropathy and cognitive changes.
4   Acute **thallium** poisoning can lead to an encephalopathy with prominent cerebellar features.
5   **Acrylamide** causes a toxic peripheral neuropathy with additional cerebellar features.
6   **Heatstroke** may be followed by permanent cerebellar damage.

Infections

1   **Acute cerebellar ataxia** is seen mainly in children and rarely in adults. There is myoclonus and a prominent eye movement disorder (opsoclonus) in some patients.

> This gives rise to a striking clinical picture with irregular multidirectional saccadic eye movements, jerking of the limbs and ataxia ('dancing eyes syndrome'). The condition may follow viral infection (especially varicella) or occasionally vaccination. In children, an underlying neuroblastoma is present in up to 50 per cent of cases.

Some cases are unexplained, but are presumed to be viral. The CSF often shows a lymphocytic pleocytosis and focal brainstem or cerebellar lesions may be seen with MRI.

2   **Post-infectious acute disseminated encephalomyelitis** is seen after measles, as well as a wide range of other infections including mumps, varicella, influenza, rubella, infectious mononucleosis and mycoplasma pneumonia. There is usually depressed consciousness and multifocal neurological signs, but cerebellar features are often prominent.
3   **Legionnaire's disease** may present with neurological features and pneumonia. Some patients are encephalopathic, but a prominent cerebellar ataxia with nystagmus, ophthalmoplegia and dysarthria is recognized. CSF and neuroimaging studies are normal.
4   **Malaria** (caused by *Plasmodium falciparum*) causes a severe encephalopathy (cerebral malaria) but a delayed cerebellar syndrome may also occur 2–4 weeks after the onset of fever. The legs are principally affected and the ataxia resolves spontaneously after a few months. An immunological mechanism is suspected.
5   **Other infections** sometimes associated with cerebellar ataxia include cysticercosis, Lyme neuroborreliosis and focal cerebellar abscess as a result of bacterial or tuberculous infection.

Hypothyroidism

Cerebellar ataxia is seen in 5–10 per cent of patients with hypothyroidism. The thyroid disorder is clinically obvious and appears before the ataxia which improves with treatment with thyroxine.

Thiamine deficiency

The manifestations of thiamine (vitamin B1) deficiency include acute Wernicke's encephalopathy, alcoholic cerebellar degeneration (see above under Miscellaneous cerebellar syndromes), Korsakoff's psychosis and peripheral neuropathy. These are often seen in combination.

1   **Wernicke's encephalopathy** is seen in alcoholics or other malnourished patients.

> **Clinical features of Wernicke's encephalopathy**
> There is a characteristic triad of **ataxia, ocular abnormalities and mental changes**. The onset is rapid over a few days with unsteadiness of gait, but minimal limb ataxia or dysarthria. The ocular abnormalities are nystagmus, abduction weakness and gaze palsies, but retinal haemorrhages and pupillary abnormalities are sometimes observed. Mentally, there is confusion and drowsiness.

Focal necrosis and haemorrhages develop in the mammillary bodies, thalamus, hypothalamus and brainstem.

The CSF is normal and the characteristic brainstem and diencephalic lesions may be detected by MRI. The thiamine deficiency may be confirmed by low red cell transketolase levels but **if the diagnosis is suspected, high dose parenteral thiamine should be administered at once**. There is often rapid improvement but some patients are left with residual deficits.

2 **Alcoholic cerebellar degeneration** is a closely related condition in which ataxia develops over weeks, months or rarely years and mainly affects the legs. Dysarthria is common, but nystagmus is rare in contrast to Wernicke's encephalopathy. Pathologically, there is cortical neuronal loss concentrated in the superior and anterior cerebellar vermis, visible with CT or MRI. Improvement may follow abstinence from alcohol and thiamine replacement, but severely affected patients rarely improve significantly.

Other nutritional ataxias

The ataxia associated with vitamin E deficiency has already been discussed. Vitamin B12 deficiency is characterized by ataxia, but is a spinal rather than a cerebellar disorder and is dealt with in Chapter 15. Ataxia can be a prominent feature of nicotinic acid (niacin) deficiency as a result of malnutrition (pellagra) or Hartnup disease (see above under Early onset metabolic ataxias).

Gluten ataxia

Some patients with cerebellar ataxia have antibodies to gluten, but no clinical signs of coeliac disease; small bowel biopsies may be negative. The frequency of this condition among 'idiopathic' adult-onset ataxia cases is unclear. The ataxia is usually of the Marie-Foix-Alajouanine type. The findings of anti-gliadin antibodies in patients with sporadic late onset ataxia have been inconsistent between studies and the nature of this association remains unclear and controversial.

Autoimmune ataxia

Some adults with late onset ataxia have been found to have autoantibodies to glutamic acid decarboxy-

lase (GAD) or anti-thyroid antibodies. Such cases are very rare and the nature of the association is uncertain.

Prion disease

Prion diseases are rare disorders caused by the accumulation of an abnormal protein (prion protein) in the brain, with subacute spongiform degeneration, gliosis and neuronal loss. There may also be aggregations of prion protein into amyloid plaques. The abnormal prion protein (PrP^{Sc}) is an isoform of a normal brain protein (PrP^{C}) and the disease occurs as a result of uncontrolled conversion of PrP^{C} to PrP^{Sc}. In about 15 per cent of cases, this is caused by an inherited or spontaneous mutation of the PrP^{C} gene. In the remainder of cases, the conversion is spontaneous except for a small number of iatrogenic cases where the disease has been transmitted by inoculation with tissue containing PrP^{Sc}. This has occurred with dural or corneal grafts, neurosurgical instruments and injections of human-derived hormones. The inoculated prion protein interacts with the host isoform, triggering a cascade of conformational change in the latter from PrP^{C} to PrP^{Sc}.

> The prion diseases characterized by a cerebellar syndrome are Creutzfeldt–Jakob disease and the Gerstmann–Sträussler–Scheinker syndrome.

Creutzfeldt–Jakob disease (CJD) may be sporadic, iatrogenic or inherited. Genetic CJD is an autosomal dominant condition caused by mutations of the prion protein (PrP) gene on chromosome 20. A variety of point mutations and insertions (abnormal expansions of an octapeptide repeat sequence) has been described. Clinically, there is often a non-specific prodromal phase with anxiety, malaise, forgetfulness and vague sensory symptoms. Severe and rapidly progressive dementia, cerebellar ataxia and multifocal myoclonus then develop. In 10 per cent of cases, the onset is with ataxia and some patients present with prominent visual symptoms. Death occurs within six months in 70 per cent of cases. Neuroimaging reveals cerebral and cerebellar atrophy and the CSF is normal. The electroencephalogram is usually strikingly abnormal with severe slow wave changes and sometimes the typical periodic complexes. PrP gene mutations can be detected by

DNA analysis in specialized laboratories. There is no effective treatment.

Gerstmann–Sträussler–Scheinker syndrome is a slowly progressive cerebellar syndrome with additional pyramidal features and less prominent dementia at a later stage. The progression of GSS is more gradual, typically over several years. The majority of cases are familial with autosomal dominant inheritance and are associated with particular PrP gene mutations.

THE HEREDITARY SPASTIC PARAPLEGIAS

Hereditary spastic paraplegias

Hereditary spastic paraplegia (HSP) is genetically and clinically heterogeneous. HSP is conventionally divided into cases with isolated spastic paraplegia 'pure HSP' and spastic paraplegia with other associated neurological features 'complex HSP'. Many genes (spastic paraplegia – SPG genes) have been described in various forms of HSP (Table 21.5). It is notable that several SPG genes can cause either a pure or complicated HSP phenotype.

Pure hereditary spastic paraplegias (Strümpell–Lorrain disease)

Pure HSP is usually inherited as an autosomal dominant disorder; autosomal recessive and X-linked forms are much less common.

---

1   **Autosomal dominant HSP** shows high penetrance, but variable expression within families. Severely affected children can have affected but asymptomatic parents. Dominant pure HSP appears to be heterogeneous with infantile, early (before 35 years of age) and later onset (after 35 years of age) variants. The early onset type is more common and typically starts between 12 and 35 years of age. A number of genes may cause autosomal dominant HSP (Table 21.5); the most common (*SPG4*) is that associated with mutations

of the **spastin** gene on chromosome 2p22; **mutations of this gene account for 40 per cent of patients with autosomal dominant pure FSP**. *SPG6* is a point mutation of the NIPA1 gene, deletions of which cause Prader-Willi/Angelman syndrome. Pathologically, there is degeneration of the corticospinal tracts with less prominent involvement of the dorsal columns and spinocerebellar tracts, motor cortex and anterior horn cells. HSP presents as a spinal cord disease with progressive spasticity of the legs. Tendon reflexes are increased and plantar responses extensor. The abdominal reflexes are often preserved. In advanced later onset cases, there may be upper limb involvement, impairment of vibration sense in the feet, ankle areflexia, distal muscle wasting and bladder dysfunction. The rate of deterioration is variable but weakness is characteristically inconspicuous. Progression in the later onset type is more rapid, with greater disability. Diagnosis of HSP must be made with caution. In many cases, the family history is incomplete or unreliable, in which case it is vital to examine both parents if possible. In doubtful cases, treatable conditions such as spinal cord compression, spinal arteriovenous malformation, vitamin B12 deficiency and multiple sclerosis will require consideration. Crucially, dopa-responsive dystonia (which may resemble HSP closely but is completely curable) must always be excluded by a therapeutic trial of levodopa even if there is a clear family history. Investigations are unhelpful and serve only to exclude other disorders, but somatosensory evoked potentials may be abnormal indicating subclinical involvement of peripheral and central sensory pathways. Treatment of HSP is limited to symptomatic management of spasticity with baclofen and physiotherapy together with management of bladder symptoms if present. Genetic counselling is essential; the recurrence risk in siblings or children of affected patients is 50 per cent and the severity is difficult to predict.

2   **Autosomal recessive pure HSP** families are rare. The distinction from the early onset form of dominant HSP is very difficult, making examination of the parents essential before diagnosing recessive HSP. The *SPG7* type on

Table 21.5 Spastic paraplegia (SPG) genes

Gene	Locus	Inheritance	Pure/complex
SPG1	Xq28 (L1CAM)	X-linked	Complex
SPG2	Xp21 (PLP)	X-linked	Either
SPG3	14q11 (atlastin)	Autosomal dominant	Pure
SPG4	2p22 (Spastin)	Autosomal dominant	Either
SPG5	8q21	Autosomal recessive	Pure
SPG6	15q11 (NIPA1)	Autosomal dominant	Pure
SPG7	16q24 (Paraplegin)	Autosomal recessive	Either
SPG8	8q23-24	Autosomal dominant	Pure
SPG9	10q23-24	Autosomal dominant	Complex
SPG10	12q13	Autosomal dominant	Pure
SPG11	15q13-15	Autosomal recessive	Either
SPG12	19q13	Autosomal dominant	Pure
SPG13	2q24-q34	Autosomal dominant	Pure
SPG14	3q27-28	Autosomal recessive	Complex
SPG15	14q	Autosomal recessive	Complex
SPG16	Xq11	X-linked	Pure
SPG17	11q12	Autosomal dominant	Complex
SPG18	8p12	Autosomal recessive	Complex
SPG19	9q33	Autosomal dominant	Pure
SPG20	13q12	Autosomal recessive	Complex
SPG21	15q22	Autosomal recessive	Complex
SPG22	Xq13	X-linked	Complex
SPG23	1q24-32	Autosomal recessive	Complex
SPG24	13q14	Autosomal recessive	Complex
SPG25	6q23-24	Autosomal recessive	Complex
SPG26	12p11-q14	Autosomal recessive	Complex
SPG27	10q22-24	Autosomal recessive	Pure
SPG28	14q21-22	Autosomal recessive	Either
SPG29	1p21-27	Autosomal recessive	Complex
SPG30	2q37	Autosomal recessive	Pure
SPG31	2p12	Autosomal dominant	Pure
SPG32	14q12-21	Autosomal recessive	Complex
SPG33	10q24	Autosomal dominant	Pure
SPG34	Xq24-25	X-linked	Pure
SPG35	16q21-23	Autosomal recessive	Complex
SPG36	12q23-24	Autosomal dominant	Complex
SPG37	8p21-q13	Autosomal dominant	Pure

chromosome 16q24 is caused by homozygous mutations of the paraplegin gene; the paraplegin protein is a mitochondrial ATPase. Friedreich's ataxia can occasionally produce a pure paraplegia phenotype.

3　**X-linked pure HSP** is genetically heterogeneous. Clinically, it is similar to early onset autosomal dominant HSP, but carrier females are normal. In some cases, there are mutations of the proteolipid protein (PLP) gene on chromosome Xq22 (*SPG2*). Mutations of the same gene can cause a **complex HSP** phenotype (see below) and X-linked sudanophilic leukodystrophy (**Pelizaeus Merzbacher disease**) indicating that these conditions and some cases of pure X-linked HSP are allelic disorders. It is important to check very long chain fatty acid levels as **adrenoleukodystrophy** may present with a pure spastic paraparesis without clinical or MRI evidence of cerebral involvement and with normal adrenal function in both affected males **and in heterozygous carrier females.**

Complex hereditary spastic paraplegias

In the complex HSP syndromes, additional neurological features are seen with the spastic paraplegia, such as mental retardation, optic atrophy, retinopathy, deafness, ataxia (especially of the upper limbs), extrapyramidal features, muscle wasting, peripheral sensory neuropathy and skin changes. The key to the diagnosis is the predominant spastic paraplegia that forms the 'core' of the syndrome.

Selected complex autosomal HSPs include:

- **Sjögren–Larsson syndrome** (autosomal recessive) presents at birth with icthyosis. Spastic paraplegia, mental retardation and retinopathy appear subsequently. Patients have mutations of the fatty aldehyde dehydrogenase (FALDH) gene on chromosome 17p11.2.
- **Behr syndrome** (autosomal recessive) is characterized by optic atrophy and HSP. A similar dominant form exists.
- **Kjellin syndrome** causes childhood mental retardation and retinal degeneration; spasticity appears later in adult life. Inheritance is autosomal recessive.
- **Complex HSP with severe sensory neuropathy** causes severe small fibre sensory loss and mutilating lower limb acropathy. This may be autosomal recessive or dominant. There is a dominant form with mild large-fibre neuropathy.
- **Complex HSP with distal muscle wasting** may be inherited as an autosomal dominant or recessive trait.
- **Complex HSP with cerebellar ataxia** usually develops in adult life with lower limb spasticity and cerebellar signs in the arms. There may be cerebellar eye movement abnormalities and dysarthria. This may be autosomal dominant or recessive and some cases are due to the autosomal recessive ataxia of Charlevoix-Saguenay.

X-linked complex hereditary spastic paraplegias

A rapidly progressive spastic paraplegia of childhood with optic atrophy is caused by a gene on chromosome Xq21. This condition, some cases of pure X-linked HSP and Pelizaeus Merzbacher disease are all caused by mutations of the PLP gene (see above). Different PLP gene mutations are associated with different phenotypes. The PLP gene encodes two proteins required for myelin synthesis, PLP and an isoform, DM-20.

Allan–Herndon syndrome comprises variable mental retardation, hypotonia, gross motor delay, ataxia and spastic paraplegia. The gene for this disorder is also on chromosome Xq13 (*SPG22*).

MASA syndrome leads to mental retardation, aphasia, shuffling gait and adducted thumbs. A spastic paraplegia develops later. A distinct form of X-linked complex HSP also maps to this locus as do X-linked hydrocephalus and X-linked corpus callosum agenesis. All are caused by mutations of the *L1* gene, which encodes the L1 neural cell adhesion molecule (L1CAM). This gene is also referred to as *SPG1*.

REFERENCES AND FURTHER READING

Burk K, Abele M, Fetter M *et al.* (1996) Autosomal dominant cerebellar ataxia type I clinical features and MRI in families with SCA1, SCA2 and SCA3. *Brain*, 119:1497–1505.

Durr A, Cossee M, Agid Y *et al.* (1996) Clinical and genetic abnormalities in patients with Friedreich's ataxia. *New England Journal of Medicine*, 335:1169–1175.

Fletcher NA (2009) Tremors and cerebellar ataxias. In: Donaghy M (ed.). *Brain's Diseases of the Nervous System*, 12th edn. Oxford: Oxford University Press, 1191–232.

Hagerman PJ, Greco CM, Hagerman RJ (2003) A cerebellar tremor/ataxia syndrome among fragile X premutation carriers. *Cytogenetic Genome Research*, 100:206–212.

Harding AE (1981) Friedreich's ataxia: a clinical and genetic study of 90 families with an analysis of early diagnostic criteria and intrafamilial clustering of clinical features. *Brain*, 104:589–620.

Marsden CD, Obeso JA (1989) The Ramsay Hunt syndrome is a useful clinical entity. *Movement Disorders*, 4:6–12.

CHAPTER 22

MULTIPLE SCLEROSIS AND RELATED CONDITIONS

Raju Kapoor

INTRODUCTION

Multiple sclerosis (MS) is an inflammatory, demyelinating condition of the central nervous system (CNS). It occurs throughout the world, but is particularly common in North America, Australasia and northern Europe, affecting at least 500 000 people in the United States and 80 000 people in the United Kingdom, where it has a prevalence of approximately one in 800. It is a major cause of chronic disability among young adults in these populations. In recent years, there have been significant advances in management and in our understanding of the epidemiology and pathology of the condition. This new knowledge has important practical implications for diagnosis, counselling and treatment.

PRESENTATION

Multiple sclerosis usually presents with an attack of neurological dysfunction which builds up over days and then improves partially or fully over weeks or months. Following optic neuritis, for example, approximately 90 per cent of patients recover a visual acuity of 6/9 or better. There tends to be an initial, rapid phase of recovery, followed by a slower but more prolonged phase, and there is electrophysiological evidence that recovery can continue for at least two years. Further attacks occur in time, and such patients have the so-called 'relapsing-remitting' subtype of the illness.

Relapses are more common in early disease, with an annual frequency of 0.8–1.2 per year falling to 0.4–0.6 per year after the fifth year. Patients with relapsing-remitting disease may later develop a gradual deterioration of neurological function, often with superimposed relapses, and are then said to have **secondary progressive MS**. Approximately 40 per cent of relapsing-remitting patients will develop secondary progressive disease ten years after onset. The time taken to convert from a relapsing to a secondary progressive course varies greatly from patient to patient, but once in the progressive phase, the rate of deterioration of function appears to be much more uniform. It is progression, rather than incomplete recovery from relapses, which dominates the development of long-term disability, although it is likely that the effects of relapses have been underestimated to some extent.

In **primary progressive MS**, which affects 10–37 per cent of patients in different studies, disability worsens gradually from onset without true relapses and remissions. Once the progressive phase begins, primary and secondary progressive patients decline at the same rate, with disability severe enough to require aid to walk occurring after a median interval of approximately six years. Patients with primary progressive disease tend to present later than those with other subtypes of the illness, men and women are affected equally (as opposed to the usual female preponderance), and pathological and magnetic resonance imaging (MRI) studies indicate that their illness has a less inflammatory nature.

Approximately 20 per cent of patients, particularly those with relapsing-remitting MS, develop little disability ten years into their illness, and the term **benign MS** is applied to this group. However, the accuracy of this term has been questioned, as the majority of these patients eventually seem to enter a progressively disabling phase of the illness.

Although most patients present between the ages of 20 and 40 years, MS can occur at either extreme of age, and patients aged below five years have been reported. Childhood MS accounts for less than 5 per cent of cases. Compared to adults, children with MS are more likely to be male, to have a relapsing onset, to have fits, to have brainstem involvement, and are less likely to have spinal cord involvement. On average, children take longer than adults to enter a progressive phase, and to reach defined disability milestones, but of course their illness begins earlier and therefore still gives rise to disability at a relatively young age. Because childhood MS is relatively rare, it has been difficult to undertake trials of treatment, and in general these children tend to be treated with disease-modifying drugs developed for use in adult disease.

PROGNOSTIC FACTORS

Among patients with a remitting course, the following suggest a more favourable long-term prognosis:
- Earlier age of onset
- Good remission from initial exacerbation
- Onset with sensory symptoms or with optic neuritis.

Five years after onset, a more favourable prognosis is associated with:
- Lower neurological deficit score
- Low relapse rate in the first two years after onset
- Long interval between the first two attacks.

Primary progressive MS has a poor prognosis because deterioration occurs from onset. This explains the poorer prognosis in men, who are more liable to this type of MS.

Magnetic resonance imaging studies provide additional prognostic information in patients seen during their first demyelinating episode. T2-weighted brain MRI shows lesions suggestive of MS in 50–70 per cent of such patients with optic nerve, spinal cord or brainstem attacks. In the cohort followed up at Queen Square, approximately 80 per cent of patients with several MRI lesions developed additional attacks (i.e. MS) within 10–20 years (versus 10 per cent of those without such lesions at ten years and 20 per cent at 20 years), and there was a degree of correlation between the T2 lesion load at presentation, its change during the initial stages of MS, and later disability. The total lesion volume increased approximately three times faster in those who developed secondary progressive disease than in those who continued to follow a relapsing course.

Less than 5 per cent of patients experience a rapidly fulminant course, and over 80 per cent of patients are alive 25 years after diagnosis. In a Canadian study, life table analysis revealed that life expectancy in MS patients at any given age was reduced by six or seven years compared to the general population. Severe disability, indicated by an expanded disability status scale (EDSS) of 7.5 or more (this equates to inability to take more than a few steps), was a major risk factor for premature death, with a case fatality ratio roughly four times the rate for controls.

The symptoms of MS (Table 22.1) depend largely on where the pathology arises in the CNS, and because any region of the white matter can be involved, the range of presentations is very diverse. Most commonly, single lesions affect the **spinal cord (50 per cent)**, leading to altered or lost sensation, weakness and upper motor neurone signs below the level of the lesion, and sphincter or sexual dysfunction, the **optic nerve (25 per cent)**, giving rise to unilateral visual loss, impaired colour perception and pain on eye movement, and the **brainstem (20 per cent)** with resulting diplopia, vertigo and ataxia.

Table 22.1 Presenting symptoms in multiple sclerosis

Presenting symptom		
Spinal cord (50%)	Sensory	Tingling, numbness, burning, tight bands, altered temperature sensation, Lhermitte's symptom
	Motor	Weakness, heaviness, clumsiness
	Sphincter	Urinary urgency, incontinence, hesitancy, constipation, faecal incontinence, impotence
Optic neuritis (25%)	Unilateral in 90% of patients	Blurred vision, 'patch' of visual loss, reduced colour perception, pain on eye movement, phosphenes
Brainstem/cerebellar (20%)	Diplopia, dysarthria, vertigo, facial numbness/weakness, deafness, paroxysmal symptoms, e.g. trigeminal neuralgia, tonic spasms	
Other (5%)	Hemiparesis, hemianopia, dysphasia, seizures, cognitive impairment	

Some demyelinating lesions can generate excessive electrical impulse activity, and consequently about 10 per cent of patients develop so-called positive or paroxysmal features. Again, the nature of these depends on the location of the lesion: cortical plaques can be associated with epilepsy (which occurs two to three times more commonly than in the general population), lesions of the cervical dorsal columns with **Lhermitte's symptom** (an electrical sensation radiating down the spine, sometimes into the arms or legs, on flexing the neck), and those in the brainstem with trigeminal neuralgia, paroxysmal limb ataxia and facial myokymia. Further manifestations include tonic spasms (painful limb contractions) and intermittent sensory disturbances.

In contrast to more focal presentations, **cognitive impairment** seems to correlate with the total T2-weighted MRI lesion load. Symptomatic cognitive impairment is rare at onset, although subtle defects can be demonstrated even then in those with a significant cerebral lesion load, using formal neuropsychological tests. Such tests show that cognitive dysfunction ultimately affects between 34 and 65 per cent of patients, but once again the effects on day-to-day life may remain modest. Recent memory, abstract thinking, attention and speed of information processing are particularly affected (and are tested only to a limited extent using standard cognitive screening), in keeping with the largely subcortical location of the pathology.

Fatigue is also a major complaint in MS, particularly before or during relapse, and about 40 per cent of patients rate it as their most disabling symptom. One of the most common and treatable causes is marked sleep disturbance due to nocturia. Fatigue is also sometimes related to depression, but in other cases electrophysiological studies link it more closely to excessive 'physiological' fatigue, which is central in origin. In other instances, rapid fatigability of gait or muscle contraction may relate to the well-known inability of demyelinated axons to transmit prolonged trains of action potentials without developing an intermittent conduction block.

Acute disseminated encephalomyelitis

In some patients, symptomatic demyelinating lesions can occur more or less simultaneously in several parts of the CNS. Such cases merge into the presentation of acute disseminated encephalomyelitis (ADEM), which often occurs after infections with agents such as *Mycoplasma pneumoniae*, Epstein–Barr virus and varicella. However, ADEM is more common in children and may be associated with features that are unusual for MS, including fever, encephalopathy and seizures.

Some patients with ADEM (Figure 22.1) have lesions in unusual sites, such as the basal ganglia, or else in a typically symmetrical distribution in the cerebellar peduncles or cerebral white matter, and furthermore oligoclonal bands may only be present transiently in their cerebrospinal fluid (CSF). Nevertheless, the distinction from an initial presentation of MS can be difficult, and in rare cases there may even be one or two further relapses in the year following presentation, before the illness settles.

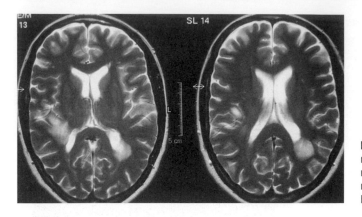

Figure 22.1 T2-weighted brain magnetic resonance image, axial view, in a patient with post-mycoplasma acute disseminated encephalomyelitis revealing large multifocal cerebral white matter lesions.

Neuromyelitis optica

Neuromyelitis optica (NMO), which is gradually replacing the label Devic's disease, refers to a group of patients presenting with optic neuritis and a complete myelitis, occurring either simultaneously or with an interval between the two, and without the clinical involvement of other parts of the CNS in its initial course.

NMO shares a demyelinating pathology with MS, but there are significant differences. NMO almost always follows a relapsing course, and compared to MS it has a higher mean age of onset (around 40 years), a much higher female preponderance (the male:female ratio is 1:9), poorer recovery from relapses, and a much poorer prognosis, with an untreated five-year survival of around 70 per cent. Typically, there are no lesions in MRI scans of the brain, and instead there are long cervical cord lesions which can extend into the low brainstem. Oligoclonal IgG bands occur in the CSF in only 15–30 per cent of cases, but there is an association with systemic autoimmune diseases, particularly systemic lupus erythematosus and Sjogren's syndrome.

The diagnosis of NMO has been revolutionized by the discovery of a specific serum autoantibody marker, NMO-IgG, which reacts with the water channel aquaporin 4. The antibody binds to astrocyte foot processes, pia and microvessels in those areas of the neuraxis which are affected clinically and radiologically by NMO. The distinction of NMO from MS is increasingly important because treatment of NMO relapses may require prolonged courses of corticosteroids or plasma exchange, and because remissions need to be induced using immunomodulatory drugs, such as azathioprine, with more recent, encouraging reports of the use of B-cell depletion using the monoclonal anti-CD20 antibody Rituximab.

Investigation and differential diagnosis

The diagnosis of MS depends on objective evidence that typical lesions have occurred within the CNS in different places and at different times (so-called 'dissemination in space and time'). Frequently, this information is clear from the history and examination. If there has only been a single clinical attack, laboratory investigations may provide evidence of lesions in unrelated parts of the CNS. These tests may be particularly useful when the clinical situation is not clear, or if there is a significant possibility of an alternative diagnosis (Tables 22.2 and 22.3). The question of an alternative diagnosis should be considered if there is any evidence of disseminated CNS disease associated with disease of the meninges (for example, a scan showing meningeal enhancement), peripheral nerves or muscles, or if there is evidence of inflammation or coincident pathology in another major organ, such as the lungs, liver, bone or skin.

Table 22.2 Differential diagnosis of progressive spastic paraparesis

Condition	Investigations
Cord compression/AVM	Spinal MRI (± angiography)
HTLV-1 associated myelopathy	HTLV-1 antibodies
Motor neurone disease	EMG
Adrenomyeloneuropathy	Very long-chain fatty acids, MRI (Figure 22.4)
Vitamin B12 deficiency	B12 level, blood count
Neurosyphilis	Treponemal serology
Hereditary spastic	Family history paraplegia

AVM, arteriovenous malformation; EMG, electromyography; HTLV, human T-cell lymphotropic virus; MRI, magnetic resonance image.

Table 22.3 Differential diagnosis of relapsing-remitting multiple sclerosis

Condition	Investigation
Systemic lupus erythematosus	Autoantibody screen
Sarcoidosis	Chest x-ray, SACE, liver biopsy
Behçet's disease	CRP, neuro-ophthalmology examination, HLA B51
Lyme disease	Borrelia serology
Neurosyphilis	Treponemal serology

MRI to exclude/confirm other pathology – also for spinal cord lesions.

CRP, C reactive protein; SACE, serum angiotensin-converting enzyme.

Magnetic resonance imaging

Nearly all patients with MS have lesions in the brain on MRI reflecting the presence of plaques of demyelination (Figures 22.2 and 22.3). These are typically present in a periventricular distribution, within the corpus callosum, in the juxta-cortical white matter (involving the subcortical u-fibres) and in the brainstem. Further evidence of ongoing disease activity is provided by the presence of lesions, which enhance with intravenous contrast (gadolinium) indicating disruption of the blood–brain barrier.

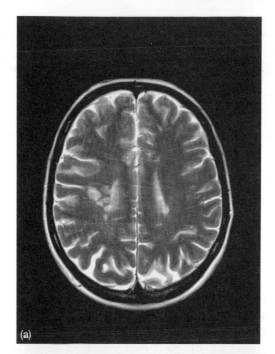

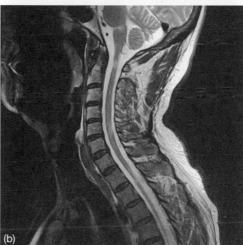

Figure 22.2 (a) T2-weighted brain magnetic resonance image (MRI) in clinically definite multiple sclerosis. There are multiple periventricular white matter lesions. (b) T2-weighted MRI of the cervical spine showing multiple hyperintense lesions within the spinal cord.

In the absence of a second definite clinical attack, MRI may show evidence of dissemination of lesions in space and, if new or enhancing lesions appear when MRI is repeated after an interval of at least three months, of dissemination in time as well. Criteria (the McDonald criteria) for diagnosing MS following a single so-called clinically isolated syndrome suggestive of demyelination depend on

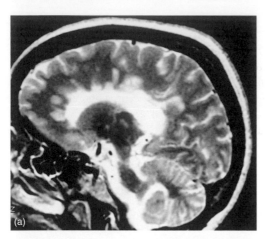

Figure 22.3 T2-weighted brain MRI, sagittal view, showing multiple high signal lesions arranged along the corpus callosum (Dawson's fingers) in a patient with MS.

MRI findings of this sort – dissemination in space is signified by the presence of a specified number of typical brain or spinal cord lesions (or oligoclonal IgG bands in the CSF), and dissemination in time by the presence of enhancing or new T2 lesions in a second scan. These criteria are still undergoing development and validation to assess their utility in day-to-day management. For example, recent work suggests that a single brain MRI scan showing both enhancing and non-enhancing lesions within three months of a single attack may indicate dissemination in time and may therefore be highly specific for predicting the early development of MS.

> **Multiple MRI lesions** also occur in other diseases associated with intermittent neurological symptoms, including cerebrovascular disease (e.g. small vessel disease, phospholipid antibody disease and cerebral autosomal dominant arteriopathy with subcortical infarcts and leukoencephalopathy (CADASIL), neurosarcoidosis and vasculitis). Cerebral lymphoma may also present with multifocal symptoms and lesions which can, at least temporarily, seem to be steroid responsive.

In MS, it is unusual for lesions to show pathological enhancement beyond two to three months, but sustained enhancement (as well as enhancement of the meninges) can occur in neurosarcoidosis. The interpretation of MRI abnormalities becomes complicated in older patients, as roughly 30 per cent of normal adults aged over 50 years have small lesions of vascular origin, often distributed peripherally in the cerebral white matter. An MRI scan of the spinal cord may be helpful in such patients, as cord lesions are rare in cerebrovascular disease, but occur in 75 per cent of patients with MS. It is also important to obtain spinal MRI in patients presenting with a progressive myelopathy, in order to exclude a compressive lesion or other pathology (Table 22.2).

Cerebrospinal fluid analysis

Lumbar puncture may be required when the clinical presentation and MRI findings are not diagnostic, and may help to show that the patient has an inflammatory disorder. An elevated CSF protein concentration or a mononuclear pleocytosis occurs in approximately 40 per cent of patients with MS, but a cell count of more than $50/mm^3$ is unusual. In addition, at least 90 per cent of patients have evidence of an intrathecal immune response, as indicated by the presence of immunoglobulin G oligoclonal bands in the CSF, which are not matched in the serum. However, the presence of such bands is not specific to MS, as they can arise in a number of other chronic neuroimmunological disorders, including vasculitis, infections (e.g. Lyme disease, neurosyphilis, subacute sclerosing panencephalitis and human T-cell lymphotropic virus-1), and possibly neurosarcoidosis. Such bands may disappear on repeat testing in conditions such as ADEM and systemic lupus erythematosus.

Evoked potentials

Slowing of axonal conduction secondary to demyelination gives rise to the characteristic delays found in visual-, auditory-, somatosensory- and motor-evoked potentials. Such abnormalities often occur in patients without a history of involvement of the relevant pathway (for example, an abnormal visual-evoked potential occurs in 70 per cent of patients suspected of having MS and in 90 per cent of those with definite disease) and may then be taken as evidence of dissemination of lesions in space.

Further tests

More detailed investigations may be required in some cases because of the wide differential diagnosis of MS (Figure 22.3). **Remitting disorders** include neurosarcoidosis, systemic lupus erythema-

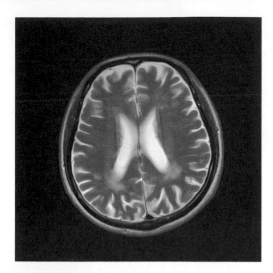

Figure 22.4 T2-weighted brain MRI in a man with adrenomyeloneuropathy. There are bilateral posterior cerebral white matter lesions.

tosus and Behçet's disease, although the remissions in these conditions are usually incomplete. Nevertheless, an autoimmune screen, chest x-ray, serum angiotensin-converting enzyme level, and serology for specific infections, may all be indicated. Progressive disorders include structural lesions (although the clinical picture can still fluctuate or occur with a stepwise progression in patients with cerebral lymphoma, spinal angiomas and meningiomas), vitamin B12 deficiency, and paraneoplastic syndromes. In younger patients, it may be necessary to consider genetic disorders such as the leukodystrophies (Figure 22.4), spinocerebellar ataxias, and hereditary spastic paraparesis, and specific biochemical or genetic testing may be available for these (Tables 22.2 and 22.3).

AETIOLOGY

Although the actual cause of MS remains unknown, the disease is thought to represent an autoimmune response to CNS antigens, possibly triggered by non-self antigens or by superantigens, in genetically susceptible individuals. Despite this autoimmune aetiology, MS only occurs in association with a limited set of immunologically determined conditions, including inflammatory bowel disease and ankylosing spondylitis.

A genetic susceptibility to MS is suggested by differences in its prevalence in different ethnic groups living in the same environment, and by studies of its occurrence in families; for example, the recurrence risk for monozygotic twins, is approximately 30 per cent, compared to a dizygotic concordance of approximately 4 per cent, a rate similar to that found in siblings. A slightly increased risk for concordance seems to exist for siblings of the same sex, with concordance rates of approximately 4 per cent for male–male pairs and 6 per cent for female–female pairs. The recurrence risk of developing MS for the children of affected individuals is approximately 2 per cent. The recurrence risk in relatives is slight if they have not manifested the illness before the age of 50 years.

Susceptibility to experimental autoimmune encephalomyelitis (EAE) in rodents depends on the animals' major histocompatability complex (MHC) background, indicating the importance of the trimolecular interaction (see below under Pathogenesis) in promoting T cell activation. T cell responses to autoantigens, such as myelin basic protein (MBP), also show restricted or limited use of T cell receptor Vβ genes. The search for human susceptibility genes has proved less fruitful, and the genes identified so far are generally related to the immune system. The most prominent genetic susceptibility factor for MS is the major histocompatibility complex, presumably through effects on both the immune repertoire and immunoregulatory circuits. Other susceptibility genes include those for interleukin (IL)-7 and IL-2. An MS-like condition is also seen in female carriers of the gene for Leber's hereditary optic neuropathy.

An environmental contribution to the aetiology of MS is likely because the prevalence of the disease generally increases with increasing latitude, and because those who migrate in youth acquire much of the local risk of MS. Apparent mini-epidemics of MS have also been reported, for example in the Faeroe Islands after the arrival of British troops during the Second World War. A number of infectious agents have been linked with MS over the years, including herpes simplex virus 2, human herpes virus 6 and *Chlamydia pneumoniae*. However, there is still no convincing evidence for their aetiological role, and it is notable that the risk of developing MS is no higher in the spouses of patients or in their adoptees. Recently, there has been considerable interest in the possible presence of Epstein–Barr virus in meningeal lymphoid follicles which are prominent in some cases of MS, and which are associated with subpial grey matter pathology (see below).

Effects of environmental factors and lifestyle
Patients often ask about the effects of environmental factors and of lifestyle on the course of the disease. In population studies, **viral infections** are associated significantly with subsequent relapse, but immunizations, anaesthesia and trauma, are not. There is also limited evidence for an association between stressful life events and relapses. However, associations may exist in small subgroups, such as those with particularly active disease; for example, influenza immunization does not increase gadolinium-enhanced MRI lesion activity in most patients with MS, but may do so in patients with the most active scans. **Because of this consideration, killed rather than live vaccines may be preferred** if immunizations are truly indicated, and elective surgery might be avoided in an active phase of the illness, even though the evidence suggests that both may well be safe in the general MS population.

Concerning **diet**, the prevalence and severity of MS are associated with both high and low levels of dietary fat intake in different populations. However, there is some evidence for a beneficial role for dietary supplementation with linoleic acid, and in general a diet that is low in saturated fats and red meat is also recommended.

There is also growing interest in a **possible disease modifying role for vitamin D**. Reduced levels of vitamin D may explain some of the increased incidence of MS at higher latitudes, and vitamin D deficiency during pregnancy and early years may increase the risk of the offspring developing MS later in life.

Recent work suggests that vitamin D may affect the risk of MS by regulating the activity of a variant of the HLA-DRB1 gene, which is known to increase the risk of developing MS roughly three-fold in heterozygotes and ten-fold in homozygotes. Although these findings suggest that it may be important to recommend vitamin D supplementa-

tion in pregnancy and childhood, the actual dose of the vitamin may well be much higher than the normal daily requirement.

Pregnancy
Pregnancy was previously said to worsen the prognosis for MS, but recent studies have shown a reduction in the relapse rate during pregnancy, which is probably compensated for by a higher relapse rate in the following three to six months. The long-term prognosis also seems no worse in those women with MS who become pregnant.

PATHOGENESIS

In MS, the immune response appears to be triggered when MHC class 2 molecules (expressed on antigen-presenting cells, such as macrophages) present antigenic peptides to the T cell receptor on CD4$^+$ T lymphocytes in the periphery, forming the so-called **trimolecular complex**. The formation of the trimolecular complex promotes T cell activation and the production of pro-inflammatory cytokines including tumour necrosis factor-α and interferon-γ. Myelin basic protein and myelin oligodendrocyte glycoprotein (MOG) are major antigens in EAE, but similar myelin antigens have not been demonstrated clearly in MS. Indeed, it seems that the T-cell repertoire broadens progressively in MS and in EAE (so-called epitope-spreading).

T-cell homing to the CNS is promoted by adhesion to molecules of the selectin family on the venular endothelial surface of venules, but also depends on the expression there of activation-dependent adhesion molecules of the immunoglobulin and integrin superfamilies. The integrins LFA-1 and α4β1 on T cells, and their complementary cell adhesion molecules ICAM-1 and VCAM-1 on vas-

---

An immunological cascade follows in which B-lymphocytes are recruited and the blood–brain barrier disrupted. Antibody secretion by B cells probably contributes to myelin injury, and a significant pathogenic role for B cells is suggested by the response of relapsing MS to treatment with the monoclonal B cell antibody rituximab.

cular endothelial cells, may be particularly important in T cell attachment and migration.

Pathogenic CD4 cells consist of at least two populations: interferon-γ secreting T helper-1 (Th1) cells, and a second subset secreting IL-17, Th17 cells. The differentiation, expansion and stabilization of Th17 cells depends on cytokines including IL-6, IL-21 and transforming growth factor β (TGF-β). The balance of pathology triggered by Th1 and Th17 cells could explain some of the clinical heterogeneity of MS.

Along with the central pathogenic role of CD4 T cells, there is also prominent infiltration of lesions by CD8 T cells, which may add to the heterogeneity of the disease process. This pro-inflammatory response is itself regulated by other aspects of the immune cascade: by Th-2 cells through the production of additional cytokines, particularly TGFβ, IL-4 and IL-10, and by the secretion of protective neurotrophic factors, such as brain-derived neurotrophic factor (BDNF).

> This rather complicated cellular and humoral response leads to the development of the characteristic demyelinating lesions, or plaques, which occur particularly in the CNS white matter in MS. Plaques are usually quite small, but can sometimes be several centimetres in diameter, and can then be confused with tumours. The plaques tend to be centred on venules, and in the acute stage they are associated with a dense perivascular cuff of lymphocytes and macrophages.

Pathologically, there are indications that plaque pathology may be heterogeneous, with different patterns of oligodendrocyte injury and immunopathology: one pattern shows similarities to T-cell mediated or T-cell plus antibody/complement-mediated autoimmune encephalomyelitis, while another is similar to a primary oligodendrocyte dystrophy, in some cases resembling the pathology of hypoxic damage. It is still not clear whether a given patient always develops plaques of a single subtype, or whether all plaques begin as a single type (for example a hypoxia-like lesion) and then evolve into different subtypes. Ultimately, however, chronic plaques generally contain little cellular infiltrate, and are composed of demyelinated axons, a low-grade inflammatory response, and astrocytic fibrillary material.

> In addition to the traditional emphasis on plaque formation in the white matter, it is also now clear that the inflammatory process in MS affects the grey matter, and secondly that it occurs in a more diffuse manner throughout the CNS. Longitudinal imaging studies indicate that there is a subtle change of tissue structure which develops over several months at sites in the so-called 'normal-appearing white matter' which then form plaques, and both pathologically and on imaging there are clear indications of a widespread abnormality of the normal-appearing white matter, associated with inflammatory activity.

There is now a growing interest in the role of the innate immune system, particularly the activity of dendritic cells and microglia, in this process, and in the transition from relapsing disease driven by adaptive immunity to progressive disease driven by innate immunity. In this respect, it is interesting that grey matter lesions, although present in all stages of MS, are particularly prominent in secondary progressive MS, and that they can occur in association with a pattern of diffuse microglial activation throughout the white matter. Subpial cortical demyelination is particularly prominent, and apart from the presence of activated microglia, these lesions are associated with meningeal B cell lymphoid follicles whose aetiology and pathological significance are under investigation. Grey matter pathology in MS can therefore be widespread and clinically relevant. Longitudinal imaging studies have suggested that whereas the rate of white matter atrophy remains roughly constant in all stages of MS, the rate of grey matter atrophy accelerates in secondary progressive disease, and that it may be associated significantly with progression of disability.

PATHOPHYSIOLOGY

The pathological changes which occur in the normal and lesional brain tissue give rise to functional effects which are transient in some cases and permanent in others. The balance between these processes, and the degree to which the pathological tissue is capable of self-repair, can explain some of the clinical manifestations of relapse, remission and permanent disability.

Immunological activation releases a number of potentially toxic proinflammatory compounds, including tumour necrosis factor-α, and free oxygen and nitrogen radicals. These agents, along with B-cell-derived antibodies that activate complement to form membrane-attack complexes, may mediate demyelination. Nearly all of the clinical deficit in MS is caused by axonal conduction block, which was explained until recently by the effects of demyelination. However, inflammation can also block axonal conduction directly, through mediators such as nitric oxide, which is capable of altering the function of axonal sodium channels, and there is also growing evidence that these mediators may inhibit oxidative phosphorylation in the brain by impairing the function of components of the mitochondrial respiratory chain, particularly complex IV. If so, inflammation may lead to neuronal dysfunction by combined effects on neuronal membrane properties and energy production, with secondary effects on ATP-dependent membrane ion pumps and ion gradients across the cell membrane.

At least some of these processes are reversible, and remission from acute relapse seems to occur when inflammation subsides and repair processes set in. These repair processes include remyelination, the acquisition of additional axolemmal sodium currents by persistently demyelinated fibres, and functional readaptation in deafferented regions of the cerebral cortex. However, patients may become disabled if these repair mechanisms fail, or if axons or their cell bodies themselves degenerate.

Pathological and imaging studies have shown that axons do degenerate from an early stage of the disease process, that the extent of axonal degeneration in a given location correlates with the extent of the inflammatory response, and that the level of clinical disability correlates well with the extent of axonal damage. Evidence is also emerging that several of the cellular and humoral components of the immune response (including cytotoxic T cells, and the direct toxicity of nitric oxide, glutamate and possibly matrix metalloproteinases) could mediate the axonal injury, in addition to the aspects of ionic imbalance and energy failure discussed earlier. Moreover, it appears that disability is related not only to white matter axonal degeneration, but also to the prominent grey matter involvement that occurs particularly in the later stages of disease. These emerging aspects of pathophysiology have implications for the sorts of treatments which could protect patients with MS from neuronal injury and long-term disability.

MANAGEMENT

The management of patients following an isolated demyelinating episode remains difficult. There is a natural reluctance to discuss the possibility of MS explicitly, because some of these patients will experience no further clinical relapses, and alterations of lifestyle probably have a limited impact on their risk of developing MS. On the other hand, the increasing availability of MRI for prognostic information after an isolated episode means that MS is increasingly being discussed at an earlier stage. In some countries, disease-modifying drugs are also used after a single attack if the imaging findings suggest a high probability of developing MS, or if the findings of a second scan a few months later indicate that the McDonald criteria for diagnosing MS have been satisfied.

Either at presentation with a single attack, or later, when a firm diagnosis of MS has been made, counselling should be tailored to the individual patient, and should recognize the anxiety engendered by the mention of MS. Patients often complain that sufficient information and support was not made available to them around the time of diagnosis.

The treatment of MS
The treatment of MS is based increasingly on the results of properly conducted clinical trials. However, the natural history of the illness, its variable expression, and the difficulties with clinical scores to quantify impairment and disability, all mean that the interpretation of these studies can be difficult.

For example, Kurtzke's extended disability status scale (EDSS), the most widely accepted measure of impairment, consists of a series of separate rank-order scales requiring non-parametric statistical analysis, has a bimodal distribution in the MS population, is relatively insensitive to change of impairment, and is heavily weighted on ambulation. On the other hand, the EDSS has a reasonable inter- and intra-rater reliability. Efforts continue to identify and to validate other sensitive, reproducible and relevant clinical outcome measures, including scales of quality of life, spasticity, dexterity and cognitive function. The Multiple Sclerosis Functional Composite (MSFC) is a more recent measure which incorporates components measuring walking time, upper limb function and speed of information processing, and efforts continue to improve it by adding measurements of vision using low contrast acuity.

A surrogate, biological measure of MS would also be very helpful. Currently, the best surrogate disease marker is MRI, particularly for relapsing-remitting disease. However, the T2-weighted lesion load does not correlate well with disability. The situation appears to be more hopeful with new magnetic resonance techniques, including magnetic resonance spectroscopy assessing axonal dysfunction using the N-acetyl aspartate signal, T1-weighted lesions, longitudinal measurements of partial or global cerebral atrophy, diffusion-weighted imaging and magnetization transfer.

Symptomatic treatment

A number of clinical problems in MS respond to treatments that do not depend on a knowledge of the underlying cause of the illness. Careful use of these measures can improve quality of life considerably.

Pain and paroxysmal symptoms

Previously regarded as uncommon, pain affects at least half of patients with MS. Back pain is common, and often arises from mechanical factors associated with weakness and immobility of the lumbar spine. Nociceptive pain of this sort can be managed effectively in the same way as in cases without MS, starting with non-steroidal anti-inflammatory drugs, transcutaneous electrical nerve stimulation (TENS) and physiotherapy.

Neurogenic pain

Neurogenic pain occurs in approximately 10–15 per cent of MS patients. Once again, management is largely the same as for patients without MS, using combinations of anticonvulsants, antidepressants and TENS, as well as pain surgery in occasional cases. However, sodium channel blocking drugs, such as carbamazepine, phenytoin and lamotrigine, have the potential to increase conduction block and to alleviate pain at the expense of increased disability, although this is often not a significant limitation in practice (see also Chapter 30).

Trigeminal neuralgia

In MS, trigeminal neuralgia is also managed pharmacologically in the same way as the idiopathic variety, and small studies suggest that microvascular decompression and percutaneous thermocoagulation can also be successful in MS (see also Chapter 11).

Paroxysmal or positive features of MS

Paroxysmal or positive features of MS, as well as true seizures, respond well to low doses of sodium channel blocking drugs, of which carbamazepine is the most widely used. A therapeutic response is often apparent using doses as low as 100 mg twice daily, although higher doses may be required, guided by measurements of blood levels.

Ataxia and tremor

Gait ataxia is best managed by physiotherapists and occupational therapists, paying particular attention to the counterproductive abnormalities of gait and posture that patients with such ataxia can adopt. Incorrect use of walking aids may contribute to these abnormalities.

Lesions of the cerebellar outflow tracts can cause a disabling upper limb tremor. Occupational therapists can provide advice on coping strategies, and some patients have benefited from wearing wrist weights, which lessen the amplitude of the tremor. Small studies have suggested that **isoniazid** (800 mg per day, building up at weekly intervals to 1200 mg per day), **clonazepam** or **propranolol** can help some patients. **Stereotactic thalamotomy or thalamic stimulation** remains an option in unilateral cases, helping approximately 60 per cent of MS patients. Unfortunately, the presence of silent, contralateral thalamic lesions means that pseudo-bulbar problems can complicate even unilateral thalamotomy. In addition, the initial benefits often disappear as the disease progresses, so that careful selection of patients with stable disease and unilateral signs and lesions remains important.

Fatigue

Depression, or nocturia causing significant sleep disturbance, should both be identified, since they are reversible factors for which treatment is feasible and likely to be successful. Fatigued patients with a normal mood and little nocturia are less easy to treat. Most learn to modify their lifestyle to cope with the problem, but in other cases graded exercise programmes can help. Pulsed steroid treatment has been advocated for episodic fatigue, assuming an inflammatory basis. **Amantadine** (100–200 mg twice daily) and **modafinil** (200–400 mg daily) have also been found to be helpful in some cases.

Bladder dysfunction

The majority of patients with MS experience bladder dysfunction during the course of their illness. This commonly arises from an interruption of the spinal pathways connecting the pontine micturition centre to the sacral spinal cord, explaining the correlation between bladder symptoms and pyramidal dysfunction in the legs, and the fact that sphincter dysfunction is rarely the sole presenting feature of MS. Detrusor hyper-reflexia results in urinary frequency and urgency, and can be treated using anticholinergic agents (**oxybutynin**, 5 mg, two to three times daily) or **imipramine** (75–150 mg at night). These drugs can exacerbate the tendency of the bladder to empty incompletely and can precipitate urinary retention, so that the post-micturition residual volume should be checked after treatment has been started.

Spinal lesions can also impair the reflex mechanism of normal relaxation of the bladder neck or sphincter before the detrusor contraction, leading to simultaneous contraction of the sphincter mechanism and detrusor, and giving rise to detrusor–sphincter dyssynergia. The resulting symptoms include hesitancy, an interrupted urinary stream and a sensation of incomplete bladder emptying. Investigation with urine culture should be accompanied by a measurement of the residual bladder volume using ultrasound or bladder catheterization. Clean (rather than sterile) **intermittent self-catheterization** improves the control of continence in approximately 90 per cent of patients with a residual bladder volume greater than 100 mL. Prophylactic antibiotics appear to be unnecessary.

Patients who complain of frequent nocturnal incontinence may be helped by the antidiuretic hormone analogue **DDAVP** (desmopressin) taken intranasally at night. This treatment appears to be safe and effective during long-term use as long as fluid overload is carefully avoided.

Severe cases of bladder disturbance resisting these treatments may be amenable to therapy with **intravesical botulinum toxin**. This renders the bladder relatively atonic, and requires intermittent self-catheterization. In some patients where severe symptoms are not helped by any of these approaches, however, it may be necessary to consider a **long-term suprapubic catheter**.

Spasticity

Spasticity is a common and often disabling problem in MS, and is related both to an increased sensitivity of the muscle stretch reflex, and to greater muscle stiffness. Effective management is available for mild to moderate degrees of spasticity, but the improvement in spasticity must be balanced against ensuing weakness and loss of function, as many patients with weak legs depend on increased tone in order to stand or to walk. There is a clear role for physiotherapy. Correction of gait abnormalities and the introduction of orthoses may be helpful, appropriate posturing and wheelchair assessment are important in more advanced cases, and passive muscle stretching twice daily may prevent contractures. There is also an increasing interest in the possibility that physical training may aid recovery by promoting the functional readaptation of distributed cortical networks in the same way that it appears to do so after stroke.

The gamma-aminobutyric acid receptor B-agonist **baclofen** has been shown to be effective in spinal spasticity and is the agent most commonly used for this in MS. Side effects include drowsiness, muscle weakness and incoordination. **Dantrolene sodium**, which is commonly used in conjunction with baclofen, acts directly on muscle contraction and is therefore associated with muscle weakness and fatigue, as well as drowsiness, weakness and bowel disturbance. Liver function tests should be monitored regularly as rare, dose-dependent hepatic toxicity can be fatal. Other anti-spasticity agents, including diazepam and **tizanidine**, have been shown in controlled studies to be as effective as baclofen.

Severely affected patients who fail to improve with oral treatment may respond to **baclofen delivered intrathecally** from a subcutaneously implanted pump. The effectiveness of intrathecal baclofen has largely abolished the need to use more destructive procedures, such as intrathecal phenol installation or rhizotomy. However, selective procedures including dorsal root entry zone ablation (DREZotomy) have been introduced recently, although they still carry a risk of permanent sensory dysfunction. Some patients continue to require assessment for orthopaedic procedures for the treatment of joint deformity and contracture, for example, using tendon-lengthening procedures. Finally, there is now considerable interest in the use of **botulinum toxin** in patients with severe spasticity, either as ongoing treatment or as an adjunct to physiotherapy.

Potassium channel blockers

The aminopyridines (**4-aminopyridine (4-AP) and 3,4-diaminopyridine (3–4 DAP)**) inhibit potassium channels and widen the nerve action potential, reversing conduction block in experimentally demyelinated axons. These agents act similarly on synaptic potassium channels. Their ability to reverse conduction block in fibres with a critically low safety factor has led to clinical studies in patients with MS, particularly those with severe and progressive disability in whom the symptoms show temperature dependence. 4-AP crosses the blood–brain barrier more easily, and has therefore been studied more intensively than 3–4 DAP. Both agents have a small but significant beneficial effect on disability, but their widespread use has been limited by a narrow therapeutic index. They are associated with significant side effects, including dizziness, paraesthesiae and abdominal pain. At higher doses, they may precipitate an encephalopathy or seizures. 4-AP is currently available for unlicensed treatment of highly selected patients. The drug is introduced at a low dose of 5 mg given once or twice daily, and dosage increments must be titrated carefully to a maximum dose of 10 mg taken three times daily. These practical difficulties with the use of potassium channel blockers have led to work using a slow release formulation of 4-AP, fampridine, and a recent trial suggested that the drug could be used relatively safely and that it was capable of improving gait in a subset of ambulant patients with established disability.

Management of acute relapses and isolated demyelinating episodes

Corticosteroids

Corticosteroids are the mainstay of treatment for disabling relapses. However, symptomatic treatment and prophylactic measures against deep vein thrombosis in patients with relapses, causing severe lower limb weakness, should not be forgotten.

Corticosteroids are known to have a number of effects on immune function. They inhibit the secretion of proinflammatory cytokines by lymphocytes and antigen-presenting cells, and alter MHC class 2 molecule expression. **Intravenous methylprednisolone** reverses temporarily the breakdown of the blood–brain barrier in acute MRI lesions.

These theoretical considerations complement the evidence from controlled trials that intramuscular adrenocorticotropic hormone, as well as oral and intravenous methylprednisolone, can shorten the duration of relapse. Intramuscular adrenocorticotropic hormone given for 14 days and intravenous methylprednisolone (i.v. MP, 1 g daily for 3 days) have comparable efficacies. However, steroids do not seem to influence the ultimate extent of the recovery from a relapse.

The majority of relapses are treated with corticosteroids given orally, yet curiously these have been subjected to fewer controlled trials. Indeed, there is considerable uncertainty about the best regimen for acute relapse, but there is a trend towards treatment with i.v. MP, followed in some centres by an oral prednisolone taper. Some centres advocate an oral regimen of high-dose methylprednisolone, 500 mg given daily for 5 days, as a more convenient alternative to intravenous therapy. In all cases, the usual precautions and contraindications applying to the use of corticosteroids should be observed. The minimum interval between courses of treatment remains unclear, although a practical lower limit of 8–12 weeks is usually adopted.

A minority of patients develop very severe disability during an acute relapse, which responds poorly to corticosteroids. Some of these patients may respond favourably to a course of plasma exchange.

Disease-modifying treatments

The greatest concern of patients with MS is that their disease will progress to the point of severe disability. Treatments that offer the potential to alter the course of the disease are therefore of enormous importance. To date, there has been increasing success in developing treatments that reduce the rate at which relapses occur, and which therefore reduce the accumulation of disability arising from such relapses. However, the licensed drugs (the β-interferons, glatiramer acetate, mitoxantrone and natalizumab) are generally expensive to use, require parenteral administration, and have side effects that reduce their overall impact on the quality of patients' lives.

It is difficult to extrapolate their long-term benefits from those found in the pivotal clinical trials, which for practical reasons can only last a few years, so it is not clear if the conversion to progressive disease can be delayed with long-term use. It is also notable that treatments for relapsing disease so far have little or no proven effects on the slow progression of disability in nonrelapsing patients with secondary or primary progressive MS, where disability may arise from different mechanisms.

β-interferon

The first interferon to be used in MS was γ-interferon, but a trial of its use was terminated rapidly because it caused a dose-dependent increase in the rate of relapse. It is now clear, of course, that γ-interferon is a central, proinflammatory cytokine in the immune response during relapse. β-Interferon is a glycoprotein with a single amino acid chain, which appears to work partly by antagonizing the effects of γ-interferon, including the upregulation of MHC class 2 molecules on the surfaces of antigen-presenting cells. Cytokine release by macrophages is also inhibited, and finally there is a broad enhancement of suppressor T cell function. More recently, modulatory effects on T cell migration and the function of Th17 cells have been reported.

In an early trial, natural β-interferon given intrathecally reduced relapse frequency.

Subsequently, β-interferon 1b (Betaferon (Schering Health)), a non-glycosylated preparation with a serine residue instead of cystine at position 17 to improve stability, was used in a controlled, double-blind trial involving 372 patients with relapsing-remitting MS, mild disability and relatively early disease. At a dose of 8 MIU given subcutaneously on alternate days, the relapse rate was reduced by approximately one-third. MRI scans of the brain obtained at annual intervals showed that, whereas the lesion area increased by 17 per cent compared with baseline in the placebo group, it actually decreased by 6.2 per cent in the treated group.

β-Interferon 1a (which has no amino acid substitution and is fully glycosylated) was subsequently shown to have similar beneficial effects to β-interferon 1b on the relapse rate, and on disease activity assessed using MRI, in large, controlled, double-blind trials. β-Interferon 1a also increases the time to conversion to MS after isolated demyelinating episodes in patients with MRI lesions at presentation. There are two preparations, Avonex (Biogen) (given as a weekly intramuscular injection of 30 mg), and Rebif (Serono) (given as a subcutaneous injection of 22 or 44 mg three times each week). There is some indication of a dose–response effect for Betaferon and Rebif, but not for Avonex. However, detailed comparisons of the effects of the different β-interferons are difficult because of the differences in the end-points used in the various trials. All three preparations have been licensed for the treatment of relapsing MS, but despite some early optimism, they do not appear to have any major effects on the rate at which disability progresses in patients with progressive forms of MS.

The side-effect profiles of β-interferon 1a and β-interferon 1b are similar, and include influenza-like symptoms, myalgia, transient nausea, injection site reactions, fever and headache, all of which diminish during the first few months of treatment. Marrow suppression and hepatotoxicity have also occurred, but are rarely serious enough to warrant cessation of therapy. However, the drugs should not be used in patients with decompensated liver disease, poorly controlled epilepsy, severe depression, or who are pregnant. Patients may also develop cross-reacting neutralizing antibodies to β-interferon, and these are likely to blunt its therapeutic benefits. However, the presence of antibodies may not indicate the need to switch treatment in patients who show a continuing clinical response, and indeed a significant number of patients found to be antibody-positive revert to a negative state at some point.

> The indications for the use of β-interferon are now generally agreed for patients with relapsing MS, and in many countries the treatment is offered in those with an initial demyelinating episode and an MRI scan suggesting a high probability of conversion to MS. In the UK, treatment is reserved for ambulant patients with relapsing-remitting MS, when at least two relapses have occurred during the preceding two years, and in whom there is clearly no progression between relapses. Patients with secondary progressive MS are also treated if their disability is advancing mainly due to the consequences of relapses occurring at least annually.

Treatment is terminated if relapsing-remitting patients enter the secondary progressive phase of the illness, unless progression of disability is due to the consequences of relapses. Alternative disease-modifying drugs are chosen if relapses continue, or if there is a marked increase in relapse frequency during follow up, compared to baseline.

Glatiramer acetate

Glatiramer acetate is a synthetic, random polymer of the four basic amino acids L-alanine, L-glutamic acid, L-lysine and L-tyrosine, with biophysical and antigenic properties intended to simulate those of MBP. Its synthesis and use arose from work showing that fragments of MBP could either exacerbate or attenuate the course of EAE. By mimicking MBP, glatiramer acetate could block antigen presentation competitively and could also induce antigen-specific suppressor T cells. Following encouraging work in the 1980s, glatiramer acetate was studied in a multicentre phase 3 trial involving 251 patients over two years, with a primary end-point of relapse frequency. Using a dose of 20 mg given by daily subcutaneous injection, treatment produced a significant, 29 per cent, reduction of the relapse rate from 0.84 to 0.59 relapses per year. Later, it was shown that glatiramer acetate has a significant effect on MRI markers of disease activity, but interestingly this effect only became evident after between four and six months' treatment, in contrast to β-interferon, where treatment effects are evident

within a few weeks. Glatiramer acetate has been licensed for the treatment of relapsing MS and after an initial attack with a high probability of developing MS. The treatment appears to be well tolerated, but side effects include injection site reactions (usually mild and transient), and in approximately 10 per cent of cases, a reaction following injection involving anxiety, flushing, palpitations, dyspnoea, chest pain or tightness. These symptoms appear to be transient and do not require specific treatment. Teratogenic side effects have not been described in animal studies.

Natalizumab

The monoclonal antibody natalizumab (Tysabri) is the first of a class of selective adhesion-molecule antagonists, and works by blocking $\alpha4\beta1$ integrin, preventing the binding of inflammatory cells to the brain endothelium, and preventing their passage into the brain. In a large phase 3 trial involving 942 participants with relapsing MS, there was a 2:1 allocation to receive natalizumab or placebo by intravenous infusion every 4 weeks for two years. Natalizumab was found to reduce the risk of sustained progression of disability by 42 per cent over two years, and that of relapse by 68 per cent over 12 months. There were 83 per cent fewer new or enlarging T_2 hyperintense lesions on MRI over two years in the treated group. Allergic reactions occurred in around 4 per cent, with serious hypersensitivity reactions in 1 per cent, generally within the first few cycles of treatment.

> These highly encouraging findings have led to natalizumab being licensed for patients with relapsing MS, but the initial enthusiasm for the treatment has been tempered to some extent by the increased risk of serious opportunistic infection. Initially, cases of progressive multifocal leukoencephalopathy (PML) were seen in people treated with a combination of β-interferon 1a and natalizumab, but cases have now occurred in those on natalizumab alone. Currently, the risk of PML is put at one per 1000 patients treated for an average of 18 months, but this figure is likely to change in either direction as experience of the drug grows.

For now, however, this risk has meant that natalizumab is used in the UK in those failing treatment with glatiramer acetate or β-interferon, and experiencing not only serious relapses on these first-line treatments, but also demonstrating new lesion activity on MRI.

Mitoxantrone

The cytotoxic anthracenedione mitoxantrone has a number of actions including a DNA-intracalating ability. In various studies, including a European phase-III trial, it has been found to have significant beneficial effects on MRI activity, on relapse freqency in relapsing-remitting patients, and on the progression of disability in secondary-progressive patients. There is evidence of a dose–response effect, and the drug is commonly infused either monthly (12 mg/m^2) for six months, or three-monthly for two years. Apart from the usual cytotoxic side effects, mitoxantrone can also cause amenorrhoea and can be cardiotoxic at cumulative doses above 140 mg/m^2. Irreversible reductions of the cardiac ejection fraction may occur in around 1 per cent of those treated, although congestive cardiac failure is much rarer with the total drug exposure used in the usual protocols. There is also a well-defined risk of approximately 0.25 per cent of acute leukaemia, with a mortality of around 50 per cent, which can present in the first few years after treatment ends. Treatment protocols include regular and ongoing assessments of haematological and cardiac function, and it is now becoming clear that these need to be continued for several years after the treatment ends.

Mitoxantrone has been licensed for relapsing and progressive MS, but these concerns about serious toxicity mean that its use (in the UK, at least) is generally restricted to patients with rapidly progressive disability, generally with superimposed relapses as assessed clinically and by MRI, and to relapsing patients who do not respond to β-interferon or glatiramer acetate. For patients with severe relapsing disease, it can be regarded as an alternative to natalizumab.

Unlicensed drugs

Apart from those drugs licensed as disease-modifying treatments, there are also a group of relatively old, unlicensed drugs for which the evidence for efficacy is more limited.

Azathioprine

Azathioprine is metabolised to 6-mecaptopurine, a competitive inhibitor of nucleic acid synthesis. It is known to suppress a range of T- and B-cell func-

tions. In a meta-analysis of the results of all published blind, randomized controlled trials, patients on treatment were twice as likely to remain free of relapse after three years. Disease progression was also reduced, but only by 0.2 EDSS points. A recent Cochrane review suggested that azathioprine reduces the risk of relapse over one to three years quite modestly, by around 20 per cent, which is less than that of the β-interferons and glatiramer acetate. Nevertheless, azathioprine is a cheap and generally well tolerated drug, and these findings have led to its use (2.5 mg/kg per day) in some patients with relapsing disease. The treatment is associated with gastrointestinal side effects, marrow suppression, hepatotoxicity, hyperuricaemia and skin rashes, and the blood count and liver function need to be monitored regularly. Moreover, there is concern about the potential risk of cancer in patients treated continuously for five or more years.

Methotrexate

The folic acid analogue methotrexate inhibits nucleotide synthesis, and interferes with the production of proinflammatory agents including prostaglandins and interleukin-1. It has been used successfully to treat autoimmune diseases, including rheumatoid arthritis, and appears to be well tolerated when administered chronically at doses of around 10 mg per week. In a controlled, blinded study, it slowed the progression of upper limb disability, but not of other aspects of disability. These results have led to its use in people with progressive forms of MS, not least because of the lack of any other competing treatment in this group of patients.

Intravenous immunoglobulin

Intravenous immunoglobulin (IVIg) has been used successfully to treat a number of disorders with an immunological basis, including neurological conditions such as demyelinating neuropathies and myasthenia gravis. The mechanism of action is not fully understood, but IVIg may contain anti-idiotypic antibodies that modulate T- and B-lymphocyte activity, and downregulate cytokine production, antigen presentation and macrophage activity. Treatment with repeated courses of IVIg has been found to reduce the rate of relapse in relapsing-remitting MS in controlled trials involving relatively small numbers of patients, and to reduce the rate at which lesions develop on MRI. Further work is under way, but the treatment is not at present licensed or in widespread use.

Emerging new treatments

Perhaps not surprisingly, the rapid advances in the understanding of the immunopathology of MS are leading to the emergence of a range of new disease-modifying drugs which may offer advantages over the existing treatments, either because of greater efficacy or because they are delivered as tablets rather than by injection. Several of these drugs are in advanced stages of development, and may well be licensed over the next few years. A general concern for all these drugs is the extent to which their greater efficacy could be associated with a greater risk of untoward effects, particularly that of opportunistic infection.

Alemtuzumab

The humanized monoclonal antibody alemtuzumab binds to the CD52 receptor on T cells, thymocytes, natural killer cells and B cells, causing cell lysis and prolonged lymphocyte depletion. It is given by infusion annually, and in controlled studies it appears to reduce the rate of relapse and of inflammatory activity on MRI to a significantly greater extent than β-interferon. There is a risk of autoimmune disease, particularly thyroiditis and idiopathic thrombocytopenic purpura.

Cladrabine

The oral agent cladrabine is an adenosine deaminase-resistant analogue of deoxyadenosine which blocks DNA synthesis, induces the mitochondrial apoptotic pathway, and causes a prolonged suppression of the peripheral lymphocyte count. It has the attraction of being an oral agent which may only need to be administered in short, intermittent courses, and a phase III trial has recently suggested that it may halve the rate of relapse.

Fingolimod

The sphingosine analogue fingolimod is an oral agent which interacts with specific G-protein-linked receptors after undergoing phosphorylation. It inhibits lymphocyte migration from the thymus and secondary lymphoid organs, with the result that lymphocytes are sequestered in those sites. Controlled trials suggest that fingolimod reduces the rate of relapse at least as effectively as existing first-line disease-modifying drugs.

In addition to these agents, there are a number of drugs which modify the immune response by interfering with lymphocyte trafficking or viability, including **rituximab**, **teriflunomide**, **laquinimod** and **fumarate**, and which are currently undergoing clinical trials. At the moment, the extent to which these and the other emerging treatments for relapsing MS can prevent long-term disability is simply not known, and there is a great deal of interest in alternative routes to so-called neuroprotection to control this major aspect of the illness.

REFERENCES AND FURTHER READING

Association of British Neurologists (2007) ABN guidelines for treatment of multiple sclerosis with β-interferon and glatiramer acetate. London: Association of British Neurologists. Available online: www.theabn.org/downloads/ABN-MS-Guidelines-2007.pdf

Compston DA, McDonald WI, Noseworthy J et al. (2008) McAlpine's Multiple Sclerosis, 4th edn. London: Churchill Livingstone.

Confavreux C, Vukusic S, Moreau T, Adeline P (2000) Relapses and progression of disability in multiple sclerosis. New England Journal of Medicine, 343:1430–148.

Filippini G, Munari L, Incorvaia B et al. (2003) Interferons in relapsing remitting multiple sclerosis: a systematic review. Lancet, 361:545–552.

Kapoor R, Miller DH, Jones SJ et al. (1998) Effects of intravenous methylprednisolone on outcome in MRI-based prognostic subgroups in acute optic neuritis. Neurology, 50:230–237.

Kutzelnigg A, Lucchinetti C, Stadelman C et al. (2005) Cortical demyelination and diffuse white matter injury in multiple sclerosis. Brain, 128:2705–2712.

Polman CH, Reingold SC, Edan G et al. (2005) Diagnostic criteria for multiple sclerosis: 2005 revisions to the 'McDonald Criteria'. Annals of Neurology, 58:840–846.

Runmarker B, Anderson O (1993) Prognostic factors in a multiple sclerosis incidence cohort with twenty-five years follow-up. Brain, 116:117–134.

Smith KJ, Kapoor R, Hall SM, Davies M (2001) Electrically active axons degenerate when exposed to nitric oxide. Annals of Neurology, 49:470–476.

Trapp BD, Peterson J, Ransohoff RM et al. (1998) Axonal transection in the lesions of multiple sclerosis. New England Journal of Medicine, 338:278–285.

Weinshenker BG, Bass B, Rice GPA et al. (1989) The natural history of multiple sclerosis: a geographically based study. 1. Clinical course and disability. Brain, 112:133–146.

CHAPTER 23

CEREBROVASCULAR DISEASE

Nick Losseff and Martin Brown

INTRODUCTION

Stroke can be defined as a focal neurological deficit resulting from a disturbance of the cerebral circulation lasting more than 24 hours (or causing early death). **Transient ischaemic attack (TIA)** is defined identically, except that the symptoms last less than 24 hours. This timing distinction is completely arbitrary and significantly out of date. An alternative description has been proposed which requires acute imaging, preferably magnetic resonance imaging (MRI), to exclude an infarct as a cause of the transient symptoms. In this definition, if the brain scan shows a relevant acute infarct, then the event is called an 'ischaemic stroke', however short the

duration of the symptoms. The latter definition is widely used in research studies, but is not currently common in clinical use.

Stroke is usually invoked to describe events with a sudden onset. Individuals may have cerebrovascular disease without symptoms (e.g. asymptomatic carotid stenosis or infarction on computed tomography (CT)) or acute symptoms without obvious imaging changes or focal signs (e.g. headache in some patients with subarachnoid haemorrhage or cerebral venous thrombosis). Cerebrovascular disease is an important cause of dementia, which may have an insidious onset. Often the cerebral symptoms of stroke or TIA result from cardiovascular or haematological disease arising outside the cranial circulation.

'**Brain attack**' is an alternative term used to describe the acute presentation of stroke and TIA, which removes the requirement for a delay of 24 hours to diagnose stroke. This term also emphasizes the need for urgent action to remedy the situation and that other diagnoses need to be considered. The term 'cerebrovascular accident' should be abandoned, because it implies that the stroke is a chance event for which little can be done.

Stroke is a massive public health problem, being the third most common cause of death in the developed world and the leading cause of adult disability. 140 000 people in the UK will have a stroke in the next year and approximately 20 per cent of these patients will die within 30 days of onset. Above the age of 45 years, one in four men and one in five women are destined to have a stroke. However, stroke can occur at any age from the perinatal period onwards. For the survivors of any age, morbidity can be considerable.

Outcome following stroke varies widely from centre to centre.

It is important to recognize that the term stroke describes the clinical presentation of the patient. It is a syndrome and 'stroke' should not be regarded as a sufficient diagnosis on its own. Accurate diagnosis requires a description of the anatomical territory involved, the underlying pathology (i.e. infarction or haemorrhage), the mechanism (e.g. embolism), the underlying aetiology (e.g. atherosclerosis) and the underlying risk factors (e.g. smoking). The task of the stroke physician is to make this accurate pathophysiological diagnosis as this will then guide appropriate acute treatment and secondary preventive measures. To accomplish this requires detailed knowledge of the clinical and radiological patterns that the different stroke syndromes may produce and familiarity with the large evidence base of clinical trials, which guide stroke treatment and prevention. The stroke physician also needs to assess the functional effects of stroke on the patient and their ability to participate in daily activities, to guide appropriate rehabilitation. The management of stroke may involve a variety of clinicians, therapists and community agencies. The stroke physician therefore needs to work as an integral part of a large multidisciplinary team.

The main subdivisions of stroke are cerebral **infarction (ischaemic stroke)** and intracranial **haemorrhage (haemorrhagic stroke)** (Table 23.1). In over 80 per cent of cases, death of brain tissue is secondary to infarction. This may affect all or part of the territory of a large intracerebral artery, occupy the border zone between arterial supplies, or

involve only a small area of white matter supplied by a penetrating vessel **(lacunar stroke)**. In 12 per cent of cases, stroke results from primary haemorrhage within the substance of the brain (intracerebral haemorrhage (ICH)). This may affect deep structures or the more superficial lobes of the brain.

In 8 per cent of stroke cases, bleeding occurs primarily within the subarachnoid space **(subarachnoid haemorrhage (SAH))**. The presentation of SAH is usually so distinct from other causes of stroke that it is not always included under this umbrella, perhaps because most patients with SAH are referred to neurosurgeons, not stroke physicians. However, SAH is frequently complicated by cerebral infarction from vasospasm and shares underlying causes with ICH, e.g. cerebral aneurysm and risk factors with both ICH and ischaemic stroke, e.g. hypertension.

Cerebral venous thrombosis is a rare cause of stroke, but can present with cerebral infarction or haemorrhage or both. Both ICH and SAH may occur together, e.g. from a ruptured middle cerebral artery aneurysm.

Differential diagnosis of stroke

The diagnosis of stroke and TIA requires a detailed history, which may need to be taken from a partner, carer, friend or relative, concentrating on the time course, rapidity of onset and location of the symptoms. The accurate timing of stroke onset has become crucial to select appropriate patients for thrombolytic treatments and often requires an independent witness. The presence of vascular risk factors needs to be established. The **sudden onset of a focal neurological deficit** is characteristic of stroke and TIA. Most strokes reach their maximum deficit over a few minutes, but they may evolve over a few hours. If the patient survives, there is a variable period from days to months of stability before the patient starts to recover. This long-term time course may be helpful in supporting the diagnosis of stroke when the patient has not been seen acutely or if the brain imaging is normal. In patients with large lesions, there may be an initial stable period, followed by deterioration on the second or third day caused by the development of cerebral oedema with mass effect and brain herniation. This should always be visible on brain imaging, although MRI, rather than CT, may be required in patients with cerebellar or brainstem infarction.

Table 23.1 Subtypes of stroke

Subtype	
Cerebral infarction	Territorial
	Border zone
	Lacunar
Intracranial haemorrhage	
Intracerebral haemorrhage	Lobar
	Deep
	Posterior fossa
Subarachnoid haemorrhage	
Cerebral venous thrombosis	

Stroke mimics need to be identified rapidly to prevent inappropriate treatment, e.g. thrombolysis. A number of different neurological and systemic disorders present to emergency departments with symptoms and signs that mimic stroke. One of the most common is **post-ictal paralysis following an epileptic seizure**. In such cases, there is usually a past history of epilepsy or focal brain injury, which may be evident on a brain scan. **Hypoglycaemia** can present with hemiparesis, and all patients with suspected stroke should have their blood sugar measured on arrival. **Migraine** is often listed as a stroke mimic, but it should be remembered that focal symptoms resulting from migraine are usually visual and very rarely last more than an hour. Migraine-like headache is commonly precipitated by stroke and this is a far more likely explanation for focal symptoms in a patient of any age who looks as though they have had a stroke, than the extremely rare condition of hemiplegic migraine. **Systemic infections, including meningitis and encephalitis**, may enter the differential diagnosis, but should be accompanied by fever and usually present with confusion rather than focal features. Neurological deficits worsen over the course of the first day in about 20 per cent of patients with stroke. However, if a patient suspected of stroke has symptoms or signs that have progressed for more than a few hours, an alternative cause, such as a space-occupying lesion, becomes increasingly likely. **Space-occupying lesions** can present with the acute onset of symptoms and up to 5 per cent of patients presenting with typical stroke-like symptoms have a **subdural haematoma, brain tumour or cerebral abscess**. The distinction is usually readily made on brain imaging, but if there is doubt, repeating the scan after an appropriate period will usually resolve the diagnosis. Occasionally, a cerebral biopsy is required.

Acute demyelination caused by multiple sclerosis or acute disseminated encephalomyelitis may occasionally present with hemiparesis, sensory impairment or brainstem symptoms that mimic stroke. Usually, the symptoms caused by inflammatory demyelination evolve over a few days. A characteristic MRI appearance and intrathecal synthesis of oligoclonal immunoglobulin may help to confirm the diagnosis. Occasionally, **somatization and dissociation disorders** may present with stroke-like symptoms ('hysterical' hemiparesis or sensory loss) and should be considered if there is marked fluctuation and signs inconsistent with 'organic' disease. The differential diagnosis of TIA is considered in more detail below.

> It is impossible to tell reliably the difference between infarction and ICH from the history or examination. Cranial imaging is therefore essential to make the distinction and exclude mimics of stroke.

In contrast, **SAH** characteristically presents with sudden, very severe headache and neck stiffness and the differential diagnosis is between other causes of acute headache and meningism, which mimics meningitis and posterior fossa mass lesions. It should be borne in mind that may occur at the same time as SAH, e.g. from a ruptured middle cerebral artery aneurysm, and then the patients may have additional focal signs.

ISCHAEMIC STROKE

Pathophysiology of ischaemic stroke

The brain is a highly metabolically active organ and even though it accounts for only 2 per cent of body weight, it uses 20 per cent of cardiac output when the body is at rest. Brain energy use is also dependent on the degree of neuronal activation. The brain uses glucose exclusively as a substrate for energy metabolism by oxidation to carbon dioxide and water. This metabolism allows conversion of adenosine diphosphate to adenosine triphosphate (ATP). A constant supply of ATP is essential for neuronal integrity and this process is much more efficient in the presence of oxygen. Although ATP can be formed by anaerobic glycolysis, the energy yielded by this pathway is small and also leads to the accumulation of toxic lactic acid. The brain needs and uses approximately 500 mL of oxygen and 100 mg of glucose each minute, hence the need for a rich supply of oxygenated blood containing glucose. Mean cerebral blood flow (CBF) in the cortex is normally approximately 50 mL/100 g per minute. The cerebral circulation maintains constant levels of CBF in the face of changing systemic blood pressure by a sophisticated process termed 'autoregulation'. However, autoregulation has upper and lower limits and in health CBF remains relatively constant over a range of mean arterial blood pressure of between 50 and 150 mmHg. The limits of autoregulation are shifted to higher values in patients with chronic uncontrolled hypertension.

The clinical manifestations of ischaemic stroke will depend to a large extent on the location and size of the vessel occluded, the duration of occlusion and the adequacy of collateral circulation. These will govern the location and extent of tissue ischaemia and infarction. If perfusion pressure falls to the lower limit of autoregulation, further falls in perfusion pressure will lead to a reduction in CBF. However, this may be tolerated without symptoms. By increasing oxygen extraction from the blood, adequate compensation can be made even if blood flow is reduced to approximately 20–25 mL/100 g per minute. As cerebral blood flow falls further, metabolic paralysis, initially without cell disruption, ensues and this may be reversible. However if prolonged, infarction is inevitable. When CBF falls below 20 mL/100 g per minute, oxygen extraction starts to fall and changes may be detected on electroencephalography. At levels below 10 mL/100 g per minute cell membrane functions are severely disrupted and the membrane cation pumps fail to maintain cell ionic integrity. Below 5 mL/100 g per minute, cell death is inevitable within a short time.

The ischaemic cascade

Severe ischaemia triggers a cascade of biochemical changes which potentiate cell death and lead to necrosis (Figure 23.1). These pathophysiological changes have been of considerable interest to those developing treatments to lessen the damage caused by ischaemic stroke. In the ischaemic brain as ion channels fail, K^1 moves out of the cell into the extracellular space, while Ca^{11} moves into the cell in extreme quantities, where it further compromises the ability of the cell to maintain ionic homeostasis and leads to mitochondrial failure. Hypoxia leads to the generation of free radicals, which peroxidize fatty acids in cell membranes, causing further cellular dysfunction. Anaerobic glycolysis results in lactic acidosis, further impairing cellular metabolic functions. Excitatory neurotransmitter activity (e.g. glutamate) is greatly increased in areas of brain ischaemia because of increased release and failure of uptake mechanisms. These neurotransmitters are themselves toxic at these increased levels by causing further Ca^{11} and Na^1 influx into cells through their actions on N-methyl-D-aspartate receptors. Hence, ischaemia triggers a vicious cascade of events leading to cell electrical failure and then death. At some point, the process becomes irreversible, even after reperfusion of tissues. Even if the severity of ischaemia is inadequate to cause necrosis it may trigger apoptosis (programmed cell death).

The ischaemic penumbra

The degree of ischaemia caused by blockage of an artery varies, partly depending on collateral supply. At the centre or core of the territory supplied by an occluded artery where blood flow is lowest, the damage is most severe. Membrane pumps fail rapidly and the damage is irreversible once infarction has occurred. However, at the periphery, collateral flow may allow continued delivery of blood, although at a lower rate sufficient to maintain membrane integrity, but not electrical activity. The neurones in this zone area will then fail to function with resulting clinical deficit, but remain alive and are then referred to as the **ischaemic penumbra**, by analogy with a lunar eclipse. The neurones in the penumbra are at risk of progression to infarction in the few hours after the onset of arterial occlusion, but also have the potential to survive, with recovery of function, if the ischaemic cascade can be halted or reversed. Sophisticated neuroimaging can now be used to define areas of irreversible brain damage and areas in which perfusion is suboptimal, but where irreversible infarction has not taken place. Reperfusion therapy, e.g. thrombolysis, and neuroprotective therapies, are designed to salvage

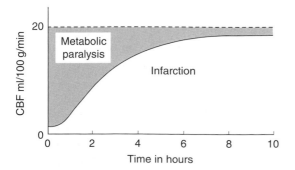

Figure 23.1 Relation of severity and duration of fall in cerebral blood flow to effect on cerebral tissue. (Redrawn from Crowell RM, DeGirolami U, Jones TH (1982) *Cerebral Ischaemia Clinical and Experimental Approach*. Tokyo: Igabu-Sharin).

the penumbra, but it is very likely that high quality simple supportive management in the acute stage also decreases the chances of this secondary brain damage in the penumbra.

Vascular anatomy

The brain is supplied by two internal carotid arteries and two vertebral arteries. The internal carotid arteries begin in the neck at the bifurcation of the common carotid artery and ascend intracranially. The first branch of the internal carotid artery is the ophthalmic artery. The former then bifurcates into the anterior and middle cerebral arteries. Both anterior and middle cerebral arteries give off other branches and deep penetrating vessels. The **anterior cerebral artery** supplies among other structures much of the '**leg**' representation of the cortex. The **middle cerebral artery** supplies the '**arm**' representation, some of the '**leg**' representation, and the **speech** areas in the **dominant** hemisphere or the areas of **spatial awareness** in the **non-dominant** hemisphere. The **penetrating vessels** supply the **deeper** portions of the hemisphere, including the **internal capsule, basal ganglia and visual radiation**.

The **vertebral arteries** are unique in that they are the only arteries in the body to anastomose to form a larger artery, the basilar artery, which overlies the brainstem. The vertebral and basilar arteries give off three **cerebellar arteries** on each side, which supply **brainstem** and **cerebellar** structures. Perforating vessels arise from the basilar artery along its length and predominantly supply the deep areas of the brainstem, particularly the cranial nerve nuclei. At the top, the basilar artery divides to form the left and right **posterior cerebral arteries**. These supply **occipital visual cortex** and the **medial inferior temporal lobes**, containing the **hippocampus and memory** areas. The anterior, middle and posterior cerebral arteries are connected via anterior and posterior communicating vessels on both sides and all these vessels together form the circle of Willis.

Causes and risk factors

Ischaemic stroke usually results from vessel occlusion from local *in-situ* thrombosis or embolism. Embolism can occur anywhere from a large artery (aorta, carotid or vertebral artery) to a smaller artery (30–40 per cent) or more proximally from the heart (30–40 per cent). Local occlusions from disease of the walls of the small penetrating blood vessels is responsible for lacunar infarction (25 per cent). Localized reduction in blood flow distal to an occluded large artery, e.g. the proximal internal carotid artery, or systemic hypotension accounts for haemodynamic infarction (in about 5 per cent).

The main underlying **pathological processes** causing stroke are **atherosclerosis, cardiac embolism and hypertensive small vessel disease** (Box 23.1). Not surprisingly, the main risk factors for stroke are also the risk factors for atherosclerosis and heart disease. **Hypertension** is a particularly important risk factor because it promotes small vessel disease, atherosclerosis and heart disease, and causes both ICH, SAH and ischaemic stroke.

Risk factors should not be regarded as causes of stroke, but rather as promoters of the underlying pathological processes responsible for vascular and cardiac disease, or increased blood coagulability. Stroke is often associated with a combination of risk factors as the combined effect of individual risk factors on stroke incidence is multiplicative rather than simply additive. The presence of one or more risk factors is insufficient to make a diagnosis of the mechanism of stroke because there is a large overlap between the syndromes associated with individual risk factors; for example, hypertension and smoking overlap as risk factors for both carotid artery stenosis and small vessel occlusion. The majority of patients with established risk factors, e.g. hypertension, never have a stroke. Thus, the presence of risk factors should not be used to make a diagnosis of stroke. The main value of

Box 23.1 Major risk factors for transient ischaemic attack and stroke

- Increasing age
- Hypertension
- Smoking
- Diabetes mellitus
- Atrial fibrillation
- Heart disease
- Hypercholesterolaemia
- Excess alcohol

identifying risk factors for stroke is in primary prevention and secondary prevention of recurrence. Although increasing age is an important risk factor, stroke can occur at any age, including in childhood. The age of the patient should not be used as a diagnostic feature. About one-quarter of all strokes occur before the age of 65 years. Some patients who have suffered a stroke have no identifiable risk factors.

Atherosclerosis of the major vessels supplying the brain is a major source of cerebral **embolism**. The emboli are usually **platelet aggregates** or **thrombus** formed on atherosclerotic plaques, but may consist of cholesterol crystals or atherosclerotic debris. It is believed that the acute occurrence of thrombosis is caused by plaque rupture, which exposes the lipid core to blood, activating the clotting cascade. Atherothrombosis may also lead to vessel occlusion, in which case stroke may result from distal propagation of thrombus, embolism or, less commonly, a reduction in distal flow (haemodynamic stroke). Symptomatic atherosclerosis is frequent at the **carotid artery bifurcation** in the neck, where it causes internal carotid artery stenosis, but also commonly affects the aorta, the carotid syphon, the common carotid artery and the vertebral and basilar arteries. Atherosclerosis may also involve the intracranial vessels, particularly the origin of the middle cerebral artery. Intracranial stenosis is more common in black and Asian populations.

Cardiac embolism causes stroke by promoting embolism of thrombus (or occasionally valve fragments or vegetations) from the **left side of the heart** to the brain, and may be divided into high risk or lower risk causes (Table 23.2). **Atrial fibrillation** remains the most important cause of cardioembolism in the elderly. Valvular heart disease, particularly mitral stenosis, and mechanical prosthetic heart valves, are other important causes. Careful examination of the pulse and cardiovascular system are essential in patients with stroke and TIA.

The term 'paradoxical embolism' is used when an embolus reaches the brain (or systemic arterial system) from the venous system, either through abnormal arteriovenous shunts in the lungs or via an abnormal communication between the right and the left hand sides of the heart. Congenital

Table 23.2 Cardiac causes of ischaemic stroke and transient ischaemic attack.

High risk	Atrial fibrillation (especially when combined with other risk factors)
	Mitral stenosis
	Prosthetic heart valves
	Bacterial endocarditis
	Cardiac surgery
Lower risk	Myocardial infarction
	Ventricular/atrial aneurysm
	Cardiomyopathy
	Patent foramen ovale

anomalies, e.g. atrial septal defects, especially when associated with pulmonary hypertension, are an important cause of paradoxical embolism. Patent foramen ovale also provides a potential route for paradoxical embolism. However, in many cases patent foramen ovale is an innocent finding and only appears to be relevant if associated with an atrial septal aneurysm.

Small vessel disease: localized occlusion of arterioles, secondary to microatheroma or degenerative disease of the walls (lipohyalinosis), is the common cause of lacunar stroke (see below under Lacunar stroke). Hypertension, diabetes mellitus and hypercholesterolaemia are the major risk factors. Lipohyalinosis is also one of the major causes of ICH.

Much rarer causes of infarction are haematological abnormalities (Table 23.3) and the non-atherosclerotic vasculopathies (Table 23.4). Some of the more important of these disorders are described in greater detail later in this chapter.

Haematological evidence for thrombophilia (inherited or acquired defects in thrombolytic proteins leading to thrombosis, Table 23.3) is commonly sought in younger patients but rarely proven as a cause of arterial stroke. **Cerebral venous thrombosis** is a far likelier mechanism of stroke associated with **thrombophilia**. The most common detectable abnormality in the population is the factor V Leiden mutation, the others are more rare. Arterial stroke can occur as part of the **antiphospholipid antibody** syndrome, in which thrombosis is associated with a history of recurrent miscarriage, thrombocytopenia and sometimes serological evidence of a connective tissue disorder. **Antiphospholipid antibodies** may also be found in association with other vasculopathies,

Table 23.3 Haematological causes of ischaemic stroke and transient ischaemic attack

	Haematological cause
Commoner	Sickle-cell disease
	Polycythaemia
	Thrombocythaemia
Rare	Antiphospholipid antibody syndrome
	Thrombotic thrombocytopenic purpura
	Paroxysmal nocturnal haemoglobinuria
	Leukaemia
Common in cerebral venous thrombosis, but of uncertain relevance in arterial stroke (except in paradoxical embolism)	Inherited thrombophilia
	Factor V Leiden polymorphism
	Protein C deficiency
	Protein S deficiency
	Antithrombin III deficiency
	Prothrombin gene mutation

including atherosclerosis, but in most cases they do not have a pathogenic role. Other important haematological causes of stroke include sickle-cell disease, polycythaemia and thrombocythaemia.

Outcome and prognosis

The average mortality within the first 7 and 30 days after stroke is approximately 12 and 19 per cent, respectively. Within the first few days, death is usually the direct result of cerebral oedema from infarction or mass effect from haemorrhage causing brainstem compression with coma and respiratory depression. Subsequently, stroke deaths are mainly caused by fatal complications of impaired swallowing and immobilization, including pneumonia and pulmonary embolism. Beyond 30 days, recurrence of stroke and myocardial infarction account for a similar proportion of late deaths.

Recovery from stroke is very variable. Some patients make a rapid and full recovery within a few days or weeks. In patients with more severe stroke, there is usually gradual spontaneous improvement.

Table 23.4 Rarer non-atherosclerotic vasculopathies

Arterial dissection	
Traumatic	
Secondary to idiopathic connective tissue disease	
Drug abuse	
CADASIL	
Mitochondrial cytopathies, e.g. MELAS	
Vasculitis	Systemic lupus erythematosus
	Polyarteritis nodosa
	Temporal arteritis
Sneddon's syndrome	
Sussac's syndrome	
Cervical or cranial irradiation	
Moyamoya syndrome	
Infections	
Acute and chronic meningitis	
Syphilis	
Herpes zoster	
HIV	

CADASIL, cerebral autosomal dominant arteriopathy with subcortical infarcts and leukoencephalopathy; HIV, human immunodeficiency virus; MELAS, myopathy, encephalopathy, lactic acidosis and stroke-like episodes.

This occurs most rapidly in the first 4–6 weeks, but may continue slowly for as long as rehabilitative input and engagement continue. Unfortunately, **approximately 50 per cent of survivors remain dependent at one year**. Mortality figures vary from location to location. Case mix is an important determinant of outcome. Large middle cerebral artery infarcts have a 30 per cent mortality at one month, while the mortality after lacunar infarction is about 5 per cent. Even after adjustment for case mix, type of bed and use of CT scan, three-month mortality has recently been shown to vary from as high as 42 per cent at some units to as low as 19 per cent at other units, depending in part on the intensity of care provided. Hence, even the crude indicator of death rate is enough to highlight major discrepancies between services.

Currently, clinical criteria do not predict indi-

Box 23.2 Poor prognostic factors for stroke recovery

- Increasing age
- Coma at onset
- Urinary incontinence at 1 week
- Large lesion on neuroimaging
- Severe motor impairment
- Cardiac failure
- Atrial fibrillation
- Persistent neglect

vidual outcome early after stroke with sufficient accuracy to be useful. However, many factors have been identified that may be associated with a high risk of death and poor functional outcome (Box 23.2). Prognostic scales have been developed, but they explain at best only about 10 per cent of the variance in disability at six months. Because clinical variables have poor predictive values in individual patients, much work has gone into developing reliable non-invasive surrogate markers of clinical outcome. These have been mostly based on imaging and biochemical markers but, like clinical factors, poorly explain the differences in outcome; for example, although visible infarction on CT does increase the relative risk of death or dependency at six months, after correction for other important prognostic variables, it only modestly predicts variation in impairment and disability. Hence, decisions about active management should not be based on any of these factors.

Individual patients may recover very well with appropriate rehabilitation despite poor prognostic factors and it is important that poor prognostic factors at onset are not allowed to become a self-fulfilling prophecy.

Box 23.3 Differential diagnosis of transient ischaemic attack

- Migraine
- Transient global amnesia
- Epilepsy
- Mass lesions
- Multiple sclerosis
- Hypoglycaemia
- Benign positional vertigo

Clinical syndromes of cerebral ischaemia

Transient ischaemic attacks

Transient ischaemic attack has for some time been arbitrarily distinguished from completed stroke (see above under Differential diagnosis of stroke), but the underlying mechanisms may be identical (e.g. severe carotid stenosis) and the main difference between TIA and stroke is only one of duration. Careful history, examination and MRI often reveal that an apparent TIA has actually resulted in a permanent deficit and would be better described as a small stroke. It is nevertheless useful to distinguish between transient and persistent symptoms and signs, because the differential diagnosis of transient events includes other causes of transient focal neurological symptoms (Box 23.3).

Symptoms of TIA

The symptoms of transient ischaemia are usually negative (loss of function), maximal at onset and last from 5 to 30 minutes.

Any cause of ischaemic stroke can also cause a TIA. Very rarely, a small cerebral haemorrhage may cause TIA-like symptoms. In general, TIAs are more likely to be embolic than local occlusion and high frequency attacks, for example, several per month (crescendo TIAs) are more likely to be caused by severe large artery stenosis.

Within the carotid circulation (Table 23.5), an embolus to the retinal circulation may lead to **transient monocular blindness (amaurosis fugax)**. This is usually described by the patient as like a curtain or shutter coming down over one eye and lasting only a few minutes. Occasionally, cholesterol emboli may be seen in a retinal vessel on fundoscopy during or after an attack. **Hemisphere ischaemia** is suggested by the sudden onset of **contralateral weakness or dysphasia** (if the dominant hemisphere is affected). The symptoms of hemisphere ischaemia usually last up to 30 minutes. Sensory loss in isolation is less common.

Transient ischaemic attacks within the **vertebrobasilar** circulation may cause **diplopia, facial or tongue numbness, dysarthria, vertigo and hemiparesis or quadriparesis** from brainstem involvement. If the top of the basilar artery is

Table 23.5 Common symptoms of transient cerebral ischaemia

Carotid territory	Monocular visual loss
	Unilateral hemiparesis
	Dysphasia
Vertebrobasilar[a]	Diplopia
	Dysarthria
	Vertigo/disequilibrium
	Bilateral visual loss
	Bilateral weakness or hemianopia
	Ataxia
	Sensory loss

[a]Various combinations of the listed symptoms.

occluded, there may also be **hemianopia or bilateral visual loss** from ischaemia in the posterior cerebral arteries. It is very unusual for transient isolated vertigo, loss of consciousness, or other brainstem symptoms to be caused by vertebrobasilar ischaemia. **Isolated transient vertigo** is usually the result of a **peripheral vestibulopathy**, for example, benign positional vertigo.

It has also become clearer that apparent transient 'ischaemic' attacks are occasionally caused by microhaemorrhages, which are not seen on conventional MRI or CT, but are visible using susceptibility-weighted MRI imaging (T2* imaging). These patients usually have poorly controlled hypertension (Figure 23.2).

Up to one-quarter of people attending specialist vascular clinics with suspected TIA turn out to have an alternative diagnosis (Box 23.3). The most common mimic of TIA is **migraine with focal neurological symptoms**. Focal migrainous symptoms may occur as an aura preceding headache (not usually confused with TIAs) or as an isolated aura without headache (commonly confused) or occasionally after or during a headache, which is extremely rare. It should be noted that stroke and transient ischaemia of any cause are often associated with headache, while some diseases may cause both migrainous symptoms and infarction (e.g. cervical artery dissection, antiphospholipid antibody syndrome, giant cell arteritis). Transient ischaemic attack or stroke should not be attributed to migraine simply because the symptoms are associated with a migraine-like headache.

The two main features in the history which point towards migraine rather than TIA are 'positive' symptoms and spread of symptoms over time. The typical **positive symptoms of migraine** consist of zigzag lines and scintillating scotomata, while migrainous sensory aura presents as tingling in one hand, often with perioral tingling. Patients may

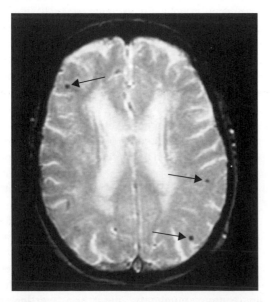
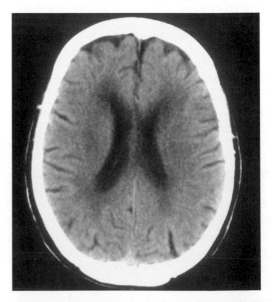

Figure 23.2 Microhaemorrhage. Gradient echo magnetic resonance image on the left shows several areas of microhaemorrhage (seen as black dots) not visible on CT in this patient with poorly controlled hypertension and recurrent transient ischaemic symptoms. This patient had been treated with increasing regimens of antiplatelet agents.

complain of weakness, but this is usually vague and not evident on examination. These **symptoms evolve slowly** – it may take several minutes for the visual disturbance to maximize, or for the tingling to spread from the hand to the face (the typical distribution). In contrast, the symptoms of TIA are sudden and maximal at onset and usually consist of 'negative' symptoms, such as loss of vision, numbness or weakness, and are distributed in a typical vascular distribution. Hemiplegic migraine is a rare familial channelopathy and quite distinct from other forms of 'migraine'. It should be diagnosed by experts only after full investigation.

Other conditions commonly confused with TIA are **transient global amnesia** and **epilepsy**. Transient **vertigo** is often wrongly attributed to transient vertebrobasilar ischaemia, rather than to a peripheral vestibular disturbance, for example benign positional vertigo, which is usually the cause. In addition, rarer serious intracranial conditions, such as subdural haematoma, tumours and multiple sclerosis, may cause transient symptoms. **Hypoglycaemia** may masquerade as all kinds of transient neurological disturbances, including hemiplegia, but is rare except in insulin-dependent diabetics.

Investigation of TIA is identical to completed stroke and is discussed later.

> Cranial CT or MRI should be performed after TIA to exclude mass lesions and rare vascular causes, for example, arteriovenous malformation.

Lacunar stroke

Lacunar infarction (Figure 23.3) is caused by occlusion of small penetrating vessels in the subcortical deep white matter, internal capsule, basal ganglia or pons.

Lacunar stroke may be preceded by TIAs in 20 per cent of cases, as in other causes of stroke. The two pathological appearances underlying small vessel occlusion are lipohyalinosis and microatheroma, but the distinction between these two pathologies cannot be made clinically. Although lacunar infarction can be associated with carotid stenosis, it does not commonly happen as a result of cardioembolism. Most patients with lacunar stroke have hypertension, diabetes and/or hypercholesterolaemia. Scans with CT and MRI and autopsy studies

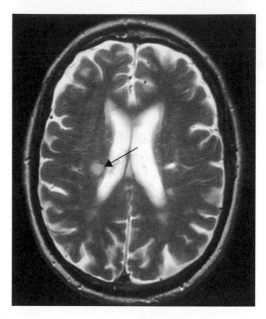

Figure 23.3 Lacunar infarction. T2-weighted magnetic resonance image showing small, deep white matter lacunar infarct.

show that occlusion of small penetrating vessels with lacunar infarction is commonly asymptomatic.

The clinical syndromes of lacunar stroke are usually easily recognized. One of the principal features is that **patients do not have cortical signs, and in particular do not have cognitive difficulties**. The latter indicate occlusion of larger branches of the cerebral arteries. Common examples of cortical signs are confusion, dysphasia, neglect, apraxia, hemianopia and conjugate eye deviation. Absence of these cortical signs with **unilateral weakness or sensory loss involving at least two of the face, hand or leg** is very suggestive of lacunar infarction, although occasionally small cortical infarcts mimic these features. It can be difficult to distinguish between lacunar infarction in the deep hemisphere structures and a lacune in the pons in the brainstem, which cause identical syndromes. There are many lacunar syndromes but the most common are listed in Box 23.4.

Computed tomography may not detect smaller lacunar infarcts, especially in the brainstem. **MRI is much more sensitive**. Often patients with lacunar infarction have widespread changes of small vessel white matter ischaemia and it can be difficult to identify the symptomatic lesion, unless diffusion-weighted imaging is available.

The mainstay of secondary prevention after

Box 23.4 Syndromes of lacunar infarction

- Pure motor hemiparesis
- Sensorimotor hemiparesis
- Pure sensory stroke
- Ataxic hemiparesis
- Dysarthria – clumsy hand syndrome
- Hemiballismus

lacunar infarction is control of hypertension and diabetes, treatment with antiplatelet agents, and statins if appropriate.

Patients should undergo evaluation for **stenosis** of the extracranial internal carotid artery. Large clinical trials have shown that patients with recent lacunar stroke and severe ipsilateral carotid stenosis benefit from endarterctomy in terms of prevention of recurrent stroke, although the benefit is less than those with large vessel stroke.

Multiple lacunar infarcts can cause subfrontal or global signs if sufficient damage from repeated penetrating vessel occlusion takes place (Figure 23.4). These include **gait apraxia** with gait ignition failure or small-stepped gait **(marche à petit pas)**, **postural instability** with a predisposition to falling backwards, and **vascular dementia** (see below under Vascular dementia).

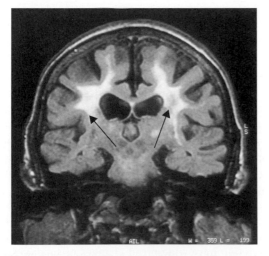

Figure 23.4 Diffuse small vessel disease. Coronal flair magnetic resonance image showing marked periventricular high signal 'caps' extending into the deep white matter and beyond in this patient with diffuse small vessel disease secondary to poorly controlled hypertension.

Rarer causes of lacunar syndromes

Antiphospholipid antibody syndrome may present with lacunar infarction and often these patients also have a history of migrainous phenomena and headaches. Such patients will need to be distinguished from small vessel vasculitides affecting the brain. **Cerebral autosomal dominant arteriopathy with subcortical infarcts and leukoencephalopathy (CADASIL)** is a rare hereditary disorder, caused by mutations in the gene coding for the notch 3 protein. Patients with CADASIL present with recurrent lacunar strokes and usually develop vascular dementia. There is often a history of migraine-like headaches. The diagnosis is suggested by a family history and florid leukoaraiosis on imaging. No effective treatment is known.

Large vessel occlusion

The pattern of infarction after **large vessel occlusion** depends on the size of the vessel occluded and the adequacy of collateral supply. Occlusion of an intracranial large vessel, such as the middle cerebral artery or its cortical branches, is more likely to be caused by thromboembolism from the heart, aortic atherosclerosis or internal carotid artery stenosis, than by local occlusive disease, in contrast to lacunar infarction. Stenosis and occlusion are distinct. Occlusion of a vessel may occur without pre-existing atheromatous stenosis, either because of embolism to the artery, or because of local injury to the vessel wall, for example, dissection after minor trauma. Hypercoagulability of the blood rarely causes local arterial thrombosis without additional vascular pathology, but is an important cause of venous thrombosis. Alternatively, occlusion may occur at the site of an atheromatous plaque or stenosis. The degree to which the brain suffers from ischaemia will depend on the duration, site of occlusion and collateral circulation.

Middle cerebral artery territory stroke

Total occlusion

The clinical features of **occlusion of the main trunk of the middle cerebral artery** with infarction of the whole territory of the artery (Figure 23.5) include **conjugate eye deviation** (frontal lobe damage), **aphasia** (in the dominant hemisphere), **hemiplegia, hemisensory loss and hemianopia** (from involvement of **the visual radiation** in temporal and parietal lobes). In middle cerebral artery occlusion (and

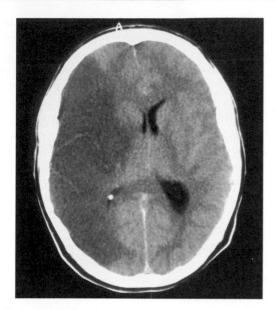

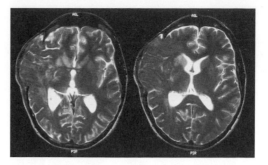

Figure 23.6 Malignant hemisphere swelling relieved by surgical decompression after complete middle cerebral artery territory infarction. Magnetic resonance imaging shows herniation of the swollen brain following decompressive craniotomy. After two months, the defect was closed. Outcome at six months was excellent (patient independently ambulant, no significant cognitive deficit), although the left arm remained plegic.

Figure 23.5 Complete middle cerebral artery territory infarction. CT at 48 hours shows infarction within the complete middle cerebral artery territory on the right with swelling of the hemisphere causing midline shift. The patient later began to develop signs of coning and decompressive surgery was carried out (see **Figure 23.6**).

most lacunar syndromes) the **hemiparesis affects the arm more than the leg,** while in anterior cerebral artery occlusion the leg is characteristically much weaker than the arm because the leg area of the motor cortex is in the anterior cerebral artery territory. **Neglect syndromes** in which the patient is unaware of, or ignores, the hemiplegic side occur acutely with both non-dominant and dominant hemisphere cortical damage, but generally are more severe and persistent with non-dominant parietal lobe damage.

The **middle cerebral artery most commonly occludes from embolism.** Occasionally, atheromatous stenosis at the origin of the middle cerebral artery leads to occlusion, particularly in Asian and African races. Rarely, patients with complete middle cerebral artery territory infarction develop severe **malignant oedema** within 48 hours, leading to brainstem compression and death by coning. In appropriate cases, surgical decompression with hemicraniectomy is required (Figure 23.6).

Branch occlusion
Branch occlusion will produce **partial syndromes** with only some of the signs of complete territory infarction described above. **Upper branch** occlusion

affecting frontal structures produces **hemiparesis, hemisensory loss, ocular deviation** and a **non-fluent expressive dysphasia** in which the patient understands speech because of an intact temporal lobe but cannot produce speech. **Lower branch** occlusions involving the temporal lobe result in **fluent receptive dysphasia,** in which the patient has difficulty understanding language, but motor production of speech is either preserved or produces a non-stop flow of nonsensical speech (jargon dysphasia).

Distal embolism
Small cortical branches are usually occluded by emboli and the patient may present only with **weakness or isolated cortical signs,** for example, dysphasia.

Deep infarction (striatocapsular infarction)
Deep infarction occurs when the trunk of the middle cerebral artery has occluded but the cortex is protected by pial collateral circulation. Deeper structures (the striatum and internal capsule) are supplied by the perforating branches, which do not have collateral supply and therefore infarct rapidly (Figure 23.7). Usually, this results from an embolus obstructing the **perforating lenticulostriate** arteries, which then breaks up spontaneously or as a result of therapeutic thrombolysis before the cortex has infarcted. The patients have **contralateral motor and sensory loss,** but also exhibit **cortical signs** (unlike pure lacunar infarction). These cortical signs resolve more quickly than when the cortex itself is infarcted.

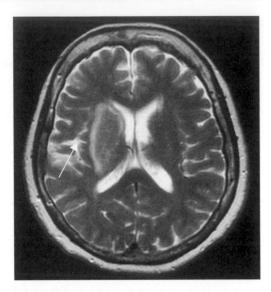

Figure 23.7 Striatocapsular infarction. This patient presented with acute right hemiplegia, neglect and dysphasia. The neglect and dysphasia resolved within a few days. The underlying aetiology was atrial fibrillation.

Anterior cerebral artery occlusion

The anterior cerebral artery is far less often affected than the middle cerebral artery, although the causes are similar. However, **anterior cerebral territory** infarction should raise the level of awareness for unusual aetiologies. It also occurs secondary to vasospasm after SAH. The clinical features of anterior cerebral artery occlusion are a **contralateral hemiplegia in which the leg is more affected than the arm**, because the cortical representation of the leg lies within its territory. Infarction of subfrontal cortex, especially if bilateral, may cause **frontal neuropsychological deficits**, particularly executive dysfunction, abulia, disinhibition and lack of insight, often without any other signs.

Carotid artery occlusion

The internal carotid artery often occludes without any clinical evidence of stroke, because of the collateral supply provided by the circle of Willis. Strokes occur after carotid occlusion only if the collateral supply is inadequate or if thrombosis spreads (or embolises) to involve the middle cerebral artery or its branches. Internal carotid artery occlusion can also involve its first branch, the ophthalmic artery, resulting in transient or persistent monocular retinal ischaemia and blindness. The picture in carotid

artery occlusion is therefore usually **identical to that of middle cerebral artery occlusion**. Infarction may be limited to a small portion of the territory or extend to involve the whole of the middle cerebral artery territory. If the carotid artery occludes from dissection, there may also be a **Horner's syndrome** on the side of the occlusion (i.e. contralateral to the limb signs). The anterior cerebral territory is often spared (via collateral flow) but may be affected in some cases. The bifurcation of the common carotid artery is the most common site of severe atheroma in the extracranial cerebral circulation and usually the internal carotid artery occludes at the origin from the common carotid. In dissection, the site of occlusion may be more distal. Rare obliterative arteriopathies, including **moyamoya disease**, may involve the terminal intracranial portion of the carotid artery and the origins of the middle cerebral artery.

Posterior cerebral artery occlusions

Occlusion of the posterior cerebral artery is commonly embolic and more patients with **posterior cerebral syndromes** are in atrial fibrillation, than with other large vessel occlusions (Figure 23.8). Emboli usually reach the posterior cerebral arteries via the vertebrobasilar system, but it should be borne in mind that in about 5 per cent of individuals, one posterior cerebral artery is supplied by a dominant posterior communicating branch of the internal carotid artery. Thus, posterior cerebral artery occlusion is occasionally caused by embolization from carotid stenosis. The posterior cerebral artery prin-

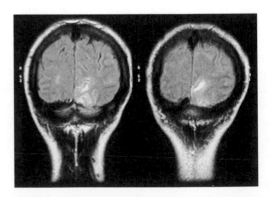

Figure 23.8 Posterior cerebral artery occlusion. Coronal magnetic resonance imaging shows acute infarction of the left occipital pole.

cipally supplies the occipital cortex, and occlusion usually causes an **isolated hemianopia**. This may spare the visual representation of the macular fibres when these may receive collateral supply from the middle cerebral artery. When infarction extends anteriorly to affect parieto-occipital areas, **neglect syndromes** may accompany the hemianopia. The posterior cerebral arteries also supply the **thalami** and the **medial posterior temporal lobes**. If these structures are involved, the patient may present with **confusion, or memory impairment** (thalamic or medial temporal amnesia). If both posterior cerebral artery territories are infarcted, as may happen when an embolus lodges at the **top of the basilar artery, cortical blindness and confusion** ensue. Sometimes, these patients may be left with tunnel vision and may recognize small but not large objects. Memory impairment following this may be severe, especially for the acquisition of new information.

Vertebral artery occlusion

The most common consequence of occlusion of the **distal vertebral artery** is infarction of the **dorsolateral medulla** within the territory of the **posterior inferior cerebellar artery (lateral medullary syndrome)**. This results in a **Horner's syndrome, temperature and pain sensory loss on one side of the face and the other side of the body, nystagmus, ataxia of the ipsilateral limbs and palatal and vocal cord paralysis**. Vertebral artery embolism or occlusion may also result in more extensive infarction of the brainstem and cerebellum and these syndromes are discussed next. The most common site for atheroma to affect the vertebral artery is at its origin from the aorta.

Basilar artery occlusion

Whereas middle and posterior cerebral artery occlusions are more often the result of embolism, the opposite is true of the basilar artery. This is because the basilar is more commonly affected by severe atherosclerosis on which in-situ thrombus may form. **Basilar artery occlusion** also commonly occurs as a result of propagation of thrombus from an occluded vertebral artery. Basilar thrombus (Figure 23.9) may obstruct blood flow into perforating vessels supplying the central brainstem structures or the two upper cerebellar arteries. A number of clinical pictures may be encountered. In

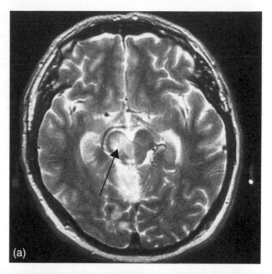

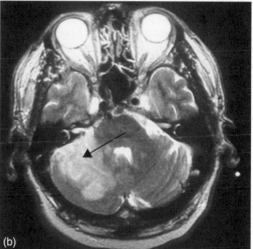

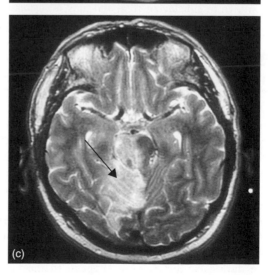

Figure 23.9 Brainstem, cerebellar and occipital infarction secondary to basilar thrombosis.

the medulla, lower cranial nerves may be affected, giving rise to a **lower motor neurone type bulbar palsy**. Upper motor neurone impairment of the same structure may cause a **pseudobulbar palsy**, with brisk facial reflexes, jaw jerk and a spastic tongue. This is often accompanied by spontaneous laughter or crying (**emotional lability**). Above the medulla, **pontine infarction** may cause a **sixth nerve palsy, gaze paresis, internuclear ophthalmoplegia and pinpoint pupils**. Emboli may lodge at the top of the basilar causing **midbrain infarction** with **loss of vertical eye movement, pupillary abnormalities and coma**. All these syndromes will be accompanied by **quadriplegia** to some degree, which may be very asymmetric. Partial brainstem or midbrain syndromes may also be caused by localized occlusion of one of the perforating arteries from small vessel disease. The posterior cerebral arteries arise from the top of the basilar artery. Thus any of these basilar artery syndromes may be accompanied by contralateral or bilateral occipital infarction with hemianopia or cortical blindness.

Subclavian artery occlusion

Subclavian artery occlusion is a rare cause of haemodynamic TIA and an even rarer cause of stroke. If the subclavian artery is occluded or severely stenosed before the origin of the vertebral artery, the arm may be supplied by blood flowing in a retrograde direction down the vertebral artery at the expense of the vertebrobasilar circulation. This is known as **subclavian steal** and may occasionally result in brainstem TIAs during exercise of the arm.

Border zone ischaemia and hypoxic ischaemic encephalopathy

The brain is particularly vulnerable to a global fall in perfusion pressure. Most often this is caused by cardiac disease (arrthymia or pump failure), especially when combined with hypoxia, although hypovolaemia alone may be sufficient to cause cerebral ischaemia. The usual circumstances in which perfusion failure leads to bilateral haemodynamic brain damage are **following cardiac arrest, severe blood loss or cardiopulmonary bypass**. Embolism is an alternative or additional cause of focal damage during cardiopulmonary bypass. In the non-anaesthetized, non-comatose patient, moderate or transient global perfusion failure results in acute

reversible non-focal brain dysfunction (confusion, attention deficits, light headedess). Following a profound insult, a number of syndromes are recognized, resulting from **border zone** or **'watershed' infarction** in the areas of the brain at the distal ends of the arterial supply (Figure 23.10). Pathological studies suggest that many such cases result from a combination of diffuse embolism and haemodynamic failure of perfusion in the border zones. The parieto-occipital cortex, which lies at the border zone between the middle cerebral artery and posterior cerebral artery territories, is particularly vulnerable. Infarction of this region results in abnormalities of behaviour, memory and vision. The visual abnormalities are complex and include inability to see all the objects in a field of vision, incoordination of hand and eye movement, such that the patient cannot locate objects in the visual field, and apraxia of gaze in which the patient is unable to gaze where desired. Other areas of vulnerability are the superficial cortical and deep subcortical border zones between the anterior and middle cerebral artery, and the hippocampi, where infarction may result in an amnesic syndrome. In severe cases, necrosis occurs in the basal ganglia, cerebellum and brainstem. Unilateral border zone infarction, often in a patchy fashion involving the subcortical white matter in the centrum semi ovale,

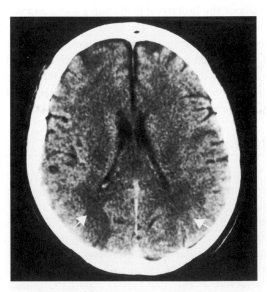

Figure 23.10 Watershed infarction following cardiac surgery. CT scan of the brain shows bilateral 'watershed' infarction more obvious on the right. This has occurred in the border zone between the middle and anterior cerebral artery territories.

may also occur in patients with ipsilateral carotid artery occlusion or severe stenosis.

Vascular dementia

Vascular dementia is an umbrella term used to describe the development of cognitive deficits in multiple domains secondary to cerebrovascular disease. This is most commonly caused by multiple cortical or subcortical lacunar infarcts (Figure 23.11). Vascular dementia can also occur after multiple intracranial haemorrhages, for example, in cerebral amyloid angiopathy, after SAH, and as a result of cerebral venous thrombosis. Typically, patients have **a stepwise deterioration** associated with other features of stroke. In **diffuse subcortical small vessel disease, (Binswanger's disease or subcortical arteriosclerotic encephalopathy) dementia** may be accompanied by **gait apraxia**, which results in failure to initiate gait, postural instability (often falling over backwards) and a **shuffling small-stepped, wide-based gait (marche à petit pas)**. This is often associated with diffuse periventricular demyelination secondary to ischaemia in the deep white matter, which causes patchy or diffuse changes, known as 'leukoaraiosis', and ventricular enlargement on CT and MRI. Urinary incontinence may occur. Characteristically, the **dementia** of small vessel disease has **subcortical features** including poor attention, slowing of mental function (bradyphrenia) and impaired executive function in excess of discrete cortical patterns of dysfunction. Occasionally, these patients present with periods of encephalopathy associated with new infarction. Multiple cortical infarcts (from large vessel occlusions) are much rarer as causes of dementia. It is important to note that older patients with cerebrovascular disease are at increased risk of Alzheimer's disease, and **mixed dementia** caused by a combination of the two disorders is common.

Asymptomatic leukoaraiosis without dementia may also be found on imaging, especially in patients over 50 years of age with appropriate risk factors. There is also an increased incidence of depression in these patients.

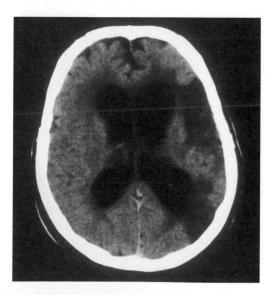

Figure 23.11 CT in vascular dementia. Atrophy, multiple lacunar infarcts and large vessel disease in a patient with vascular dementia.

INTRACEREBRAL HAEMORRHAGE

Approximately 10 per cent of stroke is caused by ICH often associated with hypertension. ICH affects a wide age range.

Intracerebral haemorrhage often has a sudden, devastating presentation. Patients who present in coma with vomiting and/or neck stiffness are more likely to have ICH than ischaemic stroke, but it is wrong to assume that patients with less severe stroke will have ischaemia. The symptoms of small cerebral haemorrhages are indistinguishable from cerebral infarction and the distinction can only be made in life by brain imaging.

This is particularly illustrated by the recognition of microhaemorrhage on T2* imaging, which reveals minute bleeds as the underlying cause of clinical syndromes previously thought clinically to have been caused by transient ischaemia or lacunar infarction (Figure 23.2).

The great majority of cases of ICH occur secondary to small vessel degenerative or hypertensive disease with rupture of small penetrating vessels in the basal ganglia, pons or cerebellum. Cerebral amyloid angiopathy is another important cause, which results in recurrent superficial lobar haematomas, usually in older patients. A ruptured cerebral aneurysm can be the reason for ICH if the bleeding occurs into the substance of the brain, rather than, or together with, SAH. Other rarer aetiologies include arteriovenous malformation and mycotic aneurysm. Non-medicinal use of cocaine and amphetamines may cause ICH, but there is often an underlying vascular malformation in these cases (Box 23.5).

One of the most important and potentially treatable causes of ICH is anticoagulation therapy, especially when poorly controlled and combined with other risk factors.

Intracerebral haemorrhage

The rupture of a vessel results in the sudden development of a haematoma. The haematoma characteristically slowly enlarges over the first few hours, and sometimes over a few days, leading to progressive focal clinical deficit and then deterioration of conscious level secondary to mass effect. Neurosurgical evacuation of haematomas or shunting of associated hydrocephalus may be lifesaving.

Any patient on an anticoagulant with new focal neurology must be assumed to have bled until proven otherwise with urgent cranial imaging. In those who have bled, anticoagulation should be immediately reversed.

Clinical syndromes

Haemorrhage may be divided into a number of categories depending on location. These are **deep (centred on basal ganglia structures), lobar, pontine and cerebellar**. In all sites, hyperten-

Box 23.5 Causes of intracerebral haemorrhage

- Hypertensive small vessel disease
- Anticoagulants
- Amyloid angiopathy
- Arteriovenous malformation
- Aneurysm
- Amphetamine/cocaine ingestion
- Infective endocarditis
- Tumours
- Disseminated intravascular coagulation
- Venous thrombosis
- Cerebral vasculitis

sion remains the most important risk factor and, although amyloid angiopathy gives rise to lobar but not deep haemorrhage, hypertension is still the most important risk factor associated with lobar haemorrhage. Hypertension may make an underlying structural cause, such as aneurysm, more likely to rupture.

Deep haemorrhage

Subcortical haematomas may be centred on the putamen, caudate or thalamus. In **putaminal** haemorrhage, the picture is of **contralateral hemiparesis and conjugate deviation of the eyes towards the side of the haematoma**. Cortical function may be impaired. If the mass becomes critical, signs of coning ensue. These haematomas may rupture into the ventricles leading to SAH. In the case of putaminal haemorrhage, the presence of ventricular blood implies a very large haematoma with a poor prognosis (Figure 23.12).

Caudate haemorrhage is much rarer and small haematomas may readily rupture into the ventricles. When the lesion is large, the picture is similar to putaminal haemorrhage, but if small, haematomas may present like SAH with acute headache and meningism, but little in the way of focal signs. **Thalamic** haemorrhage predominantly produces **sensory change in the contralateral limbs**. If local midbrain compression occurs, the eyes may be

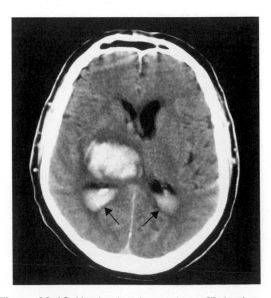

Figure 23.12 Massive deep haemorrhage. CT showing acute haemorrhage centred on the right thalamus with mass effect and intraventricular extension of blood (arrowed).

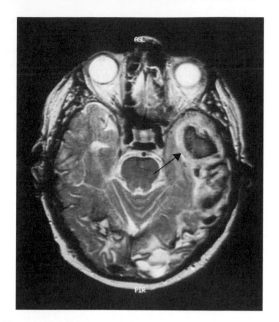

Figure 23.13 Temporal lobe haematoma secondary to poorly controlled anticoagulation. Magnetic resonance image shows cavitating haemorrhage in the left temporal lobe (arrowed). Previous left occipital infarction is also seen, which was secondary to posterior cerebral artery occlusion from atrial fibrillation.

forced into downwards gaze with small, poorly reactive pupils. Thalamic haemorrhage in the dominant hemisphere may produce dysphasia with notable naming difficulties.

Lobar haemorrhage produces signs appropriate to the location. In the frontal lobe, eye deviation and contralateral hemiparesis is common. In the central region, hemisensory loss is found associated with dysphasia in the dominant hemisphere. Parietal lobe haemorrhage causes hemisensory loss and neglect or inattention syndromes. Bleeding into the dominant temporal lobe results in a fluent dysphasia with poor comprehension, secondary to damage of Wernicke's area (Figure 23.13).

In **pontine haemorrhage**, the classic presentation is **coma associated with pinpoint pupils, loss of horizontal eye movements and quadriparesis**. Hyperpyrexia and irregular respiratory patterns ensue. Although large haemorrhage here is often fatal, the outcome may be surprisingly good.

Posterior fossa cerebellar haemorrhage accounts for 10 per cent of all primary intracerebral haematomas. It is important to recognize because it may result in secondary fatal brainstem compression and hydrocephalus (Figure 23.14). **Neurosurgical treatment can be lifesaving** and subsequently patients with cerebellar haemorrhage often make an excellent recovery. The usual presentation is with **acute headache, vomiting and unilateral ataxia**. Unilateral gaze paresis in association with ataxia or in isolation may also occur. When brainstem compression is present, the clinical features are similar to those of pontine haemorrhage.

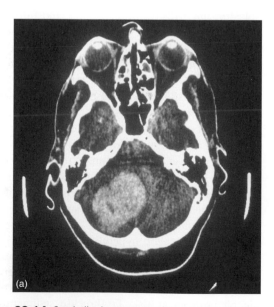

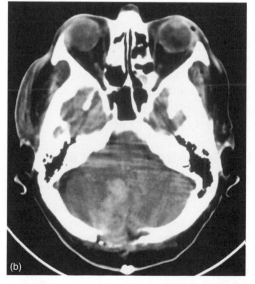

Figure 23.14 Cerebellar haematoma with secondary brainstem compression before and after surgical evacuation. Evacuation was performed in this patient because of a low conscious level associated with marked mass effect on the brainstem by the haematoma.

This clinical picture may be present from onset or the symptoms may slowly progress over the course of hours or a few days.

Intraventricular haemorrhage mimics SAH (see below under Investigation of stroke and transient ischaemic attack) with headache, vomiting, neck stiffness and depression of consciousness. There may be associated pyramidal signs. It may be caused by a subependymal region angioma or by extension of blood following deep haemorrhage. This is particularly the case with caudate haemorrhage, as this nucleus lies adjacent to the ventricular margin.

INVESTIGATION OF STROKE AND TRANSIENT ISCHAEMIC ATTACK

Investigation is aimed at:

- identifying underlying pathology (haemorrhage or infarct)
- detecting risk factors
- establishing cause and mechanism (e.g. embolism from atheromatous carotid artery stenosis)
- confirming or refuting the clinical diagnosis.

Investigation nearly always improves the clinician's understanding of the pathophysiology of the stroke or transient ischaemic syndrome. This then guides acute treatment and secondary preventive measures. 'Completed' stroke should not be separated from transient ischaemic syndromes when considering appropriate investigation, as the aetiological spectrum is identical, although management may be very different. Both are emergencies and should be investigated urgently to plan appropriate management and prevent further events.

Routine investigations for all patients

In all patients, routine **blood screening** should include full blood count to look for polycythaemia, thrombocythaemia or thrombocytopenia (Table 23.6). Anaemia of chronic disease may be a marker for endocarditis or underlying cancer. Occasional haematological malignancies may be complicated by stroke. **Basic coagulation analysis** (international normalized ratio (INR), activated partial thrombo-

Table 23.6 Investigation of stroke and transient ischaemic attack

All infarction and haemorrhage	Brain CT or MRI
	Full blood count
	Platelet count
	ESR
	Urea and electrolytes
	Blood sugar
	Cholesterol
	Chest x-ray
	ECG
All haemorrhage	Clotting screen
Selected patients	Neck ultrasound or MRA
	Autoantibody screen
	Thrombophilia screen
	Syphilis serology
	Drug screen
	Sickle-cell test
	Homocysteine
	Screening for genetic causes of stroke
	Echocardiography
	24-hour ECG
	Cerebral angiography

CT, computed tomography; ECG, electrocardiogram; ESR, erythrocyte sedimentation rate; MRA, magnetic resonance angiography; MRI, magnetic resonance imaging.

plastin time (APTT), thrombin time and fibrinogen) should be undertaken in all patients with haemorrhagic stroke and is especially important in those receiving anticoagulants. Urea and electrolytes guide homeostatic management in the acute phase and may also reveal end-organ damage from hypertension or vasculitis. Patients suffering from significant electrolyte disturbance may present with global or focal dysfunction mimicking stroke. Plasma glucose is an essential 'triage' investigation, as hypoglycaemia must be excluded in anyone with focal signs. **Hyperglycaemia** may suggest unidentified diabetes and is also found in non-diabetics with severe stroke. Rarely, hyperosmolar non-ketotic diabetic hyperglycaemia presents as a stroke syndrome. Lipid analysis for cholesterol and fasting triglycerides should be performed. There are also arguments for performing syphilis serology in all patients at risk. **Erythrocyte sedimentation rate (ESR) or C-reactive protein** is used as a non-specific screening test, principally for inflammatory arterial disease and endocarditis. Thyroid function tests should be performed in all patients with atrial fibrillation. In all patients, **chest x-ray and electrocardiography (ECG)** should also be carried out. If they are both normal, this may negate the need for echocardiography. The principal point of chest radiology is to establish the presence of a normal cardiac silhouette. The principal ECG changes of importance are left ventricular hypertrophy secondary to hypertension, previous or acute myocardial infarction (which may suggest cardiogenic embolus) and, most importantly, atrial fibrillation.

Neuroimaging is an essential investigation. Scanning with **CT or MRI should be performed in all patients immediately** to distinguish infarction from haemorrhage and to reveal mimics of the stroke syndrome, such as tumour or subdural haematoma. In the early stages, CT may be negative, depending on time to imaging, the size and severity of infarction and the skill of the interpreter. **Only 50–70 per cent of infarcts are ever visible with CT**. It has become generally accepted that CT can 'exclude' intracranial haemorrhage in the acute phase. However, CT is not always positive in SAH and there are patients with microhaemorrhages presenting with minimal impairments, in whom CT and conventional MRI will be normal. CT is a key emergency tool to assess suitability for thrombolysis.

CT or MRI brain scan

MRI is a far more sensitive investigation for both stroke and non-stroke pathology, although it is not currently available for all patients, especially in the acute phase. It is especially superior in the posterior fossa and at revealing small areas of infarction secondary to penetrating vessel occlusion. Sophisticated MRI can also be used to distinguish acute from chronic infarction using diffusion-weighted sequences (Figure 23.15a), while gradient echo sequences (T2*) may demonstrate microhaemorrhage. It is possible that in the future the combination of magnetic resonance perfusion imaging and diffusion-weighted imaging will be used more widely to select patients for treatments such as thrombolysis or neuroprotective drugs. MRI has high sensitivity for cerebral venous thrombosis and can be used in conjunction with magnetic resonance angiography (MRA) to detect dissection of the carotid or vertebral arteries. Spiral CT can also be used to perform computed tomographic angiography (CTA) or measure cerebral perfusion.

The information derived from imaging should be used to establish the pathophysiology and mechanism of stroke and guide management. **Most importantly, the imaging abnormalities must be concordant with the clinical picture**. The presence of acute or old infarcts in more than one vascular

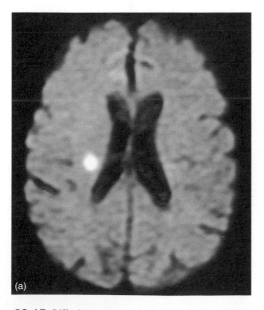
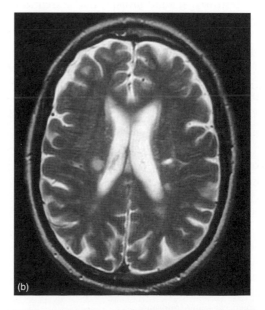

Figure 23.15 Diffusion-weighted imaging (a) shows 'light bulb' sign associated with acute infarction. On conventional T2 imaging (b), it is not as clear which area of infarction is acute.

territory should focus further investigation towards a central embolic source. Extensive asymptomatic small vessel disease, especially numerous micro-haemorrhages on gradient echo imaging, is a risk factor for haemorrhage and may refine the decision not to give anticoagulation therapy to a patient in atrial fibrillation. Similarly, lacunar infarction in a patient with carotid stenosis may tip one away from pursuing surgery in a patient with borderline severity of stenosis. Imaging also plays a critical role in identifying and managing patients with stroke who may benefit from neurosurgical intervention.

Brain imaging in acute stroke is urgent, and for thrombolysis candidates the timing should be concordant with a maximum door to needle time of around 30 minutes. The UK National Stroke Strategy calls for a maximum wait for all patients at any time of 1 hour. For high risk TIAs, investigation should be completed within 24 hours of symptoms. These guidelines are considerable improvements on the previous lackadasical approach to stroke, but it is still important to perform imaging as an emergency in specific circumstances (Box 23.6).

The initial investigations should build up a preliminary pathophysiological assessment to guide further investigation. Ischaemic stroke within the **carotid territory** should prompt the search for **carotid stenosis**. This is essential in patients in whom secondary preventive surgery would be considered. The emphasis is on non-invasive imaging,

which should always be performed as an initial screen in preference to invasive techniques such as catheter angiography. CTA, **MRA** and **colour Doppler ultrasound** are all useful. If one of these is completely normal in reliable hands, then the screen is adequate. If one suggests carotid stenosis greater than 50 per cent, or occlusion, then it is very useful to have **a repeat non-invasive test, preferably a different modality**, because if they are concordant, it is acceptable to assume that the information is accurate (Figure 23.16). In patients in whom the results of noninvasive imaging differ concerning the presence or absence of severe stenosis, it may be necessary to perform contrast-enhanced MRA or formal catheter angiography if surgery or stenting is contemplated. It should be appreciated that **catheter angiography** carries a small but significant risk of causing stroke or even death, especially in those with severe atherosclerosis, and should therefore only be carried out in specialized units.

It is necessary to exclude an arteriovenous malformation or aneurysm in patients with SAH or ICH, if the patient would be fit for neurosurgical or radiological intervention. In some with ICH, exclusion of an underlying structural cause can be

Box 23.6 Recommendations of the Royal College of Physicians for urgent imaging in stroke

Brain imaging should be undertaken as a matter of urgency if the patient has:
- Depressed level of consciousness
- Unexplained progressive or fluctuating symptoms
- Papilloedema, neck stiffness or fever
- Severe headache at onset
- History of trauma prior to onset
- Indications for thrombolysis or early anticoagulation
- History of anticoagulant treatment, or has a known bleeding tendency

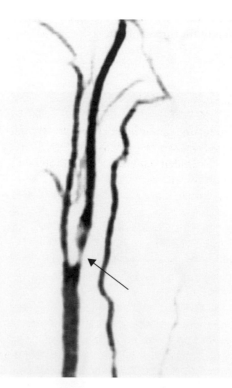

Figure 23.16 Magnetic resonance angiography showing severe stenosis at the origin of the internal carotid.

adequately achieved with MRI delayed until after resolution of the haematoma. However, many such patients will require catheter angiography and further investigation should be discussed with an expert neurovascular team.

> The yield of angiography is greatest in patients under the age of approximately 50 years. Younger patients with cerebral haemorrhage should always be considered for angiography.

In patients with suspected cardiogenic embolism, **transthoracic echocardiography** may define wall motion abnormalities or the presence of atrial or ventricular thrombus. Transthoracic echocardiography with injection of agitated saline and valsalva is now, in most hands, the optimal screening test for a patent foramen ovale. In selected patients, particularly younger patients with unexplained stroke, transoesophageal echocardiography should be performed because it provides better visualization than the transthoracic mode of aortic root disease and right to left shunts (e.g. patent foramen ovale). If cardiogenic embolus is still strongly suspected despite normal chest x-ray and ECG, then sometimes Holter monitoring may reveal paroxysmal atrial fibrillation. Holter monitoring may need to be prolonged in some cases (up to a week) to detect paroxysmal atrial fibrillation.

Special investigations

Prothrombotic abnormalities of the thrombolytic pathway, known as **thrombophilia**, such as the Factor V Leiden mutation, and Protein C, S or Antithrombin III deficiency, are rarely relevant in arterial stroke but should be sought in **cerebral venous thrombosis** and in the rare circumstance of stroke from venous paradoxical embolism to the brain through a patent foramen ovale or septal defect. **Antiphospholipid antibodies** can be associated with stroke, but the finding is often a coincidence, except in patients with other features of the antiphospholipid antibody syndrome. Autoantibodies may mark **a systemic vasculitis** or connective tissue disorder, for example, systemic lupus erythematosus. In appropriate circumstances, it is possible to screen for the common mitochondrial and NOTCH 3 mutations. MRA or CTA is useful intracranially in appropriate circumstances to screen for proximal middle cerebral artery stenosis. This is seen more often in patients with sickle-cell disease and in people of African or Asian descent. Catheter angiography may be required to delineate intracranial vascular anatomy in patients with intracranial stenosis or occlusion and to detect the enlarged lenticular basal collateral vessels characteristic of moyamoya disease. Occasionally, if an infectious aetiology or vasculitis is suspected, it may be necessary to examine the cerebrospinal fluid (CSF) by lumbar puncture and to consider a brain biopsy.

ACUTE TREATMENT OF STROKE

Treatment for stroke requires an individual approach for each patient, targeted at the individual cause and mechanism of stroke and the patient's functional impairment. Stroke is not a single entity, but there are some interventions that should be applied to the majority of patients. Treatment of some specific individual causes, including SAH, is discussed below.

Treatment of acute ischaemic stroke

Thrombolysis

Intravenous recombinant tissue plasminogen activator (rt–PA) has been licensed since 1996 for use in acute ischaemic stroke in the United States. It is likely that the scale of the benefits observed within the pivotal National Institute of Neurological Disorders and Stroke (NINDS) trial, which included a 12 per cent increase in the numbers of patients making a full recovery, only occurred because of adherence to a strict and well-defined protocol. Nevertheless, the overall benefit of thrombolysis in the NINDS trial was accompanied by an increased risk of cerebral haemorrhage of 6 per cent, compared with 1 per cent in placebo-treated patients, although not an excess mortality. The principal features of the NINDS protocol were a short time window (maximum 3 hours from onset; half were treated within 90 minutes of onset), rigorous treatment or exclusion of patients with uncontrolled hypertension, and exclusion of haemorrhage or severe stroke syndromes (who unfortunately may be made worse). It is clear from the other trials of thrombolysis that streptokinase is hazardous and that violating the protocol can have the disastrous consequences of an excess rate of intracranial haemorrhage, which negates any benefit. Increasing evidence demonstrating the benefit of thrombolysis since that pivotal trial has continued to accumulate. In particular, the pooled analysis of the major trials show an almost linear decline in the chances of making a good recovery as the stroke to needle time extends. However, the recent ECASS 3 study has shown a small benefit in selected patients treated up to 4.5 hours after onset and this time window has been adopted by most centres.

> The indication for thrombolysis is simple: ischaemic stroke when treatment can be started within 4.5 hours of onset. Knowing the onset time is therefore crucial and in those who awake with stroke this is usually unknown. The contraindications are listed in Table 23.7, but the area that requires more skill and experience are the areas in which benefit is uncertain (Table 23.7). Our current practice is to randomize these patients into the IST 3 trial whose aim is to clarify the risks and benefits of treatment in these areas.

Delivering effective thrombolysis requires a sensitive and well-oiled mechanism to ascertain, investigate and treat patients rapidly. Delays can add up across the system quickly and 'time is brain'. The aim is to deliver treatment as soon as possible and not when convenient within 4.5 hours. The issues span professional boundaries starting with public, ambulance, primary care and Accident and Emergency Department awareness. It is necessary to be oversensitive to avoid missing patients. Currently, the **FAST test** (Is there any one of **F**acial weakness, **A**rm and leg weakness, **S**peech deficit, **T**est all 3?) is a common screen used to identify patients. After the potential stroke patient has been identified, a clinical and neuroimaging response must be quickly activated. There is increasing evidence that some patients, especially those with major vessel occlusion, may benefit from intra-arterial interventional procedures, including thrombus extraction and/or intra-arterial delivery of thrombolytic agents. These treatments can only be delivered in specialized centres.

Fewer than 5–10 per cent of patients are currently being treated even in highly active centres. As the situation currently stands, thrombolysis should only be considered for use in centres with organized stroke services and considerable

Table 23.7 Contraindications and areas of uncertain benefit for intravenous thrombolysis

Contraindications	Uncertain benefit
Subarachnoid haemorrhage suspected?	Age ≥80 years
Evidence of active internal bleeding?	Severe neurological deficit (NIHSS >20)
Known bleeding diathesis including severe liver disease/known haemorrhagic retinopathy	Mild neurological deficit (NIHSS 0-5)
History of stroke or head trauma in the past 3 months?	Time from onset at start of infusion likely to be >3 and <6 hours
History of intracranial haemorrhage ever?	Systolic BP in range 185–220 mmHg
History of arteriovenous malformation or aneurysm?	Diastolic BP in range 110–130 mmHg
History of any major surgery, trauma or haemorrhage in the past 21 days? History of gastrointestinal or urinary tract bleeding?	
Traumatic external cardiac massage or obstetric delivery within 10 days?	
Lumbar puncture in the past 7 days?	
Could the patient be pregnant?	
Does the patient have acute pancreatitis?	
Does the patient have post myocardial infarction pericarditis?	
Was there any seizure activity at stroke onset?	
Symptoms likely to resolve completely in next few hours	
BM stick glucose >20 mmol/L/BM stick glucose <3.0 mmol/L	

expertise in clinical assessment and neuroimaging. It is possible that in the future sophisticated MRI or CT will allow the selection of patients most likely to benefit from thrombolysis by identifying salvageable areas of brain that have critically impaired perfusion but have not yet undergone infarction.

Aspirin

Aspirin has been extensively studied in two very large randomized clinical trials. The trials indicate that giving aspirin (150–300 mg) within 48 hours of stroke has a small but worthwhile effect by preventing early recurrence of ischaemic stroke (absolute risk reduction 0.7 per cent) and reducing death and disability at follow up by 1 per cent. There is only a very small increase in intracranial (0.2 per cent) and extracranial (0.4 per cent) haemorrhage risk with aspirin treatment in acute stroke. These modest benefits are likely to be the result of secondary prevention. In these trials, many patients received aspirin before scanning and there was no discernible early detriment to those in whom a subsequent scan showed primary ICH.

Aspirin should therefore be started (or continued) as soon as possible following stroke and certainly within 48 hours. Our view is that aspirin should only be given after neuroimaging has excluded haemorrhage (unless a scan cannot be obtained for some reason and haemorrhage appears unlikely), and that it should not be given to patients with uncontrolled severe hypertension.

Heparin

No significant reduction in death or dependency has been found in any of the large organized trials of anticoagulation in acute stroke, even in subgroups with atrial fibrillation.

This is because any reduction in recurrence of ischaemic stroke and venous thromboembolic complications is offset by an increase in intracranial and extracranial bleeding. Two small trials failed to show any benefit of anticoagulation in progressive stroke, but it should be noted that as many as 40 per cent of patients worsen after admission to hospital and the reasons for this are often systemic or multifactorial.

Anticoagulation is still used by most experts in acute ischaemia under some circumstances. These include dissection or acute thrombosis of the extracranial carotid or vertebral artery, and stroke associated with venous sinus thrombosis. In patients with a strong indication for long-term anticoagulation therapy, for example those with atrial fibrillation, immediate anticoagulation is recommended in acute stroke if the infarct is small, and the patient is normotensive and does not have significant leukoaraiosis. In patients with large infarcts, or haemorrhagic transformation, anticoagulation, if indicated, should usually be delayed for approximately 2 weeks.

Neuroprotection

A number of drugs designed to inhibit the cascade of chemical changes responsible for neuronal death after ischaemia reduce the size of infarction in animal models of stroke. However, to date, no clinical benefit has been observed in human trials of acute ischaemic stroke using a number of these neuroprotective agents, including nimodipine, corticosteroids and some N-methyl-D-aspartate antagonists. At least part of the disappointing results relate to problems with trial design.

Manipulation of physiological variables

Some units take a very aggressive approach to correcting these parameters. Fever and hyperglycaemia are risk factors for poor outcome and are associated with large stroke lesions. No trial evidence exists to support this approach as yet, but it is quite possible that manipulation of these factors contributes to the improved outcome for stroke seen when patients are treated in specialized units. We recommend the routine prescription of paracetamol for fever, early antibiotic therapy for infection and maintenance of blood glucose below 10 mmol/L by insulin if necessary.

Management of hypertension with acute stroke

The management of hypertension associated with acute stroke is controversial. Most advocate only treating acutely extremes of hypertension and hypertensive encephalopathy, because cerebral autoregulation is lost after stroke and therefore lowering blood pressure may reduce important perfusion to penumbral areas.

Perfusion through recanalized arteries into damaged capillary beds may result in haemorrhagic transformation of infarcted tissue, and rigorous treatment of hypertension is indicated if thrombolysis is planned to reduce this risk.

Neurosurgical intervention

In ischaemic stroke, hemicraniectomy is sometimes performed to decompress the brain in patients with malignant brain oedema after total middle cerebral artery territory infarction, and posterior fossa craniectomy may be indicated for cerebellar infarction with brainstem compression. This is obviously lifesaving in some cases and may improve the quality of life for survivors. Meta-analysis using randomized clinical trial data from several small trials support the value of this treatment in younger patients, with impressive figures showing a mortality rate with the malignant middle cerebral artery (MCA) syndrome in control patients of 70 per cent compared to a 50:50 chance of a good outcome after craniectomy.

Organized stroke unit care

Hyperacute stroke unit

An emerging concept in the UK is the **hyperacute stroke unit (HASU)** that can provide an intensive level of physiologic support, thrombolysis and other appropriate intervention to patients in the very acute stages of stroke (0–72 hours approximately). It is important to realise that the benefits of a HASU goes far beyond the delivery of thrombolysis. Such units aim to provide emergency assessment of all suspected acute stroke patients (whether eligible for thrombolysis or not) by specialists in acute stroke, deliver emergency brain imaging reported by neuroradiologists (including MRI if needed) and to place patients immediately into an environment of careful clinical and physiological monitoring and support provided by stroke-trained nurses and therapists, which will benefit all patients, not only those receiving thrombolysis. It is likely that only through such systems can early intensive care and investigation be implemented cost effectively. For example, immediate brain imaging has been shown to be the most cost-effective approach for all stroke patients. It would simply not be possible to provide this standard of care 24 hours a day, 7 days a week in every existing stroke unit without a massive expansion in stroke trained ward staff and consultants.

The HASU concept has not been subject to a randomized trial, but the benefits shown in the trials of stroke unit care (which are predicated on rehabilitation as the intervention) and the prescription of aspirin or thrombolysis, do not on their own explain the alarming differences observed in case mix adjusted mortality after stroke found in the studies comparing outcome in the UK with that in other European countries, such as the BIOMED project. Mortality after stroke was significantly higher in stroke units in the UK (42 per cent in one UK unit) than stroke units in other European countries (19 per cent in France). The difference was not explained by thrombolysis, but rather appeared to be associated with more active management of a wide variety of clinical and physiological parameters in the continental European centres. Within centre studies have also shown improved outcomes associated with intensive physiological monitoring compared to care on a conventional stroke unit. Although most data showing effectiveness of stroke units are from rehabilitation units, a large study from Italy demonstrated markedly improved outcome with acute stroke unit care, with most of the reduction in mortality being seen very soon after stroke.

Stroke unit

One of the most important aspects of stroke management is admission to an organized stroke unit.

There is good evidence from randomized trials that stroke unit care has substantial benefits in terms of overall prevention of death, disability and the need for institutional care. The degree of benefit is considerable when compared to individual pharmacological treatments and is similar in mild, moderate or severe disability and irrespective of age or gender. Thus, all patients with acute stroke should be admitted to a stroke unit as soon as possible after onset. Only patients who have made a good recovery by the time they are first seen do not need admission, as long as they can be seen urgently in a neurovascular clinic for investigation. Patients with intracerebral haematomas often gain considerably, and as much as ischaemic stroke, from organized care. In contrast to ischaemic stroke, haemorrhages often take much longer for recovery to begin than ischaemic stroke and need careful supportive care during this time.

The factors identified that characterize stroke unit as opposed to general medical ward care include a discreet geographical area dedicated to stroke, multidisciplinary team meetings and physicians with an interest in stroke. Specialist nursing, as well as dedicated therapists, play an important role. These are to some extent epiphenomena, exemplifying a more fundamental difference, that is, an effective team who have 'ownership' of the patient's problems and a responsibility to address them. The complex problems that affect many patients with stroke go far beyond the strict medical issues and cannot be effectively addressed by a disjointed approach. It is likely that at least part of the benefit of organized care results from better care of the acute patient, leading to less secondary brain damage. This benefit is multifactorial, for example, accurate diagnosis; appropriate use of drugs; prevention of swallowing complications, hypoxia and hypovolaemia; appropriate treatment of pyrexia, hyperglycaemia and infection; early fluid and food replacement; frequent turning and prevention of pressure sores; proper positioning and early mobilization. Second, coordinated, goal-oriented rehabilitation and discharge planning is a totally different proposition to more fragmented delivery of rehabilitation.

Treatment of intracerebral haemorrhage

In primary ICH, general supportive management, including stroke unit care, is just as important as after ischaemic stroke. **The benefits of routine surgical evacuation of cerebral haematomas are doubtful, although a randomized trial of evacuation of lobar haematomas sized between 10 and 100 mL in volume is in progress.** There are no specific drugs that have been shown to alter outcome. Neurosurgical practice varies and a 'middle of the road' approach is to carry out life-saving surgery **to evacuate large cerebellar haematomas** and **superficial lobar haematomas** that are causing **marked mass effect**. Patients can make a surprisingly good recovery from life-threatening cerebellar haematoma. Fewer neurosurgeons will tackle deep-seated basal ganglia haematomas, except in exceptional circumstances.

Haematomas related to anticoagulant therapy may present as slowly evolving lesions. It is virtually always a mistake if the haematoma is small at initial imaging not immediately to reverse warfarin, as delay may have devastating consequences. This maxim includes reversing anticoagulation in patients with prosthetic valves, because the benefit/risk ratio is much in favour of anticoagulation reversal for a period of 2 weeks, after which the rebleeding rate is considerably lower. The actual rate of systemic embolism during this period is small. In appropriate patients, it is necessary to exclude underlying vascular malformations with delayed MRI or angiography.

Prevention of secondary complications

Important preventable and treatable secondary complications are listed in Box 23.7.

Swallowing

Careful assessment of swallowing must take place in all patients with stroke; swallowing will be impaired in 50 per cent. Ideally, a speech and language therapist should assess all patients. If this assessment is delayed, and **there is doubt about the integrity of swallowing, it is better to keep patients nil by mouth and feed them via a nasogastric tube**. The gag reflex is an insensitive screen of swallowing integrity. In general, if the patient is alert and attentive, has a clear chest, normal speech and a strong, clear cough then it is safe to try sips of water, increasing to a glass and then feeding. This should be stopped if there are signs of aspiration, for example, 'wet' voice or choking, and nasogastric feeding should be instituted. If nasogastric feeding is likely to continue for more than 2 weeks, then per-endoscopic gastrostomy feeding should be considered. Per-endoscopic gastrostomy is often a

Box 23.7 Important preventable and treatable secondary complications

- Aspiration pneumonia
- Thromboembolism
- Infection
- Painful shoulder
- Depression

better option in confused patients who repetitively pull out nasogastric tubes. Stroke is associated with a massive catabolic response, but trials of oral nutritional supplementation have failed to show benefit over routine hospital diet.

> Failure to manage swallowing adequately in the early stages can result in aspiration pneumonia, which, in turn, causes fever and hypoxia, both of which are likely to exacerbate secondary brain damage.

Thromboembolism

Clinical deep vein thrombosis is rare on stroke units with active management policies because hydration, early mobilization and aspirin all contribute towards prevention. However, a small proportion of patients immobilized by stroke suffer from pulmonary embolism, usually occurring between 7 days and 6 weeks after the onset of stroke. Thigh length **compression stockings** do not benefit **immobile** stroke patients. **Low-dose subcutaneous heparin** should be considered as an option in patients at **high risk** of venous thromboembolism; for example, those with a prior history of deep vein thrombosis. However, heparin is not recommended routinely because the benefits of heparin in preventing thromboembolism are matched by the risks of promoting cerebral haemorrhage. It should be remembered that patients in atrial fibrillation are at risk of systemic embolism to the limbs and bowel, as well as recurrent stroke. However, in general, such patients should not receive anticoagulation therapy until 2 weeks after the onset of stroke, unless the patient has only had a small infarct, because the risk of causing haemorrhagic transformation negates the benefit of reduction in further embolism.

Infection

Pneumonia is common after stroke and should be vigorously treated. It is very difficult to assess prognosis at the outset in those without complicating pneumonia and even harder in those with it. Coexisting infection can make the situation appear far graver than it is. If patients are managed poorly in the acute stages because of concerns about long-term prognosis, then their poor outcome will become a self-fulfilling prophecy. Ensuring a safe swallow (see above under Swallowing) before allowing oral intake plays an important part in preventing aspiration pneumonia.

Painful shoulder

The complication of painful shoulder has become far rarer since the advent of correct positioning of the hemiplegic limb. This at the simplest level involves elevating the arm on a pillow when the patient is sitting to prevent partial subluxation of the shoulder joint.

Depression

Depression is common and readily treated. It should be distinguished from acute grief reactions, which are also common and nearly always self-limiting. It should be noted that organic brain disease predisposes to depression.

Early mobilization

Early mobilization on an active stroke unit, where all conscious patients are sat out of bed within a day, may well help to prevent many of the above complications.

REHABILITATION

The natural history of stroke is to improve over time, unless the patient succumbs to primary neurological death or secondary complications.

> **Aims of rehabilitation**
> Rehabilitation aims to enhance this spontaneous recovery and helps the patient to adjust to any residual deficit, as well as improving the patient's functional activity and participation.

Rehabilitation is a complicated and generally poorly understood process. It is not about 'popping down to the gym for a bit of physio'. One of the key factors in rehabilitation is that problems are addressed at three levels: impairment, limitation of activity (disability), and limitation of participation (handicap). Physicians often view problems solely at an impairment level and are disappointed because their patient still has a weak limb, despite several weeks of therapy. They may miss the fact that despite this, participation in the activities of daily living may have changed substantially. All therapists play a crucial role. The value of **occupational therapy** and **neuropsychological input**, in addition to **physiotherapy** and **speech and language therapy**, cannot be underestimated in a population with significant cognitive impairment. Rehabilitation must be goal-oriented and combined with active discharge planning to have maximal impact. The old style maxim 'let's see what the patient is like next week' is inefficient and incompatible with efficient use of scarce resources. Effective rehabilitation is practical proof that the brain is not hardwired, but in fact has considerable capacity to reprogramme itself through synaptic potentiation and dendritic sprouting ('brain plasticity').

MODELS OF SERVICE DELIVERY

In the past, acute stroke patients could be treated at home or in hospital; in hospital, care could be delivered within a general medical environment or a stroke unit. **Stroke units provide coordinated multidisciplinary care** within a discreet geographical area. There are now over 20 trials looking at the impact of such units compared with care on a general medical ward. Overall, stroke unit care leads to a significant reduction in the odds of death and dependency and this is seen in virtually all patient groups, irrespective of age or severity of stroke. The old maxim that aggressively managing those who seem at onset to have severe stroke syndromes is unwise, because of the likelihood that many dependent people will survive rather than die, is now untenable. While this will happen in individual cases, it will also be the case that those who would be left dependent will be shifted up a grade and leave hospital independent. There are no reliable ways of predicting outcome at presentation with stroke, therefore all patients should be admitted to a specialized stroke service.

Stroke units may provide acute care, rehabilitation or both. All three models are effective and it seems likely that a comprehensive unit (acute care and rehabilitation) will ensure the best outcome. There are new drives to set up HASU services which can deliver the first few days of care (see above under Hyperacute stroke unit), although no reason exists as to why these should not be collocated with stroke units. Acute care merges into rehabilitation

and these should not be regarded as separate entities. The outcome of patients treated on general wards, for whom regular consultation has been provided by a 'mobile' expert team, or who have been cared for at home with a domiciliary stroke team, has been shown to be less effective than admission to a geographically discrete in-patient stroke unit. Geographically discrete units not only allow concentration of expertise but also allow an effective team culture to be built. As one stroke physician commented when complemented on the good outcome seen on their unit, 'it's nothing to do with me, it's the team'.

URGENT MANAGEMENT OF TIA

The early risk of stroke following TIA or minor stroke has been underestimated and was conventionally held to be around 1–2 per cent in a month. However, population-based studies have now clearly demonstrated that the risk is much higher and that most stroke following TIA happens early with an exponential decrease across time. Hence, up to 15 per cent of patients with TIA may suffer stroke within the first 2 weeks.

Careful research has also demonstrated that it is possible to clinically stratify patients presenting with TIAs into high-risk and low-risk according to clinical criteria using the ABCD2 score (Table 23.8). Patients with a score of 4 or more are not only more likely to have a true TIA diagnosis, but also have a high risk of early stroke. These are medical emergencies warranting immediate assessment, investigation within 24 hours, and endarterectomy within 48 hours for appropriate cases. Low risk patients can be seen within an outpatient setting, provided the patient can be seen and investigated within a short time-frame of ideally 1 week or less.

'One stop' clinics provide an efficient way of providing this service. Secondary prevention can be commenced in primary care at the time of referral. There is a general trend for patients to be started liberally on antiplatelet medication, but less attention is paid to the vigorous treatment of hypertension. Lowering blood pressure too much by over-rigorous treatment of hypertension in acute stroke can considerably worsen outcome; it is, however, often the most important risk factor, certainly a far more common problem on a population basis than carotid stenosis. Hence, gradual control of

Table 23.8 ABCB2 score

High-risk TIA patients are defined as where symptoms have occurred within the last 2 weeks and the patient has a high ABCD 2 score of 4 or more, or one of the three below:	
More than one TIA within the last month	
Atrial fibrillation	
Carotid bruit	
The ABCD 2 score is determined as follows:	
Age >59 years	= 1 point
BP on presentation, systolic >139 mmHg or diastolic >89 mmHg	= 1 point
Clinical features: Unilateral weakness	= 2 points
Speech disturbance without weakness	= 1 point
All others	= 0 points
Duration: >59 minutes	= 2 points
10–59 minutes	= 1 point
<10 minutes	= 0 points
Diabetes	= 1 point

BP, blood pressure; TIA, transient ischaemic attack.

hypertension is essential and even patients with normal blood pressure benefit from blood pressure lowering therapy after recovery from stroke or TIA.

SECONDARY PREVENTION

Medical issues

The **risk of recurrence after stroke is between 5 and 15 per cent in the first year** depending on the patient's risk factors. **After five years, 30 per cent have had a recurrence**. There is also an increased risk of myocardial infarction. As well as guiding the patient through the acute phase and prospectively planning rehabilitation and discharge, it is therefore vital to ensure that modifiable risk factors for recurrent stroke are addressed early after onset of TIA and stroke (Table 23.9). This will include **smoking cessation** and **antihypertensive treatment** (target >140/80 mmHg), if appropriate. There is emerging evidence that lowering even 'normal' blood pressure (using a combination of a diuretic with an ACE inhibitor) reduces the relative risk of further vascular events as much as in those with hypertension. In addition, **statins** have been shown to reduce composite vascular outcome in patients with a history of ischaemic heart or cerebrovascular disease and normal cholesterol concentrations.

Warfarin
Anticoagulation with warfarin produces highly significant reductions in vascular events for patients in atrial fibrillation and is the only proven stroke preventive treatment for this condition.

Warfarin should therefore be considered for all patients with **atrial fibrillation** after ischaemic TIA and stroke, aiming for an INR of 2.5 (range, 2–3). However, warfarin is not beneficial in patients with other non-cardiac causes of stroke and may be harmful in older patients or in those with hypertensive small vessel disease. In patients who are not receiving anticoagulants, antiplatelet therapy should be prescribed unless stroke has been caused by ICH (Table 23.10).

Aspirin following ischaemic stroke is definitely beneficial in doses between 75 and 300 mg o.d. Addition of modified-release dipyridamole to aspirin and use of clopidogrel alone are slightly more beneficial than aspirin alone, but the differences in absolute risk reduction are small, except in those at high risk of occurrence. In the UK, the combination of aspirin and dipyridamole, or clopidogrel alone in those not tolerant of either medication, is recommended for vascular prophylaxis for two years after the onset of stroke or TIA. Ticlopidine is rarely used

Table 23.9 Secondary prevention after stroke and transient ischaemic attack

Ischaemic and haemorrhagic stroke		
	Lifestyle issues	Stop smoking
		Take regular exercise
		Reduce excess alcohol intake
		Encourage healthy diet
	Medical treatment of risk factors	Lower blood pressure
		ACE inhibition
		Optimize diabetes treatment
		Lower cholesterol with a statin
Ischaemic stroke		
	Prevention of thrombosis	Warfarin for atrial fibrillation
		Antiplatelet therapy if not receiving anticoagulation treatment
	Treatment of severe carotid stenosis	Surgery or stenting
Cerebral haemorrhage		
		Clipping or coiling of aneurysm
		Removal or obliteration of AVM

ACE, angiotensin-converting enzyme; AVM, arteriovenous malformation.

Table 23.10 Antiplatelet agents used in secondary stroke prevention

Agent	Dose	UK cost/100 tablets (£)
Aspirin	Dispersible 75 mg od	1.30
Dipyridamole	MR 200 mg bd	16.25
Clopidogrel	75 mg od	126.10
Ticlopidine	250 mg bd	166.67

nowadays because of the risk of neutropenia and the need for haematological monitoring.

Carotid stenosis

There is now considerable evidence that carotid endarterectomy is beneficial in patients with recent non-disabling ischaemic stroke or TIA associated with a concordant high-grade carotid artery stenosis. If patients with symptomatic **stenosis greater than 70 per cent** (measured by the North American Symptomatic Carotid Enderectomy Trial (NASCET) technique) are operated on by a surgeon with a resulting low morbidity and mortality rate, within a few weeks of symptoms, then the **stroke risk from**

the operation is far less than the stroke risk with medical therapy alone (Table 23.11). Carotid angioplasty and stenting is more hazardous in terms of immediate stroke risk than endarterectomy, but provides an alternative to endarterectomy in patients unsuitable for surgery. Carotid occlusion is not currently amenable to surgery.

Selecting these patients can be quite challeng-

Table 23.11 Benefits of carotid endarterectomy at various levels of stenosis, measured using the North American Symptomatic Carotid Endarterectomy Trial (NASCET) method

Percentage stenosis	Absolute risk reduction
<30	−2.9
30–49	1.2
50–59	5.2
60–69	9.6
70–79	14.2
80–89	14.3
90–99	38.1
Near occlusion	−0.3

Values taken from Rothwell P *et al. Lancet* 2003; **36**: 107–16. Negative values indicate harm from surgery.

ing and is not as simple as is suggested in Table 23.11. Particular difficulties are posed by more marginal patients with a 50–70 per cent stenosis according to the NASCET method of measurement; but this partly depends on the skill of the surgeon. This corresponds to a 70–80 per cent stenosis by European methods. Patients with isolated transient monocular blindness are at less risk from medical treatment alone and women are at higher risk from operative complications. Hence generally, men with hemisphere ischaemia are most likely to benefit and women with transient monocular blindness least likely. The longer the period free of symptoms, the less benefit from surgery, because most recurrent strokes associated with carotid surgery occur within the first three months. There is unlikely to be much overall benefit if surgery is delayed for more than six months after symptoms. Endarterectomy in appropriate high-risk TIA patients should ideally occur as soon as possible, ideally within 48 hours, but certainly within a maximum of 2 weeks. Patients with symptomatic stenosis between 50 and 69 per cent may also benefit from endarterectomy if surgery is performed rapidly after symptoms.

SUBARACHNOID HAEMORRHAGE

Subarachnoid haemorrhage (SAH) is caused by **rupture of an intracranial aneurysm** in 85 per cent, non-aneurysmal perimesencephalic haemorrhage in 10 per cent, and in 5 per cent by an arteriovenous malformation or a variety of other rare conditions. Subarachnoid haemorrhage is a devastating condition with an **overall case fatality of 50 per cent** (including pre-hospitalization deaths). Moreover, **30 per cent of survivors are left dependent** from major neurological deficits. The average age of onset is approximately 50 years, but SAH can occur at any age. In spite of many advances in diagnosis and treatment over the last decades, the case fatality rate has not changed.

Risk factors

Considerable evidence supports the role of genetic factors in the development of intracranial aneurysms. There is strong association between intracranial aneurysms and heritable connective tissues

diseases, although these only form a tiny part of any case load. Familial occurrence is marked, with reports of up to 20 per cent of patients with aneurysmal SAH having a first- or second-degree relative with a confirmed intracranial aneurysm. Unlike other forms of stroke, women form the majority of patients. Environmental factors have been extensively studied and cigarette smoking is the only factor consistently identified with SAH, raising the risk between three and ten times that of non-smokers. Hypertension is almost certainly also important, but to a lesser degree.

Clinical features

> **Headache in SAH**
> The cardinal clinical feature of SAH is a 'thunderclap headache'. This is a generalized headache of unique severity and sudden onset, often accompanied by nausea and vomiting.

Many patients give a history of unusual and acute headaches predating the definite SAH by several days to weeks. It is thought that these warning headaches may be the result of aneurysmal enlargement or minor rupture. These headaches are often not diagnosed as SAH. This is not surprising given the high incidence of primary headache syndromes. Thunderclap headache, although a cardinal feature, is non-specific and only one in ten of those presenting with sudden explosive headache will have SAH. However, there are no universal features to distinguish benign thunderclap headache from SAH, and cases with a typical history require investigation for SAH by CT scan, and lumbar puncture if CT is negative. However, in SAH, the blood characteristically irritates the meninges soon after onset.

> Signs of meningeal irritation (stiff neck, photophobia) are found in most patients and it is a common error for these not to be elicited or to be misinterpreted in patients with acute headache.

Signs of meningeal irritation are not present in all patients and occasionally SAH also presents without headache. Signs of global or focal dysfunction may also be found, depending on the severity and location of SAH. Focal deficits may be caused by intraparenchymal extension of blood, or later by vasospasm with resulting ischaemia and infarction. Patients may or may not lose consciousness briefly, or have prolonged coma at onset.

In a minority of cases, subhyaloid venous haemorrhages are visible on fundoscopy. The site of the bleeding aneurysm may be suggested by other clinical signs. A third nerve palsy suggests an aneurysm of the internal carotid or posterior communicating artery. Hemiparesis and aphasia suggests a middle cerebral artery aneurysm and leg weakness with bilateral extensor plantars, an anterior communicating artery aneurysm.

Investigation

CT scanning is mandatory in those with suspected SAH. Modern generation CT will demonstrate the presence of blood in 90–95 per cent of patients scanned within 24 hours (Figure 23.17). However, blood is rapidly cleared from the CSF and the sensitivity of **CT gradually decreases to 80 per cent at 3 days, 50 per cent at 1 week and 30 per cent at 2 weeks. If clinical suspicion is strong and the CT is normal, lumbar puncture should be performed** by an experienced operator. If clinically appropriate, this should be delayed for 12 hours after the ictus to allow xanthochromia to be detected. Negative CSF is very helpful in excluding SAH, but bloodstained CSF may result from a traumatic tap.

A decrease in the number of red cells from bottle one to three is an unreliable way of differentiating SAH from a traumatic tap.

Xanthochromia (yellow discoloration) of the supernatant indicating haemolysed red cells is, however, diagnostic of SAH, as long as the patient has not had a prior traumatic lumbar puncture.

In most laboratories, xanthochromia is determined by visual inspection rather than spectrophotometry, which is positive in all patients between 12 hours and 2 weeks. It should be remembered that patients may have SAH and a traumatic tap. Conventional MRI is not very sensitive to acute haemorrhage, but may be very useful after a delay when CT is negative.

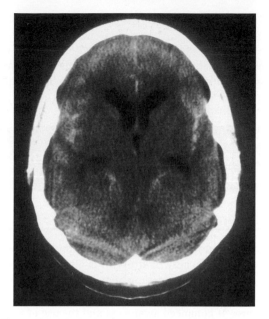

Figure 23.17 CT showing extensive subarachnoid blood and early hydrocephalus.

In patients in whom CT or LP has confirmed the diagnosis, candidates for intervention should be referred urgently to a specialist centre for neurosurgical assessment and angiography.

Management and prognosis

General supportive care should be instituted, with particular importance being placed on the avoidance of dehydration, hypotension and hypertension. Bed-rest prior to definitive treatment is conventional, but not a proven benefit. Administration of nimodipine reduces the risk of delayed ischaemia secondary to vasospasm. The **rebleeding rate from aneurysms is particularly high in the first 2 weeks** and then declines. This early high rebleeding rate, which may have devastating complications, is the reason why early intervention is favoured. In arteriovenous malformations, the risk of bleeding is lower, but in untreated cases persists indefinitely. In patients with a normal angiogram, in whom the haemorrhage is often maximal in the basal cisterns (perimesencephalic SAH), the risk of recurrence is low.

If an aneurysm is identified by angiography, this can usually then be dealt with by **neurosurgical clipping of the neck or endovascular delivery of detachable coils**, which are packed into the aneurysm to prevent further rupture. The outcomes are better after endovascular coiling in suitable patients.

Survivors of SAH have a high incidence of cognitive problems even if there are no limb signs. Assessment for rehabilitation should address this issue.

NON-ATHEROSCLEROTIC VASCULOPATHIES AND OTHER RARE CAUSES OF STROKE

Cerebral venous thrombosis

Cerebral venous thrombosis is an important treatable, but rare, cause of stroke. It is also a condition with diverse manifestations that mimic many other neurological disorders. It is increasingly recognized because of enhanced awareness and the use of MRI. **Venous thrombosis may be septic or non-septic** (Table 23.12). Septic causes are rare, but cavernous sinus thrombosis secondary to facial cellulitis, and lateral sinus thrombosis secondary to purulent otitis media or mastoiditis, are still seen from time to time. Septic thrombophlebitis of the cortical veins may also be associated with severe bacterial meningitis.

Aseptic thrombosis may affect the cortical veins, dural sinuses and deep veins. There are numerous potential causes. The most common include pregnancy, the puerperium, dehydration, thrombophilia and Behçet's syndrome. Combinations of these factors are often involved. In 20 per cent, no aetiology is uncovered.

Signs and symptoms of cerebral venous thrombosis

The clinical syndrome that manifests from cerebral venous thrombosis may be acute or subacute. The most frequent manifestations are headaches, seizures, altered consciousness, focal signs and disc swelling. Hence, cerebral venous thrombosis should be considered in the differential diagnosis of those presenting with stroke, severe headache, seizure disorders, coma, acute meningoencephalitic syndromes and idiopathic intracranial hypertension.

Venous thrombosis results in venous hypertension, which leads to raised intracranial pressure. This may simply give rise to a syndrome of headache with papilloedema and normal CT imaging. As the venous pressure rises, lobar intracranial haemorrhage or cerebral infarction, which is often haemorrhagic, results in focal neurological deficit and depression of consciousness. Occasionally, cerebral venous thrombosis presents with SAH (Figure 23.18).

A scan using CT is often normal, but may show a filling defect in one of the venous sinuses, which is more obvious after contrast injection. The diagnosis should also be suspected if there are bilateral superficial parietal infarcts or if an infarct does not respect arterial territories. Diagnosis can be made in the vast majority of cases with CTA or **plain**

Table 23.12 Causes of cerebral venous thrombosis

Septic	Facial cellulitis
	Otitis media
	Mastoiditis
	Meningitis
Non-septic	Pregnancy and the puerperium
	Contraceptive pill
	Dehydration
	Thrombophilia
	Behçet's syndrome

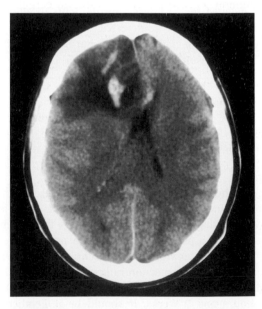

Figure 23.18 Haemorrhagic infarction secondary to cerebral venous thrombosis. The haemorrhagic infarct crosses vascular territories and is associated with generalized white matter oedema. Both these features are suggestive of venous sinus thrombosis.

MRI supplemented by flow-related MR venography images. In doubtful cases, conventional angiography may be required. The accepted treatment for cerebral venous thrombosis is anticoagulation, which has also been shown to be safe in those with haemorrhagic infarction.

Dissection

The majority of patients with stroke secondary to disease of the arterial wall will have atherosclerosis or small vessel lipohyalinosis, but there are several other important non-atherosclerotic vasculopathies to consider, including **extracranial arterial dissection**.

Cervicocephalic arterial dissection should be especially considered in young patients. There are several connective tissue diseases that are associated with dissection including Marfan's syndrome, Ehlers–Danlos syndrome and fibromuscular dysplasia. However, the vast majority occur in apparently normal subjects, either **spontaneously** or after **trivial neck trauma or manipulation**. New evidence is emerging that some of these 'normal' subjects may, in fact, have subtle underlying collagen defects. Hyperextension of the neck during hair washing in the salon or when painting a ceiling are common preceding events. Dissection can also result from more obvious trauma to the neck, as with penetrating injuries, or iatrogenically during catheter angiography. Dissection is produced by the subintimal penetration of blood as a result of a small tear in the intima with subsequent extension of the haematoma between the vessel layers. This may lead to occlusion of the vessel, but more often exposes a thrombogenic surface on which an intraluminal haematoma develops. This haematoma may then embolize and produce stroke. The vast majority of cases affect the extracranial carotid and vertebral arteries. Intracranial dissection is much rarer.

Signs and symptoms of dissection

The classic clinical scenario of dissection is a history of minor trauma to the neck followed shortly by the development of localized neck pain and headache. There is then a delay of several days (or sometimes weeks) before embolization causes TIA or stroke. Patients usually present after stroke has occurred, but occasionally present with a painful Horner's syndrome.

In some patients, dissection may never give rise to symptomatic embolization, but in others dissection may be instantly associated with devastating cerebral infarction. The association of **stroke with Horner's syndrome** should alert the clinician to the possibility of dissection. In the carotid circulation, this results from the dissecting haematoma compressing the ascending sympathetic fibres, which surround the carotid artery. In the vertebrobasilar circulation, Horner's syndrome may also result as part of lateral medullary syndrome from occlusion of the posterior inferior cerebellar artery, with resultant infarction of the dorsolateral medulla where the descending sympathetic tracts lie, and is then not specific for dissection.

MRI provides a sensitive and non-invasive means to confirm dissection. Fine-cut axial imaging with fat-suppressed sequences through the neck or cranium may reveal the characteristic crescentic vessel wall haematoma (Figure 23.19). Flow-related MRA may show luminal compromise. Conventional catheter angiography characteristically shows an eccentric tapering stenosis or occlusion and may also demonstrate underlying fibromuscular dysplasia. Ultrasound is less sensitive, especially if the dissection occurs in the high cervical carotid or vertebral artery.

A common management of dissection is to give **heparin as an anticoagulant**, followed by **warfarin for at least three months**. The rationale

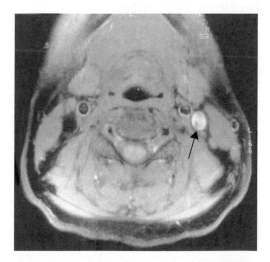

Figure 23.19 Axial magnetic resonance image showing characteristic crescentic wall haematoma secondary to dissection.

is that anticoagulation will lower the risk of embolization. However, there is no clinical trial that provides solid evidence for this practice, and antiplatelet agents may be equally effective.

Vasculitis

Vasculitis is a very rare, but important cause of stroke, because of the need for urgent immunosuppression to prevent recurrence.

Vasculitis and stroke
It is exceedingly rare for vasculitis to present as stroke without other preceding features of a systemic vasculitis.

Vasculitis causing stroke may be secondary to infections, connective tissue diseases (e.g. systemic lupus erythematosus or polyarteritis nodosa, other systemic vasculitides and giant cell arteritis.

In these conditions, cerebral infarction or haemorrhage results from true inflammation of the vessel wall, associated coagulapathies (e.g. the antiphospholipid antibody syndrome) or, more commonly, uncontrolled hypertension secondary to renal vasculitis. Occasionally, isolated central nervous system (CNS) vasculitis occurs without any systemic or extracranial features.

Infectious vasculitis

Infectious vasculitis associated with **meningitis** may occur acutely in the appropriate setting of severe bacterial, fungal, tuberculous or herpes zoster infection. There is nearly always an appropriate preceding history suggestive of a meningoencephalitic syndrome. However, in children, primary chickenpox infection can be followed by a focal vasculopathy affecting the middle cerebral artery without other features. An obliterative endarteritis affecting the small vessels of the brain may occur after primary syphilis infection, with an average latency of seven years. Headache and encephalopathy predominate in the prodrome before stroke occurs. Evidence of previous treponemal infection is easy to screen for in the blood and those with neurological involvement usually have pleocytosis and positive serology in the CSF.

Connective tissue disorders

In systemic necrotizing vasculitis, stroke is most commonly seen with **polyarteritis nodosa**, usually in association with uncontrolled hypertension. Such patients have usually been unwell for a considerable time period without treatment. The systemic features include weight loss, fever and abdominal and muscle pain. Renal involvement is common and may lead to severe hypertension. Mononeuritis multiplex secondary to peripheral nerve vasculitis may also occur. The combination of infarcts and haemorrhages on CT or MR is particularly suggestive of vasculitis, but this pattern is also seen in infectious endocarditis and venous sinus thrombosis. The diagnosis of polyarteritis nodosa is suggested by positive antineutrophil cytoplasmic antibodies. Treatment with cyclophosphamide is often necessary to induce remission.

Systemic lupus erythematosus commonly causes neurological problems. These are often neuropsychiatric and are rarely a result of vasculitis. Encephalopathy, psychosis, seizures, stroke-like focal deficits, myelopathy and neuropathy are all encountered. At pathological examination, the histology is often one of non-specific gliosis, although thrombosis may be observed, especially in those with antiphospholipid antibodies. Stroke may also occur secondary to embolism from Libman Sacks endocarditis. Management may require both anticoagulation and immunosuppression.

Giant cell arteritis

Temporal arteritis is the most important of the giant cell arteritides. The internal elastic lamina of the extracranial medium-sized arteries becomes fragmented and invaded by inflammatory cells. It virtually always occurs in those over 50 years and is accompanied by an elevated ESR in 90 per cent.

Symptoms and signs of temporal arteritis
Patients with temporal arteritis complain of headache with scalp tenderness associated with malaise, depression, myalgia and sometimes claudication of the jaw muscles while eating. Examination may reveal thickened tender temporal arteries.

Stroke is a very rare complication of the disease, but may occur from involvement of the extradural vertebral artery, leading to brainstem infarction. A far more common complication at presentation is **blindness and/or an anterior ischaemic optic neuropathy**. Diagnosis is established by temporal artery biopsy. Treatment is with high-dose prednisolone and, if the diagnosis is correct, the response of the systemic symptoms is dramatic and usually occurs within 1 day of starting treatment.

Takayasu's arteritus is much rarer. This usually affects young Asian females, and is associated with a high ESR. As well as systemic features of malaise and fever, the manifestations are a result of aortic arch inflammation, with subsequent occlusion of its branches, in particular the origin of one or both common carotid arteries.

Isolated angiitis of the central nervous system

Isolated angiitis of the CNS is a rare condition, which affects small and medium-sized intracranial vessels. It may cause a combination of infarcts and haemorrhages. The presentation is usually subacute or chronic with prominent headache, leading to encephalopathy or oedema with recurrent stroke-like focal events and the development of dementia over a few weeks or months. Angiography may reveal segmental narrowing of intracranial vessels, but is neither sensitive nor specific. The CSF often shows a pleocytosis, and imaging demonstrates multiple small vessel occlusions and haemorrhages if advanced. Diagnosis is by meningeal and brain biopsy. If patients have neither headache nor CSF pleocytosis, then biopsy rarely shows vasculitis. Treatment is with steroids and cyclophosphamide. **Lymphoma** affecting blood vessels (lymphomatous angiitis) presents in a similar fashion.

Hypertensive encephalopathy

Hypertensive encephalopathy manifests when systemic blood pressure is sustained above the upper limit of cerebral autoregulation. Oedema develops in the hyperperfused intracerebral circulation. Patients present with headache, epileptic seizures, focal TIA or stroke-like events, and, in advanced cases, depressed consciousness and cerebral infarction or haemorrhage. Examination may reveal papilloedema with proteinuria and microscopic haematuria.

> The blood pressure is often very high, for example, 250/150 mmHg.

In patients who develop hypertensive encephalopathy, the rate of blood pressure elevation has often been rapid and a result of renal disease. Occasionally, hypertensive encephalopathy can develop at lower blood pressure levels, particular in eclampsia associated with pregnancy.

Arteriovenous malformations

Arteriovenous malformations (AVM) are complex tangles of abnormal arteries and veins, which lack a capillary bed but are linked by one or more direct fistulas. They are thought to arise from developmental derangements at various stages. They may present with **SAH or ICH, epilepsy or progressive focal deficit**. With the advent of MRI, many are discovered coincidentally (Figure 23.20). They may be classified by size, location and their angioarchitecture. Advances in treatment modalities are occurring more rapidly than advances in our knowledge of the natural history of these lesions.

> The single most important fact determining prognosis is whether the AVM has bled or not. Patients with a history of intracranial haemorrhage are at a much higher risk of **rebleeding** (up to 18 per cent per year) than patients presenting without haemorrhage (1–2 per cent per year).

However, young patients without a history of haemorrhage may have a very high lifetime risk of bleeding. In any patient where treatment is considered, formal angiography in expert hands is required to define the angioarchitecture. This allows the risks of treatment or conservative management to be defined as accurately as possible. Management plans for these lesions should only be made by expert multidisciplinary teams, who can balance the risk of treatment against the risk of bleeding. Surgery is an option for treatment of accessible lesions with a single arterial supply and a single route of venous drainage. Endovascular obliteration with glue is an alternative treatment modality, which often results in partial obliteration of the AVM and may target 'high risk' elements within

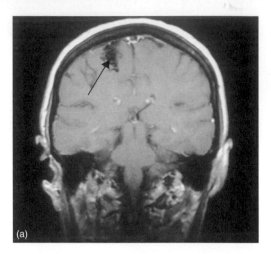
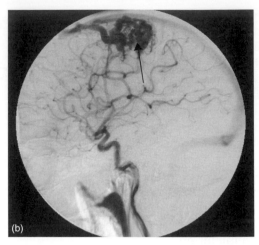

Figure 23.20 Magnetic resonance image and catheter angiogram showing an arteriovenous malformation. This patient presented with focal seizures and had no evidence of bleeding over prolonged follow up.

the malformation. It is not known whether partial obliteration is beneficial or harmful. Radiotherapy is an option for small lesions and produces obliteration in up to 80 per cent of lesions by two years, but the patient is at risk of haemorrhage during this time. Often combination therapy is necessary. Because of the uncertainty of the benefits and risks of treatment in unruptured AVMs, a trial (ARUBA) is currently randomizing patients to compare these.

Moyamoya disease

Moyamoya disease is a rare bilateral intracranial occlusive arteriopathy characterized by stenosis or occlusion of the terminal internal carotid arteries with involvement of the proximal portions of the anterior and/or middle cerebral arteries. These changes are accompanied by characteristic enlargement of basal collaterals (moyamoya vessels). A similar occlusive arteriopathy ('secondary moyamoya') can occur in response to cranial irradiation or childhood sickle cell disease, and in association with a number of genetic disorders, including neurofibromatosis and Down's syndrome. The condition usually presents with stroke or TIA and there is a high risk of recurrence. Patients may also suffer from seizures, dystonia and headache, which are often resistant to medical treatment. The arteriopathy usually presents in childhood, but increasing numbers of patients are being detected in adult life. Although endemic in Japan, it is increasingly recognized throughout the world. Treatment options include various neurosurgical

direct and indirect revascularization procedures and in adults vigorous risk factor control. Management is best undertaken by a specialized service.

Vascular disease of the spinal cord

Spinal cord infarction is a rare disorder and is usually caused by **occlusion of the anterior spinal artery**, which supplies the anterior two-thirds of the cord. Most patients with anterior spinal artery occlusion have multiple risk factors, especially hypertension and diabetes. The anterior spinal artery is also vulnerable to aortic dissection. The dorsal columns are spared by anterior spinal artery occlusion thanks to a rich plexal supply. The resultant clinical picture is therefore an acute areflexic paraplegia characterized by dissociated sensory loss: that is, striking preservation of joint position and vibration sense, with marked loss of pinprick and temperature sensation in the lower limbs and trunk. No effective acute treatment is known, but rehabilitation is very helpful to the patient.

REFERENCES AND FURTHER READING

Losseff NA, Grieve J, Brown MM (2009) Stroke and cerebrovascular disease. In: *Neurology – A Queen Square Textbook*. Oxford: Wiley-Blackwell.

Warlow CP, Dennis MS, van Gijn J *et al.* (2000) *Stroke. A Practical Guide to Management.* Oxford: Blackwell Science.

CHAPTER 24

NEUROLOGICAL REHABILITATION

Roshni Beeharry

INTRODUCTION AND CONTEXT

Neurological disorders are heterogeneous in their presentation and impact, and many have the potential to lead to long-term disability. The burden of neurological disorders to the individual, their families and society is high (40 per cent prevalence in the UK).

> The rehabilitation of an individual with a neurological disorder or any other long-term condition is complex and involves a coordinated interdisciplinary and intradisciplinary team working. Management of the long-term sequelae of neurological disability should be a partnership between primary care and secondary care specialists including neurologists, neurorehabilitation physicians, medical and surgical specialties, specialist neurotherapists and nurses. This spans the acute, post-acute (inpatient unit and outpatient clinic) and community settings.

Neurological rehabilitation is known to be beneficial in the post-acute phase of recovery from stroke, spinal cord injury and traumatic brain injury, but has also been shown to be beneficial in more chronic progressive conditions, such as multiple sclerosis and movement disorders. The needs of individuals will of course vary along the course of their life, and this is particularly salient in considering those with congenital conditions, in their transition from childhood to adolescence and then to adulthood. It is important to coordinate and manage these changing needs, and the rehabilitation physician is in a good position to do this in partnership with the general practitioner and other secondary care specialists.

In addition, palliative care input and end-of-life planning skills are increasingly needed within the long-term conditions setting, and the Royal College of Physicians, the British Society of Neurorehabilitation and National Council for Palliative Care have created national guidelines for those at the interface of care in this population.

> This chapter aims to give an overview of what rehabilitation entails, models of service delivery, and the principles behind the rehabilitation approach, with emphasis on the medical issues that neurologists and neurorehabilitation physicians will be called upon to manage in the context of neurological rehabilitation and long-term conditions. The conditions managed in the rehabilitation setting include a wide range of congenital conditions such as cerebral palsy: acquired brain injury (stroke, traumatic brain injury), spinal cord injury, multiple sclerosis, Guillain–Barré, peripheral neuropathy and myopathies.

Neurorehabilitation physicians and their teams are also involved in leading the specialist care of those with disorders of consciousness, such as minimally conscious state (MCS) and vegetative state (VS), but this is beyond the scope of this chapter.

DEFINITIONS AND TERMINOLOGY

What is rehabilitation?

> The World Health Organization (2001) defines rehabilitation as 'the use of all means aimed at reducing the impact of disabling and handicapping conditions and at enabling disabled people to achieve social integration'.

The aim is to *promote the independence* of individuals with complex disorders. The principles of rehabilitation are applied not only to neurological disorders, but to other long-term conditions, for example, amputees and those with chronic pain or musculoskeletal disorders who may also be managed by rehabilitation physicians.

The WHO Illness Model depicts the complex interaction of pathology, the individual, environment and society.

The WHO International Classification Framework (2003) lends a more positive, enabling emphasis to the previous terminology, and the newer terms are in italics:

- *Impairments*: relate to physical/structural organ damage, e.g. left hemiparesis.
- The term 'disability' is still widely used, but in this framework is more positively framed as *activity* – what the person is able to do/not do as a result of the impairment, and how this affects their interaction with the immediate environment, e.g. left hemiparesis leading to reduced ability to mobilize at home.
- *Participation* (previously termed 'handicap') relates to the person's wider role in the community and society as a whole, e.g. person with a left hemiparesis who is unable to mobilize may be unable to access the community or drive to access work, without adaptations.

The impairments and limitations of activity arising from neurological disorders stem from the physical and cognitive impact and can lead to chronic long-term disability. The rehabilitation approach compliments and extends the work of the neurologist and neurosurgical teams, in looking at the impact and consequence of the neurological disorder on the person, their family/carers, and on society as a whole.

It is important to be aware that improvements at an impairment level as a result of specialist treatment and rehabilitation do not necessarily translate into gains in functional activity or participation. For example, a patient with multiple sclerosis may show improved upper limb strength from a course of steroids, but this may not necessarily lead to improved upper limb use or function as this relies on a multitude of factors, including environmental, cognitive and psychological factors. This is a concept that individuals, their families and some health professionals struggle with, and is an important part of the rehabilitation specialist's role in managing expectations for future recovery. The converse is also true – functional gain may be realized with little change in impairment and it is through changes in function that the rehabilitation process should be viewed.

NEUROLOGICAL PRINCIPLES UNDERLYING REHABILITATION

The rehabilitation approach harnesses the **neuroplasticity** of the nervous system, that is, the ability of the brain to structurally and biochemically alter and create new pathways after injury. One can use the example of traumatic brain injury to illustrate this. Animal models reveal that within seconds to minutes after a traumatic brain injury, biochemical cascades are initiated and synaptic connections are broken and reconnected in altered ways. Indeed, the hallmarks of the traumatic mechanism of injury is diffuse axonal injury and diffuse cortical damage, leading to a wide spanning range of distributed impairments not predictable from a focal anatomic model, of both physical and cognitive, emotional and neuropsychiatric. One can contrast this to the more focal neuroanatomical damage and hence more predictable 'mapping' impairments that can arise from a stroke or tumour. The type and natural history of the disorder and its neuropathology are key when one is considering the activity, participation and further care needs aspects of rehabilitation in these individuals, as well as influence the discussion surrounding prognosis.

Prognosis in neurological rehabilitation is imprecise, multifactorial and is related to the underlying pathology. Unfortunately, there is a dearth of literature in some diagnostic categories, such as traumatic brain injury.

The rehabilitation approach

The ethos of rehabilitation is that it should be:

- person-centred
- an active, dynamic process
- educational
- empowering, encouraging self-management
- goal-focused
- holistic

Whether in hospital or community settings, the general process includes the following:

---

1 **Assessment period** – this varies from 2 to 4 weeks in most specialist inpatient units.

2 Each person is allocated a **key worker** who coordinates care and communication between the individual, family and other agencies, supported by the neurorehabilitation consultant and other members of the team.

3 **Goal setting** – this should occur within the first 10–14 days of admission to the rehabilitation unit/assessment in the community, and be reviewed at 2-weekly intervals. It should be a collaborative process **with the individual**. This may not always be possible in those who are severely impaired, and hence the team set goals based on the perceived needs of such individuals in conjunction with relevant carers/family members.
   a. Goals should follow the 'SMART framework': be **S**pecific, **M**easureable,

---

Achievable, and **R**ealistic and achieved in a **T**imely manner.
   b. Short-term goals are set every 2 weeks and reviewed as a team with the person and should be written in their own words ideally, facilitated by the team, e.g. 'to be able to brush my teeth twice a day'; 'to be able to stand with help from one person for 2 minutes'.
   c. The long-term goal and expected length of stay should be set by the specialist inpatient team, and ideally in an integrated way with the input of the community team within the multidisciplinary team meeting.

4 **Regular team multidisciplinary team meetings (MDM)** and meetings with individual undergoing rehabilitation and their family.

5 **Discharge planning** commences early on in the admission/assessment period taking into account assessment findings, prognosis and patient engagement with the rehabilitation programme, progress and participation needs.

Within the community rehabilitation setting, similar models exist, but the timings and logistics of goal setting and meetings may obviously differ.

Team structure in rehabilitation

Specialist rehabilitation is delivered by the interdisciplinary team, who are a group of highly trained individuals, including specialist medics, nurses, neurologically trained therapists, social workers who work in a coordinated way, together and alongside the patient, to help facilitate patients meeting their goals. Rehabilitation does not only occur in the hospital setting, although this is normally the setting for intensive post-acute management, e.g. post-acute stroke care after the stroke unit, and traumatic brain injury rehabilitation. It is important to highlight to patients and their families that rehabilitation can and does continue within the community, within the more realistic environment of the patient's home. It is often at this stage that the individual starts to come to terms with their new limitations and put into practice what they have learnt in the intensive rehabilitation setting, and commence reintegration into society. Ensuring the smooth transition of care from hospital settings to community is a key role of the specialist inpatient rehabilitation team.

> Intradisciplinary care involves the medical and surgical specialties that may contribute to the care of a patient with a neurological disorder. This includes neurology, neurosurgery, urology, orthopaedic surgery, pain management, palliative care and general practice.

Good coordination between interdisciplinary and intradisciplinary team relies on effective communication and rehabilitation physicians are often at the interface of the acute sector and post-acute sector. The individual with the neurological disorder should of course be at the heart of the team and care and be involved as far as possible in decision-making and care-planning.

The agencies involved in specialist rehabilitation include:

- **Medical**: GP, neurology, neurosurgery, palliative care, pain management, psychiatry services, neurorehabilitation, stroke medicine.
- **Nursing**: Rehabilitation nurses, specialist nurses, e.g. multiple sclerosis, motor neurone disease, stroke specialist nurse, continence adviser; district nurses.
- **Neurologically trained therapists, inpatient and community settings**: Occupational therapy (OT), physiotherapy (PT), speech and language therapy (SLT), neuropsychological, counsellor, rehabilitation assistants (RA), dietetics and specific to the community setting, re-enablement carers, early supported discharge (ESD) teams, community rehabilitation teams (CRT).
- **Equipment**: Orthotics, wheelchair services, assistive technology, rehabilitation engineers.
- **Support services**: Social work, stroke support worker, voluntary agencies and charities, e.g. Stroke Association, Headway.

The role of the neurorehabilitation consultant is wide ranging, and includes:
- Leading on the medical management of the sequelae of neurological disorder and preventing secondary complications, e.g. spasticity, neuropathic pain, depression.
- Disability management and coordinating multidisciplinary interventions.
- To be involved in service development, planning support and integrating care between health, social services and voluntary services.
- Managing the transitional services for adolescents with neurological disorder.
- Advising on return to work and education issues.
- Advice and support to family/carers and other specialists.
- Assessing mental capacity, working with legal services, child protection and vulnerable adult services.

Models of delivery

The smooth transition of care across secondary and primary care settings is not always made easy by the existing models of service delivery and not all specialist rehabilitation units are within district or tertiary centres. Superimposed on this, there is a stark mismatch in provision of rehabilitation services across the UK, which urgently needs to be addressed.

The National Service Framework for Long-term Conditions (Department of Health 2005) gives a structured framework to commissioners and providers and sets out 11 'quality requirements' (QR). The first three relate to diagnosis and acute management, and QR 4 and 5 pertain to early specialist rehabilitation and community rehabilitation, respectively.

Unfortunately, not every area has specialist community neurological rehabilitation services leading to a lack of continuity of care.

Clearly, the needs of the individual with chronic disability vary with time and health service models need to evolve in parallel and cater for this spectrum of needs. A good example of this is the transitional care from paediatric services to adult services which is varied nationally. The lower age limit for an adult rehabilitation unit is usually 18 years, so the 16- to 18-year-old adolescents with conditions such as cerebral palsy, acquired or congenital brain injury, remain under paediatric care and do not necessarily have recourse to specialist services which are clearly necessary given the specific needs of this age group including support in education, peer support and relationships.

However, joined-up planning across the patient pathway can be very successful as seen in the recent implementation of new stroke services in London, where awareness, prevention, hyperacute treatment (hyperacute stroke unit), acute rehabilitation (stroke unit) and post acute rehabilitation have been modelled and the acute pathway needs provided for. However, as practitioners are realizing, there is a potential mismatch between the need for post-acute specialist inpatient neurorehabilitation beds and the number of patients being discharged from the stroke units. **The Early Supported Discharge team is an exciting addition to this existing service structure, with the aims of allowing early discharge of appropriate patients from the hyperacute stroke unit (HASU) directly to the community** and supporting those further down the pathway in some cases. However, not all primary care trusts currently have access to ESD teams and pilots are ongoing. It is clear that the drive through the acute sector services and post-acute sector services will put pressure on community services to reshape service delivery rapidly.

The impact of third sector or voluntary and support agencies is increasingly important and key to both service provision and service planning so that 'user groups' can have representation at commissioning level and influence service development, e.g. stroke and cardiac networks.

REHABILITATION APPROACH AND TECHNIQUES

The mainstay of rehabilitation therapy incorporates optimizing neuroplasticity and natural recovery, that is, retraining and compensatory strategies including the use of adaptive equipment and orthosis. **However to access neural plasticity the prevention of complications is paramount, a patient locked in by contractures cannot access any functional gain.** This involves techniques such as:

- Positioning and handling of affected limbs to prevent secondary complications such as pain, contractures and optimize function
- Upper limb sensorimotor rehabilitation, e.g. constraint-induced therapy in stroke; research trials are ongoing in neurological centres into the use of robotics technology in upper limb retraining after stroke

- Working on truncal balance and transfers
- Bodyweight supported treadmill for gait re-education, used in acquired brain injury, spinal injury rehabilitation
- Spasticity management: therapy, functional electrical stimulation, oral medication, botulinum toxin, intrathecal phenol and baclofen
- Posture and mobility-specialist seating and wheelchairs
- Orthotics: ankle foot orthosis, wrist and elbow splints to optimize stretch on weakened muscles to prevent contractures, maintain normal joint range so as to optimize any senorimotor recovery for functional limb activity
- Occupational therapy improves outcome in terms of ability in personal activities of daily living
- Rehabilitation techniques for neglect and hemianopia
- Speech and language therapy techniques and communication aids for aphasia
- Cognitive rehabilitation, mood assessments and management, e.g. memory aids, errorless learning
- Work-based assessments (vocational rehabilitation)
- Assistive technology and environmental controls to allow the person to be as independent as possible in the home environment and reduce carer burden.

An approach to history taking in rehabilitation

The rehabilitation medical team is key in history taking and collating information between several specialties and it is vital for accurate and detailed information to therefore be provided by the referring neurology, neurosurgery and stroke teams to facilitate smooth and safe transfer of care.

The neurology/neurosurgical/stroke referral team transfer documents should include copies of neuroimaging, relevant blood results but most importantly a **full history of the admission and planned follow up.** Key points of the acute admission include:

- History of presenting complaint
  - In the case of traumatic brain injury:
    - o nature and timing of injury happen (e.g. road traffic accident/assault/other);

involvement of alcohol or drugs; police or legal involvement

- ○ Glasgow Coma Score at the scene and changes in this
- ○ duration of post-traumatic amnesia
- ○ documentation of nature and timing of any seizure activity and the management and planned duration of antiepileptics
- ○ any neurosurgical intervention and plans
- ○ any neurology, neurosurgical or other specialty follow up
- ○ any acute complications/co-morbidities in the acute phase
- – In the case of stroke disease:
  - ○ list the vascular risk factors
  - ○ results of investigations and those pending
  - ○ any treatment given in the acute phase and any medical complications, e.g. resistant hypertension, pneumonia, thromboembolism
  - ○ stroke follow up and recommendations
- Psychiatric co-morbidity is a major risk factor for traumatic brain injury and spinal cord injury, e.g. suicide attempt and risk-taking behaviour, so it is vital to delineate any past psychiatric history and its management, including formal mental health care admissions. Pre-morbid personality can also influence coping strategies, engagement in rehabilitation and can contribute to challenging behaviour which can negatively impact on progress.

In addition to a full medical history and examination with emphasis on neurological and psychiatric symptoms and signs, the rehabilitation assessment focuses on gaining a **picture of the person behind the disease/injury**. The history should encompass impairment–activity–participation aspects, with emphasis on the functionality and limitations of each person. Where possible, this should be from the patient, but supported with collateral history from the carer or family member who knows the person well. A full social history is integral to the personalized care of the individual. This should include details of housing including ownership status (relates to discharge planning), nature of employment, relationships, care responsibilities and financial responsibilities, any child care/protection issues, leisure pursuits and means of community access (driver, public transport user). These aspects are integral to setting goals working with the individual.

In the outpatient or community setting, when reviewing someone with any type of chronic condition, a useful technique is to ask them to describe a typical day which can help ascertain elements such as fatigue, sleep pattern, mood and activity, carer needs, and barriers to activity and participation.

ASSESSING PROGRESS AND OUTCOMES IN REHABILITATION

There are various means of assessing the effectiveness of rehabilitation, as well as the rehabilitation care needs.

One of the main outcome measures used internationally within inpatient rehabilitation settings is the 18-item Functional Independence Measure (FIM)™ devised in the United States initially for the brain injury population, but which has been further developed by UK neurorehabilitation specialists into the Functional Independence Measure + Functional Assessment Measure (FIM+FAM)™. This is a 30-item scale used to assess the baseline and changes in physical and cognitive domains of activity and participation during rehabilitation. It includes domains such as continence, mobility as well as community integration, emotional status, employment, attention, reading and writing skills.

> The Northwick Park Nursing Dependency Scores (NPDS), Northwick Park Therapy Dependency Scores (NPTDS) and Rehabilitation Complexity Scores (RCS), are well-validated tools used to assess staff–skill mix and care needs within the rehabilitation setting and in the case of NPDS give an indication of nursing care needs on discharge.

Specific outcome measures are of course used across therapy disciplines and in there are disease-specific tools for certain neurological conditions. Some examples which incorporate the key domains of impairment, activity and participation include:

- Mobility and balance:
  - – Berg balance test
  - – 10 metre walking test of speed
  - – Rivermead mobility index

- Upper limb function and dexterity:
  - 9 hole peg test
  - Frenchay Activities Index
- Mood:
  - Hospital Anxiety and Depression Score (HADS)
  - Beck Depression Inventory (BDI)
  - Depression Intensity Scale Circles (DISCS) used in aphasia
- Nursing dependency:
  - Barthel score
  - Northwick Park Dependency Score
- Aphasia:
  - Stroke Impact Scale
  - Western Aphasia Battery
  - Living with Aphasia Framework for Outcome measurement.

This is by no means an exhaustive list and the reader is referred to larger texts on stroke and neurological rehabilitation for fuller discussion of outcome measures and their limitations.

SEQUELAE OF NEUROLOGICAL INJURY

The consequences of neurological disease can be considered in the following domains:

1 Physical and medical
2 Cognitive and psychological
3 Sociological

Physical and medical sequelae managed in rehabilitation settings

There is a myriad of medical co-morbidities for which one needs to be vigilant and manage within the rehabilitation setting, in conjunction with acute specialist colleagues.

These include:

- Cardiorespiratory and vascular complications
  - obstructive sleep apnoea post-stroke
  - aspiration pneumonia
  - hemiparetic limb oedema
  - thromboembolism
- Musculoskeletal complications
  - pain
  - contractures
  - heterotopic ossification

- Gastrointestinal complications
  - neuropathic bowel: constipation and faecal incontinence
  - altered metabolism and nutritional needs
  - dysphagia
- Genitourinary complications
  - neuropathic bladder: urinary incontinence due to detrusor instability
  - renal calculi
  - sexual dysfunction
- Skin integrity issues
  - pressure areas.

The neurological medical sequelae managed within the post-acute setting include stroke recurrence, seizure activity, neuropathic pain and spasticity. The management of these requires integrated work between neurologists, pain specialists and rehabilitation teams.

This section focuses on some of the complications associated with acquired neurological injury that are commonly dealt with in the rehabilitation setting. These are spasticity, heterotopic ossification, neuropathic bladder and bowel, and pressure sores.

Spasticity

The underlying pathophysiology of spasticity is complex and readers are referred to texts listed in the reference list. The **National Guidelines – Spasticity in Adults: Management Using Botulinum Toxin (RCP and BSRM 2009)** provides a valuable overview of spasticity services and management, and highlight the fact that although there are no definitive prevalence figures, spasticity affects:

- 30 per cent of stroke patients
- 60 per cent of those with severe multiple sclerosis
- 75 per cent of those post-traumatic brain injury.

The classical definition of spasticity is:

a velocity-dependent increase resistance to passive limb movement in people with upper motor neurone syndrome (Lance, 1980).

In the clinical context, it is more helpful to consider the two components of spasticity:

1 Neurogenic component: overactive muscle contraction
2 Biomechanical component (hypertonia): stiffening and shortening of the muscle and other soft tissues.

From this definition, one can envisage that unmanaged limb spasticity can have a negative effect on function, with ongoing muscle contraction leading to abnormal limb posture, pain, soft tissue shortening and contracture. This can affect postural and seating needs, in turn leading to pressure sores, further pain, inhibit transfers and mobility, upper limb function and cosmesis.

Spasticity can be distributed as generalized, regional or focal (that is predominantly affecting particular muscle groups). One commonly finds a mixed picture of tone by virtue of the underlying pathologies. Some clinical scenarios faced in the rehabilitation setting include:

- Increased hip adductor tone in a person with, for example, cerebral palsy or multiple sclerosis, may limit access to the perineal area hence catheterization or hygiene management may be difficult. It can also affect sexual function leading to breakdown in self-esteem, body image, mood and relationships. It also can cause pain in the affected muscle group and particularly around the hips from excessive tension of the muscles. The abnormal posture can affect posture, seating and in those who are mobile lead to the classical 'scissoring gait' due to unopposed hip adductors, seen in these conditions.
- Increased tone in the the gastrocnemius–soleus complex of the calves can lead to abnormal degrees of plantar flexion of the feet, which can predispose to contracture formation, altered foot positioning for weight-bearing and hence walking, and foot placement on the wheelchair footplates.
- Increased tone in the upper limb flexors can affect limb position and function and reduce activity and participation with feeding, dressing and self-propelling a wheelchair, for example.

It is important to note that altered tonal patterns in the lower body can negatively affect upper limb and trunk tone, leading to problems such as fixed pelvic tilt, which further compound poor posture and seating, and can in turn lead to abnormal contact of bony prominences with the bed/seating which then lead to pressure sores.

It can be difficult to delineate severe spasticity from contractures and needle electromyogram

(EMG) can be useful in these circumstances as can examination under sedation or anaesthesia.

These 'negative' aspects of spasticity lead to secondary complications, increased carer burden and therefore healthcare costs. For example, it has been calculated that the cost of healing a grade 4 pressure sore is over £10 000, so if this is as a result of poorly managed spasticity one can start to appreciate the significant impact of this on care and health economics.

However, the specialist managing spasticity needs to consider in each case, to what degree patients utilize the hypertonia positively, e.g. to be able to weight-bear, transfer and mobilize. For example, **someone with cerebral palsy or hereditary spastic paraparesis may rely on hypertonia in the hip extensors and hamstrings to assist in mobility even though the underlying muscles are weak.**

This emphasizes the need for the individual with spasticity to be fully assessed by a specialist team and a detailed **functional history and examination** elicited. This has an impact on the management approaches used and hence each case must be reviewed within a multidisciplinary setting by a neurorehabilitation physician and/or neurologist, specialist neurophysiotherapist and neuro-occupational therapist with input from orthotics, as appropriate.

The history needs to include screening for triggers of increased spasms and spasticity including:
- Pain-noxious stimuli-neuropathic pain, musculoskeletal, in-growing toenail, poorly fitting footwear or orthosis
- Pyrexia and infections
- Pressure sores
- Constipation
- Urinary stones, retention and infection

The management strategy is to identify triggers, therapeutic goals for treatment and tailor treatment as related to the patient's needs.

Although the medical management of focal, regional and generalized spasticity differs, the underlying core treatment is a combination of stretching, splinting and orthotics to maintain the length of the muscle so at to maintain functional joint range and motor activity. Techniques include those applied to neurological rehabilitation in general, and include:

- **Passive stretch of affected muscles** to maintain length, using physical therapy, splinting, orthotics
- **24 hour postural management** programme: posture and handling of affected limbs in sitting, in bed posture and while upright. This includes strategies such as using pillows and appropriate supports on the wheelchair for upper limbs; T-rolls for adductor spasm to adduct the legs in supine position or a pommel in the wheelchair position.
- **Specialist seating** such as tilt-in space wheelchair
- **Medication**, such as centrally acting antispasmodics, including baclofen and gabapentin. These are widely used for generalized spasticity, but need careful titration in view of their systemic effects. They can negatively affect trunk control which could negate the benefits of reducing limb spasticity. They may also affect liver function, cause somnolence at higher doses and gastrointestinal adverse effects. The advantage of gabapentin in spasticity management is that it can also improve neuropathic pain (which itself is a trigger for spasticity) and it tends to have less negative impact on trunk control than other antispasmodics. Tizanidine and dantrolene act directly on the abnormal muscle activity, but tizandine can cause postural hypotension.

- Focal management is with intramuscular botulinum toxin, a powerful neurotoxin, which acts by blocking the release of acetylcholine from the presynaptic nerve terminals; this in turn inhibits cholinergic transmission and hence neuromuscular junction (NMJ) communication. The toxin is used therapeutically to cause dose-dependent reversible reduction in motor power and tone. The effect lasts approximately three months as the toxin degrades and the NMJ atrophies and regenerates. This needs follow up with specialist team including splinting, orthotics and an exercise/stretch programme to maintain the effect. Injections can be repeated if necessary at three-monthly intervals.

- Regional management of severe lower limb spasticity can be approached with oral medication, plus focal treatment, but more definitively with intrathecal baclofen or intrathecal phenol (in those where bowel, bladder function and mobility are irreversibly impaired). In the case of intrathecal baclofen, consideration includes the fact that this requires neurosurgery input, lifelong pump refills and pump changes every few years.
- Orthopaedic surgery can help with evaluation of the contribution of spasticity versus contracture (examination under anaesthesia will relax all muscles). Surgery may be indicated for contracture release and re-positioning limbs into more functional postures, e.g. Z-plasty of tendoachilles in pantarflexion; this needs to be carried out with specialist neurophsyiotherapy and occupational therapy input and follow up.

Heterotopic ossification

This is a condition in which periarticular mature bone forms within muscle; its aetiology remains unclear. It affects 10–15 per cent of those with spinal injury and 5–10 per cent with acquired brain injury. Various theories are postulated including that trauma to the muscle sets up microhaemorrhages which in turn calcify, but this does not account for the existence of this condition in non-traumatic conditions. The leading theory is that there is an abnormal differentiation of myoblasts to osteoblasts and osteoclasts, due to an unknown trigger. Moreover, there is a mismatch of osteoblastic and osteoclastic activity within these abnormal islands of cells which culminates in the laying down of mature lamellar bone within muscles. This occurs around joints and leads to pain, contracture formation, ankylosis and deformity and can hence predispose to pressure sores, and can exacerbate underlying spasticity.

Clinically, heterotopic ossification can be missed in its early stages as it may present with swelling of the muscle, erythema and warmth, so that differential diagnosis includes deep vein thrombosis, septic arthritis, Baker's cyst and phlebitis.

It is associated with raised alkaline phsophatase consistent with osteoclastic activity, C-reactive protein (CRP) consistent with an inflammatory process. Plain x-ray is the first-line radiological investigation and may show early signs of bony change and frank calcification. The 'gold standard' investigation is triple phase bone scan, as the newly forming lamellar bone is highly vascular.

Although the condition cannot be reversed, its progress can be delayed using indometacin and bisphosphonates (etidronate for three to six months). Medication is used with careful physiotherapy, avoiding overaggressive range of movement.

Surgery is relatively contraindicated in the acute phase as there is evidence to suggest that ossification can recur more severely, and surgery if indicated is timed for 12 to 18 months once the mature bone has formed. Radiotherapy has been shown to be effective in the preoperative phase to reduce the bulk of ossification.

Neuropathic bladder and bowel dysfunction

Bladder and bowel function is commonly affected by neurological disease including due to the disruption of pathways connecting higher micturition centres to the spinal cord and end organ. Continence issues can significantly impact on rehabilitation programmes and care needs. Loss of continence can cause secondary complications, such as recurrent infections or pressure sores due to macerated skin. Continence status influences discharge placement and carer input.

Bladder management

The bladder may be overactive, fail to empty completely or a combination of these.

It is important to enquire about symptoms of detrusor hyper-reflexia, and look for signs including charting urinary volumes and patterns, fluid intake and checking post-micturition residual volumes by means of an ultrasound bladder scan. It is important to exclude urinary tract infections via microscopy and culture. Urodynamic studies are organized via urology teams where appropriate.

Management involves a combination of bladder retraining, medication and in some cases, using different forms of catheterization to artificially empty the bladder. There are various methods of bladder retraining for example, **regular toileting** with the assistance of the nursing staff/carers where necessary, every 2 to 3 hours. This accommodates the person who lacks bladder sensation and/or the cognitive ability to independently micturate.

Anticholinergics, such as **oxybutinin** or **detrusitol**, can be trialled in detrusor instability as long as post-micturition residual bladder volumes are less than 100 mL, as these drugs have the risk of causing urinary retention. **Botulinum toxin** is now being used in certain cases, for example in spinal cord injury, to reduce the abnormal activity in high pressure bladders that can cause upper renal tract damage.

The rehabilitation team will work closely with continence nurses and urology specialists to consider the long-term bladder management of patients with neurological disorders. Urethral catheterization is avoided wherever possible, but if the individual is unable to use urinal bottles or access the toilet or commode, an alternative means such as **intermittent self-catheterization** (which relies on reasonable cognition and upper limb function dexterity) can be taught by nursing staff. This is commonly used in those with multiple sclerosis and spinal injury who are at high risk of increased bladder pressures and upper renal tract damage. Of those requiring long-term catheterization, the best method is **suprapubic catheterization**. This has the benefit of reduced risk of infection compared to urethral catheterization, avoids the risk of urinary urethral strictures, and reduces the sensation of discomfort associated with a urethral catheter and may facilitate a return of sexual function.

Bowel management

Constipation is a common complication of neurological disorders and is partly due to the underlying neurological dysfunction, reduced mobility, medication used for pain control (particularly opioids) and bladder management (anticholinergics). Diarrhoea can be a manifestation of faecal loading leading to 'overflow'. This should be avoided by a regularly reviewed bowel regime. There is risk of development of faecal impaction if constipation is inadequately managed.

It is important to review and stop where possible, any contributing medication, ensure good hydration and adequate dietary fibre in diet/gastrostomy feeds, which involves dietician input. The rehabilitation nurses and medical team establish a bowel regime for each individual and take into account the premorbid bowel regime. One example of such a therapeutic bowel regime is:

- The person is taken to the toilet/uses the commode every 2 to 3 hours as with bladder management.
- Prescribe a combination of laxatives, including stimulants (e.g. senna), stool softeners (e.g. sodium docusate) and osmotic laxatives (e.g. movicol).
- Glycerine suppositories and enemas are used after digital rectal examination if indicated.
- It is important to continually review bowel and bladder regime and record events carefully.

Gastroenterological review may be required if there is a persistent abnormality of bowel function or any abnormal symptoms or signs of structural bowel disease. Within the community setting, continence nurse advisers commonly manage both bowel and bladder monitoring in conjunction with the district nurses.

Pressure sores

Individuals with reduced mobility and sensory deficits are at greatly increased risk of skin breakdown, and this can significantly affect their general health and care needs. Skin breakdown may be compounded by other medical co-morbidities, such as diabetes mellitus and poor nutritional status.

Pressure sores are graded according to the depth from epidermis to bone, the deeper sores being associated with an increased risk of osteomyelitis. Once established, severe pressure sores can be extremely slow to heal. A major part of the rehabilitation nursing team's role is to pre-empt and prevent the development of pressure sores. This requires techniques such as daily checks of the skin, turning patients regularly if they are unable to pressure-relieve themselves, for example those with a tetraplegia or dense hemiparesis.

The tissue viability nurse's (TVN) specialist input and involvement of the dietician is vital in the care of these patients.

Established pressure sores need to be aggressively managed, to prevent deterioration. The approach is to limit weight-bearing over the affected area which means reduced sitting times in the wheelchair or bed, and this will limit full participation in the rehabilitation programme and have a severe effect on quality of life.

Cognitive and emotional sequelae managed in rehabilitation settings

Studies show that between 10 and 50 per cent of people following stroke will suffer from depression and 20 per cent from emotional lability. Between 25 and 45 per cent of those post-traumatic brain injury also suffer depression.

> Suicide rates are three times higher in those with traumatic brain injury, but as already mentioned, in some cases this may partly relate to premorbid personality.

The development of depression in this context is multifactorial. There is evidence to suggest that various biochemical changes in neurotransmitters after acquired brain injury contribute to the development of depression. Adjustment reaction to a new disability, the premorbid personality and the nature of family/social support all contribute.

A good psychiatric history and collateral history from family and friends about the individual's premorbid personality can give the team important information about the person's coping strategies and predisposing factors to mood disorders, including psychotic and affective disorders.

It also important to recognize features associated with acquired brain injury, such as apathy (common following frontal injury) or emotional lability that can mimic depression. It can often be difficult to elicit the common somatic symptoms in those with global brain injury and abnormal physical manifestations of emotional disorders.

Validated assessment tools and rating scales need to be administered by key staff, such as a neuropsychologist skilled in the assessment of acquired brain injury. The tools used include Hospital Anxiety and Depression Scale, Beck's Depression Inventory and the Depression Intensity Scale Circles (DISC) which is used in those with aphasia. The objective assessments are collated with the individual's subjective reports, mental state examination, family and team reports of observed interaction and behaviour. It is important to regularly review mood and behaviour and to discuss this at every multidisciplinary meeting.

Many antidepressants can lower seizure threshold; citalopram and sertraline are the commonly used antidepressants in acquired brain injury for depression and emotionalism, as they tend to have less effect on the seizure threshold, but the medical team should remain vigilant for seizures.

The general guidance is to continue medication for six months and then review.

Maladaptive challenging behaviour is a common feature after traumatic brain injury and in some patients with stroke, and needs to be managed using a behavioural management approach in conjunction with the psychiatry team.

Sociological impact of neurological disorders

Complex neurological disorders not only have an impact on the person with the disease/injury but also on their family, carers, working environment and social network. Altered family dynamics, for example, spouses becoming carers, can put a strain on relationships and it is unsurprising that studies have shown divorce rates 25 per cent higher than the national average in couples where one partner has had a traumatic brain injury. The burden on carers can be great, particularly on those involved in looking after those with challenging behaviour.

Voluntary support groups are a vital source of support of education, and peer support both for individuals and their families. Links can be made with these groups while the patients are in hospital and they can attend groups from here and once home.

Such groups include the **Stroke Association**, **Headway** (the national charity for a brain injury), **Different Strokes** (for the younger stroke survivors), **Connect** (providing support for those with aphasia), and the **Spinal Injuries Association** (which provides peer-support which can reach both into hospital and community settings). These groups, working alongside occupational therapists, can also provide support and advice to employers.

A significant number of those affected by neurological disorders (multiple sclerosis, spinal injury, cerebral palsy, traumatic brain injury) are working-age adults and this has an ongoing impact on the workforce and economy. Those with neurological disorders can be supported in their return to work by occupational therapists, the disability employment adviser based at Jobcentre Plus, together with occupational health teams and the employer, and Access to Work schemes. There are interagency guidelines for vocational assessment of rehabilitation after acquired brain injury and these were written as a partnership between the Jobcentre Plus, the Royal College of Physicians and British Society of Neurorehabilitation in 2004. This document is a useful guide to the processes involved and details the organizations that support people with acquired brain injury.

The community occupational therapist and clinical psychologists are particularly integral in the assessment and reintegration of those with disability back into employment, liaising with employers and relevant agencies to support people back into some form of graded work initially.

Some individuals may wish to re-enter the work arena by doing voluntary work. The occupational therapist, rehabilitation physician and general practitioners are involved in advising employers on the optimal reintegration into work, in conjunction with the specialist input of the individual's occupational health team. This would commonly involve the person returning to work in a graded fashion and adaptations made in a work environment in conjunction with the Access to Work scheme.

The Disability Discrimination Act 1995 defines a disabled person as anyone with a physical or mental impairment of substantial and long-term effect greater than one year, on his or her ability to perform day-to-day activities, and exists to protect those with disabilities from any cause.

FURTHER READING

TEXTBOOKS

Greenwood R, Barnes MP, McMillan TM, Ward CD (eds) (2003) *Handbook of Neurological Rehabilitation*. London: Psychology Press.

Lance JW (1980) Symposium synopsis. In: Feldman RG, Young RR, Koella WP (eds). *Spasticity: Disordered Motor Control*. Chicago: Year Book Medical.

Losseff N (ed.) (2004) Neurological Rehabilitation of Stroke (Queen Square Neurological Rehabilitation Series). London: Taylor Francis.

Stevenson V, Thompson A, Jarrett L (2006) *Spasticity Management – A Practical Multidisciplinary Guide.* London: Informa Press.

POLICY DOCUMENTS AND PAPERS

Department of Health (2005) Supporting people with long term conditions – NHS and social care. London: Department of Health.

Department of Health (2006) Supporting people with long term conditions to self care: A guide to developing local strategies and good practice. London: Department of Health.

Royal College of Physicians, British Society of Rehabilitation Medicine and British Geriatrics Society (2005) Concise Guidance to Good Practice. Use of antidepressant medication adults undergoing recovery and rehabilitation following acquired brain injury. National Guidelines No. 4. London: Royal College of Physicians.

Royal College of Physicians, the National Council of Palliative Care and British Society of Neurorehabilitation (2008) Concise Guidance to Good Practice. Long-term neurological conditions: management at the interface between neurology, rehabilitation and palliative care. London: Royal College of Physicians.

Frank AO, Thurgood J (2006) Vocational rehabilitation in the UK: opportunities for the health-care professionals. *International Journal of Therapy in Rehabilitation*, 13:126–132.

Royal College of Physicians and British Society of Rehabilitation Medicine (2003) National Clinical Guidelines. Rehabilitation following acquired brain injury. London: Royal College of Physicians.

PATIENT PERSPECTIVE LITERATURE

Bauby JD (2008) *The Diving-Bell and The Butterfly.* London: Harper (portrayal of locked-in syndrome).

McCrum R, Lyall S (1998) *My Year Off: Recovering Life After a Stroke.* New York: WW Norton.

USEFUL WEBSITES/JOURNALS

British Society Neurorehabilitation. Available from: www.bsrm.co.uk.

CHAPTER 25

INFECTIONS OF THE CENTRAL NERVOUS SYSTEM

Nick Davies

INTRODUCTION

In the resource-rich world, infections of the central nervous system (CNS) are rare but serious conditions; however, worldwide their cumulative morbidity and mortality is considerable. It is estimated that each year 15 000 individuals die from Japanese encephalitis in Southeast Asia; 100 000 die from tetanus worldwide and in sub-Saharan Africa between 350 000 and 560 000 children die from *Haemophilus influenzae* or *Streptococcus pneumoniae* meningitis.

Microbes can cause CNS dysfunction through a variety of direct and indirect mechanisms. Classical infection of the CNS occurs through microbial invasion of CNS tissue. However, inflammation of the CNS can occur as a remote consequence of infection; an example being the encephalitis that follows shortly after symptomatic measles infection in a minority of children. Features of inflammation without detection of measles virus in the CNS characterize the encephalitis histopathologically and it is thought to occur through virus-triggered,

immune-mediated mechanisms. Such conditions are often termed **parainfectious** or **post–infectious**. Other infections that occur outside the CNS can cause disease through the **action of a toxin**, such as occurs in botulism or tetanus. In clinical practice, the most commonly encountered infection-associated CNS dysfunction is **septic encephalopathy**. Severe systemic infection, particularly at the extremes of age, is associated with a spectrum of neurological symptoms ranging from mild disorientation or confusion to coma. Usually the neurological symptoms resolve quickly upon treatment of the underlying source of sepsis.

The CNS differs from most other organs of the body through being protected by the blood–brain barrier, which limits the passage of both cells and molecules. Furthermore, the CNS differs immunologically, often being described as 'immunologically quiet'. While there is routine surveillance of the CNS by activated T-lymphocytes there is low expression of the proteins for antigen presentation and high constitutive expression of factors with anti-inflammatory effects.

For a microbe to cause infection of the CNS it must have the requisite properties to access the CNS, to infect cells or tissues, and to cause disease. These factors respectively are named **neuroinvasiveness, neurotropism and neurovirulence**, and are best illustrated by viral CNS infections. Routes of access to the CNS include the haematogenous, neural and contiguous. Typically, bacterial infections gain access to the CNS after systemic infection via the circulation but on occasions, such as following mastoiditis or a tooth abscess, contiguous spread occurs. Some viral infections, for example mumps virus, enter the CNS via the circulation and choroid plexus, but others such as herpes simplex virus (HSV) are thought to use neuronal carriage. The cell types within the CNS that viruses are able to infect (i.e. for which they have tropism) dictate patterns of disease. For example, **poliovirus** has a specific tropism for anterior horn cells; consequently, infection can cause flaccid lower motor neurone weakness without sensory signs. Similarly, many of the **flaviviruses** can infect the anterior horn cells causing a poliomyelitis-like syndrome, but in addition they have a tropism for the basal ganglia and may manifest signs of hypo- or hyperkinetic movement disorders. The factors accounting for why a microbe can cause an innocuous infection in one individual and a devastating neurological infection in another are ill understood. Host, microbe neurovirulence and stochastic factors are likely to be important.

> The common syndromes of CNS infection are **meningitis**, when inflammation is confined to the subarachnoid space and meninges; and **encephalitis**, where the brunt of the inflammation is borne by the brain itself.

Some features of the other frequently accompany either syndrome, but for ease of discussion they are usually considered as separate entities. Neurological infections may present as acute, subacute or chronic neurological syndromes. Clinical assessment of patients with suspected CNS infections require careful history taking. Particular care should be taken to document the patient's risk factors for immunocompromise, vaccination history, travel, contact and vector exposure histories. During physical examination, care should be taken to seek evidence of meningeal irritation, rashes, lymphadenopathy and organomegaly.

MENINGITIS

Meningitis is divided into acute and chronic forms. The clinical features of acute meningitis develop over hours or days; those of chronic meningitis over weeks or months.

> One of the cornerstones of the management of meningitis is the speedy recognition of those cases that require the prompt initiation of appropriate antibiotic therapy.

Most such urgent cases are a result of acute bacterial infections and characteristically the cellular response in the cerebrospinal fluid (CSF) is predominantly polymorphs, producing purulent meningitis. The other traditional group of meningitis cases are those where the CSF pleocytosis is predominantly lymphocytes. Although most of the latter group have a viral aetiology, there are a number of other treatable causes that should always be considered.

Initial assessment of the patient

Meningitis from whatever cause is characterized by:
- Headache, often severe and described as bursting in nature, and worsened by jolt accentuation (turning the head horizontally two or three times/second)
- Fever
- Photophobia
- Nausea and vomiting
- Spinal muscle spasm, detected by neck stiffness and positive Kernig's sign (pain from hamstring spasm provoked by attempting to extend the knee with the hip flexed)
- In severe bacterial meningitis, there may also be cerebral oedema and raised intracranial pressure leading to confusion or declining consciousness and seizures.

> Some or all of such classical features of meningitis are found in nearly 90 per cent of patients with bacterial meningitis but, in some patients, notably neonates and infants, immunocompromised patients and the very old, the signs are

often much more subtle. In neonates, apathy, irritability, lethargy, a strange cry and refusal to feed may be the only features. In the elderly or immunocompromised patient, fever and confusion may develop without any specific evidence of meningeal irritation and be mistakenly ascribed to some concomitant illness or other infection.

Once the possibility of meningitis has been recognized, then the next step depends upon an assessment of the patient's condition and the speed of progression of the illness (Figure 25.1). Most patients will not have any specific clinical findings and will have experienced symptoms for more than 24 hours by the time they are first seen by a doctor. Any of the organisms listed in Table 25.1 may be responsible for the illness in this group and a decision regarding therapy depends upon the results of lumbar puncture (LP). In contrast, about **25 per cent of patients with bacterial meningitis will have a very acute and rapidly progressive illness**. In these cases, whatever the time course of their illness, in neonates, and in those with a rash suggestive of meningococcal infection, then providing an initial brief examination fails to reveal papilloedema or focal neurological signs, an LP, blood cultures, an EDTA blood sample for polymerase chain reaction (PCR) (and a coagulation screen for those with possible meningococcaemia) should be obtained and empirical therapy directed at the likely pathogens started before the CSF result is available (see below under Investigations).

Papilloedema and focal neurological signs are found in <1 per cent of cases of meningitis at initial presentation and should prompt an

Table 25.1 The predominant microbial causes of meningitis

		Pathogen
Acute meningitis	Common pathogens	Neisseria meningitidis
		Streptococcus pneumoniae
		Haemophilus influenzae
		Enteroviruses
		Herpes simplex viruses types 1 and 2
		Varicella zoster virus
	Rarer causes	Listeria monocytogenes
		Staphylococci
		Mycobacterium tuberculosis
		Gram-negative bacilli
		Leptospira
		HIV
		Other viruses
	In the newborn	Escherichia coli
		Other Gram-negative bacilli
		Group B streptococci
		Listeria monocytogenes
Chronic meningitis		Mycobacterium tuberculosis
		Borrelia burgdorferi (Lyme disease)
		Brucella species
		Treponema pallidum
		Leptospira
		Cryptococcus neoformans
		Other fungi
		Parasites

HIV, human immunodeficiency virus.

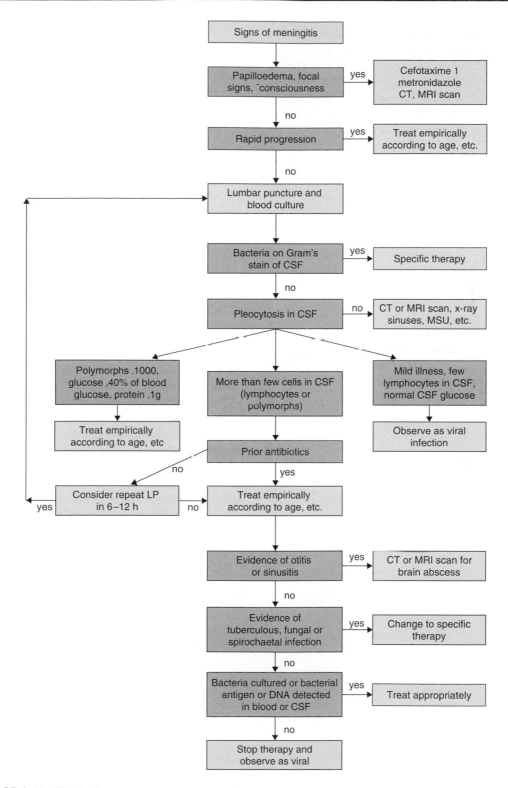

Figure 25.1 Algorithm for the management of acute meningitis. LP, lumbar puncture; MSU, midstream urine test.

urgent search for an intracranial space-occupying lesion by computed tomography (CT) scan or magnetic resonance imaging (MRI) before LP can be contemplated. In addition, imaging before LP is recommended in patients with new onset seizures, an immunocompromised state, or moderate-to-severe impairment of consciousness. Immediate treatment with antibiotics is recommended for those patients where the LP is delayed in order that imaging is performed first. The microscopic and biochemical examination of the CSF will usually give a clear indication of the type of organism causing the meningitis (Table 25.2), but there is a good deal of overlap between the findings in the various categories. A Gram's stain of the CSF is mandatory in all cases.

Acute bacterial meningitis

Epidemiology

The annual incidence of bacterial meningitis is between 4 and 6/100 000 adults, but the incidence is highest in the first month of life and nearly 75 per cent of sporadic cases occur in children under 15 years old.

Almost any bacterium is capable of causing meningitis but, for many species, this is only as part of a generalized illness. There are, however, a few bacteria that consistently cause meningitis as a primary manifestation of disease (Table 25.1) and, in most instances, the likely aetiology of purulent meningitis can be further narrowed down by a consideration of the patient's age and previous health (Table 25.3).

Pathophysiology

In most cases of bacterial meningitis, the immediate source of the pathogen is the nasopharynx; the bacteria colonize the mucosal surfaces and then cross the epithelium and spread via the bloodstream to the choroid plexus where they cross the blood–brain barrier into the subarachnoid space. The principal pathogens are capsulated bacteria and the capsule enables them to counter phagocytosis and complement-mediated bactericidal activity in the bloodstream, but the major factors that facilitate meningeal invasion are poorly understood.

The inflammatory response that begins in the subarachnoid space within a few hours of bacterial arrival has profound effects. Bacterial products trigger the release of inflammatory cytokines that upregulate adhesion molecules on endothelial cells and promote granulocyte penetration into the CSF, leading to release of further inflammatory mediators. Vascular permeability causes vasogenic cerebral oedema: cellular damage induced by toxins released from bacteria and granulocytes results in

Table 25.2 Lumbar puncture findings in meningitis of different aetiologies

	Normal	Acute bacterial meningitis	Viral meningitis	Tuberculous meningitis
Appearance	Clear	Turbid/purulent	Clear/opalescent	Clear/opalescent
Pressure	<21 cmH2O	>21 cmH2O	<21 cmH2O	Usually >21 cmH2O
Cells	0–5/mm^3	5–2000/mm^3	5–500/mm^3	5–1000/mm^3
Polymorphs	0	>50%	<50%	<50%
Glucose	2.2–3.3 mmol/L[a]	Low (<40% of blood concentration)	Normal[b]	Low (<40% of blood concentration)
Protein	<0.4 g/L	Often >0.9 g/L	0.4–0.9 g/L	Often >1 g/L
Other tests		Bacteria on Gram's stain	Viral nucleic acid by PCR	Bacteria on Ziehl-Neelsen or fluorescent stain
		Bacterial DNA by PCR		

[a]Approximately 60% of blood concentration.
[b]May be low in mumps meningitis.
PCR, polymerase chain reaction.

Table 25.3 Principal causes of purulent meningitis under specific circumstances

Historical data	Organism
Age	
Neonate	Group B streptococcus, *Escherichia coli*, Listeria
Under 6 years old	Meningococcus, Pneumococcus, *Haemophilus influenzae*
6–50 years old	Meningococcus, Pneumococcus
Over 50 years old	Pneumococcus, Listeria
Co-morbidity	
Diabetes mellitus	Pneumococcus, Gram-negative bacilli, Staphylococci
Alcoholism	Pneumococcus, Listeria
Asplenism	Pneumococcus
Critical-care patient	Gram-negative bacilli, *Staphylococcus aureus*
Intracranial shunt	Staphylococci, Gram-negative bacilli
Immunosuppression	Listeria
Pregnancy	Listeria
Associated findings	
Petechial	Meningococcus purpuric rash
Otitis, sinusitis	Pneumococcus, anaerobes
Pneumonia	Pneumococcus, Meningococcus
Neurosurgery	Gram-negative bacilli, staphylococci
CSF leak	Pneumococcus
Other factors	
Recurrent	Pneumococcus

CSF, cerebrospinal fluid.

Investigations

The diagnosis of bacterial meningitis is made by culturing the blood and by examination of the CSF (Table 25.2). **A difficult dilemma arises when the CSF examination suggests a bacterial cause (Table 25.2), but no organism can be seen on a Gram stain.** This often results from outpatient antibiotic therapy, which has partially treated the bacterial meningitis; viral meningitis, however, is also associated with polymorphs in the CSF during the first few hours of infection and occasionally it also produces a reduced glucose level, particularly when caused by mumps virus. Distinguishing between the two is not always easy.

The PCR may be used to amplify meningococcal DNA and may enable a more specific diagnosis to be made earlier than the culture results or when prior antibiotics have been used. However, care should be taken when interpreting the results of latex bacterial antigen CSF tests as these may give false-positive results and their sensitivity is only comparable to that of Gram's stain. In acute meningitis, the finding of a CSF lactate level of ≥3.5 mmol/L is highly suggestive of a pyogenic aetiology. Post-neurosurgery, a CSF lactate ≥4.0 mmol/L is suggestive of bacterial infection as opposed to a chemical meningitis and has greater diagnostic specificity in this setting than elevation in CSF white cell count or fall in the CSF plasma glucose ratio.

Treatment

The treatment of bacterial meningitis requires the prompt administration of antibiotics that achieve high levels in the CSF. This requires parenteral administration.

loss of cellular homeostasis and development of cytotoxic oedema.

The purulent exudate obstructs the normal flow of the CSF and reduces CSF reabsorption by the arachnoid villi; hence hydrocephalus (obstructive or communicating) is produced. Vasculitis and thrombosis of the superficial meningeal vessels cause major changes in cerebral perfusion and, ultimately, infarction.

Furthermore, the penetration of most antibiotics is proportional to the degree of meningeal inflammation and therefore the dose should generally not be reduced as irritation diminishes and the patient improves. Except in neonates and certain other special instances (see below), in the UK the vast majority of cases of bacterial meningitis are caused by pneumococci and meningococci. The antibiotic regimens discussed incorporate current recommendations for the UK. However, anti-microbial resistance patterns evolve and vary across the globe. Therefore, physicians are urged to acquaint themselves with local antimicrobial guidelines and patterns of bacterial resistance.

For patients presenting with bacterial meningitis acquired within the UK, a **third-generation cephalosporin** (in adults intravenous cefotaxime (2 g every 6 hours) or ceftriaxone (2 g every 12 hours)) is suitable empirical therapy against these two pathogens. However, in many parts of the world (such as North America, Africa and Spain), the rates of penicillin-resistant pneumococcus are much higher and the combination of **vancomycin** with a **third-generation cephalosporin** is advised. If the patient is aged over 50 years or has specific risk factors for **Listeria monocytogenes** meningitis (see Table 25.3) then **ampicillin** should be added. Chloramphenicol with or without vancomycin can be given to the patient with a history of anaphylaxis from β-lactam antibiotics.

Dexamethasone, given 10–15 minutes before or with the first dose of antibiotics, has been shown to reduce the neurological sequelae from childhood meningitis caused by *H. influenzae* or *Streptococcus pneumoniae*. In adults with bacterial meningitis, dexamethasone reduces the risk of unfavourable outcome and halves mortality.

> Therefore, empirical administration of **dexamethasone** (0.15 mg/kg every 6 hours for 4 days) is recommended in all cases of presumed bacterial meningitis in children over 6 weeks of age and similarly for adults without evidence of immunocompromise.

General supportive measures are also important and some patients will require fluid replacement, anti-emetics, anticonvulsants and treatment of raised intracranial pressure.

Fever usually settles within a few days and any recurrence of pyrexia during antibiotic therapy is likely to be caused by drug fever, subdural effusion or empyema, thrombophlebitis (cerebral or leg vein), or an unrelated infection.

Outcome

> Overall, there is a mortality of about 5 per cent from bacterial meningitis and 16 per cent of survivors have at least one major adverse outcome (severe intellectual disability, spasticity, paresis, epilepsy, deafness) when assessed two years

later. More subtle long-term complications, particularly cognitive and behavioural impairment in childhood, are common following bacterial meningitis in infancy.

Particular forms of bacterial meningitis

Neisseria meningitidis (meningococcus)

Epidemiology

There are 13 different serogroups of this Gram-negative diplococcus, six of which are associated with severe invasive disease. It is the most common cause of bacterial meningitis in the UK, occurring most frequently in the winter months. Group B is the most common serogroup seen in the UK; smaller numbers of groups A, C and W 135 are reported. A dramatic reduction in serogroup C meningococcal disease was seen in the UK following the introduction conjugate serogroup C vaccine. Groups A and C dominate in the developing world. Meningococcal disease may occur at any age, but is predominantly found in children and young adults. Occasionally, small clusters of cases occur in susceptible populations and in parts of sub-Saharan Africa large epidemics of type A occur annually.

Clinical features

The organism is carried asymptomatically in the nasopharynx and is transmitted by droplets. The incidence of carriage is about 10 per cent of the general population (25–37 per cent in those 15–24 years old) but only occasionally is acquisition followed by bacteraemia and meningitis. **There are two different forms of meningococcal disease. There is always a bacteraemic phase and in some patients this leads to fulminant meningococcal septicaemia (FMS), often without meningeal involvement, within a few hours. In others, the bacteraemia is initially controlled and meningitis develops over a period of 18–36 hours.**

The bacteraemic phase is usually heralded by an abrupt onset of fever, chills and myalgia. Generalized vasculitis, resulting from disseminated intravascular coagulation and consumption coagulopathy, is a hallmark of meningococcal disease.

The visual manifestation of this is skin haemorrhages: two-thirds of patients have a rash (characteristically petechial or purpuric (Figure 25.2), but erythematous and macular in the early stages). Widespread skin lesions, disseminated intravascular coagulation, adrenal haemorrhages, circulatory collapse and rapid progression to multi-organ failure, coma and death characterize FMS. **This is the Waterhouse–Friderichsen syndrome.** Metastatic infection in the joints, pericardium and lungs may also occur.

Mortality from FMS is 20–70 per cent (often in the first 24 hours) and limb amputations are necessary in many survivors. The prognosis in cases of meningococcal meningitis without circulatory collapse is excellent; the mortality is 1–5 per cent and neurological complications are infrequent. Immunologically mediated complications, notably reactive arthritis, pericarditis and fever sometimes appear 10–14 days after the onset of the disease.

Investigations

Consideration of the possibility of meningococcal disease is required in all patients with fever and a rash and antibiotics should be administered without delay to those in whom the clinical suspicion is high. Demonstrating *N. meningitidis* in the CSF or blood makes the diagnosis; but previous antibiotics may reduce the yield and PCR testing or antigen detection may be used for confirmation.

Treatment

Treatment is intravenous with a third-generation cephalosporin (cefotaxime or ceftriaxone) given for 5–7 days. Chloramphenicol (15–25 mg/kg bodyweight 6-hourly) should be used in patients with a history of an anaphylactic reaction to penicillin.

There is no convincing evidence of any specific benefit from steroids, heparin, fresh frozen plasma (FFP), plasmapheresis or leukopheresis for FMS. However, use of activated recombinant protein C is recommended in adults with septicaemia and multiple organ failure. Patients should be isolated for the first 24 hours of treatment.

Prevention

Close contacts of the patient within the previous 7 days (household, daycare and 'kissing' contacts) are at a 1000-fold increased risk of cross-infection and all such contacts should be given rifampicin (600 mg those >12 years; 10 mg/kg for 1–12 year olds; and 5 mg/kg if <1 year) twice daily for 2 days to eliminate the organism from the nasopharynx. A single dose of ciprofloxacin (500 mg) or ofloxacin (400 mg) may be used when a large number of adolescents or adults require prophylaxis. Unconjugated polysaccharide vaccines are available against meningococci of groups A, C, W 135 and Y, but not group B. In the UK, a conjugate vaccine against serotype C is now part of the childhood vaccination schedule. Documented vaccination with the combined A, C, Y and W 135 vaccine is required for travellers to the annual Haj to Mecca.

Streptococcus pneumoniae (pneumococcus)

Epidemiology

Individuals are at increased risk of this important form of meningitis at the two extremes of age. Other predispositions to infection include splenic

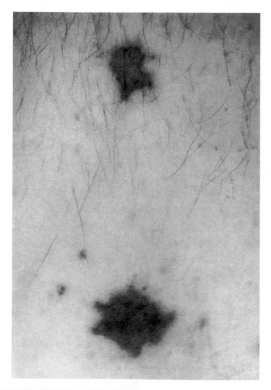

Figure 25.2 Photograph of the rash of meningococcal meningitis.

dysfunction (including sickle-cell disease), alcoholism, abnormal humoral immunity (e.g. patients with multiple myeloma) and CSF leaks following skull fractures. Repeated attacks may occur. In half the cases, the source of infection cannot be determined and meningitis is presumed to follow primary bacteraemia from nasopharyngeal colonization; in others, it is associated with pneumonia or infection in the middle ear or paranasal sinuses.

Symptoms and signs

Pneumococcal meningitis is often the most severe of the common forms of meningitis, with coma and seizures frequently developing early in its course.

Neurological complications (venous sinus thrombosis, hemiplegia, ventriculitis, hydrocephalus) are frequent after pneumococcal meningitis and the mortality remains between 20 and 40 per cent.

Treatment

Antibiotic resistance has modified recommendations for the empirical therapy of suspected pneumococcal meningitis. The frequency of **penicillin resistance** in pneumococci is increasing in many countries; it is 10 per cent in some areas of the UK, more than 25 per cent in some US centres and Iceland and more than 50 per cent in South Africa and Spain. **Cefotaxime or ceftriaxone** can be used to treat most such strains and are now recommended for empirical therapy. **Vancomycin with or without rifampicin** is needed for treatment of meningitis caused by a cephalosporin-resistant strain.

> Susceptibility testing must be performed for all isolates of *S. pneumoniae* from CSF and blood and, in areas where cephalosporin resistance is reported, all patients with presumed pneumococcal meningitis should receive high-dose cefotaxime (or ceftriaxone) plus vancomycin until the isolate is proved susceptible to penicillin or cephalosporins. Treatment should be continued for 10 days or 2 weeks.

In the UK, routine vaccination is recommended, using the 23-valent polysaccharide vaccine, of all those aged 65 years or over and younger adults or children aged over two years who are immunosuppressed or have chronic diseases. The UK childhood vaccination programme ensures children under two years receive the 7-valent conjugate vaccine, which since its introduction has led to a 50 per cent decrease in childhood invasive pneumococcal disease.

Haemophilus influenzae

Epidemiology

Bacterial meningitis caused by *Haemophilus influenzae* is almost exclusively a disease of children between the ages of four months and six years and is caused primarily by capsulated, type b strains of the small, Gram-negative bacillus. Although there has been a 90 per cent decline in the incidence of *H. influenzae* meningitis in many countries since the introduction of conjugate *H. influenzae* type b vaccines, there are still 400 000 cases annually in the developing world.

Symptoms and signs

> Meningitis is often a complication of a primary respiratory or ear infection, which is frequently acquired from another family member with a similar illness, and begins insidiously with drowsiness or irritability. Inappropriate antidiuretic hormone secretion, deafness, cortical vein thrombosis and sterile subdural effusions are common complications. The latter may require repeated aspiration or surgical drainage.

Treatment

Cefotaxime or ceftriaxone are the antibiotics of choice; **ampicillin resistance** is common among *H. influenzae* and ampicillin should only be used once the organism is known to be sensitive. The duration of therapy should be for 10 days. In the resource-poor world, the mortality is nearly 30 per cent and another 30 per cent have major sequelae.

Prevention

The polysaccharide vaccine against *H. influenzae* type b is given to infants in the UK and in many other resource-rich countries. Unvaccinated household, playgroup or nursery school contacts under the age of five years are at increased risk of secondary disease and rifampicin prophylaxis (600 mg (20 mg/kg bodyweight) daily for 4 days) should be given to all family members if there is such a young child in the house, and is recommended for all attendees and staff of playgroups, etc.

Neonatal meningitis

Epidemiology

Meningitis in the newborn is a serious problem, with a high mortality and morbidity. In the UK, its incidence is about 1/2500 live births and it is particularly seen in low birthweight and premature infants (below 2.5 kg). The organisms that are responsible are chiefly **group B streptococci and Escherichia coli**, particularly strains carrying the K1 capsular antigen. Other less common organisms include *L. monocytogenes, Pseudomonas aeruginosa* and *Staphylococcus aureus*. Although the majority of infecting bacteria arise from the mother's genital tract and colonize the infant during birth, others are introduced from environmental sites as a result of invasive procedures.

Symptoms and signs

The classical features of meningitis are often absent in the newborn and the signs are usually non-specific. Fever, poor feeding, lethargy, apathy and irritability may predominate. Diarrhoea, apnoea, respiratory distress or jaundice may suggest disease of another system and brief tonic spasms may not be recognized as convulsions. Neck stiffness is rare and the diagnosis of neonatal meningitis requires a high index of suspicion.

Meningitis caused by group B streptococci presents in two distinct ways, depending upon its time of onset after birth:

1 **Early onset** (first week of life). This is frequently associated with prematurity or obstetric complications and the organism is from the maternal birth canal. The infant has a fulminant illness with a high mortality. Septicaemia and respiratory symptoms (often confused with respiratory distress syndrome) are prominent.
2 **Late onset** (after the first week of life). This is a more insidious illness, with meningitis a prominent feature and a mortality of only about 15 per cent. Infection is often acquired from hospital personnel or equipment.

Investigations

The diagnosis of neonatal meningitis depends upon the CSF findings, but it should be remembered that in the neonate, normal CSF has up to 30 cells/mm^3 (often neutrophils) and a protein concentration up to 1.5 g/L.

Treatment

The treatment usually recommended for neonatal meningitis is immediate empirical administration of a combination of **ampicillin and gentamicin**. The penetration of aminoglycosides into the CSF is variable and levels should be measured. An alternative is to use cefotaxime, which penetrate well into the CSF and are effective against most of the likely organisms when combined with ampicillin. For premature neonates, a combination of vancomycin and ceftazidime (to cover staphylococci and *P. aeruginosa*) can be used empirically. Treatment can be modified upon the basis of Gram's stain or culture of the CSF.

The prognosis of neonatal meningitis remains poor, particularly in premature infants, with mortality of 10–30 per cent; neurological and cognitive sequelae are found in one-third of the survivors.

Other types of purulent meningitis

Shunt-associated meningitis

Historically, up to 25 per cent of patients with ventriculoatrial or ventriculoperitoneal shunts for hydrocephalus developed meningitis, although more contemporary studies show an infection rate between 5 and 10 per cent. Risk factors for infection include: postoperative CSF leak, the presence of intraventricular haemorrhage, young age, shunting for neurocysticercosis, site of drainage, breach of sterile field and operator experience.

Most cases are caused by **coagulase-negative staphylococci**; many of the remainder are the result of infection with *Staphylococcus aureus* or Gram-negative bacilli. The route of infection is usually by direct inoculation at the time of shunt implantation and 70 per cent of infections occur in the two months after surgery. Diagnosis relies upon culture of the organism from CSF or blood. CSF obtained from the shunt has the highest rate of positive culture. Unfortunately, CSF white cell count and protein levels are less diagnostically helpful as these are often elevated following the surgical intervention. Systemic and intraventricular therapy with antibiotics (intraventricular vancomycin and systemic rifampicin for staphylococci and an aminoglycoside with or without a cephalosporin, or meropenin, for aerobic Gram-negative bacilli) must often be combined with removal of the shunt and temporary external ventricular drainage.

Gram-negative enteric bacilli

Other than during the neonatal period, meningitis caused by Gram-negative enteric bacilli is primarily seen in patients with head injuries, alcoholics, elderly diabetics and those who have had neurosurgery. Therapy should be with a third-generation cephalosporin (e.g. cefotaxime or ceftazidime) until the responsible organism and its antibiotic sensitivity are known.

Listeria monocytogenes

Meningitis from *Listeria monocytogenes* infection is chiefly a disease of neonates or pregnant, debilitated or immunocompromised adults (especially recipients of renal transplants).

The organism is a Gram-positive bacillus, but as it is motile it may appear coccoid on Gram's stain and not infrequently is mistaken for pneumococcus. Meningitis or a diffuse or focal meningoencephalitis, with predilection for the brain stem, may occur and, despite the name of the organism, polymorphs usually predominate in the CSF. Ampicillin, given for 3 weeks with or without gentamicin, is the best therapy. Co-trimoxazole should be used in penicillin-allergic patients.

Lymphocytic meningitis

Lymphocytic meningitis
If examination of the CSF shows an excessive number of lymphocytes and a raised protein but no organisms are seen on Gram's stain, then the likeliest cause is a viral infection. There are, however, other causes of this CSF picture and many of them require specific therapy. These other possibilities must, therefore, always be considered before assuming that the illness is viral in aetiology (Figure 25.1).

Tuberculous meningitis

Epidemiology

Tuberculous meningitis can occur at any age, affecting approximately 1 per cent of patients with active tuberculosis (TB). In children or adolescents, it is usually a manifestation of primary tuberculosis, but in adults it is frequently the result of rupture into the subarachnoid space of a subependymal tubercle that has lain quiescent for many years. Risk factors include HIV, alcoholism, diabetes mellitus, malignancy and treatment with immunosuppressive agents: particularly corticosteroids and drugs that block the action of tumour necrosis factor.

Symptoms and signs

The clinical presentation is very variable and depends upon a number of factors: the thick meningeal exudate, vasculitis, cerebral oedema and the presence of tuberculomas. **The illness often begins with a period of general ill health and malaise, which lasts for a week or two before, a slowly progressive headache and signs of meningitis appear.** Changes in consciousness and focal neurological signs, particularly sixth cranial nerve palsies, then develop. Seizures are far more common in children than adults. Fever is recorded in only 40–60 per cent of patients by the time of presentation.

Investigations

Diagnosis can be confirmed in 10–20 per cent of cases by finding *Mycobacterium tuberculosis* in the CSF on Ziehl–Neelsen stains (in adults at least 6 mL of CSF should be examined for mycobacteria), but treatment often has to be given on suspicion when the other CSF results, particularly the glucose level, are suggestive (Table 25.2). In children, the chest x-ray often shows evidence of pulmonary tuberculosis, but in adults is often normal. However, the presence of features of miliary tuberculosis on a chest x-ray is strongly supportive evidence for tuberculous meningitis. The Mantoux test is negative in at least 50 per cent of cases of CNS TB and a similar sensitivity is found with interferon gamma release assays. CSF PCR tests to detect *M. tuberculosis* should be performed, but although specific are insensitive and cannot be used to rule out the diagnosis. CSF mycobacterial culture remains the gold standard laboratory test. CT and MRI brain scans frequently demonstrate enhancement of the basal meninges often accompanied by hydrocephalus. Tuberculomas often develop during treatment, but are usually asymptomatic unless they affect an eloquent area of the CNS. All patients with suspected CNS tuberculosis should be tested for HIV.

Treatment

In the UK, four anti-tuberculous drugs are advised for the treatment of tuberculous meningitis. The two anti-tuberculous drugs that attain the best CSF levels, pyrazinamide and isoniazid, are given together with rifampicin and ethambutol, for the first two months. Treatment is then continued with isoniazid and rifampicin for a further ten months. Patients receiving ethambutol should be monitored for drug-induced optic neuropathy. Pyridoxine must also be given to prevent isoniazid toxicity. All patients with tuberculous meningitis should receive adjunctive steroids. In adults with coma, a daily dose of dexamethasone (0.4 mg/kg per day to a maximum of 24 mg tapered over 8 weeks) or without coma (0.3 mg/kg per day to a maximum of 24 mg tapered over 6 weeks) should be used.

Most patients will recover completely if therapy is started before the level of consciousness is reduced, but some will develop hydrocephalus, spinal arachnoiditis, and cerebral infarctions – particularly affecting the middle cerebral artery. Therefore, the patient needs to be closely monitored during the early stages of therapy, with frequent CSF examinations and CT scanning to detect progressive changes. **Even with early diagnosis the mortality is 10 per cent and another 10–30 per cent of cases have residual neurological damage.**

Cryptococcal meningitis

Epidemiology

Meningitis caused by the yeast *Cryptococcus neoformans* is usually seen in patients whose cellular immunity is depressed by steroids, diabetes, lymphoproliferative disorders or the acquired immunodeficiency syndrome (AIDS) (see Chapter 26).

The organism is widely distributed in nature and infection is acquired by inhalation. Normal hosts are able to contain the infection in the lungs, but in those with abnormal T-lymphocyte function, dissemination to the meninges and other organs is frequent. Increasingly another species of Cryptococcus – *C. gatti* – is recognized to cause severe fungal meningitis among the immunocompetent.

Symptoms and signs

The symptoms of cryptococcal meningitis tend to be intermittent over several weeks and meningism is less common than fever, confusion, memory loss and depressed consciousness. Visual disturbances and cranial nerve palsies may be present.

Investigations

The organism may be seen in the CSF using either Gram's stain or an India ink preparation, but **the most accurate diagnostic test is the detection of cryptococcal antigen in the** CSF **or blood** using latex agglutination or enzyme-linked immunosorbent assay.

Treatment

Patients who are acutely ill with cryptococcal meningitis should be treated with intravenous **amphotericin B combined with 5-flucytosine.** Recommended drug doses and duration of therapy vary dependent upon whether the patient is co-infected with HIV. In HIV-negative patients, treatment usually needs to be continued for at least 6 weeks, during which time the CSF should become sterile to culture. In all patients, a consolidation phase of therapy then follows with oral **fluconazole.** Patients are at particular risk of development of communicating hydrocephalus and should be carefully monitored for headache and papilloedema. Those that have CSF opening pressures >25 cm of water should have repeat lumbar punctures to control intracranial pressure.

Parameningeal suppuration

A suppurative process adjacent to the meninges (see below) may be associated with the CSF changes of aseptic meningitis – a history of sinusitis or ear infection should suggest the possibility and indicates the need for a CT scan.

Spirochaetal infection

Leptospirosis

Leptospirosis is a biphasic illness contracted from mammals and is typically a disease of agricultural or abattoir workers. Initially, there is a systemic illness with chills, conjunctivitis and *Leptospira* in blood and CSF. Lymphocytic meningitis, often in conjunction with abnormal liver and kidney function, is part of the second, immune-mediated, phase. **Penicillin** is the usual treatment.

Lyme disease

See below under Lyme disease.

Syphilis

See below under Syphilis.

Viral meningitis

A wide variety of different viruses have been implicated in meningitis but **80 per cent of cases are caused by enteroviruses** (coxsackie, ECHO (enteric cytopathic human orphan) and polio-viruses). The clinical features of meningitis are not specific, although clues to the aetiology may be obtained from the epidemiological history. Enterovirus infections are spread by the faecal-oral route and are more common in the late summer when small epidemics occur. A macular rash (and occasionally other rashes) is not unusual. Parotitis would favour mumps; a shingles rash implicates varicella-zoster virus; genital herpes, herpes simplex type 2; and a history of exposure to small rodents, lymphocytic choriomeningitis virus. Not infrequently HIV seroconversion illness is accompanied by aseptic meningitis and the diagnosis of HIV should therefore be considered in such cases.

The responsible virus should be sought from cultures of the CSF, stools and throat swabs; PCR is the gold standard for herpesviruses and entero-viruses, but serological tests are the main means for laboratory confirmation of other viral infections. Whatever the cause, the management of viral meningitis (without evidence of encephalitis) is purely symptomatic and recovery is usually rapid and complete within a few days.

ENCEPHALITIS

Often, meningitis is complicated by some degree of inflammation of the brain, so that the term **meningoencephalitis** probably more correctly reflects the extent of the pathological process.

There are, however, some forms of CNS infection in which widespread involvement of brain tissue regularly occurs so that disturbances of consciousness, personality, thought and motor function predominate. Whereas HSV or rabies virus encephalitis are caused by **direct invasion** of brain cells, other acute encephalitides can result from an immune-mediated process secondary to infection or immunization (**parainfectious** or **post-infectious encephalitis**). Acute infectious encephalitis histopathologically is characterized by the presence of inflammation, neuronophagia and the detection of microbial antigen; post-infectious encephalitis shares the same histopathological features of acute disseminated encephalomyelitis – perivenous inflammation and acute demyelination.

Clues to the aetiology can sometimes be found in the epidemiological history or clinical examination (Table 25.4). In the UK, among the immunocompetent, the most frequent causes of acute infectious encephalitis are herpes simplex viruses types 1 and 2, varicella zoster virus and the enteroviruses.

Table 25.4 Clues to the aetiology of encephalitis

History	Microbial agents to be considered
Recent travel, mosquito or tick bites	Cerebral malaria, arboviruses
Seasonality	Arboviruses, enteroviruses
Animal bite	Rabies
Other present illness	Herpes zoster, infectious mononucleosis, *Mycoplasma pneumoniae*, mumps, etc.
Preceding illness or immunization	Measles, influenza, varicella
Immunocompromised host	Cytomegalovirus, *Toxoplasma gondii*, JC virus (a papovavirus named after the initials of the index patient)

Without any obvious clue to aetiology, all cases of encephalitis should be treated as resulting from HSV infection until proven otherwise.

Herpes simplex encephalitis

Epidemiology

In the neonate, CNS disease caused by HSV infection is usually part of a disseminated HSV type 2 infection contracted from maternal genital lesions. At all other ages, HSV type 1 is the most common form of sporadic encephalitis in the UK. There is no clustering and it is not seasonal. The encephalitis is only rarely a primary HSV infection, although there is still debate as to whether it is usually caused by reactivation of latent HSV (from the trigeminal ganglion or the brain) or by reinfection with a different exogenous HSV strain.

Symptoms and signs

The disease typically has an acute onset with fever, behavioural abnormalities, an early deterioration in consciousness, seizures and rapid progression. The virus has a particular predilection for the temporal and frontal lobes and the necrosis and oedema often produce focal symptoms (anosmia, olfactory or auditory hallucinations, etc.).

Investigations

Focal abnormalities are also commonly detectable clinically or on electroencephalography, CT or preferably MRI scans (Figure 25.3). Currently, the most sensitive imaging modality is MRI with acquisition of diffusion-weighted sequences. Normal CT or MRI scans cannot be used to exclude the diagnosis. The finding of periodic lateralized epileptiform discharges (PLED) (see Chapter 5) on the electroencephalogram is not specific for herpes simplex encephalitis; rather it is indicative of severe damage to a temporal lobe from any cause. Typically in herpes simplex virus encephalitis (HSE), the CSF contains a mononuclear cell pleocytosis with elevated protein level. **The diagnosis can be confirmed by detection of viral DNA by PCR within the CSF; which in HSE has a sensitivity of over 95 per cent.** Very occasionally, CSF sampled early in the disease process can be negative and caution should be exercised before halting treatment after a negative result where the patient's clinical picture strongly resembles HSE. Should diagnostic uncertainty remain, convalescent CSF and serum can

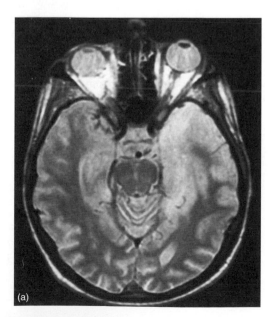 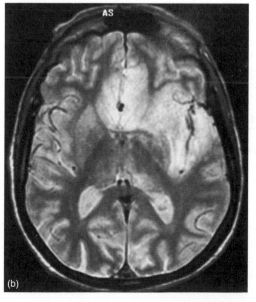

Figure 25.3 Magnetic resonance imaging brain scans, axial view, showing high signal in the right temporal lobe as a result of herpes simplex encephalitis.

be studied for the presence of production of local HSV-specific antibody, which if present confirms the diagnosis retrospectively.

Treatment

The drug of choice for the treatment of HSE is **intravenous aciclovir** (in adults: 10 mg/kg bodyweight 8-hourly; in neonates: 20 mg/kg bodyweight 8 hourly), which is clearly beneficial, providing treatment is started before severe brain necrosis has occurred. **Aciclovir should be started whenever the clinical picture suggests HSE** (i.e. any form of encephalitis for which an alternative aetiology is not evident), but investigations aimed at other treatable causes of the symptoms should be continued until the patient responds or proof of HSV infection is obtained.

The duration of treatment with aciclovir is not well established. Most authorities would treat for at least 2 weeks, but others would recommend repeating the lumbar puncture and ensuring the HSV can no longer be detected by PCR before halting treatment.

While the use of aciclovir has dramatically reduced mortality from HSE from ~70 per cent to <20 per cent, survivors frequently suffer severe sequelae related to parenchymal damage at the sites of infection. Common morbidities include epilepsy, memory disorders and behavioural abnormalities. Good outcome from HSE is associated with commencing aciclovir early after the onset of neurological symptoms.

Arbovirus encephalitis

In many parts of Asia and the Americas, encephalitis is caused by various **arboviruses (*ar*thropod-*bor*ne viruses)** transmitted by mosquito or tick bites. Cases are only very rarely seen as importations into the UK, although occasionally a related virus is transmitted from sheep to farm workers in the UK causing Louping illness. **Important arboviral encephalitides worldwide include many flaviviruses – Japanese encephalitis virus (South East Asia), West Nile virus (North America, Africa, Mediterranean, and Middle East), St Louis encephalitis virus (North America), Murray Valley encephalitis virus (Australia), Tick-borne encephalitis virus (central Europe and Scandanavia), and Russian spring-summer encephalitis virus (Russia and central Asia).** Currently, there are no specific treatments for flavivirus encephalitis. Effective vaccines exist for Japanese encephalitis virus and Tick-borne encephalitis virus, which in endemic areas should be administered to children and travellers whose duration of stay or activities place them at particular risk. Otherwise, reducing mosquito and tick exposure and use of repellents can lessen risk.

Rabies

Epidemiology

Rabies is an almost inevitably fatal encephalitis, which is transmitted in the saliva of infected mammals by bites, scratches or licks of open wounds or mucous membranes. Dogs, wolves, cats and bats are the animals that most often transmit the virus to man. There are very few areas of the world where rabies is not endemic and even within the British Isles a rabies-related lyssavirus infects bats.

Symptoms and signs

The virus binds to and enters the peripheral nerves via nicotinic acetylcholine receptors and is transported along the axons to reach the CNS. The site of the inoculation largely determines the incubation period, which can be many months following distal bites, such as to the legs. The first symptoms are often non-specific, but include itching or paraesthesiae at the inoculation site (often long after the wound has healed). After 2–10 days, frank CNS signs of furious or paralytic rabies develop. Excitability and spasms of the pharyngeal and laryngeal muscles induced by draughts of air or the sight of water (hydrophobia) are typical of the former. The illness is rapidly progressive and, despite intensive care, paralysis, coma and death from cardiorespiratory failure are the rule. No treatment is effective.

Diagnosis

Diagnosis in life is by virus isolation from saliva, tears or CSF or by immunofluorescent detection of viral antigen in full thickness skin biopsies from hairy areas at the nape of the neck.

Prevention

Effective vaccines are available: pre-exposure prophylaxis is recommended for certain occupations or travellers, and post-exposure vaccination and immunoglobulin should be given as soon as possible after exposure to the saliva of a potentially rabid animal. Specialist advice should be sought.

Chronic and progressive viral encephalitis

In addition to these acute infections, there are several chronic and progressive neurological conditions resulting from viral infections. These chronic infections are exemplified by **subacute sclerosing panencephalitis (SSPE)**, which is a very rare fatal infection caused by a form of measles virus and which becomes manifest as a progressive neurological deterioration developing several years after an apparently uncomplicated attack of measles. Since the introduction of routine vaccination of children against measles, the incidence of SSPE has fallen markedly, although worryingly there has been an increase in reported cases in those countries with lower uptake of the mumps, measles and rubella (MMR) vaccine. Progressive multifocal leukoencephalopathy is discussed below.

Trypanosomiasis

African trypanosomiasis or sleeping sickness is caused by species of *Trypanosoma brucei*, which are protozoal parasites transmitted by the tsetse fly. Trypanosomiasis may produce a myriad of neurological symptoms, including an encephalitic illness. It is acquired in areas of Africa south of the Sahara and north of the river Zambesi. West African trypanosomiasis is associated with late involvement of the CNS, sometimes mimicking dementia, whereas East African trypanosomiasis has early acute CNS disease. Specialist advice should be sought to facilitate diagnosis and appropriate treatment.

BRAIN ABSCESS, EPIDURAL ABSCESS AND SUBDURAL EMPYEMA

Epidemiology

Collections of infected pus can occur within the parenchyma of the brain (**brain abscess**), between the vertebral periosteum and spinal dura mater

(**epidural abscess**), and within the skull between the dura and arachnoid mater (**subdural empyema**). The incidence of brain abscesses in resource-rich countries is approximately 0.3–1.3 per 100 000 people per year. The frequency of epidural abscesses and subdural empyema is lower, but all three conditions share a male preponderance. The infections can occur through seeding from the circulation, contiguous spread from another infected structure (such as the mastoid), or as a result of a penetrating injury or surgery. The most common microbe isolated in epidural abscesses is *Staphylococcus aureus*, whereas for brain abscesses and subdural empyema streptococci especially of the *Streptococci milleri* group are more frequently found. Brain abscesses resulting from contiguous spread from the ear often contain a mixed growth of Gram-negative bacilli and anaerobic bacteria. Abscesses caused by fungi or protozoa are rare and are particularly found in the immunosuppressed.

Symptoms and signs

Brain abscesses and subdural empyema typically present with symptoms of fever, headache and focal neurological signs. Seizures are more frequent in those with subdural empyema than brain abscesses. Epidural abscesses present initially with localized back pain followed by radicular symptoms and then myelopathy as the lesion develops.

Investigations

Blood cultures should be obtained from all patients with suspected pyogenic CNS infections. Often blood markers of systemic infection (such as blood white cell count and C-reactive protein (CRP)) are unremarkable and cannot be used to exclude the diagnoses. Imaging of the CNS, ideally MRI, with contrast enhancement is required. In the case of suspected epidural abscesses, imaging should be obtained urgently to exclude significant spinal cord compromise and to guide surgical intervention.

Treatment

Management of these conditions requires the combined skills of the neurologist, microbiologist and neurosurgeon. Community-acquired infections should be treated intravenously with a **third-generation cephalosporin and metronidazole** until more specific microbial sensitivities are available. Epidural abscesses and most subdural empyema require surgical intervention.

> Brain abscesses can be aspirated stereotactically for culture; but multiple abscesses <2.5 cm in diameter usually can be managed conservatively or with only the largest lesion being aspirated.

In cases where a haematogenous source for infection is thought likely, a careful screen for underlying infection or evidence of right-to-left circulatory shunt should be undertaken.

NEUROCYSTICERCOSIS

Cysticercosis results from infection with the helminth *Taenia solium* – a pork tapeworm. Worldwide, this organism causes considerable morbidity and in many countries it is the most common cause for adult-onset epilepsy. *T. solium* has a complex life-cycle involving infection of both humans and pigs. Humans may develop the tapeworm through eating infected undercooked pork. However, to develop cystercercosis they must have contact with *T. solium* proglottids, found in material contaminated with the faeces of a human tapeworm carrier.

Cystercerci can form in any organ, but neurocysticercosis occurs when they develop in the CNS, **where lesions can act as an epileptogenic focus** or obstruct the ventricular system causing hydrocephalus. Diagnosis is usually dependent upon identifying the typical neuroimaging finding of one or more calcified or cystic lesions with a scolex often with ring enhancement. On occasions, cysticerci can be identified elsewhere in the body, such as in the retina or through evidence of calcification of dead cysticerci in muscle. Unfortunately, current serological tests have low sensitivity. Hydrocephalus should be treated surgically; however, it is controversial as to which patient groups clearly benefit from anti-helminthic agents. It is important to note that dying cysticerci can illicit a marked immune reaction and therefore drug treatment may worsen neurological status.

CEREBRAL MALARIA

> ## Epidemiology of malaria
> Approximately 2000 cases of malaria are imported into the UK every year resulting in 10–20 deaths. Although four species of *Plasmodium* infect man, only *P. falciparum* causes cerebral malaria. Falciparum (malignant tertian) malaria is endemic in much of the tropical and subtropical world and malaria should **always** be suspected as the cause of any neurological symptoms in a patient who has returned from an endemic area within the previous two months. It is a medical emergency.

Symptoms and signs

Malaria is transmitted by the bite of an infected mosquito and after a short intrahepatic cycle the parasites invade red blood cells. Fever always occurs and often it is not periodic. **Non-specific influenza-like symptoms are frequent.** In severe disease, endothelial damage and sludging of the parasitized red cells lead to blockage of capillaries and hence ischaemia of vital organs. Cerebral malaria leads to lethargy, drowsiness, coma and almost any CNS symptoms and signs; it can progress to death with frightening rapidity. Haemolysis and disseminated intravascular coagulation compound the severity of the illness.

Investigations

The diagnostic test is examination of a peripheral blood smear. Rapid diagnostic antigen tests should only be used as an adjunct to the blood smear, not as a substitute. It can sometimes be difficult to differentiate between the species of *Plasmodia*, but if over 1 per cent of the red cells are parasitized or ring forms are seen then *P. falciparum* infection should be assumed.

Treatment

> For cerebral malaria **intravenous quinine** therapy should be used and specialist advice obtained. In many countries, **intravenous artesunate** is advocated for severe malaria as it appears superior to intravenous quinine. This agent is not yet widely

available in Europe, but it may be obtained in the UK from tropical disease hospitals. During treatment for all severe malaria, vigilance for hypoglycaemia is required as this can manifest as neurological deterioration and may occur secondary to quinine-induced hyperinsulinaemia.

CENTRAL NERVOUS SYSTEM INFECTION IN THE IMMUNOCOMPROMISED PATIENT

Infections of the CNS are not uncommon in patients with compromised host defences and are often caused by pathogens that do not usually infect the normal host. Abnormalities of immune function are normally classified under one of four headings, each of which is associated with a predisposition to infection of the CNS by certain opportunistic pathogens (Table 25.5):

1 **Defects in polymorph function**. Patients with inadequate polymorph function, typically those with severe neutropenia, are prone to infection with Gram-negative aerobic bacteria (*E. coli*, *Klebsiella*, *P. aeruginosa*, etc.) and certain fungi.
2 **Defects in humoral immunity**. Defects in the ability to mount an antibody response are accompanied by an increased risk of infection by encapsulated bacteria and by a rare chronic encephalitis caused by enteroviruses. Such defects are seen in patients with B-cell lymphoma and leukaemia, or myeloma.
3 **Defects in cellular immunity**. Patients with defects in cell-mediated immunity (organ transplant recipients, patients with Hodgkin's disease and other lymphomas, those receiving steroid therapy and patients with AIDS) are highly susceptible to intracellular microorganisms.
4 **Splenic dysfunction**. Loss of splenic function, whether by disease or surgery, is associated with abnormal phagocytic function and lack of opsonizing antibodies and predisposes the individual to infection with encapsulated bacteria.

It should be appreciated that, as a result of surgery or therapy with cytotoxic or immunosuppressive drugs or corticosteroids, many patients have abnormalities of their immune system that fall into several of these categories and are thus prone to a wide range of opportunistic pathogens.

The features of meningitis caused by *Listeria* and *Cryptococcus* have already been described. Brief mention of some other opportunistic pathogens is given below, but for all such infections specialist advice is recommended.

Table 25.5 Major opportunistic pathogens causing syndromes of central nervous system infection in immunocompromised patients

Immune defect	Meningitis	Encephalitis	Brain abscess
Polymorph defect	Gram-negative bacilli Candida	Gram-negative bacilli Candida	Aspergillus
Antibody defect	Pneumococcus *Haemophilus influenzae*	Enteroviruses	
Cellular immune defect	Listeria Cryptococcus Tuberculosis Toxoplasma	Listeria Cryptococcus Toxoplasma Varicella/zoster virus Cytomegalovirus (CMV) Papovaviruses (JC virus)	Nocardia Aspergillus
Splenic dysfunction	Pneumococcus *H. influenzae*		

CMV, cytomegalovirus.

Candida

Meningitis from *Candida* infection is usually part of disseminated disease in a patient with neutropenia or following parenteral hyperalimentation. It is a subacute or chronic infection similar to cryptococcosis.

Nocardia

The branching bacterium *Nocardia* typically causes a single brain abscess as part of a disseminated infection.

Aspergillus

Central nervous system infection with *Aspergillus* occurs in neutropenic patients and those with defects in cellular immunity. Single or multiple brain abscesses are found, often in conjunction with a CSF pleocytosis and signs of meningitis.

Toxoplasma gondii

Cerebral toxoplasmosis has become of major importance in patients with AIDS, in whom it is the most common opportunistic infection of the CNS.

Varicella zoster virus

Visceral dissemination of chickenpox or shingles is not uncommon in the immunocompromised patient and CNS infection. There may be a period of several months between the rash and onset of neurological symptoms. The CNS complications of varicella zoster virus (VZV) result from an infectious vasculopathy that may affect either, or both, small and large vessels. VZV small vessel vasculopathy presents similarly to viral encephalitis; whereas the large vessel vasculopathy, which can also occur in the immunocompetent, presents as ischaemic stroke. **VZV large vessel vasculopathy typically follows shingles in the distribution of the trigeminal nerve, affecting one or more of the ipsilateral intracranial arteries.** Aciclovir should be given in both conditions, and steroids should be considered in cases of VZV large vessel vasculopathy.

Progressive multifocal leukoencephalopathy

Progressive multifocal leukoencephalopathy (PML) is a rare progressive demyelinating disease caused by a **papovavirus – JC virus**. JC virus (JCV) is ubiquitous and after innocuous primary infection in childhood it establishes latency in the kidneys. Following systemic reactivation among those with impaired cell-mediated immunity, JC virus in a minority of individuals can infect oligodendroglia causing demyelination. PML can present with cognitive or more focal signs and often affects the occipital cortex causing cortical blindness. It never affects the optic nerve and less commonly the spinal cord. The frequency of PML increased substantially with the advent of AIDS.

However, in the last five years, it has been recognized as a rare complication of treatment with certain immunosuppressive monoclonal antibodies used to treat immune-mediated diseases (such as rituximab, natalizumab or alemtuzamab).

Diagnosis is based upon the white matter MRI findings that characteristically show little enhancement or mass effect. Without immune reconstitution, PML relentlessly progresses to death within a few weeks (see Chapter 26). However, if the immune deficit can be reversed, then improvement can occur. No JCV-specific antiviral therapy has yet been demonstrated to be clinically useful, although clinical trials of agents are currently underway.

POLIOMYELITIS

The three strains of polioviruses are enteroviruses and, like others in this genus (see above under Viral meningitis), usually produce an asymptomatic or mild, non-specific infection. Aseptic meningitis also occurs and in a small minority of cases extensive neuronal necrosis, especially of the anterior horn cells in the spinal cord, causes paralytic disease.

Epidemiology

Indigenous transmission of poliomyelitis has now been eradicated in the Western world and, following the World Health Organization's global initiative, by 2008 only in Afghanistan, India, Nigeria and Pakistan does the virus remain endemic. Polioviruses are spread by the alimentary route, either via faeces or oral secretions, and, even without vaccination, where poor sanitation and overcrowding exist almost all people over the age of five years have antibodies to all three strains. Poliomyelitis-like syndromes occasionally occur following infection with non-polio enteroviruses or certain flaviviruses including West Nile virus and Japanese encephalitis virus.

Symptoms and signs

The vast majority (90–95 per cent) of infections are not clinically apparent. In the remainder, 2–5 days after exposure there is a 'minor illness': fever, headache, sore throat, vomiting and malaise are common complaints but resolve within a day or two, a self-limiting viral meningitis. In a minority of cases (1–2 per cent overall) the 'major illness' follows several days later. In about 0.15 per cent of all poliovirus infections, muscle pains herald the development of paralysis a few days later.

The paralysis is of the lower motor neurone type with flaccidity and absent tendon reflexes. Characteristically it is asymmetrical, proximal more than distal, affects the legs more than the arms, and progresses over 24–48 hours.

Bulbar polio

In a small number of cases, the nuclei of the cranial nerves, particularly the IXth and Xth, are involved. Dysphagia, nasal speech and respiratory difficulties follow. Very rarely, the respiratory and vasomotor centres in the medulla are involved.

Investigations

In any form of neurological poliovirus infection, the CSF findings are those of aseptic meningitis (see above) and this can be helpful in distinguishing the condition from Guillain–Barré syndrome. The virus can be cultured from the stools or throat washings (but seldom from the CSF).

Treatment

No form of treatment will affect the neurological outcome once paralysis has become established. In the acute stage of the disease, exercise should be avoided as this can increase disease risk and severity. Management consists of respiratory support if there is bulbar or respiratory muscle disturbance, avoidance of deep vein thromboses, prevention of contractures and rehabilitation.

Prevention

Paralytic polio can be prevented by immunization with either inactivated poliovirus (IPV) or live oral poliovirus (OPV) vaccines. Occasionally, vaccine-associated paralysis has been reported with the OPV. Therefore, in many resource-rich countries, where the very small risk of OPV complications are felt to outweigh the benefits, national vaccination programmes now utilize only the IPV.

Post-polio syndrome

Stabilization occurs after the acute phase, but many patients develop new weakness, fatigue and pain 25–35 years later. These symptoms may affect muscles not obviously involved in the original attack. Such patients require careful multidisciplinary assessment particularly to ascertain whether the initial diagnosis of poliomyelitis was correct and to exclude other causes for weakness and pain such as compression neuropathies. There are no specific treatments for the post-polio syndrome, but supervised exercise training can help improve strength in mildly or moderately weak muscles, as well as reducing fatigue.

TETANUS

Epidemiology

The clinical manifestations of tetanus result from the effects of an exotoxin (tetanospasmin) produced by *Clostridium tetani*, a spore-forming, strictly anaerobic, Gram-positive bacillus that exists primarily in the soil. Contamination of a wound by bacterial spores, which then vegetate and elaborate toxin, results in disease. Tetanus has become rare in developed countries as a result of vaccination.

Symptoms and signs

The incubation period is between 3 and 21 days (usually 5–10 days), during which tetanospasmin is transported along axons to the CNS. Tetanospasmin has its major effect upon the spinal cord, where it causes presynaptic blockade of inhibitory synapses. This produces **muscle rigidity** and **spasm**, and **sympathetic overactivity**. Many cases have masseter spasm and **trismus** as the presenting symptom. This produces the characteristic sardonic smile (**risus sardonicus**). Stiffness of the spinal and abdominal muscles also occurs and **opisthotonos** can result. As the disease progresses, severe spasms of muscles occur and may result in apnoea and choking. Sweating, tachycardia, profound fluctuations in blood pressure and other signs of autonomic dysfunction may appear. The shorter the incubation period and the faster the progression of the disease, the more severe the illness is likely to be. Milder localized forms of tetanus can occur, affecting just muscles adjacent to the site of injury or being confined to the lower cranial nerves.

Investigations

There are no specific diagnostic tests for tetanus, and diagnosis is based on the overt clinical signs. The CSF is normal and often there is no evidence of the original wound.

Treatment

Specific treatment should be given with a single dose of **human hyperimmune immunoglobulin** (150 units/kg i.m.) and **metronidazole** (500 mg qds i.v. for 10 days). Benzylpenicillin, although traditional, is probably best avoided, because it may enhance the antagonism of gamma aminobutyric acid by tetanospasmin. Surgical excision of the injured tissue is sometimes needed.

The mainstay of treatment of tetanus is expert nursing and medical care in an intensive care unit. The number of spasms should be minimized by keeping the patient quiet and the use of benzodiazepines and, in the most mild cases, this and sedation may be all that is needed. In more severe cases, paralysis and intubation are necessary. Continuous infusion of magnesium sulphate has been shown to reduce the use of drugs to control autonomic dysfunction, but does not reduce the frequency of artificial ventilation. Aggressive nutritional support, control of autonomic dysfunction and prevention of pneumonia and venous thromboembolism are all vitally important.

An attack of tetanus does not confer immunity to further attacks and all patients should be given a course of immunization.

Prevention

Everyone should receive a complete basic course of toxoid given as part of the normal childhood immunizations, with further routine boosters given every ten years thereafter. The use of toxoid and hyperimmune globulin should be considered in all patients with wounds and depends upon the immunization history and the type of wound (Table 25.6).

BOTULISM

Epidemiology

Botulism is the rare clinical syndrome resulting from the action of the most poisonous substance known to humankind – botulinum neurotoxin. Spore-forming bacteria of the genus *Clostridium*, that includes *Clostridium botulinum*, as well as other species produce it. Seven neurotoxins are known of which four cause naturally occurring botulism. They act intracellularly to inhibit normal synapse and vesicle fusion inhibiting release of acetylcholine, which results in neuromuscular blockade and disruption of the autonomic nervous system. Humans can be exposed to the toxin by consuming contaminated food, clostridial wound infection, infantile infection or adult intestinal colonization, inadvertently following therapeutic use, or intentionally through acts of bioterrorism. Contaminated food usually results from home canning of foods or home curing of meat. The toxins are heat labile, but clostridial spores can withstand temperatures of 100°C.

Table 25.6 Guidelines for tetanus prophylaxis in wound management

History of tetanus toxoid administration	Clean minor wounds[a]		All other wounds[a]	
	Tetanus toxoid vaccine[b]	Immunoglobulin	Tetanus toxoid vaccine[b]	Immunoglobulin
Fully immunized, i.e. total of 5 doses at appropriate intervals	No	No	No	Only if high risk[c]
Primary immunization complete, boosters incomplete but up to date	No	No	No	Only if high risk[c]
Primary immunization incomplete or boosters schedule not up to date	Yes and complete schedule	No	Yes and complete schedule	Yes
Not immunized or immunization status not known or uncertain	Yes and complete schedule if records confirm this is needed	No	Yes and complete schedule if records confirm this is needed	Yes

[a]A clean minor wound is less than 6 hours old and is clean and non-penetrating. All other wounds are tetanus prone.
[b]Given as Td/IPV (i.e. with the low adult dose of diphtheria toxoid and inactivated polio vaccine) for adults and adolescents.
[c]High risk is defined as a wound with a significant degree of devitalized tissue, puncture-type wound, contact soil or manure likely to harbour tetanus organisms, or clinical evidence of sepsis.

Wound botulism was exceedingly rare, but is increasingly recognized as a complication of parenteral illicit drug abuse, particularly in those who develop chronic abscesses through 'skin popping'.

Symptoms and signs

The clinical features of botulism result from impairment of cholinergic neurotransmission. The pattern of neuromuscular transmission usually is of acute onset with weakness of the cranial nerves causing diplopia and bulbar dysfunction followed in more severe cases by descending weakness, respiratory failure and tetraparesis. Prominent autonomic dysfunction including fixed dilated pupils, hypotension without compensatory tachycardia and constipation is frequently noted.

Milder forms of botulism can occur.

Investigations

The diagnosis of botulism is primarily through recognition of the clinical syndrome, although nerve conduction studies can help localize the neurophysiological deficit to the neuromuscular junction presynatic membrane. A mouse bioassay can be used in specialist laboratories to demonstrate the presence of the neurotoxin in human serum.

Treatment

Treatment of botulism requires early administration of equine botulinum anti-toxin coupled with careful patient monitoring and intensive care. Patients who have developed profound weakness may require a prolonged period of intensive care as anti-toxin is not effective once the toxin has entered neurones. Those with wound-related botulism should undergo debridement and be given antibiotics.

LYME DISEASE

Epidemiology

Lyme disease is caused by *Borrelia burgdorferi*, a spirochaete transmitted to humans from a reservoir in small mammals by the bite of hard-bodied ticks, common in many parts of northern Europe and North America.

Symptoms and signs

Infection may be asymptomatic, cause only the specific rash **(erythema chronicum migrans (ECM))** at the site of the bite, or disseminate to many organs, including the CNS.

Primary disease

The first, and often only, manifestation of Lyme disease is ECM, an area of expanding erythema (sometimes with central clearing) at the site of a tick bite, which typically occurred 7–10 days earlier. At this stage, treatment with doxycycline (100 mg bd), amoxycillin (500 mg tds) or oral cefuroxime axetil (500 mg bd) for 14 days is recommended.

Secondary disease

Some weeks or months later, bacteraemic spread of the spirochaete may cause disseminated disease, including **migratory arthritis, carditis and neurological manifestations. The latter include meningoencephalitis with facial and other cranial nerve palsies, and a painful sensorimotor radiculitis.** Symptoms can be relapsing or chronic. Treatment of neurological disease is with a high-dose intravenous third-generation cephalosporin (e.g. ceftriaxone 2 g i.v. for 14 days).

Tertiary disease

Chronic Lyme arthritis, a peripheral sensory neuritis and subacute or chronic encephalopathy may occur. The neurological symptoms are of subtle memory and cognitive dysfunction. The brain MRI findings can include white matter lesions similar to those found in multiple sclerosis. Therapy is the same as for the secondary phase of infection, but the antibiotics are generally given for up to 6 weeks.

Investigations

The diagnosis of ECM is based upon clinical judgement and a history of exposure to ticks. For extracutaneous Lyme disease, laboratory support is essential. Culture of the organism is the gold standard, but is insensitive. A positive enzyme-linked or immunofluorescence serological assay requires confirmation by an immunoblot for antibodies to individual *B. burgdorferi* antigens. Reliance on laboratory tests such as PCR leads to overdiagnosis in endemic areas.

SYPHILIS

Syphilis is the result of infection with *Treponema pallidum*, a slender spirochaete between 5 and 15 μm in length. It cannot be cultured on artificial media and diagnosis therefore depends upon direct visualization, serological testing, or detection by PCR of *T. pallidum* DNA from a clinical sample.

Epidemiology

Transmission is almost always venereal, although infection can occur *in utero* or as a result of blood transfusion. The true incidence in the UK is unknown, but it is more common in urban areas and has increased recently among men who have sex with men.

Symptoms and signs

The clinical features of syphilis reflect a complex interaction between the organism and the immune system.

Primary disease

Between 1 and 6 weeks after infection, a papular lesion develops at the site of inoculation. This develops into a shallow, painless, indurated ulcer (the **chancre**) accompanied by regional lymphadenopathy. If left untreated, it heals within 2–3 weeks.

Secondary disease

Multisystem involvement occurs 6–8 weeks later, corresponding to the time of maximal antigenic load. There is a generalized polymorphic non-itchy rash, often involving the palms and soles, moist, highly infectious, **condyloma lata** around the genitalia, and **mucocutaneous lesions**. There is a bacter-aemia and the nervous system becomes infected. Central nervous system symptoms are rare, but occasionally lymphocytic meningitis may develop. Secondary disease spontaneously heals after 4–6 weeks, but in one-quarter of patients relapses occur at some time over the next four years.

Latent syphilis

During this stage, there are no clinical symptoms and the infection can only be detected by positive serological tests. Latent syphilis is classified as early if infection occurred within the preceding two years, and thereafter it is described as late.

Symptomatic late syphilis (tertiary syphilis)

Approximately one-third of patients will develop clinical evidence of late disease as a result of continuing destructive inflammation. This may only become manifest several decades after infection. The cardiovascular system (aortitis), musculoskeletal structures and the **nervous system** (20–30 per cent of cases) are commonly involved. There are a number of varieties of neurosyphilis and more than one can occur in any individual.

Gumma

Gumma is a nodule of granulomatous inflammatory tissue, which may produce the neurological signs of a progressive space-occupying lesion.

Meningeal syphilis

Meningeal syphilis occurs between five and ten years after the primary infection and produces subacute or chronic meningitis. There may also be focal signs as a result of endarteritis of the cerebral vessels. The CSF is abnormal with a mononuclear pleocytosis, raised protein and sometimes a reduced glucose concentration.

General paralysis of the insane

Ten or more years after infection, about 5 per cent of untreated syphilitics develop general paralysis of the insane (GPI) characterized by progressive dementia, speech and thought disorders, long tract signs and exaggerated tendon reflexes.

Tabes dorsalis

The syndrome of tabes dorsalis may be delayed by 20–30 years and results from progressive demyelination of the posterior columns and dorsal nerve roots. It is characterized by ataxia, paraesthesiae, sensory loss and clusters of severe instantaneous pains in the legs or trunk (lightning pains). The loss of sensation leads to Charcot's joints and trophic ulceration. Disturbance of bladder and bowel function is common and urinary retention may be an early feature. Optic atrophy and Argyll Robertson pupils (small, irregular pupils that react to accommodation but not to light) occur in tabes dorsalis and general paralysis of the insane.

Investigations for syphilis

The demonstration of *Treponema pallidum* by darkfield microscopy is the method of choice for a suspected syphilitic chancre or condyloma lata, although PCR-based tests are now increasingly used.

In the other forms of disease, diagnosis is based upon serological tests, which fall into two groups: the non-specific (reaginic) antibody tests and those for specific treponemal antibodies (Table 25.7). The reaginic antibody tests are useful as screening tests or for monitoring the response to treatment, but false-positive results are common and any positive result in the serum therefore needs further confirmation.

Table 25.7 Serological tests for syphilis

Non-specific (reaginic) tests	Venereal Diseases Research Laboratory (VDRL)
	Carbon antigen test/rapid plasma reagin test (RPR)
Specific tests	Treponemal enzyme immunoassay (EIA) for IgG, IgG and IgM, or IgM
	Treponema pallidum haemagglutination assay (TPHA)
	T. pallidum particle agglutination assay (TPPA)
	Fluorescent treponemal antibody absorption test (FTA-abs)

The specific tests recommended for screening are the enzyme immunoassay (EIA) for IgG and IgM and the TPPA. The IgM EIA is recommended if primary syphilis is suspected. Once positive, the specific tests usually remains so for life, with or without treatment, and the test cannot therefore be used to document the adequacy of therapy. The majority of patients with neurosyphilis have abnormal CSF white cell counts and/or protein levels. A positive CSF Venereal Disease Research Laboratory (VDRL)/rapid plasma reagin (RPR) test is diagnostic of neurosyphilis in a non-blood contaminated sample; however, CSF VDRL/RPR is not sensitive and a negative test cannot exclude neurosyphilis, whereas a negative CSF syphilis antibody test excludes the diagnosis. Detection of *T. pallidum* DNA in CSF by PCR is more common in early than late syphilis; and therefore the role of this test in neurosyphilis remains to be clarified.

Treatment

Penicillin remains the treatment of choice for all stages of syphilis. The recommended regimens and follow up are summarized in Table 25.8. Corticosteroids are used in cardiovascular and neurological syphilis to prevent tissue injury after starting treponemicidal therapy. Follow-up VDRL/RPR should be performed monthly for the first three months, then at six and 12 months, and thereafter at six-monthly intervals until it is negative or stable (serofast). In addition to the reappearance of signs or symptoms a four-fold rise in VDRL/RPR suggests reinfection or recurrence. In patients who fail to show a four-fold decrease in VDRL/RPR 6–12 months after therapy, CSF examination and retreatment is indicated.

EMERGING INFECTIONS

Emerging infections are infectious diseases that have either not previously been recognized by medical science, have jumped a species barrier, have altered characteristics of their pathogenesis or have translocated to a discrete geographical area in which the disease was not previously found. Of all emerging infections recently described, approximately half have presented with syndromes due to infection of the CNS. Many emerging infections have environmental reservoirs and are transmitted to humans by vectors. The increasing recognition of these illnesses in part may relate to environmental changes.

The most well-studied emerging infection is that of the translocation of **West Nile virus** to North America. Cases of neuroinvasive West Nile virus were first noted in New York in 1999 when concurrently an epidemic was also found among birds and horses. The virus had not previously been found in the United States and Canada, but over the following years it spread rapidly to reach the western

Table 25.8 Treatment and follow up of syphilis

Stage	Treatment
Primary, secondary or early latent (mU) IM daily for 10 days	Procaine penicillin[a] 0.6 million units or benzathine penicillin[a] 2.4 mU i.m. single dose
Late latent, cardiovascular or gumma[b]	Procaine penicillin[a] 0.6 mU i.m. daily for 17 days or benzathine penicillin[a] 2.4 mU i.m. on days 1, 8 and 15
Neurosyphilis (including neurological / ophthalmic involvement in early syphilis)[b]	Procaine penicillin[a] 1.8–2.4 mU i.m. daily plus probenecid 500 mg qds for 17 days or benzylpenicillin 3–4 mU i.v. every 4 hours (18–24 mU/day) for 17 days
Penicillin allergic patients	
Primary or secondary	Doxycycline 100 mg bd or erythromycin 500 mg qds for 14 days
Tertiary (all types)	Doxycycline 200 mg bd for 28 days

[a]Procaine penicillin and benzathine penicillin are unlicensed in the UK, but can be obtained by special order.
[b]Steroids are recommended to start 24 hours prior to treatment with antibiotics (prednisolone 40–60 mg od for 3 days).

seaboard, with approximately 3000 neuroinvasive cases per annum reported in 2002 and 2003.

Also in 1999, a novel paramyxovirus was identified in the Malay Peninsula as a cause of encephalitis – **Nipah virus**. In this case, the virus was transmitted from pigs to farmers. Nipah virus originates from fruit bats being transmitted to pigs through consumption of fruit contaminated through contact with the bats.

Worldwide, the majority of patients with suspected viral encephalitis have no aetiology identified for their illness. Therefore, it is important that the physician recognizes the possibility of emerging infections in patients with presumed CNS infections and in particular follow national guidelines for statutory public health notification of cases.

FURTHER READING

Johnson RT (1998) *Viral Infections of the Nervous System*, 2nd edn. Philadelphia: Lippincott-Raven.

Scheld WM, Whitley RJ, Marra CM (2004) *Infections of the Central Nervous System*, 3rd edn. Philadelphia: Lippincott Williams & Wilkins.

Solomon T, Hart IJ, Beeching NJ (2007) Viral encephalitis: a clinician's guide. *Practical Neurology*, **7**:288–305.

Thwaites G, Fisher M, Hemingway C *et al.* (2009) British Infection Society guidelines for the diagnosis and treatment of tuberculosis of the central nervous system in adults and children. *Journal of Infection*, **59**:167–187.

Van de Beck D, de Gass J, Tuskel AR, Wijdicks EF (2006) Community-acquired bacterial meningitis in adults. *New England Journal of Medicine*, **354**:44–53.

HIV

Carolyn Gabriel

INTRODUCTION

Patients with disease caused by the human immunodeficiency virus (HIV) may present with both the full spectrum of general neurological conditions, as well as a more specific range of HIV-related illnesses. When the first edition of this book was published in 1989, treatments for HIV were in their infancy and young patients often presented with advanced disease, frequently with opportunistic infections and tumours, which were invariably fatal. Patients with HIV in the developed world are now often well, living long lives and frequently present with neurological syndromes unrelated to their HIV status. Headache in a patient with HIV these days is more often due to migraine than to intracranial infection.

Of course, patients do still present with neurological manifestations of HIV/acquired immune deficiency syndrome (AIDS). Although presentation still occurs over the whole spectrum of the disease, there have been considerable changes in recent years in communities with widespread availability of antiretroviral therapy, and in the developed world the patient presenting with untreated advanced disease is now less common.

Highly active anti-retroviral therapy (HAART) is now standard therapy in many countries. HAART comprises a combination of three or more antiretroviral drugs, usually two nucleoside-analogue reverse-transcriptase inhibitors (nRTIs) and one or more protease inhibitors (PIs). This has dramatically altered the disease course, controlling viral replication and vastly reducing the development of drug resistance. In effectively treated patients, there have been significant reductions in the incidence of opportunistic infections and tumours, and dramatic reductions in associated mortality.

Unfortunately, not all patients infected with HIV have the benefit of HAART. Access to treatment is poor in many developing countries – by late 2008 only 42 per cent of people needing treatment were receiving it (although this was a significant improvement on the 33 per cent from 2007). Ninety-five per cent of new infections with HIV occur in the developing world, and in the United Kingdom, neurologists continue to encounter this group of patients migrating from outside Europe. The patient cohort is different; these patients are often heterosexual and unfortunately often still present with late stage HIV infection.

The HIV pandemic

The statistics for HIV are stark. In 2007, the latest date for which figures are available, 33 million people worldwide were infected with HIV, with 2.7 million new infections that year.

The annual number of deaths from AIDS was 2 million, although there was some cause for hope given that this was a decline from 2.2 million in 2005. The decline was thought to be in response to both access to treatment and marked changes in sexual behaviour, and has resulted in a stabilization of the global epidemic. **The disease has caused 25 million deaths to date, perhaps worth comparing to the 75 million worldwide who died from Black Death in the mid-1300s.**

In the UK, Health Protection Agency data suggest that the number of people living with HIV in the UK was 83 000 by late 2008, of whom it is estimated a quarter were unaware of being infected. During 2008, there were 7298 new diagnoses of HIV in the UK, a slight decline on previous years. However, there were increases in the number of new diagnoses in those who acquired their infection via homosexual and via heterosexual contact within the UK, with the decline representing those who become infected via heterosexual contact abroad. The number of patients dying from HIV-related illness has remained fairly stable over the last ten years – 525 people died in 2008.

At present, the Department of Health in the UK estimates the cost of treating an individual with HIV at about £16 000 per annum. As described above, most patients are taking HAART, a combination of three or more antiretroviral drugs. As newer and better drugs become available, and drug resistance continues, costs will increase.

The CD4 count and viral load

The blood CD4 lymphocyte count and viral load (the number of 'copies' of HIV ribonucleic acid (RNA)/mL of blood) give an indication of the current level of infection and guide the timing of initiation of treatment. Prior to the availability of HAART, the CD4 count was useful in guiding the neurologist to the likely group of diagnoses at particular stages of the disease and this remains useful in untreated patients (Table 26.1).

At seroconversion, usually a month or two after infection, HIV replicates within CD4 cells, the viral load rises, the CD4 count begins to fall and a febrile systemic syndrome is common. A mild aseptic meningitis – sometimes manifesting simply as a severe headache lasting several days, or as a more florid meningitic illness, is fairly common. Bell's palsy also occurs not infrequently at seroconversion. Occasionally, other immune-mediated neurological disorders occur (Box 26.1).

Early disease (CD4 count >500 cells/mm³), in general, is particularly associated with immune activation syndromes – inflammatory conditions affecting both the central and peripheral nervous systems. In moderately advanced disease (CD4 count 200–500 cells/mm³), infections and other immune syndromes predominate, and in advanced disease (CD4 count <200 cells/mm³), opportunistic infections and tumours are more common as are direct consequences of HIV invasion of the nervous system.

In the UK in 2008, one-third of newly diagnosed adults developed a CD4 count <200/mm³ within three months of diagnosis (and this group has a worse prognosis overall). A CD4 count <350/mm³ is the threshold at which treatment is recommended according to British HIV Association guidelines.

Box 26.1 Opportunistic infections in the nervous system

- Toxoplasmosis
- Herpes encephalitis (HZV, HSV)
- CMV encephalitis, radiculopathy, retinitis, neuropathy
- Cryptococcal meningitis
- JCV-related PML
- TB meningitis, tuberculomas, abcesses, neuropathy
- Atypical mycobacteria
- Candida/nocardia abscesses
- Histoplasmosis
- Coccidiomycosis
- Aspergillosis

CMV, cytomegalovirus; HSV, herpes simplex virus; HZV, herpes zoster virus; JCV, JC virus; PML, progressive multifocal leukoencephalopathy; TB, tuberculosis.

Single/multiple enhancing lesions.

Table 26.1 Neurological complications in HIV

	Complication	
Early disease (CD4 count >500 cells/mm³)	Meningitis Encephalitis ADEM Myelitis Guillain–Barré syndrome (AIDP) Mononeuropathies (especially facial palsy, trigeminal, optic neuropathy) Brachial neuritis Myositis	
Moderately advanced disease (CD4 count 200–500 cells/mm³)	CIDP Meningitis Polymyositis DILS Syphilitic and HC radiculopathy Herpes viruses	
Advanced disease (CD4 count <200 cells/mm³)	Opportunistic infections:	Toxoplasmosis Cryptococcal meningitis PML CMV retinitis, radiculopathy, encephalitis Atypical mycobacteria and TB
	Lymphoma HIV-associated dementia Vacuolar myelopathy HIV neuropathy Myopathy	
Medication-related	Neuropathy Myopathy IRISs:	PML, myelitis, neuropathy, meningitis, encephalitis

ADEM, acute disseminated encephalomyelitis; AIDP, acute inflammatory demyelinating polyradiculoneuropathy; CIDP, chronic inflammatory demyelinating polyradiculoneuropathy; CMV, cytomegalovirus; DILS, diffuse infiltrative lymphocytosis syndrome; HC, hepatitis C; IRIS, immune reconstitution inflammatory syndrome; PML, progressive multifocal leukoencephalopathy; TB, tuberculosis.

NEW PROBLEMS IN HIV NEUROLOGY

Although HAART has undoubtedly had a very positive contribution to controlling HIV, the body's response to immune restoration can result in aggressive inflammatory syndromes, some of which involve the nervous system. These reactions have been called immune reconstitution syndromes (IRIS) and include inflammatory activity against antigens, including those of opportunistic agents, causing atypical manifestations of these infections, which are often culture-negative. The nervous system seems to be particularly affected by IRIS in the months after initiation of HAART, particularly in those with initially very low CD4 counts.

In the longer term, the sustained use of antiretroviral drugs has not been without problems. Side effects are often mild, but neurological consequences such as neuropathy can have a major impact on quality of life and level of functioning. Effects are frequently unpredictable and there is considerable variation between patients. Although usually improving when treatment is switched or stopped, not infrequently some of these complications are irreversible.

Drug resistance is also an issue, usually due to viral mutations, both complicating HIV therapy and contributing to deaths.

Late diagnosis remains a problem for a large minority of newly diagnosed people with HIV, and occurs particularly in heterosexual men. If patients' CD4 counts are low at diagnosis (as it was in about a third of those diagnosed in the UK in 2008), they are less likely to respond to antiretroviral therapy.

OPPORTUNISTIC INFECTIONS

As the immune system weakens, and CD4 cells are damaged or killed by viral replication, these cells are no longer able to fight infections as usual. **If HIV-infected subjects have any of the particularly prevalent infections in those with low CD4 activity, they are considered to have AIDS.** Many opportunistic infections are from reactivation of previous, often asymptomatic, infections, and many are non-neurological. However, opportunistic infections of the nervous system are common enough to merit particular consideration.

Cryptococcal meningitis

Cryptococcus neoformans, the most common cause of meningitis in AIDS in the UK, and the most common lethal fungus in AIDS, is commonly found in soil contaminated by avian excreta. Transmission occurs via inhalation of fungal spores and upper respiratory colonization, with the central nervous system (CNS) the most common site of dissemination, either via haematogenous spread or by reactivation. Cryptococcal IRIS may occur in up to 20 per cent of patients with advanced HIV disease treated with HAART, often culture-negative.

Presentation is typically subacute, over weeks, with headache, fever and increasing confusion with or without meningism, often with papilloedema. Complications include seizures, hydrocephalus and motor or sensory deficits. The main differential diagnoses are toxoplasmosis, tuberculous meningitis (TBM), cytomegalovirus (CMV) encephalitis and lymphoma.

The organisms spread through the Virchow–Robin spaces, which may become dilated by mucoid material, giving a punctate appearance in the basal ganglia on magnetic resonance imaging (MRI), although imaging may be normal. **The cerebrospinal fluid (CSF) may also be normal, although the pressure is raised in 75 per cent and the constituents are abnormal in 40 per cent.** Pleocytosis, high protein and low sugar are the most common findings. **India ink staining is positive in 75 per cent but the most reliable test is the cryptococcal antigen (CrAg) titre (>95 per cent positive in HIV-related cryptococcal meningitis) in blood and CSF.** Titres over $1:10^{24}$ are associated with a poor outcome, as are visual abnormalities, altered mental status and a low CSF white cell count and higher CSF opening pressures.

Treatment is with high-dose amphotericin B (via a central line) plus oral flucytosine for 2 weeks, then oral fluconazole consolidation for 8 weeks or until the CSF is sterile, then fluconazole maintenance therapy. When the intracranial pressure is >25 cm CSF and there are signs of cerebral oedema, repeated lumbar puncture to lower pressure may be necessary, sometimes daily. Patients may require a lumbar drain or ventriculoperitoneal shunt. Restoration of immune function by HAART allows prophylaxis to be discontinued.

Toxoplasmosis

Toxoplasmosis (Figure 26.1) in immunocompetent people is often a benign self-limiting flu-like syndrome, with associated lymphadenopathy. Exposure to the protozoan parasite *Toxoplasma gondii* is generally acquired via its animal host, either by eating raw or undercooked meat (mainly pork or lamb) containing cysts, or from food or water contaminated by cat faeces. Transmission can also be vertical, and via organ transplantation or blood donation. About half the UK population are seropositive. In HIV, manifest disease is generally due to reactivation (and therefore seropositivity is the rule) and it is the most common cause of focal brain lesions. Up to 30–50 per cent of patients with advanced disease are affected worldwide, although in the UK widespread use of HAART has resulted in rates falling markedly and the prognosis improving significantly.

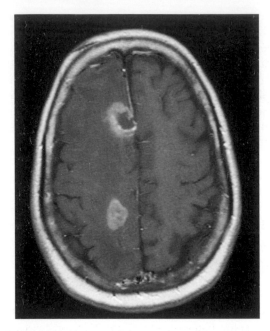

Figure 26.1 Post-contrast axial T1-weighted magnetic resonance imaging (MRI) brain scan. There are two enhancing lesions in the right cerebral hemisphere, one ring shaped, with surrounding oedema and right cerebral swelling. The appearance is non-specific and the radiological differential diagnosis includes other infections and lymphoma. Biopsy confirmed toxoplasmosis (image courtesy of Dr Phillip Rich, Consultant Radiologist, St George's Hospital Trust).

Headache, fever and malaise are the usual non-specific initial symptoms, then confusion, drowsiness, seizures and focal neurological deficits, the pattern determined by the distribution of abscess formation, but hemiparesis, hemianopia and aphasia are common presentations.

MRI (Figure 26.1) usually shows multiple ring enhancing lesions with a predilection for the grey–white interface. Tuberculous abscesses appear very similar, and chest x-ray should always be done. Primary CNS lymphoma is also a differential diagnosis, although a single lesion is usual, rather than multiple lesions. Positive serology for acute infection with high IgM titres may be helpful, but its interpretation is limited by the prevalence in the general population. Response to treatment at 2–3 weeks is often used to aid diagnosis (see below). Lumbar puncture is contraindicated with mass lesions.

Treatment with sulfadiazine, pyrimethamine and folinic acid (to reduce pyrimethamine-induced bone marrow suppression) should continue at high dose for 6 weeks, then at lower lifetime maintenance doses, unless the CD4 count is restored to >200. Clindamycin is the second-line treatment if there is drug allergy or intolerance. Failure of clinicoradiological improvement within 2–3 weeks should prompt diagnostic review and biopsy of brain lesions if necessary.

Cytomegalovirus infection

Cytomegalovirus can affect the peripheral nervous system (PNS), with **painful radiculopathy** and less commonly **neuropathy**, and the CNS, with **encephalitis** and **myelitis**, often with concurrent **retinitis** (Figure 26.2), usually occurring in advanced disease.

The radiculopathy is almost always lumbosacral, presenting as a painful cauda equina syndrome with paraesthesia over the perineum and legs and a progressive flaccid paraparesis. Severe back pain is common and usually prompts a lumbosacral MRI which frequently shows contrast enhancement of the cauda equina, although MRI may be normal. The CSF is usually cellular with a polymorphonuclear pleocytosis, raised protein and low glucose, although non-specific changes may be present. The polymerase chain reaction (PCR) for CMV DNA is usually positive, culture mostly negative.

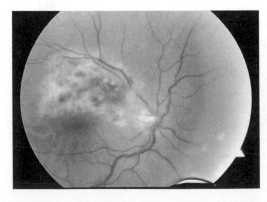

Figure 26.2 Fundus photograph showing the haemorrhagic appearances of cytomegalovirus retinitis (illustration kindly provided by Dr P Frith).

CMV encephalitis is occasionally subacute, but more commonly causes rapidly progressive confusion and drowsiness which is often fatal, usually without focal neurological signs. Pathologically, there are two main forms, one with diffuse microglial nodular encephalitis especially affecting the grey matter, the other with ventriculoencephalitis with destruction of the ependymal lining and necrosis of periventricular tissue. CMV ventriculoencephalitis was not described in adults before AIDS. MRI scan may show patchy white matter hyperintensity with or without ventricular enhancement and hydrocephalus.

Treatment is with i.v. ganciclovir and foscarnet; prophylaxis can be discontinued if CD4 counts increase above 150. Unfortunately, prognosis remains poor.

Progressive multifocal leukoencephalopathy

JC virus is a ubiquitous polyomavirus latent in the bodies of 70 per cent of healthy adults, which may reactivate with immunosuppression and destroy brain oligodendrocytes causing demyelination. PML is also seen in the setting of an IRIS in the months after HAART is commenced when response to early steroids is reported. Incidence has decreased more slowly than other opportunistic infections since HAART, from about 4 to 1–2 per cent.

Progressive hemiparesis and hemianopia are most common, usually in clear consciousness initially (unlike other focal brain syndromes in HIV) and without systemic inflammatory or infective symptoms. With disease progression and widespread demyelination, cognitive impairment develops and seizures may occur.

MRI typically shows asymmetrical hemispheric white matter signal change with little mass effect or contrast enhancement (Figure 26.3), sometimes affecting the brainstem or cerebellum and occasionally the spinal cord. JC virus PCR in the blood is not useful, and although PCR in the CSF is usually positive, it can be negative. Biopsy of the

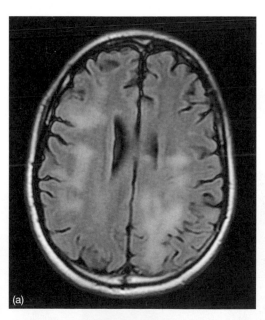
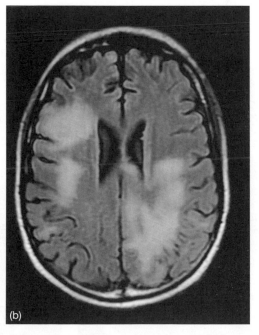

Figure 26.3 Axial FLAIR magnetic resonance imaging (MRI) brain scans. The first scan (a) shows bilateral, asymmetrical signal abnormality in cerebral white extending to the corticomedullary junction without involving the overlying cortex. There is no mass effect and there was no enhancement on post-contrast scans (not shown). The appearance is typical of progressive multifocal leucoencephalopathy (PML), confirmed at biopsy. The corresponding scan (b), the same patient 18 days later, showing increase in extent of signal abnormality with mild swelling. The clinical diagnosis was PML in the setting of an immune restoration inflammatory syndrome (IRIS). (Image courtesy of Dr Phillip Rich, Consultant Radiologist, St George's Hospital Trust.)

abnormal areas shows multiple foci of demyelination with associated bizarre giant astrocytes, and abnormal oligodendrocytes with intranuclear inclusions. The virus can be demonstrated in these cells.

Survival times have increased with HAART, from 0.4 years pre-HAART in 1995, to 1.8 years in 2006. Patients with a relatively high CD4 count, or with PML as the presentation of AIDS, tend to do better. PML IRIS may respond to steroids although overall, the development of PML IRIS has no effect on mortality. Other treatments are all experimental to date.

Other infections

Tuberculosis

Tuberculosis (TB) is the most common cause of death in AIDS patients worldwide, often develops insidiously, and may be difficult to diagnose, so that treatment often needs to be started presumptively.

Meningitis, brain and spinal **epidural abscesses** and **tuberculomas** (Figure 26.4) may occur. Target lesions, with a zone of low attenuation between higher central and peripheral attenuation, are more suggestive of brain tuberculomas than toxoplasmosis or lymphoma. Patients with tuberculous meningitis are usually extremely unwell. CSF rarely shows a positive staining for acid fast bacilli, although prolonged culture may be positive and PCR may also be positive. CSF typically contains a high protein and raised leukocyte count (predominantly lymphocytes), with low glucose, or may be non-specifically abnormal (due to suppression of the immune response to TB in patients with HIV).

Treatment complexities include interactions between antituberculous therapies and antiretroviral treatment, and multidrug resistance. Adjunctive corticosteroids are given for TB meningitis and sometimes in other conditions where there is significant mass effect. Treatment is preferably in specialist units where there is close liaison between HIV and TB specialists. The introduction of HAART may be associated with an exacerbation of the

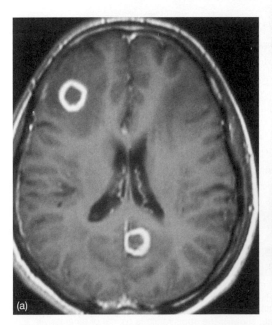
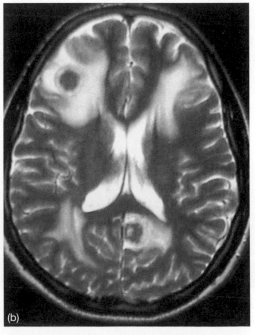

Figure 26.4 Axial T1-weighted post-contrast magnetic resonance imaging (MRI) brain scan. (a) Ring-enhancing lesions surrounded by oedema in the right cerebral hemisphere. The lesion cavities return uniformly low signal on the corresponding T2-weighted scan (b), typical of tuberculomas. (Image courtesy of Dr Phillip Rich.)

symptoms of tuberculosis in the initial weeks of treatment.

Syphilis

Between 1997 and 2007, there was a ten-fold increase in the number of syphilis cases diagnosed in the UK, the focus of the epidemic being in homosexual men, and this resurgence continues. Meningitis and meningovascular disease may occur as well as **painful polyradiculopathy**. Less common features include ocular infections, optic neuritis and other cranial nerve lesions, such as facial palsy or sensorineural hearing loss. Late manifestations of neurosyphilis (usually manifesting during the tertiary stage of syphilis) occur when there is extensive damage to brain and spinal cord parenchyma and include dementia, tabes dorsalis and general paresis. Although these are rare, they are still seen occasionally in patients presenting late with HIV.

A symptomatic patient with positive syphilis serology, should, like patients not infected with HIV, have a CSF examination. In non-HIV-infected individuals, the serum RPR (rapid plasma reagin) or venereal disease research laboratory (VDRL) tests are usually done as screening tests. In people with HIV, these may be falsely positive due to polyclonal stimulation, and the FTA-ABS (fluorescent treponemal antibody absorption) test is regarded to be more specific in this group.

In people without HIV, a cellular CSF or a positive treponema pallidum particle agglutination (TPPA) or VDRL test in a clear (i.e. non-blood-stained) CSF is then probably diagnostic, in association with the appropriate clinical syndrome. In the HIV-infected population, interpretation of CSF is more challenging: A positive CSF-VDRL or TPPA is still confirmatory for neurosyphilis, but the sensitivity is lower. HIV itself often causes a mild elevation in CSF white cell and protein counts, so the cut-off for presumptive neurosyphilis is usually higher. Many HIV physicians would not regard a CSF cell count of less than 10/mm³ to be diagnostic.

Penicillin remains the treatment of choice for neurosyphilis in patients with HIV, preferably intravenously for 10–14 days. If this is not possible for practical reasons, intramuscular penicillin for 14 days is an alternative, with oral probenecid. Neurological relapses are extremely uncommon in patients without HIV who are treated for neurosyphilis, but unfortunately do occur more commonly in those infected with HIV. HIV-infected patients also have slower resolution of serum and CSF syphilis tests after treatment. Most now recommend three doses of intramuscular penicillin at weekly intervals after the completion of the initial 14 day course for HIV-infected patients. No oral treatment alternatives are recommended.

Herpes viruses

Dermatomal zoster (shingles) is common and occasionally progresses to affect the nerve roots, spine and brain. Herpes simplex may cause an encephalitis or, rarely, myelitis (Figure 26.5) and both zoster and simplex can cause retinitis.

CSF PCR is very helpful and treatment is with aciclovir, famciclovir or valacyclovir, sometimes with corticosteroids.

Hepatitis B and C

Both hepatitis B and C are associated with peripheral neuropathy in patients with and without HIV. The estimate for coinfection with HIV in the UK is 5–10 per cent for hepatitis B, and more than 50 per cent of HIV-infected drug users are also affected with hepatitis C.

Hepatitis B can cause a multiple mononeuropathy due to a florid vasculitis in both infected and non-infected groups. Treatment is with alpha interferon and lamivudine (3TC) with a protease inhibitor such as tenofovir (both lamivudine and tenofovir have anti-HIV and anti-hepatitis B activity) or similar antiretroviral agents. Patients with HIV who are not affected should be vaccinated against hepatitis B.

Hepatitis C is more complex. Neuropathy is uncommon in subjects without HIV and, if present, is usually a multiple mononeuropathy, with about 75 per cent being associated with cryoglobulinaemia. In those coinfected with HIV,

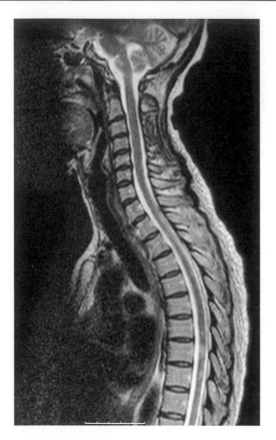

Figure 26.5 Sagittal T2-weighted magnetic resonance imaging (MRI) scan of the spinal cord. The lower thoracic spinal cord returns abnormal high signal in a patchy distribution without obvious cord swelling. The diagnosis was herpes zoster myelitis, although vacuolar myelopathy would show a similar appearance. (Image courtesy of Dr Phillip Rich.)

hepatitis C-related neuropathy is of two types – a distal symmetrical neuropathy or a mononeuropathy/multiple mononeuropthy, and cryoglobulinaemia is almost universal. One-third of patients affected will also have an ill-defined encephalopathy, and nephrotic syndrome is also seen in a proportion. Neurophysiologically, the syndrome is predominantly axonal, although conduction block (similar to that seen in inflammatory demyelinating neuropathies) may be seen. Hepatitis C-related neuropathy is treated now with pegylated interferon-alpha and ribavirin. In patients coinfected with HIV, treatment choices are difficult, as the toxicity of HAART agents is increased with interferon-ribavirin.

TUMOURS

Primary CNS lymphoma

After toxoplasmosis, primary CNS lymphoma (PCNSL) is the most common cause of mass lesions in HIV disease, and is particularly common in children.

PCNSL is usually a high-grade B-cell lymphoma, multifocal in 50 per cent. It has been reported in 6–20 per cent of HIV-infected patients, virtually all (more than 95 per cent) males, and is particularly prevalent in intravenous drug users. PCNSL can originate within the brain, in the spinal cord, in the meninges or in the eye. It usually remains confined to the central nervous system and therapy is hampered therefore by the blood–brain barrier. Epstein–Barr virus (EBV) DNA can be demonstrated in the CSF in virtually all patients with PCNSL, presumably because EBV drives increased B-cell turnover, especially in the immunosuppressed.

Presentation is usually with headache, confusion, lethargy and seizures. Alternatively, presentation may be with subacutely progressive focal neurological symptoms, although this is less common than in immunocompetent patients with PCNSL. However, by presentation, focal neurological symptoms and signs are usually found, determined by the site of the tumours.

Imaging may be indistinguishable from other mass lesions in the brain, particularly toxoplasmosis (Figure 26.6), with multifocal enhancing lesions, although periventricular enhancement is particularly suggestive, as is spread across the corpus callosum. Single photon emission computed tomography (SPECT) may help to distinguish these. CSF is often not examined if the lesions are space-occupying, but when possible shows EBV DNA, and cytology may reveal lymphoma cells. It is worth performing slit-lamp examination for vitrous lymphoma. The decision whether to proceed to biopsy for confirmation of the diagnosis depends on the degree to which other aspects of the patient's illness limit chances of deriving advantage overall from any treatment.

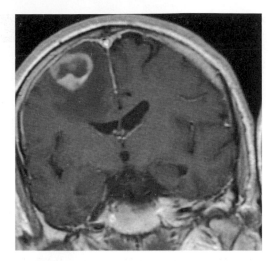

Figure 26.6 Coronal T1-weighted magnetic resonance imaging (MRI) brain scan post-contrast. There is a ring-enhancing lesion peripherally in the right frontal lobe surrounded by oedema causing brain swelling and slight subfalcine herniation. The radiological differential diagnosis includes infection. Lymphoma was diagnosed at biopsy. (Image courtesy of Dr Phillip Rich.)

Whole brain radiotherapy and steroids may increase survival a few months, but the prognosis is very poor (with a median survival in HIV-infected patients of approximately four months) with this alone. In immunocompetent patients with PCNSL, chemotherapy has extended survival to 44 months, but only a subgroup of HIV-infected patients have been shown to tolerate both chemotherapy and radiotherapy, and in them median survival may be up to 18 months. As with opportunistic infections, it now appears that HAART improves the prognosis.

Other tumours

Systemic AIDS-related non-Hodgkin's lymphoma involves the nervous system uncommonly, and when it does, shows a predilection for cranial nerves, meningeal and epidural involvement rather than the brain parenchyma. Multicentric Castleman's disease is associated with human herpes virus 8 (HHV-8) and is increasingly reported. This is essentially a lymph node hyperplasia which may progress to non-Hodgkin's lymphoma. It usually presents systemically with lymphadenopathy and fever. Peripheral neuropathy occurs in 20 per cent of cases, sometimes as POEMS (polyneuropathy, organomegaly, endocrinopathy, mono-

clonal paraprotein, skin changes) syndrome. Rarely, Burkitt's lymphoma and Kaposi's sarcoma may involve the nervous system.

DISORDERS DIRECTLY CAUSED BY THE HIV VIRUS

HIV-associated neurocognitive disorders

HIV-associated dementia is invariably a late-stage manifestation of HIV, associated with a low CD4 count. However, milder neurocognitive impairments are now recognized in earlier disease (distinct from mood disorders), particularly when HIV is longstanding, and the prevalence of these has increased as individuals live longer with disease.

These more minor syndromes may progress to HIV dementia over years, so where once HIV dementia represented a group with fairly rapidly fatal disease, **HIV-associated neurocognitive disorders (HAND) are now more often a chronic problem requiring multispecialty input.**

Some studies suggest neurocognitive impairment in more than 50 per cent of HIV-positive subjects. The mini-mental test score has been found to be insensitive to detecting HAND and an HIV dementia scale has been developed composed of four components: memory registration and recall, attention, psychomotor speed and construction, with a total score of 16; a score of less than 10 is considered to be more sensitive for HAND.

Though HIV dementia is thought to be a direct consequence of infection with the virus, HIV does not appear to infect neurons directly. When the CD4 count is low, replication of HIV in the brain may proceed unchecked, although this is predominantly in perivascular macrophages and microglia. This results in the release of potentially neurotoxic factors (cytokines, chemokines and other inflammatory mediators), causing neuronal damage. Beta-amyloid may also be detected in brains affected by HIV, and this seems to be neuronal, as compared with the extracellular plaques of beta-amyloid found in Alzheimer's disease. Histopathologically, microglial nodules, a fusion of HIV-infected and non-infected cells, are seen.

HIV-associated dementia usually develops insidiously over months with cognitive, affective, behavioural and motor manifestations (Table 26.2), often mimicking depression. Increasing forgetfulness, neglect of usual activities, personality change and deteriorating motor skills and gait then typically occur. MRI (Figure 26.7) helps exclude other causes but is usually non-specific, with atrophy and diffuse white matter change. CSF is also non-specific, but helps exclude other aetiologies (Box 26.2).

Box 26.2 Differential diagnosis of HIV-associated dementia

- Depression/anxiety
- Drugs
- Metabolic encephalopathy
- Lymphoma
- Toxoplasmosis
- Cryptococcosis
- PML
- CMV encephalitis

CMV, cytomegalovirus; PML, progressive multifocal leukoencephalopathy.

Table 26.2 Manifestations of HIV dementia

Domain	Symptoms/problems
Cognitive	Impaired concentration and attention
	Bradyphrenia (mental slowing)
	Visuospatial memory and coordination deficits
	Sequencing problems
	Verbal memory impairment
Affective	Apathy
	Irritability
Behavioural	Personality changes
	Social exclusion
Motor	Gait unsteadiness
	Leg weakness
	Hand coordination difficulty and fine motor deficits
	Tremor

Despite the low CNS penetration of some of the components of HAART, the introduction of drug combination regimens has led to further improvements in both prevention and treatment of dementia. A CNS penetration effectiveness score for antiretroviral drugs has been developed to help

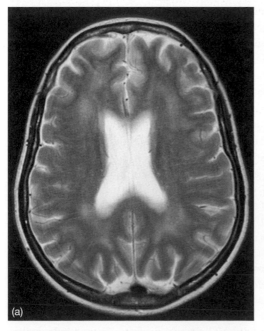
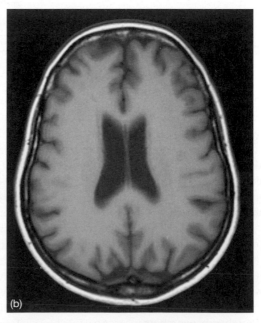

Figure 26.7 Axial T2-weighted magnetic resonance imaging (MRI) brain scan. There is diffuse, ill-defined abnormal signal returned from deep cerebral white matter (a). This is not visible on the accompanying T1-weighted scan as would usually be the case in PML (b). (Image courtesy of Dr Phillip Rich.)

Table 26.3 Antiretroviral drugs with high CNS penetration

Type of drug	Drug name
NRTI	Abacavir, Zidovudine
NNRTI	Nevirapine, Delavirdine
PI	Indinavir, Lopinavir, Amprenavir, Atazanavir, Fosamprenavir

CNS, central nervous system; NNRTI non-nucleoside analogue reverse transcriptase inhibitor; NRTI, nucleoside analogue reverse transcriptase inhibitor; PI protease inhibitor.

Box 26.3 Differential diagnosis of vacuolar myelopathy

- Epidural abscess
- Herpes virus myelitis (CMV, VZV, HSV)
- Subacute combined degeneration of the cord
- Tuberculosis
- Human T-cell lymphotropic virus (HTLV)
- Syphilis
- Lymphoma
- Toxoplasma

CMV, cytomegalovirus; HSV, herpes simplex virus; VZV, varicella zoster virus.

guide therapy (Table 26.3). However, outcome is variable, some failing to respond and others relapsing after initial improvement. Numerous trials of specific agents have been largely unsuccessful to date.

Vacuolar myelopathy

Before HAART, autopsy studies suggested 20–55 per cent of patients with HIV had evidence of vacuolar myelopathy, clinically apparent in 10 per cent, usually with an insidiously developing spastic paraparesis, and often found in association with neurocognitive disease. Histologically, the myelin sheath is separated from the underlying axon to create vacuoles, thought to be due to dysregulated cytokine release in response to local HIV. The dorsolateral white matter tracts of the middle and lower thoracic cord are particularly affected. Similarities with the cord changes found in vitamin B12 deficiency led to suggestions that a metabolic mechanism interfering with transmethylation may be responsible, but this remains unconfirmed. The finding of vacuolar myelopathy in small numbers of immunosuppressed HIV-negative patients raises the possibility of alternative causes, including a possible unidentified infective agent (Box 26.3).

Clinically, early disease may present simply as hyper-reflexia, but the condition usually progresses as a painless spastic paraparesis with bladder dysfunction and sensory ataxia. MRI may show thoracic cord atrophy, sometimes with intrinsic cord signal change. CSF is usually inactive, but is helpful in excluding other causes (Table 26.3). Myelopathy is substantially less frequent in the era of HAART. Other than this preventive effect of HAART, no specific treatments for the myelopathy have been found to be effective.

Others

HIV within the CSF may directly cause radiculopathy which may mimic that seen with CMV (although it is usually less painful). Demyelination affecting the brain is also increasingly reported, which may improve with HAART. HIV itself has also been reported to cause myopathy.

DISORDERS DIRECTLY CAUSED BY THE HIV VIRUS OR BY HIV THERAPIES

Peripheral neuropathy

Peripheral neuropathy may be caused by various pathologies in HIV, broadly related to the stage of disease (Table 26.4). For instance, a distal sensory polyneuropathy (DSPN) directly due to the virus affects about one-third of patients with advanced disease, whereas inflammatory neuropathies generally occur earlier in the course of HIV disease.

Neuropathy is a frequent toxic effect of antiretroviral medication, although the newer drugs less commonly lead to neuropathy (Table 26.5). This can be difficult to distinguish from DSPN. Usually, drug-induced symptoms improve on drug withdrawal, but not always immediately – the 'coasting period' is a time of up to 8 weeks following drug withdrawal when symptoms may continue or increase, before improvement begins. Some toxic

Table 26.4 Types of peripheral neuropathy in HIV disease

Early disease (seroconversion illnesses)	Guillain–Barré syndrome (AIDP) Mononeuropathies Brachial neuritis
Moderately advanced disease (CD4 count 200–500 cells/mm³)	CIDP Multiple mononeuropathies VZV-related radiculopathy DILS Syphilitic and HC radiculopathy Motor neuron disease-type syndrome
Advanced disease (CD4 count <200 cells/mm³)	CMV lumbosacral radiculopathy/ multiple mononeuropathy DSPN
Medication-related	Neuropathy IRIS

AIDP, acute inflammatory demyelinating polyradiculoneuropathy; CIDP, chronic inflammatory demyelinating polyradiculoneuropathy; CMV, cytomegalovirus, DILS, diffuse infiltrative lymphocytosis syndrome; DSPN, distal sensory polyneuropathy; HC, hepatitis C; IRIS, immune reconstitution inflammatory syndrome; VZV, varicella zoster virus.

Table 26.5 Drugs used in HIV that cause neuropathy

	Drug
nRTI antiretrovirals	ddC (zalcitabine), ddI (didanosine), d4T (stavudine) Possibly 3TC (lamivudine), fialuridine
Other agents	Isoniazid, ethambutol Vincristine, vinblastine Dapsone, metronidazole Thalidomide Statins Alcohol and solvents

nRTI, nucleoside analogue reverse transcriptase inhibitor.

effects, particularly distal numbness and foot pain seem, in the author's experience, to have a significant degree of irreversibility, indicating that recovery is often only partial.

Because patients now survive in the long term on HAART, in theory other complications, such as diabetes, related to protease inhibitors with associated diabetic neuropathy are possible, although this does not seem to be an issue yet in practice.

Both DSPN and drug-induced neuropathy tend to have a gradual onset, with numbness or paraesthesiae in the toes and soles of the feet, which spread slowly proximally. In some patients, neuropathic pain is a prominent feature, sometimes with severe allodynia (pain in response to light touch; see Chapter 30). Ankle reflexes are usually absent, although knee jerks may be brisk if there is coexistent vacuolar myelopathy. Abnormalities of autonomic function may also occur, although are less common.

Nerve conduction studies may be normal or show typical axonal neuropathy (reduced amplitude of sensory action potentials with normal nerve conduction velocities). Thermal thresholds are generally abnormal, indicating that small fibres are affected, which can be confirmed if necessary by skin punch biopsy and assessment of the epidermal nerve fibre density. If there are atypical features, CSF examination and sural nerve biopsy may be necessary to exclude the other causes listed in Table 26.4.

Treatment of those with DSPN not yet taking an antiretroviral agent involves starting such therapy, and for drug-related neuropathy involves changing the drug regime to non-toxic agents. Symptomatic treatment for the neuropathic pain is very limited. Some drugs shown to be effective in neuropathic pain from other causes, have proved to be ineffective in controlled trials of HIV-associated neuropathy, notably tricyclic antidepressants and gabapentin. Topical capsaicin (8 per cent) was effective in one double-blind controlled trial (see also Chapter 30). A number of open-label studies have reported response of pain to the anti-oxidant acetyl-carnitine.

In addition to direct effects of the HIV virus and its therapies, peripheral neuropathy can occur due to various perturbations of the immune system. **Early HIV disease may be associated with acute inflammatory demyelinating neuropathy (AIDP, the most common type of Guillain–Barré syndrome**

in the UK). The condition is symptomatically and electrophysiologically indistinguisable from that in patients without HIV, usually with raised CSF protein, although the CSF may also show a raised white cell count. Guillain–Barré syndrome has also been described as an IRIS, sometimes in association with the antiretroviral drug, stavudine, but also with a variety of therapies.

> A syndrome similar to chronic inflammatory demyelinating neuropathy (CIDP) may also occur, most often in moderately advanced HIV disease, with similar CSF features to AIDP in HIV (as above). Treatment is complicated by the risks of further impairing immune function and intravenous immunoglobulin is generally preferable, although steroids and sometimes other immunosuppressants may be required.

A sensory neuropathy, frequently painful, is reported in association with diffuse infiltrative lymphocytosis syndrome (DILS), a condition with similarities to Sjögren's syndrome, with dry eyes and dry mouth. There is usually evidence of systemic involvement – parotidomegaly, lymphadenopathy or splenomegaly, with a CD8 cell lymphocytosis and CD8 cell infiltration of the nerve. HAART appears to be the most effective treatment, with or without steroids.

Myopathy

Skeletal muscle disorders are seen at all stages of HIV infection (Table 26.6) including at the time of seroconversion. As with peripheral neuropathy, most commonly muscle disease occurs either as a direct effect of the HIV virus or as an adverse effect of anti-retroviral treatment.

HIV can cause several types of muscle disease, the most common being polymyositis. HIV polymyositis may occur at any stage of HIV disease and is characterized by proximal painful muscle weakness usually developing over weeks. Creatine kinase (CK) is usually raised. Electromyography (EMG) generally shows typical features of myositis (although they may be normal) and muscle biopsy is inflammatory with CD8+ cell infiltration. Treatment is with steroids and other immunosuppressant drugs, as with non-HIV polymyositis. Rarely, HIV is associated with a myopathy similar to inclusion body myositis, and a painless progressive myopathy with electron microscope characteristics of nemaline (rod) myopathy has also been described.

Table 26.6 Muscle disease in HIV

HIV-associated myopathies	HIV Polymyositis
	Inclusion body myositis
	Nemaline myopathy
	DILS
	HIV-wasting syndrome
	Vasculitis
Anti-retroviral myopathies	NRTIs: AZT (zidovudine), d4T (stavudine), ddC (zalcitabine), ddI (didanosine), 3TC (lamivudine)
	NNRTIs: nevirapine, efavirenz, delaviridine
	PIs: ritonavir, saquinavir, indinavir, nelfinavir, amprenavir
	HIV-associated lipodystrophy syndrome
	HAART-related IRIS
Opportunistic infections and tumours	Toxoplasmosis
	Staphylococcus aureus
	CMV
	Cryptococcus
	Mycobacterium avium intracellulare
	non-Hodgkin's lymphoma
	Kaposi's sarcoma
Rhabdomyolysis	

CMV, cytomegalovirus; DILS, diffuse infiltrative lymphocytosis syndrome; HAART, highly active anti-retroviral therapy; IRIS, immune reconstitution inflammatory syndrome; NNRTI, non-nucleoside analogue reverse transcriptase inhibitor; NRTI, nucleoside analogue reverse transcriptase inhibitor.

> Zidovudine (AZT) myopathy is thought to result from disordered muscle mitochondrial function and mimics HIV polymyositis; most patients improve when treatment is stopped. It usually follows high cumulative doses of AZT.

A syndrome called HIV-associated lipodystrophy syndrome is increasingly common with the use of HAART. The syndrome comprises two components: a change in body fat distribution with peripheral fat atrophy and central fat accumulation, together with metabolic abnormalities of hyperlipidaemia and insulin resistance. The syndrome is thought to be a combination of the effects of PIs causing fat accumulation, high lipids and insulin resistance, and nRTIs causing lipoatrophy.

Muscle disease may also occur as an IRIS, usually as a polymyositis, and rarely in association with opportunistic infections and tumours of muscle. Rhabdomyolysis, with painful weakness, very high CK and myoglobinuria, may also occur due to HIV, either as a consequence of treatment or as an end-stage process. DILS may affect muscle as well as peripheral nerve in HIV, with CD8 cell infiltration of muscle fibres. Again HAART, with or without steroids (usually with) is most effective.

CEREBROVASCULAR DISEASE

HIV-associated vasculopathy is recognized as a cause of young-onset stroke and may respond to HAART. The pathophysiology is uncertain, but it is probably wise to consider HIV a relatively prothrombotic state and test for HIV in young patients with stroke. Cortical venous sinus thrombosis is also more common, possibly due to changes in clotting factors and the development of anticardiolipin antibodies in HIV, and usually occurs in advanced disease.

As with many of the neurological conditions already described, vascular disease is also described consequent to treatment, and a vasculitis occurs after commencing HAART which is thought to be an inflammatory IRIS. Meningovascular syphilis, zoster vasculitis and, rarely, CMV vasculitis may also occur, and cardiogenic embolism, particularly from bacterial endocarditis in intravenous drug users must not be forgotten.

IMMUNE RESTORATION INFLAMMATORY SYNDROMES

Immunocompromised patients treated with HAART may develop a paradoxical inflammatory response as their immune system is reconstituted, related either to infections or to non-infectious inflammation (Table 26.7). **The risk of developing IRIS is linked to the duration and extent of immunocompromise (patients usually have an initial CD4 count less than 50), the speed and pattern of immune reconstitution and some form of genetic susceptibility in the host.** Onset is usually within 6 weeks of initiating antiretrovirals, but it may occur several months later. Similar exacerbations are described in non-HIV patients following treatment of, for example, TB or syphilis, but the condition

Table 26.7 Immune restoration inflammatory syndromes (IRIS)

Infectious inflammatory processes	Silent opportunistic pathogens:	TB meningitis or abscess PML (often JCV negative) CMV retinitis Cryptococcal meningitis HZV, HSV
	Human herpes virus-8 (HHV-8)-associated disease:	Castleman's disease Kaposi's sarcoma
Non-infectious inflammatory processes	Autoimmune diseases: polymyositis, SLE, rheumatoid arthritis Allergic reactions Sarcoidosis Atherogenic chronic inflammation/vasculitis	

CMV, cytomegalovirus; HSV, herpes simplex virus; HZV, herpes zoster virus; JCV, JC virus; PML, progressive multifocal leukoencephalopathy; SLE, systemic lupus erythematosis; TB, tuberculosis.

seems to be more frequent in those infected with HIV.

The pathophysiology of IRIS remains poorly understood, but it seems that HAART-induced restoration of the immune system results in an abnormal immune response to the antigens of certain dying infectious agents or to other non-infectious antigens.

> Clinically, IRIS manifests either as a worsening of an underlying infection, or the development of new symptoms and signs. The condition is particularly well recognized in patients taking treatment for TB or other mycobacteria who, on commencement of HAART, may develop an exacerbation of symptoms, signs or radiological findings of TB without any evidence of recurrence or relapse of the infection. As described above, the syndrome may cause apparent recurrence of cryptococcus and wosening of JC virus-induced progressive multifocal leukoencephalopathy (PML). IRIS also occurs with CMV, herpes and hepatitis viruses and HHV-8 (Kaposi's sarcoma and Castleman's syndrome).

Autoimmune diseases may also be exacerbated as part of an IRIS, such as Gullain–Barré syndrome.

No prospective treatment trials have been performed in IRIS to date. The manifestations are highly variable and there is no test available to establish the diagnosis, impeding the development of treatment strategies. The management recommended, from small numbers of case reports in the literature and from personal experience, is to treat infection, to maintain treatment with antiretroviral drugs unless the condition is life-threatening, and to give steroids or other anti-inflammatories.

FURTHER READING

Authier F-J, Chariot P, Gherardi RK (2005) Skeletal muscle involvement in human immunodeficiency virus (HIV)-infected patients in the era of highly active antiretroviral therapy (HAART). *Muscle and Nerve*, 32:247–260.

Brew BL (2003) The peripheral nerve complications of human immunodeficiency virus (HIV) infection. *Muscle and Nerve*, 28:542–552.

Carr A, Cooper DA (2000) Adverse effects of an antiretroviral therapy. *Lancet*, 356:1423–1430.

Clifford DB (2008) HIV-associated neurocognitive disease continues in the antiretroviral era. *Topics in HIV Medicine*, 16:94–98 (original presentation available as webcast at www.iasusa.org).

Cutfield NJ, Steele H, Wilhelm T, Weatherall MW (2009) Successful treatment of HIV asociated cerebral vasculopathy with HAART. *Journal of Neurology, Neurosurgery and Psychiatry*, 80:936–937.

Falco V, Olmo M, Villar del Saz S *et al.* (2008) Influence of HAART on the clinical course of HIV-1-infected patients with progressive multifocal leukoencephalopathy: results of an observational multicenter study. *Journal of Acquired Immune Deficiency Syndromes*, 49:26–31.

Health Protection Agency. HIV in the United Kingdom: 2009 Report. Available from: www.hpa.org.uk.

Manji H, Miller RF (2000) Progressive multifocal leukoencephalopathy: progress in the AIDS era. *Journal of Neurology, Neurosurgery and Psychiatry*, 69:569–571.

McCombe JA, Auer RN, Maingat FG *et al.* (2009) Neurologic immune reconstitution inflammatory syndrome in HIV/AIDS: outcome and epidemiology. *Neurology*, 72:835–841.

Murdoch DM, Venter WDF, Van Rie A, Feldman C (2007) Immune reconstitution syndrome (IRIS): review of common infectious manifestations and treatment options. *AIDS Research and Therapy*, 4:9.

Tan K, Roda R, Ostrow L *et al.* (2009) PML-IRIS in patients with HIV infection. Clinical manifestations and treatment with steroids. *Neurology*, 72:1458–1464.

CHAPTER 27

NEUROLOGICAL MANIFESTATIONS OF MEDICAL DISORDERS

David Werring and John Scadding

INTRODUCTION

Historically, neurology developed apart from general medicine and other specialties. However, it is clear that disease of any body system can cause disturbance of function in the nervous system. Neurologists, general physicians and other specialists need to be familiar with the many neurological manifestations of medical disorders. This is especially important because the complications of medical disorders include some of the most readily treatable neurological presentations. This chapter summarizes the clinical neurological manifestations of the disorders of other body systems, outlining basic elements of pathophysiology, diagnosis and management.

CARDIOVASCULAR DISORDERS

The neurological consequences of cardiovascular disease include stroke and transient ischaemic attack (TIA), which are considered in detail in Chapter 23. Some additional aspects relating to aortic, great vessel and spinal cord arterial diseases are considered here, as are neurological complications of cardiac surgery and some acquired cardiac diseases.

Cerebral ischaemia due to aortic disease

Aortic atherosclerosis, aortitis or aneurysm, can cause ischaemic stroke, transient ischaemic attack and hypoperfusion syndromes.

Aortic atheroma is increasingly recognized as a cause of embolism to the brain and can be well-visualized by transoesophageal echocardiography. **Steal syndromes** are due to stenosis of the innominate or subclavian vessels proximal to the origin of the vertebral artery, three times more often on the left than the right. Reverse flow in a vertebral artery is typically exacerbated by exercising the ipsilateral arm, thus increasing blood flow to the arm or, less commonly, by neck movement. The great majority of cases of steal are asymptomatic. The term '**subclavian steal syndrome**' should only be used if symptoms are present; these are those of posterior circulation ischaemia including vertigo, visual disturbances and ataxia, and may respond to endovascular treatment of stenosis.

Spinal cord ischaemia due to aortic disease

About one in 100 strokes affect the spinal cord. The most important vascular syndrome is infarction in the territory of the anterior spinal artery, with loss of pain and temperature (spinothalamic) sensation and paraparesis below the lesion; preserved vibration and joint position (carried in the dorsal columns which are supplied by the posterior spinal arteries); and loss of sphincter control. Symptoms may develop abruptly, or evolve over several hours, typically following severe, radicular-type thoracic pain at the onset.

The mid to lower thoracic region is most vulnerable to ischaemia. Anterior spinal infarcts are often due to aortic disease or surgery, but in about half of cases no cause is identified; there is an association with conventional vascular risk factors (hypertension, smoking, diabetes and hypercholesterolaemia). The diagnosis of spinal infarction is clinical, although magnetic resonance imaging (MRI) usually shows signal abnormalities. Atherosclerosis, aortitis, dissection, aneurysms and coarctation can all cause spinal cord ischaemia, but generally only if the suprarenal aorta is involved.

Dissection of the thoracic aorta classically causes searing interscapular pain, hypotension and asymmetric arm pulses, with a thoracic sensory level. Cardiac or aortic surgery requiring prolonged clamping of the aorta, and aortic angiography can also cause anterior spinal infarction; the risk for suprarenal procedures is up to 10 per cent; infrarenal interventions are safer.

Aortitis can cause neurological symptoms via the development of aneurysms, aortic stenosis or atherosclerosis. **Syphilitic aortitis** is now rare, but typically causes aneurysms of the thoracic aorta. By contrast, atherosclerosis causes abdominal aneurysmal dilatation. **Takayasu disease** is a rare cause of aortitis, typically in female patients under 30; a 'pre-pulseless phase' with fever, weight loss, arthralgia, myalgia, night sweats and chest pain develops into the 'pulseless phase', in which there is occlusion of the major vessels of the aortic arch with aortic regurgitation, aneurysm formation and hypertension. Cerebral ischaemia is uncommon.

Neurological complications of cardiac surgery

Coronary artery bypass grafting (CABG) is still a common operation in developed countries, and peri-operative stroke occurs in up to 5 per cent of patients. A more subtle late encephalopathy may develop. These complications result from microemboli and hypoperfusion during surgery, and from postoperative atrial fibrillation. Embolism accounts for most (up to 60 per cent) cases of stroke; previous cerebrovascular disease increases the risk.

Carotid stenosis is associated with an increased risk of postoperative stroke, but this is probably because it is a marker of generalized vascular disease, rather than a direct cause. In symptomatic patients with carotid stenosis of greater than 70 per cent, intervention (carotid endarterectomy or stenting) prior to cardiac surgery is recommended. Treatment of asymptomatic carotid stenosis remains controversial and is generally avoided unless the stenosis is very severe.

Neurological complications of acquired cardiac disease

Cardiac embolism

About 80 per cent of cardiac emboli enter the anterior cerebral vessels; an anterior circulation branch occlusion is suggestive of a cardioembolic source. Although cardioembolism to the posterior circulation is less common, certain stroke syndromes are

> Cardiac embolism accounts for up to one-quarter of all ischaemic strokes. Clinical and radiological findings suggestive of cardiac embolism include: abrupt and maximal deficit at onset (rather than stepwise); haemorrhagic transformation, due to rapid reperfusion; or multiple vascular territory infarcts on imaging, with an identified potential cardiac source on echocardiography (ECG).

characteristic, including the 'top of the basilar syndrome' (reduced conscious level, visual field loss, limb sensory or motor symptoms), and unilateral posterior cerebral artery occlusion causing isolated hemianopia and striatocapsular infarction. Of course, none of these features is specific, and it must be remembered that a confident diagnosis of cardiac embolism can be difficult in the presence of coexisting large vessel atherothrombotic or cerebral small vessel disease.

Rhythm disturbances

Sick sinus syndrome

Sick sinus syndrome is idiopathic dysfunction of the sinus node in older people. Although often asymptomatic, cardioembolic stroke occurs in up to 20 per cent of patients, especially those with tachyarrhythmias. Other rhythm disturbances include sinus bradycardia, sinus arrest, sinoatrial block, and bradycardia–tachycardia syndrome; these may cause syncope, palpitations or dizziness. Pacemakers do not definitively reduce the risk of stroke. If atrial fibrillation occurs, anticoagulation reduces the future stroke risk.

Cardiomyopathies

> Primary cardiomyopathies, i.e. not secondary to acquired diseases like ischaemic heart disease, are associated with arrhythmias and a tendency for blood stasis, increasing the risk of left ventricular thrombus formation and embolism to the brain. Dilated or restrictive types are far more likely to be a cause of embolism than hypertrophic cardiomyopathies, in which cerebral embolism is rare.

Primary cardiomyopathies have a genetic component, and family screening may be indicated.

In stroke considered due to cardiac embolism and where the ejection fraction is low, anticoagulation is often recommended to prevent recurrent events, but the evidence for this approach is limited.

Valve disease

> Infective endocarditis causes embolism to the brain in about one-fifth of cases, usually during active infection, clinically characterized by fever, malaise and evidence of emboli to other organs (e.g. the skin, eyes and kidneys).

Patient groups at particular risk of endocarditis include those with immunosuppression, intravenous drug use, prosthetic heart valves or structural heart valve disease. Emboli may cause infection or vasculitis of vessels where they impact, with or without the development of mycotic aneurysms (typically in distal branches of the middle cerebral artery). Anticoagulation is not recommended in native valve endocarditis because of the high risk of haemorrhagic complications, but in the case of prosthetic valve endocarditis anticoagulants may need to be continued (although it is probably safe to discontinue them for 1–2 weeks acutely). Early cerebral angiography is generally advised in the case of areas of symptomatic haemorrhage to exclude mycotic aneurysm, which can be treated by endovascular methods. Conversely, angiography is probably not necessary in cases of asymptomatic unruptured mycotic aneurysms.

> Because endocardtitis may often remain undetected by blood cultures and even echocardiography, a high index of suspicion is needed in any patient with unexplained haemorrhagic or ischaemic stroke and a cardiac murmur.

Meningeal involvement is common: cerebrospinal fluid (CSF) analysis, if safe following careful clinical and radiological assessment, may suggest the diagnosis if a markedly high polymorph count is found (>100 cells/mm^3). Rheumatic fever can also cause valvular damage leading to embolism to the brain, particularly if the mitral valve is affected, or if atrial fibrillation develops during the illness.

Atrial myxoma

The diagnosis of atrial myxoma is difficult and often delayed. About 30 per cent of atrial myxomas cause cerebral emboli – accounting for about 0.4 per cent of all strokes. Nevertheless, stroke is the most common neurological presentation of this disease. The majority of patients with atrial myxoma (up to 90 per cent) present with constitutional symptoms of fatigue, fever, myalgia, arthralgia and weight loss. Cardiac symptoms are often present and include breathlessness in association with congestive failure and syncope. Investigations show elevated erythrocyte sedimentation rate (ESR) and C-reactive protein (CRP), anaemia, thrombocytosis or thrombocytopenia. Chest x-ray may show left atrial or ventricular enlargement and occasionally intracardiac tumour calcification. Echocardiography is the investigation of choice, but transthoracic studies have a false-negative rate of about 20 per cent. For this reason, if the clinical suspicion is high, transoesophageal echocardiography must be performed.

Stroke may result from embolic tumour fragments rather than fibrin thrombus, so anticoagulation may not be helpful and is probably best avoided, particularly as delayed cerebral aneurysm formation, often fusiform, in distal branches, can lead to cerebral haemorrhage. The treatment of atrial myxoma is optimization of cardiac function and urgent surgical removal. Follow up with transoesophageal echocardiography is recommended as recurrence may occur, especially within the first two years – but occasionally more than ten years later.

ENDOCRINE DISORDERS

The thyroid gland

Thyroid disorders can impact on the function of any part of the central nervous system (CNS), peripheral nerves or muscle, mainly via high or low levels of circulating T4 and T3 or immune-mediated damage. It is especially important to recognize neurological manifestations of thyroid disease, as the symptoms are usually treatable. About 20 per cent of patients with myasthenia have a thyroid disorder, more commonly hyperthyroidism than hypothyroidism; this link is probably due to an underlying autoimmune susceptibility in some individuals.

Hyperthyroidism

Hyperthyroidism is most often due to immune mechanisms (termed **Grave's disease**), but other causes include **thyroiditis**, **multinodular goitre** or, rarely, **pituitary tumours**. Some degree of **myopathy** is present in almost all patients with hyperthyroidism, but may be asymptomatic. Subacute painful proximal limb weakness is typical, causing difficulty climbing stairs, rising from a chair and raising the arms. Bulbar involvement is less common. Clinical findings are proximal wasting of the shoulder and pelvic girdle muscles (including quadriceps), with hyper-reflexia but normal tone. Tremor is nearly always found in hyperthyroidism, most often a postural upper limb tremor, but myoclonus, chorea and even parkinsonism have been described.

Investigation findings usually include a normal creatine kinase (CK), in contrast to the raised CK of hypothyroid myopathy. Electromyogram (EMG) abnormalities include polyphasic motor potentials (see Chapter 5).

Hyperthyroidism can cause an **upper motor neurone syndrome**, particularly affecting the legs, with spasticity, clonus, weakness and extensor plantars. This can cause diagnostic confusion by mimicking spinal cord compression. **Lower motor neurone** features may also be present, leading to an amyotrophic lateral sclerosis-like presentation. Peripheral neuropathy is uncommon in hyperthyroidism, but a flaccid paraparesis with areflexia may rarely occur (Basedow paraplegia).

Thyroid eye disease is a common feature of Graves' disease, occurring in up to 70 per cent of patients, especially middle-aged women. The clinical features are lid retraction; inflammation of orbital soft tissues, causing redness and swelling of the lids and conjunctivae; proptosis (exophthalmos); extraocular muscle involvement causing diplopia and often pain on attempted eye movement (a restrictive ophthalmopathy); corneal damage; and occasionally, optic nerve compression at the orbital apex. The conjunctiva may appear oedematous and injected.

Thickened and infiltrated eye muscles can be demonstrated by a forced duction test (showing that the eyeball is restricted in its range of movements). MRI or computed tomography (CT) imaging

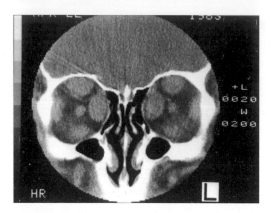

Figure 27.1 Coronal orbital CT scan, showing grossly enlarged extraocular muscles in a 58-year-old man with thyrotoxicosis (thyroid eye disease). Reproduced from Souhami R.L. and Moxham J. (eds.), *Textbook of Medicine, Fourth Edition*, Churchill Livingstone, 2002, with permission.

can help to show the enlarged extraocular muscles, particularly the medial and inferior recti (Figure 27.1). The increase in volume of the extraocular muscles may impair venous drainage from the orbit, causing papilloedema. Although both eyes are usually involved, the condition may be markedly asymmetric.

Neuropsychiatric symptoms are common in hyperthyroidism, and include anxiety, altered mood and behaviour, with restlessness and clinical signs of sympathetic overactivity. Full-blown hyperthyroid encephalopathy is now rare, but may occur either in untreated patients, or after radio-iodine treatment, or during intercurrent illness or following surgical procedures. Florid signs of thyrotoxicosis, confusion, agitation, fever, seizures and upper motor neurone signs may all be present. Mortality from this disorder remains high.

Conventional thyroid function tests, including TSH level, free T3 and free T4 assays, will usually confirm the diagnosis. Treatment is with drugs, carbimazole and propranolol, therapeutic doses of radio-iodine, and sometimes, thyroid surgery. Corticosteroids are indicated in severe eye disease, particularly when there is papilloedema and visual impairment. Other treatments for ophthalmopathy include botulinum toxin, radiotherapy or surgery.

Hypothyroidism

Hypothyroidism, resulting from immune-mediated mechanisms or following surgical or radiotherapy-induced thyroid ablation can affect any

part of the nervous system, and must be recognized because it is so readily treatable.

The history reveals weight gain, cold sensitivity, constipation, a dry skin and a hoarse voice. On examination, patients typically show coarse features, thinned hair, evidence of physical and mental slowing, sometimes sensory-neural deafness, and ankle jerks with slow relaxation. There may be bradycardia and swollen legs. Commonly, older women may be affected and the complication of hypothermia is a real risk in the winter.

An **encephalopathy**, characterized by slowness, lethargy and impaired attention is common. The most severe form, **myxoedema coma**, often follows a precipitating event such as sepsis or trauma, and has a substantial mortality if not recognized early and treated. In this situation, early recognition and treatment with thyroid replacement (T4 and T3), antibiotics and corticosteroids are often life-saving.

Other neuropsychological features can also occur, including confusion, delusions, hallucinations and paranoid suspicions. Rarely, this presents as an acute psychosis with paranoia and hallucinations – **myxoedema madness**. Hypothyroidism should therefore be carefully excluded in all patients presenting with dementia, because it is so readily amenable to treatment: indeed, it is the most common treatable cause of dementia, arising in some 2–4 per cent of elderly patients, with a 3:1 female to male ratio.

Cerebellar ataxia occurs rarely in hypothyroidism, involving the gait and the limbs, with normal eye movements. Muscular weakness is a common and sometimes early clinical feature.

Hypothyroid myopathy presents with weakness, usually fairly mild, accompanied by depressed or slow-relaxing reflexes (pseudomyotonia), and typically involves the pelvic and shoulder girdles. Percussion of the muscle may cause a slow rippling effect termed 'myoedema'. Pain during or following muscle activity is typical of hypothyroid myopathy, and all patients presenting with unexplained muscle pains, especially related to exertion, should be screened for hypothyroidism. Prompt treatment prevents development of more severe symptoms. By contrast with hyperthyroid myopathy, the CK level is usually raised, sometimes markedly so (>10 times normal). Treatment with thyroxine usually produces rapid improvement, but in severe myopathy, full recovery may take a year or longer.

In the peripheral nervous system, an **entrapment neuropathy**, most frequently **carpal tunnel syndrome**, is seen in approximately 10 per cent of hypothyroid patients. Treatment is restoration of the euthyroid state rather than surgical decompression. Hypothyroidism can cause a peripheral polyneuropathy in up to two-thirds of patients. This is usually a mild, predominantly sensory neuropathy.

Hashimoto's encephalopathy

The term 'Hashimoto's encephalopathy' describes a subacute, sometimes relapsing encephalopathy, responding well to corticosteroids, associated with a high titre of antithyroid peroxidase antibodies. Patients present with confusion, dementia, ataxia, seizures and myoclonus, extrapyramidal rigidity and sometimes stroke-like focal deficits. The onset may be abrupt, and occasionally there is a relapsing course. The encephalopathy is not explained by thyroid status, which may be normal. Although it is implied that the antibodies are causal, there is little clear evidence that this is the case. Indeed, it has been suggested that the antibodies may represent an epiphenomenon, as they may be found in encephalopathies known to have an alternative cause. It is therefore important to investigate thoroughly any patient with an encephalopathy associated with antithyroid antibodies, to exclude other causes. For example, the recently described syndrome of encephalopathy (typically a limbic encephalitis syndrome) with antibodies to voltage-gated potassium channels may also need to be considered.

Diabetes mellitus

Diabetes mellitus can cause many effects on the nervous system. Rare congenital causes of diabetes include mitochondrial cytopathies, particularly patients with sensorineural deafness, but also those with MELAS or Kearns–Sayre syndrome, Friedreich ataxia and Wolfram syndrome (type 1 diabetes, diabetes insipidus, optic atrophy and deafness; DIDMOAD). The other situations in which diabetes is important for neurologists are acute metabolic disturbances (related to hyperglycaemia or hypoglycaemia) and the diabetic neuropathies (see Chapter 16 and Chapter 18).

Acute metabolic disturbances

Hypoglycaemia

Low blood glucose must be considered in any acute neurological emergency, as it is easily treatable, and can lead to irreversible damage if it is not quickly recognized and treated (Table 27.1). Hypoglycaemia most often occurs in known diabetics, from excessive doses of oral hypoglycaemics, or, more commonly, insulin. Very rarely insulin-secreting tumours (insulinomas) are the cause. As the glucose drops below about 2.5 mmol/L, there is often a warning prodrome, including sweating, trembling, tingling hands and palpitations; this may allow the patient to correct the problem. However, in some patients with type 1 diabetes, the warning is absent, placing them at much greater risk of prolonged hypoglycaemia. Hypoglycaemia causes confusion, dysarthria, altered behaviour and agitation, seizures and occasionally, focal neurological signs (e.g. hemiplegia) which can mimic a TIA or stroke. If hypoglycaemia is not treated promptly, conscious level will deteriorate, leading to coma.

Table 27.1 Symptoms and signs of hypoglycaemia

	Sign
Sympathetic (adrenaline)	Anxiety
	Tremor
	Tachycardia
	Pallor
	Sweating
Neuroglycopenia (low glucose)	Hunger
	Weakness
	Behaviour change (confusion, aggression)
	Slurred speech, unsteady
	Focal signs, e.g. hemiplegia
	Epileptic seizures
	Coma

When hypoglycaemia is suspected, blood should be taken for glucose estimation, and 20–30 mL of 50 per cent glucose given intravenously. It is essential to combine this with thiamine 50 mg intravenously in all patients in whom the presenting complaints and past history are not fully known, and thus in all emergency situations. The indications for doing this are that Wernicke's encephalopathy can sometimes present with impaired consciousness, without obvious focal signs typical of the condition (see later in this chapter); or more commonly, in those at risk of developing Wernicke's encephalopathy, a glucose load increases the metabolic demand for thiamine and so may precipitate the encephalopathy.

The therapeutic response to intravenous glucose should be immediate unless hypoglycaemia has been prolonged or the diagnosis is incorrect.

Plasma glucose levels less than 2.0 mmol/L confirm the diagnosis. Diagnosis of insulinomas can be difficult, but a prolonged fast with estimation of glucose, insulin and plasma-C peptide levels will usually establish the diagnosis.

Hyperglycaemia

Hyperglycaemia may cause a deteriorating conscious level leading to coma from:

- Diabetic ketoacidosis
- Hyperosmolar non-ketotic hyperglycaemic coma.

Diabetic keto–acidosis occurs in patients with type 1 diabetes, usually because of undertreatment with insulin or its omission, with or without intercurrent illness such as sepsis. Occasionally it can be a dramatic first presentation of diabetes, but more often a known diabetic patient becomes ill over a few days with complaints of headache, weakness, vomiting and abdominal pain. There is dehydration with acidotic breathing and ketones may be present on the breath. Increasing drowsiness, accompanied by confusion, precede coma. Often the blood pressure is low and the pulse rapid. Rarely, cerebral oedema develops during treatment because of over-rapid correction of hyperosmolality, especially in children. This can cause death from raised intracranial pressure.

Ketotic patients have glycosuria and ketonuria. The blood glucose is usually very high, the pH low with a low bicarbonate, the potassium high and sodium normal. The urea may be raised if there is moderate or severe dehydration.

Treatment is to rehydrate with intravenous saline, intravenous insulin and correction of acidosis if severe. The electrolytes (especially potassium) must be monitored regularly to maintain normal values. The insulin dose will need to be titrated against plasma glucose levels, using a sliding scale. Unconscious patients will need a nasogastric tube and aspiration of gastric contents. Any precipitating cause for the ketoacidosis requires appropriate treatment.

Hyperosmolar non-ketotic coma occurs mainly in patients with type 2 diabetes and may lead to very high blood glucose (40–65 mmol/L), with high sodium levels and high plasma osmolality. Reduced conscious level or seizures may occur. Some patients present in shock with features of dehydration.

Diabetic neuropathies

The neuropathies caused by diabetes are described in Chapter 16. The most common type is a distal sensorimotor polyneuropathy, affecting over 50 per cent of patients with long-standing disease. Less common neuropathies include diabetic autonomic neuropathy, acute painful neuropathy, acute cranial neuropathies (especially oculomotor), thoraco-abdominal neuropathy and painful proximal neuropathy (diabetic amyotrophy).

The pituitary gland

In all patients with suspected pituitary tumours or disturbed pituitary function, particular attention should be paid on examination to visual acuity and the visual fields. MRI is the imaging of choice, but failing that, CT scanning should be performed. Appropriate endocrine assessment should be undertaken (Box 27.1).

Prolactin-secreting tumours

Prolactinomas cause very high prolactin levels (Table 27.3) resulting in secondary amenorrhoea, infertility and impotence. Occasionally, a raised prolactin is not associated with symptoms. Galactorrhoea occurs in 30–80 per cent of patients. Other clinical features include anxiety, depression and sometimes hostility. Many prolactinomas are

Pituitary tumours are common, discovered incidentally in about a quarter of all autopsies. Many are asymptomatic small **microadenomas** (<10 mm), but larger tumours (**macroadenomas**) can cause symptoms by mass effect including headache and visual disturbances. As the tumour extends upwards out of the sella, there is compression of the optic chiasm, typically producing a bitemporal hemianopia, although this is often asymmetrical. Lateral tumour extension can affect structures in the cavernous sinus (cranial nerves III, IV, Va and VI). Very large pituitary tumours can result in an obstructive hydrocephalus with signs of raised intracranial pressure. Pituitary adenomas are hormone-secreting in about two-thirds of cases. Of these, 60–70 per cent secrete prolactin, 10–15 per cent growth hormone and a few secrete adrenocorticotropic hormone, gonadotropins or thyroid-stimulating hormone. The symptoms depend on the hormones secreted by the tumour, and any mass effect on remaining pituitary function. The disturbances associated with excess of different pituitary hormones are shown in Table 27.2. Anterior pituitary hormones are secreted in a pulsatile fashion, so serial estimations may be necessary to make a correct diagnosis. In some 30 per cent of pituitary tumours, there may be a failure of endocrine function (panhypopituitarism (see below under Hypopituitarism)). Non-secreting tumours may cause hypopituitarism, with secondary amenorrhoea, infertility or impotence, loss of secondary sexual characteristics or hypothyroidism.

Box 27.1 Investigation of patients suspected of having a pituitary lesion

- Measurement of visual acuity
- Charting of visual fields
- Endocrine assessment
- Imaging of pituitary gland: MRI preferable, but CT if MR not possible

CT, computed tomography; MRI, magnetic resonance imaging.

macroadenomas and so may also cause headache and visual disturbance. Prolactinomas show a tendency to increase in size during pregnancy.

Investigation reveals prolactin levels usually greater than 3600 mIU/L, which do not increase after thyrotropin-releasing hormone (TRH) stimulation or in response to domperidone.

Dopamine agonists inhibit prolactin release and may shrink the gland without recourse to surgery. Bromocriptine was the first to be used, but others have followed and cabergoline treatment results in some 92 per cent of patients showing a response. Surgery is indicated for large tumours causing visual impairment, and those unresponsive to medical treatment.

Growth hormone secreting tumours (acromegaly)

Growth hormone excess causes gigantism before skeletal maturation and **acromegaly** in adults. Clinical features relate to bony overgrowth, with a characteristic facial appearance, and large hands and feet. Arthralgia and backache are common. There may be excess sweating and carpal tunnel symdrome is frequent. One-third of patients with acromegaly are hypertensive and some two-thirds have abnormal glucose tolerance. Patients with acromegaly have a shortened lifespan.

The best screening test is the serum IGF-1 level, which is significantly raised in acromegaly. Levels of growth hormone (GH) fluctuate, due to pulsatile secretion, but some 50 per cent of cases show a raised level. During a glucose tolerance test, there is either a paradoxical rise in GH or no fall. Stimulation of TRH and gonadotropin-releasing hormone (GnRH) may cause an elevation of GH levels. Treatment is often surgical, via a transsphenoidal approach. Treatment with somatostatin analogues, such as octreotide and lanreotide, will produce a clinical response in some 70 per cent of patients, although a higher number are left with raised GH levels. Levels of IGF-1 are used to monitor the effects of treatment. The somatostatin analogues may initially cause some tumour expansion, so the visual fields need to be carefully monitored in the early stages. Surgical treatment is sometimes combined with radiotherapy.

Adrenocorticotropin-secreting tumours (Cushing's syndrome)

Cushing's syndrome is caused by adrenocortical hormonal excess. Some 70 per cent of naturally occurring Cushing's syndrome is caused by corticotrophin-secreting pituitary tumours, usually

Table 27.2 Pituitary hormones and associated disturbances

Excess hormone secretion	Stimuli	Clinical condition	Clinical symptoms
GH	GHRH and S+	Acromegaly	Coarsened facial features, enlarged hands and feet, hypertension, impaired glucose tolerance
IGF-1		Acromegaly	
ACTH	CRH	Cushing's disease	Centripetal obesity, hypertension, impaired glucose tolerance, abdominal striae, amenorrhea, myopathy, neuropsychiatric symptoms
Prolactin	PRH? TRH, VIP	Prolactinoma	Headache, visual loss, galactorrhea, amenorrhea, infertility
TSH	TRH	TSH- and TRH-secreting tumours	Goitre, headaches, field defects, hyperthyroidism
LH	GnRH	Gonadotropinoma	Headaches, visual disturbance, altered testosterone in men. Often asymptomatic, particularly in women
FSH	GnRH	Gonadotropinoma	

FSH, folicle-stimulating hormone; GH, growth hormone; GnRH, gonadotropin-releasing hormone; LH, luteinizing hormone; PRH, TRH, thyrotropin-releasing hormone; TSH, thyroid-stimulating hormone; VIP, vasoactive intestinal peptide.

Table 27.3 Causes of raised prolactin levels

Cause		
Pregnancy, lactation, oestrogens		
Pituitary tumours – prolactinoma		
Parapituitary tumours and granulomas – gliomas, sarcoidosis		
Pituitary stalk damage		
Hypothalamic disease – tumours, granulomas		
Drugs	Dopamine receptor antagonists	Phenothiazines – chlorpromazine
	Butyrophenones	Haloperidol
	Anti-emetics	Metoclopramide, domperidone
	Antidepressants	Imipramine, amitriptyline
	Hypotensives	Methyldopa, reserpine
		Cimetidine
Endocrine – acromegaly, hypothyroidism, Cushing's disease		
Nipple stimulation		
Stress		
Major epileptic seizure		

microadenomas (this is Cushing's disease). A few cases are due to ectopic production of adrenocorticotropic hormone (ACTH), most commonly from a small cell lung carcinoma. Some cases are ACTH-independent, most often arising from an adenoma or carcinoma of the adrenal gland. However, the most common cause of mild to moderate Cushing's syndrome is iatrogenic, resulting from therapeutic use of corticostroids. or iatrogenic from corticosteroid excess. Pseudo-Cushing's syndrome may arise from major depressive illness and from chronic alcoholism.

The clinical features caused by adrenocortical excess include weight gain, with central obesity, a moon face and buffalo hump, oedema, prominent skin striae, hypertension, glucose intolerance, oligomenorrhoea or amenorrhoea, impaired potency, hirsutism, acne, proximal muscle wasting and weakness, osteoporosis and psychiatric disturbances, such as depression, lethargy and insomnia.

Investigations in patients with suspected Cushing's syndrome include measurement of 24-hour urinary-free cortisol levels (preferably on three successive days), 09.00 h and 24.00 h plasma cortisol levels (normally plasma cortisol levels are highest in the early morning) and ACTH levels. Dexamethasone suppression, using low dose (0.5 mg 6-hourly for eight doses) or a midnight injection of 1 mg, in normal subjects will suppress ACTH levels and so result in low cortisol levels. Failure of suppression indicates Cushing's syndrome and the need for more detailed tests to elucidate whether the pituitary, ectopic ACTH or adrenal excess is the cause.

Gonadotropin-secreting tumours

Gonadotropinomas secrete excess GnRH, which is responsible for the pulsatile secretion of luteinizing hormone (LH) and follicle-stimulating hormone (FSH), so single measurements may be unreliable. They often present as large, non-functioning macroadenomas with accompanying visual field defects, rather than endocrine symptoms. They may also result in hyposecretion of ACTH and TSH.

Hypopituitarism

The causes of **hypopituitarism** are listed in Table 27.4. Hypopituitarism has varied presentations, ranging from sudden life-threatening adrenal insufficiency (pituitary apoplexy) to slowly progressive, non-specific symptoms, such as tiredness or loss of libido. When hypopituitarism is due to macroadenomas or other mass lesions, headache and visual loss occur. The effects of hypopituitarism relate to endocrine failure of target glands: adrenal insufficiency, hypothyroidism or hypogonadism. Hypogonadism manifests clinically as secondary amenorrhoea, infertility or impotence. There may be loss of secondary sexual characteristics with

Table 27.4 Causes of hypopituitarism

Cause	
Pituitary tumours	Usually macroadenomas
Non-pituitary tumours	Craniopharyngiomas
	Meningiomas
	Gliomas
	Chordomas
	Ependymomas
	Metastases
Infiltrative processes	Sarcoid, histiocytosis X, haemochromatosis
Infections	Brain abscess, meningitis, encephalitis, tuberculosis
Ischaemia and infarction	Subarachnoid haemorrhage
	Post-partum haemorrhage (Sheehan's syndrome)
	Pituitary aplplexy (acute infarction of a pituitary adenoma)
Iatrogenic	Irradiation, neurosurgery
Empty sella syndrome	Radiological absence of normal pituitary within the sella turcica. Usually benign and asymptomatic but may develop hypopituitarism
Head injury (may have occurred up to several years before)	
Congenital: Kallman's syndrome (congenital hypogonadotropic hypogonadism)	
Lymphocytic hypophysitis	
Pituitary hypoplasia or aplasia	
Congenital causes	e.g. septo-optic dysplasia

reduced beard growth, skin pallor, cold intolerance and lethargy, due to lack of TSII and ACTH. Posterior pituitary function may also be affected, leading to diabetes insipidus producing polydipsia and polyuria.

Hypopituitarism may result from ischaemic damage, for example due to post-partum haemorrhage; from pituitary apoplexy; or from infection, granulomas, or occasionally, metastatic deposits.

Pituitary apoplexy describes a dramatic clinical syndrome of abrupt onset of severe headache, nausea, vomiting and often hypotensive collapse with sudden bilateral visual loss. The most common cause is haemorrhage into a pituitary macroadenoma.

Evaluation of pituitary function

Modern radioimmunoassays allow basal measurements of cortisol, ACTH, TSH, free tri-iodothyronine (FT3), free thyroxine (FT4), LH, FSH, prolactin and GH, and insulin-like growth factor (IGF-1) levels (Box 27.2). Plasma and urine osmolalities assess posterior pituitary function, and sometimes levels of oestradiol, progesterone and testosterone may also be appropriate. Dynamic tests of anterior pituitary function are based on the sequential administration of four hypothalamic-releasing hormones (GnRH, TRH, corticotropin-releasing hormone (CRH), growth hormone-releasing hormone (GHRH)); these are injected intravenously, and measurements of LH, FSH, TSH, ACTH, GH and prolactin levels are made at intervals. Baseline measurements are also made of oestradiol, testosterone, thyroxine, cortisol and IGF-1. An absent response suggests loss of function in the anterior pituitary cells.

Box 27.2 Evaluation of basal pituitary function

- Diurnal cortisol levels – midnight and 09.00
- Plasma ACTH
- TSH
- FT4, FT3
- LH
- FSH
- Prolactin
- GH
- IGF-1
- Plasma and urine osmolalities

ACTH, adrenocorticotropic hormone; FT3, free tri-iodothyronine; FT4, free thyroxine; FSH, follicle-stimulating hormone; GH, growth hormone; IGF-1, insulin-like growth factor; LH, luteinizing hormone; TSH, thyroid-stimulating hormone.

To assess the pituitary gland reserve for GH and ACTH, insulin-induced hypoglycaemia (0.15 units/kg) is used. Blood is taken at intervals for measurement of glucose, GH, ACTH, prolactin and cortisol levels. In normal subjects, the insulin-induced neuroglycopenia causes a rise in GH and ACTH (hence cortisol), but no such rise occurs in patients with hypopituitarism. This insulin stress test should not be used in patients with a history of epilepsy or ischaemic heart disease, or in patients who are clearly hypothyroid or hypoadrenal in endocrine function. Patients undergoing insulin-induced hypoglycaemia must be monitored closely during the test.

Posterior pituitary function

The posterior pituitary secretes two peptides, arginine vasopressin (AVP), the antidiuretic hormone (ADH) and oxytocin. Plasma osmolality (normally 285–288 mosmol/kg) is maintained through AVP secretion from the osmoregulation of thirst. AVP causes increased water reabsorption in the renal tubules, thus reducing urine output. In **diabetes insipidus**, there is commonly thirst with polydipsia and polyuria (urine output of >3 litres per 24 hours). Diabetes insipidus results from dysfunction of the posterior pituitary. Reduced secretion of arginine vasopressin and antidiuretic hormone cause symptoms of thirst, polyuria and polydipsia. The common causes are trauma, tumours, sarcoidosis and other granulomatous conditions, and infections. If water is restricted, dehydration follows. In diabetes insipidus, the water deprivation test causes the urine osmolality to rise, but the urine volume remains high and the plasma osmolality rises, often to more than 295 mosmol/kg.

The parathyroid glands

In cases of **hypoparathyroidism** (or pseudohypoparathyroidism, a rare familial form with skeletal and developmental anomalies), the reduction in serum ionic calcium causes clinical features that include sensory disturbances, tetany, chorea and seizures; basal ganglia or cerebellar calcification may also occur. **Hyperparathyroidism** resulting from parathyroid adenoma or hyperplasia causes muscle weakness, fatiguability and amyotrophy with preserved reflexes, and has been reported on occasion to produce a clinical picture resembling motor neurone disease.

The adrenal glands

Cushing's disease

Cushing's disease results from pituitary hyper-secretion of ACTH and thus high plasma cortisol, most often from a pituitary microadenoma (see above under The pituitary gland). The distinction between Cushing's disease and Cushing's syndrome is described above under Adrenocorticotropin-secreting tumours (Cushing's syndrome), the latter being a result of treatment with exogenous steroids or primary hyperadrenalism. Clinically, the disease and the syndrome are indistinguishable, both being characterized by centripetal obesity, hyperten-sion, hirsutism, abdominal striae, acne, menstrual irregularity, immunosuppression, myopathy and psychosis. Cushing's disease is usually caused by a microadenoma that typically does not cause visual symptoms.

Addison's disease

> The term **Addison's disease** is usually used to refer to the clinical syndrome caused by adrenal insufficiency. In the past, tuberculosis was a common cause, but now an autoimmune mecha-nism underlies the majority of cases.

The onset may be acute or insidious depending on the cause. The important features of Addison disease are hypotension, with a tendency to faint, weight loss, apathy and vomiting, with pigmenta-tion of the skin and mucous membranes (due to chronic ACTH hypersecretion). The condition can be life-threatening, especially during an additional intercurrent illness.

> Acute Addisonian crises, often precipitated by infection or surgery, lead to anorexia, vomit-ing, diarrhoea, abdominal pain, cramps, postural hypotension, dehydration, lethargy and weight loss.

There is sodium and water depletion from min-eralocorticoid deficiency, causing a low sodium, raised urea and potassium and, in a few patients, a raised calcium level. The plasma cortisol is low and the ACTH raised. An ACTH stimulation test with an injection of 250 mg i.m. of soluble ACTH (tetracos-actide) normally shows a rise in cortisol level unless there is adrenal failure.

Acute treatment involves rehydration with saline, glucose and the intravenous injection of 100–200 mg of hydrocortisone with subsequent doses adjusted down until a maintenance dose is used, often hydrocortisone 20 mg in the morning and 10 mg at night. Mineralocorticoid replacement with small doses of fludrocortisone 0.05–0.20 mg daily is sometimes necessary. The steroid dose will need to be increased with any intercurrent infection or proposed surgery.

Phaeochromocytoma

Phaeochromocytoma is a neuroendocrine catecho-lamine secreting tumour of the adrenal medulla. It is an important cause of hypertension, especially in younger people. Tumours are often multiple and sometimes extramedullary (paragangliomas). Other clinical features include panic, anxiety, palpita-tions, headaches and weight loss. Neurological fea-tures are rare, but can include those of accelerated hypertension, including intracranial haemorrhage and hypertensive encephalopathy.

NEUROLOGICAL COMPLICATIONS OF ELECTROLYTE IMBALANCES

> The effects of electrolyte imbalances range from being asymptomatic to causing profound disturbance of function in the central and/or peripheral nervous system. Generally, the clini-cal severity of electrolyte disturbance is greatest when the abnormality has developed rapidly. Treatment is aimed at not only correcting the electrolyte disturbance itself, but also identify-ing and treating the cause.

The central nervous system effects of electrolyte imbalance, often including altered consciousness and seizures, are related to fluid shifts and brain volume changes. Plasma hyperosmolality causes brain volume loss, while hypo-osmolality causes brain swelling. Other mechanisms include disor-dered transmembrane potentials and neurotrans-mission. The clinical features of abnormalities in serum sodium, potassium, calcium and magnesium are summarized in Table 27.5 and are briefly dis-cussed here.

Table 27.5 Causes and features of electrolyte imbalances

Electolyte disturbance	Common causes	Clinical features
Hyponatraemia	Excessive water intake SIADH Cerebral salt wasting Diuretic use Addison's disease Drugs (e.g. carbamazepine, acetazolomide, diuretics) Excess fluid losses (e.g. vomiting, diarrhoea) replaced by hypotonic fluids Liver disease Cardiac failure	Confusion) Coma Convulsions (if <115 mmol/L
Hypernatraemia	Diabetes insipidus HONK Diarrhoea Dehydration	Reduced conscious level Seizures Tremor Movement disorders
Hypokalaemia	Diarrhoea Vomiting	Generalized muscle weakness
Hyperkalaemia	Renal failure Drugs (e.g. ACE inhibitors) Excessive intake may contribute but rarely causes hyperkalaemia on its own	Generalized muscle weakness ECG changes Cardiac arrest
Hypercalcaemia	Hyperparathyroidism Malignancy – bone metastases, myeloma, other Immobility Sarcoidosis Vitamin D intoxication	Anorexia, abdominal pain Nausea Fatigue Reduced conscious level Constipation Myoclonus, rigidity Elevated CSF protein
Hypocalcaemia	Metabolic bone disease Hypoparathyroidism Renal failure Pancreatitis Drugs, e.g. serotonin reuptake inhibitors, proton pump inhibitors	Paraesthesias Tetany Seizures, chorea Encephalopathy Papilloedema and $\uparrow$ICP Coma
Hypermagnesaemia	Renal failure Iatrogenic (e.g. treatment of eclamptic seizures)	
Hypomagnesaemia	Reduced intake or absorption Rarely isolated - usually part of complex electrolyte derangement	

ACE, angiotensin-converting enzyme; CSF, cerebrospinal fluid; HONK, hyper-osmolar non-ketotic coma; ICP, intracranial pressure; SIADH, syndrome of inappropriate ADH secretion.

Sodium

Hyponatraemia

Hyponatraemia is defined as a serum sodium value of less than 130 mmol/L, but does not always cause symptoms (particularly if it is chronic). Plasma sodium of less than 120 mmol/L is usually symptomatic, usually causing confusion. As the level falls, other symptoms develop, including muscle cramps, seizures, decline in conscious level and facial or limb oedema. Hyponatraemia may arise from excessive fluid intake (water intoxication) without a sodium deficit, but sodium may also be lost from the intestines (from diarrhoea and vomiting) or due to disturbed renal function. Most water intoxication occurs in sick patients who are either being fed by nasogastric tube or intravenously. Hyponatraemia may also follow inappropriate secretion of ADH (SIADH), reducing renal water loss. The rapid correction of serum sodium may cause the distinct syndrome of central pontine myelinolysis (see below under Central pontine myelinolysis) – in the fully developed syndrome causing a quadriparesis with brainstem signs; it carries a high mortality. This syndrome is more common in high risk groups such as alcoholics.

SIADH

The causes of this syndrome are listed in Table 27.6. SIADH (syndrome of inappropriate ADH secretion) can only be diagnosed when:

- secretion of antidiuretic hormone is inconsistent with the low plasma osmolality and volume status is normal (no hypovolemia or hypotension);
- renal function is normal; and
- there is no disturbance of adrenal or thyroid function.

The diagnosis of SIADH can be made only when the serum is dilute and the urine inappropriately concentrated, so serum and urine osmolality measurements are essential.

Most patients with SIADH can be managed initially by restricting water intake to between 800 and 1000 mL per day. This results in net water loss and a progressive rise in serum sodium and thus plasma osmolality. Weight and serum sodium should be monitored daily. When hyponatremia is associated with severe neurological symptoms, it may be necessary to infuse a small amount of hypertonic saline (e.g. 200–300 mL of 3 or 5 per cent sodium chloride solution intravenously over 3 to 4 hours) to cautiously elevate the serum sodium concentration. Studies have shown that oral or intravenous urea is highly effective and safe to use for the same indication. The possibility of inducing congestive cardiac failure is reduced by administering furosemide and continuing fluid restriction.

The rapidity with which the serum sodium concentration should be normalized depends on the degree of hyponatraemia, its duration, and the severity of the patient's symptoms. In severe hyponatraemia, especially if accompanied by evidence of central nervous system dysfunction, prompt but cautious correction of electrolyte abnormalities is required. There is a link with the speed of correction of hyponatraemia and the development of **central pontine myelinolysis**. Too rapid correction may precipitate this severe type of brainstem damage. As a general rule, correction of serum sodium should not exceed 0.5 mmol/L per hour or 10 mmol/L in 24 hours. Close monitoring of electrolyte status with appropriate adjustments of therapy is necessary. If over-rapid correction is suspected, reversal using desmopressin and water may be appropriate. The underlying cause must always be sought (Table 27.6) and treated once identified.

Central pontine myelinolysis

In **central pontine myelinolysis**, a focus of demyelination develops, usually within the centre of the pons. This is not associated with any inflammatory changes and the axons are usually preserved. Although this was originally considered to be a specific effect of chronic alcoholism, subsequently it has been shown to arise in the context of a severe metabolic or general medical disorder, the most common setting being hyponatraemia that is corrected too rapidly. In addition to alcoholism, it has been linked with cirrhosis, malnutrition, malignancy and hyperemesis gravidarum. Regions of extrapontine myelinolysis can also occur, for example in the basal ganglia or corpus callosum. The clinical spectrum varies from minimal symptoms with ataxia to a profound tetraplegia and pseudobulbar

Table 27.6 Causes of the syndrome of inappropriate ADH secretion (SIADH)

	Causes of SIADH	
1	Malignant disease	Particularly carcinoma of the lung and lymphomas
2	Nervous system disorders	Trauma, head injuries, subarachnoid haemorrhage
		Meningitis, tuberculous meningitis
		Strokes
		Central nervous system tumours
		Polyneuritis, e.g. Guillain-Barré, porphyria
		Limbic encephalitis associated with voltage-gated potassium channel antibodies
3	Infections	Pneumonia
4	Drugs	For example, carbamazepine, chlorpropamide, cyclophosphamide, phenothiazines, tricyclics

palsy. The signs may appear a few days after the hyponatraemia has been corrected. MRI shows a characteristic focus of high signal on T2-weighted images and low signal on T1-weighted images in the central pons. Mortality is high in central pontine myelinolysis, and permanent, often severe, neurological deficits in survivors are common.

The importance of slow correction of hyponatraemia is emphasized above.

Potassium

Hyperkalaemia or hypokalaemia are features of **periodic paralysis** (see Chapter 18). Indeed, the main neurological effect of low (or sometimes high) serum potassium is generalized muscle weakness, so serum potassium must always be checked in anyone with unexplained new muscle weakness. A serum potassium of less than 3 mmol/L may be associated with complaints of fatigue, myalgia and muscle weakness. With values between 2.0 and 2.5 mmol/L, there may be a flaccid paralysis with depressed or absent reflexes. There may be associated bowel smooth muscle involvement leading to ileus. Hypokalaemia may precipitate life-threatening cardiac arrhythmias. Thirst and polyuria are occasionally symptoms of hypokalaemia.

Certain medical conditions causing hypokalaemia may present with muscle weakness. These include **aldosteronism (Conn's syndrome), Cushing's disease and some forms of periodic paralysis**. Other causes of potassium loss include diuretics, renal causes, and gastrointestinal upsets (diarrhoea and purgative abuse, pyloric stenosis and vomiting).

The agents used to reduce intracranial pressure, such as mannitol or urea, by inducing a diuresis may also lead to potassium loss. Treatment involves correction of the cause and potassium supplements.

Calcium and magnesium

Disturbances of calcium metabolism sometimes present to a neurologist and should be sought in cases of tetany, seizures or occasionally chorea. Hypercalcaemia may cause calcification of the basal ganglia, usually found coincidentally on imaging. Hypomagnesaemia may be a feature of eclamptic seizures and requires treatment in this context.

Hypocalcaemia

Hypocalcaemia is most often due to parathyroidectomy (often as a result of thyroid surgery), severe malabsorption, renal failure, prolonged use of anticonvulsants and from primary failure of the parathyroid glands.

Hypocalcaemia produces neuromuscular irritability with a calcium level of less than 2.0 mmol/L, accompanied by symptoms of lethargy, tingling in the extremities and around the mouth, twitching, carpopedal spasm, tetany and occasionally epileptic seizures. Psychotic features and stupor occur rarely. Examination reveals dry skin with brittle nails. Cataracts, and occasionally papilloedema, develop. Tapping over the facial nerve may provoke twitching of the facial muscles (Chvostek's sign) and inflation of a pneumatic cuff around the arm above arterial blood pressure may provoke a *main d'accoucheur* from carpal spasm (Trousseau's sign).

Investigations show a low serum calcium and the electrocardiogram may show a prolonged QT interval. CT of the brain may demonstrate cerebral calcification, particularly in the basal ganglia and cerebellum. Treatment is with calcium and vitamin D supplements. In the acute situation, 20–30 mL of 10 per cent calcium gluconate injected intravenously over 10 minutes is effective.

Hypercalcaemia

Hypercalcaemia characteristically presents with 'stones, bones, abdominal groans, and psychic moans'. Renal stones occur in about 50 per cent of patients, and bone pain (particularly back pain) and abdominal pain are common. However, approximately one-third of patients found to have hypercalcaemia are asymptomatic. Hypercalcaemia may cause anorexia, nausea and vomiting, constipation, polyuria and thirst. Headaches and depression are common symptoms. Fatigue, a proximal myopathy, confusion and behaviour disorders may herald neurological upsets. In a few patients, very high calcium levels may be associated with increasing confusion, drowsiness and eventual coma. Conjunctivitis from corneal calcification is sometimes a feature.

The serum calcium will be high, usually >3 mmol/L, but it should be remembered that venous sampling below an inflated tourniquet may give an erroneously high calcium value.

Hypercalcaemia most often occurs in **primary hyperparathyroidism** (with high levels of parathyroid hormone), in patients with **widespread bony metastases**, **sarcoidosis** or with **vitamin D intoxication**. Treatment depends on the cause. With symptomatic patients, a forced saline diuresis will increase the urinary excretion of calcium, which can be augmented by the addition of frusemide. For hypercalcaemia due to bony metastases, the bisphosphonate disodium pamidronate given intravenously or sodium clodronate (which can be given orally) are effective. Calcitonin given intravenously may also result in a short-lived fall in calcium level.

HAEMATOLOGICAL DISORDERS

Haematological disorders and stroke are discussed fully in Chapter 23.

Anaemias

Anaemias usually cause non-focal symptoms including fatigue, dizziness, impaired concentration, syncope, irritability and headache.

A full blood count should always be performed to exclude anaemia as a cause of any of these symptoms, including unexplained chronic daily headache. Occasionally, severe anaemia can cause focal neurological deficits, especially if there is significant atherosclerotic stenosis in an extracranial or intracranial vessel. **Iron deficiency anaemia** is occasionally associated with idiopathic intracranial hypertension; this responds to anaemia treatment. Iron deficiency is also associated with restless leg syndrome; serum ferritin is reduced, even if the haemoglobin is normal.

Vitamin B12 deficiency, one cause of megaloblastic anaemia is an important and potentially treatable cause of neurological symptoms and signs. B12 deficiency can cause many neurological syndromes, including a peripheral neuropathy with or without myelopathy (together known as **subacute combined degeneration of the cord**), encephalopathy, dementia, optic neuropathy and ophthalmoplegia. Folic acid can mask the anaemia without preventing the neurological sequelae. Before the discovery of vitamin B12, subacute combined degeneration of the cord was fatal. Treatment is with life-long hydrocobalamin injections. Measurement of serum homocysteine should be carried out if the serum vitamin B12 level is non-diagnostic and there is clinical suspicion of deficiency. Low serum copper is a rare cause of a syndrome resembling subacute combined degeneration of the cord.

Sickle cell disease causes neurological symptoms via mechanisms including large vessel arteriopathy, small perforating vessel occlusion, haemolysis, abnormal vasomotor tone and promotion of a hypercoaguable state. The incidence of stroke in sickle cell disease is much higher than in the general population.

Sickling is exacerbated by low oxygen saturation and/or intercurrent illness. Small vessels may be occluded leading to subcortical infarction (often not acutely symptomatic), while large vessels (especially the supraclinoid intracranial internal carotid and proximal middle cerebral arteries) can develop intimal proliferation causing stenosis and thrombo-embolism (often symptomatic). In patients with overt large artery stroke, there is commonly distal collateral formation (secondary Moyamoya changes). Subacute or chronic symptoms include headaches, which can be migrainous, and cognitive impairment caused by the accumulation of ischaemic damage. Haemorrhagic complications of sickle cell disease can occur in adults, especially subarachnoid haemorrhage. **Neurological symptoms have been found to occur in some 25 per cent of patients with sickle cell disease, while up to one-third have imaging evidence of cerebrovascular disease.** Treatments available to prevent the neurological consequences of sickle cell disease include partial-exchange transfusion, hydroxyurea and bone marrow transplantation.

Thalassaemia is a rare cause of neurological symptoms. Haematopoeisis outside the marrow may occur in lymphoid tissue, spleen, liver and bone. Myelopathy has been described and attributed to haematopoietic tissue in the epidural space. Corticosteroids, radiotherapy, blood transfusions and surgical decompression have been used in this situation.

Proliferative conditions

Leukaemias

Leukaemia can cause neurological symptoms by direct infiltration of nervous tissue or indirectly by haemorrhage related to low platelets, from infection resulting from impaired immunity, electrolyte disturbances or hyperviscosity. Leukaemic cells enter the nervous system via the blood circulation, along lymphatics, or direct invasion by spread along the meninges.

Meningeal leukaemia is most commonly associated with acute lymphocytic leukaemia (ALL) and presents as a subacute meningitis, with headache, drowsiness, neck stiffness, irritability, papilloedema and cranial neuropathies, especially affecting the optic, oculomotor, abducens, facial and vestibulo-cochlear nerves. There may be hydrocephalus. The CSF contains leukaemic cells and has a high protein. Solid leukaemic deposits may occur in any part of the CNS, although the brain is more commonly affected than the spine.

Plasma cell dyscrasias

Plasma cell dyscrasias are due to the proliferation of a single clone of immunoglobulin-secreting plasma cells (activated B cells). The antibodies secreted are classified into immunoglobulin M (IgM), IgG and IgA types according to their heavy-chain class, from which are derived various terms including monoclonal gammopathy, M-protein and other paraproteins. These disorders have increasingly been linked to peripheral neuropathies, so all patients with an unexplained neuropathy should be screened for a paraprotein.

The plasma cell dyscrasias include myeloma (multiple myeloma and osteosclerotic myeloma), Waldenstrom's macroglobulinaemia, monoclonal gammopathy of undetermined significance (MGUS), plasmacytoma and plasma cell leukaemia.

Multiple myeloma affects bones, causing pain, fractures and sometimes compression of neural tissue, especially the spinal cord, when a paraparesis is usually preceded by back pain for several months. The cauda equina and nerve roots may be infiltrated directly. Myelomatous meningeal involvement can cause cranial neuropathies. A peripheral neuropathy may result from either a paraneoplastic mechanism, amyloid deposition compromising nerve vascular supply, or direct infiltration.

Waldenstrom's macroglobulinaemia may lead to a hyperviscosity syndrome, associated with an IgM gammopathy. It involves the nervous system in about 25 per cent of cases. A progressive sensorimotor neuropathy results from IgM antibody binding and/or lymphocytic infiltration. Hyperviscosity may cause focal deficits including strokes, or an encephalopathy with headache. Patients also have a bleeding tendency and may develop bruising, purpura and subarachnoid haemorrhage. MGUS is a benign condition, but some patients ultimately develop a malignant plasma cell dyscrasia; the paraprotein level should be monitored once or twice a year. A chronic inflammatory demyelinating peripheral (CIDP) neuropathy may be associated.

Lymphomas

Both **Hodgkin and non-Hodgkin lymphomas** can affect the nervous system. Usually patients will have lymphoma elsewhere, which spreads directly to the CNS. Spinal cord tumours and meningeal infiltration are common. Extradural deposits may cause a myelopathy by compressing the spinal cord. The cauda equina and lumbosacral roots may be infiltrated causing painful radicular syndromes. Meningeal lymphoma can run a chronic clinical course sometimes with spontaneous temporary remission. A number of **lymphoma–associated paraneoplastic syndromes** have been described, including peripheral neuropathy, necrotizing myelopathy, leukoencephalopathy and polymyositis (see below under Scleroderma).

Primary CNS lymphomas are rare, constituting only 1 per cent of primary brain tumours. They are typically of B-cell origin and affect individuals with impaired immunity, including transplant recipients, patients with HIV and inherited immunodeficiency disorders. The tumours are usually ill-defined lesions in the cerebral hemispheres, ventricles, corpus callosum, basal ganglia and cerebellum. Lymphoma may respond dramatically but temporarily to corticosteroids in the early stages. Lymphoma may also present with focal symptoms or encephalopathy and/or seizures and nodular enhancing lesions in the ventricular wall. The differential diagnosis of cerebral lymphoma is wide and includes metastatic carcinoma, glioma, tuberculosis, toxoplasmosis, neurocysticercosis and sarcoidosis. A tissue diagnosis is usually essential. For further discussion of primary CNS lymphoma, see Chapter 14.

Polycythaemia

Polycythaemia is an increased red cell mass causing a raised haematocrit. It may be primary (**polycythaemia vera**) or secondary to another condition (e.g. chronic hypoxia). The symptoms of polycythaemia are varied: they may be generalized and rather ill-defined (including poor concentration, feelings of cephalic fullness, tinnitus, paraesthesias); or focal acute vascular syndromes, either permanent or transient, due to arterial or venous events. Chorea is associated with polycythemia vera (now known to be related to a mutation in the erythropoietin receptor gene, *JAK2*) and may respond to treatment of the polycythaemia. Polycythaemia vera can transform into other haematological malignancies (leukaemias, myelofibrosis). The mainstay of treatment of polycythaemia is repeated venesection.

Thrombocythaemia

Thrombocythaemia (platelet count >800 000/mm^3) is associated with an increased risk of thrombosis and haemorrhage within the CNS. It may be associated with leukaemia or myelodysplasia. Thrombosis can occur in arteries, veins or venous sinuses and is related to hyperviscosity. Haemorrhage of any type can be found (subdural, extradural, intracerebral, subarachnoid), the mechanism involving abnormal platelet function. Treatment with hydroxyurea is usually recommended to prevent neurological symptoms.

Bleeding disorders

Thrombotic thrombocytopenic purpura

Thrombotic thrombocytopenic purpura (TTP) is a rare disorder of early adulthood which, despite the low platelet count, causes recurrent and wide spread occlusion of small vessels. The pathophysiology involves microangiopathic haemolysis and formation of platelet microthrombi. TTP may be familial or acquired, but in both cases endothelial cells secrete abnormally large von Willebrand factor multimers; these are not degraded because of the lack of the cleavage enzyme ADAMTS-13. This causes the formation of platelet thrombi in small vessels. The clinical hallmarks are fevers, hepatic and renal disease, and a low platelet count. Fragmented red cells on the blood film, elevated lactate dehydrogenase, bilirubin and reticulocyte count are typical laboratory clues. Fluctuating neurological symptoms of altered conscious level, seizures, headache or encephalopathy may herald disease onset in half of the patients, sometimes provoked by intercurrent illness; and most patients have neurological symptoms at some stage of the illness. Low platelets can lead to intracerebral haemorrhage, but ischaemic stroke from large or small vessel occlusion may occur. The mainstay of treatment is plasma exchange. Antiplatelet agents or anticoagulants are usually used in ischaemic stroke, although evidence for efficacy is lacking. Other immunomodulatory treatments have been used, including ciclosporin and rituximab. Haemophilia, disseminated intravascular coagulation and von Willebrand disease are also rare causes of intracerebral haemorrhage.

Coagulation disorders

The **antiphospholipid antibody syndrome**, although characterized by venous thromboses, is also an important although rare cause of arterial cerebrovascular events, sometimes in association with skin rashes, migraine and recurrent miscarriage. **Thrombophilias including protein C and S deficiency, antithrombin III deficiency, factor V Leiden and the *MTHFR* mutation** are associated with an increased risk of cerebral venous thrombosis and deep vein thrombosis, but not strongly with arterial events.

GASTROINTESTINAL DISORDERS

Malabsorption

About 3 per cent of patients with inflammatory bowel disease, ulcerative colitis or Crohn's disease have neurological complications, most often a demyelinating peripheral neuropathy. Less commonly, a chronic progressive or acute inflammatory myelopathy may appear: these are more common in Crohn's disease. Vascular complications associated with inflammatory bowel disease may result from hypercoagulability and include cerebral venous sinus thromboses and ischaemic strokes.

In **coeliac disease** (gluten-sensitive enteropathy), about 10 per cent of patients have neurological complications, probably due to immunological mechanisms. Many syndromes affecting the central and peripheral nervous systems have been reported, including epilepsy, myoclonus, ataxia, multifocal leukoencephalopathy, dementia and peripheral neuropathies, both axonal and demyelinating. The key syndromes in which to consider coeliac disease are cryptogenic ataxias and neuropathies – the latter often associated with sensory ataxia linked to disturbed posterolateral column function in the spinal cord. Initially, it was thought that the neurological features might be caused by malabsorption, especially of vitamin B12, folate and vitamin E, but subsequent studies and replacement therapy have not reversed the deficits. Substantial neurological features can occur in the absence of clinically overt coeliac disease. The diagnosis of coeliac disease is supported by the presence of antigliadin and anti-endomysial antibodies and anti-tissue transglutamate, although the typical villous atrophy of the intestinal mucosa on biopsy still gives the definitive histological proof.

Whipple's disease is rare, but can produce striking and characteristic neurological features in a minority of cases. It is a chronic multisystem granulomatous disease largely affecting middle-aged males, due to bacterial infection with *Tropheryma whippelii*. It usually presents with intestinal symptoms – diarrhoea and steatorrhoea – accompanied by weight loss and abdominal pain. Other systemic features include fever, hyperpigmentation, lymphadenopathy and cardiac involvement. Neurological complications appear in approximately 5 per cent, most often including dementia with myoclonus and a supranuclear ophthalmoplegia. A curious oculomasticatory myorhythmia has been described, comprising pendular oscillations of the eyes accompanied by rhythmic contractions of the jaw muscles. Seizures, cerebellar ataxia, pyramidal and extrapyramidal signs, as well as a peripheral neuropathy have also been reported.

The CSF is normal or shows a mild protein rise with a lymphocytic pleocytosis. MRI may show scattered high signal lesions in the brainstem, hypothalamus and cerebral hemispheres. Periodic acid–Schiff (PAS)-positive macrophages may be seen in a jejunal biopsy specimen and similar PAS-positive material may be present in scattered granulomatous nodules in the brain. A polymerase chain reaction test may be useful. Making the diagnosis is important, as long-term treatment with trimethoprim and sulfamethoxazole or tetracycline is helpful.

Hepatic failure

The most important neurological presentation of liver disease is **hepatic encephalopathy**. This results when toxins, including ammonia, aromatic amino acids, mercaptans, short-chain fatty acids and endogenous benzodiazepines, are not removed from hepatic portal blood, so enter the systemic circulation. The speed of onset of encephalopathy parallels that of the underlying hepatic failure; this may vary from hours (as in acute paracetamol poisoning) to days (as in acute hepatitis), to very slow progression over months (as in cirrhosis). Patients with cirrhosis are the most commonly affected by encephalopathy, which may decompensate acutely in response to an infection, a gastrointestinal haemorrhage (most often from oesophageal varices), to certain drugs, potassium loss or to protein excess. Initial mild symptoms, such as restlessness, anxiety, fluctuating confusion and inverted sleep patterns, are easily missed.

Once established, **delirium typically fluctuates during the day** and may be accompanied by euphoria and neurological signs including a flapping postural tremor of the hands (asterixis) and constructional apraxia. Hepatic foetor is the sickly sweet odour on the breath found in many cases; hepatic enlargement, spider naevi, jaundice, ascites, and peripheral oedema are other important clinical stigmata of liver disease, which should be actively sought in any unexplained encephalopathy. Untreated, delirium progresses to stupor and coma; seizures may also occur. Focal or bilateral pyramidal signs, rigidity, primitive reflexes and extensor plantar responses may be present. In coma, the pupils may dilate.

A progressive spastic paraparesis, portocaval encephalomyelopathy, is a rare complication of liver failure, which may follow episodes of portosystemic encephalopathy or even surgery in patients with cirrhosis. Many patients show high blood ammonia levels; normally this is less than 50 mmol/L, but with hepatic failure it may rise to well above 100 mmol/L. In addition, liver function tests show elevated enzyme levels, and a prolonged prothrombin time (which may lead to bruising and haemorrhagic complications). The blood glucose may be low. The CSF may be normal or show a slight protein rise. The EEG may show paroxysmal slow wave activity mirroring the depressed conscious level; sometimes triphasic delta waves appear in stuporose patients (see Chapter 5). A CT brain scan may be normal or show a swollen brain; this investigation is indicated to exclude haemorrhagic complications.

Treatment involves the elimination of any precipitating cause, the maintenance of a correct fluid balance with restriction of dietary protein and its replacement by intravenous glucose. Coagulation defects will need correction. The treatment is aimed at reducing the nitrogen burden in the bowel and includes a low protein diet, regular large doses of lactulose and sometimes neomycin to reduce

nitrogen-producing organisms. In selected patients, haemodialysis may be life-saving, although transplantation may ultimately be required.

Reye's syndrome

Reye's syndrome is a rare form of encephalopathy arising in children aged between five and 15 years, characterized by acute brain swelling with fatty infiltration of the liver. It appears often to be triggered by an acute viral infection, and there is an association with salicylate use. The onset is acute, with preceding symptoms of an upper respiratory tract infection, then profuse vomiting and a deteriorating conscious level ending in coma, seizures, rigidity and signs of cerebral damage. There may be a low blood and CSF glucose, abnormal liver enzymes, a prolonged prothrombin time and raised blood ammonia. The EEG shows diffuse slow activity. The brain may become very swollen and this can be detected by imaging. The CSF is usually under increased pressure and is acellular. Many children die, but prompt recognition of the condition accompanied by treatment to lower the raised intracranial pressure, intravenous glucose and correction of associated metabolic disturbances, leads to survival, although some show signs of residual deficits.

VITAMIN DEFICIENCY

Many vitamin deficiencies result from the effects of widespread malnutrition, usually from starvation or severe malabsorption. A few may reflect dietary fads or the substitution of food in the diet by alcohol.

Vitamin B1 deficiency

Vitamin B1 (thiamine) deficiency causes Wernicke encephalopathy, Korsakoff syndrome and beri-beri.

Although classically a result of chronic alcoholism, Wernicke encephalopathy and Korsakoff syndrome are well known to result from other causes, such as intractable vomiting (including anorexia nervosa and hyperemesis gravidarum). One of the three patients originally reported by Wernicke suffered from severe vomiting from pyloric stenosis induced by ingestion of sulphuric acid.

Multiple small areas of necrosis and haemorrhage are found in the midbrain, the periaqueductal

Wernicke encephalopathy is a subacute illness causing delirium, nystagmus – with or without ophthalmoplegia – and ataxia, typically of gait more than limbs. The ocular signs include unilateral or bilateral abducens palsies (54 per cent), disturbances of conjugate gaze (44 per cent) including an internuclear ophthalmoplegia, and horizontal and vertical nystagmus (85 per cent). The ataxia is a reflection of cerebellar damage and may be so severe as to prevent walking unaided. In over 80 per cent, there are also signs of a peripheral neuropathy. The syndrome is underdiagnosed and potentially treatable.

Korsakoff syndrome (psychosis) can follow Wernicke encephalopathy and is characterized by a more restricted syndrome of anterograde and retrograde amnesia without delirium. There is often striking confabulation. Many patients appear apathetic, muddled and drowsy. A few may show the more florid hallucinations of alcoholic withdrawal.

region, the paraventricular areas of the thalamus, the hypothalamus, the mammillary bodies and around the fourth ventricle. These abnormalities may be seen on MRI. The cerebellum may also show neuronal loss. This damage is a result of thiamine deficiency and, if treated early, many of the clinical features can be reversed.

Thiamine deficiency can be confirmed by a significant reduction in the red cell transketolase level. In severe cases, some irreversible damage occurs and, if left untreated, the condition is fatal. Many patients are left with memory deficits (amnesic syndrome).

Treatment is a neurological emergency. The diagnosis is made on clinical grounds and should not depend upon the results of investigations. A high index of suspicion is needed, and it is better to treat patients who turn out not to be suffering from this condition, than to miss the diagnosis. Intravenous thiamine 50–100 mg daily for 5 days is the specific treatment, accompanied by the restoration of a normal diet (or adequate parenteral feeding where indicated). As mentioned above, glucose administration, by itself, can dramatically worsen or precipitate the effects of thiamine deficiency.

The extent of recovery is influenced by the time to diagnosis and treatment with thiamine. Some of the eye signs and ataxia often resolve, but the residual amnestic syndrome (Korsakoff) is common. In any patient with cognitive disturbance or delirium in the context of heavy alcohol use, prompt treatment with high-dose intravenous B vitamins is recommended.

Vitamin B12 deficiency

Vitamin B12 (cobalamin) has a vital physiological role in nervous system function; up to 40 per cent of those with B12 deficiency have neurological manifestations.

B12 deficiency should be suspected in any patient with otherwise unexplained:
- peripheral neuropathy
- myelopathy
- optic neuropathy (with centrocaecal scotoma)
- dementia, or psychiatric disturbances.

The most common early sign is paraesthesiae, typically first noticed in the feet. Although at first objective neurological signs may be absent, subsequently symptoms and signs of a myelopathy involving the dorsal and lateral columns develop – termed subacute combined degeneration of the cord. A mild, predominantly sensory peripheral neuropathy is also often present. Weakness is usually not found, but dorsal column involvement causes impaired vibration and joint position sense; there may be ataxia. The vacuolar myelopathy of HIV infection may resemble subacute combined degeneration (Chapter 26).

Deficiency of vitamin B12 may arise after a total gastrectomy, in vegans, after some parasitic infestations or inflammatory intestinal disorders, and from pernicious anaemia. Pernicious anaemia is an autoimmune-mediated atrophic gastritis, causing failure of B12 absorption in the stomach due to lack of intrinsic factor; it causes the vast majority of cases of symptomatic B12 deficiency. Gastrectomy removes parietal cells, the source of intrinsic factor. Disease of the distal ileum can impair absorption of the intrinsic factor–cobalamin complex, explaining the B12 deficiency found in Whipple's disease, ileal tuberculosis, tropical sprue and ileal surgical resection. Infestation by the tapeworm Diphyllobothrium latum causes deficiency by competing with the host for cobalamin. Nutritional deficiency can develop in vegans.

The serum B12 level should be determined in any patient with an appropriate clinical syndrome. Although a macrocytic megaloblastic anaemia is typically found, abnormal blood cell indices are not sufficiently sensitive or specific to reliably diagnose B12 deficiency. In patients with borderline low B12 levels, finding elevated serum methylmalonic acid and homocysteine levels may confirm a physiological deficiency. Nerve conduction studies usually show neuropathic changes and some patients may show abnormal visual evoked potentials. MRI may demonstrate hyperintensities on T2-weighted images in the posterior columns; in cases of cognitive disturbance, high signal lesions may also be found in the cerebral white matter. A Schilling test measuring the absorption of radioisotope-labelled B12, with and without intrinsic factor, confirms the diagnosis and its mechanism. Antibodies to intrinsic factor are present in those with pernicious anaemia.

Treatment is injections of hydroxocobalamin daily for ten days, then monthly for life. Providing severe damage has not occurred, symptoms usually improve over the first few months of treatment. However, several clinical trials have now failed to show a therapeutic effect of B12 supplementation in treating dementia associated with low B12, or a benefit of B12 and other B vitamin supplementation in preventing stroke or coronary ischaemic events.

Recent randomized trial data have suggested an effect of B vitamin supplements, including B12 on reducing progressive cerebral atrophy in patients with mild cognitive impairment, but it is too early to know if this will be clinically helpful in preventing dementia.

Vitamin D deficiency

Proximal muscle weakness can develop as a result of vitamin D malabsorption. The symptoms usually start in the legs, affecting hip movements but with preservation of distal power, reflexes and sensation. EMG may show myopathic features with short duration polyphasic potentials. The degree of muscle weakness is not correlated with plasma calcium concentration and the underlying mechanism is unclear. Vitamin D treatment is generally helpful.

Vitamin E deficiency

Vitamin E deficiency results from cholestatic liver disease, fat malabsorption, abetalipoproteinaemia or as a familial absorption disorder. The clinical features include neuropathy, ataxia, ophthalmoplegia and muscle weakness. A familial condition with poor conservation of plasma alpha-tocopherol in very low density lipoproteins is characterized by ataxia, cerebellar signs, dysarthria, leg areflexia, impaired proprioception, bilateral extensor plantar responses, pes cavus and scoliosis. These signs are strikingly similar to those seen in Friedreich's ataxia (Chapter 21). All patients presenting with an unexplained spinocerebellar syndrome or tremor should have vitamin E concentrations measured, as the symptoms may respond to treatment.

Pellagra (niacin deficiency)

Niacin (also termed vitamin B3 or nicotinic acid) deficiency is characterized by dementia, dermatitis and diarrhoea (the three Ds). There may also be damage to the pyramidal tracts, producing a spastic weakness of the legs, or more widespread neurological disturbance with extrapyramidal and peripheral nerve signs.

Occasionally, an acute confusional state with deteriorating conscious level occurs. Many patients show skin changes with a dermatitis (often photosensitive), mucocutaneous lesions and gastrointestinal disturbances, particularly diarrhoea, and even malabsorption. A scarlet painful tongue is common.

Pellagra, rarely seen in developed countries, was originally described in vegans from poor maize-eating countries and in deprived prisoners. It is probable that many of the latter were suffering from multiple vitamin deficiencies as well as an inadequate diet. The most common cause of pellagra now is **chronic alcoholism**, which usually presents with acute and isolated delirium. There can also be generalized rigidity (sometimes cogwheeling), dysarthria and myoclonus.

Nutritional and toxic amblyopia

Some specific deficiency states can cause optic nerve damage leading to visual failure and optic atrophy. These include **vitamin B12 deficiency** (see above) and **thiamine deficiency**; the latter may have some links with the toxic effects of alcohol and/or tobacco to which many of these patients are also exposed, and a poor general nutritional state may contribute.

There is an insidiously progressive impairment of vision affecting both eyes. The acuity falls and the optic discs appear pale. Examination reveals centrocaecal scotomas, most easily detected with a red target. Electroretinograms and visual evoked potentials may aid diagnosis. Some patients may show low red blood cell folate levels.

Treatment is abstinence from tobacco and/or alcohol, and most patients are also given hydroxocobalamin injections and folic acid, although it is equally important to ensure a good diet, including adequate thiamine and other B vitamins.

Tropical amblyopia and neuropathies

Tropical amblyopia and neuropathies arise from the combined effects of malnutrition and vitamin deficiency, most often found in deprived areas associated with starvation, or in prisoners. Many have combinations of beriberi, pellagra and their neurological manifestations. These include a peripheral neuropathy with complaints of sensory symptoms and sometimes 'burning feet', with weakness and clumsiness of the extremities: in some, this may be combined with a spastic paraparesis. Other patients show signs of a sensorimotor neuropathy with marked muscle wasting and prominent ataxia. There may also be visual disturbance associated with optic atrophy, and sometimes deafness. Many patients may develop mucocutaneous lesions and some complain of abdominal pain. In some cases, a toxic mechanism has been suggested, including excess ingestion of *Lathyrus sativus* or cassava.

However, the differential diagnosis includes **tropical spastic paraparesis**, arising from an inflammatory necrotic myelitis caused by infection with the human T-cell lymphotropic virus (HTLV-1) virus. In many such patients, symptoms include back pain, paraesthesiae, sphincter upset and leg weakness from the spastic paraparesis. Antibodies to the HTLV-1 virus can be detected by blood tests.

RENAL DISORDERS

Renal diseases are relevant to neurologists in two ways. First, some conditions affect both the kidneys and the nervous system – these include the vasculitides and connective tissue diseases, as well as genetic disorders (Anderson–Fabry disease, Wilson disease, von Hippel–Lindau disease), and infections and plasma cell dyscrasias. Second, renal failure, dialysis and renal transplantation can all affect neurological function in a variety of ways.

Conditions affecting both renal and neurological function

These conditions are mainly described in other chapters. In its early stages, renal disease causes few or no symptoms, so renal function must be investigated when there is clinical suspicion of a multisystem disorder. Vigilance is important because the consequences of progressive renal disease are severe and potentially avoidable. Routine biochemistry (urea and creatinine) will only pick up already advanced renal dysfunction. Thus, if renal disease is suspected, for example in a patient with mononeuritis multiplex, renal investigation should include urine microscopy for casts and detailed urinalysis, close monitoring of blood pressure, renal ultrasound and occasionally additional investigations.

Neurological consequences of renal disease

In **uraemic encephalopathy**, as the blood urea and creatinine rise, patients become increasingly confused, drowsy and eventually comatose. Other symptoms associated with the deteriorating conscious level include hallucinations, twitching, tremors, asterixis, restlessness, tetany, myoclonic jerking and tonic-clonic seizures. Commonly, such symptoms fluctuate. Patients with a depressed conscious level may show acidotic breathing, which later may wax and wane (Cheyne–Stokes breathing). Associated systemic features include anorexia, nausea, vomiting, fatigue, pruritus, a haemorrhagic state and, in acute renal failure, oliguria.

Electrolyte disorders are common and include hyperkalaemia, hyponatraemia, a rising blood urea and creatinine. In addition, hypocalcaemia and hypomagnesaemia may develop.

Specific treatment will depend on the underlying cause. Dialysis relieves the uraemia, and effects reversal of many of the neurological symptoms. Convulsions can usually be controlled with low doses of anticonvulsants. Hypertensive encephalopathy may also arise in patients with renal failure.

Patients with chronic uraemia often develop a peripheral sensorimotor neuropathy; **uraemic neuropathy** is a distal axonal degeneration with secondary myelin loss. This occurs in the majority of patients with chronic renal failure; the severity is related to the extent and duration of renal failure. Onset is often with periodic limb movements or restless legs, and established neuropathy is characterized by distal paraesthetic sensory disturbance. The neuropathy is reversible with treatment of the renal failure.

Dialysis-associated neurological problems

Two neurological syndromes are recognized in dialysis patients: these are often termed 'dialysis dementia' and 'dialysis disequilibrium'.

Dialysis dementia

Dialysis encephalopathy (dialysis dementia) is the rare but potentially fatal condition that previously complicated chronic dialysis and is still occasionally seen. Patients develop subacute progression of fluctuating symptoms in the early stages which either become fixed or progress. The condition is characterized by dysarthria, dysphasia and progressive metabolic encephalopathy with myoclonus and asterixis culminating in generalized seizures and intellectual decline.

The syndrome is caused by the aluminium content in gels and dialysate solution. Purified dialysate has led to the almost total disappearance of this condition. Chronic haemodialysis can also lead to Wernicke encephalopathy, sensorimotor axonal polyneuropathy and occasionally subdural haematoma.

Dialysis dysequilibrium syndrome

Dialysis dysequilibrium syndrome is related to changing osmotic gradients between plasma and brain during rapid dialysis. It can present with non-specific symptoms of nausea, visual blurring and headache prior to development of worsening mental confusion, clouding of consciousness, seizures and tremor. The symptoms come on within 3–4 hours of starting dialysis and last for some hours.

The symptoms are usually mild and can be alleviated with slow flow rates during dialysis and the addition of osmotically active solutes to the dialysate. It is accompanied by a diffuse EEG disturbance. Either water intoxication, from over-rapid dialysis, or aluminium toxicity from the dialysate may be responsible for the acute or subacute encephalopathy.

Following renal transplantation, patients taking immunosuppressive treatment are more prone to unusual infections, for example cryptococcus or listeriosis (see Chapter 25). Ciclosporin used as an immunosuppressant in transplant patients may provoke tremor and epileptic seizures. It may also produce 'burning' extremities, headache, weakness, ataxia and symptoms suggestive of a myopathy.

VASCULITIDES, CONNECTIVE TISSUE DISEASES AND RELATED DISORDERS

General overview

In **vasculitides and connective tissue diseases** (Table 27.7), the pathogenesis remains uncertain, but they are associated with an inflammatory disturbance of connective tissue and often blood vessels (vasculitis). Vasculitis causes ischaemic damage (usually irreversible) in the brain, spinal cord, peripheral nerve or muscle. All these disorders are considered to have an immunological basis, and are characterized by the presence of various humoral antibodies, which are often helpful in diagnosis and disease monitoring. Many may cause an aseptic meningitis, with a CSF pleocytosis and mild protein rise. There are also some **secondary causes of vasculitis** affect-

Table 27.7 Vasculitides and related disorders affecting the nervous system

Disorder	Key neurological features
Polyarteritis nodosa	Peripheral neuropathy (mononeuritis multiplex). Central nervous system complications rare – include encephalopathy, seizures
Churg–Strauss syndrome	Peripheral neuropathy (mononeuritis multiplex)
Wegener's granulomatosis	Hearing loss, cranial nerve palsies (ophthalmoplegia, trigeminal, facial) Mononeuritis multiplex
Sjögren's syndrome	Axonal sensory neuropathy Myelopathy Cognitive disturbance Imaging findings may resemble multiple sclerosis
Rheumatoid arthritis	Entrapment neuropathies Mononeuritis multiplex
Scleroderma	Rare – reported associations include peripheral or cranial neuropathies, headache, seizures, stroke
Dermatomyositis	Pain, muscle weakness (shoulder and hip girdles)
Systemic lupus erythematosis	Neuropsychiatric – mood, cognitive disturbances, stroke
Isolated angiitis of the central nervous system	Encephalopathy Multiple sclerosis-like illness with optic neuropathy and stroke-like episodes Intracranial mass with focal signs and/or raised intracranial pressure
Giant cell arteritis	Monocular blindness Strokes

ing the nervous system to bear in mind, including **infections** (fungi, tuberculosis, bacteria, spirochaetes, viruses including varicella zoster virus (VZV), HIV); **drugs** (including amphetamine and cocaine); and **malignancy**, either via direct involvement, such as in lymphoma, or as part of a paraneoplastic vasculitis.

Histologically, there is typically a necrotizing arteritis with a transmural infiltrate, initially comprising polymorphs, lymphocytes and eosinophils. The proportions, subtypes and behaviour of these cells vary depending on the type of vasculitis: for example, granulomas (a nodular aggregation of mononuclear inflammatory cells) are more common in **Wegener's granulomatosis (WG)** and **giant cell arteritis (GCA)**. It is these various inflammatory cells which reduce blood flow through the affected vessel leading to nervous tissue ischaemic damage. On angiography, vessel walls commonly show multifocal thickening (beading) and occlusions.

Tissue damage in vasculitis results from thrombosis with distal embolism, or directly from thrombotic occlusion of arteries, capillaries or veins. Thus, anticoagulation may theoretically be appropriate in some situations. In peripheral nerves,

arteritis usually affects the precapillary arteries. In the CNS, the calibre of blood vessel affected is associated with disease type, but overlaps are common. Although classification has traditionally used vessel size, therapy is not yet at the stage where different populations of inflammatory cells can be targeted.

Neurological involvement in systemic vasculitic disorders is common, but in most cases, patients are already known to have a particular rheumatological or systemic vasculitis, and so may be receiving immunomodulatory therapy. GCA and primary CNS vasculitis are exceptions, where the first presentation is almost always neurological.

In vasculitides, there are three main mechanisms underlying neurological dysfunction, each of which requires a different treatment approach:

1   The neurological problems are due to active increased underlying systemic disease activity, needing prompt escalation of immunomodulatory therapy.
2   The symptoms are related to adverse effects of disease treatment, for example, proximal myopathy due to corticosteroids. The

treatment here will usually involve stopping or adjusting the dose of the relevant agent.

3 The symptoms may be caused by a separate, but possibly associated disease process requiring its own treatment, for example ischaemic stroke in a patient with GCA and diabetes.

4 The symptoms may result from mechanical effects of the disease or its treatment. Compressive spinal cord or root pathology can occur in any of the systemic disorders, especially as steroid-related osteopenia has a predilection for the vertebral bodies. However, this is most commonly seen in patients with rheumatoid arthritis (RA). Entrapment neuropathies can be caused by nodule formation in RA (typically ulnar or median nerve) or granulomas (typically cranial nerves).

General principles of treatment of vasculitides involving the nervous system

Immunosuppressive therapies for vasculitis are relatively toxic, so the decision to administer them should be supported by a tissue diagnosis, if at all possible. When neurological symptoms and signs occur alongside multisystem disease activity, a diagnostic biopsy may well be obtained from affected skin, kidney or lung. However, if the neurological syndrome occurs while disease remains quiescent in other organs then brain, nerve or muscle biopsy may be the only reasonable option. Immunosuppressive treatment of neurological involvement in systemic disorders is unlikely to be based directly on prospective randomized trials, due to the relative rarity of these conditions. However, indirect evidence is available from controlled trials of patients with systemic vasculitis. Given that the underlying pathology is similar in non-neurological organs, extrapolation of results is reasonable. In general, the majority of vasculitic disorders can be reversed or controlled in some 90 per cent of patients with a combination of high-dose oral corticosteroids and oral cyclophosphamide. Cyclophosphamide is usually given for approximately three months with less toxic drugs, such as azathioprine, then used to sustain remission, while corticosteroid dosage is gradually reduced. Newer agents or non-pharmacological treatments, such as plasma exchange, may need to be used in resistant or persistently relapsing conditions. Some of the important immunosuppressive drugs and their associated adverse-effect monitoring variables are included in Table 27.8.

Polyarteritis nodosa and related conditions

Polyarteritis nodosa

Polyarteritis nodosa (PAN) is the prototype necrotizing vasculitis. Medium-sized vessels are usually affected, with irregular 'beading' seen on angiography, sometimes leading to occlusion or multiple aneurysm formation. Middle-aged men are most commonly affected. Many organs are involved: the kidney in some 75 per cent (often associated with hypertension), the lungs (asthma), the heart (80 per cent), the skin and the nervous system. Systemic symptoms include abdominal pain (from hepatic or other visceral infarcts), hypertension (from renal involvement), fever and weight loss and arthralgia.

Diagnosis is based on the clinical features and either positive angiography or biopsy of affected tissue (skin, kidney or peripheral nerve). The only serological marker clearly associated with PAN is hepatitis B infection (20–40 per cent HbsAg-positive). PAN is considered to be an antineutrophil cytoplasmic autoantibodies (ANCA)-negative syndrome. The most common neurological problem is a progressive mononeuritis multiplex (MNM), which occurs in up to 50 per cent of patients with PAN. In common with other causes of vasculitic mononeuritis, this often presents with a painful sensory or sensorimotor picture, or a mononeuritis multiplex. More central involvement occurs in other cases, in a variety of patterns – headache, encephalopathy, psychosis, seizures, stroke, aseptic meningitis, rarely an ischaemic myelopathy and sometimes cranial nerve palsies. Ocular involvement is also common and may result in retinal infarcts, haemorrhages, exudates and ischaemic optic nerve damage.

Abnormal blood investigations include neutrophilia with eosinophilia in about one-third of patients, a raised ESR and CRP, and a posi-

Table 27.8 Immunomodulatory treatments for vasculitis

Drug	Class/action	Side effects	Monitor (prophylaxis)
Acute or induction			
Methylprednisolone	Corticosteroid	Diabetes, neuropsychiatric, osteoporosis with regular use	Glucose, blood pressure. Dip urine to rule out infection before treatment
Cyclophosphamide	Alkylating agent	Haemorrhagic cystitis (Mesna prophylaxis), bone marrow suppression, neutropenia, sepsis	FBC
IVIg	Pooled antibodies	As for blood products, headache, aseptic meningitis (rare), renal failure (rare)	Check IgA levels pretreatment (absent IgA = absolute contraindication), U&E
Infliximab	Monoclonal anti-TNF antibody	Hypersensitivity (delayed), atypical infections especially TB, induction of dsDNA antibodies	FBC, U&E, LFT and pre-Rx. CXR (exclude TB), ANA and dsDNA. Use prophylactic isoniazid in patients at high risk for TB
Rituximab	Monoclonal anti-CD20 antibody	Infusion related (flu-like), neutropenia (may be late), anaemia	FBC, B lymphocytes.
Long term			
Prednisolone	Corticosteriod	Diabetes, osteoporosis, adrenal suppression, infections	DEXA scan (bisphophanates for osteoprophylaxis)
Mycophenolate mofetil	Inhibitor of inosine monophosphate dehydrogenase	Bone marrow suppression, gastrointestinal intolerance, chronic viral infections	FBC; (ideally) monitor mycophenolic acid levels
Methotrexate	Folate antagonist/ adenosine agonist	Pulmonary fibrosis, liver failure, bone marrow suppression	FBC, U&E, LFT (folate prophylaxis)
Azathioprine	Blocks purine synthesis	Bone marrow suppression, squamous cell carcinoma, chronic viral infections, hypersensitivity	FBC + (ideally) check thiopurine methyltranferase (TMPT) pre-Rx. (absent TMPT = absolute contraindication; reduced level = reduce dose)
Tacrolimus	Calcineurin inhibitor	Diabetes, hypertension	FBC, U&E, glucose, tacrolimus levels

FBC, full blood count; LFT, liver function test; U&E, urea and electrolysis.

tive ANA. Antineutrophil cytoplasmic antibodies (pANCA, cANCA) may be present: the perinuclear pattern (pANCA) refers to the autoantigen link with myeloperoxidase, and the diffuse cytoplasmic pattern (cANCA) links with autoantigen proteinase 3. These antibodies are more likely to be present with microscopic polyarteritis.

Churg–Strauss syndrome

Churg–Strauss syndrome is a necrotizing vasculitis commonly affecting the lungs, with asthma, fever, an eosinophilia and systemic vasculitis. Nasal polyps are common. There may be purpura and skin nodules. A patchy, often painful, mononeuritis multiplex is very common and less often a polyneuropathy.

Cerebral vessels may rarely be affected, resulting in memory impairment and seizures. There is a weak association with ANCA, but there is nearly always a peripheral eosinophilia ($>1.5 \times 10^9\,L^{-1}$). Cardiac, gastrointestinal and skin involvement are also common. Histology of affected tissue usually shows three cardinal features: necrotizing vasculitis, granulomas and infiltration by eosinophils. ANCA are usually present. Raised serum levels of immunoglobulin E are commonly found.

Wegener's granulomatosis

Wegener's granulomatosis is characterized by upper respiratory tract granuloma (typically affecting the nasal mucosa and/or inner ear), lower respiratory tract granuloma (typically pulmonary nodules) and a necrotizing glomerulonephritis. The **neurological effects** are from proximity of neurological structures to active lesions, or ischaemia/haemorrhage due to the vasculitis. There is often aggressive spread through the **sinuses, orbits and base of the skull**. This may cause cranial nerve, brainstem, and ocular involvement, especially an arteritic anterior ischaemic optic neuropathy. Acute or subacute hearing loss is associated with WG; this is often because of a combination of conduction hearing loss (otitis media or otitis interna) and sensorineural loss (granuloma or vasculitic processes affecting the auditory nerve).

There is a **peripheral neuropathy** (usually mononeuritis multiplex) in up to 50 per cent of cases; the most common nerve affected is the common peroneal nerve, followed by the tibial, ulnar, median, radial and femoral nerves. There is often an associated fever, and generalized skin and joint symptoms; laboratory tests frequently show anaemia, a raised ESR and CRP. **Antineutrophil cytoplasmic antibodies (cANCA)** in high titre are strongly suggestive of WG, with specificity of 95 per cent and sensitivity of 80 per cent. Circulating levels are used as an indirect disease marker against which immunomodulatory therapy can be titrated. The diagnosis may also be supported by biopsy (the highest yield being from the lung). The development of neurological features of WG is an indication for an increase in immunomodulatory therapy.

Sjögren's syndrome

Sjögren's syndrome (SS) is characterized by lymphocytic infiltrates and destruction of epithelial exocrine glands. Up to 40 per cent of patients develop neurological complications. Several different **neuropathies** have been described; the most common pattern (approximately 50 per cent) is an asymmetric, segmental or multifocal sensory neuropathy, starting with distal paraesthesia, but often progressing to involve the trunk or face. A large proportion of these patients have an associated sensory ataxia, which can be severe; high signal intensity in the posterior columns of the spinal cord on T2 MRI is sometimes seen. In some subjects, ataxia is less prominent but neuropathic pain more so; progression of symptoms tends to occur months or years. A less common pattern is a mononeuritis multiplex, which can be more acute. Autonomic features are common, especially abnormalities of pupillary function (Holmes–Adie pupils), sweating and orthostatic hypotension.

Cranial neuropathies in SS include a sensory neuropathy affecting one or both trigeminal nerves, and a cranial polyneuropathy that can affect any nerve with little discrimination between motor and sensory nerve populations. Hearing loss is sensorineural because of a lesion of the VIIIth nerve and this may develop acutely or progressively.

An **acute or subacute myelopathy** (transverse myelitis) is also described. MRI of the brain and spinal cord may show focal high signal abnormalities that are indistinguishable from those seen in multiple sclerosis. Other CNS features include subcortical cognitive impairment, seizures or focal deficits, such as hemiplegia. Patients thus affected commonly show hyperglobulinaemia with positive non-organ-specific antibodies, such as rheumatoid factor or ANA. Extractable nuclear antigens, particularly anti-Ro and anti-La are regularly found in Sjögren's syndrome. Schirmer's test (measuring the wetting of a standardized strip of filter paper inserted into the corner of the eye) will objectively confirm dry eyes. A minor salivary gland biopsy showing focal lymphocytic sialadenitis (usually of the lip) can be helpful in confirming the diagnosis. Systemic involvement is characterized by chronic fatigue, arthralgia, oesophageal hypomotility, haematological disorders and rarely a cutaneous vasculitis, alopecia and vitiligo.

If there is involvement of the peripheral or central nervous system, aggressive treatment for the underlying vasculitis is indicated. First-line treatment is intravenous corticosteroid, but if progression continues an alternative immunosuppressant may be indicated. The sensory axonal ganglioneuropathy responds poorly to immunosuppression. Other agents used with corticosteroids include azathioprine and hydroxychloroquine.

Rheumatoid arthritis

Rheumatoid arthritis is a multisystem disorder usually presenting with a symmetrical distal polyarthropathy. Morning joint stiffness is prominent, and the diagnosis is usually supported by the presence of rheumatoid nodules, rheumatoid factor in serum and characteristic juxta-articular changes on x-rays of affected joints. The neurological manifestations are listed in Table 27.9. Inflammatory or vasculitic neurological complications also occur, but are rare. More common are entrapment neuropathies and, most worrying, spinal cord or lower brainstem syndromes secondary to erosive skeletal involvement of the atlanto-axial, odontoid or other vertebral components. The cervical spine is most often affected by erosive disease, but extradural pannus can cause compression at any spinal level, including the cauda equina.

Peripheral nerve involvement

Peripheral nerve involvement is also common, arising from:

- Entrapment neuropathies (approximately 45 per cent), e.g. carpal tunnel syndrome
- Mononeuritis multiplex

- Symmetrical neuropathy:
  - digital sensory neuropathy
  - sensorimotor neuropathy – may be severe.

Magnetic resonance scanning is the best way to demonstrate changes in the cervical spine or at the craniocervical junction. Blood tests include a raised ESR and CRP, a positive rheumatoid factor, a positive ANA (some 40 per cent), and a normal or raised complement level. Nerve conduction studies and EMG will confirm peripheral nerve involvement. Spinal cord compression may require neurosurgical intervention.

Scleroderma

In addition to skin and gastrointestinal tract changes, scleroderma may be associated with muscle weakness from an inflammatory polymyositis or a non-inflammatory myopathy. Rare neurological complications include peripheral neuropathy, entrapment neuropathies and cranial neuropathies. Headache, seizures, stroke, radiculopathy, and myelopathy have all been reported rarely. In some of these patients, extractable nuclear antigens may be present.

Dermatomyositis

This is considered in Chapter 18.

Mixed connective tissue diseases

A group of rheumatological disorders overlap with RA, the mixed connective tissue diseases (MCTD) comprising RA, scleroderma, SS, systemic lupus erythematosus (SLE) and myositis. Patients with

Table 27.9 Neurological complications of rheumatoid arthritis

Anatomical region affected	Clinical complications
Spine (malalignment, cord compression)	Atlanto-axial subluxation, other levels particularly cervical
Peripheral nerves	Peripheral neuropathy
	Entrapment neuropathy CTS
	Mononeuropathy multiplex
	Symmetrical neuropathy
	Digital sensory
	Sensorimotor
Muscle	Myositis (rare)
Central nervous system	Cranial nerve palsies, seizures, vasculitis with stroke (rare)

CTS, carpal tunnel syndrome.

this disorder are often positive for the U1-RNP antibody which is itself associated with the main threat to life: pulmonary hypertension. Neurological manifestations are similar to those seen in RA or SLE; an inflammatory myopathy is present in up to 50 per cent of cases. Evidence suggests that MCTD-associated myopathy is particularly responsive to corticosteroid treatment.

Systemic lupus erythematosus

SLE is a multisystem disorder which commonly affects the joints and almost any other organ system, although mucocutaneous involvement is especially common. In part, the pathogenesis of SLE is vascular, including a hypercoagulable state, and in part results from immunological mechanisms. Antiphospholipid antibodies may be found, linked with an increased thrombotic risk. Immunological changes include a high ESR, often with a normal CRP. The antinuclear antibody (ANA) test has a high false-positive rate and detection of more specific antibodies to intracellular antigens is often required (e.g. double- and single-stranded DNA).

Neurological manifestations occur in at least 20 per cent of patients. These include neuropsychiatric symptoms, seizures, TIAs, focal neurological signs including hemiplegia, chorea, cerebellar ataxia and cranial nerve lesions. Spinal cord involvement presents with paraparesis. Peripheral neuropathy and myositis also occur.

Commonly, these manifestations are associated with joint and skin changes (butterfly facial rash), fever, renal and pulmonary involvement. Of these manifestations, **neuropsychiatric disturbances** are especially frequent; about a third of SLE patients have so-called neuropsychiatric lupus. Mood disorders, strokes and cognitive disorders each occur in 10–15 per cent of patients, seizures, psychosis and acute confusional states are less common.

Current evidence favours a primary thrombotic/occlusive cerebral vasculopathy over a vasculitis, with antiphospholipid antibodies, particularly those directed at cardiolipin, present in 55 per cent of patients with neuropsychiatric SLE compared to 20 per cent with SLE alone. The therapeutic implication is that neuropsychiatric SLE should be treated with anticoagulation rather than immunosuppressive therapy. However, it should also be remembered that the development of conventional atherosclerosis seems to be accelerated in SLE, especially in premenopausal women. The incidence of myocardial infarction and stroke may be higher in patients with SLE, even after controlling for the usual risk factors, making SLE an important cause of premature vascular death. Disease activity is related to risk of stroke.

Isolated cerebral angiitis

Isolated cerebral angiitis (ICA) or primary cerebral vasculitis is very difficult to diagnose as there are no clear diagnostic criteria or specific tests. Unlike most of the diseases mentioned above, there are neither diagnostic clues from involvement of non-neurological organ systems, nor specific serological or CSF tests. ICA can present in a wide variety of ways with an acute or subacute, relapsing or chronic time course. Three main patterns of presentation are recognized: encephalopathy with headache, confusion and coma; intracranial mass with a mixture of focal and non-specific CNS signs and raised ICP; and an atypical multiple sclerosis (MS)-like syndrome with a relapsing-remitting course, optic nerve involvement, sometimes with stroke-like episodes and seizures.

Brain MRI is usually abnormal in patients with ICA, but there are no specific findings; intra-arterial cerebral angiograms have poor specificity and sensitivity, of the order of 30 per cent. Thus, brain biopsy is the only reliable diagnostic test, and leads to a diagnosis in over 75 per cent of cases. Importantly, about half of positive biopsies show an alternative, unsuspected cause, such as infection, lymphoma or MS.

Treatment of ICA is with immunosuppression using high-dose intravenous corticosteroids, combined with other agents, including azathioprine or cyclophosphamide.

Giant cell arteritis

Giant cell arteritis (GCA), also widely known as temporal arteritis, is the most common primary vasculitis in those aged over 50 years. Typically, the extracranial branches of the aorta and the aorta itself are involved; intracranial disease is less common because these vessels lack the internal elastic lamina that harbours the inflammatory response.

Headache is the most common symptom, but can be absent. Other symptoms, caused by involvement of extracranial arteries, include jaw claudication and scalp tenderness (**Box 27.3**). Constitutional symptoms are present in at least one-third of cases (weight loss, fever and myalgia). Blindness is the most common serious neurological sequel and either causes a monocular or homonymous deficit. The former is caused by arteritic involvement of the posterior ciliary arteries, leading to optic nerve head infarction which may be partial typically causing altitudinal field defects. Sequential ischaemic optic neuropathies or bilateral occipital infarction can lead to permanent blindness.

Sometimes, the arteritis is clinically apparent to palpation of the temporal artery or other extracranial branches of the external carotid artery, such as the facial artery as it runs under the mandible, or the occipital arteries as they pass over the inion.

Box 27.3 Features of giant cell arteritis

- Patients nearly always aged 50 years or more
- Headache in 80–90%
- Systemic upsets – fever, malaise, fatigue, weight loss, scalp ulceration
- Overlap with polymyalgia rheumatica in 40% – girdle muscle aching and weakness
- Pain on chewing – jaw claudication in approximately 40%
- Visual loss in ~20% – total loss or altitudinal defect: amaurosis fugax may precede this in 45%. If one eye is blind, there is a very high risk that the second eye will be affected – so do not delay steroid treatment!
- Neurological manifestations in ~30% – peripheral and cranial nerves, transient ischaemic attacks, ischaemic stroke (posterior circulation)
- Elevated ESR 50 mm/hour or more – often near 100 mm. CRP is a more sensitive index. Liver function tests abnormal in ~30%
- Temporal artery biopsy may be diagnostic – but may have 'skip' areas
- Treatment with steroids produces rapid symptom relief if the diagnosis is correct – typically with 40–60 mg/day prednisolone

CRP, C-reactive protein; ESR, elevated sedimentation rate.

Affected arteries feel thickened, pulseless and cord-like, and may be tender. The ESR is almost always raised as is the CRP; anaemia is present in two-thirds of cases with a leukocytosis and raised transaminases in one-third. Temporal artery biopsy is the most specific finding, but often a diagnosis will have to be made without this confirmation, as 'skip lesions' occur.

It cannot be overemphasized that treatment of GCA is a neurological emergency. High-dose prednisolone (initially 60 mg daily) should be given as soon as the diagnosis is suspected. Institution of this treatment takes precedence over temporal artery biopsy. Failure to give prompt treatment can result in unilateral or bilateral permanent loss of vision. It should be recalled that biopsy of an affected artery will show arteritic changes for up to 72 hours following initiation of corticosteroid treatment. When clinical suspicion of the diagnosis is high, corticosteroid treatment should never be delayed.

Patients started on corticosteroid are not completely protected from ischaemic events; it is sensible to also give low-dose aspirin to patients with GCA.

SARCOIDOSIS

Sarcoidosis is a multisystem granulomatous disorder of unknown aetiology that affects the nervous system in about 5 per cent of patients. Its pathological hallmark is non-caseating epitheloid cell granulomas with associated infiltration of the affected tissues by T-lymphocytes and other mononuclear cells associated with macrophage aggregation. The last form either epithelioid or multinucleated giant cells. Later lesions may go on to develop fibrosis and irreversible tissue damage. The incidence varies between 1 and 40/100 000 and the disease usually presents in younger patients. In the United States, there is a nearly three-fold increased incidence in the black population. Over 90 per cent show respiratory system involvement, most commonly enlargement of the hilar lymph glands. If there is bihilar lymphadenopathy, the diagnosis may be confirmed by bronchoscopy, broncho-alveolar lavage or tissue biopsy. Some 20–50 per cent present with Löfgren's syndrome – erythema nodosum, hilar lymphadenopathy and polyarthralgia. Some 25 per cent have skin involvement (erythema nodosum, skin nodules, lupus pernio), approximately 25 per cent eye involvement (uveitis, conjunctival nodules), approximately 40–70 per cent show liver granulomas, and approximately 5–10 per cent cardiac involvement. The salivary and lacrimal glands may be involved. Systemic symptoms may include fatigue, anorexia, weight loss and fever. As a result of the many manifestations of the disease, the clinical presentation may be protean (Box 27.4).

Nervous system involvement in sarcoidosis

The neurological effects of sarcoidosis are listed in Box 27.4. It can be seen that although there are some characteristic presentations (e.g. cranial neuropathies, meningeal or parenchymal involvement), many manifestations are non-specific. This, together with the lack of reliable non-invasive tests, makes this one of the most challenging neurological disorders in which to establish a definite diagnosis. Neurological involvement is uncommon but carries a worse prognosis than pulmonary disease, and is associated with ocular and cardiac involvement. In approximately 15 per cent of patients with neurosarcoidosis, the presenting features of the disease

are neurological, but in the remainder presentation is systemic and neurological involvement develops within two years of presentation.

Chronic neurosarcoidosis includes multiple cranial nerve palsies, parenchymatous cerebral involvement, hydrocephalus and encephalopathy, and peripheral nervous system and muscle manifestations.

Cranial neuropathy

The most common neurological manifestation is isolated cranial neuropathy. Up to 75 per cent of neurosarcoid patients present with an isolated or bilateral facial palsy. This may be associated with dysgeusia, indicating a proximal lesion affecting the chorda tympani. Deafness from VIIIth nerve involvement occurs in 10–20 per cent of cases; bilateral, often consecutive, involvement strongly suggests neurosarcoidosis. Optic neuropathy occurs in up to 40 per cent of patients and is often subacute, presenting with a progressive visual field defect, impaired acuity and pupillary dysfunction. Examination may show anterior uveitis, papillitis, papilloedema or optic atrophy secondary to granulomatous infiltration or compression of the optic nerve. Oculomotor abnormalities or bulbar weakness may occur as a result of diffuse meningeal infiltration. Basal meningeal infiltration is common and may lead to hydrocephalus in 6–30 per cent of patients with neurosarcoidosis, which may be either obstructive or communicating. CSF diversion procedures may be necessary but tend to fail.

Meningeal and parenchymatous sarcoid

Meningeal involvement commonly presents as an aseptic meningitis or occasionally as a meningeal mass lesion. The CSF shows a mononuclear pleocytosis with an elevated protein and a reduced glucose level. Parenchymal lesions are unusual. Clinical manifestations depend on their location and size. They can mimic tumours or demyelination, cause raised intracranial pressure with headache and papilloedema, seizures or focal involvement of the brainstem, basal ganglia or cerebellum. Isolated spinal lesions may present as a progressive myelopathy with paraparesis, hemiparesis and sphincter dysfunction. Pituitary and hypothalamic involvement occurs and can result in neuroendocrine disorders, including diabetes insipidus, panhypopituitarism and hyperprolactinaemia.

Box 27.4 Some characteristic neurological features of sarcoidosis

- Cranial nerve palsies (50%) – often bilateral including cranial nerves VII, V, VIII, IX and X
- Involvement of the optic nerves and chiasm
- Peripheral nerves – most often a mononeuritis multiplex, less commonly a symmetrical polyneuropathy
- Aseptic meningitis
- Myelopathy with intramedullary granuloma
- Hydrocephalus
- Pituitary dysfunction or hypothalamic disturbance (diabetes insipidus)
- Seizures
- Neuropsychiatric deficits
- Intracranial mass lesions (granulomas)
- Proximal myopathy

Sarcoid encephalopathy

A diffuse or relapsing sarcoid encephalopathy presents with cognitive impairment or a confusional state often associated with memory disturbance. T2-weighted MRI shows diffuse contrast enhancement of the meninges with increased signal. Encephalopathy may coexist with a diffuse vasculopathy characterized by arteritis, external compression of arteries by an inflammatory mass lesion or multiple cardiac emboli. Rarely, dural venous thrombosis occurs. Neuropsychiatric features are also well described, patients presenting with psychosis or bipolar affective disorder. There may occasionally be an isolated progressive amnesia or dementia without evidence of other neurological or systemic involvement. These patients appear to respond well to corticosteroids.

Peripheral neuromuscular sarcoidosis

Peripheral neuromuscular involvement occurs in some 20 per cent of patients with neurosarcoidosis. Peripheral nerve involvement may be either an isolated mononeuritis, or a mononeuritis multiplex caused by granulomatous vasculitis or compression from granulomas. A symmetrical chronic axonal neuropathy occurs in approximately 25 per cent of patients with neurosarcoidosis. This is usually a mild mixed sensorimotor pattern, but a more acute form indistinguishable from Guillain–Barré syndrome with demyelinating features can also develop. Muscle involvement is common, but usually asymptomatic with non-caseating granulomas found on biopsy in more than 25 per cent of patients. Symptomatic involvement varies from acute to chronic myopathy with an inflammatory component and occasionally palpable intramuscular nodules.

The presence of elevated serum angiotensin-converting enzyme (SACE) and characteristic imaging appearances may help, but these have limited specificity. CSF ACE may be elevated. Gallium scans may show characteristic increased uptake in parotid salivary glands. However, in the absence of tissue evidence of non-caseating granulomas the diagnosis can be extremely difficult to make and is often one of exclusion. Acute presentations are associated with a better prognosis. Poorer prognostic features include a later age of onset, Afro-Caribbean extraction, the presence of lupus pernio, chronic uveitis, chronic hypercalcaemia, progres-sive pulmonary pathology, nasal mucosal disease and cardiac involvement.

Diagnosis

Diagnosis can be challenging and whenever possible, a tissue diagnosis should be sought. This is most often from lymph glands, the skin, liver or muscle. Biopsy of cerebral lesions and the meninges is occasionally necessary. Chest x-ray may show enlarged hilar glands and pulmonary infiltrates. Respiratory function tests may show restricted lung volumes and abnormal gas exchange. Blood tests may confirm an inflammatory process with an elevated ESR and CRP. The serum calcium may be raised and liver function tests may be abnormal. A raised serum angiotensin-converting enzyme level is found in up to 70–80 per cent of patients, but this is not specific. MRI brain may show parenchymatous mass lesions – hyperintense lesions on T2 sequences, with linear enhancement of thickened meninges and focal nodular enhancement. CSF findings are non-specific, but may be helpful if there is meningeal involvement. There may be a pleocytosis of up to 100 cells/mm^2, and elevated protein. Glucose is occasionally reduced in active aseptic meningitis, CSF pressure is increased and oligoclonal bands are variably present.

Prognosis

The prognosis is variable and difficult to predict in individual patients. However, neurosarcoidosis is a often a serious disease. In some patients with mild involvement, there may be relapses and remissions with good recovery. Involvement of the peripheral nervous system tends to carry a better prognosis than central involvement. One-third of patients with neurosarcoidosis have progressive disease despite immunosuppression with steroids and other agents.

Extensive nervous system involvement also indicates a poor outcome.

Corticosteroids are the mainstay of treatment, with dose and duration determined by the disease location, severity and response. Treatment aims to reduce the inflammatory component and prevent progression to fibrosis and ischaemia. Steroids should be built up rapidly to high doses (usually with a short course of intravenous methylprednisolone), with reduction of the dose only after a good clinical response has been established. Occasionally, it is possible to withdraw steroids completely, but many patients require long-term steroids and some require additional immunosuppressive agents, including azathioprine, methotrexate, ciclosporin or mycophenolate.

BEHÇET'S DISEASE

Behçet's disease (BD), first described by the Turkish dermatologist Professor Hulusi Behçet (1889–1948), is a multisystem disease comprising recurrent orogenital ulceration, skin lesions and ocular lesions (including uveitis) and a positive pathergy test. The diagnostic criteria are shown in Table 27.10. BD usually presents in the third decade and is seen most commonly in regions along the Silk Route, extending from the Eastern Mediterranean to Japan; the prevalence in Turkey and Japan is 20 times higher than in the UK. Men are more commonly affected than women.

Neurological involvement occurs in two distinct patterns which rarely overlap: parenchymal CNS lesions, most commonly (but not exclusively) affecting the brainstem; and cortical venous sinus thrombosis (CVST). Pathologically, there is perivascular and meningeal infiltration with lymphocytes, plasma cells and macrophages, with multiple foci of softening and necrosis in the white and grey matter often found in relation to blood vessels. Skin lesions are also common with erythema nodosum and a tendency to furunculosis.

The typical patterns of nervous system involvement in BD are listed in Table 27.10 and briefly discussed below.

Patterns of nervous system involvement

Of patients with BD and neurological involvement, about 80 per cent present with parenchymal disease, while the remaining 20 per cent have CVST. Headache is the most common neurological symptom in BD, even given its high prevalence in the general population, but is clearly not specific enough to be of diagnostic value on its own; both migraine and tension-type patterns are seen. New or severe headache in patients with known BD should have prompt imaging to exclude CVST or parenchymal lesions.

CNS involvement: parenchymal

Parechymal involvement in BD is usually multifocal, with complex symptoms and signs. The most common pattern is a subacute brainstem syndrome that may be associated with lesions elsewhere in the CNS or, more rarely, cranial neuropathies (V, VII or VIII). Corticospinal tract and hemispheric presentations are also common. Cerebellar signs and a progressive course can occur, and carry a poor prognosis. Symptoms not easily localizable are also seen (impaired consciousness, epilepsy, neuropsychiatric BD). Isolated optic neuropathy is rare (>1 per cent), as are peripheral neuropathies. Whether neurological manifestations can occur without any of the systemic features is doubtful; patients who present with neurological symptoms generally have a history of recurrent oral ulcers at least. Neurological BD may cause diagnostic confusion with multiple sclerosis, but optic neuritis is

Table 27.10 Diagnostic criteria for Behçet's disease

Major diagnostic criteria	Minor diagnostic criteria
Oral ulcers recurring at least three times per year (essential for the diagnosis)	Arthritis or arthralgia
Genital ulcers or scars	Deep venous thromboses
Eye involvement	Subcutaneous thrombophlebitis
Skin lesions (erythema nodosum, folliculitis, acneiform lesions)	Epididymitis
Pathergy skin test observed by a physician	Family history
	Gastrointestinal, central nervous system, or vascular involvement
Oral ulcers and two other major criteria are required for the diagnosis.	

much rarer and headaches much more common in BD than in MS.

Cerebral venous sinus thrombosis

CVST is discussed in Chapter 23. The management in BD is similar: anticoagulation (low molecular weight heparin, then warfarin for at least several months), although the optimum duration is uncertain. In BD, pulmonary artery aneurysms can develop, which should be sought by CT pulmonary angiography, before starting anticoagulation therapy; they can be treated with immunosuppression, endovascular intervention or surgery.

Diagnosis

The CSF shows a lymphocytic pleocytosis, with a raised opening pressure in 20 per cent of patients. The protein level may be elevated and oligoclonal bands may be present in a minority. However, in some 30 per cent, the CSF may be normal. The opening pressure is increased if there is venous sinus thrombosis. The pathergy test (the formation of a sterile pustule at the site of a needle puncture) has been suggested as a diagnostic observation, but has variable sensitivity. MRI in the acute stage may show lesions that appear iso- or hypointense on T1 images and hyperintense on T2 and FLAIR, due to venous thrombosis with reversible oedema. Lesions, which can be single or multiple, are seen most commonly at the mesodiencephalic junction, in the cerebellar peduncle, basal ganglia and brainstem, but can also occur in the optic nerves and hemispheres. In chronic disease, brainstem atrophy with gliosis can develop.

Treatment

Treatment in acute neurological relapses, particularly where there has been multifocal CNS involvement, is usually with pulsed corticosteroids and then oral immunosuppressive drugs, usually ciclosporin. However, these have only limited success. Major CVST is be treated with anticoagulation, often combined with steroids. Azathioprine, methotrexate or pulsed cyclophosphamide, with or without added prednisolone may be used for relapsing or progressive neurological disease. Newer immunomodulatory therapies, such as tacrolimus, infliximab and anti-TNF-alpha, have been advocated. Thalidomide and colchicine are widely used for the mucocutaneous manifestations. Neurovascular

disease (stroke) is managed conventionally, usually with antiplatelet agents.

NEUROLOGY AND PREGNANCY

The physiological changes in hormone levels in pregnancy can either change the presentation or severity of pre-existing neurological diseases, including migraine, epilepsy, multiple sclerosis and myasthenia gravis; or they may be associated with a conditions arising *de novo* during pregnancy, in particular cerebrovascular disorders. The management of epilepsy in women of child-bearing age is of particular importance and is dealt with in some detail here.

Epilepsy and women of child-bearing age

This topic is considered in Chapter 13.

Cerebrovascular disorders in pregnancy

Ischaemic stroke, cerebral venous sinus thrombosis, and cerebral haemorrhage are considered in Chapter 23.

Pre-eclampsia

Pre-eclampsia is defined by pregnancy-associated proteinuria and hypertension, with evidence of multisystem involvement: renal, hepatic and neurological. The neurological manifestations include seizures (usually generalized), visual disturbances and reduced conscious level. These symptoms arising in pregnancy always require urgent investigation, to exclude venous sinus thrombosis, intracranial haemorrhage or other vascular causes.

Once pre-eclampsia is confirmed, urgent treatment of hypertension and of seizures (with intravenous magnesium and sometimes conventional anticonvulsant drugs) is needed.

Specific neurovascular syndromes associated with pregnancy include the reversible cerebral vasoconstriction syndromes. These have a multitude of names, including **posterior reversible leukoen-**

cephalopathy syndrome (PRES) and **cerebral vaso-constriction syndrome (Call–Fleming syndrome)**. They have a shared mechanism, with abnormality of vascular tone (reversible multifocal segmental vasoconstriction) and imaging abnormalities, sometimes with stroke (infarction or haemorrhage).

Posterior reversible encephalopathy syndrome

This characteristically occurs in the first postpartum week, and may present with seizures, uncontrolled hypertension and visual symptoms. The pathophysiology is thought to be disruption of the blood–brain barrier, perhaps because perfusion exceeds the autoregulation threshold. The predilection for the posterior circulation is suggested to result from a reduced sympathetic innervation compared to the anterior circulation. The symptoms can mimic those of cerebral venous sinus thrombosis and eclampsia, and imaging, preferably with MRI, is essential to make an accurate diagnosis. Urgent treatment is required for the hypertension and seizures, and good recovery is the rule if treatment is started promptly. It has been suggested that the term PRES be abandoned because the condition is not only posterior in location, not always reversible and not always associated with encephalopathy.

Call–Fleming syndrome

This is also commonly observed in the postpartum period and presents with a thunderclap headache, followed by focal neurological deficit. Definitive diagnosis requires the demonstration of vasospasm on angiographic imaging. Areas of ischaemic change may be seen on MRI as infarction may result from vasospasm. There is clearly clinicoradiological overlap, and lack of firm diagnostic criteria for differentiation of PRES and Call–Fleming syndrome, emphasizing a need for further understanding of the pathophysiology and clarification of these diagnostic terms.

Pregnancy and other neurological diseases

Pituitary disorders

Pregnancy causes the pituitary gland to enlarge. **Sheehan syndrome** is a rare condition of pituitary infarction, usually caused by postpartum

hemorrhage and systemic hypotension, or by the vascular demands of an enlarging pituitary gland exceeding the available vascular supply. Infarction may transform into haemorrhage. Infarction or haemorrhage can result in acute pituitary insufficiency and shock, hence the term **pituitary apoplexy**. Lymphocytic hypophysitis is thought to be of autoimmune origin and is usually self-limiting. Treatment with corticosteroids is indicated if there is visual impairment due to chiasmal compression.

Headache and pregnancy

Migraine is reported to improve in four out of five cases during pregnancy, probably due to altered oestrogen levels. However, because migraine is so common, there are still a large number of women with persistent or worsening migraine requiring treatment during pregnancy. Headache arising for the first time in pregnancy is of greater concern and may require further investigation. If migraines are frequent and disabling, then propranolol can be safely used in pregnancy. Paracetamol is the safest acute treatment for migraine in pregnancy. Ergotamine is contraindicated; there is insufficient information on the safety of triptans to recommend them in pregnancy. Overall, however, the most common type of headache in pregnancy is tension-type headache.

Neuromuscular disorders

Bell's palsy is several times more common during pregnancy and the puerperium than at other times. **Carpal tunnel syndrome** affects about one-fifth of patients in the third trimester and is likely to resolve after delivery. **Meralgia paraesthetica** can occur late in pregnancy because of stretch of the lateral cutaneous nerve of the thigh, and usually resolves gradually following delivery. **Gestational polyneuropathy** may be related to nutritional deficiency because of general malnourishment or hyperemesis gravidarum. In extreme cases, the latter can also cause **Wernicke's encephalopathy**. **Damage to the nerves of the lumbosacral plexus** is a rare complication of delivery, particularly if there are complicating factors including cephalopelvic disproportion, shoulder dystocia or instrumentation with forceps. **Restless leg syndrome** affects up to 30 per cent of women during the third trimester. There is evidence that oral folic acid reduces the frequency of symptoms. Pregnancy has no consistent effect on the natural history of myasthenia gravis. Neurological complications of epidural anaesthesia are rare.

Multiple sclerosis

Multiple sclerosis in pregnancy is considered in Chapter 22.

Chorea gravidarum

The term **chorea gravidarum (CG) (chorea in pregnancy)** describes a clinical syndrome, but does not imply a specific cause. About one-third of patients who develop CG have a history of rheumatic fever or Syndenham's chorea. It is speculated that CG results from the reactivation of previous subclinical basal ganglia damage, the mechanism involving ischaemia or increased dopamine sensitivity, mediated by elevated hormone levels during pregnancy. CG may be secondary to other known causes of chorea, including Syndenham's chorea, SLE or Huntington's disease. CG seldom requires drug treatment. If CG is mild, the patient may even be unaware of the involuntary movements. Drug treatment is only used if the severity of the chorea puts the mother or fetus in danger, from poor nutrition, disturbed sleep or injury. If treatment is necessary, dopamine blockers including haloperidol are used.

Tumours

Overall, CNS tumours are no more common in pregnant than non-pregnant women of similar age. However, **meningiomas** present more often than expected by chance during the second half of pregnancy as they may enlarge because of the effects of changes in circulating oestrogen levels on tumour oestrogen receptors. The symptoms of meningiomas may improve spontaneously postpartum, so that treatment can often be delayed until after delivery. However, surgery for large or aggressive brain tumours during pregnancy may be needed urgently if there are signs of raised intracranial pressure or papilloedema. Most women with brain tumours presenting in pregnancy are managed by caesarean section to avoid the risk of cerebral herniation during labour.

Choriocarcinoma occurs in pregnancy and often metastasizes to the brain. **Pituitary adenomas** are slightly more common in pregnancy and large tumours may be associated with the onset of visual failure. Careful visual field assessment is therefore mandatory in any woman presenting with new headache during pregnancy.

Idiopathic intracranial hypertension

Idiopathic intracranial hypertension (benign intracranial hypertension (BIH) occurs more commonly during pregnancy, often presenting in the second trimester. If already present, it usually deteriorates in pregnancy. Treatment is guided by close monitoring of visual function and serial measurement of CSF pressure. Weight control (a challenge in pregnancy) is recommended. A short course of corticosteroids may be considered, together with serial lumbar puncture to lower pressure. More invasive procedures, including lumboperitoneal shunting or optic nerve fenestration, are occasionally needed if vision is seriously threatened. The teratogenic potential of acetazomlamide is unknown, but the drug should probably be avoided in the first trimester.

TOXIC AND PHYSICAL INSULTS TO THE NERVOUS SYSTEM

Alcohol and the nervous system

Most doctors are familiar with some of the effects of alcohol, particularly acute self-poisoning. Alcohol is a CNS depressant, explaining the clinical features of **acute intoxication**. Alcohol is absorbed rapidly, reaching a maximum blood concentration 30–90 minutes after ingestion. At 50 mg/100 mL, there may be mild incoordination and impaired learning and by 100 mg/100 mL slurring dysarthria and obvious clumsiness. With higher concentrations, there is depression of the conscious level, resulting in coma (often 300–400 mg/100 mL). This can be fatal. There will be an accompanying peripheral vasodilation and tachycardia.

Chronic habituation and abstinence syndromes

Subjects habituated to alcohol will develop **acute withdrawal** symptoms if their intake stops suddenly, and are at risk of developing **delirium tremens (DT)**. Cessation may be precipitated by injury, acute infection or surgical emergency leading to admission to hospital, with the loss of a regular intake. The first stage ('the shakes') consists of irritability, restlessness and tremor, with an exaggerated startle response. Patients appear overactive, are inattentive, have a tachycardia and are sometimes febrile. Such symptoms commonly start the morning after alcohol cessation and last 24–48 hours. They may be relieved by drinking further alcohol. The next stage includes confusion and auditory and visual hallucinations accompanied by considerable amnesia.

So-called **alcoholic blackouts** consist of gaps in memory, often lasting hours, for which the patient later has no recall, but during which may show some automatic behaviour. Mild hallucinatory states may be described as 'bad dreams'.

Alcohol withdrawal seizures ('rum fits'), occur 8–48 hours after cessation of drinking, most often after 12–24 hours. The seizures are usually generalized tonic-clonic attacks, either single or a cluster in series. Such seizures occur after single episodes of binge drinking, as well as in chronic alcoholics.

In the final stage of withdrawal, **delirium tremens**, there are vivid hallucinations, often frightening (seeing animals or insects), marked confusion, anxiety and overactivity, leading to insomnia. DTs usually start 2–4 days after stopping drinking, and usually last 2–3 days, but occasionally may last much longer. Treatment of DTs includes adequate sedation, rehydration and usually parenteral feeding with glucose solutions and thiamine given intravenously. Any concomitant infection or injury should be treated appropriately. Sedatives used include benzodiazepines, such as lorazepam, chlordiazepoxide or diazepam. Paraldehyde is effective treatment to sedate and control seizures, but is now rarely used.

Alcoholic permanent damage

Alcohol may produce damage to the nervous system by its direct toxic effects.
This can include:

- **Peripheral neuropathy** (see also Chapter 16)
- **Cerebellar degeneration** (see also Chapter 21)
- **Cerebral degeneration with dementia** (see also Chapter 19)
- **Myopathy and cardiomyopathy**

Other disturbances include **central pontine myelinolysis** (see above under Central pontine myelinolysis) and **Marchiafava–Bignami disease** (primary degeneration of the corpus callosum). Alcohol may also precipitate the **Wernicke–Korsakoff syndrome** (see above under Vitamin B1 deficiency).

Cerebellar degeneration

In cerebellar degeneration, there is gradual loss of cerebellar neurones, leading to atrophy, particularly involving the cerebellar vermis. This presents with ataxia, affecting the gait more than the limbs (midline ataxia) and dysarthria, which may be difficult to differentiate from the effects of acute intoxication, although persistence of these signs after 'drying out' signifies the presence of permanent damage. CT or magnetic resonance scanning reveals cerebellar atrophy, most marked in the vermis.

Cerebral degeneration and alchohol-related dementia

Long-standing chronic alcoholics frequently develop a degree of a diffuse global dementia, which is sometimes severe. Imaging with CT or MRI demonstrates cerebral atrophy, with ventricular dilatation and cortical atrophy. However, there is a poor correlation of the imaging findings with the presence and severity degree of dementia. In chronic alcoholic patients with dementia, particularly those aged over 45 years, abstinence may not lead to improvement of cognitive function.

The management of alcohol dependence is discussed in Chapter 31.

Toxic effects of drugs

Many drugs may affect the nervous system. Drug toxicity includes the unwanted (adverse) effects of those used in therapy, for example, a **peripheral neuropathy** (Box 27.5) or **myopathy** (Box 27.6); or those resulting from self-poisoning, for example, a depressed conscious level leading to coma as a result of overdosing with **tranquillizers or antidepressants**. These effects are dose-dependent. The effects of habituation to opiates and other powerful analgesics are described below.

Habituation to barbiturates and other sedatives, such as **benzodiazepines**, produces physical and mental slowing, apathy, slurred speech, clumsiness and ataxia, the symptoms and signs mimicking acute alcohol intoxication. These features may be accompanied by emotional lability and personal neglect. Such signs may fluctuate greatly.

Withdrawal states from such habituation may lead to restlessness, tremor, insomnia, agitation and

Box 27.5 Drug causes of neuropathy

- Alcohol
- Amiodarone
- Amitriptyline
- Chloroquine
- Cimetidine
- Cisplatin
- Dapsone[a]
- Didanosine (ddi)
- Disulfiram[a]
- Ethambutol
- Gold salts
- Griseofulvin
- Hydralazine[a]
- Indometacin
- Isoniazid[a]
- Lithium
- Metronidazole[a]
- Nitrofurantoin[a]
- Phenytoin[a]
- Propafenone
- Stavudine (d4t)
- Sulfasalazine
- Sulphonamides
- Taxanes
- Thalidomide
- Tricyclic antidepressants
- Tryptophan
- Vinca alkaloids[a]

[a]Common causes.

Box 27.6 Drug causes of myopathy

- Alcohol
- Amiodarone
- Amphetamines
- Beta-blockers
- Chloroquine[a]
- Cimetidine
- Cocaine
- Ciclosporin
- Emetine
- Fibric acid derivatives (bezafibrate, ciprofibrate, fenofibrate, gemfibrozil)
- Heroin
- HMG-coa reductase inhibitors (atorvastatin, fluvastatin, pravastatin, simvastatin)
- Hydralazine
- Isoniazid
- Isotretinoin
- Lithium
- Methadone
- D-penicillamine
- Procainamide
- Rifampicin
- Salbutamol
- Steroids[a]
- Thyroxine
- Tryptophan
- Vincristine
- Zidovudine (AZT)[a]

[a]Common causes.

occasionally, withdrawal seizures. Habituation may also occur to **analgesics**, and many chronic headache sufferers may experience a further headache unless another analgesic dose is given (medication misuse headaches, see Chapter 10).

Phenothiazines and butyrophenones, used particularly in the long-term treatment of schizophrenia, including depot injections of long-acting preparations, may lead to the development of extrapyramidal symptoms and signs (see Chapter 20). These are predominantly parkinsonian in type, with rigidity, slowed movements and a shuffling gait. Such symptoms may be reduced by the use of anticholinergic drugs, such as benzhexol. Phenothiazines and butyrophenones also commonly provoke involuntary movements, dyskinesias, dystonic postures and restlessness (akathisia). Many

of these symptoms reverse with cessation of therapy (although this is not always feasible) and the use of anticholinergics. Tardive dyskinesias, particularly affecting the muscles of the face, mouth, neck and trunk, may prove very resistant to treatment.

The **malignant neuroleptic syndrome (MNS)** (see Chapter 20) is a rare complication of treatment with neuroleptic drugs, most commonly provoked by haloperidol and depot injections of fluphenazines. In this condition, rigidity and akinesia develop relatively acutely accompanied by fever, autonomic disturbances, instability of the blood pressure and a depressed conscious level. It is associated with a massive rise in the serum creatine kinase level, a raised white count and often abnormal liver function. Treatment with bromocriptine and dantrolene sodium is effective, combined with withdrawal of the offending drug, but MNS is associated with significant mortality.

Drug misuse

The effects of some neurological toxins are listed in Table 27.11.

Narcotics

Alkaloid derivatives of opium, either natural opiates or synthetic analogues, act at opiate receptors concentrated in the limbic system, periaqueductal grey matter and spinal sensory pathways. These modulate central pain perception and its transmission, affording pain relief.

Diamorphine (heroin) and morphine

Diamorphine and morphine are very potent analgesics, which, in high dose, can cause euphoria, miosis, constipation, cough suppression, orthostatic hypotension and increasing cardiorespiratory depression, resulting in coma. Pulmonary oedema may develop. In acute poisoning, patients

Table 27.11 Effects of some neurological toxins

Amphetamines	Insomnia, hypertension, tremor, haemorrhagic stroke
Opiates (heroin, morphine)	Cerebral infarction, rhabdomyolysis (SBE, HIV infection – dangers of i.v. use)
Cocaine	Hyperpyrexia, haemorrhagic stroke, vasculitis
Organic solvents	Acute encephalopathy
	Chronic – dementia, ataxia, pyramidal signs, optic atrophy, deafness
Acrylamide	Neuropathy
Trichlorethylene	Trigeminal sensory neuropathy
Heavy metals	
Lead	Encephalopathy, motor neuropathy
Cisplatin	Sensory neuropathy, deafness
Gold	Peripheral neuropathy
Organophosphates	Peripheral neuropathy

SBE, subacute bacterial endocarditis.

are likely to require ventilatory support and intravenous naloxone. More chronic use results in drug dependence and tolerance. Drug withdrawal results in cravings, anxiety, profuse sweating, lacrimation, rhinorrhoea, dilated pupils, goose flesh, tachycardia, abdominal cramps and limb pains, diarrhoea and vomiting, restlessness and twitching. Such symptoms can last 7–10 days. Chronic users are more liable to develop strokes, a vasculitis, infections (including HIV), myelopathies, leukoencephalopathies, pressure palsies and epileptic seizures.

Cocaine

Cocaine is an alkaloid derived from coca leaves that was introduced medicinally as a local anaesthetic. It is also a stimulant. It may be taken intranasally, or by intramuscular or intravenous injection. The smoking of the free alkaloid base **'crack' cocaine** results in very rapid penetration into the nervous system with a resulting 'high'. Cocaine produces a rapid euphoria with sympathetic features including tachycardia, hypertension and pupillary dilatation, which may be followed by a 'down' phase accompanied by craving. Long-term cocaine abuse may cause hallucinations and paranoia.

Cocaine use carries an increased risk of vascular complications – hypertension, subarachnoid haemorrhage, haemorrhagic and ischaemic stroke. Young patients with stroke should always have blood and urine toxicology for recreational drugs, including cocaine. There is also risk of infections and occasional rhabdomyolysis. Epileptic seizures are particularly common. Severe cerebellar damage has been reported in some patients smoking 'crack' cocaine.

Amphetamines

Amphetamines are stimulants and have been used therapeutically in narcolepsy and related conditions, and in former years, to suppress appetite. In excess, they produce a sympathomimetic syndrome with delusions, paranoia, sometimes mania, hyper-reflexia, seizures, tremors and occasionally chorea. Prolonged use may cause hypertension. Amphetamines may also provoke strokes, both from intracerebral and subarachnoid haemorrhage and from cerebral vasculitis. Ecstasy is a substituted amphetamine, 3,4-methylenedioxyamphetamine, which may cause depletion of serotonin (5-HT) and also affect dopaminergic neurones, producing a combination of a serotonin syndrome (myoclonus, agitation, hyper-reflexia, incoordination) with some features of the malignant neuroleptic syndrome (see above).

Heavy metals and organophosphates

Heavy metals have a strong propensity to damage the nervous system. They are used therapeutically, for example **gold** injections in rheumatoid arthritis, which may cause a thrombocytopenia and bleeding resulting in peripheral and central nervous system damage. **Cisplatin** used in cancer treatment can cause deafness and a peripheral neuropathy (Table 27.11).

Lead poisoning is now uncommon since its removal from paint and modern water pipes. Previously, children were more commonly affected, presenting with irritability, confusion, clumsiness and seizures from a relatively acute encephalopathy causing a deteriorating conscious level and a grossly swollen brain. There was often anorexia, vomiting and abdominal pain. In adults, a peripheral neuropathy, predominantly motor with a bilateral wrist drop, was the common presentation. This was often associated with anaemia and abdominal pain. Plasma lead levels will be raised, usually greater than 50–70 mg/dL. There will be an associated anaemia with basophilic stippling of red cells and 'lead lines' may be present on the x-rays of long bones in children.

Treatment is with chelating agents.

Other metals are also toxic: **manganese** poisoning may produce an encephalopathy and extrapyramidal signs. **Mercury** poisoning produces tremor, confusion and cerebellar disturbance.

Organophosphates, used as insecticides, in certain mineral oils and in sheep dip, are also highly toxic. They produce a peripheral neuropathy with axonal degeneration. Acute poisoning will produce headache, vomiting, pinpoint pupils, profuse sweating and abdominal cramps (anticholinesterase effects), which can be relieved by atropine.

Physical insults

Anoxia

The brain requires a rich oxygen supply. If the circulation is arrested, within 2–3 minutes normal function fails. Consciousness is lost more rapidly, so that in asystolic cardiac arrest, consciousness is lost within 15 seconds. Over the ensuing 5 seconds there may be twitching, rigidity or clonic jerks which may be mistaken for an epileptic seizure. Within 4–5 minutes of circulatory arrest, cyanosis appears, the pupils dilate and become unreactive, the plantar responses become extensor and the breathing appears stertorous. Providing oxygenation and the circulation are restored to the brain within 5 minutes, recovery usually occurs: beyond this short time, irreversible damage may follow. A respiratory arrest or an obstructed airway may produce acute respiratory failure, but more often the picture is a combination of hypoxia and ischaemia with concomitant circulatory failure. The causes include heart attacks with ventricular arrest or fibrillation, acute respiratory failure, for example in drowning or asthmatic crises, severe trauma and anaesthetic mishaps. A fall in cerebral perfusion may occur during operations, particularly on the open heart, or where there is massive blood loss leading to shock.

More gradually progressive chronic hypoxia may arise from ventilatory muscle weakness, as in Guillain–Barré syndrome, certain myopathies and obstructive airways disease or pulmonary fibrosis. With a slower onset, hypoxic symptoms include restlessness, agitation, tremors, headache, clumsiness and confusion (see also Chapter 29).

Post-anoxic brain damage

Survivors of anoxic brain damage show a variable picture, with depressed conscious level often with some preservation of brainstem reflexes, but commonly twitching or myoclonic jerking of the limbs, sometimes repeated seizures, decerebrate or decorticate postures and extensor plantar responses. A variety of deficits may persist in less severely damaged survivors. These include cognitive and behavioural disturbances, extrapyramidal and pyramidal signs, visual field defects, involuntary movements, ataxia and action myoclonus.

Electric shock

Electric shock may cause immediate death, from cardiac arrest. Commonly, at the site of contact, whether from an electric cable or lightning, there will be extensive burns with tissue destruction. The nervous system can be damaged directly, for example a shock to the head producing a hemiplegia, or the damage may involve the spinal cord or peripheral nerves. In survivors of acute shocks, a delayed myelopathy can develop, with slowly progressive damage leading to muscular atrophy, or the clinical picture of a transverse myelopathy. Instances of motor neurone disease have been described following electric shocks

Hypothermia

Prolonged exposure to cold can cause damage, although under experimental conditions, very low body temperatures are necessary to produce a conduction block in peripheral nerves. Core body temperatures of less than 35°C, which may follow cold exposure, particularly in the elderly, or in patients with hypothyroidism, or after drug overdoses, may lead to impaired cerebral function – confusion, stupor and coma. Breathing becomes shallow and the respiratory rate is slowed, together with an overall slowing of metabolic rate. Treatment is by gradual rewarming, but there is an appreciable mortality, largely accounted for by cardiac arrhythmias and persistent metabolic disturbances.

Heat stroke

Heat stroke most often follows vigorous exercise in very hot temperatures. It may be aggravated by impaired sweating, as in patients with Parkinson's disease taking anticholinergic drugs, or in patients with tetanus and autonomic disturbance. As the body temperature rises (rectal temperature of more than 41°C), agitation and confusion may appear, followed by a deteriorating conscious level. Convulsions occur, and the development of status epilepticus may itself lead to hyperpyrexia, producing further brain damage. Death is usually caused by circulatory collapse and renal failure. Survivors may be left with cognitive deficits, spastic weakness and a sometimes severe persistent cerebellar deficit.

Malignant hyperthermia

Hyperthermia as part of neuroleptic malignant syndrome is described in Chapter 20.

Decompression sickness

Decompression sickness is also known as the 'bends'. Too rapid decompression causes nitrogen under pressure in the blood to produce gas emboli and microinfarcts. The typical presentation is acute pain in the limbs and trunk. The thoracic spinal cord is most often affected, producing a paraparesis or posterior column disturbance, but brain damage may also occur, leading to a hemiplegia, vertigo or visual disturbance. These deficits usually recover slowly, but chronic persistent deficits are common following severe acute decompression sickness. Recognition of decompression symptoms, with recompression and then much slower decompression, may help to prevent this. Patent foramen ovale (PFO) has been suggested to be a risk factor for decompression syndrome, the mechanisms being that with a high venous nitrogen gas bubble load, the PFO may allow paradoxical arterial nitrogen gas emboli to the brain and so cause damage. PFO closure is therefore sometimes recommended for regular divers, but this remains a controversial area with little clear guiding evidence.

Mountain sickness

Symptoms of acute mountain sickness develop as low-altitude dwellers climb to considerable heights quickly, with onset usually at 24–48 hours after the ascent. The symptoms include headache, nausea, vomiting, lethargy, dizziness, impaired balance, irritability and insomnia. In some cases, acute pulmonary oedema develops, and cerebral oedema with papilloedema, stupor and a flaccid paralysis, is also well recognized. The acute symptoms can be relieved by breathing oxygen. Slow acclimatization to height allows a gradual increase in the haemoglobin concentration, which will largely prevent such symptoms. Dexamethasone and acetazolamide may help to relieve symptoms of acute mountain sickness.

REMOTE EFFECTS OF CANCER ON THE NERVOUS SYSTEM – PARANEOPLASTIC SYNDROMES

These syndromes are discussed in Chapter 14. Tables 27.12 and 27.13 summarize the major syndromes and the associated antibodies, respectively.

NEUROLOGICAL COMPLICATIONS OF CANCER TREATMENT

The neurological effects of cancer treatment are described in Chapter 14.

Table 27.12 Paraneoplastic syndromes affecting the nervous system

Central nervous system	Peripheral nervous system
Multifocal encephalomyelitis	Sensory neuronopathy/ ganglionopathy
Cerebellar degeneration	Vasculitis
Limbic encephalitis	Sensorimotor polyneuropathy
Opsoclonus-myoclonus	Motor neuropathy
Extrapyramidal syndrome	Neuromyotonia
Brainstem encephalitis	Autonomic failure
Myelopathy	Lambert–Eaton myasthenic syndrome (LEMS)
Motor neuron disease	Myasthenia gravis
Stiff-person syndrome	Polymyositis/ dermatomyositis
Optic neuritis	Necrotizing myopathy
Retinal degeneration	

NEUROLOGICAL COMPLICATIONS OF ORGAN TRANSPLANTATION

Organ transplantation is now widely undertaken, including kidney, liver, heart, lung, pancreas and bone marrow. The number of operations continues to increase, and up to 50 per cent of allograft recipients will develop some form of neurological complication. These may be related to the surgical procedure, **immunosuppression (adverse effects of the drugs used, or opportunistic infection), graft rejection**, or to the **underlying disorder** that led to the need for transplantation.

The most important complication is **opportunistic infections**, a particular hazard more than a month after surgery. The more intensive the degree of immunosuppression, the greater becomes the risk of both opportunistic infection and neurotoxicity, but aggressive immunosuppression may be indicated to prevent organ rejection.

CNS infections develop in less than 10 per cent of transplant recipients, but can be severe and carry a high mortality. In the first month after transplantation, infection is unrelated to immunosuppression and is usually caused by hospital-acquired organisms, such as Gram-negative bacteria and staphylococci. *Listeria monocytogenes* can cause meningoencephalitis, often with a brainstem emphasis, multiple abscess formation or myelitis. Mycobacteria cause pulmonary tuberculosis, tuberculous meningitis or atypical CNS infection. Patients are predisposed to these infections by contamination of vascular access or drainage catheters, prolonged intubation, stents, other foreign bodies and fluid collections. More than one month after transplantation, as effective immunosuppression develops, the patient develops increased risk of infection with viruses (cytomegalovirus, Epstein-Barr virus, herpes viruses and fungi (*Aspergillus* and *Candida*).

Seizures may be caused by drug toxicity (e.g. ciclosporin), metabolic derangements, hypoxic ischaemic injury, cerebrovascular disease and sepsis. **Encephalopathy** is a recognized complication of transplantation, varying from a mild confusional state to psychosis with obtundation and coma. In the acute postoperative period, it is often due to a surgical complication (including hypoxic-ischaemic insult), the development of a metabolic encephalopathy, acute allograft rejection, isolated or multiple organ failure, sepsis, seizures or drug toxicity (particularly ciclosporin). **Stroke** may be related to the underlying disease process, for example accelerated cerebrovascular atherosclerosis in diabetes mellitus, but may also be a consequence of cardiac emboli after heart or lung transplants. CNS infections can cause ischaemic or haemorrhagic stroke. Cerebral venous thrombosis occurs as a consequence of a hypercoagulable state, dehydration or CNS infection.

There is an increased incidence of **CNS malignancy** in allograft recipients who are immunosuppressed. Intracerebral B-cell lymphoma affecting the brain and spinal cord and glioblastoma multiforme are the most common, and are associated with previous EBV infection.

Drug adverse effects from immunosuppressants (for example tacrolimus and ciclosporin) include cortical blindness, complex visual disturbances and hallucinations, and are often dose-related and reversible. Ciclosporin and tacrolimus are associated with a high incidence of tremor. Occasionally, parkinsonism has been described in bone marrow transplant recipients.

Table 27.13 Paraneoplastic neurological syndromes and associated autoantibodies

Neurological syndrome	Associated tumours	Selected associated autoantibodies
Cerebellar degeneration	Breast, ovarian, others	Anti-Yo, anti-Ma1, anti-Ri
	SCLC, others	Anti-Hu, antiamphiphysin, anti-VGCC, anti-Ri
Opsoclonus-myoclonus	Breast, ovarian	Anti-Ri, anti-Yo, antiamphiphysin
	SCLC	Anti-Hu, anti-Ri, antiamphiphysin
	Neuroblastoma (children)	Anti-Hu
	Testicular, others	Anti-Ma2
Multifocal encephalomyelitis	SCLC	Anti-Hu, antiamphiphysin, anti-Ri
Limbic encephalitis	SCLC	Anti-Hu, antiamphiphysin, anti-VGKC, anti-VGCC, anti-glur
	Testicular, breast	Anti-Ma2, anti-glur
	Thymoma	Anti-VGKC, anti-glur
	Ovarian teratoma	Anti-NMDA receptor
Myelopathy	SCLC, thymoma, others	Anti-CV2, antiamphiphysin, NMO-igg
Extrapyramidal syndrome	SCLC, thymoma, testicular	Anti-Hu, anti-VGKC, anti-Ma2
Brainstem encephalitis	SCLC, breast, others	Anti-Hu, anti-Ri
	Testicular	Antl-Ma2
Paraneoplastic retinal degeneration	SCLC, others	Antirecoverin, others
	Melanoma	Antibipolar cell
Stiff-person syndrome	Breast, SCLC, others	Antiamphiphysin, anti-Ri, anti-GAD
Motor neuron disease	SCLC, others	Anti-Hu
Sensory neuronopathy	SCLC, others	Anti-Hu, anti-CV2, ANNA-3, anti-Ma1, antiamphiphysin
	Plasma cell dyscrasias	Antigangliosides
Neuromyotonia	Thymoma, SCLC	Anti-VGKC
Sensorimotor polyneuropathy	SCLC, others	Anti-Hu, ANNA-3
	Plasma cell dyscrasias	Anti-MAG
Autonomic insufficiency	SCLC, thymoma	Anti-Hu, antiganglionic achr, anti-VGKC
Lambert–Eaton syndrome	SCLC	Anti-VGCC
Myasthenia gravis	Thymoma	Anti-achr, anti-striated muscle

AchR, acetylcholine receptor; GAD, glutamic acid decarboxylase; GluR, glutamate receptor; MAG, myelin-associated glycoprotein; NMO, neuromyelitis optica; SCLS, small cell lung carcinoma; VGCC, voltage-gated calcium channel; VGKC, voltage-gated potassium channel.

Mononeuropathies follow surgery and anaesthesia and may occur as a consequence of positioning, traction or the mechanical complications of surgery. Phrenic nerve damage can follow cold plegia of the heart (induced hypothermia) during cardiac transplantation.

REFERENCES AND FURTHER READING

Aminoff MJ (ed.) (1999) *Neurology and General Medicine*, 3rd edn. New York: Churchill Livingstone.

Austin S, Cohen H, Losseff N (2007) Haematology and neurology and the blood. *Journal of Neurology, Neurosurgery and Psychiatry*, **78**:334–341.

Baughman RP, du Bois RM, Lower EE *et al.* (2003) Sarcoidosis. *Lancet*, **361**:1111–1118.

Goodin DS (1992) Neurological complications of aortic disease and surgery. In: Aminoff MJ (ed.) *Neurology and General Medicine.* New York: Churchill Livingstone, 27–52.

Hughes GRV (1994) *Connective Tissue Diseases.* Oxford: Blackwell Scientific Publications Ltd.

McAllister LD, Ward JH, Schulman SF, DeAngelis LM (2002) *Practical Neuro-Oncology.* Boston, MA: Butterworth-Heinemann.

Newman LS, Rose CS, Maier LA (1997) Sarcoidosis. *New England Journal of Medicine*, **336**:1224–1234.

Nishino H, Rubino FA, DeRemee RA *et al.* (1993) Neurological involvement in Wegener's granulomatosis: an analysis of 324 consecutive patients at the Mayo Clinic. *Annals of Neurology*, **33**:4–9.

Nowak DA, Widenka DC (2001) Neurosarcoidosis: a review of its intracranial manifestations. *Journal of Neurology*, **248**:363–372.

Perkin GD, Murray-Lyon I (1999) Neurology and the gastrointestinal system. In: Hughes RAC, Perkin GD (eds) *Neurology and Medicine.* BMJ Books, 185–209.

Posner JB (1995) *Neurologic Complications of Cancer.* Philadelphia, PA: FA Davis.

Sawle GV, Ramsay MM (1998) The neurology of pregnancy. *Journal of Neurology, Neurosurgery and Psychiatry*, **64**:717–725.

Siva A, Kantarci OH, Salp S *et al.* (2001) Behçet's disease: diagnostic and prognostic aspects of neurological involvement. *Journal of Neurology*, **248**:95–103.

Siva A, Altintas A, Saip S (2004) Behçet's syndrome and the nervous system. *Current Opinion in Neurology*, **17**:347–357.

Victor M, Adams RD, Collins GH (1971) *The Wernicke-Korsakoff Syndrome.* Philadelphia, PA: FA Davis.

Watkins PJ, Thomas PK (1998) Diabetes mellitus and the nervous system. *Journal of Neurology, Neurosurgery and Psychiatry*, **65**:620–632.

Younger DS (2004) Vasculitis of the nervous system. *Current Opinion in Neurology*, **17**:317–336.

Zajicek JP, Scolding NJ, Foster O *et al.* (1999) Central nervous system sarcoidosis: diagnosis and management. *Quarterly Journal of Medicine*, **92**:103–117.

Zandi MS, Coles AJ (2007) Notes on the kidney for the neurologist. *Journal of Neurology, Neurosurgery and Psychiatry*, **78**:444–449.

CHAPTER 28

PAEDIATRIC NEUROLOGY

Elaine Hughes and Helen Cross

INTRODUCTION

Neurological disorders in childhood fall into two broad groups: those in which there is a disorder of central nervous system (CNS) or peripheral nervous system development, which may be genetically driven or result from an insult in fetal life; and those in which there is an acquired abnormality after initially normal development, such as occurs with neurodegenerative disorders or following brain infection or injury. An awareness of normal processes in terms of anatomical, neurological and developmental pathways is a crucial part of paediatric practice, and increasingly, an awareness of the control exerted by specific genes in these pathways.

DISORDERS OF CNS DEVELOPMENT

Normal development

Developmental event	Timing (gestation)
Primary neurulation	3–4 weeks
Secondary neurulation	4–7 weeks
Prosencephalic development	1–2 months
Proliferation	2–4 months
Migration	3–5 months
Organisation	5 months – postnatal
Myelination	mainly postnatal

In normal development, the term **primary neurulation** refers to the appearance of a region of special-ized dorsal ectoderm (the neural plate), which then folds, elevates and then fuses in the midline to create a neural tube. This process is then dependent on the activity of specific surface receptors to ensure adhesion and closure of the neural tube. Interaction of the neural tube with associated mesoderm results in formation of the dura and axial skeleton. **Secondary neurulation** starts around the future upper sacral level. The neural tube here forms in the tail bud – the remnant of the regressing primitive streak – without folding being required, culminating in the gradual canalization and regression of caudal structures. The vertebral columns grow faster than the spinal cord so that the latter travels cranially in fetal life. At birth, the conus is opposite L3/L4 and by adulthood at L1.

Prosencephalic (forebrain) development occurs in three phases: prosencephalic formation from the rostral end of the original neural tube, followed by cleavage (to divide the telencephalon from the diencephalon, to form the optic expansions and to create the paired cerebral hemispheres, lateral ventricles and basal ganglia) and then midline development. This last event results in the appearance of the commissural structures (including the corpus callosum), the optic chiasm and the hypothalamus.

Cerebral cortical development can also be divided into three main stages, but it is important to recognize that these overlap. **Cellular proliferation** takes place in the germinal zones of the developing prosencephalon between weeks 10 and 18 of gestation with the full neuronal complement achieved by 20 weeks. The brain increases in size over the next 20 weeks, with the occurrence of sulcation to accommodate this. **Neuronal migration** mainly occurs in a radial fashion along microglial extensions that extend from the ventricular ependyma to the pial surface of the neural tube and resulting structures. It occurs in an 'inside out' sequence with neurones destined for the deepest cortical layer migrating first followed by those destined for more superficial layers. Migration continues as **organization** commences with formation of discrete lamina and development of synaptic connections.

Neural tube disorders

Disorders of primary and secondary neurulation include all forms of failure of the neural tube to fuse completely, with secondarily abnormal development of related mesenchymal structures (Figure 28.1). Adequate periconceptual folate supplementation is known to reduce the risk of a further affected infant in a family, but remains difficult to achieve in low risk groups. Specific teratogens, such as sodium valproate and retinoic acid, increase the risk of these defects.

Disorders of neurulation
- Primary neurulation
  - anencephaly
  - myeloschisis
  - encephalocele
  - myelomeningocele
- Secondary neurulation
  - occult dysraphic conditions

In **anencephaly**, there is a failure of anterior neural tube closure which usually results in absence of the skull vault, no optic nerves (although eyes are usually present) and absent or deficient pituitary. The condition is incompatible with prolonged survival: the majority of infants are stillborn or die in the neonatal period. This is distinct from **hydranencephaly** in which cerebrospinal fluid (CSF)-containing sacs replace most of the cerebral hemisphere structures. This is thought most likely to be a consequence of a vascular catastrophe in the territory supplied by the internal carotid arteries.

Encephaloceles, in turn represent selective or segmental failure of anterior neural tube closure. They may be anterior – sphenoidal or frontoethmoidal – or more commonly posterior, where they may be associated with other anomalies, such as brainstem and skull base deformities and hydrocephalus. The swelling contains brain tissue in most cases and the outcome in general otherwise relates to the position of the defect and to the associated anomalies. Syndromic forms exist such as in Meckel–Gruber syndrome, a rare, autosomal recessive condition, where multicystic kidney dysplasia and post-axial polydactyly occur with an occipital encephalocele.

Whereas anterior neural tube defects have a high mortality, posterior neural tube defects of which the classical lesion is the **myelomeningocele**, are compatible with prolonged or normal lifespan. The majority of lesions occur in the lumbar region and may be several centimetres in diameter. The axial skeleton is uniformly deficient with a variable dermal covering – typically a thin translucent membrane or sometimes no covering at all. Management relates to the treatment of the primary lesion, detection and treatment of any associated hydrocephalus and of genitourinary, orthopaedic and neurological consequences. A multidisciplinary approach is essential. As the incidence of children being born with this condition declines with improved antenatal detection, and ideally with pri-

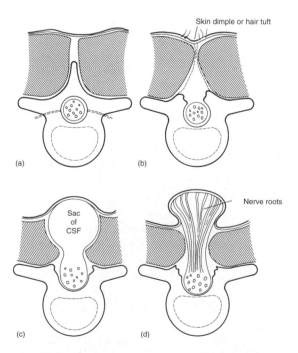

Figure 28.1 Spina bifida, transverse sections through the lumbar region; (a) normal; (b) spinal bifida occulta; (c) meningocele; (d) myelomeningocele. CSF, cerebrospinal fluid.

mary prevention, expertise in the management of these complex children may decline.

Management of myelomeningocele
- Multidisciplinary approach essential
- Early closure of primary lesion may reduce infection and improve
- Neurological outcome
- Detection and intervention with regard to hydrocephalus: ventriculoperitoneal shunt or third ventriculostomy
- Assessment and appropriate intervention for neuropathic bladder and bowel
- Orthopaedic management of limb deformity, scoliosis, provision of appropriate orthotics, seating, etc.
- Psychological support.

In the mildest form of **spinal dysraphism** there is a bony abnormality only – spina bifida occulta – that is usually of no functional significance. In more major forms of 'occult dysraphic disorders' the main features, that may be seen, are:

- an abnormally low conus;
- a thickened filum terminale, tethered to a dermoid, fibrous band, lipoma or dermal sinus extension;

- an associated vertebral defect in 85–90 per cent and on occasions the cord may be split in two (diastematomyelia) and there may be a bony spur between;
- associated cutaneous markers typically a tuft of hair, a dimple or tract, haemangioma or superficial lipoma as a clue to the underlying defect.

Spinal dysraphism may also present with
- Delayed bladder control;
- Gait abnormality sometimes with asymmetric weakness or muscle deficiency;
- Foot deformity such as pes cavus or talipes;
- Scoliosis or back pain;
- (Recurrent) meningitis.

Definitive investigation is now with magnetic resonance imaging (MRI) and plain x-ray films, as well as bladder studies (urodynamics), the latter even where overt symptoms are absent.

Hydrocephalus

It is difficult to determine an accurate figure for the incidence of hydrocephalus (Figure 28.2); figures quoted generally being between 0.4 and 0.8 per

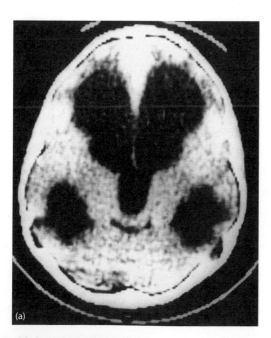
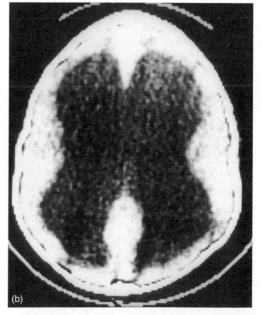

Figure 28.2 Computed tomography brain scan showing gross hydrocephalus caused by aqueduct stenosis. Note the enlargement of the lateral and third ventricles.

1000 births. Antenatal ultrasound has allowed early detection of anomalies. Malformations are the most common causes of antenatal onset hydrocephalus and not surprisingly increase the likelihood of a poor outcome. However, in terms of postnatal acquired hydrocephalus, prolonged survival of extremely preterm infants has led to increased numbers of infants with hydrocephalus secondary to perinatal intraventricular haemorrhage.

CSF is produced mainly in the choroid plexus, circulating through the foramina of Monro, via the third ventricle, through the aqueduct to the fourth ventricle. It leaves the latter to enter the subarachnoid space in the cisterna magna, which is continuous with the spinal subarachnoid space. It is generally considered that CSF is absorbed through the arachnoid villi into the venous sinuses, but there is some evidence from flow studies that the main route of absorption may be through the blood capillaries.

There are three mechanisms for development of hydrocephalus:

1 obstruction of CSF pathways
2 overproduction of CSF
3 failure of reabsorption.

Congenital malformations resulting in obstruction include aqueduct stenosis (usually sporadic but may occur in X-linked form often with adducted thumbs) and Chiari malformations (often associated with a myelomeningocele and Dandy–Walker association). Bony defects at the skull base may also cause obstruction, as, rarely, may a vascular aneurysm of the vein of Galen. In the preterm infant, hydrocephalus may follow intraventricular haemorrhage (IVH). Congenital infections, or postnatally acquired infections, leading to meningitis may cause adhesions and so obstruction to CSF flow or reabsorption. A choroid plexus papilloma produces excessive CSF rather than obstruction.

In infants, hydrocephalus presents with increasing head size (head circumference deviating away from the original centile), splaying of cranial sutures and fullness of the anterior fontanelle. Superficial scalp veins may be distended and later 'sunsetting' of the eyes is seen with failure of upgaze. There may be delayed acquisition of milestones, especially poor head control – sometimes a specific finding of 'head bobbing' may occur early with hydrocephalus secondary

to a third ventricular cyst as in aqueduct stenosis. Once irritability, vomiting and other symptoms of raised intracranial pressure are evident, there is likely to have been considerable progression of the disorder. In the older child, signs are similar to those in adult patients.

The differential diagnosis of a large head in infancy is outlined in Table 28.1. MRI has made discrimination between major subgroups much more straightforward.

Chiari malformation

Abnormalities of the craniocervical junction may cause significant neurological disturbance in infants and children (Figure 28.3 and Table 28.2). In Chiari I malformations, there is caudal cerebellar tonsillar ectopia so that the tonsils are below the foramen magnun. Significant ectopia is >5 mm, although greater degrees may be normal in school age children. This condition may be associated with congenital and acquired craniocervical anomalies.

Table 28.1 Causes of macrocephaly

	Cause
Due to increased cerebrospinal fluid volume	Hydrocephalus
	Glutaric aciduria type 1
Due to increased cerebral volume	Neurocutaneous syndromes especially NF1, haemangiomatosis
	Dysmorphic syndromes, such as Sotos, Beckwiths
	Primary megalencephaly in cortical dysgenesis
	Diffuse infiltrative tumour
	Abnormal storage as in Tay-Sachs, Sandhoff's
	Abnormal white matter in Canavan's and Alexander's
Of extracerebral origin	Subdural effusions
	Vein of Galen aneurysm
	Skeletal dysplasias, such as achondroplasia
	Familial macrocephaly

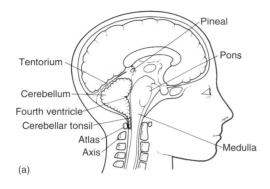

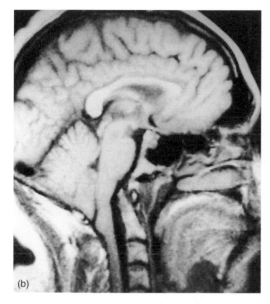

Figure 28.3 (a) Diagram of median sagittal view to show a Chiari malformation. (b) Sagittal view MRI scan of the craniocercival junction showing cerebellar ectopia.

Table 28.2 Chiari malformation

Type/ classification	Details
Type I	Caudal displacement of cerebellar tonsils below plane of foramen magnum (±syringomyelia in 20-75%)
Type II	Caudal displacement of cerebellar tonsils or vermis, fourth ventricle and lower brainstem (±myelomeningocele in >95%)
Type III	Herniation of cerebellum into cervical encephalocele
Type IV	Cerebellar hypoplasia

The **Arnold–Chiari type or Chiari II** malformation involves posterior fossa structures, skull base and spinal column. There is herniation of the cerebellum through the foramen magnum, caudal descent of the brainstem with a cervicomedullary kink in more than two-thirds of patients. The low and narrowed fourth ventricle may become trapped and may herniate, posteriorly and inferiorly. The majority of affected patients (>95 per cent) have an associated myelomeningocele and presenting features are related to the primary lesion or to the associated hydrocephalus and much less often to the Chiari malformation. Occasionally, however, signs of cervical compression and lower brainstem involvement may be evident, with difficulty feeding and respiratory distress.

In **basilar impression**, there is upward displacement of the cervical spine, invaginating the base of the skull at the foramen magnum. This may arise as a developmental defect, or be acquired, as in osteogenesis imperfecta. A narrow foramen magnum (without basilar impression) occurs in a number of skeletal dysplasias – the best known of which is achondroplasia. Abnormalities of the odontoid peg – either congenital or acquired – may exist. In Down's syndrome and Morquio's, atlantoaxial dislocation may occur more frequently as a consequence of increased ligamentous laxity. Cervical vertebral blocks are a feature of several syndromes, especially Klippel–Feil. Patients may be asymptomatic even though the deformity is a congenital one. A short neck, low hairline and restricted mobility at the neck are common. Neurologically, when deterioration occurs, characteristic features are:

- ataxia, pyramidal signs, loss of proprioception in upper limbs, nystagmus and lower cranial nerve signs manifest as swallowing difficulties
- occipital pain
- with or without signs of associated hydrocephalus.

Trauma may precipitate symptoms. This is a particular issue in Down's syndrome where atlantoaxial instability is very common, but dangerous instability is unusual. Patients considered to be at high risk should be cautioned against activities such as trampolining or somersaulting. In symptomatic cases of basilar impression, surgical decompression of the cranial–cervical junction is indicated.

Disorders of cortical development

With advances in neuroimaging techniques, disorders of brain development have increasingly been identified. They form a heterogeneous group with clinical features ranging from severe developmental delay and epilepsy to the asymptomatic. Emerging information about the genetic basis for a number of malformations of cortical development may be of major significance when counselling patients. Current classification schemes take as their basis the stage at which cortical development was affected, combined where available with information from genetics, neuroimaging and pathology (see Table 28.3).

Cerebral malformations will result from disruption of any part of the normal developmental process, that is ventral induction, proliferation or apoptosis, migration or organization of the cortex. Some of the disorders have been found to have a genetic basis; for example, **lissencephaly/ subcortical band heterotopia spectrum**; whereas others, such as **polymicrogyria** may occur either on the background of a genetic abnormality or in the context of an antenatal infection or presumed vascular insult. Cerebral malformations have also been increasingly recognized as part of established syndromes and metabolic disorders.

Failure of ventral induction

Failure of ventral induction refers to the malformations that result from failure of induction involving the three germ layers. This inductive interaction

Table 28.3 Classification of cerebral malformations

Embryological event	Examples (gene and/or locus)
Failure of ventral induction	Holoprosencephaly
Abnormal proliferation or apoptosis	
1. Reduced proliferation/increased apoptosis	Microcephaly
2. Increased proliferation/reduced apoptosis	Megalencephaly
3. Abnormal proliferation (abnormal cell types)	
Non-neoplastic	Tuberous sclerosis (TSC1/2)
	Cortical dysplasia with balloon cells
	Hemimegalencephaly
Neoplastic	Dysembryoplastic neuroepithelial tumours (DNET)
Abnormal neuronal migration	Gangliocytoma
1. Lissencephaly/SBH spectrum	X-linked lissencephaly and abnormal genitalia (ARX)
	Isolated lissencephaly or SBH (DCX, TUBA1A, LIS1)
	Miller-Dieker (LIS1)
	With cerebellar hypoplasia (RELN)
2. Cobblestone complex	Fukuyama muscular dystrophy or Walker–Warburg syndrome (FCMD)
	Muscle–eye–brain disease (several)
3. Heterotopia	Periventricular nodular (FLNA)
Subcortical	
Abnormal cortical organization	
1. Polymicrogyria	Bilateral perisylvian syndrome
	With schizencephaly
	With rolandic szs, oromotor dyspraxia (SPRX2)
2. Cortical dysplasia without balloon cells	
3. Microdysgenesis	
Unclassified	1. Secondary to inborn errors of metabolism
	2. Other unclassified malformations

not only controls forebrain development, but also the formation of much of the face so that facial abnormalities are commonly associated. The most common disorder is **holoprosencephaly** where the anterior part of the brain is undivided, but the severity of the resulting abnormality is highly variable. In the most severe forms, death occurs in the first year of life. In less severe presentations, most infants develop seizures and have severe mental retardation.

Abnormal neuronal and glial proliferation or apoptosis

It has now been recognized that apoptosis also has an important part to play in cortical development. An abnormal brain size may therefore be a consequence of disorders of proliferation or apoptosis. **Microcephalies** may result from reduced proliferation and/or increased apoptosis. **Megalencephalies** may be due to increased proliferation and/or reduced apoptosis. These findings may occur in isolation or as part of a syndrome in association with other congenital anomalies. A large or small head does not invariably indicate an underlying cerebral malformation. The majority of children with large heads and normal or near-normal development have genetically determined macrocephaly. This stresses the importance of measuring parental head sizes as part of the paediatric neurological examination.

Focal malformations thought to result from interference with neuronal and glial proliferation are now commonly encountered in children with drug-resistant epilepsy being assessed for possible surgical treatment of their epilepsy. Pathologically, balloon cells are a marker for non-neoplastic malformations due to abnormal proliferation. Hemimegalencephaly is an MRI and pathological diagnosis, although classified as a disorder of proliferation, abnormalities of migration and organization coexist. It may be an isolated condition or be associated with neurocutaneous disorders including neurofibromatosis and tuberous sclerosis. The 'tumour' group consists of **gangliogliomas, gangliocytomas and dysembryoplastic neuroepithelial tumours (DNETs)**. These benign lesions are characterized by the presence of mature neuronal and glial cells. Many will be missed or misinterpreted on computed tomography (CT) scan and will only be fully elucidated on MRI.

Abnormal neuronal migration

Interference with the process of neuronal migration may occur as a consequence of an infective or vascular insult in pregnancy (see Figures 28.4 and 28.5). Congenital cytomegalovirus infection in particular may manifest as a combination of calcification and abnormal gyral pattern, such as pachygyria. However, a significant proportion of these disorders are now recognized to have a genetic basis, with a spectrum of severity from the most severe lissencephaly to subtle band or focal heterotopias.

Lissencephaly (literally 'smooth brain') refers to a disorder where there is a lack of gyral and sulcal development. It has now been recognized that **subcortical band heterotopia (SBH)** form part of the classical lissencephaly spectrum with a common genetic basis. Mutations in several genes, LIS1, DCX (doublecortin) or XLIS, and RLN (reelin) have been identified as producing different patterns of abnormality, the latter being associated with additional cerebellar hypoplasia. On occasions, it is these additional abnormalities either in the CNS or outside that may define the disorder.

In classical lissencephaly, there are areas of the brain with agyria (absence of gyri) and pachygyria (few broad thick gyri). In one subtype, **Miller–Dieker**

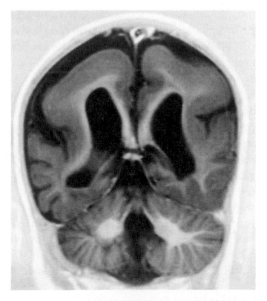

Figure 28.4 Coronal section of an MRI brain scan showing lissencephaly (lack of gyral and sulcal development).

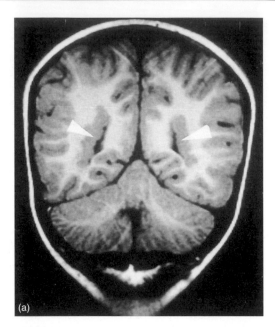 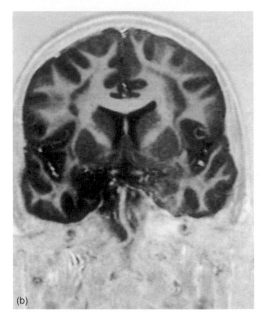

Figure 28.5 Coronal sections of MRI brain scans to show (a) subependymal heteropias (arrowed); (b) band heterotopias.

syndrome, a chromosomal deletion at 17p13.3, also produces characteristic facies with a narrow forehead, long philtrum and upturned nares, along with digital abnormalities and hypervascularization of the retina. Affected individuals usually have severe learning difficulties and often difficult to treat epilepsy. In a form of X-linked lissencephaly with abnormal genitalia (XLAG), mutations in the Aristaless-related, homeobox gene (ARX) have been found. Mutations in this same gene have now been identified in a variety of neurological presentations.

In **Walker–Warburg syndrome**, the cortex is thickened, sulci are shallow, meninges thickened and the cerebellum is small with an absent vermis. Hydrocephalus is commonly associated along with eye malformations – retinal dysplasia and microphthalmia. This condition and Fukuyama congenital muscular dystrophy are members of the **cobblestone complex** in which the glial limiting membrane fails to prevent migration of neurones into the subpial space.

Heterotopic nodules may occur as isolated abnormalities often presenting with seizures. A particular pattern of X-linked dominant, **periventricular nodular heterotopia**, has been identified as resulting from mutations in FLNA (filamin A). A range of other disorders has also been associated with mutations in this gene, including cardiac valvular abnormalities, tendency to premature stroke, and with joint hypermobility producing an Ehlers–Danlos variant.

Abnormal cortical organization

Polymicrogyria and **schizencephaly** often occur together and may be a consequence of a number of genetic and environmental causes. In schizencephaly, clefts lined with grey matter extend through the cerebral hemisphere from the ependymal lining of the lateral ventricles to the pial lining of the cortex. Clefts may be unilateral or bilateral and may present with seizures, variable degree of learning difficulties or hemiparesis, depending on the extent and location of the malformation. Several bilateral polymicrogyria syndromes are now well described of which the best known is the bilateral perisylvian syndrome. Patients present with a pseudobulbar palsy – usually with significant feeding difficulties – and epilepsy. It is now well recognized that some children with polymicrogyria will develop electrical status in sleep (ESES), which has a good prognosis for resolution but not without cognitive impairment.

Associated disorders

Some developmental brain malformations may be associated with inborn errors of metabolism, in particular peroxisomal disorders such as Zellwegers, but also disorders of mitochondrial function, and of pyruvate metabolism, as well as a number of other conditions. **Agenesis of the corpus callosum** is a common association, but this is also often seen in isolation or as part of a syndrome such as that of **Aicardi**. Its true incidence is unknown as many cases are asymptomatic.

CEREBRAL PALSY

The term cerebral palsy (CP) refers to **a group of permanent disorders of the development of movement and posture, causing activity limitation, that are attributed to non-progressive disturbances that occurred in the developing fetal or infant brain.**

The consequences for motor development will vary with the timing of the insult, as well as its extent and localization, and while the underlying lesion may be static, the clinical picture is an evolving one and secondary musculoskeletal problems are often a feature. While the term 'cerebral palsy' refers to the motor disorder, it should be recognized that co-morbidities are common, especially communication, learning and behavioural difficulties, sensory impairments and epilepsy. Conventionally, children in whom a mild motor abnormality is overwhelmed by other difficulties, such as profound learning disability, tend to be excluded.

In developed countries, the incidence of cerebral palsy remains relatively consistent at between 1.5 and 2.5 per thousand live births. While increasingly sophisticated, neonatal care has improved the outcome for many infants, it has also led to better survival of extremely low birthweight infants (400–1000 g), and more often multiple births, with increased incidence of major motor disability.

Almost any pathological process in the developing brain can produce a motor deficit. Aetiologically, it is more helpful to look at risk factors (Table 28.4) for the development of CP. It is now clear that prenatal are numerically much more important than perinatal factors and in particular that 'birth asphyxia' is an uncommon cause of cerebral palsy. However, a fetus that is already compromised prenatally may also be more vulnerable to the process of labour. In this regard, fetal monitoring with pH

Table 28.4 Risk factors for cerebral palsy

Prenatal factors	Preterm birth
	Intrauterine growth retardation
	Brain malformations
	Fetal circulatory disorder
	Genetic factors (uncommon except in ataxic form)
Prenatal factors	Hypoxic ischaemic injury
	Infections
Postnatal factors	Vascular trauma including non-accidental injury
	Infections
	Prolonged seizure (vary rare)

sampling and continuous fetal monitoring have proved poor predictors of outcome. Apgar scores (a theoretically objective measure of a newborn's well-being and assessment of need for intervention) are only strongly predictive of the development of CP when they remain low (<3) for 20 minutes or more after delivery. In the immediate neonatal period, increasingly sophisticated brain imaging is helping in the early identification of 'at risk' infants.

Hemiplegic CP remains the most common pattern in term infants in whom it is prenatally acquired in 75 per cent, although overt structural lesions are not always apparent. Hypoperfusion events in the third trimester are most commonly implicated. It is rarely diagnosed at birth but usually evident at around six months, when the child begins to show abnormally early hand preference when reaching for toys. Fisting of the affected upper limb and altered tone may then be apparent. Since the lower limb is less affected in term infants, delay in walking may not be marked and is usually achieved by 18 months unless there are associated learning difficulties. Hand function is most compromised. An acquired hemiplegia may occur in the context of vascular disease, migraine or status epilepticus. Facial involvement is probably present even in most prenatal onset cases, but is more prominent in postnatally acquired cases. In preterm infants, leg involvement is generally more severe. 'Preterm' hemiplegia has a non-specific association with perinatal events, such as impaired autoregulation of cerebral blood flow, acidosis and hypoglycaemia.

Classification of cerebral palsy

The classification of CP has been the subject of extensive debate, but there is general agreement that the following components need to be included:

- A description of the **type of motor disorder** with division as before into predominantly **spastic**, **ataxic** and **dyskinetic** categories, with the latter further subdivided into **choreoathetoid** and **dystonic** groups. During the evolution of the disorder, the predominant motor pattern may change, so that involuntary movements may not become prominent until the second year of life, while hypotonia may precede the development of spasticity in the acute phase.
- The **anatomical distribution of the disorder**, describing the pattern of trunk, limbs and any oromotor involvement, moving away from the terms 'diplegia' and 'quadriplegia' because they are insufficiently discriminating, but retaining the term 'hemiplegia'.
- The **extent of functional impairment**, ideally through a system such as the GMFCS (Gross Motor Classification System). This was developed in response to the need for a standardized system for assessing severity across a series of age bands and enables clear communication between professionals clinically and for research purposes. It uses five levels, with children at level 1 able to carry out activities appropriate to their age group, but with limitations in speed or coordination, while those at level 5 have a profound limitation of all aspects of voluntary control of head and trunk in most positions.
- A description of **additional impairments**.
- Information regarding **aetiology**, with imaging findings and other relevant information contributing, for example, history of prematurity, meningitis, etc.

In children born preterm, the most common pattern is one of predominantly lower limb involvement (previously termed 'spastic diplegia'). The distribution of involvement correlates with the involvement of periventricular white matter. Progressive ventricular dilatation (hydrocephalus) may follow intraventricular haemorrhage (IVH) – initially secondary to impaired CSF absorption caused by blood debris, and subsequently by an obliterative arachnoiditis in the posterior fossa where blood tends to collect. Additional learning difficulties may be mild depending on the extent of cortical involvement.

Dyskinetic CP occurs most often in term infants – motor patterns are disorganized either by superimposed unwanted movements or by fluctuating tonal abnormalities. Inability to organize or execute intended movement results in major disability in concert with preservation of primitive infant reflex patterns. The dystonic version is characterized by abnormal postures and fluctuating but increased tone, while the choreoathetoid version has hyperkinesis and mainly reduced tone. The latter condition is now less common because of a reduction in the occurrence of kernicterus (bilirubin encephalopathy), and the pattern is now seen most often following perinatal difficulties in the term baby.

True **ataxic CP** typically with coordination difficulties, and often tremor, on the background of low tone, is a difficult condition to diagnose with certainty in the early stages. Both progressive neurodegenerative disorders and potentially treatable conditions may present in this manner (see Box 28.1).

Box 28.1 Differential diagnosis of cerebral palsy

- Variants of normal development, e.g. bottom shufflers
- Transient tonal abnormalities in preterm infants
- Hypotonia as apart of syndromic disorder, e.g. Prader-Willi, or weakness as part of congenital myopathy or dystrophy
- Ataxia as part of a progressive disorder including posterior fossa and cervical cord tumours, leukodystrophies, DNA repair disorders, such as ataxia telangiectasia, hereditary ataxias, such as Freidreich's
- Dystonia as part of dopa-responsive dystonia
- Choreoathetosis as part of decompensation of neurometabolic disorder, e.g. glutaric aciduria type 1, glucose transporter disorder (GLUT1)
- Gait disturbance secondary to poorly controlled epilepsy

Management

It must be recognized that for many children their motor disability is only one aspect of their special needs. Other problems that may need to be addressed include: **feeding difficulties** (whether due to posture, palatopharyngeal incoordination, oral hypersensitivity or gastro-oesophageal reflux) and **respiratory difficulties**, which may be a consequence of recurrent microaspiration. Intervention by a speech therapist may be very helpful to devise appropriate feeding strategies, but anti-reflux measures and in some instances insertion of a feeding gastrostomy may be required.

Motor difficulties – spasms, contractures, hip dislocation, scoliosis – may be reduced or sometimes eliminated by the appropriate use of physiotherapy, provision of adequate seating and sometimes lying boards, by drug treatment including baclofen, nitrazepam and botulinum injections. Gait analysis allows more objective assessment of walking patterns, especially before considering orthopaedic or other procedures (e.g. dorsal rhizotomy).

Educationally, the need for effective communication tools cannot be over-emphasized and the paramount importance of appropriate positioning for the child so that they can perform to the best of their abilities. Cognitive and sensory deficits and seizures are highly relevant when determining functional outcome. A multidisciplinary approach is crucial not only to provide an assessment of the child's condition and associated difficulties, but also to plan appropriate intervention and support.

LEARNING DISABILITY

Intellectual functioning is usually measured using a cognitive scoring system, such as the Wechsler Intelligence Scale for Children (WISC) or developmental tests in younger children such as the Griffith's or Bayley's developmental scales that have been tested for reliability and validity on large populations. A resulting intelligence (or developmental) quotient is obtained, made up of many subscores of selected abilities. Although the overall score allows a comparison of an individual child's performance with others of the same age, it is also useful when monitoring an individual

child's progress over time. Variations in scores on individual subsets may allow identification of specific areas of difficulty. It must be remembered that impaired intellectual functioning may be compounded by a delay in maturation and impaired social adjustment.

Learning disability (synonymous with mental retardation) is not a disorder but is a descriptive term, allowing grouping of individuals whose common feature is an IQ score below 70 points on a standardized test. Within this group, those with severe learning difficulties have IQs below 50. In functional terms, the presence or not of other problems such as epilepsy, sensory or motor impairments, or especially social communication difficulties (autism) are of major significance. Although the prevalence of severe learning disability is accepted to be 3–4/1000, the prevalence of mild learning disability is harder to define, but is generally considered to be between 1 and 3 per cent with an increased prevalence in males.

The causes of learning disability can be broadly divided based on the assumed timing of the insult into prenatal (e.g. genetic or developmental), perinatal and postnatal aetiologies. Most studies suggest that the aetiology of severe learning disability can be established in around 80 per cent with two-thirds of cases having a prenatal origin. However, despite advances in genetics and neuroimaging in particular, a large number of children with mild learning problems do not have a recognized cause of their difficulties. A full history, including pregnancy, delivery, developmental milestones, the presence or absence of seizures and family history is important. Examination may also give clues especially in the form of neurocutaneous stigmata, dysmorphism, large or small head, or other congenital anomalies.

Chromosomal and other genetic disorders

Cytogenetic studies have an important role in evaluation. Clues to finding abnormalities from prior history and examination include a history of recurrent miscarriage or family history of learning difficulties, other congenital anomalies, microcephaly and other dysmorphic features. Array CGH (microarray comparative genomic hybridization) allows detection of microdeletions and duplications at a higher resolution level than previous techniques. Gains and losses in the genome in the test sample relative to the control are identified. There are limitations, in the first instance, failure to detect balanced translocations and second, the finding that copy number variants occur not infrequently in the otherwise normal population so that identification of such may not necessarily be aetiologically significant.

In trisomy 21 (Down's syndrome), there is characteristic facial dysmorphology, and increased incidence of cardiac defects (usually anteroventral septal defects), duodenal atresia and Hirschsprung disease, and later of autoimmune disorders, leukaemia and hypothyroidism. Neurologically, affected individuals have motor delay and learning disability, but also increased incidence of epilepsy, especially infantile spasms and reflex seizures; increased incidence of early dementia, usually Alzheimer-like, but rarely with recurrent stroke secondary to moyamoya. Other trisomies are less common and usually incompatible with prolonged survival as in the case of trisomies 13 (Patau's) and 18 (Edward's).

Fragile X is the most common cause of X-linked learning disability. It affects approximately one in 4000 males and one in 6–8000 females. Dysmorphic features of this condition are hard to recognize in prepubertal children. Common features apart from the learning disability are: attention deficit hyperactivity disorder (ADHD), anxiety, gaze avoidance and other autistic traits, and seizures in approximately 25 per cent. Physical features include a long face with prominent jaw, large ears, flat feet and joint hypermobility with post-pubertal macroorchidism. A proportion of women (perhaps 30–50 per cent) have some intellectual difficulties. Fragile X is a trinucleotide repeat disorder, the endpoint of which is a blocking of production of the fragile X mental retardation protein (FMRP). A full mutation is defined as having at least 200 CGG repeats on Southern blot analysis. Pre-mutations are defined as having 60–200 repeats, typically without observable effects but some older adults have now been described with fragile X associated tremor/ataxia (FX-TAS). In **Klinefelter's** (XXY), affected males are tall, with hypogonadism and low verbal IQ.

Prader–Willi syndrome is thought to be under-diagnosed, with rates quoted between one in 10 000 and one in 25 000. It most often occurs as a consequence of deletion of a segment of paternally derived chromosome 15 in the region 15q11-13. The early picture is one of severe hypotonia and feeding difficulties, with subsequent speech delay and motor in-coordination. Characteristic hyperphagia emerges in early childhood and will produce marked obesity if intake is not carefully controlled, alongside delayed puberty with short stature and hypogonadism. Learning disability is generally mild or borderline with strengths in visual organization including reading, but poorer spoken language and auditory processing. Compulsive behaviours with skin picking and anxiety are common. Prader-Willi and **Angelman's** syndrome are examples of imprinting, the expression of the gene being determined by parental origin. In Angelman's, a similar deletion is generally maternally derived. A percentage of patients have either no detectable deletion or a mutation of the UBE-3A, gene with risk of recurrence. Children with Angelman's have severe learning disability, including marked language impairment and jerky ataxia (with underlying cortical myoclonus). Epilepsy is common and the EEG may show posterior slow wave activity, which may be notched or associated with true spikes, this activity enhanced by eye closure, along with fast bursting cortical myoclonus.

Other chromosomal disorders include the **velo-cardio-facial syndrome** (sharing a 22q11 deletion with DiGeorge syndrome) in which there are congenital cardiac anomalies, cleft palate and learning disability.

Of the disorders with autosomal dominant inheritance, **neurofibromatosis 1 (NF1)** affects about one in 3000 individuals, and **neurofibromatosis 2 (NF2)** around one in 35 000 people. There is almost complete penetrance for NF1, but 30 per cent of cases are new mutations. Both disorders are characterized by growth of neurofibromas, in NF1 in skin and on the optic nerve and in NF2 within the spinal cord and brain, with a predilection for the 8th nerve. NF1 maps to chromosome 17, NF2 to chromosome 22. Specific learning difficulties and attention deficit disorder are common in NF1 with IQ typically lower than unaffected siblings. Epilepsy is more common but probably occurs in less than 5 per cent. Brain imaging in children and adolescents with NF1 frequently identifies 'unexplained bright objects' of uncertain significance especially as they may change in size and even disappear over time.

Diagnostic criteria for NF1: needs two or more criteria for diagnosis

- Prepuberty: >6 café-au-lait patches >5 mm
- Postpuberty: >6 café-au-lait patches >15 mm
- Two or more neurofibromas or one plexiform neurofibroma
- Axillary or inguinal freckling
- Optic gliomas
- Two or more Lisch nodules (best seen on slit-lamp examination)
- Typical bony lesion, e.g. Sphenoid dysplasia
- First-degree relative with NF1

Cognitive difficulties and autistic features in **tuberous sclerosis complex (TSC)** are closely correlated with early onset epilepsy. Presentation in childhood may be with seizures, especially infantile spasms, or with skin stigmata, or later with hypertension or other renal complications. Subependymal astrocytomas located at the foramen of Monro may cause ventricular obstruction. Early diagnosis of TSC may be made on the basis of antenatal identification of cardiac nodules which usually then regress without needing treatment. It is the result of a mutation in the TSC1 (9q34, encoding hamartin) or TSC2 (16p13, encoding tuberin) genes, both of which are critical to the normal functioning of the mTOR pathway. Loss of inhibition of this pathway leads to unchecked cell growth and cell proliferation; inhibitors of this pathway such as rapamycin may have a role in treatment. **Incontinentia pigmenti**, an X-linked condition, is lethal in males but girls present with a blistering rash in the neonatal period, with later development of linear pigmentation. CNS involvement with learning disability is seen in up to a third of cases.

Rett syndrome is a disorder, affecting girls, associated with mutations in the *MECP2* gene. Mutations are not entirely specific for this disorder and have been identified in a number of phenotypes including a severe neonatal encephalopathy in boys. Initial mild delay with hypotonia may not have been appreciated and is followed by a period of decelerating head growth, loss of previously acquired purposeful hand function, accompanied by an autistic withdrawal with loss of language and the emergence of hand stereotypies. Bruxism and respiratory irregularities emerge and epileptic seizures are frequently reported, but may be over-diagnosed. Pyramidal signs and musculoskeletal problems with scoliosis and trophic changes in the hands and feet contribute to increasing immobility.

Metabolic causes of learning disability may easily be overlooked and may have autosomal recessive inheritance. **Phenylketonuria (PKU)** is screened for in newborn infants in the UK (along with congenital hypothyroidism) and prompt diagnosis allows early dietary intervention. This has resulted in a fall in the incidence of severe learning difficulties in these children, although early treated subjects still have a mean IQ about half a standard deviation lower than their unaffected siblings.

Developmental and environmental causes

Brain MRI, particularly in children with severe learning disability, may provide valuable diagnostic information through the identification of forms of cerebral dysgenesis or other structural abnormalities. It may also suggest exposure to *in-utero* infections or an underlying metabolic disorder. Positive findings are more likely in the presence of a motor disorder, abnormal head size, epilepsy or neurocutaneous markers. **Congenital infection** refers to any viral infection sustained in pregnancy, but those most commonly recognized include herpes, rubella, toxoplasmosis and cytomegalovirus (CMV). Although there may be suggestive features on neuroimaging, these require confirmation with serology and this may be difficult or impossible outside the neonatal period. Exposure to **toxins** such as alcohol or drugs (both prescribed medicines and substances of abuse) puts the fetus at increased risk of an adverse outcome.

Perinatal causes

There is some epidemiological evidence that perinatal hypoxic ischaemic events are associated with later learning disability, but there have been no prospective studies and there is no definite evidence to suggest that perinatal 'asphyxia' alone causes learning disability in the absence of a motor disorder.

Postnatal causes

Congenital hypothyroidism causes irreversible mental retardation if not treated within the first three months of life and is also associated with hypotonia, prolonged jaundice and delayed closure of the anterior fontanelle. Head injury which may be accidental or non-accidental may result in permanent sequelae and, in the case of non-accidental shaking injuries, there is now evidence that learning and behavioural difficulties may become evident after an apparently 'symptom-free' interval. Meningitis in the newborn period is a major risk factor for motor, sensory and cognitive sequelae.

Miscellaneous causes

Sturge–Weber syndrome is a phakomatosis, also called 'encephalofacial angiomatosis' because patients show an extensive angioma (port wine stain or naevus flammeus) involving one side of the face including the eye. There may be an associated overgrowth of soft tissues on the affected side with involvement of the eye. This may lead to the development of glaucoma. There is usually extensive intracerebral calcification affecting the underlying brain (see Figure 28.6), which may become atrophic. The cerebral changes are associated with the development of epilepsy, hemiplegia and learning difficulties. Familial cases are rare and cause is unknown.

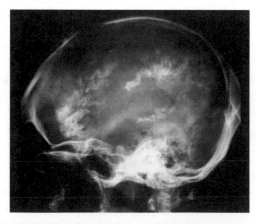

Figure 28.6 Lateral skull x-ray to show intracranial calcification. This pattern outlining the gyri is typical of Sturge–Weber syndrome.

NEUROMETABOLIC DISORDERS

Neurometabolic and other neurodegenerative disorders in children constitute a significant proportion of the paediatric neurology workload. Recognition of the progressive nature of many of these conditions is vital for accurate counselling about that child's long-term outcome and also because of the

Certain features unique to the paediatric population are relevant here:

- The progressive nature of the disorder may not be readily apparent. This is because the progressive brain disturbance is superimposed on continuing maturational processes so that there is a period in the disease course when developmental progress outstrips the rate of deterioration. Occasionally, with disorders of prenatal onset, damage already evident at birth may be so profound that no developmental progress is observed, suggesting initially a severe static encephalopathy.
- The age and therefore cooperation of the child may limit formal examination and observed performance of language and fine motor tasks especially may improve markedly as confidence in the examination setting and the examiner grows. An accurate developmental history from parents is therefore crucial in determining progress.
- Developmental maturation may unmask new problems without indicating progressive pathology – the appearance of hemiplegic posturing at around six months in congenital hemiplegia and of surplus or dystonic movements in the second year of life exemplifies this. A growth spurt may hinder previously acquired walking or sitting, as may scoliosis or hip dislocation. Seizure disorders are not specific to the paediatric age group, but epileptic encephalopathies of early onset such as West syndrome, Dravet's syndrome or Lennox–Gastaut syndrome, may produce a pseudodementia. This may be exacerbated by inappropriate and often ineffective drug therapy, by behavioural disorder or occasionally by secondary damage following a prolonged seizure.

genetic implications. Many of the known disorders have autosomal recessive inheritance.

This diverse and often confusing group of disorders may be grouped according to:

- the underlying biochemical abnormality where known;
- age of onset – prenatal, neonatal, infancy, childhood;
- predominant clinical features.

Disorders predominantly affecting muscle or nerve have been considered in other chapters so that this section will concentrate on those disorders with central nervous system involvement. Given the large number of conditions under this heading only the major groups of disorders are considered here. While the majority of disorders described have their onset in childhood – many in the newborn period or infancy – adult phenotypes of a number of the disorders are increasingly being recognized.

Aminoacidopathies and related disorders

Disorders of intermediary metabolism do not result in storage, but have a profound impact on brain development (Table 28.5). In some cases, this is already apparent at birth – evidenced by the association of callosal agenesis or hypoplasia with non-ketotic hyperglycinaemia (NKH) – or of macrocephaly in glutaric aciduria type 1. For a number of conditions, neonatal screening allows early dietary or other intervention. In other conditions, early diagnosis may allow supportive treatment until the infant is old enough for other procedures, such as liver transplantation, to be considered.

A number of clinical features are common in these conditions – vomiting, seizures and encephalopathy. Tachypnoea is a marker of either metabolic acidosis, found in the branched chain aminoacid disorders, or hyperammonaemia in the urea cycle disorders, in propionic acidaemia and methylmalonic acidaemia. Ophthalmoplegia is seen in both NKH and maple syrup urine disease (MSUD). Fluctuating eye movement disorders with sparing of pupillary function should always raise suspicion about an underlying metabolic disorder – this may easily be missed and the infant labelled instead as having a hypoxic-ischaemic encephalopathy.

In children presenting outside the neonatal period, intermittent drowsiness, vomiting, ataxia or psychiatric disturbance have been reported. Recurrent attacks are usually precipitated by a protein load, either dietary or catabolic, as with an intercurrent infection.

Disorders characterized by energy failure

Glucose transporter type 1 disorders (GLUT1) are increasingly being identified as a cause of neurological disorders in infancy and childhood. While the initial reports were of early onset and difficult to control epilepsy, associated with acquired microcephaly, motor disorders and cognitive difficulties, milder phenotypes are now being reported without seizures. The diagnosis is suggested by finding a low ratio of CSF glucose concentration to blood glucose concentration, and can now be confirmed in the majority by identification of mutations in the *SLC2A1* gene. The importance of this diagnosis is that the ketogenic diet allows alternative energy delivery with benefit for seizure control and usually some improvement in movement disorders, cognition and behaviour, although some difficulties typically persist.

Similarly, **disorders of creatine metabolism**, may be partly amenable to treatment. There are two known creatine biosynthesis disorders: (1) guanidinoacetate methyltransferase (GAMT) deficiency and (2) l-arginine glycine amidinotransferase (AGAT) deficiency, as well as one transporter defect, SLC6A8-related creatine transporter (SLC6A8) deficiency which is X-linked. Seizures and variable degrees of learning disability are a feature of GAMT deficiency, typically with speech delay and behavioural disorder. Creatine supplements, in the case of GAMT deficiency combined with dietary manipulation with restriction of arginine and supplementation of ornithine may improve seizure control, but not appreciably modify the other features.

Disorders of mitochondrial energy metabolism (Table 28.6) have a heterogeneous presentation. Detection relies on a high index of clinical suspicion based on a number of recurring phenotypes, supported by biochemical evidence such as lactic acidosis, characteristic neuroimaging and tissue-specific findings, such as ragged red fibres in muscle. The latter may also be used as a source of

Table 28.5 Aminoacidopathies and related disorders (main types)

Disorder	Biochemistry	Clinical features
Urea cycle disorders carbamyl phosphate synthetase deficiency, ornithine trans-carbamylase deficiency (OTC)	Hyperammonaemia variable depending on site of block; raised orotic acid in OTC	Vomiting, drowsiness leading to coma, seizures. In late onset forms, vomiting, anorexia, failure to thrive; later still behavioural disturbance, nocturnal restlessness overactivity, learning difficulties, psychosis. Spastic diplegia (arginase deficiency)
Phenylketonuria (PKU)	Raised plasma phenylalanine	Learning difficulties, microcephaly
Branched chain amino acid disorders, MSUD, propionic acidaemia, methylmalonic aciduria	Raised plasma branched chain aminoacids (valine, leucine isoleucine), raised ketoacids	Coma, ketoacidosis, hyperammonaemia (not in MSUD) Late onset cases: recurrent encephalopathy with vomiting, ataxia, drowsiness, possible cognitive decline, movement disorder
Glutaric aciduria type 1	Raised glutaric acid, 3 OH, glutaric acid	Macrocephaly, movement disorder often after acute illness
Homocystinuria	Raised total homocysteine + plasma methionine, reduced urinary homocystine	Learning difficulties, stroke, lens dislocation
Isolated sulphite oxidase/ molybdenum cofactor deficiency	Positive urinary sulphite, low plasma urate	Neonatal onset: seizures, feeding difficulties, spasticity, later lens dislocation renal stones
Tyrosinaemia	Raised succinyl acetone in urine	Hepatic failure, peripheral neuropathy, proximal renal tubulopathy
Non-ketotic hyperglycinaemia (NKH)	Raised CSF/plasma glycine ratio	Neonatal onset encephalopathy with hiccups, respiratory insufficiency hypotonia, myoclonus, coma. EEG shows burst suppression pattern (late onset cases with spinocerebellar degeneration)

MSUD, maple syrup urine disease.

mitochondria for DNA analysis in addition to other molecular genetic studies.

Neonatal phenotypes include a fulminant lactic acidosis with hypotonia, seizures, tachypnoea and coma. This picture may be seen in a number of respiratory chain disorders, as well as in disorders of pyruvate utilization. In disorders of the pyruvate dehydrogenase complex, craniofacial dysmorphism may also be evident with underlying cortical dysgenesis – callosal agenesis and subependymal heterotopias. A fatal infantile myopathy, sometimes associated with a Fanconi-type picture or with cardiomyopathy, may occur with complex 1V (cytochrome oxidase) deficiency. In Alper's syndrome, there are very refractory seizures including focal motor status (epilepsy partialis continua) with developmental regression and often liver impairment. Hepatic decompensation may occur with sodium valproate. Children are often found to have mutations in POLG (polymerase gamma A), but these mutations are not specific for Alper's.

In childhood, syndromes resemble those in adulthood and clinical features may include hypotonia, muscle weakness, ataxia, spasticity, seizures and developmental delay. Non-neurological features include failure to thrive, liver disease, renal dysfunction, short stature, cardiac defects, retinopathy or ophthalmoplegia and deafness. Leigh's syndrome was originally a neuropathological diagnosis based on findings of changes in the basal ganglia (especially putamen) and brainstem. It is now recognized that these changes may occur in the context of a

Table 28.6 Disorders of mitochondrial energy metabolism in childhood

1. Transport defects	Primary carnitine deficiency
	Carnitine palmitoyl transferase (CPT) deficiency
2. Defects of substrate utilization	Pyruvate dehydrogenase complex deficiency
	Pyruvate carboxylase complex deficiency
	Fatty acid oxidation defects: MCAD, LCAD, LCHAD, SCAD, multiple acy1 CoA dehydrogenase deficiency (GA11)
3. Krebs cycle defects	Fumarase deficiency
	Alpha ketoglutarate decarboxylation defects
4. Respiratory chain disorders	Complex I-V

number of different biochemical abnormalities, including respiratory chain disorders.

Other disorders of energy supply including **defects of beta-oxidation of fatty acids** of which the best known is **MCAD** (medium chain acyl CoA dehydrogenase deficiency), tend to appear later, either as a Reye-like illness or as a cause of sudden infant death. The long chain defects tend to be more severe and so present earlier. Later presentations may be with predominantly muscle involvement with myoglobinuria, painful muscle crises and cardiomyopathy. Transport defects may appear similarly.

Peroxismal disorders

Peroxisomes are responsible for a number of enzyme functions. For diagnostic purposes, their main roles are in beta-oxidation of **VLCFAs (very long chain fatty acids – C24 and C26)**, bile acid and plasmalogen synthesis.

Disorders of peroxisomal function fall into two main groups, those in which peroxisome biogenesis is defective so that peroxisome numbers are reduced or absent and there is generalized enzyme dysfunction, and those in which there is a single enzyme defect.

The classical example of a generalized disturbance of peroxisomal activity is **Zellweger's syn-**drome; that of a single enzyme defect, **X-linked adreno-leukodystrophy (ALD)**. In Zellweger's syndrome, there is striking craniofacial dysmorphism with a large fontanelle and high forehead. Infants are profoundly hypotonic and inactive at birth. Neonatal seizures are common and there is visual failure with a pigmentary retinopathy, cataracts and sometimes glaucoma, auditory impairment, hepatomegaly, renal cysts and calcific stippling of the epiphyses best seen at the patellae. Imaging and neuropathology reveal extensive neuronal migrational abnormalities and death occurs in the first year of life. Milder variants include infantile Refsum's and neonatal adrenoleukodystrophy (ALD).

X-linked ALD (gene maps to Xq 28) presents in boys with gait disturbance or school failure or occasionally with adrenal insufficiency. There is marked phenotypic variability in families – late onset adrenomyeloneuropathy presenting as a spastic paraparesis may be seen in families with classical ALD. Women heterozygous for X-ALD may also develop a spastic paraparesis.

Confirmation of the diagnosis requires estimation of VLCFA levels, although normal levels in plasma do not preclude the diagnosis and require assay of VLCFAs in fibroblasts.

Lysosomal disorders

This group of conditions are characterized by abnormal accumulation of substrate due to a variety of lysosomal enzyme deficiencies. They can be classified into two main groups – those in which lipid storage occurs and the mucopolysaccharidoses.

Lipid storage disorders

A number of terms are used for this group of disorders (sphingolipidoses, gangliosidoses, neurolipidoses), which may cause confusion. Sphingolipids are normal constituents of all cell membranes, the simplest consisting of a base (sphingosine) and a fatty acid. The resulting compound is called 'ceramide'. In more complex sphingolipids, different side chains are added to the ceramide. Gangliosides are complex sphingolipids present in high concentration in neurones. They consist of a ceramide + sugar(s)

+ sialic acid residue(s). Storage occurs when the normal enzymatic degradation of sphingolipids fails to occur.

Clinically, while there is wide variation in the age of onset and rate of progression, there are features in common. In particular, ocular signs (visual failure with a cherry red spot at the macula), cognitive deterioration, seizures (especially myoclonic seizures) and motor disturbance with ataxia or spasticity. Hepatosplenomegaly and bony changes signal extra CNS involvement. Late onset cases may present with an atypical phenotype with survival into adulthood.

Table 28.7 outlines features of a number of the lipid storage disorders. **Tay Sachs disease** is the most common of the gangliosidoses. It is inherited in an autosomal recessive manner (with a marked increase in gene frequency in Ashkenazi Jews). It is characterized by loss of motor milestones from around three to six months of age, initially with hypotonia, then spasticity. An exaggerated startle response, progressive macrocephaly and cherry red spot at the macula are typical, but as already noted, non-specific. **Sandhoff's** is very similar in presentation, although in this case hexosaminidase A and B are deficient, just hexosaminidase A in Tay-Sachs. A 'juvenile' form exists, misleading terminology since the onset is usually in the preschool-age child

Table 28.7 Main lipid storage disorders

Disorder	Lipid storage	Clinical features (enzyme involved)
Disorders characterized by mainly neuronal storage		
Niemann Pick disease (NPD)	Ceramide phosphorylcholine = sphingomyelin (sphinogomyelinase)	Type A (classical) early onset with hepatic failure, developmental delay, then regression with spasticity, seizures, blindness
Gaucher's	Ceramide glucose = glucocerebroside (glucocerebroside-β-glucosidase)	Type 1 (adult – non-neuronopathic
		Type 2 (acute infantile) motor and social regression. Spasticity, bulbar involvement, splenomegaly
		Type 3 (juvenile) hepatosplenomegaly, oculo motor apraxia, myoclonic epilepsy, dementia, spasticity
GM1 gangliosidosis	GM1 ganglioside (b-galactosidase)[a]	Type 1 (generalized) hepatosplenomegaly, bony changes, dementia
		Type 2 (juvenile) spasticity, ataxia, dementia
GM2 gangliosidosis	GM2 ganglioside (hexosaminidase A±B)	Type 1 (Tay Sachs)
		Type 2 (Sandhoffs)
		Macular red spot, visual failure, macrocephaly, dementia, startle
Fabry's (X-linked)	Ceramide – trihexoside (α-galactosidase)	Skin lesions, painful crises, fevers, strokes renal involvement
Disorders involving predominantly white matter		
Metachromatic leukodystrophy (MLD)	Ceramide-galactose-sulphate = sulphatide (cerebroside sulphatase, measure arylsulfatase A)	Gait disturbance, spasticity, peripheral neuropathy, dementia – late in early onset forms prominent in late onset + psychiatric disturbance
Krabbe's	Ceramide β-galactose = galactocerebroside (galactocerebroside β-galactosidase	Irritability, startle, spasticity, neuropathy seizures

[a]G refers to ganglioside; M, D, T to the number of attached sialic acid residues; 1, 2, 3 to the number of hexosides (1, tetra; 2, tri; 3, di).

with gait disturbance followed by ataxia, spasticity and dementia. A 'chronic' or 'adult' form is more often heralded by speech disturbance (dysarthria), then motor deterioration and psychiatric disorder and may simulate Freidreich's ataxia. Numerous gene mutations have been identified. The spectrum of phenotypes in GM2 gangliosidosis highlights the relevance of the disorder to paediatric and adult neurological practice.

Niemann Pick disease (NPD) refers to a group of conditions in which sphingomyelinase activity is deficient. Neurological involvement is prominent in type A, but rarely seen in type B. Type C is now considered to be a consequence of defective cholesterol esterification with normal sphingomyelinase activity in most tissues, often presenting with later onset seizures with a slow cognitive decline, and the later emergence of cataplexy and extrapyramidal signs.

In **metachromatic leukodystrophy (MLD)**, diagnostic assays of arylsulfatase A activity are complicated by finding a low level of activity in up to 2 per cent of the apparently healthy population. This pseudodeficiency may also present problems for prenatal diagnosis. Clinical presentation is characterized by neurodevelopmental regression and peripheral neuropathy. Other leukodystrophies exist without lipid storage, but with another identified metabolic defect as in Canavan's, where acylaspartase deficiency has been found in a large proportion of cases.

Mucopolysaccharidoses

Storage of mucopolysaccharides (glycosaminoglycans (GAGS)) occurs in a group of disorders characterized by dysmorphic features (coarse facies), corneal clouding, short stature with joint abnormalities and kyphoscoliosis. Mental retardation is a feature of MPS 1-H (Hurler's) and MPS111 (San Filippo's) in which it is severe, and progressive deterioration occurs. Nerve entrapment disorders especially carpal tunnel syndrome are common and craniocervical problems a feature of type 1V (Morquio) and V1 (Maroteaux–Lamy).

Phenotypes of the mucolipidoses and sialidoses overlap the mucopolysaccharidoses and lipid storage disorders. Myoclonus is a prominent feature of sialidosis 1 (cherry red spot myoclonus syndrome) and sialidosis 11.

Neuronal ceroid lipofuscinoses

The neuronal ceroid lipofuscinoses (NCLs) are a family of autosomal recessive disorders, usually with onset in childhood, characterized by abnormal storage in neurones and other cells. Progressive myoclonic epilepsy, cognitive deterioration and visual failure are markers of these disorders with death in childhood or early adulthood. An expanding number of variants are being identified and diagnosis arises from the characteristic clinical and neurophysiological features, enzyme analysis and identification of vacuolated lymphocytes or inclusion bodies, and subsequent genetics. Of the more common forms, the **juvenile type** is heralded by visual failure, with emerging educational difficulties, later seizures, mental health difficulties, speech and gait disturbance. Diagnosis is often first suggested following ophthalmology review, with identification of retinal changes and early loss of ERG, leading to the finding of vacuolated lymphocytes and then genetic confirmation. **Classical late infantile NCL** usually presents with seizures in early childhood, often with background of some speech delay. There is steady deterioration with loss of developmental skills and onset of motor difficulties with ataxia and pyramidal signs. Visual failure is a later feature. Clues may come from the abnormal response on EEG to slow photic stimulation. Lysosomal enzyme studies show low activity of tripeptyl peptidase 1 (TPP1), vacuolated lymphocytes are not found, but there are curvilinear inclusion bodies in white cells seen on electron microscopy. Again mutation analysis provides confirmation and is crucial for genetic counselling.

REFERENCES AND FURTHER READING

Aicardi J (2009) *Diseases of the Nervous System in Childhood*, 3rd edn. London: MacKeith Press (with Wiley Publishers).

Barkovich AJ, Kuzniecky RI, Jackson GD *et al.* (2005) A developmental and genetic classification for malformations of cortical development. *Neurology*, **65**: 1873–1887.

Chumas P, Tyagi A, Livingston J (2001) Hydrocephalus – what's new? *Archives of Disease in Childhood*, **85**:F149–F154.

Gray RGF, Preece MA, Green SH *et al.* (2000) Inborn errors of metabolism as a cause of neurological disease in adults: an approach to investigation. *Journal of Neurology, Neurosurgery and Psychiatry*, **69**:5–12.

Palisano R, Rosenbaum P, Walter S *et al.* (1997) Development and reliability of a system to classify gross motor function in children with cerebral palsy. *Developmental Medicine and Child Neurology*, **39**:214–223.

Rosenbaum P, Paneth N, Leviton A *et al.* (2007) A report: The definition and classification of cerebral palsy. *Developmental Medicine and Child Neurology*, **49** (Suppl. 109):S8–11.

CHAPTER 29

RESPIRATORY ASPECTS OF NEUROLOGICAL DISEASE

Robin Howard and Nicholas Hirsch

INTRODUCTION

The care of patients with neurological critical illness may differ significantly from that for those with general medical disorders in neurological units. The principle areas of concern include the short- and long-term management of coma, encephalopathy, autonomic failure and neuromuscular weakness causing ventilatory failure and impaired bulbar control. Furthermore, patients with neurological critical illness may differ from those with general medical disorders because the nature of the illness leads to an increased mean length of stay, but a potentially better prognosis.

This chapter will deal mainly with neurological conditions causing respiratory insufficiency which may require ventilatory support.

RESPIRATORY INSUFFICIENCY

Respiratory insufficiency is the inability to maintain adequate ventilation to match acid-base status and oxygenation to metabolic requirements. The initial abnormality may be intermittent nocturnal hypoventilation leading to hypercapnia and hypoxia during sleep. This eventually persists while the patient is awake and symptoms may develop concurrently. Respiratory insufficiency may develop during the course of many neurological disorders. It occurs most commonly as a consequence of neuromuscular weakness, but may also accompany disturbances of brainstem function or interruption of descending respiratory pathways. Previously unsuspected respiratory insufficiency may present as failure to wean from elective, perioperative mechanical ventilation.

Symptoms

Respiratory insufficiency may develop insidiously. There may be exertional dyspnoea, but, in neurological disease, symptoms may be present only after the development of nocturnal hypoventilation and sleep apnoea develop. Established nocturnal respiratory insufficiency is chartacterized by insomnia, daytime hypersomnolence and lethargy, morning headaches, reduced mental concentration, depression, anxiety or irritability. The symptoms of obstructive sleep apnoea are similar, but the patient or their partner often complains of snoring, abnormal sleep movements and disturbed sleep with distressing dreams. Patients with progressive diaphragm weakness develop orthopnoea which may be severe, and prevent the patient lying flat. Nocturnal orthopnoea is usually severe and can mimic paroxysmal nocturnal dyspnoea due to heart failure. A careful history is crucial in identifying the cause of generalized weakness or failure to wean in the intensive treatment unit (ITU). Evidence of pre-existing sensory and motor dysfunction should be sought from careful questioning of the patient or the patient's family. A thorough history of exposure to medications or other toxins should also be taken.

Examination

Clinical signs are often absent in the early stages of ventilatory failure and this can lead to the condition being missed. With progression, signs include unexplained tachycardia, an accentuated second heart sound over the pulmonary valve area and **signs of polycythemia**. Obesity is often present in patients with obstructive sleep apnoea, and there is increased accessory muscle activity. Diaphragmatic weakness or paralysis leads to paradoxical movement of the abdominal wall, with inspiratory indrawing of the lower lateral rib margin when the patient is supine or near supine. As the condition progresses, the full picture of respiratory failure is present and sudden unexpected death can occur. Coexisting bulbar dysfunction is revealed by clinical signs of lesions of the IXth and Xth cranial nerves, including loss of posterior pharyngeal wall sensation, reduced palatal movement and pharyngeal reflex, poor cough, impaired speech and ineffective swallowing. However, clinical signs of bulbar dysfunction are not always a good guide to the development of aspiration. Muscle weakness may be difficult to recognize in critically ill patients because the clinical examination is often limited by the presence of encephalopathy or due to sedation.

Investigations

Imaging studies (computed tomography (CT) or preferably magnetic resonance imaging (MRI)) may allow identification and characterization of a wide range of central nervous system (CNS) disorders. Electrodiagnostic studies are needed to define lesions of the peripheral nervous system in critically ill patients. Occasionally, nerve or muscle biopsy is indicated to exclude vasculitis or to distinguish an inflammatory or axonal neuropathy. Muscle biopsy may be helpful to make a diagnosis of inflammatory myopathy (polymyositis, inclusion body myositis), vasculitis and structurally distinct myopathies (glycogen storage disorders and acute quadriplegic myopathy).

Assessment

In progressive neuromuscular disease, **vital capacity (VC) falls** both because of respiratory muscle weakness and/or fatigue and reduced chest wall and lung compliance, due to micro-atelectasis and restriction of chest wall movement.

Diaphragm weakness is associated with a marked fall (greater than one-third) in VC when sitting or lying. Regular measurements of VC (both erect and supine) allow assessment of the extent and progression of respiratory muscle weakness.

Chest x-rays may show clinically unsuspected unilateral or bilateral diaphragmatic paresis, aspiration pneumonitis or bronchopneumonia. Fluoroscopic screening performed when supine may show paradoxical upward movement of the paralysed diaphragm during inspiration or, preferably, during short, sharp submaximal sniff.

Waking arterial blood gas tensions are often virtually normal during the early stages of neurological respiratory insufficiency, even when significant nocturnal hypoventilation is occurring. As the condition progresses, daytime $PaCO_2$ becomes elevated. Oximetry, however, is the measurement of choice to detect periodic sleep apnoea. However, detailed analysis of the mechanisms of sleep-induced respiratory failure require full polysomnography.

Pathophysiology

Respiratory muscle weakness, bulbar failure or disturbance of the central control of respiration contribute to nocturnal hypoventilation and may precipitate respiratory insufficiency. Although the effects of respiratory failure due to neuromuscular disease can become obvious, the initial abnormality is disordered breathing during sleep and this remains the critical period for respiratory compromise and sudden death.

Respiratory muscles

Adequate ventilation during rapid eye movement (REM) sleep is largely dependent on diaphragm function, and episodic hypoventilation or central sleep apnoea is inevitable if the diaphragm is paralysed. The consequences of respiratory muscle weakness, which may be exacerbated by scoliosis, include widespread atelectasis, reduced compliance, ventilatory perfusion inequality and impaired airway patency. Weakness of abdominal muscles also reduces the capacity to cough, as does abdominal distension caused by ileus, constipation or bladder distension. Other factors may precipitate respiratory deterioration in patients functioning with reduced reserve include obesity, anaesthesia, sedative drugs, surgery, tracheostomy complications and general medical disorders.

Sleep apnoea and alveolar hypoventilation

Periodic apnoea is conventionally divided into obstructive sleep apnoea, central sleep apnoea and nocturnal hypoventilation. In **obstructive apnoea**, there is upper airway obstruction despite normal movement of the intercostals and diaphragm. In **central apnoea**, all respiratory phased movements are absent. **Alveolar hypoventilation** is characterized by a reduced ventilatory response to CO_2 and consequent CO_2 retention in the absence of primary pulmonary disease. There is progressive reduction in the tidal volume and reduced hypoxic and hypercapnic drive which may culminate in central apnoea. These effects occur primarily during sleep, but hypercapnia may persist while awake with the development of respiratory failure.

Central control

Neural control of respiration in man may be considered to depend on three largely anatomically and functionally independent pathways, although it is clear that these systems must interact with one another.

1 Automatic (metabolic) respiration is the homeostatic system by which ventilation may be altered to maintain acid–base status and oxygenation to the metabolic requirements. It originates in localized areas of the dorsolateral tegmentum the pons and medulla in the region of the nucleus tractus solitarius and retroambigualis, descending via pathways in the ventrolateral columns of the spinal cord. It has been suggested that the abnormal patterns associated with brainstem lesions may be

of localizing value. Certainly, variations in respiratory rate and rhythm may be associated with dysfunction of the automatic or voluntary system, but there is considerable overlap in patterns and it is often impossible to exclude coexisting pulmonary pathology in the acutely ill.

2 Voluntary (behavioural) respiration operates during consciousness and allows modulation of ventilation in response to voluntary actions such as speaking, singing, breath-holding and straining. This system originates in the contralateral cortex, descending via the corticospinal tract to the segmental level. Voluntary control may be impaired by bilateral lesions affecting the descending corticospinal or corticobulbar tract and is particularly seen in association with destructive lesions of the basal pons or of the medullary pyramids and adjacent ventromedial portion which may result in the 'locked-in' syndrome.

3 Limbic (emotional) control accounts for the preservation of respiratory modulation to emotional stimuli, including laughing, coughing and anxiety, despite loss of voluntary control. This implies that descending limbic influences on automatic respiration are anatomically and functionally independent of the voluntary respiratory system. These systems appear to be largely distinct and in man, destructive lesions have occasionally enabled the study of one or other of them functioning in isolation.

PATTERNS OF RESPIRATORY IMPAIRMENT DUE TO NEUROLOGICAL DISORDERS

Cortex

Periods of apnoea are common during **complex partial and generalized seizures** (Tables 29.1 and 29.2). They may be associated with upper airway obstruction, laryngospasm and masseter spasm leading to hypoxaemia and cyanosis. Isolated apnoea may be an ictal phenomenon requiring prolonged ventilation and may contribute to sudden unexpected death in epileptics. **Convulsive status epilepticus** may be associated with prolonged

Table 29.1 Central causes of ventilatory insufficiency or failure

Cortical	Epilepsy	
	Vascular	
	Tumour	
Brainstem	Congenital (Ondine's curse)	Primary alveolar hypoventilation
		Tumour
		Vascular
		Multiple sclerosis and acute disseminated encephalomyelitis
		Motor neurone disease
	Infection	Borrelia
		Listeria
		Post-varicella encephalomyelitis
		Poliomyelitis
		Encephalitis lethargica
		Western equine encephalitis
		Paraneoplastic
		Leigh's disease
		Reye's syndrome
		Hypoxaemia
Formen magnum and upper cervical cord	Arnold Chiari malformation – cerebellar ectopia	
	Achondroplasia, osteogenesis imperfecta	
	Rheumatoid arthritis – odontoid peg compression	
	Trauma	
	Vascular	
Disorders of the spinal cord	Acute epidural compression due to neoplasm or infection	
	Acute transverse myelitis	
	Cord infarction	
	Other myelopathies (including traumatic)	
	Tetanus	
Autonomic	Multisystem atrophy	
Extrapyramidal	Idiopathic Parkinson's disease	
	Dystonia	

hypoxia which contributes to the development of cardiac arrhythmias and secondary cerebral damage. Intubation and ventilation are mandatory to prevent the development of these complications.

Hemispheric **ischaemic strokes** influence respiratory function to a modest degree. Both reduced chest wall movement and reduced contralateral diaphragmatic excursion, particularly during voluntary breathing, contralateral to the stroke have been reported. The latter association correlates well with the localization of the diaphragm cortical representation found by transcranial magnetic stimulation and positron emission tomography scanning. Patients with bilateral hemispheric cerebrovascular disease show an increased respiratory responsiveness to CO_2 and are liable to develop Cheyne–Stokes respiration suggesting disinhibition of lower respiratory centres. Such a response may persist months to years after the stroke.

Diffuse cortical vascular disease may also lead to a selective inability of voluntary breathing (respiratory apraxia). Intermittent upper airway

Table 29.2 Peripheral causes of ventilatory insufficiency or failure

Anterior horn cell	Motor neurone disease
	Poliomyelitis or post-polio syndromes
	Rabies
Multiple radiculopathies	Carcinomatous meningitis
AIDS polyradiculitis	
Polyneuropathy	Acute inflammatory demyelinating polyneuropathy (AIDP)
	Acute motor and sensory axonal neuropathy (AM SAN)
	Acute motor axonal neuropathy (AMAN)
	Critical illness polyneuropathy
	Other polyneuropathies:
	Hereditary motor-sensory
	Acute porphyria organophosphate poisoning
	Herpes zoster/varicella
	Neuralgic amyotrophy
Neuromuscular transmission defects	Myasthenia gravis
	Lambert–Eaton myasthenic syndrome
	Neuromuscular blocking agents
	Other:
	Botulism
	Toxins
	Hypermagnesaemia
	Organophosphate poisoning
Muscle	Dystrophy:
	Duchenne, Becker, limb girdle, Emery Dryfuss
	Inflammatory
	Myotonic dystrophy
	Metabolic:
	Acid maltase deficiency
	Mitochondrial myopathies
	Myopathies associated with neuromuscular blocking agents and steroids
	Acute quadriplegic myopathy
	Myopathy and sepsis
	Cachectic myopathy
	HIV-related myopathy
	Sarcoid myopathy
	Hypokalaemic myopathy
	Rhabdomyolysis
	Periodic paralysis

obstruction and apnoea due to periodic fluctuations in the position of the vocal cords is associated with cortical supranuclear palsy due to bilateral lesions of the operculum.

Brainstem

The effects of brainstem dysfunction on respiration depend on the pathology, localization and speed of onset of the lesion. In patients with bulbar lesions, particularly vascular or demyelinating, the combination of impaired swallow, abnormalities of the respiratory rhythm, reduced vital capacity and reduced or absent triggering of a cough reflex all increase the risk of aspiration pneumonia. Nocturnal upper airway occlusion may also contribute to respiratory impairment.

The most common cause of brainstem lesions which disrupt respiration is **cerebrovascular disease**. Unilateral or bilateral lateral tegmental infarcts in the pons (at or below the level of the trigeminal nucleus) leads to apneustic breathing and impairment of the CO_2 responsiveness, while similar lesions in the medulla (e.g. lateral medullary syndrome) may result in acute failure of the automatic respiration. Infarction of the basal pons (locked-in syndrome) or of the pyramids and the adjacent ventromedial portion of the medulla may lead to complete loss of the voluntary system with a highly regular breathing pattern, but a complete inability to initiate any spontaneous respiratory movements.

Respiratory abnormalities may be associated with **encephalitis** involving the brainstem. A variety of patterns occur during the acute phase and following recovery including alveolar hypoventilation, central sleep apnoea and respiratory dysrrhythmias, such as tachypnoea, myoclonic jerking of the diaphragm, apneustic, ratchet and cluster breathing. Respiratory failure has also been described as a result of **post–rubeolar** and **varicella encephalomyelitis** and **acute disseminated encephalomyelitis**.

Brainstem tumours may lead to automatic respiratory failure or central neurogenic hyperventilation. Although aspiration and bronchopneumonia are common complications of **acute bulbar demyelination**, multiple sclerosis has only rarely been associated with central disorders of respiratory rate and rhythm. Acute loss of the automatic system has been associated with large demyelinating lesions in the region of the medial lemniscus and loss of the voluntary control system with evidence of an acute demyelinating lesion at the cervicomedullary junction.

Other clinical causes of automatic respiratory failure due to brainstem disorders include other CNS infections, such as Borrelia and Listeria, post-infectious encephalomyelitis, malignant disease, either primary or secondary, or as a paraneoplastic brainstem encephalitis with anti-Hu antibodies which may cause central alveolar hypoventilation and central sleep apnoea culminating in respiratory failure.

Involuntary movements of the respiratory muscles

In **idiopathic Parkinson's disease** respiratory impairment is associated with upper airflow obstruction, reduced tidal volume, respiratory muscle weakness, restrictive defect due to respiratory muscle rigidity, abnormalities of central CO_2 sensitivity and impairment of voluntary control. Patients with primary and secondary dystonic syndromes occasionally develop severe episodes of generalized dystonia and rigidity (status dystonicus) which may be refractory to standard drug therapy. The most severe cases may develop bulbar and ventilatory failure necessitating intubation and ventilation.

Autonomic failure

Multisystem atrophy is a global term which includes many neurodegenerative disorders (see Chapter 20). A characteristic feature is paresis of the vocal cord abductors (posterior cricoarytenoids); the cords lie closely opposed leading to severe upper airway limitation during sleep and giving rise to the characteristic presenting feature of severe nocturnal stridor. Other factors also contribute to the development of respiratory insufficiency. These include abnormalities of rate, rhythm and amplitude during sleep, a reduction in central respiratory drive leading to **obstructive sleep apnoea** due to upper airway occlusion and **central sleep apnoea** due to loss of automatic control. A further important factor is the accompanying autonomic failure which contributes to impaired cardiorespiratory control mechanisms.

Foramen magnum lesions

Lesions at the foramen magnum frequently cause acute or subacute respiratory insufficiency. **Cerebellar ectopia and syringomyelia** may present with either progressive nocturnal hypoventilation, obstructive sleep apnoea or sudden respiratory arrest, usually precipitated by some intercurrent event. In patients with **rheumatoid atlantoaxial subluxation**, clinically unsuspected hypoventilation and sleep apnoea are common if there is severe medullary compression and this may contribute to the high mortality of the condition. Similar respiratory abnormalities may be associated with **achondroplasia, osteogenesis imperfecta** and **foramen magnum meningioma**.

Cervical cord

Traumatic, **demyelinating** or **vascular** lesions of the spinal cord, particularly at high cervical levels, may selectively affect respiratory control. Lesions of the anterior pathways lead to loss of automatic control and sudden nocturnal death from apnoea. The respiratory effects of traumatic or vascular lesions of the spinal cord depend on the timing of onset and the extent of involvement of the phrenic nerve supply (C3–C5). Complete lesions usually lead to sudden respiratory arrest and death unless immediate resuscitation is available. Patients with lesions at or above C3 and some patients with lesions at a lower level may require prolonged or even permanent ventilator support. Quadriparesis with levels below C4 lose intercostal and abdominal muscle function while maintaining diaphragm and spinal accessory muscles. Progressive diaphragm fatigue is an important factor in predisposing to intercurrent respiratory infection. Other complications leading to respiratory problems include impaired cough effectiveness, increased physiological arteriovenous shunting and ventilation-perfusion mismatching.

Anterior horn cell

During **acute poliomyelitis**, respiratory insufficiency occurs as a result of respiratory muscle weakness or involvement of the central respiratory control mechanisms. Respiratory insufficiency may develop many years after poliomyelitis, even in the absence of any obvious respiratory involvement during the acute illness or convalescent phase. Respiratory insufficiency is the common terminal event in **motor neurone disease** either due to respiratory muscle or bulbar weakness leading to hypoventilation, aspiration bronchopneumonia or pulmonary emboli. However, an important proportion of patients with motor neurone disease may develop respiratory insufficiency early in the course of the disease and may present with respiratory failure or even respiratory arrest.

Neuropathies

Acute idiopathic demyelinating polyneuropathy (Guillain–Barré syndrome (GBS)) (see Chapter 16) develops 1–4 weeks after an infectious illness, as a progressive weakness in the arms and legs with areflexia. The onset is relatively symmetrical and mainly motor. There may be unilateral or bilateral facial weakness. The autonomic nervous system may be affected and respiratory insufficiency requires mechanical ventilation in approximately one-third of patients.

The incidence of respiratory failure requiring mechanical ventilation in GBS is approximately 20 per cent. Ventilatory failure is primarily due to inspiratory muscle weakness, but weakness of the abdominal and accessory muscles of respiration, retained airway secretion leading to aspiration and atelectasis are all contributory factors. The associated bulbar weakness and autonomic instability contribute to the necessity for control of the airway and ventilation.

Acute motor and sensory axonal neuropathy (AMSAN) is the acute axonal form of GBS which usually presents with a rapidly developing paralysis developing over hours and rapid development of respiratory failure requiring intubation and ventilation.

There may be total paralysis of all voluntary muscles of the body, including the cranial musculature, the ocular muscles and pupils. This variant of GBS may be related to precipitating enteral infection from *Campylobacter jejuni*, and probably elevation of anti GM1 antibodies. The condition has a relatively poor outcome.

Critical illness polyneuropathy (CIP) is a sensorimotor axonal neuropathy. CIP develops in the setting of the systemic inflammatory response syndrome (SIRS). This is a severe systemic response that occurs in up to 50 per cent of those in a critical care setting in response to infection or other insults, such as burns, trauma or surgery. There is distally predominant limb weakness, atrophy and reduced reflexes. Sensory loss can be demonstrated in patients who are able to cooperate with the examination. However, the signs are variable and difficult to elicit because of sedation or coexistent encephalopathy, an even more common complication of SIRS. Nearly half of the patients affected by CIP die of their critical illness. Of those who survive, recovery mirrors that seen in most axonal neuropathies. Those who survive with mild to moderate neuropathy recover fully over months. Those with severe neuropathy either have no recovery or a significant persistent deficit.

Phrenic neuropathies

Neuralgic amyotrophy (acute brachial neuritis) may present with dyspnoea and orthopnoea due to selective or isolated involvement of the phrenic nerve causing unilateral or bilateral diaphragm paresis. Predominant phrenic nerve involvement may occur in neuropathies associated with underlying **carcinoma, diphtheria, herpes zoster-varicella, and following immunization**. Acute respiratory failure is also a feature of **vasculitic, acute porphyric and toxic neuropathies**. Similarly diaphragmatic weakness has also been described in **hereditary sensorimotor neuropathy** and this is associated with reduced transdiaphragmatic pressures and undetectable phrenic nerve conduction. However, phrenic nerve involvement occurs most commonly as a result of **trauma during thoracic surgery, hypothermia or direct involvement by neoplasm**.

Neuromuscular junction

Respiratory failure in **myasthenia gravis** often results from a myasthenic crisis (usually precipitated by infection), but is also associated with cholinergic crisis, thymectomy or steroid myopathy. Associated bulbar weakness predisposes to aspiration and acute respiratory failure necessitating urgent intubation and ventilation.

Expiratory and inspiratory intercostal and diaphragm weakness is common even when there is only mild peripheral muscle weakness. Respiratory impairment is also an important feature in **Lambert–Eaton myasthenic syndrome** where it may be precipitated by anaesthesia. In **botulism**, respiratory muscle weakness and aspiration leading to arrest is common and urgent and prolonged ventilatory support may be necessary as the prognosis is generally good.

Persistent neuromuscular blockade is associated with the use of neuromuscular blocking agents used increasingly in the intensive care unit (ICU) to improve lung compliance and allow more efficient mechanical ventilation. Other neuromuscular transmission disorders which may require admission to a critical care unit includes **organophosphate poisoning and botulism**.

Muscle

Respiratory muscle weakness is a common cause of morbidity and mortality in muscular dystrophies. In **Duchenne muscular dystrophy**, diaphragmatic weakness is not prominent but chronic respiratory insufficiency is due to intercostal weakness, scoliosis, reduced lung compliance, aspiration and repeated infections. Respiratory involvement in **Becker's muscular dystrophy** is rare and associated with global respiratory muscle weakness. In **limb girdle dystrophy (LGD)**, the major pattern of respiratory involvement is gradual, progressive global weakness of the respiratory muscles is compounded by scoliosis. However, in both LGD and **facio-scapulohumeral dystrophy**, there may be selective diaphragm involvement and respiratory tract infections are common despite the absence of clinically overt bulbar weakness. In contrast, **acid maltase deficiency** is characterized by early and selective diaphragm weakness, often with minimal involvement of other respiratory and bulbar musculature.

Congenital myopathies including mitochondrial and nemaline myopathy may present with respiratory insufficiency or develop alveolar hypoventilation early in the course of the disease. Progressive scoliosis and restrictive ventilatory insufficiency is an important complication of **Emery–Dreifuss muscular dystrophy** and the **rigid spine syndrome**.

In **dystrophia myotonica**, respiratory involvement is multifactorial. Respiratory muscle weakness may affect both the diaphragm and expiratory muscles leading to a poor cough, restrictive lung defect and alveolar hypoventilation. There is little evidence that myotonia of the respiratory muscles is a significant factor. A central abnormality contributes to alveolar hypoventilation, as may a reduced ventilatory response to CO_2 in the absence of CO_2 retention, hypersomnolence and an undue sensitivity to anaesthetics and sedatives.

Acute quadriplegic myopathy (AQM) is a myopathy seen in adult patients admitted to critical care units, and appears to be associated with exposure to high doses of glucocorticoids and non-depolarizing muscle-blocking agents to treat acute pulmonary disorders, such as asthma.

AQM can occur with other diseases. Major organ transplantation also requires the combined use of these drugs in patients with a complicated course in critical care units. Patients may present when it becomes apparent that they are quadriparetic as the acute illness resolves. Some patients have only mild weakness, but many are severely affected and weaning from the ventilator is often delayed, due to the myopathy. Extraocular muscles are often spared, but have occasionally been involved. Sensation is spared and reflexes are decreased.

MANAGEMENT OF RESPIRATORY FAILURE DUE TO NEUROLOGICAL DISEASE

It is clear from the preceding account that a diverse number of neurological conditions may result in acute or chronic respiratory failure. Often the resulting ventilatory inadequacy requires treatment in the form of assisted ventilation. The manner by which this is achieved depends on the underlying cause and its severity.

Patients with **acute neurological diseases affecting the respiratory muscles** (e.g. Guillain–Barré syndrome) are nursed in an intensive care unit and require conventional mechanical intermittent positive pressure ventilation (IPPV). If the underlying disease is readily reversible within a short period, IPPV can be delivered via a tracheal tube. However, in the majority of cases, prolonged respiratory support is needed until adequate respiratory muscle function returns. In this situation, IPPV is delivered via a **tracheostomy** which affords greater patient comfort, easier and more effective tracheobronchial suction and results in less tracheal trauma. As respiratory muscle function improves, the patient is gradually weaned from mechanical ventilation using a variety of weaning techniques.

In contrast, patients with **chronic neuromuscular disease** are often managed at home with the choice of various methods of assisted ventilation.

For reasons already stated, patients with respiratory muscle weakness may exhibit adequate ventilation while awake and upright, but develop respiratory insufficiency while asleep and supine. This group of patients derives benefit from **assisted ventilation at night**. The respiratory assistance may be delivered using negative pressure or positive pressure techniques.

Negative pressure ventilation was, for many years, the mainstay of treatment for patients with chronic neuromuscular respiratory failure. Although there are many methods described for delivering negative pressure ventilation, all rely on the principle of enclosing the chest and abdomen in an airtight rigid chamber from which air is intermittently evacuated. The resulting subatmospheric pressure around the thorax and abdomen causes air to be drawn into the lungs through the mouth and nose. Examples of negative pressure devices include tank (iron lung), jacket (Tunnicliffe) and cuirass ventilators. Unfortunately, these devices are rather cumbersome, require the patient to sleep on his back and may produce indrawing of the soft tissues of the neck resulting in upper airway obstruction. Their use tends to be confined to a small number of specialist units.

Until recently, **positive pressure ventilation** required the presence of a tracheostomy through which simple bellow-type ventilators delivered a preset tidal volume at a preset respiratory rate. Patients with normal bulbar function are managed with an uncuffed tracheostomy tube (often silver) which allows normal speech. Those patients with poor bulbar function require cuffed tracheostomy tubes to decrease the risk of pulmonary aspiration. However, more recently, methods of augmenting ventilation using **nasal positive pressure ventilation (NIPPV)** have been introduced and provide an alternative to IPPV via a tracheostomy. NIPPV is applied via a tightly fitting nasal mask, facial mask or nasal 'pillows' and requires a ventilator capable of delivering twice-normal tidal volumes since dead space is very high and the facial tissues are very compliant. Ventilators used for this purpose may deliver a set volume or more commonly a set pressure. During inspiration, the soft palate moves against the tongue and prevents the escape of air through the mouth. The newer NIPPV machines are compact and portable and have revolutionized the lives of patients with chronic neuromuscular respiratory failure.

REFERENCES AND FURTHER READING

Bolton CF (1994) Muscle weakness and difficulty in weaning from the ventilator in the critical care unit. *Chest*, **106**:1–2.

Chokroverty S (1992) The assessment of sleep disturbance in autonomic failure. In: Bannister R, Mathias CJ (eds) *Autonomic Failure*, 3rd edn. Oxford: Oxford Medical Publications, 442–461.

Ellis ER, Bye PTB, Bruderer JW, Sullivan CE (1987) Treatment of respiratory failure during sleep in patients with neuromuscular disease. *American Review of Respiratory Disease*, **135**:148–152.

Howard RS, Hirsch NP (2000) The neural control of respiratory and cardiovascular function In: Crockard A, Hayward R, Hoff JT (eds). *Neurosurgery – The Scientific Basis of Clinical Practice.* Oxford: Blackwell Scientific Publications, 289–309.

Howard RS, Wiles CM, Hirsch NP, Spencer GT (1993) Respiratory involvement in primary muscle disorders: assessment and management. *Quarterly Journal of Medicine*, **86**:175–189.

Munschauer FE, Mador MJ, Ahuja A, Jacobs L (1991) Selective paralysis of voluntary but not limbically influenced automatic respiration. *Archives of Neurology*, **48**:1190–1192.

Plum F (1970) Neurological integration of behavioural and metabolic control of breathing. In: Parker R (ed.). *Breathing: Hering-Breuer Centenary Symposium.* London: Churchill, 314–326.

Plum F, Posner JR (1983) *Diagnosis of Stupor and Coma.* Philadelphia: FA Davis.

Ropper AH (1985) Guillain–Barré syndrome: management of respiratory failure. *Neurology*, **35**:1662–1665.

Smith PEM, Edwards RHT, Calverley PMA (1991) Mechanisms of sleep disordered breathing in chronic neuromuscular disease: implications for management. *Quarterly Journal of Medicine*, **81**:961–973.

CHAPTER 30

PAIN IN NEUROLOGICAL DISEASE

John Scadding

NEUROPATHIC PAIN

Nociceptive and neuropathic pain

Pain signalled by an intact somatosensory system serves an essential protective biological function. This is **nociceptive pain**. Rapid localization and identification of the nature of a painful stimulus is required to take appropriate action to avoid injury. This normal function is emphasized by the tissue destruction that may occur in conditions in which pain pathways are severely impaired, for example, in the peripheral neuropathies of leprosy and diabetes, or in the loss of spinothalamic tract function in the spinal cord in syringomyelia.

> **Neuropathic pain** is defined as pain arising as a direct consequence of a lesion affecting the somatosensory system.

It is paradoxical that the very conditions affecting the somatosensory system, leading to loss of pain sensation, are also those that may lead to the development of neuropathic pain (NP). NP has no protective biological function, is often severe and is always difficult to treat. The purpose of this chapter is to review the features and causes of NP, and outline approaches to treatment.

Terminology

Several terms are commonly used to describe NP, some with overlapping meaning:

- **Neurogenic pain** refers to all neurological causes of pain and although differently defined in the past, to all intents and purposes it now has the same meaning as neuropathic pain in clinical practice.
- **Neuralgia** describes pain arising in the distribution of a nerve or nerves. It is usually restricted to describe NP due to a lesion of a single nerve, for example intercostal, sciatic, femoral or trigeminal, or a sensory spinal nerve root, in the case of postherpetic neuralgia.
- **Central pain** describes NP caused by lesions within the central nervous system – either spinal cord or brain.

In the peripheral nervous system, NP is caused particularly by conditions affecting small nerve fibres, and in the central nervous system by lesions of the spinothalamic tract and thalamus, and rarely by subcortical and cortical lesions. The clinical feature common to virtually all conditions leading to the development of NP is the experience of pain in an area of sensory impairment, although sensory loss may be mild and difficult to detect, often being overshadowed by abnormal skin sensitivity (allodynia – see below under Stimulus-dependent pain: allodynia, hyperalgesia and hyperpathia). In the great majority of cases of trigeminal neuralgia, there is clinically no detectable sensory loss, and this is, for practical purposes, the only exception to this rule (see Chapter 11).

Classification and causes of neuropathic pain

It is not yet possible to classify NP in terms of mechanism, and the classification remains anatomical and aetiological (Tables 30.1 and 30.2). The mechanisms of NP are still only partly

Table 30.1 Painful peripheral neuropathies

Peripheral neuropathies	
Traumatic mononeuropathies	
Entrapment neuropathies	
Amputation stump pain (nerve transaction, partial or complete)	
Causalgia	
Intercostal neuralgia (post-thoracotomy)	
Morton's neuralgia (plantar digital nerve entrapment)	
Painful scars	
Other mononeuropathies and multiple mononeuropathies	
Postherpetic neuralgia	
Diabetic mononeuropathy	
Diabetic amyotrophy (proximal diabetic neuropathy)	
Malignant plexus invasion	
Radiation plexopathy	
Neuralgic amyotrophy (inflammatory brachial plexopathy)	
Trigeminal and glossopharyngeal neuralgia	
Borrelia infection	
Connective tissue disease (vasculitis)	
Herpes simplex	
Polyneuropathies	
Metabolic and nutritional	Diabetes mellitus
	Alcohol
	Amyloid
	Beriberi (vitamin B1 deficiency)
	Burning feet syndrome
	Pellagra (nicotinic acid deficiency)
	Strachan's syndrome (Jamaican neuropathy)
	Tanzanian neuropathy
	Cuban neuropathy
Drugs	Antiretrovirals
	Vincristine
	Cisplatin
	Ethambutol
	Isoniazid
	Disulfiram
	Nitrofurantoin
	Thalidomide
	Thiouracil
Toxins	Acrylamide
	Thallium
	Arsenic
	Clioquinol
	Dinitrophenol
	Ethylene oxide
Hereditary	Amyloid neuropathy
	Fabry's disease

	Charcot–Marie–Tooth disease type V, type 2B
	Hereditary sensory and autonomic neuropathy, type I, type IB
Malignant	Paraneoplastic
	Myeloma
Infective/postinfective/immune	Acute inflammatory polyradiculoneuropathy (Guillain–Barré syndrome)
	Borreliosis
	HIV (human immunodeficiency virus)
Other polyneuropathies	Idiopathic small fibre neuropathy
	Trench foot (non-freezing cold injury)
	Erythromelalgia

Table 30.2 Causes of central neuropathic pain

Anatomical site	Cause of central neuropathic pain
Spinal root/dorsal root ganglion	Prolapsed disc
	Arachnoiditis
	Trigeminal neuralgia
	Glossopharyngeal neuralgia
	Root avulsion
	Tumour
	Post-herpetic neuralgia
	Surgical rhizotomy
Spinal cord	Trauma, including compression
	HIV
	Multiple sclerosis
	B12 deficiency
	Syphilis
	Syringomyelia
	Spinal dysraphism
	Infarction, haemorrhage, AVM
	Surgical anterolateral cordotomy
Cranial nerve root/ganglion	Trigeminal neuralgia
	Glossopharyngeal neuralgia
Brain stem	Lateral medullary syndrome
	Syrinx
	Multiple sclerosis
	Tumours
	Tuberculoma
Thalamus	Infarction
	Haemorrhage
	Tumours
	Surgical thalamotomy
Subcortical and cortical	Infarction
	AVM
	Trauma
	Tumour

AVM, arteriovenous malformation.

understood, but there are numerous pathophysiological properties that develop following damage to the peripheral or central sensory pathways, and which are likely to be the basis for NP (see below under Pathophysiology of NP).

Clinical features of neuropathic pain

NP comprises ongoing stimulus-independent pains and evoked stimulus-dependent pains (allodynia, hyperalgesia and hyperpathia) (Table 30.3). These stimulus-dependent pains are frequently major symptoms of the overall pain complaint. In addition, NP is often associated with comorbidities that can have a major impact on quality of life, and which also require careful assessment.

Stimulus-independent, ongoing pain

NP, being produced by abnormal sensory mechanisms, has qualities that patients find difficult to describe, as it is outside their previous experience of 'normal' (nociceptive) pain. The most usual descriptions of the ongoing pains are deep aching in the

Table 30.3 Clinical features of neuropathic pain

	Clinical feature
Ongoing pain (stimulus independent)	Abnormal character: burning, stinging, pricking, shock-like
	Paroxysmal pains common
	May radiate beyond expected anatomical extent
Stimulus-dependent pain	Allodynia
	Hyperalgesia
	Hyperpathia
Sensory loss	Usually in an anatomical distribution
Associated sympathetic changes	Vascular
	Temperature
	Sweating
Comorbidities	Depression
	Anxiety
	Disturbed sleep

extremities and a superficial burning, stinging or pricking pain. Other words used include electric shocks, stabbing pain, tingling and unpleasant itching. NP is often poorly localized and may be continuous, intermittent or paroxysmal.

Paroxysmal pains are characteristic of some NPs, for example trigeminal neuralgia, the lightning pains of tabes dorsalis and the painful crises of the neuropathy in Fabry's disease. Paroxysmal pains may also occur in NP due to almost any cause, both peripheral and central.

Stimulus-dependent pain: allodynia, hyperalgesia and hyperpathia

Evoked, stimulus-dependent pains include allodynia, hyperalgesia and hyperpathia, to mechanical, thermal or chemical stimulation.

- **Allodynia** is pain resulting from a stimulus that does not normally provoke a painful sensation.
- **Hyperalgesia** is an increased response to a stimulus that is normally painful. In hyperalgesia, normally noxious stimuli are often associated with a lowering of the pain threshold, together with an exaggerated perception of pain. In clinical practice, the term 'hyperalgesia' tends to be loosely used to describe abnormally painful responses to stimuli that are normally not painful, so that strictly speaking, these fall into the category of allodynia rather than hyperalgesia.

In **static hyperalgesia**, gentle pressure on the skin causes pain. In **punctate hyperalgesia**, stimuli such as pinprick evoke pain. In **dynamic hyperalgesia**, light brushing of the skin evokes pain (as mentioned above, this is really a form of allodynia). In **heat and cold hyperalgesia**, warm and cool stimuli respectively evoke pain. In the physical examination to elicit these signs, hot and cold stimuli are used that are not normally painful, at 40 and 20°C, so again these are further examples of allodynia. Dynamic hyperalgesia is a particularly unpleasant component of NP for many patients, caused by the friction of clothes brushing against the skin.

In **hyperpathia**, there is a raised sensory threshold, delay in perception of a stimulus, an abnormally painful reaction, with summation (increasing pain) to repetitive stimuli, and a painful after-sensation, sometimes longlasting. Hyperpathia is often severe and may have an explosive character, due to rapid summation. The raised sensory threshold of hyperpathia results from partial loss of afferent input, and the summation and after-sensation are due mainly to central sensitization.

Radiation of neuropathic pain

NP may be localized to the anatomical area corresponding to the causative neurological lesion, either peripheral or central, and this is useful in neurological diagnosis. However, NP often radiates well beyond the distribution of the expected neural anatomical territory. This is true particularly for the stimulus-dependent components of NP. Furthermore, the more severe the NP, the more likely it is to radiate widely.

Non-neurological pain in patients with neuropathic pain

It is important to recognize that NP and nociceptive pain often coexist, and it is necessary to characterize the different components of a patient's pain by careful clinical assessment, leading to appropriate investigation, accurate diagnosis and correct treatment.

A common example serves to illustrate this: in cervical and lumbar spine disease, pain described by patients is often of both musculoskeletal (nociceptive) and neuropathic types (radicular and/or myelopathic in the case of cervical disease). In these situations, the description of the pain and its distribution may not clearly discriminate between the two types, particularly when the pain is unilateral. Careful examination, both neurological and musculoskeletal, together with the results of electrophysiological testing and imaging are often needed. Even so, in some patients there can be continuing doubt about the relative contributions of the different types of pain. Matters are further complicated when there has been previous cervical or lumbar surgery.

Other painful consequences of neurological disease include arthropathies, postural abnormalities, skeletal deformities, spasticity, contractures and dystonia. For example, in patients with painful diabetic peripheral neuropathy, there is NP in a distal distribution in the legs and feet, but there

may also be pain due to vascular insufficiency, foot and ankle arthropathies, or diabetic skin ulceration. This emphasizes the need for clinical awareness and careful diagnostic assessment.

Sensory loss in patients with NP

Sensory loss is usually found in a distribution that is anatomically appropriate to the lesion causing the NP, but as described above, in NP the symptoms and signs may radiate beyond the expected anatomical area. In addition, sensory impairment can be subtle, particularly when overshadowed by allodynia, hyperalgesia or hyperpathia. The degree of sensory loss and the severity of ongoing and evoked NP are not closely related. Trigeminal neuralgia (Chapter 11) is the only neuropathic pain in which cutaneous sensation is usually normal on routine physical examination.

Loss of pain and temperature sensations, due to selective small fibre involvement, is often found in peripheral neuropathies causing NP. In the case of central lesions in the spinal cord or brain causing NP, it is likely that sensory loss is of spinothalamic type will be found.

Sympathetic activity and NP

While there is substantial animal experimental evidence of a role for sympathetic efferent adrenergic activity in the initiation and maintenance of pain after neural injury, there is little evidence of its importance in man. This is discussed further below under Complex regional pain syndrome.

Sensory examination in patients with NP

From this account of the symptoms and signs associated with NP, it can be appreciated that the sensory examination in patients suspected of having NP requires care. Thresholds and suprathreshold responses to light touch and pin-prick stimulation are assessed, followed by dynamic (brushing) and repetitive stimulation to assess the presence of allodynia and hyperpathia.

Cold and heat are best tested either with metal rollers kept at 20 and 40°C, or with water-filled tubes, although these also test touch and dynamic mechanical stimulation, respectively. To overcome this, radiant heat sources or lasers can be used for selective thermal testing in selected patients. Thermal threshold testing using a thermocouple with a Peltier element is now performed routinely in many neurophysiological laboratories, supplementing clinical examination (see Chapter 5).

Examination of vibration and joint position sensations as usual aids anatomical localization, and together with cutaneous sensory modalities, provides information about the density and selectivity of sensory modality loss.

Comorbidities of NP

Comorbidities are particularly common in patients with NP. They contribute to suffering and loss of function, and can markedly impair quality of life. The major comorbidities include depression, anxiety, altered sleep patterns, social isolation and loss of employment.

It is worth noting that pain may be a symptom of primary psychiatric disease, particularly depression (for example atypical facial pain; see Chapter 11) and somatization disorders (see Chapter 31).

Anxiety is related to pain severity, delay in making an accurate diagnosis, poor response to treatment, fear of disease progression and worsening of pain, and the social and financial consequences of the illness.

Substance abuse can be an important cause of comorbidity in patients with chronic pain, and the adverse effects of prescribed medications also frequently cause problems, including sedation, fatigue, dysphoria and depression.

Routine clinical assessment will uncover the presence and severity of these comorbidities, and an array of measurement tools and scales is available for use in selected patients (see Further reading).

Pathophysiology of NP

The symptoms and signs of NP cannot yet be tightly linked with cellular, physiological and neuropharmacological changes. However, data derived mainly from studies in animals show the multitude of changes that occur following peripheral or central nervous system damage. Increasingly, investigative techniques, such as microneurography and skin biopsy in peripheral neuropathies, positron emission tomography (PET) and functional magnetic resonance imaging (MRI) are contributing data of direct relevance to human disease.

The major pathophysiological changes can be categorized under five main headings:

1 Ectopic impulse generation in damaged sensory fibres
2 Central sensitization, resulting from an abnormal primary afferent input
3 Disinhibition, due a failure or reduction of normal peripheral and central inhibitory mechanisms
4 Degenerative and regenerative processes (plasticity), leading to altered connectivity in the central nervous system (CNS)
5 Imbalance of activity in central pathways

Tables 30.4 and 30.5 summarize these properties in the peripheral and central nervous system, respectively, and attempt to relate underlying pathophysiological properties to the symptoms and signs of NP. The reader is referred to Further reading for a fuller account of this complex subject.

TREATMENT OF NEUROPATHIC PAIN

General considerations

NP is more difficult to treat effectively than most nociceptive pains and the range of specific therapies is still limited. NP and its comorbidities impose a substantial burden for many patients, often compounded by other neurological deficits, such as motor and sensory loss.

When NP is due to compression of peripheral nerves, spinal roots and sometimes of the spinal cord, surgical decompression can partly or completely relieve pain. However, this cannot be guaranteed, particularly if compression has been prolonged.

The place of other surgical interventions for neuropathic pain is very limited. Ablative operations that produce new lesions in the somatosensory system to relieve NP, may do so temporarily, but are themselves potent causes of NP, with onset at variable latency following surgery, ranging from days to years (see below under Surgical neuroablative treatment).

When NP is anatomically limited in extent and particularly when it is associated with allodynia,

Table 30.4 Mechanisms of peripheral neuropathic pain

	Sensory fibre type	Mechanism
Stimulus-independent pain		
Ongoing pain	A delta and C fibres	Ectopic impulse generation in damaged and regenerating peripheral axons and dorsal root ganglion cells
Sympathetically maintained pain	A beta, A delta and C fibres	Sensitization due to expression of alpha-adrenergic receptors in regenerating axons
Deafferentation pain	None, generated centrally in spinal cord	Loss of primary afferent fibres leading to disinhibition of dorsal horn cells in spinal cord Partial, e.g. postherpetic neuralgia Complete, e.g. brachial plexus avulsion
Radiation of pain	A beta, A delta or C fibres	Recruitment of dorsal horn neurons over several spinal cord segments
Stimulus-dependent pain		
Light touch	C fibres	Sensitized C fibres
Light brush/stroking- dynamic hyperalgesia and allodynia	A beta fibres	Sensitization of dorsal horn neurons by nociceptor input and maintained by a low threshold (A beta) fibre peripheral input
Pinprick hyperalgesia	A delta fibres	Central sensitization initiated, but not maintained by nociceptor input
Cold hyperalgesia	Cold sensitive C fibres	Central disinhibition and probably also peripheral sensitization
Heat hyperalgesia	C fibres	Sensitization of peripheral nociceptors
Hyperpathia	Nociceptors or A beta fibres	Recruitment of dorsal horn wide dynamic range neurons over several segments of the spinal cord

hyperalgesia or hyperpathia, the focus should be on trials of local measures. Such measures are often partly effective, and they may obviate the need for systemic drug treatment, which is frequently associated with adverse effects, particularly in older patients.

The majority of patients with chronic NP will benefit from a multimodality approach to their treatment, including measures for the pain itself and the associated comorbidities, such as depression. Management in integrated multidisciplinary pain clinics with input from neurologists, anaesthetists, psychologists, psychiatrists, physiotherapists and occupational therapists represents best practice and is increasingly becoming the norm.

Local treatments

Local anaesthetic injections

Local anaesthetic blocks of peripheral nerves, plexuses or spinal roots can sometimes be helpful diagnostically, although an effective sensory spinal root block may mask a more peripheral lesion. The effect of local anaesthetic is short-lived and so of limited use in the treatment of chronic NP. The addition of corticosteroid may prolong the effect in some nerve blocks, but the effect is unpredicatable.

Topical local anaesthetic

In patients with limited areas of allodynia, skin patches impregnated with local anaesthetic are sometimes highly effective. A cheaper alternative is the application of simple 5 per cent lignocaine ointment. Topical local anaesthetic has been shown to be beneficial in painful polyneuropathy (for example due to diabetes), post-herpetic neuralgia and a variety of other NPs.

Topical capsaicin

Capsaicin, the pungent ingredient of chilli peppers, binds to vanilloid receptors and causes depolarization of afferent C fibres, with release of substance P. This agonist action leads to burning pain on first

Table 30.5 Mechanisms of central neuropathic pain

Site	Pathology and pathophysiology	Central pain symptoms
Spinal cord	Deafferentation disinhibition (see **Table 30.4**)	Ongoing pain
	Development of inappropriate neural connections, resulting from aberrant regeneration	Innocuous peripheral stimuli cause pain in partial lesions. Border zone allodynia and hyperalgesia; below-lesion pain
	Loss of inhibitory neurons in the dorsal horn, resulting from peripheral lesions	Reduced effectiveness of local and descending inhibitions in spinal cord: ongoing and evoked pain
	Inflammatory changes in dorsal horn neurons, with increased intracellular calcium, synthesis of nitric oxide and prostaglandins	Sensitization of dorsal horn neurons to afferent peripheral input: ongoing and evoked pain
	Increased excitatory amino acid receptor activation, particularly glutamate	Central sensitization (spinal cord generation of pain): ongoing and evoked pain
	Abnormal expression of sodium and calcium channels	Central sensitization: ongoing and evoked pain
	Imbalance in central pathways: dorsal columns and spinothalamic tract spinothalamic and spinoreticulothalamic	Ongoing and evoked pain
	Thalamic reorganization secondary to spinal changes: altered thalamic neuron receptive fields bursting activity in disinhibited thalamic neurons	Ongoing and paroxysmal pains
Brain	Thalamic lesions:	Lesions in these nuclei most likely to cause ongoing central pain (including central post stroke pain (CPSP))
	ventroposterior nuclei reticular nucleus medial/intralaminar nuclei	
	Thermosensory disinhibition: loss of cold activated spinothalamic tract projections that normally inhibit burning sensations	Ongoing pain – following thalamic and spinal lesions
	Thalamocortical lesions	Occasional cause of ongoing central pain
	Reactivation of 'memory' of deafferented region and long-term potentiation; possibly due to N-methyl-D-aspartate (NMDA) receptor and calcium channel activation	Delayed onset of central pain (e.g. CPSP)

application, and this frequently limits the clinical use of capsaicin. With repeated topical application, there is prolonged depletion of substance P and it is probably this action that leads to desensitization of afferent C fibres and reduction in allodynia and hyperalgesia. Topical capsaicin 0.075 per cent has been demonstrated in clinical trials to be effective in painful diabetic neuropathy, postherpetic neuralgia and post-surgical pain, but is not effective in HIV neuropathy.

Topical amitriptyline

The systemic effect of tricyclic antidepressants in NP is well established (see below under Systemic drugs), but topical application has recently been shown to be also effective, partly due to local and partly to systemic (CNS) actions. This has been demonstrated in both peripheral and central causes of NP. Trials of other drugs, applied topically, are underway. The benefits of achieving analgesia by this route, with reduction in the adverse effects of systemic medication, are obvious.

Systemic drug treatment

Interpretation of drug trials for NP

The quality of trials of drug treatment for NP has improved considerably over the past two decades, with better trial design and the measure of multiple outcomes, in recognition of the multidimensional nature of NP.

A widely used metric of the effectiveness of treatments for NP in clinical trials with dichotomous data is the number needed to treat (NNT), defined as the number of patients who have to be treated to produce pain relief in one patient. The degree of analgesia required for a positive effect is usually set at 50 or 30 per cent, the latter figure equating to a value patients describe as at least 'moderate' pain relief. Conversely, the number needed to harm (NNH) provides a clinically useful measure of safety and acceptability of a drug. This is defined as the number of patients who need to be treated for one patient to stop taking medication due to adverse effects.

Comparison of data from different trials remains difficult, and interpretation of NNTs calculated from pooled data needs to be cautious. This is due to a number of methodological factors, including trial design (parallel or crossover), different drug dosages, variation in the scales and instruments used for assessment of pain severity, baseline pain scores at the time of entry to the trial, variable inclusion of comorbidity data, clinically heterogeneous patient inclusion, incomplete reporting of results including adverse effects, variable magnitude of placebo effects in different trials, and under-reporting of trials producing negative results.

It should be emphasized that many mechanisms contribute to the development and maintenance of NP (Tables 30.4 and 30.5), so it is not surprising that a single drug usually produces only partial analgesia. In NP, there is a tendency to use multiple drugs in combination and this inevitably leads to a high incidence of adverse effects.

Table 30.6 summarizes NNT values for systemic drug treatment of peripheral, central and mixed neuropathic pain, together with some NNH values from trials where these have been calculated.

Actions of different drug classes used for treatment of NP

Antidepressant drugs

Tricyclic antidepressant drugs (TCAD) have a serotoninergic action, enhancing the inhibitory effect of descending pathways from brain stem to the dorsal horn of the spinal cord. However, this is unlikely to be the only mechanism of action in NP, because the selective serotonin reuptake inhibitors (SSRI) have a greater such action, but are less effective in relieving NP. TCAD also block the uptake of noradrenaline, and may also produce analgesia by potentiating the effect of descending noradrenergic inhibitory pathways to the dorsal horn of the spinal cord.

TCAD may also help the frequent comorbidity of NP, depression. The mechanisms of action of TCAD in chronic pain and depression are different and distinct, as the analgesic effect is achieved before an antidepressant effect. Furthermore, an analgesic effect may occur without relief of associated depression, and an analgesic effect may occur in patients with NP who are not depressed.

The lesser effectiveness of the SSRI is reflected in the higher NNTs listed in Table 30.6. Selective serotonin and noradrenaline reuptake inhibitors (SNRI) have an effect that appears to be superior to SSRI.

Neuroleptic drugs

The use of neuroleptic drugs in the treatment of NP, both alone or more commonly in combination with TCAD, was once popular. However, evidence of effectiveness of this class of drug is limited. This, together with the serious adverse effects of long-term therapy has resulted in the demise of neuroleptic treatment for NP.

Anticonvulsant drugs

Carbamazepine and **phenytoin** are sodium channel blockers that stabilize neural membranes via this action.

The discovery of the specificity of the effect of carbamazepine in trigeminal neuralgia in the 1960s (see Chapter 11) led to widespread use of carbamazepine and phenytoin for treatment of all other types of NP, without support from well-conducted clinical trials. More recent trial data have

Table 30.6 Drug treatment of neuropathic pain

Drug	Peripheral neuropathic pain NNT	Central neuropathic pain NNT	Mixed neuropathic pain NNT	NNH
Antidepressants:				
TCAD	2.1–2.8	4.0	–	14.7
SSRI	6.8	–	–	–
SNRI	5.5	–	–	–
Combined	3.3	4.0	1.6	16.7
Anticonvulsant drugs:				
Phenytoin	2.1	–	–	–
Carbamazepine	2.3	–	–	–
GBP and PGB	3.9–4.6	–	–	–
Lamotrigine	4.0–5.4	–	–	–
Valproate	2.1–2.4	–	–	6.3
Topiramate	7.4	–	–	10.6
Combined	4.2	–	10.1	
Opioids:				
Strong opioids	2.3–3.0	–	2.1	17.1
Tramadol	3.5–4.8	–	–	9.0
NMDA antagonists:				
Dextromethorphan	2.5–3.4	–	–	8.8
Antiarrhythmics:				
Mexiletine	2.2–7.8	–	–	–
Topical lignocaine	4.4	–	–	–
Cannabinoids	–	3.4	9.5	–
Topical capsaicin	3.2–11.0	–	–	11.5

Pooled data, adapted from Finnerup *et al.* (2005).

GBP, gabapentin; NMDA, N-methyl-ᴅ-aspartate; NNH, number needed to harm (see text); NNT, number needed to treat (see text); PGB, pregabalin; SNRI, selective noradrenaline and serotonin reuptake inhibitors; SSRI, selective serotonin reuptake inhibitors; TCAD, tricyclic antidepressant drugs.

demonstrated the ineffectiveness of both drugs in peripheral and central NP.

Gabapentin and **pregabalin** bind to the alpha-2-delta subunit of voltage-dependent calcium channels, modulating neurotransmitter release from primary afferent terminals, via an action on interneurones in the dorsal horn of the spinal cord. Both drugs have been shown to be effective analgesics in painful diabetic neuropathy and postherpetic neuralgia.

Lamotrigine has an inhibitory effect on voltage-sensitive sodium channels, and inhibits release of the excitatory amino acids glutamate and aspartate, stabilizing neuronal membranes. It has been shown to be effective in painful diabetic neuropathy, with a weak effect in HIV neuropathy and central post-stroke pain, but no effect in myelopathic pain due to spinal injury.

Sodium valproate has several actions by which it might have an analgesic effect in NP. These include increased synthesis and release of GABA, sodium channel blockade and reduced neuronal excitability to glutamate. However, the results of clinical trials have been inconsistent. Valproate may have a weak analgesic effect in patients with diabetic neuropathy and postherpetic neuralgia, but not in other types of NP.

Topiramate stabilizes neuronal membranes

by several mechanisms, including anti-glutamate effects, sodium channel blockade, and enhancement of GABA-mediated inhibitory actions. However, only one trial has demonstrated a weak effect in painful diabetic neuropathy, and all trials have shown a high incidence of unacceptable adverse effects.

Opioids

Although it was previously taught that opioids were ineffective in NP, recent trials have shown an analgesic effect in peripheral NP, including diabetic neuropathy, postherpetic neuralgia and phantom limb pain. The potential adverse effects of opioid treatment need to be recognized and carefully monitored. The effect of a weak opioid, such as dihydrocodeine, should be assessed before progression to a medium strength opioid, such as tramadol, and finally, with caution, to strong opioids, such as morphine or fentanyl. Unless there is clear benefit, these drugs should be withdrawn at an early stage.

NMDA antagonists

NMDA antagonists such as ketamine block the afferent C fibre 'wind-up' of dorsal horn neurons (see Table 30.3). Intravenous ketamine and other NMDA antagonists produce transient pain relief in NP lasting minutes or hours at most. However, serious adverse effects include sedation and hallucinations. Overall, the majority of clinical trials have shown no long-term benefit in either peripheral or central NP.

Antiarrhythmics

Lignocaine, a non-specific sodium channel blocker, relieves NP for a few minutes when given intravenously. Trials of mexiletine, the oral analogue of lignocaine, have been disappointing in NP, showing an absence of effect in the majority of trials.

Cannabinoids

Cannabinoid receptors (CB1) are present in the thalamus, periaqueductal grey and rostroventromedial medulla. In the spinal cord, receptors are expressed in the superficial dorsal horn and dorsolateral funiculus; and several endogenous ligands have been found, the so-called 'endocannabinoids'. Trials of natural and synthetic cannabinoids are ongoing. In summary, there is evidence of a modest

analgesic action in NP, together with a clinically important incidence of adverse effects.

> **Recommendations for drug treatment of NP**
>
> On the basis of currently available evidence, the following schedule is suggested for systemic drug treatment of **peripheral NP**:
>
> - TCAD, or gabapentin or pregabalin if TCAD are contraindicated
> - Gabapentin or pregabalin. There is currently no evidence to indicate superiority of one of these drugs above the other
> - SNRI.
> - Tramadol
> - Oxycodone or other strong opioid
>
> For **central NP**, in which there is evidence from fewer controlled clinical trials, the following order is suggested:
>
> - Gabapentin or pregabalin
> - TCAD, if not contraindicated
> - Lamotrigine, tramadol, cannabinoids and strong opioids (insufficient evidence at the moment to rank these drug classes further).

Epidural drug treatment

The scope for spinal drug treatment of chronic NP is limited, the principal indication being severe spinal root pain that is resistant to all other measures. Single injections of local anaesthetic and corticosteroid may relieve chronic root pain refractory to other treatments, sometimes for days or even weeks, and this may be a useful form of treatment in a few patients.

Lignocaine and opioids, such as fentanyl, act synergistically when given via the epidural route, and the analgesic action is prolonged by the addition of adrenaline, which reduces the absorption and clearance of both drugs, without reducing spinal cord blood flow. Although epidural infusions can be very effective for the treatment of severe root pain, there is a tendency for epidural fibrosis and adhesions to develop, limiting the long-term usefulness of the treatment.

Accurate placement of the epidural catheter is essential in achieving good analgesia, and loss of an initial therapeutic effect is often the result of catheter tip migration. The technique is not without serious adverse effects: these include haemodynamic disturbances, sensory loss and motor paralysis, loss of bladder function, respiratory problems due to rostral spread of the infused opioid in the epidural space, infection, granuloma formation, and intraspinal bleeding with haematoma formation leading to cord compression.

As a result, epidural treatment is used only in carefully selected patients, in whom all other less invasive measures have failed.

Sympatholysis and sympathectomy

The rationale for and place of sympathetic block and sympathectomy is considered later, together with the treatment of complex regional pain syndrome (CRPS).

Neural stimulation

The therapeutic effects of physical measures, including various forms of electrical stimulation and acupuncture, have been recognized since ancient times. The gate control theory of Melzack and Wall, in 1965, proposed that non-painful large fibre stimulation in the periphery would inhibit the activation of cells in the dorsal horn of the spinal cord by C fibre, noxious inputs.

Acupuncture, transcutaneous electrical nerve stimulation (TENS) and other forms of peripheral counterstimulation, and electrical stimulation of the CNS, are difficult to study in clinical trials, due to the obvious problems of adequate blinding and placebo control. However, neurophysiological mechanisms for the production of analgesia have been established for each of these treatments in experimental situations, and there is a limited evidence base for efficacy in patients with both nociceptive and neuropathic pains.

Transcutaneous electrical nerve stimulation

TENS inhibits nociceptive transmission in the spinal cord and possibly also by inducing inhibition in the thalamus. Recruitment of these inhibitions is dependent on stimulus frequency and intensity.

Trials have shown limited efficacy of TENS in patients with various types of nociceptive pains. Trials have also demonstrated some effectiveness in patients with peripheral NP, although in central NP the evidence is weaker.

Although unpredictable in its effect, a trial of TENS should be considered in patients with NP, particularly when the pain is relatively localized, which is more likely to be the case with NP due to peripheral nerve, plexus or root lesions than with CNS causes of NP. TENS is not advisable in patients with cardiac pacemakers, and is generally considered to be contraindicated in pregnancy, particularly during the first trimester.

TENS and some other forms of counterstimulation give patients active personal involvement and some control over the treatment of their pain, and this may help to counter feelings of helplessness that are frequently associated with chronic NP.

Acupuncture

Acupuncture (ACP) activates sensory A delta and C fibres and is thus itself usually painful to some extent. Evidence suggests that ACP analgesia is mediated by stimulation of endogenous opioid mechanisms. ACP produces an increase in cerebral spinal fluid (CSF) endorphin concentrations, and ACP-induced analgesia can be blocked or reversed with naloxone.

Unfortunately, there have been few well-controlled clinical trials of ACP, because convincing sham ACP is difficult to achieve. ACP may have a place in the treatment of tension-type headache. A Cochrane systematic review of ACP for the treatment of non-specific low back pain found no convincing evidence of benefit. A trial in patients with painful diabetic neuropathy indicated some effect, but there is currently no evidence in other peripheral or central causes of NP.

Vibration, heat and cold stimulation

There is some evidence that vibration relieves nociceptive pain of musculoskeletal origin. Vibration has been shown in a single controlled trial to relieve amputation stump and phantom limb pain. Other types of counterstimulation, including hot and cold packs and massage, are sometimes reported to be helpful by patients with NP, particularly cold packs in postherpetic neuralgia. However the use of these methods is not supported by strong evidence from clinical trials.

Peripheral nerve stimulation

Direct stimulation of peripheral nerves, requiring operative placement of electrodes, has been suggested as a treatment for NP due to lesions of single peripheral limb nerves and in occipital neuralgia.

However, there are technical difficulties with this technique and it is rarely used in clinical practice.

Spinal cord stimulation

Spinal cord stimulation (SCS) can be performed either by percutaneous epidural insertion of an electrode stimulating the dorsal aspect of the spinal cord, or by open operation. Stimulation produces both ascending activity and retrograde descending activity in the dorsal columns. Both ascending and descending stimulation may be important in producing analgesia, at spinal (dorsal horn) and supraspinal (thalamic) levels, respectively.

SCS is effective in pain relief and restoration of the microcirculation in chronic limb ischaemia, and has found a place in the treatment of NP, particularly the failed back surgery syndrome (FBSS), in which there is usually a mixture of nociceptive and neuropathic pains. However, a large systematic review concluded that there was limited evidence of efficacy.

Given the limited evidence base, a reasonable recommendation currently is that SCS should only be considered for patients with FBSS and other intractable radicular pains, including postherpetic neuralgia, and stump and phantom limb pain, when all other less invasive measures have been tried and have failed. Technical problems due to electrode migration are common with SCS, leading to loss of an initial analgesic effect after weeks or months, and it is thought that physiological adaptation to the SCS may be an additional reason for loss of an initial analgesic effect.

Brain stimulation

Reports of pain relief from stimulation of deep sites within the brain emerged in the 1960s, but although many studies have been reported, the technical difficulties, expense, variations in clinical assessment and problems of conducting well-controlled studies in sufficient numbers of patients have all contributed to inconsistent results. Three brain sites have been particularly targeted: the sensory thalamus, the periaqueductal and periventricular grey matter, and more recently, the motor cortex.

Clear indications for **thalamic stimulation** have not been established, and as with SCS, an initial good effect of stimulation may be lost after weeks or months.

Periaqueductal or periventricular grey matter stimulation in the upper midbrain and medial thalamus produces a strong analgesic effect in experimental animals, by an endogenous opioid-mediated mechanism, reversible with naloxone. Adverse effects include dysphoria and diplopia.

There has been a recent resurgence of interest in this technique for the treatment of chronic pain, but its place, either for nociceptive pain or NP, remains to be established.

Motor cortex stimulation (MCS), at a strength that does not lead to motor activation, has recently been reported to be effective in the treatment of central post-stroke pain and trigeminal anaesthesia dolorosa and results from further trials are awaited with interest. Based on the results of PET studies, the mechanism of action may be an inhibitory action in several brain areas of importance in pain processing and perception, including the ventral lateral thalamus, cingulate gyrus, insula and brainstem.

Surgical neuroablative treatment

Surgical treatment to decompress peripheral nerves, plexuses, spinal roots and sensory cranial nerves for the treatment of NP and associated neurological deficits is well established. However, although frequently advocated in past years, ablative neurosurgery for the treatment of NP has very limited indications, not least because surgical lesions in the somatosensory system, designed to relieve pain, may often themselves be the cause of NP.

Peripheral neurectomy for painful peripheral nerve lesions, such as neuromas, will be followed by the inevitable reformation of a neuroma. The only indication for resection of a peripheral nerve is the treatment of Morton's neuralgia, in which NP results from a severe compressive lesion of a plantar digital nerve between two metatarsal heads. However, the terminal neuroma that develops postoperatively leads to continuing pain in about one-third of patients.

Dorsal rhizotomy and **ganglionectomy**, which were performed for chronic intractable pains, for example postherpetic neuralgia and severe root compression and scarring, are operations no longer performed. Rhizotomy interrupts large sensory fibres as well as small nociceptive afferents, leading to unwanted sensory loss, including proprioceptive, and in the sacral segments may also lead to impaired bladder and bowel function. In addition, surgical deafferentation may cause the later development of central NP. Rhizotomy may have a very limited place in the relief of severe pain due to malignant disease, where life expectancy is very limited and other measures fail to relieve pain.

Dorsal root entry zone lesioning (Nashold procedure) ablates the dorsal horn of the spinal cord. In patients who already have extensive peripheral deafferentation, associated with severe central NP, this operation can be very effective. The main indication is NP due to brachial plexus avulsion injury, most often the result of motorcycle accidents in young men. It has also been used in the treatment of NP due to Pancoast tumours of the lung. Results in the treatment of postherpetic neuralgia have been mixed, and there is a risk that the pain may be altered and exacerbated by surgery.

Anterolateral cordotomy, either surgical or by percutaneous radiofrequency heat lesioning in the cervical cord interrupts the spinothalamic tract, leading to contralateral loss of pain and temperature sensation. The only indication for the procedure is intractable cancer pain, although with improved methods of pain control it is now performed infrequently. It is contraindicated for the treatment of chronic pain of non-malignant origin because of the limited duration of analgesia (usually not longer than two or three years), and because of the development of central NP due to the surgical lesion itself, after months or years. It is difficult to control the extent of the lesion, so that other spinal cord deficits are sometimes caused by the operation.

The operation of **mesencephalotomy** involves making lesions of the ascending spinothalamic tract and the quintothalamic tract from the face. These surgical targets are small and thus difficult to target selectively. Other unwanted neurological deficits are common, and so even for pain due to malignant disease, where prognosis is limited, the procedure has been largely abandoned.

Thalamotomy for pain has involved numerous targets within the thalamus. Lesions in the intralaminar group of nuclei are most likely to lead to analgesia, and minimize the risk of producing loss of tactile and proprioceptive sensory deficits. However, review of many reports of operations in the medial thalamus for pain demonstrates a high incidence of temporary analgesia, unwanted neurological deficits, and the late development of

NP resulting from the procedure. For these reasons, thalamotomy is no longer performed.

Other brain areas targeted for the treatment of intractable pain include the dorsomedian nucleus, which projects to the cingulum, the frontal lobes and limbic system, and the medial and lateral pulvinar nuclei. Lesions in these structures tend to produce only transient analgesia. Lesions of the frontothalamic projections and the frontal lobes themselves will lead to reduced suffering from pain, but are associated with a change in personality, although this may be mild.

Cognitive behavioural therapy

The common comorbidities of chronic pain have already been described. Patients who are distressed and functionally incapacitated by their pain are those most likely to benefit from psychological interventions. Psychological measures are often used together with other treatments, and it is important that psychological intervention is not delayed until all other treatments have been tried, as a last resort.

A common progressive sequence for patients with NP is that the pain shows limited response to a variety of drug and other treatments, it is accompanied by reduced physical activity, fatigue, poor sleep, social and family isolation, depression, anger, frustration and a fear of the pain worsening, particularly through physical exertion, leading to an increasing dependence on medical services. It is important to recognize this worsening symptom complex at an early stage, before it becomes entrenched and intractable, so that psychological intervention can be initiated.

The aims of treatment should always be geared to the individual patient's situation and needs, but are likely to include relief of depression and anxiety, pacing, improved physical activity and fitness, reduction in fear, improved adaptive and coping behaviour; and eventually, return to work.

Of the many psychological techniques advocated, the best evidence is in favour of **cognitive behavioural therapy (CBT)**, although further research in this area is needed.

Well-informed understanding, sympathy and a long-term commitment and supportive approach from the doctor and all others involved in treatment (ideally in a multidisciplinary pain clinic setting) goes a long way to helping those with chronic NP.

COMPLEX REGIONAL PAIN SYNDROME

Complex regional pain syndrome (CRPS) is the term now used to embrace a number of conditions previously known as reflex sympathetic dystrophy, causalgia, algodystrophy, Sudeck's atrophy and several other conditions listed in Box 30.1.

The clinical features common to all these conditions include chronic pain associated with allodynia and hyperalgesia, autonomic disturbances, trophic changes, oedema and loss of function of the affected part, usually a limb.

The term causalgia means 'burning pain' and was coined to describe the severe burning pain, hyperaesthesia, glossy skin and colour changes in the limbs of soldiers following injury to major peripheral nerves, sustained in the American Civil War. Subsequently, it became apparent that injuries to limbs, such as fractures, not involving peripheral nerves, could sometimes lead to the same symptoms and signs. This became known as 'reflex sympathetic dystrophy'.

The definition and classification of these conditions remains difficult, because their pathophysiology is poorly understood. The term CRPS is descriptive of a clinical state and, in distinction to some of the previous diagnostic labels (Box 30.1), makes no attempt to attribute an underlying pathophysiological basis to the condition.

Box 30.1 Complex regional pain syndrome, older diagnostic terms

- Reflex sympathetic dystrophy
- Post-traumatic sympathetic dystrophy
- Algodystrophy
- Causalgia major
- Causalgia minor
- Sudeck's atrophy
- Transient osteoporosis
- Post-traumatic painful osteoporosis
- Acute bone atrophy
- Shoulder-hand syndrome
- Post-traumatic vasomotor syndrome

Definition of CRPS

CRPS describes a variety of painful conditions that usually follow injury, occur regionally, have a distal predominance of abnormal findings, exceed both in magnitude and duration the expected clinical course of the inciting event, often result in significant impairment of motor function, and show variable progression over time. CRPS is divided into types 1 and 2.

In CRPS type 1:
- There is an initiating noxious event.
- Ongoing pain and/or allodynia and hyperalgesia occur beyond the territory of a single peripheral nerve, and are disproportionate to the inciting event.
- There is or has been evidence of oedema, skin blood flow abnormality, or abnormal sudomotor activity, in the region of the pain since the inciting event.
- The diagnosis is excluded by the existence of conditions that would otherwise account for the degree of pain and dysfunction.

CRPS type 2 follows nerve injury and is synonymous with causalgia. It is similar in other respects to CRPS type 1, with the following features:
- It is a more regionally confined presentation about a joint or area, provoked by a nerve injury.
- Ongoing pain and/or allodynia and hyperalgesia are usually limited to the nerve area involved, but may spread distally or proximally, outside the territory of the affected peripheral nerve.
- Intermittent and variable oedema, skin blood flow change, abnormal sudomotor activity and motor dysfunction, disproportionate to the inciting event, are present about the area involved.

Being descriptive of symptoms and signs, these definitions suffer from lack of clarity about the definable limits of the conditions, particularly CRPS type 1, but they do have the advantage of avoiding unjustified assumptions about pathophysiology. Confusion also results from making CRPS type 2 and causalgia synonymous, emphasizing the difficulty arising from the use of a word originally intended to refer to a single symptom (burning pain), to a clinical descriptive syndrome. However, this is the widely accepted current terminology.

Causes

The many causes of CRPS are listed in Table 30.7. The majority are CRPS type 1, resulting from peripheral tissue injury such as fractures and soft tissue injury. The incidence of CRPS type 2 is much lower. CRPS is a rare complication of lesions affecting the CNS.

Clinical features

Table 30.8 lists the major symptoms and signs, with relative frequency, from a large prospective study of patients with CRPS, at two time intervals. As the diagnosis depends on a qualitative assessment of symptoms and signs, there is understandably some uncertainty and difference between clinicians in agreeing the threshold at which the diagnosis should be made. However, it is likely that less

severe cases of CRPS are under-recognized. There have been very few prospective studies, so the true incidence of CRPS is unknown. The point at which symptoms and signs are judged to be dispropor-

Table 30.7 Causes of complex regional pain syndrome

Location	
Peripheral tissues	Fractures
	Tendon and ligament injury
	Fasciitis
	Arthritis
	Deep vein thrombosis
	Prolonged immobilization (an important contributory factor)
Peripheral nerve and dorsal root	Peripheral nerve injury (type 2 CRPS)
	Brachial plexus lesions
	Spinal nerve root lesions
	Postherpetic neuralgia
Central nervous system	Spinal cord trauma
	Head injury
	Cerebral infarction
	Cerebral tumour
Viscera	Myocardial infarction
	Abdominal disease
Idiopathic	No initiating cause identifiable

CRPS, complex regional pain syndrome.

Table 30.8 Clinical features of complex regional pain syndrome

Clinical feature	Patients with symptom or sign (%) (CRPS duration 2–6 months)	Patients with symptom or sign (%) (CRPS duration >12 months)
Inflammatory		
Pain	88	97
Colour difference	96	84
Temperature difference	91	91
Limited movement	90	83
Exacerbation with exercise	95	97
Oedema	80	55
Neurological		
Allodynia/ hyperalgesia	75	85
Hyperpathia	79	81
Incoordination	47	61
Tremor	44	50
Involuntary spasms	24	47
Muscle spasms	13	42
Paresis	93	97
Pseudoparesis	7	26
Dystrophic		
Skin	37	44
Nails	23	36
Muscle	50	67
Bone	41	52
Sympathetic		
Hyperhidrosis	56	40
Abnormal hair growth	71	35
Abnormal nail growth	60	52

Adapted from Veldman et al., 1993 with permission from Elsevier.

tionate in severity and duration to the inciting event is often a matter of genuine clinical uncertainty, emphasizing the imprecision of the current diagnostic criteria.

Spontaneous and evoked pains are experienced by all patients at some time during the course of CRPS. Pain is most often described as burning, aching or throbbing. In CRPS type 2, additional paroxysmal pains are common. Allodynia, hyperalgesia and hyperpathia often lead to avoidance of any skin contact or pressure on the affected limb. The resulting immobility contributes to muscle wasting and joint stiffness, in addition to the dystrophic changes that frequently occur as part of the condition.

Autonomic signs are variable in CRPS, ranging from very obvious to subtle. Symptoms of abnormal colour, temperature and sweating in the affected limb are frequent, and oedema is also common.

Examination is usually limited by the ongoing pain and pain provoked by touching or moving the limb. Motor signs include wasting and weakness, tremor, incoordination, muscle spasms and sometimes dystonia.

Dystrophic changes include skin atrophy with a shiny appearance, but sometimes there is skin thickening with flaking. Nails may become thickened and there may be hair loss or coarsening. Osteoporosis is common, and in its worst form leads to **Sudeck's atrophy**.

Other less common clinical features include recurrent skin infections associated with chronic oedema, increased skin pigmentation, fasciitis of the palmar or plantar skin and nail clubbing.

Psychological factors and pathogenesis of CRPS

Psychological factors in the pathogenesis and maintenance of the symptoms of CRPS have often been postulated, in part a reflection of the very limited understanding of the pathophysiology of the condition. However, there is no evidence that CRPS is a primarily psychologically determined illness.

Many patients with CRPS face delay in diagnosis, and this is often associated with anxiety, fear and depression. This psychological comorbidity may be compounded by an ill-founded sceptical attitude of medical staff, and when issues of secondary gain are raised.

Staging of clinical features in CRPS

Three clinical stages of CRPS can be recognized: an acute warm phase, in which oedema is a major feature; a dystrophic phase characterized by muscle wasting and vasomotor instability; and a later atrophic phase, characterized by bone and skin changes. However, not all patients develop all these signs or follow this course.

Diagnosis of CRPS

As already stated, the diagnosis of CRPS is based on clinical features and there are no diagnostic investigations. Three phase isotope bone scans are frequently abnormal, but a normal scan does not exclude the diagnosis.

Pathophysiology of CRPS

As already mentioned, the pathophysiology of CRPS is poorly understood. Full discussion is beyond the scope of this chapter and the reader is referred to fuller accounts listed in Further reading. Current research is focused in five main areas:

1 Involvement of the sympathetic nervous system in the periphery
2 Central autonomic dysregulation
3 Peripheral tissue inflammation and immune stimulation
4 Central sensory sensitization
5 Abnormal CNS mechanisms underlying the motor abnormalities of CRPS

Involvement of the sympathetic nervous system: sympathetically maintained pain

In 1916, the relief of causalgia in a patient with a brachial plexus injury and thrombosis of the brachial artery, by periarterial surgical sympathectomy was described. In other patients also treated with sympathectomy, relief of pain was associated with improvement in discoloration and sweating changes. As a result, pre-ganglionic sympathectomy became established as standard treatment for painful nerve injuries.

In experimental studies of nerve injury, there is evidence of an interaction between sympathetic efferent noradrenergic and sensory afferent fibres, which develops at the site of injury, in undamaged fibres distal to the injury, and in the dorsal root ganglion. Limited human studies have also indicated that an abnormal sympathetic–sensory interaction develops. However, treatment of patients with CRPS type 1 or type 2 gives very variable results, and as described below, carefully controlled studies have not shown a therapeutic effect of sympathetic blockade.

CRPS type 1 develops in the absence of an initiating nerve injury, and as described below, there is emerging evidence of the importance of inflammation in pathogenesis. Some aspects of cutaneous inflammation and hyperalgesia are increased by alpha-adrenoreceptor stimulation, and noradrenaline causes release of prostaglandins, which mediate inflammatory responses. Furthermore, an increase in alpha-adrenoreceptor density in skin biopsies has been reported in patients with CRPS type 1.

These and other experimental findings indicate a role for the sympathetic nervous system in CRPS, but the lack of a demonstrable therapeutic effect of sympathetic blockade in controlled studies has led many to question the existence of 'sympathetically maintained pain'.

Central autonomic dysregulation

In patients with CRPS type 1, hyperhidrosis is often found, and studies of centrally mediated sympathetic reflexes have demonstrated abnormal responses, suggesting that there may be central autonomic dysregulation.

Inflammation and immune stimulation

There are often signs of inflammation in CRPS (see Table 30.8), and a therapeutic effect of corticosteroid in the early stages of the condition has been reported. However, CRPS of longer than 13 weeks' duration is unresponsive to this treatment.

Neurogenic inflammation occurs in CRPS, causing oedema, vasodilatation and increased sweating. It has been suggested that the inflammatory features of CRPS type 1 might represent a chronic post-infectious state, stimulated by intestinal pathogens including *Campylobacter jejuni*, or by *Borrelia* infection. In support of this hypothesis, preliminary trials have indicated a therapeutic effect of intravenous human immunoglobulin, though the outcome of a large-scale controlled trial is awaited. At the moment, it is not possible to conclude more

than that inflammatory and immune processes may be important in the pathogenesis of CRPS.

Central sensitization

As described earlier in relation to peripheral NP, prolonged noxious inputs from peripheral tissues in CRPS type 1 will lead to central sensitization. In addition, functional MRI studies have shown adaptive changes in the thalamus and cortex, which resolve with effective treatment of the pain.

Central motor abnormalities in CRPS

Table 30.8 indicates the frequency of motor abnormalities in CRPS. These include tremor, paresis and dystonia. There is evidence that abnormal central motor processing may underlie these clinical features.

Treatment of CRPS

The treatment of causalgia (CRPS type 2), a type of peripheral NP, has already been outlined, and the following paragraphs describe treatment approaches for CRPS type 1.

Early recognition and treatment

Early recognition of CRPS remains difficult, and while it seems intuitively correct that early treatment would improve outcome, there is no clinical study that demonstrates this. Particularly because immobilization is likely to contribute to the development of CRPS type 1, the management of fractures and soft tissue limb injuries, conditions known to have the potential to provoke the development of CRPS, should include early mobilization and restoration of function.

Sympathetic blockade and sympathectomy

Although in past years there were many reports of a therapeutic effect of sympathetic blockade, achieved either by the peripheral Biers block technique (intravenous regional blockade) or by local anaesthetic ganglion block, to the extent that sympathetic block became the established treatment of choice, systematic review of controlled trials conducted in more recent years, for the treatment of pain due to both CRPS type 1 and peripheral NP indicates a lack of effectiveness. Similarly, there is no reliable evidence demonstrating effectiveness of surgical sympathectomy.

Systemic drugs

There have been few controlled trials of systemic drug treatment for CRPS type 1, and further research is needed. On the basis of present evidence, the following observations and recommendations can be made.

- **Mild analgesic drugs**, such as paracetamol, have only marginal effect. Non-steroidal anti-inflammatory drugs are often used and reported to be helpful by some patients, but neither type of drug has been investigated in controlled trials.
- **Corticosteroids**. If a diagnosis of CRPS type 1 can be made with confidence at an interval of less than three months following the initiating event, a trial of prednisolone, initially at high dose, is justifiable. Treatment at later times is not indicated.
- **Opioids** have not been investigated in controlled trials. However, due to the severity of the pain in CRPS, they are frequently used and may be partially pain relieving. Trials of tramadol, then either slow release morphine or fentanyl patches, is appropriate for severe intractable pain.
- **Bisphophonates and calcitonin**. There is limited evidence that both these calcium regulating drugs may be helpful: bisphophonates via the oral route and calcitonin given intranasally.
- **Gabapentin** has been shown to have an analgesic effect in CRPS type 1 in two trials.

In addition, there are reports of beneficial effects in uncontrolled studies using phenoxybenzamine, tricyclic antidepressants, phenytoin and nifedipine.

Clinically, the pain and associated sensory signs of CRPS type 1 are very similar to those found in patients with NP. For this reason, it is justifiable to undertake open clinical trials in CRPS type 1 of the drugs listed earlier in this chapter for the treatment of NP, particularly given the severity and debilitating nature of the pain. However, such trials must be undertaken with close monitoring, on the clear understanding by both clinician and patient that the drugs are being prescribed for an unlicensed indication.

Epidural and intrathecal treatments

Intrathecal morphine and epidural clonidine have both been reported to reduce pain in CRPS. Intrathecal baclofen is advocated as a treatment for CRPS-associated dystonia.

Electrical counterstimulation

Uncontrolled observations suggest that both TENS and SCS are sometimes effective.

Physiotherapy

Mobilization and attempts to restore normal function are of paramount importance in the treatment of CRPS, the symptoms and signs of which are almost certainly perpetuated by immobilization.

Psychological measures: CBT

A combination of physiotherapy and CBT has been shown to have some effect in the treatment of CRPS.

Amputation

Patients with intractable pain in a limb due to CRPS type 1 may enquire about amputation, as a means of ridding themselves of the severe pain and a useless limb. Although this may successfully relieve the pain, there is a substantial risk that amputation of a painful limb will lead to the development of stump and phantom limb pain, which can be as troublesome as the pain of CRPS, or even worse. Attempts at pain relief and restoration of function are preferable to amputation.

Prognosis of CRPS

There have been few studies, but in one investigation, more than half of patients with CRPS had persistent severe pain at an interval of 5.5 years. It is clear that for some patients, pain is likely to be lifelong. Poor prognostic factors include pain severity, female gender and CRPS involving the leg, and these patients are most likely to experience the serious complications, including skin ulceration, infection, chronic oedema and dystonia.

FURTHER READING

Baron R (2005) Chapter 64. Complex regional pain syndromes. In: McMahon SB, Koltzenburg M (eds). *Wall and Melzack's Textbook of Pain*, 5th edn. Amsterdam: Elsevier, 1011–1027.

Boivie J (2005) Chapter 67. Central pain. In: McMahon SB, Koltzenburg M (eds). Wall and Melzack's Textbook of Pain, 5th edn. Amsterdam: Elsevier, 1057–1074.

Bonica JJ (1991) Introduction: semantic, epidemiologic, and educational issues. In: *Pain And Central Nervous System Disease. The Central Pain Syndromes.* New York: Raven Press, 13–30.

Breivik H (2005) Chapter 33. Local anaesthetic blocks and epidurals. In: McMahon SB, Koltzenburg M (eds). *Wall and Melzack's Textbook of Pain*, 5th edn. Amsterdam: Elsevier, 507–520.

Devor M (2005) Chapter 58. Response of nerves to injury in relation to pain. In: McMahon SB, Koltzenburg M (eds). *Wall and Melzack's Textbook of Pain*, 5th edn. Amsterdam: Elsevier, 905–28.

Finnerup NB, Otto M, McQuay HJ *et al.* (2005) Algorithm for neuropathic pain treatment: an evidence based proposal. *Pain*, 118:289–305.

Fishbain DA, Steele-Rosomoff R, Rosomoff HL (1992) Drug abuse, dependence, and addiction in chronic pain patients. *Clinical Journal of Pain*, 8:77–85.

Gybels JM, Tasker RR (2005) Chapter 36. Supratentorial neurosurgery for the treatment of pain. In: McMahon SB, Koltzenburg M (eds). *Wall and Melzack's Textbook of Pain*, 5th edn. Amsterdam: Elsevier, 553–61.

Morley S, Eccleston C, Williams ACdeC (1999) Systematic review and meta-analysis of randomized controlled trials of cognitive behaviour therapy for chronic pain in adults, excluding headache. *Pain*, 80:1–13.

Meyer-Rosberg K, Kvarnstrom A, Kinnman E *et al.* (2001) Peripheral neuropathic pain – a multidimensional burden for patients. *European Journal of Pain*, 5:379–389.

Scadding JW, Koltzenburg M (2005) Chapter 62. Painful peripheral neuropathies. In: McMahon SB, Koltzenburg M (eds). *Wall and Melzack's Textbook of Pain*, 5th edn. Amsterdam: Elsevier, 973–1000.

Scadding JW (2006) Chapter 26. Clinical examination. In: Cervero F, Jensen TS (eds). *Handbook of Clinical Neurology*, vol. 81. Amsterdam: Elsevier, 385–395.

Sindrup SH, Finnerup NB, Otto M, Jensen TS (2006) Chapter 57. Principles of pharmacological treatment. In: Cervero F, Jensen TS (eds). *Handbook of Clinical Neurology*, vol. 81. Amsterdam: Elsevier, 843–54.

Veldman PJHM, Reynen HM, Arntz IE, Goris JA (1993) Signs and symptoms of reflex sympathetic dystrophy: prospective study of 829 patients. *Lancet*, 342:1012–1016.

Williams ACdeC (1999) Chapter 18. Measures of function and psychology. In: Wall PD, Melzack R (eds). *Textbook of Pain*, 4th edn. Edinburgh: Churchill Livingstone, 427–444.

CHAPTER 31

PSYCHIATRY AND NEUROLOGICAL DISORDERS

Simon Fleminger

NEUROLOGY AND PSYCHIATRY: BRAIN AND MIND

It has been suggested that neurologists deal with disorders of the brain, whereas psychiatrists see people with disorders of the mind. Whereas the brain may be considered like any other organ of the body, the **mind** is generally seen as indivisible from the person as an individual and is closely linked to concepts like soul and freewill. Thus, a mind, a person, can be energetic, or lazy, or morally good or bad.

On the other hand, the **brain** can get damaged and despite the person's best intentions cause them to behave in an inconsiderate way. For example, damage to the medial orbital frontal surface of the brain may result in the person becoming thoughtless and violent. Diffuse brain injury, as well as more localized damage to basal ganglia, often results in problems initiating activity and a lack of drive; the patients are described as having an amotivational state.

Because behaviour may be attributed to the mind on the one hand and to disorders of the brain on the other, different words may be used to describe similar behaviours. For example a person may be described as 'lazy' if their lack of activity is attributed to the mind, but suffering an 'amotivational state' if it is attributed to a disorder of the brain. Similarly, different words may be used to describe the same movement disorder; a **grimacing mannerism** in a treatment-naive patient with **schizophrenia** may look very similar to an **orofacial dyskinesia** in a patient with **dystonia**.

Many neuropsychiatric conditions arise from an **interaction** between cerebral disease and psychological processes. For example, in delusional misidentification, in which people or places are believed to have been replaced by duplicates, it is often the combined effects of both brain disease and suspiciousness that produces the symptom. Antisocial behaviour is particularly likely if there is a combination of birth injury, causing brain damage, and poor parenting.

> Therefore, it is not possible to make an absolute distinction between mental symptoms which arise from disorders of the brain from those which arise in the absence of manifest organic brain disease. The mental symptoms of organic brain disease overlap considerably with symptoms to be found in the absence of brain disease. While it is useful to understand the importance of the cardinal symptoms of organic brain disease (see below under The cardinal mental symptoms of disorders of the brain), it is equally important to realise that the absence of such symptoms does not rule out brain disease. For example, a brain tumour may present with mania indistinguishable from that seen in someone with manic-depressive disorder.

BRIDGING THE GAP BETWEEN NEUROLOGY AND PSYCHIATRY

This chapter will discuss the overlap between neurology and psychiatry, before going on to consider psychiatric diagnosis and management, particularly where it is relevant to neurology.

Biological psychiatry and **behavioural neurology** are bridging the gap between neurology and psychiatry. **Functional imaging techniques** enable us to see which parts of the brain may be involved in functional mental illness, for example, when a patient with schizophrenia experiences a hallucination.

These studies demonstrate how hallucinations involve the corresponding sensory association cortex, but may in addition involve areas of the cortex involved in higher order processing; for example, auditory verbal hallucinations in schizophrenia are likely to involve auditory association cortex, as well as language areas and cingulate cortex. Musical hallucinations, frequently associated with acquired deafness but not with other psychotic symptoms,

tend to demonstrate a more discrete involvement of auditory processing in the right hemisphere known to be the site of music processing.

Advances in psychopharmacology

Those interested in understanding the biological foundations of psychiatry have also relied heavily on improved understanding of **neurotransmitter systems and receptors**. In the dopamine system, the ventral striatal (mesolimbic) system projects to the nucleus accumbens and is involved in reward systems, whereas the dorsal striatal (nigrostriatal) system, well known for its role in movement, has been shown to influence cognitive tasks. It has been proposed that **new 'atypical'** (because they produce fewer extrapyramidal side effects) **antipsychotics**, such as clozapine and risperidone, act preferentially on dopamine receptors in the ventral system and this explains their relative lack of motor side effects. The basis for this selectivity may be that atypical antipsychotics are selective for D_3 dopamine receptors, which are more abundant in ventral striatum, rather than D_2 receptors, which are more likely to be involved in dorsal striatum. Neuroimaging *in vivo* of dopamine receptor blockade in the basal ganglia (largely dorsal striatum) has demonstrated that atypical drugs produce much less blockade of dopamine receptors, despite good antipsychotic effects, than, for example, haloperidol. However, the antipsychotic effect of atypical drugs may, in fact, be explained by their activity at other receptors, in particular serotonin (5HT), rather than as a result of selectivity for D_3.

Serotonin (5HT), in addition to any role it may play in psychotic illness, undoubtedly is involved in depression. **Selective serotonin reuptake inhibitors (SSRIs)** have become the standard treatment for depression. A more specific role for serotonin in impulse control disorders, including temper control, gambling and eating disorders, is less definite. SSRIs have now been joined by selective **noradrenaline reuptake inhibitors (NRIs)**, and while there is no good evidence of a differential effect of NRIs, it does mean that if depression has not responded to an SSRI then it may be worth trying an NRI.

Advances in the field of dementia are of interest to both neurologists and psychiatrists; **new** cholinergic agents that slow cognitive decline, and advances in molecular biology and genetics, have revitalized this area (see Chapter 14).

Transcranial magnetic stimulation (TMS) is one of several new therapeutic techniques involving direct stimulation of the central nervous system. Transcranial magnetic stimulation over the frontal lobes appears to have an antidepressant effect, and may even be an alternative to electroconvulsive therapy (ECT). There is some evidence that TMS over the left temporal lobe may inhibit auditory hallucinations. Because it can selectively interfere with cerebral cortical function, TMS is increasingly being used to study brain behaviour relationships; for example, TMS can selectively inhibit detection of visual movement when delivered over the appropriate area of visual association cortex.

LIAISON PSYCHIATRY

Up to one-third of patients attending a neurology clinic have symptoms that are largely unexplained by neurological disease. Those with neurological disease, e.g. multiple sclerosis or Parkinson's disease, have high rates of psychiatric illness, especially anxiety, depression and psychosis. Alcohol dependence may be found in up to 20 per cent of general hospital inpatients. On average, those with psychiatric disorders accompanying their medical problem utilize medical services more than those without.

Therefore, there is good reason to have a good liaison between a neurology service and psychiatry. In many hospitals, this will rely on the general liaison psychiatry service serving the Accident and Emergency Department and the rest of the hospital. However, neuropsychiatry services have developed over recent years and most large neuroscience centres should expect to have a specific liaison with a neuropsychiatrist. If possible, this should be on the basis of a consultation–liaison model with a specific link between the neuropsychiatrist and the clinical neuroscience services. In this way, the neuropsychiatrist becomes known to the neurology and neurosurgery teams, and easy channels of communication are created. This raises awareness of mental health issues in the neurology/neurosurgery

services. For some high risk areas, for example head injury clinics, then joint clinics may be useful.

THE CARDINAL MENTAL SYMPTOMS OF DISORDERS OF THE BRAIN

Disturbance of conscious level or orientation indicates organic brain disease until proved otherwise. It is for this reason that the neurologist's mental state concentrates on whether or not the patient is 'alert and orientated'. In addition, the presence of specific disorders of cognition and memory may indicate disruption to the normal function of the cerebral cortex.

Delirium, often called an acute confusional state, is characterized by a primary disturbance of conscious level. The patient is obtunded, or drowsy, or highly distractible. Attention and concentration are impaired, e.g. as demonstrated by poor performance on a digit span. The patient is likely to be agitated and frightened. Psychotic symptoms with hallucinations, often visual, and fleeting delusions may be elicited. Delirium may also present as a hypoactive withdrawn state akin to stupor. Management consists of making the patient safe and then finding the cause. Those conditions which cause coma may produce delirium.

In dementia, there is generally no disturbance of conscious level, yet the patient is usually disorientated, as well as showing evidence of a global acquired impairment of cognitive function. Personality change, often with a coarsening of social behaviour, mood disturbance, particularly depression, and psychotic symptoms, both delusions and hallucinations, are also very common.

Patients with dementia are very prone to episodes of delirium precipitated by systemic factors on a lowered cognitive reserve.

PSYCHIATRIC DIAGNOSIS

Psychiatric diagnosis, although relying often on subjective data, for example a patient describing their mental state, is nevertheless valid. Psychiatric diagnoses show good inter-rater reliability and predict outcome and treatment responsiveness. More recently, functional neuroimaging has provided objective evidence of abnormalities of brain function to match the subjective descriptions of symptoms.

It is useful to think of a **hierarchy of diagnosis** with all psychiatric diagnoses being trumped by organic mental disorders (Figure 31.1).

Therefore, if a patient has both depression (level 3) and schizophrenia (level 2), their course and management are determined more by the schizophrenia. Symptoms of depression may be produced by schizophrenia, but not vice versa. Organic mental disorders (level 1) may result in psychoses, neuroses (depression, anxiety, somatization disorder) or changes in personality.

> **Mental disorders** in the absence of brain disease are crudely classified into **mental illness** (the psychoses and neuroses) and **personality disorders**. A key criterion for diagnosis of a **mental illness** is that the **normal functioning** of the person should be **impaired**.

There are many ways in which this can be manifest, most frequently difficulties working, or a decline in personal care or social relationships. On the other hand, people with a **personality disorder** may continue to function normally; the critical criterion is that they or others should **suffer** as a result of their personality traits.

In the following sections, psychiatric diagnoses will be discussed in hierarchical order starting with the personality disorders, then the neuroses, including anxiety disorders and somatoform disorders, and finally psychoses. Affective disorder will be discussed with the psychoses. The addictions, which do not fit comfortably in the hierarchy, will be discussed last.

PERSONALITY DISORDERS

Personality comprises the characteristic patterns of thinking and behaviour of an individual, and is made up of numerous personality traits, for example a tendency to be impulsive, or obsessional, or assertive. **Personality disorders** are distinguished by the fact that traits are present to an abnormal degree and fairly consistently from early adult life, and that suffering results. Under stress, many patients with conspicuous personality traits or disorders develop a corresponding mental illness, for example somebody who is obsessional develops symptoms of obsessional compulsive disorder.

Personality disorders are classified according to the outstanding traits. In **paranoid** personality disorder, the person is excessively suspicious and sensitive. People with **schizoid** personality disorders are emotionally cold and distant. Indecisiveness and doubt and rigidity are typical of **anankastic** personality disorders. Other categories include **antisocial** personality disorder with aggression and lack of concern for others, and **borderline** personality disorder in which the patient tends to over-idealize,

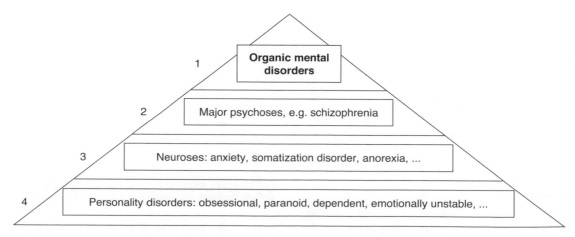

Figure 31.1 A hierarchy for psychiatric diagnosis.

is inclined to repeated self-harm, and has periods of altered conscious level akin to dissociation (see below under Somatization and dissociation: patients with physical symptoms not due to organic disease) with 'borderline' psychotic symptoms.

> Personality disorders have tended to be regarded as untreatable. However, psychodynamic and cognitive behaviour therapy (CBT), as well as psychotropic medication may help, particularly for those with borderline personality disorder.

ANXIETY DISORDERS

> The anxiety disorders consist of several conditions in which anxiety is the major problem; anxiety disorder, obsessive-compulsive disorder (OCD), and phobic disorder including agoraphobia and social phobia.

The symptom of anxiety is common to all these conditions. Many people have problems describing their symptoms of anxiety, and will describe instead not feeling quite right, or restless. The physician needs to be alert to the possibility that strange feelings in the head may be symptoms of anxiety. Some patients describe a sense of their head being full of cotton-wool, or that their head is going to explode.

> Anxiety is a normal human emotional response to threatening events. It can be useful and help to improve performance. On the other hand, it becomes morbid if it occurs regularly in the absence of any significant stressor or starts to interfere with function.
>
> Anxiety is related to fear and commonly coexists with depression. Chronic anxiety causes fatigue, irritability and poor sleep. High levels of anxiety may precipitate psychotic illness and dissociative states.

Free floating anxiety is fairly continuous and independent of the situation or circumstance the person finds themselves in. The person is not aware of why they are feeling anxious.

Panic attacks are short-lived crescendos of anxiety such that the person experiences terror or extreme discomfort. Catastrophic thoughts, e.g. of impending death or going crazy, are present. Symptoms are aggravated by hyperventilation often related to a sense of suffocation. Panic attacks tend to build up over a few minutes, may last up to 2 hours but rarely longer, and then subside. They are common, with the majority of the population experiencing a panic attack at some point.

Anxiety may produce various somatic symptoms (Table 31.1). **Globus hystericus** is the sensation that one is going to choke on one's tongue. **Hyperventilation may result in paraesthesiae in the hands and around the mouth, or carpo–pedal spasm.** Fatigue or headaches are a common symptom of chronic anxiety.

Phobic anxiety disorders

In **agoraphobia**, the patient typically feels anxious when they feel trapped and unable to return to a place of safety. Such situations are more threatening when they are alone. As a result, the patient may avoid going into anxiety-provoking situations. These include crowded supermarkets, sitting in an auditorium, queuing, being in large crowds, travelling on trains or buses. In severe agoraphobia, the patient avoids leaving their house.

Social phobia, on the other hand, is precipitated by situations in which the patient feels under scrutiny. Public speaking, or even talking in small groups, will cause anxiety. They are likely to find it difficult eating in public. The patient is very self-conscious and anxiety is reinforced by blushing or sweating. Many patients suffer both social phobia and agoraphobia.

Specific phobias include fear of spiders or thunderstorms or flying. Even thinking about the object of the phobia causes anxiety, and extreme fear may occur at the prospect of the being exposed to the feared situation or object.

A key feature of all the situationally dependent anxiety disorders is **avoidance**. If the avoidance interferes with normal function, then treatment is likely to be necessary.

Obsessive-compulsive disorder

Many of us have obsessive personality traits and these are helpful in certain jobs where errors are potentially dangerous; a degree of perfectionism

Table 31.1 Content of typical obsessions and compulsions

	Obsession	Corresponding compulsion
Contamination	e.g. My hand touched the carpet which was contaminated with faeces	Wash hands repeatedly after contact with anything that may have had contact with carpet
Physical violence	e.g. I will take knife and attack my baby	Throw away all knives, avoid being alone with baby
Anti-social behaviour	e.g. I am going to swear out loud and make crude sexual jokes	Avoid public speaking, repeat a magic word in ones head to stop such thoughts, ask for reassurance that did not swear
Orderliness/ perfectionism	e.g. Have to read all the books of a particular author	Avoid reading any of his books
	Hall has to be painted with the same batch of paint	Repeatedly check the batch numbers, take back paint without number on
	Have to drive out of the garage 'just right'	Repeatedly drives back into garage to get it just right
Accidental harm	I have forgotten to turn the gas off	Repeatedly go back to check the gas tap
Visions of destruction and death	Images of child being killed	

and checking is reassuring. On the other hand, a person may find that recently they have had to check over and over again, or get things just right, to the extent that it interferes with their ability to function effectively; they would now be diagnosed as suffering from obsessive-compulsive disorder.

Obsessional thoughts are unwelcome, intrusive and cause anxiety. They are recognized by the person as their own thoughts, and this distinguishes them from some psychotic disorders of possession of thought. Often, the obsessional thought is relieved by carrying out a **compulsion**, which is generally a motor act, but can be a ritualistic thought (see Table 31.1). OCD is often quite responsive to life events, relapsing at times of stress. In some, however, it becomes chronically very debilitating.

OCD is associated with Gille de la Tourette's syndrome. OCD needs to be distinguished from organic orderliness seen in patients with dementia.

Adjustment and bereavement reactions

After severely traumatic or distressing life events, it is common to find symptoms of anxiety lasting days or weeks. In this situation, benzodiazepines may be used, but physical dependence starts within days of starting medication so great care is necessary.

Psychological response to trauma

It is necessary to distinguish between events that are psychologically traumatic from those which result in physical trauma, particularly if there is head injury. If there is physical injury, then the psychological reaction has to be interpreted in the light of any physical disability and damage to the central nervous system (CNS).

Post-traumatic stress disorder (PTSD) occurs following exposure to life-threatening events. In the aftermath, but sometimes after a latent interval of a few days or weeks, the characteristic syndrome of flashbacks, nightmares, hyperarousal and avoidance of situations which act as reminders of the event, appear. The syndrome may be seen in those who lost consciousness at the time of the event; implicit unconscious memories may still be activated.

Assaults are particularly likely to result in PTSD. PTSD is often complicated by depression and substance abuse, and is more common in women. Neuroendocrine studies find evidence of a chronic stress reaction, and the reduced hippocampal volume found in veterans with PTSD has been attributed to chronic high levels of corticosteroids.

> The majority of those who develop PTSD will recover within a year, but a substantial proportion go on to develop chronic disabling symptoms. SSRI antidepressants and cognitive-behaviour therapy have been shown to be effective, but the effect size is not large. Debriefing immediately after a trauma has not been shown to be effective and may even have deleterious effects.

Travel anxiety or phobia is a common symptom after road traffic or other transport accidents. The person experiences intense anxiety travelling, particularly when using the same method of transport as was involved in the accident. They become hypervigilant and see danger at every opportunity.

> **Post-concussion syndrome** is seen following head injury. Common symptoms include headaches, poor concentration and memory, fatigue, dizziness, noise and light sensitivity, double vision, irritability, depression and anxiety. These symptoms overlap heavily with those seen in the somatization disorders, including chronic fatigue syndrome. However, depending on the severity of the head injury, it is likely that a proportion of the symptoms are related to brain injury.

To what extent the symptoms are organic is often the subject of intense debate. Some clinicians go so far as to suggest that head injury not producing loss of consciousness is nevertheless a frequent cause of brain injury. Other clinicians may assume that there are major psychological factors at play, despite the presence of good evidence of brain damage. A fair compromise is to suggest that persistent symptoms of post-concussion syndrome are often due to **anxiety interfering with healthy recovery** from physiological damage to the brain.

The whole picture is complicated several-fold by **litigation**; many of those with surprisingly severe symptoms years following a mild head injury are seeking compensation because somebody was to blame for the injury. A reasonable estimate is that being involved in compensation increases symptoms after a head injury by 25 per cent. The figure is greater in those with mild injuries, and probably with chronic symptoms. This excess of symptoms has been attributed to '**compensation neurosis**'. This label draws attention to the fact that symptoms may be influenced by secondary, financial, gain.

Even in the absence of conscious exaggeration or fabrication of symptoms or disability, it is easy to understand that being involved in seeking compensation has a deleterious effect on outcome after injury. This may reflect the anger and bitterness experienced by patients in this situation; it is easier to come to terms with one's loss if it is an act of God, than if it is due to someone else's incompetence. It may reflect the process of being involved in a lengthy claim; numerous doctors are seen, each one demanding the patient goes back over the history. The normal process of recovery, involving symptoms disappearing from memory, is impeded. The process is usually stressful.

Nevertheless, a more sceptical approach by the physician may be required for the patient who is involved in litigation, even if the patient is being seen for clinical management. It is possible that **secondary gain** is driving the maintenance of symptoms. **Malingering** is probably not very common, but many compensation-seeking patients give an impression that the potential for secondary gain undermines their motivation for recovery. In a proportion of patients, detective work demonstrates quite clearly that they are consciously and fraudulently fabricating the evidence.

Reporting bias complicates the picture. Patients and their family and friends overestimate the patient's health and well-being before the injury. However, this rose-tinted glasses effect is not particular to those involved in compensation, it is seen in all patients with head injury, and indeed in all patients with disability. People are inclined to attribute all their problems to the illness.

The **chronic whiplash syndrome** is bedeviled by issues related to compensation.

Treatment of the anxiety disorders

Response prevention is the psychological treatment strategy which is central to treatment of the anxiety disorders. The response the patient uses to reduce anxiety is identified; this almost always involves avoiding the situation that causes anxiety, for example by not going travelling or by getting off the train early. The patient is then, with negotiation, prevented from making the response. Anxiety initially increases, but with treatment over a few sessions, many will find that they are less anxious in the feared situation.

General **relaxation techniques** may be used. These usually involve progressive muscle relaxation techniques, along with relaxing imagery and suggestion.

Panic attacks are likely to need a specific cognitive approach in which catastrophic thoughts are challenged and replaced by more realistic thoughts. The mainstay of treatment of OCD is cognitive-behaviour therapy with response prevention.

> Although benzodiazepines are very effective anxiolytics, they are not recommended for anxiety treatment in view of the risk of dependence. SSRIs are the treatment of choice, although it needs to be acknowledged that in some with generalized anxiety disorders, SSRIs may initially exacerbate the symptom.

If SSRIs fail, other classes of antidepressant that may be tried include tricyclic antidepressants, particularly those with serotoninergic effects, the selective noradrenergic and serotinergic reuptake inhibitors, e.g. venlafaxine, and mono-amine oxidase inhibitors. Propranolol is effective for some patients.

THE SOMATOFORM DISORDERS: HYPOCHONDRIASIS, SOMATIZATION AND DISSOCIATIVE DISORDERS

Somatoform disorders
These are all disorders in which physical symptoms and complaints are not due to organic disease. There is debate as to how the somatoform disorders should be classified. What is important is that they overlap heavily with one another and are all varieties of abnormal illness behaviour. They are associated with anxiety and depression and psychological stress.

The conditions that need to be considered are:

- **Hypochondriasis**: the emphasis is on *fear of illness*. The patient may or not have symptoms (most do), but they are frightened that they have a serious illness.
- **Somatization disorders**: symptoms and signs are present in the absence of organic disease sufficient to explain them. If symptoms and signs involve the nervous system then it is likely that they will be labeled as conversion disorder (see below under Dissociation: conversion disorders).
- **Dissociative disorders**: this classification has recently been introduced to cover conversion disorders and dissociative states. In both, psychological processes are considered to be dissociated from one another. In the **conversion disorders**, synonymous with **hysteria**, typical symptoms and signs include hemiplegia, hemianaesthesia or blindness. The **dissociative states** consist of psychogenic amnesia, fugue and stuporose states and pseudoseizures.

Anxiety is a theme common to all these conditions (see Table 31.2).

> The diagnosis of a conversion disorder, unlike the diagnosis of most mental disorders, depends on the physician attributing the symptoms to a specific psychological process. However this requires care; diagnostic classification systems in psychiatry are much more reliable and valid if they do not rely on interpretations about psychological mechanisms, but rely merely on operational criteria based on symptoms and signs.

Therefore, it may be better to use the diagnostic terms **unexplained medical symptoms**, or **physical symptoms not due to organic disease** (see below under Somatization and dissociation: patients with physical symptoms not due to organic disease).

Hypochondriasis

> The core symptom of hypochondriasis is the patient's **fear that they have a disease**; usually a life-threatening or severely disabling disease, despite a reasonable history, examination and investigation indicating that they do not.

Table 31.2 Anxiety – the master mimic

Process	Symptom
Subjective experience of anxiety	A feeling of pressure/'cotton wool' in the head
	The head is going to burst
	Tension in the body
	Motor restlessness
Panic	Light headedness/sense of imminent loss of consciousness
	Terror of imminent death/heart attack
	Shortness of breath/sense of suffocation
	Globus hystericus – difficulty swallowing
Interferes with concentration and the normal integration of conscious experience	Poor memory and cognitive impairment
Focuses attention on bodily sensations causing a sense of dysfunction	Depersonalization/derealization
	Altered feeling in body/anaesthesia
	Déjà vu
	Altered visual or auditory sense
	Tinnitus, vertigo, dizziness
Muscle tension and increased excitability	Pain in the muscles
	Headaches
	Chest pains
	Muscle twitches/myokimia
	Trembling/shaking
Increased autonomic activity	Palpitations/flushing
	Sweating/night sweats
	Upper abdominal symptoms – butterflies
	Diarrhoea
	Urinary urgency and frequency
	Dry mouth
	Peripheral vascular changes
Hyperventilation	Paraesthesiae – especially perioral and hands
	Muscle contractions, especially muscles of hands and feet; carpopedal spasm
	Light headedness/epilepsy
Non-specific	Fatigue
	Poor sleep

Anxiety may produce symptoms through a variety of routes. The symptoms often result in referral to a neurologist.

Patients may worry that they have cancer or heart disease. Hypochondriasis is therefore a phobia: a fear of illness. Hypochondriacal concerns that may be seen by a neurologist include the fear of having a brain tumour or multiple sclerosis. Usually, the fear is based on symptoms, for example headaches or visual disturbance. However, a small proportion of patients with hypochondriasis will have no physical symptoms, yet are troubled by fear of illness and demand increasingly sophisticated investigations to rule out the possibility.

Dysmorphophobia, a fear of being deformed or ugly, may be regarded as a variant of hypochondriasis. Concerns about body shape tend to occur in early adult life, whereas concerns about health occur later. Correspondingly, dysmorphophobia has an earlier mean age of onset than hypochondriasis.

A key element to the diagnosis is that there

is a **mismatch** between the patient's view of their health and their doctor's. As a result, they may demand numerous consultations and second opinions. As with all mental illness, a diagnosis is only made if the symptoms have an impact on normal functioning. The patient with hypochondriasis is likely to lose time off work, alienate their friends and neglect themselves as a result of their constant preoccupation with their health.

They also **demand reassurance**. A model of hypochondriasis that is useful for guiding treatment is that the patient develops increasing anxiety as they experience catastrophic thoughts of impending disease. Physical symptoms may deteriorate as the anxiety increases. Reassurance that they are alright, particularly from a doctor but also from family and friends, reduces symptoms of anxiety. A vicious cycle may be created so that the only way they can rid themselves of anxiety is by seeking reassurance.

This model is akin to other models of specific phobias in which a response alleviates anxiety (see above). **Response prevention**, in the case of hypochondriasis, prohibits the patient obtaining reassurance; family and friends are taught not to reassure the patient. Cognitive therapy will focus on enabling the patient to **challenge the catastrophic thoughts** of impending illness and replace them with more appropriate thoughts (cognitions).

Some patients with hypochondriasis develop frank delusions. The diagnosis of **hypochondriacal delusions** is made when the beliefs are florid and firmly held and go beyond any evidence to support them. Enquiry may reveal a systematization of the delusional beliefs; for example, the patient may have persecutory delusions of a conspiracy involving their doctors. Hypochondriacal and dysmorphophobic delusions are classified as delusional disorders (see below under Delusional disorders).

Somatization and dissociation: patients with physical symptoms not due to organic disease

The classification of conditions in which the patient has symptoms of physical disease, with no evidence of organic disease, is clumsy. **Somatization** refers to the process whereby somatic symptoms are produced in the absence of physical disease. **Dissociation** is a more specific explanation of how either somatic symptoms (conversion disorder) or altered states of conscious awareness (dissociative states) may be produced.

> A significant proportion of patients who are referred to neurology clinics do not have organic disease to explain their symptoms. In one study, 10 per cent were rated as 'not at all explained' by organic disease, with a further 20 per cent whose symptoms were 'only somewhat explained' by organic disease. Those with lower organicity were more likely to suffer anxiety or depression.
>
> However, faced with a patient with somatic symptoms but no evidence of physical disease, the physician should never close the door on the possibility that physical disease may be present or evolving. The fact that symptoms and signs cannot be explained by organic disease does not mean that organic disease is not present. Follow up of patients diagnosed as having hysteria has demonstrated that a few, though far less than described 40 years ago, go on to develop manifest organic illness. Multiple sclerosis, for example, is known to occasionally present with symptoms and signs that are clearly 'non-organic'. Organic illness, particularly if it involves the CNS, may predispose to hysterical reactions.

These conditions are all weakly associated with alcohol dependence and with antisocial personality disorder. Childhood experience seems to be relevant; many have poor memories of childhood, some will have experienced illness either in themselves or others, while the dissociative states are associated with sexual abuse as a child. Women are at greater risk.

The **psychological origins** of the symptoms are suggested by observations that the symptoms are responsive to life events and other stressors, may go hand in hand with other mental symptoms, particularly anxiety and depression. The occasional patient may show *belle indifférence*. A poor prognostic sign is reluctance on the part of the patient to consider a psychological explanation, or part explanation, for their symptoms. Many come with fixed ideas about causation, for example patients with **chronic fatigue syndrome** who believe their symptoms are due to persistent viral infection of muscles and nerve.

Symptoms often appear in early adult life and a proportion of patients go on to run a chronic fluctuating course. Symptoms may remain restricted to one bodily system, or spread to involve many systems.

Disorders involving somatization include somatization disorder itself, as well as chronic pain syndromes, including chronic tension headache and chronic fatigue syndrome. The dissociation disorders consist of the conversion disorders and the dissociative states, as well as one or two rare conditions. Finally, it is necessary to discuss factitious disorders in which the patient consciously fabricates symptoms.

Somatization disorder

Somatization disorder is used to describe a condition characterized by multiple, recurrent physical symptoms involving different bodily symptoms. Patients are usually women who often have sexual dysfunction and may have menstrual problems. Many will develop drug dependence, for example, steroids or analgesics or anti-diarrhoeal agents.

Patients with fewer symptoms, perhaps restricted to one bodily system and with symptoms that are understandable as arising from the autonomic nervous system (Table 31.2) are labelled as having **somatoform autonomic dysfunction**. However, there is no certain value in distinguishing the various conditions, and they all overlap with chronic fatigue syndrome.

A more pragmatic approach is to acknowledge that some people are vulnerable to developing somatic symptoms which they select from a core collection of symptoms which are common in the normal population. Whether this involves one system or many may be related to idiosyncratic factors. Somatoform syndromes are, for example, labeled cardiac neurosis, irritable bowel syndrome, gastric neurosis, atypical facial pain or chronic fatigue, depending on which are the most prominent symptoms. However, they tend to have more symptoms in common than set them apart.

Core symptoms include fatigue, muscle aches and pains and tenderness, headaches, difficulty concentrating, sleep problems, irritability, tension, dizziness, indigestion, constipation, abdominal pain, diarrhoea and regional pain.

Chronic pain syndromes

In many patients with chronic pain, there is no definite organic explanation, although there may have originally been an acute cause, for example injury. Such patients are often distressed and it can be difficult to distinguish cause and effect in the relationship between pain and depression. Analgesic abuse and dependence is often a major issue in managing these patients, with some patients demanding narcotics. Most patients do better by not taking analgesics. The worst regime is 'as required' use of strong quick acting, particularly intramuscular narcotics; this is likely to reinforce pain behaviour and to create dependence.

Regional pain syndromes are likely to be seen by neurologists. While there is some continuing debate about the psychological contributions to **complex regional pain syndrome** (see Chapter 30), there is more of a consensus that **atypical facial pain** should be regarded as a somatoform disorder (see Chapter 11).

Chronic tension headache

Tension-type headache is specifically excluded from the somatoform disorders in ICD-10, and classified as a neurological disorder. Nevertheless, most would accept that the psychological processes behind tension headache are similar if not identical to many other physical symptoms unexplained by 'organic' disease. Up to 4 per cent of the population suffer chronic daily headaches which tend to decline with age. Precipitants include caffeine, eye strain and alcohol.

Amitriptyline, at doses of about 75 mg/day, has been shown to be effective, but no study has looked at longer-term efficacy of amitriptyline. Citalopram has been shown to be effective in one study, but anecdotal evidence suggests that some SSRIs may make headache worse.

CBT and relaxation therapy is likely to be beneficial. Electomyographic (EMG) biofeedback therapy where the patient learns to reduce the EMG signal in scalp muscles has been shown to be effective.

Chronic fatigue syndrome

Chronic fatigue syndrome (CFS) is characterized by severe disabling fatigue that is mental and/or physical. Other common symptoms include muscle aches and pains, concentration and memory problems and sleep disturbance. An influenza-like illness may have precipitated the syndrome, and the role of organic physical disease in maintaining symptoms is poorly understood. **Exercise avoidance** is typically seen; the patient has a marked exacerbation of symptoms after taking exercise, and as a result avoids doing so.

In ICD-10, chronic fatigue syndrome is not classified as a somatoform disorder, but as 'neurasthenia'. However, the marked overlap with other somatoform disorders, in terms of shared symptomats, suggests that this may not be a useful nosology. Myalgic encephalomyelitis (ME) is another term that is probably best avoided, suggesting as it does a definite pathophysiological process underlying the symptoms.

The focus of treatment is **graded increased moderate exercise**. Many patients have an 'all or nothing' attitude to activity; when they feel a little better they are active, but then the next day get severe symptoms of fatigue and muscle pains, and so rest. The period of rest is then prolonged for fear of exertion, causing low levels of fitness and increased symptoms following exertion. Cognitive therapy aimed at challenging assumptions, enabling the patient to feel less helpless, and problem solving, usually is incorporated into a CBT treatment package.

CBT and **exercise programmes** have been shown to be effective for chronic fatigue. There is less evidence to support the use of other treatments. Antidepressants should be used if depression is present, but there is no evidence of a specific effect of antidepressants on CFS.

Dissociation: conversion disorders

Conversion disorders, a specific form of somatization disorder, usually present to the neurologist who may label the symptoms and signs as **hysterical**. Typical symptoms include blindness, hemi-anaesthesia, paralysis and aphonia. Problems with balance may be seen; astasia–abasia describes the extravagant wobble that is seen on standing and walking.

It is dangerous to assume that because a neurological symptom is bizarre or unusual or situationally dependent, it is due to a conversion disorder. For example, patients with Huntington's chorea may have a bizarre gait disturbance, and be able to walk backwards better than forwards. It would be easy to label paroxysmal kinesogenic choreoathetosis as hysterical.

On the other hand, certain patterns of symptoms are almost pathognomonic of conversion disorder. Tunnel vision in which the same physical area, e.g. a circle two feet in diameter, is the limit of the visual field whether at three feet or ten feet from the patient, is almost certainly due to conversion disorder. Likewise hemi-anaesthesia, which involves the whole body from head to toe right down the midline. The **Hoover sign** may be telling in a patient with psychogenic paralysis of a leg; when lying on the couch and asked to raise the paralysed leg, there is no downward force exerted by the healthy side as would be found in somebody with a hemiplegia due to neurological disease. On the other hand, when the patient is asked to lift the healthy leg, a normal downward force, hip extension, is produced by the paralysed leg.

The conversion disorders may be understood as an attempt to relieve the mind of anxiety by production of a physical symptom. For this reason '**belle indifference**' may be seen; the patient, rather than being upset and distressed by their symptoms, has found relief from their anxiety. However, some patients will complain of anxiety symptoms or be upset by their disability.

Once an organic illness has been reasonably confidently ruled out, the mainstay of treatment is to encourage a return to normal activity. Some clinicians advocate enabling the patient to have an 'excuse' for recovery without ever confronting the patient with their diagnosis. This may involve enrolling the patient in a rehabilitation programme, for example, alongside patients with stroke. Suggestion during hypnosis, or an interview while under the influence of amytal (amylobarbitone) may be tried for more stubborn symptoms. Some patients become wheelchair bound and remain disabled for months or years; for these patients, a period of in-patient care in a specialist unit experienced in the treatment of conversion disorders can produce dramatic results.

Patients may be labelled as being hysterical if they are attention seeking and emotionally labile or theatrical. It is probably better to use the less pejorative term **histrionic**.

Dissociation: dissociative states

In the dissociative states, there is a failure to integrate conscious life, particularly with autobiographical memory.

In **psychogenic amnesia**, autobiographical memories for a period of time, lasting seconds to years, are lost without any organic disease to explain the amnesia. Often, there is a psychologically traumatic event related to the amnesic gap. Reported loss of memory for criminal offending may be factitious and for secondary gain, but many people without obvious secondary gain do report loss of memory at times of extreme arousal. Personal identity is retained, so that at no stage does the patient not know who they are. Prolonged retrograde amnesia, for example for years leading up to the injury, after a minor head injury raises the suspicion of psychogenic amnesia, but has been described following bilateral temporal lobe damage. Psychogenic amnesia needs to be distinguished from transient global amnesia (see Chapter 2).

In **fugue states**, personal identity is lost. As the name implies, the person in a fugue state is typically found at some distance from home, having been missing for a day or two, and taken to a police station not being able to say who they are. During the fugue, the person is usually able to interact normally with others. Precipitants include psychosocial stressors, e.g. a marriage which is breaking down or serious financial debt. Fugue states are also precipitated by alcohol and depression and probably by altered brain function, for example, incipient dementia. Occasionally, they occur repeatedly.

Psychogenic stupor is diagnosed when no physical cause is found for a reduced level of consciousness. There appears to be a constriction of conscious awareness and unresponsiveness to external stimuli. The patient may lie motionless and mute and it may only be the presence of tracking eye movements that indicates that the patient is neither asleep nor unconscious. A normal sleep–wake cycle is usually maintained. There is usually a psychological stress triggering the stupor. The differential diagnosis includes severe catatonic states associated with manic-depressive illness or schizophrenia, and an encephalopathy. So, for example, the autoimmune encephalopathies may present with unusual changes in mental state, with the patient remaining conscious, but no longer interacting socially. Such unresponsive states are easily mistaken for psychogenic stupor but may be the first symptom, for example, of an anti-NMDA receptor encephalitis. An EEG is a critical investigation to help rule out the possibility of an organic cause for the change in mental state.

Pseudoseizures are brief ictal episodes with altered conscious level not due to epilepsy or other recognized causes of syncope. They may be referred to as non-epileptic attack disorder (NEAD). Many patients have both epilepsy and pseudoseizures (see Table 31.3). Other evidence of abnormal illness behaviour may well be present, with evidence of a propensity to seek medical help. There is an association with a history of sexual abuse in childhood.

The seizures themselves may be so florid, for example with gyratory movements of the arms and legs, as to immediately suggest a non-organic cause. However, epileptic seizures arising from medial orbital frontal lobe can have a bizarre appearance.

Pseudo status epilepticus is occasionally seen in patients who abuse benzodiazepines; they have learnt that a prolonged pseudoseizure is a quick way to obtain diazepam.

In many patients, doubt about the diagnosis remains until a seizure, obtained during an EEG recording, shows a normal background rhythm. This may require telemetry, with continuous EEG and video recording of the patient and over several days (see Chapter 13, Epilepsy and sleep disorders).

Because a significant proportion of patients who present with epileptic-like symptoms do not have epilepsy, it is important to diagnose pseudoseizures early. However, even if only the occasional seizure is due to epilepsy, then the patient may

Table 31.3 Characteristics of epilepsy and pseudoseizures

	Epilepsy	Pseudoseizures
Semiology	Full range of seizure disorders with distinctive patterns, e.g. petit mal, partial complex fits with an aura tonic–clonic pattern tend to be highly stereotyped	Highly variable both across patients and even within an individual patient may vary from one fit to the next
Cyanosis	May be seen	Very rare
Incontinence	May be seen	Rare
Tongue biting	May be seen	Rare
Burns and other injuries	May be seen	Rare
Plantar reflexes	Extensor after tonic–clonic	Flexor
Eyes	Easy to open	Flicker and may be held firmly shut
Duration	Seconds to minutes	Very variable, may last up to an hour
Arise from sleep as demonstrated using EEG	Frequently	Never
Ictal EEG	Abnormal	Normal
Post-ictal EEG	Quite often shows alteration of amplitude and rhythm	Unchanged by seizure
Blood	>1000 U/L	May be slightly raised prolactin
Responsive to psychological events	Frequently	Very frequently

benefit from anticonvulsants. Therefore, a cautious approach is necessary. The pseudoseizures should be treated with cognitive behavioural treatment, which will enable the patient to look for psychological precipitants, and manage anxiety symptoms that may play a role. An important part of management is to help the patient accept that the seizures may not all be due to epilepsy. Reattribution techniques are useful (see below under Management of the somatoform disorders).

Other conditions involving dissociation

Ganser syndrome and multiple personality disorder are generally regarded as dissociative states. In the **Ganser syndrome**, the patient offers 'approximate answers' that are so nearly correct, or so exactly opposite to being correct, as to imply an underlying knowledge of the correct answer. The syndrome is typically seen in forensic settings where secondary gain may be present and sometimes conscious fabrication or malingering is suspected.

Multiple personality disorder is another condition in which there may be uncertainty about how genuine the patient is being. Some suggest that it is iatrogenic, and only occurs in response to overzealous questioning by the clinician in a suggestible patient. The patient behaves as though they are more than one person. The two or more personalities usually are unaware of each other's existence. Quite often the personality change is triggered by a psychologically traumatic event. They sometimes occur in forensic settings, raising the possibility of fabrication for secondary gain.

Factitious disorders

Some patients, usually with evidence of other personality disorder, particularly narcissistic personality disorder, make up stories of ill-health, or make themselves ill. This is associated with **pseudologia fantastica**, a tendency to tell big stories, lies, about their own prowess, for example dramatic athletic feats, or connections with royalty. Probably the most important management task in the factitious disorders is to prevent unnecessary operations and other interventions.

Management of the somatoform disorders

Patients with somatoform disorders usually attribute their problems to physical illness, and therefore expect physical treatments. Given that the treatment is going to be psychological, it is important that they are helped to reattribute their symptoms to psychological causes. This is particularly important if the general physician is going to refer them to a psychiatrist for treatment.

> The first principle in management is to ensure you are confident in the diagnosis. Possible organic causes should be excluded, particularly if there may be functional overlay. Investigations need to include as a minimum a full blood count, and basic biochemistry including thyroid function. Explain what investigations have been done and the findings.

This is then the foundation for working on the **reattribution** of physical symptoms. The reattribution model consists of three stages:

1 **Feeling understood.** The doctor is much more likely to be successful in helping a patient to change their attribution about the cause of their symptoms if the patient feels understood. This cause is helped by taking a take a full history and examination and not relying on others for the diagnosis. It is also helpful, during the interview, to respond to mood cues, for example the patient saying 'I was really troubled by that', and to explore family and social factors, and the patient's health beliefs.
2 **Changing the agenda.** Acknowledge the reality of the physical symptoms, but feedback the negative findings. Introduce into the discussion the psychological factors that the patient has described, for example life events and mood changes.
3 **Making the link**. This stage enables the patient to understand how psychological stress or disorder may result in their physical symptoms or concerns. Therefore in a patient with tension headache, one might describe how anxiety and depression can produce muscle tension and therefore pain. In a patient with pseudoseizures with episodes of loss of awareness, one might draw their attention to observations of people having no recollection of an extremely frightening event. If possible, illustrate the theme with observations the patient has made about the psychological responsiveness of their own symptoms.

The reattribution model is likely to be complemented by **anxiety management**, for example relaxation therapy, and **cognitive behaviour therapy** (CBT) targeted at the particular symptom. CBT will usually begin with a detailed diary of symptoms, noting antecedent events or situations that may act as triggers, as well as the consequences of the behaviour. This will be used to drive a behavioural programme, while cognitive therapy will help the patient identify and challenge negative thoughts, as well as increase a sense of control. General measures may be necessary to improve quality of life and reduce disability, possibly through a rehabilitation programme.

Clinically significant anxiety and depression should be treated with appropriate psychotropic drugs if necessary.

Some incorrigible patients remain fixed in their beliefs about the physical origin of their symptoms and refuse, or fail to respond to, psychological treatments. In some cases the target will be to reduce the patient's utilization of medical services by good liaison with GP and the local hospitals.

ANOREXIA NERVOSA

> Anorexia is characterized by an intense **fear of gaining weight** or becoming fat, dieting such that weight is maintained at 15 per cent less than normal healthy weight, and a disturbed body image feeling themselves to be fat. Other characteristics include abnormal eating behaviour, for example eating only very low calorie food, not eating with others, excessive exercise or laxative use to curb weight gain, and amenorrhoea. The median age of onset is 17 years, and over 90 per cent of those affected are female.

Body changes include thin hair and skin with easy bruising. Complications of dietary restriction have been described, including Wernicke's encephalopathy due to thiamine depletion. Mild cerebral atrophy develops in some. Very occasionally, anorexia nervosa may be caused by a brain tumour, particularly if it involves right sided temporofrontal circuits.

Treatment includes refeeding to reach normal weight, as well as family support. Associated mental symptoms, in particular OCD, may need treatment with SSRIs.

Prognosis is poor if the illness extends into the 20s and 30s, with a significant percentage of patients dying from suicide or complications of anorexia.

In **bulimia nervosa**, dieting alternates with binge eating. After bingeing, the person usually induces vomiting. Weight is likely to be in the normal range, and the patient is sometimes overweight. Compared with anorexia nervosa, bulimia tends to have a later age of onset, late teens to 20s, and a poorer prognosis. It is associated with other impulse control disorders, for example shop lifting.

PSYCHOSES

The psychoses are those conditions in which some aspect of reality testing is disturbed as a result of delusions, hallucinations or thought disorder. Insight into the condition is generally lacking.

Delusions are false beliefs that are held with conviction. Empirical evidence or argument against the belief is dismissed. To be regarded as a delusion, the belief must be outside of cultural and religious norms. It may be difficult to distinguish from an overvalued idea or confabulation.

Overvalued ideas are for example seen in anorexia nervosa where the patient is convinced that they are thin; this is a value judgement and not open to verification. Hypochondriasis is often associated with overvalued ideas; for example the conviction that a particular diet is essential to health.

Confabulations involve false memories and are seen in confusional states. They are generally fleeting and changeable, but if persistent and firmly held are indistinguishable from delusions.

Delusions in mental illness are usually paranoid, that is, self-referential; the patient may believe they themselves to have special powers, or believe that someone is trying to kill them. As such, delusions often have to be distinguished from ideas of reference; this is the common experience of thinking that things happening around one refer to oneself;

for example hearing a car hooting and thinking it is hooting at you. More pathological are **sensitive ideas of reference** in which the person is convinced that somebody is making fun of, or criticizing them.

Hallucinations are false perceptions in the absence of a sensory stimulus. All sensory modalities may be involved but the most common are auditory verbal hallucinations.

Visual hallucinations are more often found in the organic psychoses. It is important to determine whether insight is preserved. Insight is likely to be preserved in elderly patients with poor eyesight who develop visual hallucinations; the patient will realize that their mind is playing tricks on them.

Thought disorder describes the disorganized language of some patients with schizophrenia. It is not easy or possible to follow their train of thought. Sometimes, the language is so disorganized that the grammatical construction of sentences, and therefore any meaning, is lost.

Thought disorder is indistinguishable from what is observed in some patients in delirium, and is easy to confuse with the word salad that may be produced by patients with a severe dysphasia, particularly if fluent (Wernicke's). Thought disorder may involve expression of language more than comprehension, but when severe it is very likely that the patient will have little understanding of what is going on around them.

The major psychoses are **schizophrenia** and **manic–depressive psychosis**. However, there are large overlaps between the two conditions and many patients have symptoms of both disorders, particularly over the course of a lifetime.

Schizophrenia

Schizophrenia is characterized by a chronic illness which is usually relapsing–remitting. Onset is early in adult life, particularly in men; as a result it is rare for a patient with schizophrenia to get a university degree. The lifetime risk is about 1 per cent, and is much greater (10–15 per cent) in first degree relatives of a patient with schizophrenia. Several putative genes that render a person susceptible to schizophrenia, possibly through effects on synaptic plasticity or NMDA receptor activity, have been identified over the last decade.

> **Symptoms**
>
> Delusions, hallucinations and thought disorder, in the absence of affective disorder sufficient to explain the psychosis, are the core symptoms. Some depressive symptoms are not uncommon, particularly after treatment of an acute relapse.

It is important to determine the mood congruence of any delusions or hallucinations. For example, derogatory auditory verbal hallucinations in somebody who is severely depressed, suggests the diagnosis may be a psychotic depression, rather than schizophrenia. However, if the patient is fatuously describing how somebody is trying to kill them, then this suggests schizophrenia.

> A lack of emotional responsiveness is characteristic of schizophrenia; patients show a reduced range of emotional expression. At interview, they may lack any emotional warmth or rapport.

> Some 'first rank' symptoms are particularly important for the diagnosis of schizophrenia, though they are not diagnostic. They include auditory verbal hallucinations which talk about the patient in the third person, or provide a running commentary. Disorders of the ownership of one's thoughts, for example the experience that one's thoughts are broadcast and can be received at a distance. And passivity phenomena, that one's actions or thoughts are under another person's control.

Motor symptoms

Catatonia is used to describe disorders of movement in the absence of any obvious neurological explanation. A variety of motor symptoms are seen. General activity may be increased or reduced. Mutism is common. Unusual postures may be adopted and waxy flexibility occurs when the patient maintains a posture which they have been placed in by the examiner. The patients may be negativistic; **gegenhalten** describes the sense that the harder the examiner pushes or pulls, the harder the patient pushes or pulls to stop a limb being moved. Mannerisms and stereotypies, movements without a purpose, are also seen.

Over the last few decades, catatonic symptoms are encountered less frequently, perhaps because they are particularly sensitive to antipsychotics. They are seen in schizophrenia and affective disorder, but importantly may herald a neurological disease, particularly if it involves the basal ganglia.

Negative symptoms

Most of the symptoms described above are 'positive'. They are usually fairly sensitive to antipsychotic medication. However, perhaps more disabling in the long term are negative symptoms including **lack of ambition and drive**, social withdrawal and lack of emotional warmth.

Treatment of schizophrenia

Antipsychotic drugs are effective both to treat an acute psychotic episode and to prevent relapse. Long-term treatment is recommended if there is a history of relapses off treatment. There is some evidence that delay in treating the first episode of schizophrenia results in worse outcome in the long term, but the evidence is not conclusive.

Depot antipsychotics, which are given by intramuscular injection once every 1–4 weeks, have the advantage of ensuring compliance. However, they should only be started after a small test dose has been given and when the diagnosis is reasonably firm.

Atypical antipsychotics, for example quetiapine, olanzapine or risperidone, probably have less likelihood of producing extrapyramidal side effects (EPSE) (see Chapter 20). However, some recent pragmatic studies have called into question the assertion that these drugs are better tolerated. It has also been suggested that subdividing all antipsychotic drugs into two discrete classes, conventional or atypical, with the latter distinguished by their lesser extrapyramidal side effects, is in fact unhelpful. It would be better to acknowledge the individual differences of antipsychotic drugs, regardless of whether they are 'atypical' or not, in terms of the balance of side effects and benefits based on their pharmacological profile.

Clozapine, an atypical antipsychotic, is recommended for treatment-resistant schizophrenia, as well as seeming to produce fewer EPSE. However, its potential to cause agranulocytosis, particularly in the elderly, means that its use has to be closely monitored with frequent blood counts. Side effects include sedation, hypersalivation, hypotension, myoclonus and epilepsy.

Psychological therapies may be effective, but should never be given in isolation, without antipsychotic medication. **Family therapy**, aiming at reducing expressed emotion, for example overt criticism of the patient by their family, may be effective. Recently, **cognitive techniques**, to help patients challenge delusions or cope with hallucinations, have been studied. **Compliance therapy**, helping the patient to take their medication regularly, probably has a role for some patients.

Psychosocial measures, aimed at reducing social isolation and other stressors that result from the illness, are essential. Patients with severe chronic schizophrenia are likely to need residential care.

Prognosis

Insidious onset, lack of acute psychotic attacks with affective symptoms and negative symptoms, and poor treatment compliance predict a poor prognosis. Many will end up in residential care. A proportion, perhaps 10 per cent, of patients with chronic schizophrenia, develop dementia. More than 10 per cent of patients with schizophrenia commit suicide. Homicide is very rare.

Delusional disorders

These differ from schizophrenia in as much as the only symptom of psychosis is **paranoid delusions**. These are invariably well **systematized**, that is, all related to the same theme. For example, a patient may become convinced that they are at the mercy of some huge international conspiracy against them, that started as a result of a small argument at work many years ago. Chronic grandiose delusions may be seen. **Erotomania** is an example in which the patient is convinced that another person, usually famous, loves them. As a result, they may stalk and pester the subject of the delusion. Hypochondriacal and dysmorphophobic delusions (belief that one's body is ugly or misshapen) are also seen (see above under Hypochondriasis).

Personality tends to be well preserved, in contrast to schizophrenia, and some patients function quite well despite their delusions. Antipsychotic medication is not always successful, partly because of poor compliance.

Hallucinoses

Chronic auditory verbal hallucinosis, in the absence of other psychotic symptoms suggesting schizophrenia, is occasionally seen. **Alcohol dependence** is the most common cause in which case the voices are often derogatory, for example swearing obscenities at the patient. **Deafness or impairment of sight** may be associated with auditory and visual hallucinations, respectively. In the elderly, delusions of infestation may appear to arise from somatic hallucinations of insects crawling over the skin.

Organic psychoses

Chronic epilepsy, particularly temporal lobe epilepsy, may result in a psychotic illness that is indistinguishable from schizophrenia.

The natural history of the illness may be different with a later age of onset, relative preservation of personality and a failure to develop negative symptoms over time.

Psychotic symptoms occur in about a third of patients with **Alzheimer's disease**, and in **Lewy body dementia** they are even more common.

Of particular interest is the observation that psychotic symptoms in these dementias may be responsive to **donepezil** or **rivastigmine**, drugs which increase cholinergic transmission. This is particularly useful given that antipsychotics are likely to produce severe EPSEs in Lewy body dementia.

Psychotic symptoms may be seen in **Parkinson's disease**, particularly when dopaminergic treatment is increased.

Visual hallucinations are common but often with preserved insight and are not particularly troublesome. However, persecutory delusions may demand treatment. Very low doses of the atypical antipsychotic drugs **clozapine** or **olanzapine** may improve the psychosis without exacerbating the parkinsonism.

Drug dependence may result in psychosis (see below).

AFFECTIVE DISORDERS: MANIC-DEPRESSIVE PSYCHOSIS

When somebody suffers episodes of depression and episodes of mania they are described as suffering **bipolar affective disorder**, or manic-depressive psychosis. The word 'psychosis' is used even though they may never have suffered psychotic symptoms. Such illnesses are usually classified together with depression that tends to relapse and remit without obvious psychological precipitants, in which biological symptoms and severe mood disturbance are prominent. The classification acknowledges the fact that they are at high risk of suffering a manic illness in the future, and may well have a first degree relative with bipolar disorder. **Bipolar 1 disorder** refers to those patients with a combination of both depression and mania, whereas patients with **Bipolar 2 disorder** only have hypomanic episodes rather than manic, that is, the symptoms of mania are less severe.

In the absence of a history of mania, depression is diagnosed as **major, moderate or minor depression**, and this is qualified by saying whether the depression is recurrent or associated with psychotic symptoms.

Short-lived depression, which occurs only in response to a major stressor, is usually classified as an **adjustment disorder** (see above under Adjustment and bereavement reactions).

Depression involves subjective and objective evidence of mood disturbance, with alterations in behaviour, thought content and cognition, and biological symptoms (Table 31.4). Psychotic symptoms are seen in more severe depressive illness, and are mood congruent.

The terms **mania** and **hypomania** refer to the same symptom complexes, but in mania the disorder results in admission to hospital. Numerous symptoms may be found with a core elevation of mood and sense of well-being and energy. Insight is lost early and this, along with the tendency to irritablity and aggression, makes management difficult. The patient often refuses medication and continues to put themselves at risk and jeopardize their social and vocational network. They are quite likely to need to be admitted under a section of the Mental Health Act.

Often, a mixture of manic and depressive symptoms is present in the same episode; a mixed affective state. Irritability is common to both depression and mania, but usually more troublesome in manic patients. Mania is often immediately followed by depression, as insight returns.

> The major risk of depression is **suicide** (see Box 31.1), while patients with mania place themselves in the way of all sorts of untoward events, including injury.

Causes of manic-depressive illness and differential diagnosis

Depression is common, especially in women; some community surveys have identified clinically significant depression in over 20 per cent of the population. It tends to increase with age and is associated with a family history of depression, having a physical illness, and recent life events, especially 'loss events', for example the death of a spouse, or loss of a job.

Depression needs to be distinguished from disorders of the brain which can produce similar biological symptoms, but without any core mood disturbance, for example Parkinson's disease or brain injury. Metabolic conditions, in particular hypothyroidism, may mimic depression. Anorexia may be part of anorexia nervosa, or due to a neoplasm. If the latter, the general lethargy and malaise may be mistakenly regarded as confirming the diagnosis of depression.

> Most neurological disorders are associated with depression. For example, there are increased rates in multiple sclerosis, Parkinson's disease, epilepsy and traumatic brain injury. A systematic review of **depression after stroke** concluded that although stroke is associated with

Table 31.4 Symptoms and signs of affective disorder

	Depression	Mania
Appearance and behaviour and objective mood symptoms	Psychomotor retardation/poverty of speech, poor self-care, poor eye contact, tearfulness, agitation	Increased motor and mental activity. Jocular. Irritated by what they perceive as attempts to frustrate their plans. Spends money, promiscuous, family and work ignored, thoughtless. Pressure of speech, loosening of associations. Over-familiar
Subjective mood symptoms and thought content	Low mood, hopelessness, low self esteem, helplessness, worthlessness. Self-blame, guilt, feelings that life is not worth living. Suicidal thoughts. Anxiety symptoms common	Cheerful, elated or euphoric. A sense of having lots of things to do and lots of energy. A sense of well-being. Grandiose and full of themselves. Irritable and angry if demands not met
Biological/somatic symptoms of mood disturbance	Anhedonia (reduced ability to experience pleasure), fatigue, diurnal variation of mood, sleep disturbance usually with insomnia and early morning wakening but occasionally excessive sleep, appetite disturbance, reduced libido and very occasionally constipation and amenorrhoea	Does not need sleep, lots of energy, increased libido
Psychotic symptoms	Delusions of guilt or persecution, and auditory hallucinations, often derogatory or command hallucinations to injury themselves. Nihilistic delusions of rotting or being dead	Delusions, usually of a grandiose theme
Cognitive	Poor concentration and complaints of poor memory especially in the elderly	Attention and concentration are usually disrupted
Insight	May be preserved till late	Insight is lost early

depression there is no evidence for an effect of lesion location; the review strongly disconfirmed previous suggestions that depression is particularly associated with frontal left-sided strokes. For all these neurological conditions, the increased prevalence of depression is not simply due to a psychological reaction to disability; patients with non-CNS disorders, but with equivalent disability, tend to show less depression.

Some drugs may induce depression, particularly older antihypertensive agents. **Alcohol abuse** and **steroids** may lead to mania or depression.

Mania is much less common than depression. A family history of affective disorder is quite likely to be found. Manic illness may be precipitated by life events including those that would be expected to be followed by depression.

Brain injury and infections may precipitate mania. It is now rare to see general paresis of the insane (GPI) due to syphilis which sometimes presented with mania; on the other hand, it may be observed in brain lesions, particularly if in the right hemisphere or involving the frontal lobes.

Some patients with damage to the frontal lobes appear very similar to manic patients; they may be overfamiliar, jocular, thoughtless, irritable and slightly pressured in their speech. They are more likely to be fatuous, rather than distinctly elated. Euphoria with lack of insight and concern about their illness, is found in some patients

Box 31.1 Suicide assessment and management

- **High risk**. Previous attempts, family history, suffers depression, schizophrenia or drug dependence, recent loss, recent diagnosis of physical illness, access to method (guns, farmers; drugs, anaesthetists), recent discharge from psychiatric hospital
- **Immediate risk requiring urgent management**. Threats to commit suicide, especially if recent attempt (i.e. within weeks or months), if dangerous method and good evidence of intent, especially if at the time they are confused/distressed/psychotic. Command hallucinations to harm

Management
- Assess for risk factors above, get history from notes and informants
- Don't be afraid to ask for suicidal thoughts – start by asking about mood generally, then enquire about feelings of life not being worth living, then ask directly if they are having/have had suidical thoughts. If 'yes', then explore frequency and whether they feel they will act on their thoughts.
- Never assume a threat to commit suicide is an idle threat
- Make safe:
  - Is there a carer? Are they reliable? Who will look after medication? Admission to hospital required?
  - If in hospital, observe with one-to-one nursing? Access to open windows, balconies, knives, other methods of self-injury?
- Keep others informed of concerns, e.g. GP
- Get psychiatric opinion urgently, if any uncertainty
- Consider detention under Mental Health Act
- Document what you have done and why

with severe damage to the CNS, for example due to multiple sclerosis. Patients after traumatic brain injury may well show frequent dramatic shifts of mood, lasting a day or two, and therefore be described as showing 'rapid cycling' mood disorder.

Drugs, particularly amphetamines, can produce mania. In some patients, antidepressants precipitate mania.

Treatment of affective disorders

Antidepressants, antipsychotics and mood stabilizers are used to manage the affective disorders.

Newer antidepressants have the advantage of having fewer cholinergic and sedative side effects. They are much safer in overdose than the older tricyclic antidepressants and are therefore the first line of treatment. There are several different classes (see Table 31.5) related to selective pharmacological effects. There is little good evidence that drugs of different classes have selective clinical profiles. The most important consideration in selecting an antidepressant, other than its potential toxicity in overdose, is whether or not it is sedative, in which case it is useful for insomnia or anxiety symptoms, but not if fatigue is a prominent symptom.

If one antidepressant has not worked, then it is better to choose a drug from another class as the next line of treatment. First, ensure that the patient has been compliant and has achieved adequate dosage for long enough (at least 6 weeks). For severe treatment-resistant depression, adjuvant therapy with lithium may be necessary, although this runs the risk of producing a serotinergic crisis. Combinations of antidepressants need expert management.

Electroconvulsive therapy (ECT) may be useful for difficult to treat severe depression, particularly if a quick response is needed, for example if the patient is refusing food and drink. **Predictors of a good response to ECT** include psychomotor symptoms, including agitation or retardation, other biological symptoms, and psychotic depression. CNS disease is generally not a contraindication, because the main risk of the ECT is the brief anaesthetic. ECT may be particularly useful in Parkinson's disease; it has been shown to improve both the depression and the parkinsonism.

For the **prophylactic** treatment of manic-depressive illness, **lithium, valproate or the antipsychotics olanzapine and quetiapine** are all recommended options. Lithium is probably still the first choice, but the therapeutic window is quite narrow and neurotoxicity, particularly cerebellar signs, is a recognized complication when blood levels are too high; thyroid and renal function need to be monitored. More recent studies have demonstrated

Table 31.5 Antidepressant drugs

Antidepressant class	Examples	Comments
Tricyclic antidepressants (all have increased risk of cardiac toxicity in overdose)	Amitriptyline	A standard highly effective drug, quite sedative
	Imipramine	As above, but less sedative
	Dosulepin	Sedative with less cardiac side effects
	Trazodone	Less anticholinergic side effects, sedative, quite selective for serotonin, good in the elderly
Monoamine oxidase inhibitors (MAOI)	Phenelzine	Potentially dangerous, dietary (tyramine) and drug interactions produce hypertensive crisis
	Moclobemide	Reversible inhibitor of MAO A (RIMA) few, if any, dietary restrictions
Selective serotonin reuptake inhibitors (SSRI)	Fluoxetine	Not sedative, quite alerting
	Citalopram	Both quite 'neutral' and with little enzyme induction
	Sertraline	
Serotonin and noradrenaline reuptake inhibitors (SNRI)	Venlafaxine	Risk of hypertension, avoid if cardiac arrythmia
Selective noradrenaline reuptake inhibitors (NRI)	Reboxetine	
Presynaptic β_2 antagonist	Mirtazapine	Increases central noradrenergic and serotinergic transmission

the value of olanzapine and quetiapine, both in terms of treating manic relapses, but also preventing further relapses whether manic or depressed.

ALCOHOL AND OTHER DRUG ADDICTIONS

Drug dependence, addiction and abuse are, for all intents and purposes, synonymous. It is of course possible to abuse a drug without becoming dependent, but this is rare.

Drug dependence is both **physical**, that is, the body becomes physiologically dependent on the drug, and **psychological**. For some drugs, for example cocaine, ecstasy and cannabis, there is very little physical dependence. For others, for example benzodiazepines, physical dependence may develop long before psychological dependence.

Physical dependence is demonstrated by tolerance (increased doses of drug are needed to produce the same effect) and withdrawal symptoms (Table 31.6). Cross-tolerance to benzodiazepines, alcohol and barbiturates occurs, probably largely explained

by their common agonist effects on the GABA receptor.

Psychological dependence consists of craving and an increased **saliency** for drug taking; drug taking becomes more important than anything else in the person's life and as a result, work, family, leisure and social life suffer.

Fast acting, short half-life **opiates** are highly addictive. The opiate withdrawal syndrome, though very unpleasant, is not dangerous. Of much greater danger is overdose, producing coma with pinpoint pupils. The other great danger is infection from intravenous drug use, ranging from local abscesses to systemic and CNS infection with opportunistic organisms. Intravenous drug users are at high risk of HIV and hepatitis.

Amphetamine produces a sense of well-being and energy, as well as anorexia and lack of sleep. Long-term use will often induce paranoia and hallucinations.

Cocaine produces a sense of euphoria as a result of its effects on reuptake of catecholamines, including dopamine and serotonin. It is highly addictive, partly due to its very quick onset if taken intranasally, or by smoking the free alkaloid base 'crack'. Dangerous effects are related to sympathetic stimulation and possibly direct effects on cerebral

Table 31.6 Drug dependence withdrawal syndromes

Alcohol	Delirium tremens	1–4 days after stopping, delirium with visual hallucinations, other psychotic symptoms and fear, epilepsy
Opiates	'Cold turkey'	Piloerection (goose flesh), rhinorrhoea/lacrimation, sweating, stomach cramps, diarrhoea, dilated pupils, shivering, yawning, fatigue
Benzodiazepines		Muscle tension and twitching, anxiety/panic/depersonalization, rebound REM (nightmares) hyperacuity, metallic taste in mouth, other abnormal sensations, convulsions
Amphetamines		Fatigue, dysphoria, anhedonia, hyperphagia

blood vessels. Cardiac, pulmonary and cerebrovascular problems occur.

MDMA (Ecstasy) promotes the release of brain monoamines. However, it is probably also directly neurotoxic for serotoninergic neurons. Chronic use is associated with cognitive impairment.

Cannabis acts on cannabinoid receptors in the CNS. Its main effect is to induce a sense of calm, but in a significant minority the effects are directly opposite, with panic attacks, depersonalization, and sometimes persecutory delusions with hallucinations. Chronic use may be associated with increased risk of schizophrenia, but it is difficult distinguishing cause and effect, that is, patients with schizophrenia may be more likely to take cannabis. Cannabinoids do not cause a physical dependence syndrome.

Volatile substance abuse (glue sniffing) is most common in teenagers. It rapidly induces an altered state of consciousness, often with euphoric mood. Death from cardiac arrhythmias and respiratory depression may occur. Long-term use is associated with cerebellar atrophy and probably cognitive impairment.

Alcohol dependence

Alcohol dependence is of great importance to the neurologist; it is common and alcohol is neurologically highly toxic (see Chapter 27). Clinically, a high index of suspicion is needed and the CAGE is a useful symptom screening test: have you ever felt the need to **C**ut down your drinking, felt **A**nnoyed by criticism of your drinking, felt **G**uilty about how much you drink, or needed an **E**ye-opener? Blood tests may suggest the diagnosis with a raised

serum gamma glutamyl transpetidase or mean corpuscular volume (MCV). High risk professions include publicans, doctors and journalists.

Healthy drinking limits are 21 unit of alcohol per week (1 unit = 10 mL pure alcohol) for men and 14 for women, that is about a pint of normal strength beer a day for a woman.

Depression and anxiety are commonly associated with alcohol dependence. Some patients develop **persecutory delusions**. **Reduced anger control**, particularly when drunk, is a very troublesome effect. **Suicide** and **alcoholic hallucinosis**, chronic auditory verbal hallucinations that usually consist of a voice hurling abuse at the patient, are less frequent psychiatric complications.

Patients who are alcohol dependent often present to the Accident and Emergency Department where they may be difficult to assess if drunk or agitated. It is important to be alert to other causes of impairment of conscious level, over and above intoxication. Chronic subdural haematomas and other intracranial space-occupying lesions, post-ictal states, Wernicke's encephalopathy, delirium tremens, hepatic encephalopathy, hypoglycaemia, and infection, both systemic and intracranial, are all easy to miss. It is essential to give thiamine, remembering that alcohol-dependent patients are at particular risk of developing Wernicke's encephalopathy when glucose or another source of carbohydrate is given. It is better to give thiamine when it is not necessary, than to miss the emergency indication for this treatment – Wernicke's encephalopathy. Failure to give thiamine in the early stages of Wernicke's encephalopathy will result in death or the development of Korsakoff's psychosis (see Chapter 27).

Cognitive impairment is common. Classical Wernicke–Korsakoff syndrome, with a selective anterograde amnesia, is uncommon but devastating for the patient. It is more usual to find a gradual cognitive decline, selective for memory. Early signs may be the appearance of 'memory blackouts'; the person has no recollection of events that happened while they were drunk, but were nevertheless conscious at the time.

Treatment for alcohol dependence is largely aimed at education about the harmful effects of alcohol, with support to reduce and stop drinking. However, success rates are not good. Brief interventions, for example given by general practitioners, are almost as effective as intensive programmes of detoxification followed by psychotherapy. Detoxification programmes involve substitution of alcohol with a benzodiazepine, and then weaning off the benzodiazepine over the course of a few days. This is unlikely to be successful at home because of the risk of abusing both the prescribed benzodiazepine and alcohol.

Management of aggression and agitation

Aggression in the Accident and Emergency Department is often caused by **intoxication** with alcohol and other drugs, particularly in somebody with a **personality disorder**. On the other hand, most agitation and aggression on hospital wards is related to **drug withdrawal**, especially alcohol, and/or **fear** and **acute confusional states (delirium)**. Agitation is also associated with anxiety and akathisia. Poor sleep, pain, constipation, systemic illness and side effects of prescribed drugs, may be playing a part. Unexplained agitation and restlessness may be prodromal symptoms to delirium.

Therefore, the first priority, after making sure of the immediate safety of the patient and others, is to consider what physical illness may be present, particular one involving the CNS.

Safety, for a patient with severe agitation or assaultativeness, requires **plenty of staff**, preferably men. The security staff should be called and if necessary police. One-to-one and sometimes two-to-one nursing may be required once the acute situation has been treated.

Some patients will settle with reassurance and explanation. Relatives may be able to help. Others will need medication and the psychiatry liaison team should be called. The standard rapid tranquillizer protocol consists of **haloperidol and lorazepam**. The patient should be regularly observed by the nurses, with monitoring of breathing and neurological state. If sedation is required for more than 1 or 2 days, it is worth starting regular atypical antipsychotic medication, for example olanzapine, which has less chance of producing extrapyramidal effects. Every opportunity should be taken to review evidence of physical illness.

Much of the management is common to that of delirium. Nursing should be in a side room with consistent staff and plenty of light and things to occupy the patient. On the other hand, it should be a calm environment with opportunities for rest.

CAPACITY, CONSENT, THE MENTAL HEALTH ACT, MENTAL CAPACITY ACT AND COURT OF PROTECTION

'**Capacity for what?**' is the retort when you are asked to assess a patient's capacity. Patients may be quite capable in one area of decision making, but entirely incompetent in another.

Consent to treatment

Capacity to make a decision requires a person to:

- **understand** the information relevant to making the decision;
- **retain** the information long enough to make the decision;
- **use and weigh** the information in the balance to make a decision, taking into account the options;
- **communicate** the decision.

If the patient fails any one of these steps then they will be deemed to lack capacity for the decision in question. Lack of capacity may only be temporary, for example in somebody with a delirium, and the **Mental Capacity Act 2005**, which defines in England and Wales how a person who may lack capacity should be managed, notes that if there is a reasonable likelihood of capacity returning in the near future decisions should, where possible, be postponed until the patient has regained capacity.

In British law, nobody can consent to treatment on behalf of another adult. If an adult patient lacks capacity to consent then **medical/surgical treatment decisions** rest with the clinical team, acting in the patient's **best interests**. In England and Wales, the rules for decision making are defined by the **Mental Capacity Act**. This essentially codifies good practice and for example allows emergency treatment of an unconscious patient. Moreover, people are assumed to have capacity until proved otherwise; in a patient with cognitive impairment, their capacity to consent to treatment should be explicitly assessed and where appropriate documented.

When a patient who has been assumed capable of consenting then **refuses essential treatment**, then their capacity should be assessed. This should be done by a psychiatrist because if they are found to be lacking capacity it is likely to be because refusal was the result of mental illness. However, if found incapable of consenting due to a mental illness, yet the treatment itself is for a **medical/ surgical** condition, then the treatment can go ahead in the patient's best interests under the Mental Capacity Act (in England and Wales). An example would be when a patient refuses operation on a burst appendix, believing that the pain in their stomach is due to rats gnawing their intestines.

Consent to treatment for mental disorders, at least in England and Wales, falls under the remit of the **Mental Health Act**. Patients with mental disorders can be detained in hospital under the Mental Health Act for treatment of their mental disorder. To be detained

- they must have a mental disorder of such severity as to warrant detention;
- they must be at risk of harm to themselves or others if they were not detained;

- and there is no suitable alternative to hospital treatment.

Two doctors must recommend detention, at least one of whom is a specialist in mental disorders. A social worker then makes the application if they agree detention is warranted. The patient's next of kin must be consulted. Patients can be detained to a general hospital, as well as a mental hospital but need to be under the care of a clinician trained in the Mental Health Act, an approved clinician, for the purposes of their detention. Emergency powers to detain for up to 3 days can be authorized by a doctor or nurse.

Mental symptoms due to intoxication with alcohol or other drugs do not constitute grounds for detaining someone. However, mental disorders due to alcohol or drugs, e.g. delirium tremens, are grounds for detention.

It has been standard practice not to detain patients with dementia who do not resist treatment or demand to leave hospital, despite the fact that they lack capacity to consent and that if they did try to leave they would be kept on the ward for their own safety. The argument is that their consent can be inferred from their behaviour and that it is in their best interests to remain in care. This practice has been called into question by the European Court of Human Rights. It is seen to breach a person's right to liberty (Article 5 of the European Convention on Human Rights) in as much as the detention is considered to be arbitrary, that is without a formal procedure documenting and describing the detention, and without any recourse to a court or independent review to determine that the detention is lawful.

Because of these findings, patients in England and Wales who lack capacity to consent to treatment and who are being effectively detained in a hospital or nursing home, that is, if they tried to leave they would be prevented from doing so, now have to be assessed to determine if **Deprivation of Liberties safeguards** need to be put into place. If the patient is found to be being deprived of their liberties then an authorization from the body commissioning their care has to be completed and subsequently reviewed.

Capacity to administer one's finances and affairs

In the UK, a **Power of Attorney** enables a person, the donor, to authorize another, the attorney, to act on their behalf to administer their financial affairs. The limits of the attorney's authority are defined in the Power of Attorney. For example, it might be to collect rent and manage a property, while the donor is travelling. Should the donor become incapable of managing their affairs, the Power of Attorney is immediately annulled.

If a person wants a Power of Attorney to extend beyond the time that they lose capacity then they can set up a **Lasting Power of Attorney**. This is typically for patients who have recently developed a dementing illness. To set up a Lasting Power of Attorney, the patient must have capacity to authorize the Power, that is, to understand the implications of handing over authority to another person to act on their behalf. Once they have lost the capacity to administer and manage their finances and affairs then the Court of Protection has to be notified.

The **Court of Protection** is usually called in when it becomes apparent that somebody is not capable of administering and managing their own finances and affairs, for example after a severe brain injury. To be registered with the Court of Protection, the patient must suffer a mental disorder. The Court of Protection will appoint a deputy, for example the spouse, who will be accountable to them. In British law, the spouse or next of kin is not able to administer a patient's finances on their behalf without the authority to do so.

FURTHER READING

Carson AJ, Ringbauer B, Stone J *et al.* (2000) Do medically unexplained symptoms matter? A prospective cohort study of 300 new referrals to neurology outpatient clinics. *Journal of Neurology, Neurosurgery, and Psychiatry*, **68**:207–10.

Creed F, Mayou R, Hopkins A (1992) *Medical Symptoms Not Explained by Organic Disease.* London: Royal College of Psychiatrists and Royal College of Physicians.

Gelder MG, López-Ibor JJ, Andreasen NC, Geddes JR (2009) *New Oxford Textbook of Psychiatry*, 2nd edn. Oxford: Oxford University Press.

David A, Fleminger S, Kopelman M *et al.* (2009) *Lishman's Organic Psychiatry*, 4th edn. Oxford: Blackwell Science.

Moore DP (2001) *Textbook of Clinical Neuropsychiatry.* London: Arnold.

Owens DC (2008) How CATIE brought us back to Kansas: a critical re-evaluation of the concept of atypical antipsychotics and their place in the treatment of schizophrenia. *Advances in Psychiatric Treatment*, **14**:17–28.

Rogers D (1985) The motor disorders of severe psychiatric illness: a conflict of paradigms. *British Journal of Psychiatry*, **147**:221–232.

Ron MA, David AS (1998) *Disorders of Brain and Mind.* Cambridge: Cambridge University Press.

Stone J (2009) Functional symptoms in neurology. *Practical Neurology*, **9**:179–189.

Taylor D, Paton C, Kapur S (2009) *The Maudsley Prescribing Guidelines*, 10th edn. London: Informa Healthcare.

Wessely S, Nimnuan C, Sharpe M (1999) Functional somatic symptoms: one or many? *Lancet*, **354**:936–939.

INDEX

The index entries appear in word-by-word alphabetical order.